Dual-Process Theories in Social Psychology

Dual-Process Theories in Social Psychology

Edited by

SHELLY CHAIKEN

YAACOV TROPE

THE GUILFORD PRESS
New York   London

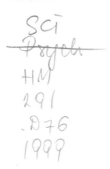

©1999 The Guilford Press
A Division of Guilford Publications, Inc.
72 Spring Street, New York, NY 10012
http://www.guilford.com

Printed in the United States of America

This book is printed on acid-free paper.

Last digit is print number: 9 8 7 6 5 4 3 2 1

Library of Congress Cataloging-in-Publication Data

Dual-process theories in social psychology / edited by Shelly Chaiken,
    Yaacov Trope.
        p. cm.
    Includes bibliographic references and index.
    ISBN 1-57230-421-9
    1. Social psychology. I. Chaiken, Shelly. II. Trope, Yaacov.
HM291.D76 1999
    302—dc21   98-54248
                                                          CIP

About the Editors

Shelly Chaiken received her PhD in 1978 from the University of Massachusetts at Amherst before teaching at the University of Toronto and then Vanderbilt University. She has been Professor of Psychology at New York University since 1985. Dr. Chaiken has published *The Psychology of Attitudes* with Alice H. Eagly and is also the author of numerous theoretical, review, and empirical articles on attitude structure, formation, and change.

Yaacov Trope received his PhD in 1974 from the University of Michigan at Ann Arbor before joining the Hebrew University of Jerusalem. Since 1991, he has been Professor of Psychology at New York University and Tel-Aviv University. Dr. Trope has edited, with Tory Higgins, a special issue of the *Personality and Social Psychology Bulletin* entitled "Inferring Personal Dispositions from Behavior" and has published theoretical and empirical articles on the cognitive and motivational mechanisms underlying biased and unbiased search and processing of information about self and others.

From 1997 to 1998, Shelly Chaiken was a fellow at the Center for Advanced Study in the Behavioral Sciences, with financial support provided by National Science Foundation Grant SBR 9601236. The Center experience—uninterrupted time for scholarship in an idyllic environment—greatly facilitated work on this project. Preparation of this book was also supported by the National Institute of Mental Health Grant HH 45557 to Yaacov Trope.

Contributors

Icek Ajzen, PhD, Department of Psychology, University of Massachusetts at Amherst, Amherst, MA

John A. Bargh, PhD, Department of Psychology, New York University, New York, NY

Reuben M. Baron, PhD, Department of Psychology, University of Connecticut, Storrs, CT

Ute Bayer, PhD, Department of Psychology, University of Konstanz, Konstanz, Germany

Denise R. Beike, PhD, Department of Psychology, University of Arkansas, Fayetteville, AR

Herbert Bless, PhD, Fachbereich I, Psychologie, Universität Trier, Trier, Germany

Galen V. Bodenhausen, PhD, Department of Psychology, Northwestern University, Evanston, IL

Marilynn B. Brewer, PhD, Department of Psychology, Ohio State University, Columbus, OH

Serena Chen, PhD, Department of Psychology, University of Michigan, Ann Arbor, MI

Jamie DeCoster, PhD, Department of Psychological Sciences, Purdue University, West Lafayette, IN

Patricia G. Devine, PhD, Department of Psychology, University of Wisconsin, Madison, WI

Carol S. Dweck, PhD, Department of Psychology, Columbia University, New York, NY

Seymour Epstein, PhD, Department of Psychology, University of Massachusetts, Amherst, MA

Russell H. Fazio, PhD, Department of Psychology, Indiana University, Bloomington, IN

Amy S. Harasty Feinstein, PhD, Research Analyst, Goldberg Moser O'Neill Advertising, San Francisco, CA

Susan T. Fiske, PhD, Department of Psychology, University of Massachusetts, Amherst, MA

Adam D. Galinsky, PhD, Department of Psychology, Princeton University, Princeton, NJ

Ruth Gaunt, PhD, Department of Psychology, Harvard University, Cambridge, MA

Richard J. Gerrig, PhD, Department of Psychology, State University of New York at Stony Brook, Stony Brook, NY

Daniel T. Gilbert, PhD, Department of Psychology, Harvard University, Cambridge, MA

Roger Giner-Sorolla, PhD, Department of Psychology, University of Virginia, Charlottesville, VA

Julie H. Goldberg, PhD, Department of Psychology, University of California at Berkeley, Berkeley, CA

Peter M. Gollwitzer, PhD, Department of Psychology, University of Konstanz, Konstanz, Germany

David L. Hamilton, PhD, Department of Psychology, University of California at Santa Barbara, Santa Barbara, CA

E. Tory Higgins, PhD, Department of Psychology, Columbia University, New York, NY

Larry J. Jacoby, PhD, Department of Psychology, New York University, New York, NY

Colleen M. Kelley, PhD, Department of Psychology, Florida State University, Tallahassee, FL

Asher Koriat, PhD, Department of Psychology, University of Haifa, Haifa, Israel

Arie W. Kruglanski, PhD, Department of Psychology, University of Maryland, College Park, MD

Ziva Kunda, PhD, Psychology Department, University of Waterloo, Waterloo, Ontario, Canada

Jennifer S. Lerner, PhD, Department of Decision Sciences, Carnegie Mellon University, Pittsburgh, PA

Melvin J. Lerner, PhD, Department of Psychology, University of Waterloo, Waterloo, Ontario, Canada

Sheri R. Levy, PhD, Department of Psychology, Columbia University, New York, NY

Ravit Levy-Sadot, BA, Graduate Student, Department of Psychology, University of Haifa, Haifa, Israel

Monica Lin, MA, Department of Psychology, University of Massachusetts, Amherst, MA

C. Neil Macrae, PhD, Department of Experimental Psychology, University of Bristol, Bristol, United Kingdom

Keith B. Maddox, PhD, Department of Psychology, Tufts University, Medford, MA

Brian D. McElree, PhD, Department of Psychology, New York University, New York, NY

Stephen J. Misovich, PhD, Department of Social Sciences, Hillyer College, University of Hartford, West Hartford, CT

Margo J. Monteith, PhD, Department of Psychology, University of Kentucky, Lexington, KY

Gordon B. Moskowitz, PhD, Department of Psychology, Princeton University, Princeton, NJ

Steven L. Neuberg, PhD, Department of Psychology, Arizona State University, Tempe, AZ

Rosemary Pacini, PhD, Department of Psychology, University of Massachusetts, Amherst, MA

Richard E. Petty, PhD, Department of Psychology, Ohio State University, Columbus, OH

Jason E. Plaks, MA, Department of Psychology, Columbia University, New York, NY

Deborah A. Prentice, PhD, Department of Psychology, Princeton University, Princeton, NJ

Kenneth R. Ryalls, PhD, Department of Psychology, College of Saint Mary, Omaha, NE

Norbert Schwarz, PhD, Department of Psychology, University of Michigan; Institute for Social Research, Ann Arbor, MI

James Sexton, PhD, Department of Psychology, University of Massachusetts at Amherst, Amherst, MA

Jeffrey W. Sherman, PhD, Department of Psychology, Northwestern University, Evanston, IL

Steven J. Sherman, PhD, Department of Psychology, Indiana University, Bloomington, IN

Ian Skurnik, PhD, Department of Psychology, Princeton University, Princeton, NJ

Eliot R. Smith, PhD, Department of Psychological Sciences, Purdue University, West Lafayette, IN

Scott Spiegel, MS, Department of Psychology, University of Maryland, College Park, MD

Philip E. Tetlock, PhD, Department of Psychology, Ohio State University, Columbus, OH

Erik P. Thompson, PhD, Department of Psychology, Washington University, St. Louis, MO

Tamara Towles-Schwen, MA, Department of Psychology, Indiana University, Bloomington, IN

James S. Uleman, PhD, Department of Psychology, New York University, New York, NY

Duane T. Wegener, PhD, Department of Psychological Sciences, Purdue University, West Lafayette, IN

Wendy Wood, PhD, Department of Psychology, Texas A & M University, College Station, TX

Preface

During the past two decades, researchers in various areas of social and cognitive psychology have developed dual-process models of social information processing. The intellectual seeds of this family of psychological theorizing date back even farther (see Chapter 2). Dual-process models have been applied in a variety of areas, including social attitudes, stereotyping, person perception, memory, judgment, and decision making. Although these theories differ on a number of dimensions, including domain of application and specific definitions, they all share the basic assumption that two qualitatively different modes of information processing operate in making judgments and decisions and in solving problems. In essence, the common distinction in dual-process models is between a fast, associative information-processing mode based on low-effort heuristics, and a slow, rule-based information-processing mode based on high-effort systematic reasoning. Related dual-process perspectives distinguish between controlled versus uncontrolled, conscious versus unconscious, and affective versus cognitive modes of processing. The present volume reviews basic assumptions of dual-process theories and the numerous areas of social, personality, and cognitive psychology in which these models have been applied and tested.

The purpose of this book is to integrate existing theory and research on alternative modes, or systems, of processing information about the social world. We feature theorizing that incorporates alternative processing modes, rather than theorizing that (while it may acknowledge alternative systems) aims mainly to explicate a single system of information processing. The contributions to this volume thus go beyond providing alternative theories of a process, such as the additive versus configural explanations of impression formation that were popular in the 1950s and 1960s, and the dissonance versus self-perception explanations of induced compliance that were in vogue in the 1970s. Instead of alternative theories of a process, then, the present contributions explicate theories of alternative processes.

In planning this project, we hoped for a volume that would provide a forum for study, discussion, and potential integration of the nature, antecedents, and consequences of the alternative systems implicated in current dual-process theorizing. An essential question that our contributing authors address concerns the defining properties of the alternative processing modes they postulate. As suggested above, many of our authors distinguish between a fast, low-effort, associative processing mode and a relatively slow, high-effort, rule-based processing mode (e.g., Chapters 4, 5, 6, 11, 12, 13, 16, and 24). As readers will see, this distinction is then used to understand phenomena as diverse as attitude change (e.g., Chapter 3), stereotyping and prejudice (e.g., Chapters 11, 17, and 21), the predictability of behavior from attitudes (Chapters 5 and 6), overconfident attributional inferences (Chapter 8), inferences about personality traits (Chapter 7 and 9), and metacognition (Chapter 24). Some of these authors, and others, emphasize other questions about processing modes: their intentionality (e.g., Chapters 4, 7, 12 and 20), their controllability versus uncontrollability (e.g., Chapters 17, 18, 19, and 21), their conscious versus unconscious nature (e.g., Chapters 4, 8, 13, 18, and 22), their affective versus cognitive nature (e.g., Chapters 10, 22, 23, and 24), and their serial versus parallel nature (e.g, Chapters 1, 15, and 19).

Another important set of issues addressed by many of our contributors concerns the relationship between alternative processing modes. Do the alternative processing modes postulated in these theories operate simultaneously or in a stage-like manner, or are they mutually exclusive (e.g., Chapters 1, 3, 4, 8, 15, 19, and 20)? Do alternative processing modes lie along a continuum, or are they more or less dichotomous (e.g., Chapters 11, 12, and 30)? Do the alternative modes of processing operate independently, or do they interact, and if so in what forms (e.g., Chapters 3, 4, 5, 6, 12, and 25)?

A third general issue concerns the antecedents and consequences of alternative processing modes. What are the motivational factors (e.g., affect, goals; e.g., Chapters 3, 4, 20, 27, 28, and 31); and cognitive factors (e.g., expertise, processing demands; e.g., Chapters 4, 8, 11, and 12) that activate or exacerbate each mode or system of processing? Can we identify personality factors, in addition to situational factors, that regulate the selection and utilization of processing mode (e.g, Chapters 3, 9, 23, and 25)? Are different processing modes differentially associated with different types of social stimuli (e.g., Chapters 10, 26, and 30)? Finally, what outcomes ensue from alternative processing modes? For example, does processing mode differentially affect the likelihood of cognitive biases and errors (e.g., Chapters 8, 10, 11, 12, 15, 19, 21, 28, 29, and 31), subjective confidence (Chapters 4 and 8), and the perseverance and behavioral impact of judgments and decisions (e.g., Chapters 3, 5, and 6)?

Finally, although the majority of our contributors articulate or endorse the merits of qualitatively distinguishable modes of processing, this assumption is itself an issue of scholarly attention (see Chapter 1). In particular, some contributors argue that such distinctions are unnecessary (Chapters 14 and 15). For these contributors, only one reasoning process (e.g., syllogistic reasoning) is necessary to account for the variety of findings observed in the current dual-process literature.

The present volume thus provides the first comprehensive summary of theory, research, and criticism about multiple modes of processing in social and cognitive psychology. As such, the book provides a useful source for researchers in many areas of social, cognitive, and personality psychology. Because of the breadth of phenomena covered by dual-process theories, the book should also prove useful as a primary text or secondary reading for graduate-level and advanced undergraduate-level courses in psychology.

As we hope readers will discover, the last two decades of research on dual-process theories have produced a wealth and variety of important insights about social thought, judgment, and behavior. Thus we feel that the time is particularly ripe for a volume such as this one. Of course, such a book would have been impossible to produce without the enthusiastic cooperation of our contributors. These authors are an especially prominent and dedicated group of scholars who have successfully conveyed in their chapters the excitement and importance of their work, which in many cases reflects years of programmatic research.

SHELLY CHAIKEN
YAACOV TROPE

Contents

V APPLICATIONS AND EXTENSIONS
OF DUAL-PROCESS THEORIZING

I

Overview

1

What the Mind's Not

DANIEL T. GILBERT

Do I contradict myself?
Very well then I contradict myself,
(I am large, I contain multitudes.)
—WALT WHITMAN, *Song of Myself* (1855/1959)

Like Walt Whitman, this book contains multitudes. It is a collection of roughly 30 chapters, most of which describe dual-process models of some interesting and important psychological phenomena. With roughly 30 chapters on dual processes before them, some readers may be tempted by arithmetic to conclude that the human mind is characterized by roughly 60 psychological processes that are conveniently paired and explicated in these pages. Others may be suspicious of a number that is so perfectly round and that so coincidentally approximates the number of authors. Those readers may suspect that the human mind is actually characterized by a somewhat smaller number of processes—as small a number as, say, two—and that the authors of these chapters must therefore be describing different functions, consequences, or features of this fundamental pair.

PLATO'S GAME

So which is it? Two, roughly 30, or something between? It depends, of course, on how one counts. The neuroscientist who says that a particular phenomenon is the result of two processes usually means to say something unambiguous—for example, that the inferior cortex does one thing, that the limbic system does another, and that together the electrochemical activities of these two anatomical regions produce a feeling of ennui, the aroma of stale cabbage, or the sneaking suspicion that one's spouse has been replaced by a replica. In such instances the phrase "dual processes" refers to the activities of two different brain regions that may be physically discriminable, and the neuroscientist says there are "two processes" because the neuroscientist is talking about things that can be counted. But few of the psychologists whose chapters appear in this volume would claim that the dual processes in *their* models necessarily correspond to the activity of two distinct brain structures (cf. Smith & DeCoster, 1997). What, then, could these dry psychologists mean when they say "two"? Are such claims to be taken literally and tested? Could anyone do an experiment whose results would convince us that an embarrassing calculation error had been made and that, as it turns out, there are actually *11* processes underlying persuasion, or stereotyping, or person perception, or attitude formation?

Probably not. And the reason why not is that while the word "dual" is a stolid descendant of the Latin *duo* or "two," "process" is a friskier term derived from the Latin *processus*, meaning "a moving forward" or "an unfolding in time" or, roughly speaking, "an event." Surely a herd of philosophers could spend the happier part of eternity debating and never deciding whether a wink and a nod constitute one or two events for a blind horse. Because there are generally no tangible referents for the "processes" specified by dry psychology's talk of dual processes, there is generally no proper way to count them, and hence no way to know whether they have been counted properly. Not to fear, because dry psychologists who champion dual-process models are usually not stuck on two. Few would come undone if their models were recast in terms of three processes, or four, or even five. Indeed, the only number they would not happily accept is one, because claims about dual processes in dry psychology are not so much claims about how many processes there *are*, but claims about how many processes there *aren't*. And the claim is this: There aren't one.

And why not? Because people are capable of too many different things—capable of being foolish one moment and wise the next, capable of behaving intransigently and then credulously in turn, capable of believing the right thing with their whole hearts while saying precisely the wrong thing with their whole mouths, and so on. The sheer variety of an individual's behavior is perhaps the first and most inescapable observation one can make about a person, and such variety seems to cry out for explanation. "How could you be so stupid?" we ask—never of those who are stupid, but rather of those whose momentary stupidity stands in stark relief against the background of their typical cleverness. What could possibly give rise to the diversity of thought, feeling, and action of which most people are naturally possessed? Plato suggested that complex behavior is best understood as the product of the interaction of less complex faculties (Hundert, 1995) and some form or another of this "homuncular functionalism" (Lycan, 1991) has been the favorite explanatory strategy of philosophers and psychologists for the roughly 2,000 years since. Indeed, it is almost a truism in modern

psychology that "the *explanation* of mental phenomena must always reside in the interaction and organization of multiple parts" (Bateson, 1979, p. 103; emphasis in original). An inventory of those multiple parts—cognition and emotion, reason and intuition, automaticity and control, consciousness and unconsciousness, ego and id—provides a natural history of psychology's attempts to explain the complexity of the individual (see Moskowitz, Skurnik, & Galinsky, Chapter 2, this volume).

A NOISE IN THE BOX

Like this book, then, the mind is also a container of multitudes. But how can a list of simple parts explain the complex behavior of wholes? Parts execute processes, and through their interaction, these processes give rise to complex behavior. Consider, for example, how four elementary "interior designs" might be used to explain the complex behavior of the soft drink machine at the refreshment counter in the cinema lobby (see Figure 1.1).

Selective Designs

The first thing one notices about a system is its overt behavior. For example, while standing in the popcorn line we may notice that when the underemployed teenager in the paper hat thumps the button on the side of the soft drink machine, the machine delivers a cup of cola. When the teen exhibits a somewhat lighter touch, the machine delivers a cup of water. How might we explain the complex behavior of the machine? The behaviorist would map the historical relations between the teenager's taps and the machine's spurts and offer these regularities as explanations of the machine's reactions. But this is rather like explaining an automobile's performance by avoiding all mention of things under the hood, and it naturally leaves modern psychologists hungry. Although we cannot see the soda machine's interior from where we are standing, we might pass the time by speculating that deep inside the machine are two nozzles, one of which draws water from a hidden reservoir and spurts it into the output tube and the other of which does the same with cola. We might speculate further that the in-

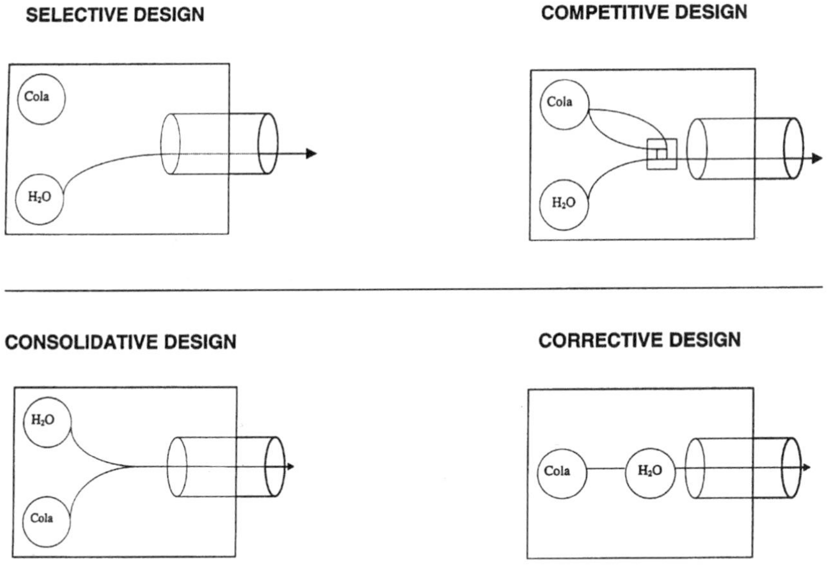

SELECTIVE DESIGN

COMPETITIVE DESIGN

CONSOLIDATIVE DESIGN

CORRECTIVE DESIGN

FIGURE 1.1. Four elementary interior designs for a soda machine.

tensity of the button press causes one or the other of these inner nozzles to spurt its particular brand of liquid into the output tube. An imaginary interior of this sort seems to do a fine job of explaining how a machine with just one output tube can behave "water-ishly" and "cola-ishly" in turn. Similarly, psychologists often explain the fact that people behave differently at different times by positing two inner processes that are activated by different stimuli. Chaiken's (1987) heuristic–systematic model, Petty and Cacioppo's (1986) elaboration likelihood model, Schwarz's (1990) mood-as-information model, and Tesser's (1986) self-evaluation maintenance model are just a few of the well-known social-psychological models that use selective designs to explain the behavioral variety of individuals. In each case, people do one thing on one occasion and another thing on another occasion because they are on all occasions inhabited by two qualitatively distinct processes, one of which is active and one of which is dormant in any given instance.

Competitive Designs

If the popcorn line is especially long, we might find ourselves dreaming up even fancier architectures. For example, we might imagine an interior design in which a button press causes *both* of the invisible inner nozzles to send their liquids surging toward the output tube. Upon arriving at the output tube, the faster or more forceful stream pushes up against a gate that allows the flow into the output tube, while simultaneously closing another gate that reroutes the slower or less forceful stream back to its original reservoir. We could even weave into our story something about how the force of the button press gives a hydraulic advantage to one or the other stream, thus determining which stream will hit the gate first and thus be funneled down the output tube. Or perhaps we would rather imagine that the humidity in the room, the magnetic fields generated by the nearby nacho-making machine, or even some random quantum event determines the position of the gate, and hence determines which of the two streams will win or lose. In any case, the two streams compete, the victor earns the right to send its stuff sliding down the output tube, and the loser returns home to wait for another opportunity. This architecture, like the one before it, explains how a machine with one output tube can behave "water-ishly" and "cola-ishly" on different occasions.

Although social psychologists enjoy a

good competition as much as anyone, they rarely call on the competitive design, which is for them a relatively minor variant of the selective design. In both cases, one process controls behavior and one does not. In the selective design, the noncontrolling process is dormant, and in the competitive design it is active but ultimately ineffective. Because social psychologists are generally in the business of explaining observable behavior, they tend to worry more about the nature of the controlling process than about that of the noncontrolling process. The noncontrolling process has no readily observable consequences, and thus social psychologists have no compelling reason to postulate its occurrence. Cognitive psychologists, on the other hand, are often more concerned with the nature of mental events than with the observable behaviors to which they give rise, and thus their models often do include competitive designs. For example, when people hear polysemous words such as "bank" (which can mean "riverside" or "financial institution"), they seem to experience only one of the word's meanings. But Marcel (1981) suggests that both meanings are initially activated by the utterance, and that a gating mechanism then quickly considers the appearance of the word "boat" in an earlier sentence, allows "riverside" into consciousness, and sends "financial institution" back from whence it came. The fact that a process is launched may be quite important, even if that process fails to control behavior.

Consolidative Designs

Both the selective and competitive designs can explain why a soda machine (or a soda jerk) acts one way on some occasions and a very different way on others. In the first case, the selection happens early, before one of the processes ever gets started. In the second case, the selection happens later, after the processes are initiated but before they eventuate in a behavioral output. But inner processes need not battle for control of the output tube. Rather, inner processes may be simultaneously activated by a single stimulus, and the system's behavior may be understood as a joint function of both processes. Consider, for example, a soda machine that does not deliver just two kinds of drinks, but instead delivers an array of drinks ranging from a cupful of oozing syrup to a tasty cola to a somewhat watery cola to a glass of stale tap water. How might such behavioral variety be explained? One possibility is that the machine has two inner nozzles, and that in response to the push of a button, one nozzle spurts a very stout cola and the other nozzle spurts carbonated water. The two spurts then merge and are directed into the output tube, so that when all goes well, a perfectly balanced stream of cola is extruded. When all does not go well (e.g., when the machine is tilted, or when one of the nozzles is a bit clogged with airborne dust, or when the tapping sequences is like this rather than like that), the result is a soft drink that is too hearty or too thin.

In the last few decades, philosophers, psychologists, and neuroscientists alike have come to think of the brain as a massively parallel system that "generates reality" by integrating the results of computations that are performed by discrete, distributed modules (e.g., Fodor, 1983; Gazzaniga, 1988; McClelland & Rumelhart, 1986). The identity and location of an object in space may be computed by different neural systems (Ungerleider & Mishkin, 1982), but fortunately for us, those computations are consolidated before they reach consciousness. As such, we see "a toaster on the table" rather than "a something on the table" or "a toaster everywhere at once." In social psychology, consolidative designs are so plentiful that we often don't recognize them as designs at all. For example, no theorist suggests that our impressions of others are based on either their verbal behavior, their nonverbal behavior, or their category membership. Rather, different processing mechanisms are thought to make sense of these different kinds of information and then to consolidate the results of their computations before sending an integrated impression to consciousness (e.g., Carlston, 1992). Just as a soda machine may blend the water and the cola somewhat differently across instances, such that some cups of soda are a bit more watery than others, so the informational outputs of different modules may be blended slightly differently across instances and hence may give rise to a smooth continuum of inferences and actions. Sometimes our impressions are dominated by a person's nonverbal behaviors; sometimes they are merely tinged by it. A consolidative design can give rise to the full spectrum of possibilities.

Corrective Designs

Soda machines with consolidative interior designs are usually preset to blend the two inner streams according to the manufacturer's recipe for *le cola magnifique*, and the occasional cup of goop is generally regarded as a disappointment rather than an innovation. One way to reduce such disappointments is to reengineer the machine so that its design is corrective rather than consolidative. Imagine a machine that has a reservoir filled with perfect cola. A button press directs a stream of the substance from the reservoir to the output tube. Alas, because even the most perfect beverage undergoes subtle changes as it sits in its reservoir waiting for a customer to order it, the machine has a sensor located between the reservoir and the output tube. After it receives a button press, this sensor quickly samples and measures the sugar content of the cola stream as it surges forward. If the sensor determines that the surging cola is too sweet, it signals a second nozzle (located just in front of the output tube) to squirt just a tad of water into the surging cola stream before it hits the output tube. In both the corrective and the consolidative machines, the outputs of the two inner nozzles are being blended. But the corrective machine's blends are especially well balanced because the output of one process serves as the input for the other.

Just as the competitive design is a variant of the selective design, the corrective design is a variant of the consolidative design. In both the consolidative and corrective designs, the system's output is a mixture of the products of its inner processes. But there are two important differences between these designs. First, in the case of the consolidative design, some initiating event (such as a button press) activates both processes simultaneously, and each process's contribution to the final output is determined by the formula for their admixture. Second, although the mixture may vary from occasion to occasion, this variability is always the unanticipated consequence of some annoying external condition, such as the tilt of the machine, random fluctuations in the teenager's thumb pressure, or the amount of dust in the air. In the case of the corrective design, the initiating event activates just one process, and that process activates a second process. The second process modifies, adjusts, or corrects the first, but it does so *sensitively*; that is, on each occasion it uses information about the state of the first process to determine the proper mixing formula. The corrective design is in this sense a "smart consolidator" that can hold a system's behavior relatively constant by using the second process to compensate for momentary variations in the product of the first process. Corrective designs are among social psychology's favorites: The sequential-operations model (Gilbert, Pelham, & Krull, 1988), the Spinozan model (Gilbert, 1991), Fiske and Neuberg's (1990) continuum model, Devine's (1989) model of stereotyping, and Wegener and Petty's (1997) flexible-correction model are just a few examples.

	ARE BOTH PROCESSES ACTIVATED?	DO BOTH PROCESSES CONTROL OUTPUT?
Selective Design	NO	NO
Competitive Design	YES	NO
Consolidative Design	YES	YES
Corrective Design	SOMETIMES	SOMETIMES

FIGURE 1.2. Features of the four elementary interior designs.

THINNING THE MULTITUDES

Three things should be clear from this tour de guts. First, there are many more than four ways to hook up a dual-process system. The selective, competitive, consolidative, and corrective designs are among the most familiar to psychologists, but gates and sensors and nozzles can always be added, removed, and rearranged to produce any number of other equally amazing machines. Second, it should be clear that a good detective may often use a machine's behavior to learn something about the machine's interior design. For example, if every time a machine delivers a delicious cup of cola it also emits a gurgling sound from somewhere in the vicinity of the water reservoir, then the good detective can be fairly certain that the water reservoir is being affected in some way by the cola-inducing button press, and that the selective design is therefore not a plausible architecture for this machine. Similarly, if over many occasions the machine's output comprises a smooth continuum of beverages that range from syrup to water, then both the selective and competitive designs may be effectively dismissed, because each produces just two distinct drinks and not a rainbow of blends.

But the third and most important clear thing is this: Although a talented detective may be able to rule out one or more architectures, no detective can rule in just one (Anderson, 1978). When inferences about architecture are informed only by knowledge of inputs (tap tap) and outputs (spurt spurt), then the conceptual Erector Set of gates, sensors, and other optional accessories affords the creative tinker an endless number of ways to link the tapping to the spurting (see Braitenburg, 1984). To be sure, there are behaviors that a particular architecture cannot possibly perform, and hence behaviors that can be used to rule out that particular architecture. But there is no behavior that can be performed by only one architecture, and hence no behavior that can unequivocally determine the nature of the machine's design. If we learn that an animal flies, then we know it cannot be designed like a turtle or a Chevrolet. Nonetheless, it could well be designed like any one of the known or unknown varieties of birds or insects, or like something else entirely. The ability to fly tells us how an animal is not designed, but it can never tell us precisely how an animal is designed, because there will always be more than one design that can do flying. Extending the list of criterial behaviors does not solve the problem ("It flies, lays eggs, has teeth, and votes Republican"), because the talented tinker can always design two slightly different animals, both of which can accomplish everything on the list.

The conclusion should be sobering: If dry psychology is an attempt to deduce a machine's true interior design by observing its behavior, then dry psychology is a game with no winning moves. And getting dry psychology all wet won't solve that problem. Emerging technologies are now allowing us to peek inside the head, and we might naively hope that someday soon we will find ourselves *looking* at the designs that until now we have merely *inferred* from behavior. But that won't happen. Because when we look inside the container of multitudes, we do not find ourselves looking at designs, but at the marvelous meatloaf that implements the designs—which are not, after all, real, meaty things that can be looked at, but *descriptions* in "Erector Set language" of how real meat makes real behavior. The microscopic behaviors of the wet gray stuff that constitutes the system (like the macroscopic behaviors of the system itself) provide much useful information, which allows us to rule out more designs more effectively than ever before. But if we are to avoid being disappointed at the end of a long day of brain science, we need to recognize at its dawn that knowledge of a brain's doings cannot reduce the number of plausible designs to one, any more than knowledge of inputs and outputs can. Just as different designs may underlie a single pattern of taps and spurts, so a single pattern of electrochemical activity or nervous connections can be the foundation for many different designs. Behaviors are real, brains are real, and designs are ways of thinking about and talking about—and hence understanding—the relation between these real things.

Now most of us don't like to play games they we can't possibly win, and if we buy the foregoing arguments, we may be tempted to give up the design game altogether and concentrate our efforts instead on the mapping of macroscopic and microscopic spurts: "When Jacob thinks about whitefish, this brain region lights up. When he doesn't, it doesn't. Next question?" Alas, that's not a winning move either. Neural behaviorism is no more interesting than the full-body behaviorism that psychologists abandoned several decades ago, and a psychological science that specializes in design-free descriptions of neural activity, bodily movements, words, deeds, or social interactions is a science whose intellectual achievements are destined to be no deeper than "The shin bone is connected to the thigh bone." Psychology tried giving up the design game once, and the results were a generation of disaffected cognitive revolutionaries and an extraordinary number of well-trained pigeons. Psychology-as-We-Know-It *is* the design game, and if we find that we can't make the winning move, then we need to change our minds about what it means to win. Specifically, rather than defining dry psychology as a game in which players win by deducing the mind's One True Design, we might think of it instead as a game in which players earn points by making observations that eliminate one false design after another—a game in which we measure molar and molecular human activity with our scanners, chronometers, rating scales, and eyes, and then use these measurements to say what the human mind cannot possibly be. For instance, if our measurements allowed us to conclude that the mind cannot possibly be a device that, say, represents information before believing it, or has conscious intentions before it acts on them, or knows the causes of its own reactions to events in the world, then those measurements could eliminate certain designs and hence eliminate myths about the mind that we might otherwise be tempted to embrace. There would still be an infinite number of plausible designs, of course, but in each case, one design would be discredited and gone for good.

Is that progress? If our experiments rule out some implausible designs but leave an infinite number of plausible alternatives, do they accomplish anything at all? Yes, they do, and to understand how they do requires that we consider two different conceptions of scientific progress. Most of us think of science as a long, slow journey from ignorance to certainty, which can be represented as movement along a fragment with a fixed origin and a fixed endpoint. (See the top panel in Figure 1.3, but don't look at the bottom panel.) When one moves along a fragment, one may estimate one's progress by the distance one has traveled from the origin or by the distance remaining until the endpoint. Both ways of reckoning produce the same estimate of progress because the two distances are perfectly reciprocal, and one can measure the journey by asking, "How far have we come?" or "Are we there yet?" The latter question makes perfectly good sense because there is a "there" to get to, and if any distance remains between it and one's present position, then one is most certainly not yet "there." The fragmentary view of the design game suggests that one may measure one's progress by counting the number of plausible designs that remain when an experiment is finished. If the number is more than one, then the traveler has every right to be crabby.

But if we accept the notion that there are *always* several plausible designs that can account for a particular set of behavioral observations, then we are acknowledging that we can be perfectly ignorant of—but never perfectly certain about—the mind's true design. In that case, scientific progress is best construed as a journey along a vector—a line with a fixed origin but no endpoint. (Now see the bottom panel of Figure 1.3 and pretend you didn't peek earlier.) As our experiments teach us more and more about what the mind's not, we move further and further from the origin. If we use the "Are we there yet?" heuristic and calculate our progress in terms of the distance remaining, then we will mistakenly conclude that we have not moved because we are, as we were, infinitely far from our final destination. Indeed, no matter what kinds of experiments we do, we cannot see progress in the design game if we insist on measuring the distance between here and eternity. After a few such measurements, even the most devoted among us would probably give up such a journey and send out for pigeons.

What a shame. Because if for just a moment we had glanced backward instead of forward, we would have noticed something wondrous. Although perfect knowledge was drawing no closer, our perfect ignorance was disappearing at a pulse-pounding rate. Indeed, the vectorian view of science suggests that the only meaningful way to measure progress in the design game is to count the

Fragmentary Science

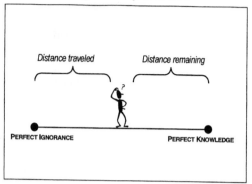

Vectorian Science

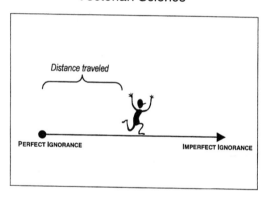

FIGURE 1.3. Two ways of thinking about scientific progress in psychology.

number of implausible designs that have been eliminated by a day of honest work, and not to calculate the distance remaining to some final solution. Just as adventurers evaluate their journeys by the lands they have visited and not by the worlds without end that they've yet to explore, so psychologists may evaluate their progress by the myths they've dispelled and the ignorance they've vanquished, rather than by their proximity to a complete understanding of the human mind.

CONCLUSION

The vectorian view suggests that an essay does not have a conclusion so much as it has one brief section that just happens to be fur-

thest from the title. This chapter has done the easy work by arguing that the mind can profitably be thought of as a container of multitudes, and that the goal of dry psychology is to invent plausible descriptions of the relations between these multitudes without anointing one of them. But abstract argument is cheap, and the chapters that follow this one do the much more difficult work of describing in detail how particular parts might interact by design and give rise to particular complexities. The authors of these chapters are all good detectives who have gathered considerable evidence of the mind's doings and then constructed compelling accounts of how the mind might do them. Each chapter tells us something valuable about what the mind's not, and thus leaves us less ignorant than we were before. In this world, at least, who could ask for more?

ACKNOWLEDGMENTS

The writing of this chapter was supported by research Grant No. RO1-MH56075 from the National Institute of Mental Health. I am grateful to the members of the Harvard University Emotion, Cognition, Brain, and Behavior Group for their insightful comments on an earlier version of this chapter.

REFERENCES

Anderson, J. R. (1978). Arguments concerning representations for mental imagery. *Psychological Review, 85,* 249–277.

Bateson, G. (1979). *Mind and nature: A necessary unity.* New York: Bantam.

Braitenberg, V. (1984). *Vehicles: Experiments in synthetic psychology.* Cambridge, MA: MIT Press.

Carlston, D. E. (1992). Impression formation and the modular mind: The associated systems theory. In L. L. Martin & A. Tesser (Eds.), *The construction of social judgments* (pp. 301–341). Hillsdale, NJ: Erlbaum.

Chaiken, S. (1987). The heuristic model of persuasion. In M. P. Zanna, J. M. Olson, & C. P. Herman (Eds.), *Social influence: The Ontario Symposium* (Vol. 5, pp. 3–39). Hillsdale, NJ: Erlbaum.

Devine, P. G. (1989). Stereotypes and prejudice: Their automatic and controlled components. *Journal of Personality and Social Psychology, 56,* 5–18.

Fiske, S. T., & Neuberg, S. E. (1990). A continuum of impression formation, from category-based to individuating processes: Influences of information and motivation on attention and interpretation. In M. P. Zanna (Ed.), *Advances in experimental social psychology* (Vol. 23, pp. 1–74). San Diego, CA: Academic Press.

Fodor, J. A. (1983). *The modularity of mind.* Cambridge, MA: MIT Press.

Gazzaniga, M. S. (1988). Brain modularity: Towards a philosophy of conscious experience. In A. J. M. E. Bisiach (Ed.), *Consciousness in contemporary science* (pp. 218–238). Oxford: Clarendon Press.

Gilbert, D. T., Pelham, B. W., & Krull, D. S. (1988). On cognitive busyness: When persons perceive meet persons perceived. *Journal of Personality and Social Psychology, 54,* 733–740.

Gilbert, D. T. (1991). How mental systems believe. *American Psychologist, 46,* 107–119.

Hundert, E. M. (1995). *Lessons from an optical illusion.* Cambridge, MA: Harvard University Press.

Lycan, W. G. (1991). Homuncular functionalism meets PDP. In W. Ramsey, S. P. Stich, & D. E. Rumelhart (Eds.), *Philosophy and connectionist theory* (pp. 259–286). Hillsdale, NJ: Erlbaum.

Marcel, T. (1981). Conscious and preconscious recognition of polysemous words: Locating the selective effects of prior verbal context. In R. Nickerson (Ed.), *Attention and performance VIII* (pp. 435–457). Hillsdale, NJ: Erlbaum.

McClelland, J. L., & Rumelhart, D. E. (Eds.). (1986). *Parallel distributed processing: Explorations in the microstructure of cognition* (Vol. 2). Cambridge, MA: MIT Press.

Petty, R. E., & Cacioppo, J. T. (1986). The elaboration likelihood model of persuasion. In L. Berkowitz (Ed.), *Advances in experimental social psychology* (Vol. 19, pp. 123–205). New York: Academic Press.

Schwarz, N. (1990). Feelings as information: Informational and motivational functions of affective states. In E. T. Higgins & R. M. Sorrentino (Eds.), *Handbook of motivation and cognition: Foundations of social behavior* (Vol. 2, pp. 527–561). New York: Guilford Press.

Smith, E. R., & DeCoster, J. (1997). *Heuristic–systematic and other dual process models in social and cognitive psychology: An integration and connectionist interpretation.* Unpublished manuscript, Purdue University.

Tesser, A. (1986). Some effects of self-evaluation maintenance on cognition and action. In R. M. Sorrentino & E. T. Higgins (Eds.), *Handbook of motivation and cognition: Foundations of social behavior* (pp. 435–464). New York: Guilford Press.

Ungerleider, L. G., & Mishkin, M. (1982). Two cortical visual systems. In D. J. Ingle, M. A. Goodale, & R. J. W. Mansfield (Eds.), *Analysis of visual behavior* (pp. 549–586). Cambridge, MA: MIT Press.

Wegener, D. T., & Petty, R. E. (1997). The flexible correction model: The role of naïve theories of bias in bias correction. In M. Zanna (Ed.), *Advances in experimental social psychology* (Vol. 29, pp. 141–208). San Diego, CA: Academic Press.

2

The History of Dual-Process Notions, and the Future of Preconscious Control

GORDON B. MOSKOWITZ
IAN SKURNIK
ADAM D. GALINSKY

If I say that I see a book before me on my desk, I shall be criticized, because nobody can *see* a "book." . . . Even the character of being an "object," or "thing," which I have tacitly attributed to the experiences I have called "book" and "desk," is improper in correct psychological description . . . we must learn to make the all-important distinction between *sensation* and *perception*, between the bare sensory material actually given to us and the host of other items which since childhood have become associated with it. You cannot see a book, I am told, since this term involves some knowledge about a class of objects to which this specimen belongs, and about their use, etc., whereas in pure seeing such knowledge cannot enter. . . . Objects cannot exist for us before sensory experience has become imbued with meaning.
—WOLFGANG KÖHLER (1930, pp. 54–55; emphasis in original)

In the quotation above, Köhler asserts that even the simplest forms of knowing, such as knowing that the thing on the desk is a "book," require the individual to make inferences that are not directly revealed by the properties of the thing (book). Such inferences represent a leap beyond what is objectively revealed by the stimuli, and this inferential leap becomes far more elaborate when the stimuli are social in nature—such as interpreting what others are like. A basic principle of human social-psychological functioning is that a person's understanding of self and others is transformed and "constructed" according to the specifications that the perceiver brings to meet the world of stimuli that bombard his or her senses (Gollwitzer & Moskowitz, 1996).

People are biased by their particular views; they see what they want to see, that which they already believe to be true. Certainly, this epistemological canon predates its exposition by psychologists such as Köhler (1930). Shakespeare invoked this principle when Hamlet, after likening Denmark to a prison, responds to his friend Rosencrantz's disagreement by retorting "Why then 'tis none to you; for there is nothing either good or bad, but thinking makes it so. To me it is a prison." Kant (1781/ 1990) stated this more formally: "Without the sensuous faculty no object would be given to us, and without the understanding no object would be thought" (p. 45). Instead of tracing this epistemological dictum through Hegel to Socrates and down through the ages to the

Talmud (where it is written: "We do not see things as they are; we see things as we are"), we focus on the final 100 years of the millennium—on empirical examinations of the psychological mechanisms through which social cognition is regulated and controlled.

How people negotiate their sense of meaning and understanding of the social world by making inferential leaps from sensory stimulation is the theoretical domain of social cognition and the dual-process models that inhabit the domain. If even a book is not immediately perceived, how do people come to arrive at a sense of knowing when perceiving other people and forming beliefs? Dual-process models in social psychology have approached questions of this type by conceiving of information processing as happening along a continuum. The anchors of this continuum reflect the "duality" invoked by these models. On the one hand, people can utilize little cognitive effort, elaboration, or capacity in thinking about the social world. They can lean on prior knowledge, heuristics, stereotypes, expectancies, scripts, and schemas to impose structure and order on new situations. In each of these cases, people act in a somewhat "mindless" fashion, arriving at their sense of knowing through a "top-down" process whereby a preconception is imposed on new information. On the other hand, people can expend a great deal of time, effort, and mental energy in systematically building decisions, beliefs, and a sense of knowing. This more "mindful" strategy is a "bottom-up" process that requires the exertion of cognitive effort to reflect on and examine the stimulus. Neither strategy guarantees a bias-free response; the two are just distinctive paths to arriving at knowledge—paths that individuals have the cognitive flexibility to choose between.

Dual-process models share a subset of beliefs about the quest for knowledge, opinions, and understanding. Each section of this chapter explores a theme that is common to these models, and traces some of the historical roots of the assumptions made concerning human epistemology.

THE CONSTRUCTION OF KNOWLEDGE

We have already seen the first theme emerging from the passage by Köhler that begins this chapter—that perception and knowing are never simply given to a perceiver by stimuli, but are constructed by the perceiver. Even a pencil cannot exist for an individual before the sensory experience of the object has been transformed through an interface with the individual's prior knowledge about writing utensils. As Bruner (1957, p. 123) put it, a perceiver's use of prior categories in inferring the identity of a perceived object "is as much a feature of perception as the sensory stuff from which percepts are made." This process in which the individual helps determine the identity of a stimulus (moving one from receiving a sensory cue to having a sense of knowing what the sensory cue actually is) was described as a process of forming *inferences* about identity. Bruner (1957, p. 133) labeled this "the most ubiquitous and primitive cognitive activity," where the person goes beyond the information given in order to imbue the stimulus with meaning (consistent with Köhler, 1930).

Constructing Knowledge Can Occur Unconsciously

The sense of "knowing" that inferential processes provide is experienced as something immediate—the identity of an object "pops" into our heads because the meaning seems to be a natural part of the object itself (we simply "know" that this is a pencil, he is a priest, etc.). But this "phenomenal immediacy" is actually mediated by a categorization process that occurs through a series of stages, and at each stage the interpretation of the sensory stimulus is subjected to being influenced by the perceiver. Bruner (1957, p. 124) believed that all perceptual experience occurs through a process whereby the thing (or person) being perceived "is placed in and achieves its 'meaning' from a class of percepts with which it is grouped." When the process is complete, the perceiver has moved from an unidentified sensory stimulation to an inference that categorizes the stimulus, producing knowledge of what it is: "That is a pencil" we state. The immediacy of this process led Bruner (1957) to believe that as "Helmholtz long ago suggested, the process is a silent one. If you will, the inference is often an 'unconscious' one" (p. 129).[1]

Thus, although we are influenced by internal processes of inference and categorization in understanding the social world, these processes proceed unconsciously, without our awareness. The "silence" of this process is dependent on how much overlap there is between the cue and our categories. As a consequence, even inferences about another person's disposition could "silently" pop into our heads through unconscious inferential processes. However, the overlap between cue (the other person's behavior) and our categories often is less complete in the case of categorizing interpersonal behavior, making the silence of the inference less likely. But given clear and diagnostic behavior (Moskowitz & Roman, 1992), perceivers do passively infer qualities in others and accept them as something inherent to the perceived person (Uleman, Newman, & Moskowitz, 1996). An important consequence of a silent (or spontaneous) inference is its phenomenal immediacy: A perceiver does not experience the judgment as a construction, built through the aid of expectancies, needs, and heuristics. Instead, there is what Asch (1952) called a "naïve realism," a belief that one's inferences accurately reflect, without mediation or bias, an external reality. Ichheiser (1943) articulated this view that subjectivity in perceiving others is so commonplace that it proceeds unconsciously:

> [A person] is not aware of the fact that certain processes [of misinterpretation] are at work within him [sic], which distort and falsify his experience of other people even on the level of immediate observation. It remains concealed from him that what he considers as "facts" is permeated by . . . unnoticed and unconscious but nevertheless systematically proceeding misinterpretations . . . we automatically interpret manifestations of other persons in specific ways without being aware of our doing so and without noticing that our observations are based on, and guided by, those unconscious interpretations. What we consider to be "objective facts" are actually products of our unnoticed interpretative manipulations. (pp. 145–146)

The Passive versus the Active Mind

Bruner's model of perception is consistent with Köhler's (1930, p. 61) view that "no experience escapes from the influence of meaning" and that psychology's task is to separate meaning from "pure" sensation. The notion that perception and sensation are distinct, and that the mind actively imposes meaning on

sensory data, is by no means universally accepted. Indeed, Köhler and his fellow Gestalt psychologists were a minority at the time they stressed the active and constructed nature of object perception. The behaviorist movement dominated during that period and did not deem speculations regarding the nature of cognition to be proper for the domain of psychological inquiry. The focus instead was on observed behavior as the only true form of psychological data. The behaviorists, instead, reflected the philosophical position of the 18th-century empiricist school (e.g., Berkeley, Hume, Locke), which stressed the role played by pure sensation in shaping perception. The empiricists rejected the notion of abstract or unobservable "causes" in favor of laws that are not predicated on the assumption of some unseen entity. It is simply enough to know that objects fall to the ground at a constant rate and to use the word "gravity" to describe this, rather than to believe in the notion of an entity called "gravity" that somehow "pulls" things and causes them to move at a constant rate. Empiricists regarded observable facts as the domain of reality; in their view, unseen entities are nice metaphors, but they have no place in science or philosophy.

For example, Locke (1690/1844, p. 75) presumed that the mind starts out like white paper—"void of all characters, without any ideas; How comes it to be furnished?" The one-word answer was "experience." All knowledge was said to be founded through two sources that together account for all of one's experience: "sensation" and "reflection." Locke described sensation as the understanding one achieves when the senses convey to the mind how an external object of stimulation affects the senses. Knowledge of coldness comes through experiencing the way in which an object labeled as "cold to the touch" affects the sense of touch. This basic type of knowledge was labeled a "simple idea," and Locke claimed that (1) "the mind is wholly passive in the reception of all its simple ideas" (p. 110), and (2) such ideas served as the material and foundation for more complex ideas. Reflection (e.g., thinking, doubting, believing, and willing) was described as the understanding one achieves when the mind operates on the simple ideas it already has. Through reflection, the mind has the power to repeat, compare, unite, and associate ideas, forming new and complex thoughts. "All this creative power of the mind amounts to no more than the faculty of compounding, transposing, augmenting, or diminishing the materials afforded us by the senses and experience" (Hume, 1788, p. 30).

Whereas the philosophical stance of behaviorism, with its emphasis on concrete experience and principles of association, followed from empiricism, Gestalt psychology adopted its philosophical stance from links to pragmatism and back to Kant and Hegel. Thus, though the early part of the 20th century presented a debate between Gestaltists and behaviorists, this debate had a character similar to that which epitomized James's (1890/1950, p. 403) and other pragmatists' stance toward the empiricists:

> These writers are bent on showing how the higher faculties of the mind are pure products of experience; and experience is supposed to be of something simply given. . . . [They] regard the creature as absolutely passive clay upon which experience rains down. The clay will be impressed most deeply where the drops fall thickest, and so the final shape of the mind is moulded. . . . These writers have, then, utterly ignored the glaring fact that subjective interest may, by laying its weighty index finger on particular items of experience, so accent them as to give to the least frequent associations far more power to shape our thought than the most frequent ones possess. . . . [Interest] *makes* experience more than is made by it. (Emphasis in original)

Gestalt Psychology and the Construction of Knowledge

The conflicting philosophical moorings of Gestalt psychology and behaviorism resulted in a dispute over the proper subject matter for psychological study. In one corner was Köhler's (1930) description of "direct experience" or the naive experience of reality (e.g., a feeling of warmth at family gatherings, memories of the Rhine's serenity along the German–Swiss border). Behaviorists labeled such experiences as impervious to and unavailable for scientific study, equating them with terms like "spirituality," which they saw as reflecting a "prescientific mythology." Instead, they took physics as their template, emphasizing how a system reacts under certain conditions, and how the reaction changes under different conditions. Such in-

formation is gained by objective observation and measurement. Behaviorism held this to be the proper form of experimentation in psychology, with observable behavior as the *only* subject matter.

Köhler (1930) believed that behaviorists wrongly equated studying experience with the psychology of introspection and its limited methodology. According to Köhler, psychology was driven to embrace behaviorism as a reaction against the introspectionists (e.g., Ebbinghaus, Wundt), whose approach (1) utilized reports about one's own mental experiences rather than experimentation, and (2) excluded external stimuli from the domain of interest. Gestalt theorists rejected both introspectionists' attempts to ignore external stimuli and behaviorists' reactionary belief that naive experience is outside the realm of study because such experience is not directly observable. They applied the scientific method espoused by behaviorists to the content area (mental experiences) focused on by introspectionists.

> As a scientific attitude the Homeric assault of behaviourism against "direct experience," "consciousness" and so forth appears very strange to me. . . The behaviourist forgets, however, that it is a truism in epistemology that I shall never be able to "prove" conclusively the existence of an independent physical world. As an extreme purist I might argue this point exactly as the behaviourist disputes the assumption of direct experience in others. Somehow it does not occur to the behaviourist to apply his epistemological criticism to the assumption of the physical world . . . he assumes the reality of this world with all the healthy naivete which he lacks in psychology. . . . Of course, personally and practically I am as convinced of [the physical world's] existence as any behaviourist has ever been, and I am fully aware of the fact that sciences may and must believe and postulate where the epistemologist, if he likes, may doubt. But then I shall believe and postulate the direct experience of others. (Köhler, 1930, pp. 23–24)

Postulating such experience, and believing that sensory data are altered into a perception by the mind's use of meaning and prior learning, reflect the fundamental assumptions of Gestalt psychology: The parts of a mental representation interact to make up a structure, and those interacting parts are dynamic in that they exert influence on one another. Understanding a structure cannot be achieved by examining the individual elements; it is achieved by examining the nature of the relationship between the parts and the emerging properties that the dynamic system reveals. A *gedanken* experiment illustrates this. Imagine a man walking toward you; he is 10 yards away, then 5. The image on the retina informs you that as the man approaches, he grows in size. But you do not perceive an emerging giant. Although the physical object remains constant, the stimulation that strikes the sensory apparatus varies. Yet your experience agrees with the constancy of the object. This apparent constancy illustrates that the organism does not respond to local stimuli as a series of mutually independent events, but to a constellation of stimuli as a functional "whole" (Köhler, 1930).

Gestalt psychology posed a dynamic view of perception, implying that the perceptual field is structured into *meaningful and understandable units* that are built through relationships among the parts, including the prior knowledge and needs of perceivers. This perspective influenced social psychology through two directions: first, through the Austrian and German researchers (e.g., Fritz Heider, Kurt Lewin) who emigrated to the United States at about the time of Hitler's rise to power; second, through the brand of pragmatism that emerged from the "metaphysical club" at late 19th-century Harvard (e.g., Charles Peirce, William James, Oliver Wendell Holmes), which influenced Allport and Bruner at Harvard in the 20th century. We now turn to social psychology's adoption of the idea that knowledge is a "construction."

Field Theory and the Life Space

The Gestalt movement was so nested in the hard-wired world of the psychology of perception that it was not uncommon to hear Gestalt psychologists reject the idea of studying such things as interpersonal judgments and motivation. But the general point that perceiving and knowing are not equivalent to pure sensory stimulation is especially true in the realm of social perception, where the stimulus behaviors observed are open to many interpretations, and perceivers are equipped with biases/expectations they are ready to impose.

Kurt Lewin worked during the early part of this century in Berlin (the center of Gestalt psychology) and applied Gestalt principles to a level of analysis that included the social sphere. Lewin believed that to discover the basic principles guiding behavior, we cannot reduce the elements being studied to neurophysiology. Rather, behavior can be understood only within the entire field of stimuli, as an interaction of a person within a situation. His general approach was labeled "field theory" (e.g., Lewin, 1936), and a person and his or her environment together made up a unit known as the "life space." The notion of life space was meant to capture both the physical and psychological (conscious and unconscious) environment. It emphasized a dynamic systems approach (combinations of elements in a stimulus field yield a product that is more than the sum of the qualities of the individual parts) and reflected the Gestalt principle of holism, in that action can be understood only within the context of the entire field:

> Every action one performs has some specific "background," and is determined by that background. A statement or a gesture which may be quite appropriate between companions in a swimming pool may be quite out of place, even insulting, at a dinner party. Judgment, understanding, perception are impossible without a related background, and the meaning of every event depends directly upon the nature of its background . . . the background itself is not often perceived, but only the "figure." (Lewin, 1935, p. 175)[2]

Another way Lewin's model leaned on the Gestalt notion that perception is subjective, is that needs were said to play a central role in structuring experience; wants of the individual operate like forces that guide perception of and movement within the life space. Of course, there are many forces operating at a given time on an individual, as the individual has many wants and desires simultaneously competing with one another. Behavior is as much a function of which of these internal wants is strongest as it is a function of which environmental opportunities (or obstacles) are present for promoting movement toward obtaining (or blocking obtaining) a desired object that would satisfy one of the individual's wants. Important in this thesis is the idea that the forces that direct perception and action are joint products of the individual and the environment. Lewin conceived of these forces as being like vectors between the individual and the environmental stimuli. The strength of each of these vectors, and in turn their ability to direct behavior, is dependent on the extent to which the environmental stimulus attracts or repels the individual. Through this ability of the stimulus to "speak" to the individual, the vector between the stimulus and a particular need of the individual develops what Lewin called *aufforderungscharakter*, which is translated as "valence." Thus, vector-like forces guide behavior by providing both a direction to act and a strength associated with that direction. In their ecological approach, McArthur and Baron (1983) similarly discussed the ability of stimuli to "speak to" one's needs, labeling the ability of the environment to draw out a specific behavior unique to that situation (and the individual's needs within that situation) as "affordance."

As an example, a person studying for an exam in his or her room may be enticed by the bed to lie down or by a novel on the bookshelf to procrastinate. This is not meant to imply that the person mechanically responds to stimuli; the bed alone does not trigger sleeping, the novel reading, or the exam notes studying. Whether the person sleeps, reads, or studies depends on his or her goals within that situation and which environmental stimulus speaks to those goals most clearly.

In addition, the model states that motives direct perception and movement in the life space latently, even if such motives were initially consciously chosen: "A goal can play an essential role in the psychological situation without being clearly present in consciousness" (Lewin, 1936, p. 19). Lewin referred to consciously chosen motives and goals that nonetheless operate unconsciously as "quasi-needs." To illustrate, when a person who usually walks to work adopts the goal of driving there, objects relevant to driving that normally go unnoticed begin to "appear" to the individual. Thus, signs along Nassau Street in Princeton that forbid a U-turn and appear every 20 yards went unseen while the person walked past them every day, but they now entice him or her to attend to them. The signs have not suddenly appeared; only their ability to speak to the person's current needs has, so that they no

longer fade into the background of the perceptual field. Furthermore, a sign's ability to capture attention (the intensity of the valence) depends on the strength of the quasi-need. Does the person need to make a U-turn? If not, he or she may drive past the sign, as oblivious to it as when the individual is on foot. Finally, valence exerts its influence even though the person is not consciously "looking" for signs. The goal is operating passively: An environmental cue is linked to and can trigger the goal, initiating an intended response (despite the person's not *consciously* intending the response at the time it occurs). Thus, people are not mechanically controlled by stimuli; goals operate preconsciously and surrender control over attention, perception, and action to the environment, so that the goal can be activated by relevant cues (See Moskowitz, Gollwitzer, Wasel, & Schaal, in press).

Construction That Draws from One's Culture

Much as Lewin did, Sherif brought the Gestalt emphasis on the dynamic and holistic nature of perception to social psychology. Sherif's focus, however, was not on needs and motives, but on culture and norms as a frame of reference used in constructing perception.

> Experience appears to depend always upon *relations*. . . . Perception, conceived as a case illustrative of experience in general, is the result of the organization of external and internal stimulating factors that come into functional relationship at a given time. Factors that come into such functional relationships are interdependent; they affect each other and the properties of any factor are determined partly by the properties of other factors. . . . This relational whole in our perceptions, judgments, and other experiences, involves definite frames of reference. These frames of reference prove to be not an arbitrary abstraction from the experience but a fundamental characteristic of every situation consisting of external and internal factors which form a functional whole. (Sherif, 1936, pp. 32–33; emphasis in original)

Sherif discussed two ways in which frames of reference guide the construction of knowledge. First, each time a stimulus is perceived, it may not arouse the same effect on the person: "There is no point-to-point correlation between a physical stimulus and the experience and subsequent behavior it arouses; the experience and the behavior may be, to a large extent, a function of the state of the organism at that time" (1936, p. 28). Second, different individuals perceive the same information in different ways: "Different persons may notice different characteristics of the same stimulus field . . . each culture emphasizes different aspects of the field, so that the field may take on altogether different modes of organization" (1936, p. 31). Such variations in perception both within and between individuals occur whether the external information is highly structured and well defined or not. But in ambiguous situations, where the physical stimuli do not impel an obvious meaning, the state of the organism, attitudes and anticipations, culture, and so forth exert a particularly large effect; a person does not experience confusion, but form, "total structures."

This point is made by Sherif's classic experiment utilizing the autokinetic effect to create an ambiguous situation in which a light, though stationary, was perceived as moving. When participants were asked to estimate the distance the light moved (the ambiguous judgment), their responses demonstrated how in ambiguous situations people rely on frames of reference, or norms, provided (in this case) by the responses of others to help achieve structure and meaning.

> In the course of the life history of the individual and as a consequence of his contact with the social world around him, the social norms, customs, values, etc., become interiorized in him. These interiorized social norms enter as frames of reference among other factors in situations to which they are related, and thus dominate or modify the person's experience and subsequent behavior in concrete situations. (Sherif, 1936, pp. 43–44)

Phenomenal Causality

Sherif's work stresses that in ambiguous situations, where the stimuli are not highly structured, we don't experience confusion; instead, units or wholes are formed that are structured and perceived as meaningful through their order. The perceptual system moves away from random groupings, open systems, irregular patterns, seeking instead closure (Gestalt-

mehrdeutigkeit). This was the starting point for Heider's (1944, 1958) examination of the processes involved in interpersonal perception.

Heider (1944) asserted that when we have an experience of any sort, the psychological situation has changed, and the cause for the change must be ascertained. The origin of the changed state can be attributed either to ourselves, to others, or to some environmental force. In attaining phenomenal causality, "causal effects often play the role of data and can be thought of as stimuli through which are mediated to us properties of the origin which belong to the stable relevant psychological environment" (p. 359). Adopting the Gestalt perspective, Heider assumed that the origin of the behavior (the other person) and the change (the person's behavior and its effects) form a perceptual unit, such that the two are believed to belong together. As a consequence, the behavior is then seen as a property of the person, and the person as the cause of the change.

Heider believed that this tendency to form units between people and their actions leads to a tendency to overattribute the causes of actions to the inherent qualities (personality) of the persons performing them—"to see the cause of their successes and failures in their personal characteristics and not in other conditions. When Nietzsche says, 'success is the greatest liar,' he refers to this error in attribution" (p. 361). This attributional bias occurs despite the fact that perceived behavior is almost always caused by a combination of factors (e.g., a perceived person's disposition, situational forces, and our own actions that could have provoked the behavior; see Heider, 1958). The result, as Ichheiser (1943, pp. 151–152) put it, is that "in interpreting individual behavior as an expression and consequence of personal traits, with disregard to the all-important role played by the (social) situation, we usually misinterpret the real underlying motivation of behavior."

Heider was proposing that our perception of others is an active construction, in that we have cognitive processes that promote unit formation, which affects the manner in which a stimulus is categorized. But he further believed that we subjectively determine the meaning of a stimulus through the filter of our wants, or the value in the life space of the person we are perceiving. "If we are inclined to disparage him we shall attribute his failures to his own person, his successes to his good luck or unfair practices" (p. 361).

Perceptual Readiness and Values

Rather than describing people as making attributional errors, Heider (1958) felt that wants, needs, expectancies, and meaning guide perception because they create "a general readiness to perceive" (p. 58). Bruner (1957) defined such readiness in interpreting a stimulus as

> the accessibility of categories for use in coding or identifying environmental events. Accessibility is a heuristic concept ... we measure the accessibility of the category apples [for example] by the amount of stimulus input of a certain pattern that is necessary to evoke the perceptual response "there is an apple" ... The likelihood that a sensory input will be categorized in terms of a given category is not only a matter of fit between sensory input and category specifications. It depends also on the accessibility of a category. To put the matter in an oversimplified way, given a sensory input with equally good fit to two nonoverlapping categories, the more accessible of the two categories would "capture" the input. (pp. 129–132)

Accessibility leads perceivers to interpret relevant information in line with what they are perceptually ready to see, rather than some competing interpretation. If a situation is ambiguous or overly complex, and its features are difficult to fit into a category (as is often the case for perceiving people), then accessible categories guide categorization. This interpretive influence is exerted by providing a frame of reference for the stimuli to be eased into. Thus, if a stereotype of a Jewish man is activated, the behavior of that man will be seen in line with the stereotype. The greater this perceptual readiness is, according to Bruner, "(a) the less the input necessary for categorization to occur in terms of this category, [and] (b) the wider the range of input characteristics that will be 'accepted' as fitting the category in question" (1957, p. 129). Thus, the minutest of actions, and a wide range of such actions by the man, will be interpreted as being consistent with the stereotype of Jews.

But how do people become perceptually ready? Heider spoke of "perceptual styles," indicating an emphasis on chronic states of readiness that guide a person from situation to situation (see also Higgins, King, & Mavin, 1982). Bruner noted that readiness often reflects a learned probability of events—the probability that a given category frequently occurring in a given context will come to be activated in the presence of that context. But Bruner also focused on the role played by the subjective needs and values of the perceiver, in relation to a given object of perception, in structuring the interpretation of the situation.

> In short, the accessibility of categories I employ for identifying the objects of the world around me must not only reflect the environmental probabilities of objects that fit these categories, but also reflect the search requirements imposed by my needs, my ongoing activities, my defenses, etc. (1957, p. 132)

Much as Lewin saw needs as operating passively to direct attention to environmental cues that facilitate movement toward achieving one's goals, Bruner believed that the role of values and needs in structuring perception is pervasive. Postman, Bruner, and McGinnies (1948) demonstrated this point by focusing on attention:

> What one sees, what one observes, is inevitably what one selects from a near infinitude of potential percepts. Perceptual selection depends not only upon the "primary determinants of attention" but is also a servant of one's interests, needs, and values. (p. 142)

They demonstrated that value-laden words had different thresholds of perceptivity, depending on whether the words were valued or disliked by an individual. James (1890/1950) eloquently put forth this idea that values and needs determine what, and how easily, attention is captured by determining what we are prepared (perceptually ready) to see. James asserts that the object we wish to capture with our attention may be very weak, a small noise in the midst of a crowd, and the way not to miss it is to prepare for it by either rehearsing it mentally or actually coming into contact with an exemplar. In doing so, this allows one to stand ready to receive the outward impression.

Watching for the distant clock to strike, our mind is so filled with its image that at every moment we think we hear the longed for or dreaded sound. So of an awaited footstep. Every stir in the wood is for the hunter his game; for the fugitive his pursuers . . . the image in the mind is the attention, the preperception is half of the perception. (p. 442)

Bruner and Goodman (1947) demonstrated that needs affect not only attention, but judgment as well. They asked participants to judge the size of coins, using a knob that controlled a circle of light. They found that the value of the coins distorted judgment, so that a 5-cent coin was less distorted in size than a 25-cent coin. The greater the value of the coin, the more likely participants were to distort their perception of how big it was; and the distortion due to value of the coin was even greater for poor participants, for whom money would be especially valued.

Construction as Integration

What distinguishes modern social cognition (and dual-process models) from the models of early researchers in the field (described above) is the emphasis in the modern models on examining the processes through which judgments are produced. Solomon Asch's (1946) pioneering experiments in person perception helped bridge this transition from theorizing that employed Gestalt principles to examinations of the processes utilized in social perception. The Gestalt focus is evidenced in Asch's belief that we must "look at the facts as they interpenetrate, as they complete or fit each other, or as they clash and move away from each other. We must see what kinds of units they form, what kind of center the units have, and what principle governs the whole" (Asch, 1946, p. 60).

The focus on process is evidenced in Asch's belief that the goal in person perception is to provide a unified and coherent image of the person—one in which the perceived traits are integrated together and make sense in describing the person.[3] Asch examined trait integration through presenting lists of traits about a target. An elementalistic perspective suggests that the perception produced should be a summary of the individual traits. However, a Gestalt perspective, where the individual integrates traits, suggests that the relationship between the traits should affect one's final judgment. Asch assumed that some traits are "central," in that they serve an organizing function that integrates one's impression into a coherent Gestalt. Thus, even when diverse traits are applied to the same individual, the traits are seen in a lawful relation that produces a coherent impression. When one is cognizing about others, their "characteristics seem to reach out beyond the merely given terms of the description . . . the final account is completed and rounded. Reference is made to characters and situations which are apparently not directly mentioned in the list, but which are inferred from it" (Asch, 1946, p. 261; see also Bruner's [1957] "going beyond the information given," or what Markus [1977, p. 64], in discussing the impact of schemas, called "going beyond the information available"). Asch and Zukier (1983, p. 1240) pointed out that seeking unity should not be equated with describing perceivers as simplistic in their processing: "Persons are not simple. (However, because unity implies patterning and order, it greatly enhances the possibilities of comprehension.) It follows also that unity is not equivalent to homogeneity, nor is it at odds with contradiction and conflict."

This section began with Köhler's belief that "sensory fields are replete with qualities and properties which one neglects if one takes 'sensations' as their sole content" (1930, p. 144). It ends with Asch's bringing this principle to a process-oriented study of social cognition. Person perception is not the forming of an exact mental representation of sensations impinging on the sensory apparatus; rather, it is a dynamic process of subjectively determining how other people are to be categorized, known, and understood. Asch (1952) remarked about studying such phenomena that "it is dangerous to concentrate on the parts and to lose sight of their relations" (p. 60), as the perceptual system does not produce inferences and meaning by transcribing the environment in the way a video camera reproduces the external world. Knowledge is developed through a lens of subjectivity.

PRODUCING MEANING AND CLOSURE THROUGH REMOVING DOUBT

Doubt is an unhappy and dissatisfied state from which we struggle to free ourselves and pass into a state of belief, while [the feeling of believing] is a calm and satisfactory state which we do not wish to avoid, or change into a belief in anything else. On the contrary, we cling not merely to believing, but to believing just what we do believe ... The irritation of doubt causes a struggle to attain a state of belief. I shall term this struggle inquiry.... With the doubt, therefore, the struggle begins, and with the cessation of doubt it ends.

—PEIRCE (1877, p. 66)

In the preceding section, we have outlined the support for the belief that people construct knowledge. But this raises the issue of why it is that meaning is pursued both so relentlessly and so subjectively. From Jones and Thibaut's (1958) discussion of the interaction goals that guide interpersonal perception, to Smith and Mackie's (1995) overview of social psychology, various social needs that direct action and cognition have explicitly been examined by social psychologists. Jones and Thibaut classified these goals as "maximizing beneficent social response," "securing motivational and value support," and "gaining cognitive clarity." Maximizing beneficent social response describes the human need to receive approval and to have high self-identity and social identity. Securing motivational and value support describes the human need to affiliate with others.

Social cognition focuses mostly on the final need, gaining cognitive clarity, which describes the drive to attain meaning. Bartlett (1932) spoke of the role cognitive structures play in pursuing meaning, describing people as exerting "effort after meaning." Bruner, Goodnow, and Austin (1956) described a "motive to categorize" that impels a search for meaning (invoking Tolman's [1951], notion of a "placing need"). Heider (1944, p. 359) described attribution as having "its roots in the individual's pursuit of meaning.... Some authors talk of a general tendency toward causal explanation, a causal drive. Oppenheimer (1922) considers it as a third basic drive beside the drives for self conservation and for conservation of the species." Allport (1954) described people as having an "insatiable hunger for explanations" (p. 170),

and as being "under constant pressure to obtain definite meanings ... intent upon the task of organization" (p. 316).

This motive is also central in the research by Lewin's doctoral student, Zeigarnik. Zeigarnik (1927) noted a tendency for people to perseverate on interrupted tasks, and suggested that this occurs because the goal of completing the task is unfulfilled. This creates a state of tension due to lacking closure, which leads people to strive toward closure by continuing to devote mental energy to the task. Lewin believed that a system that has closure is stable or at rest—frozen. A system that lacks closure instigates what he likened to a cognitive thaw: There is an "unfreezing," in which effort is exerted until the system is brought back to closure.

The Dissatisfaction of Doubt

Though the belief in the search for meaning as a fundamental drive is a commonly held assumption in dual-process models, it was also a central component of the cognitive consistency models that preceded them, such as Festinger's (1957) cognitive dissonance theory. Aronson (1992, p. 304) described dissonance theory as being about "how people try to make sense out of their environment and their behavior—and thus, try to lead lives that are sensible and meaningful." The logic was that if a person holds two cognitions that are inconsistent, he or she will experience dissonance and will need to reduce that state of discomfort by producing a coherent sense of understanding. The use of the word "need" was deliberate in this model, as it likened dissonance reduction to the pursuit of drives such as hunger and thirst. Lacking meaning produces an intolerable state—one that the individual is driven to reduce through attaining new, consistent meaning. This idea was expressed by James (1907/1991, p. 29) when he stated:

> The individual has a stock of old opinions already, but he [*sic*] meets a new experience that puts them to a strain. Somebody contradicts them; or in a reflective moment he discovers that they are incompatible; or desires arise in him which they cease to satisfy. The result is an inward trouble to which his mind

till then had been a stranger, and from which he seeks to escape by modifying his previous mass of opinions. He saves as much of it as he can, for in this matter of belief we are all extreme conservatives.

Striking is the similarity between Festinger's proposal of the dissonance reduction drive, James's discussion of an "inward trouble," and Peirce's description of "inquiry" in the quotation that opens this section. Each invokes the notion of a tension state created by the existence of an unsettled opinion; each describes a process of seeking to reduce that state; and, finally, each notes the individual's wish to avoid returning to that state (preferring instead the relative calm of having a system in balance, without tension).

> The existence of dissonance, being psychologically uncomfortable, will motivate a person to try to reduce the dissonance by achieving consonance. When dissonance is present, in addition to trying to reduce it, the person will actively avoid situations and information which will likely increase the dissonance. (Festinger, 1957, p. 3)

Thus, central to both Lewin's and Festinger's models (along with subsequent cognitive consistency theories) was the pragmatist dogma articulated by Peirce (1877), and later by John Dewey (1929). People actively avoid having their knowledge upset and faced with contradiction; the arousal of doubt shakes them from the calm and satisfactory state of firmly knowing what they feel to be the "truth." From this perspective, the experience of having truth is not a reflection of the actual external realities, but a state of mind whereby people are secure in their beliefs, free of doubt: "The true conclusion would remain true if we had no impulse to accept it; and the false one would remain false though we could not resist the tendency to believe in it" (Peirce, 1877, p. 64). People do not seek meaning by discerning absolute truth—by objectively examining and accurately representing the data. They simply seek to terminate doubt in a manner that produces sufficient closure, allowing them to experience having arrived at meaning.

The sole object of inquiry is the settlement of opinion. We may fancy that this is not enough for us, and that we seek not merely an opinion, but a true opinion. But put this fancy to the test and it proves groundless; for as soon as a firm belief is reached we are entirely satisfied, whether the belief be false or true. (Peirce, 1877, p. 66)

Assimilation: Constancy in the Mind's Meanings

We now see one consequence of conceiving of the quest for meaning as a process of eliminating, and actively avoiding the return of, doubt: Individuals accept any sufficiently held belief to be a reflection of truth. James (1907/1991, pp. 88–90) put this in the ultimate pragmatic terms, defining truth not as an accurate reflection of reality, but as those ideas that

> *we can assimilate, validate, corroborate and verify* . . . the truth of an idea is not a stagnant property inherent in it. Truth *happens* to an idea. It *becomes* true, is *made* true by events. Its verity *is* in fact an event, a process: the process namely of its verifying itself, its *verification* . . . from this simple cue pragmatism gets her general notion of truth as something essentially bound up with the way in which one moment in our experience may lead us toward other moments which it will be worth while to have been led to. (Emphasis in original)

But there is an additional consequence of conceiving of the attainment of meaning and the "experience" of truth in this fashion. Because people feel sufficiently confident that the beliefs they have are correct, they cling tenaciously to these beliefs, despite the presence of contradicting evidence. The process of inquiry leads people to transform the data, assimilating them to fit with and maintain prior structures. This is how Aronson (1992) described the dissonance reduction process, stating that in trying to produce meaning "we frequently get ourselves into a tangled muddle of self-justification, denial, and distortion" (p. 304).

James described the act of fitting new information to be consistent with what we already believe as the most important of all the features of our mental structure. He referred to this tendency toward assimilation and perceptual unity as "the principle of constancy in the mind's meanings." We do not merely construct what we see; we see what we already believe.

> [The] sense of sameness is the very keel and backbone of our thinking . . . we do not care whether there be any real sameness in things or not, or whether the mind be true or false in its assumptions of it. Our principle only lays it down that the mind makes continual use of the *notion* of sameness . . . the outer world might be an unbroken flux, and yet [we] perceive a repeated experience. (1890/1950, pp. 459–460)

Thus, contradictory evidence is dealt with in a manner that allows the structure to be maintained (e.g., ignoring, subtyping, and manipulating new data). "Observe the part played by the older truths . . . their influence is absolutely controlling. Loyalty to them is the first principle . . . for by far the most usual way of handling phenomena so novel that they would make for a serious rearrangement of our preconceptions is to ignore them altogether" (James, 1907/1991, p. 30). This position was very much tied to James's pragmatic conception of truth, whereby beliefs and judgments that we hold to be true can "pass" as true as long as they are functional; they produce good results. James (1907/1991, p. 92) asserted that beliefs arrived at through assimilation and reliance on prior constructs "pass" because they typically work:

> All things exist in kinds and not singly . . . so that once we have verified our ideas about one specimen of a kind, we feel free to apply them to other specimens. . . . A mind that habitually discerns the kind of thing before it, and acts by the law of the kind immediately, without pausing to verify it, will be a "true" mind in ninety-nine out of a hundred emergencies.

Although keeping old knowledge unaltered, to be utilized time and again, is functional, James did not believe that people were incapable of breaking from their set knowledge. This is simply a default strategy, that, barring contradiction, will be followed. But, as James (1907/1991) told his audience at Co-lumbia University, contradictory evidence could be perceived:

> You listen to me now with certain prepossessions as to my competency, and these affect your reception of what I say, but were I suddenly to break off lecturing, and begin to sing "We won't go home till morning" in a rich baritone voice, not only would that new fact be added to your stock, but it would oblige you to define me differently. (p. 74)

Given an inability to hold to a prior set, the tension of doubt gets reintroduced, setting people off on a quest for greater certainty and new beliefs. But the point at hand is not that people are incapable of altering beliefs; they simply avoid doing so, preferring to see sameness.

Assimilation in Person Judgment

Gestalt psychologists proposed, in their notion of "holism," that pieces of information fit together and make sense. When they do not, there is confusion, which needs to be removed so that coherence and closure can be achieved. The idea that this is accomplished through assimilating new information to prior structures is captured by the principle of *prägnanz*: The products of perceptual organization tend to be structured in the clearest, least ambiguous way. There is a tendency toward perceptual rigidity, toward intolerance of ambiguity, and toward viewing new experiences from the standpoint of an existing set (e.g., Block & Block, 1951; Frenkel-Brunswik, 1949).

Heider (1944) directly incorporated into the groundwork for attribution theory the idea that a lack of closure and simple structure produces tension, which the perceiver is motivated to reduce. Earlier we have outlined Heider's belief that people seek to form perceptual units that serve to link an actor with an action; this causes them to impute causal responsibility for the act to the actor, and to tend to see the two as corresponding (Jones, 1979, referred to this as the "correspondence bias"). We have detailed how this perceptual bias grew out of the Gestalt principle of closure—the perceptual system's tendency to parse the life space into coherent units, to seek structure. We have described this earlier as if it were relatively void of motivational influences—as a function of Gestalt ideas about how the cognitive system operates.

However, Heider believed that the reason people seek closure is to illuminate the life space with meaning, to alleviate the discomfort of doubt. When behavior is observed, it requires an explanation. According to Heider, a situation once comprehended has now been changed to some extent, and this upset system is in a state of imbalance—lacking meaning. Attributing the cause for an event as lying in the dispositional qualities of others is one type of resolution to this tension and doubt, enabling a person to achieve meaning and closure: "The organism is enabled to reinstate an equilibrium even when otherwise irreversible changes have disturbed it" (1944, p. 361). Heider (1958) believed that equilibrium is reinstated (meaning is achieved) by forming person–action units not only because this transforms behavior into disposition, thus successfully providing meaning (by placing causal weight on the person), but because this is the simplest way to achieve closure: "Persons, as absolute causal origins, transform irreversible changes into reversible ones. . . . The person can represent the disturbing change in its entirety" (p. 5).

Heider (1944) further posited that the tendency toward unit formation creates a reliance on *assimilation*, whereby an act is seen as consistent with some "perceptually ready" interpretation. Expectations surrounding a perceived person color the interpretation of the behavior of that person.[4] Allport (1954) described a similar process in explaining the ubiquity of stereotyping: People rely on stereotypes to assimilate information about groups, and in so doing are constantly supporting and maintaining the stereotypic categories while using them to structure the world (for a more recent review of the effects of stereotypes on judgment and recall, see Stangor & Lange, 1994). He described stereotypes as stubborn, resistant to change, even resistant to contradictory evidence. People can avoid such inconsistencies by a process of "refencing," or subtyping, creating separate categories for members of groups who break the mold. They selectively admit new information to a category only if it confirms their prior beliefs.

Our experience in life tends to form itself into clusters, and while we may call on the right cluster at the wrong time, or the wrong cluster at the right time, still the process in question dominates our entire mental life. . . . Open-mindedness is considered to be a virtue. But, strictly speaking, it cannot occur. A new experience must be redacted into old categories . . . categorization assimilates as much as it can to the cluster. There is a curious inertia in our thinking. We like to solve problems easily. We can do so best if we can fit them rapidly into a satisfactory category and use this category as a means of prejudging the solution. (p. 20)

Warranted Assertibility: Producing Sufficient, Rather Than Accurate, Knowledge

Aside from pointing out the tendency toward assimilation that accompanies the drive to avoid doubt, our discussion of the pursuit of meaning as a process of inquiry raises a separate issue. The manner in which people pursue knowledge was described by Peirce as not the most accurate method possible, but a process of accepting any belief that seems "enough" to remove doubt. Jones and Davis (1965) stated that "the perceiver seeks to find sufficient reason why the person acted. . . . Instead of a potentially infinite regress of cause and effect . . . the perceiver's explanation comes to a stop when an intention or motive is assigned that has the quality of being reason enough" (p. 220). As discussed above, what one will deem to be "reason enough" will vary according to one's goals and expectancies. A prejudiced person might accept seeing a member of an ethnic minority giving an ambiguous shove as reason enough to come to the conclusion that the minority individual is violent (e.g., Duncan, 1976). As Allport (1954, p. 7) stated, "It is not easy to say how much fact is required to justify a judgment. A prejudiced person will almost certainly claim that he has sufficient warrant for his views."

The idea that people seek "sufficient" rather than accurate knowledge, attempting to alleviate a tension state instigated by doubt, is implicit in dual-process models. The very notion of accurate, individuated, systematic processing as one extreme of the processing continuum (and not the default level of processing people use) signifies that absolute accuracy is not what these models view people as typically striving for. For example, the heuristic–systematic model describes a "sufficiency threshold," whereby people stop processing once they have attained a sufficient level of confidence in their judgment (see also Chen & Chaiken, Chapter 4, this volume; Bohner, Moskowitz, & Chaiken, 1995). Because it is effortful, systematic processing is not likely to occur in the absence of specific motivating circumstances (e.g., Thompson, Roman, Moskowitz, Chaiken, & Bargh, 1994). The default processing strategy is the heuristic route. But such economy-minded processors become motivated to process systematically when a feeling of insufficiency arises, such as when heuristics produce an actual confidence that falls short of the sufficiency threshold (their desired confidence). Later in the chapter, we return to discuss factors that lead people to abandon a reliance on heuristics and exert the cognitive effort to overturn beliefs.

PREPARING FOR ACTION AND EXPERIENCING CONTROL

Let me begin by reminding you of the fact that the possession of true thoughts means everywhere the possession of invaluable instruments of action; and that our duty to gain truth, so far from being a blank command from out of the blue, or a "stunt" self imposed by our intellect, can account for itself by excellent practical reasons. . . . We live in a world of realities that can be infinitely useful or infinitely harmful. Ideas that tell us which of them to expect count as the true ideas. . . . The possession of truth, so far from being here an end in itself, is only a preliminary means towards other vital satisfactions.
—JAMES (1907/1991, p. 89)

It has been posited above that in person perception we seek to end doubt; the goal is to give meaning to the action of others. But why do we desire meaning? Why is this a fundamental drive? James's (1907/1991) pragmatic definition of "truth" has the answer to this question built in. To pragmatists, truth is the arrival at meaning that has *practical use*[5] for us: "All realities influence our practice . . . and that influence is their meaning for us" (p. 24). Truth is conceived of as something *instrumental*—an idea that is capable of carrying us from one experience to the next, linking things in a satisfactory fashion. Without attaining this type of practical meaning, we are ill prepared to act in our environment. With it, as is seen in the quotation that begins this section, we are armed with invaluable instruments of action. As James stated, we seek meaning because "beliefs are really rules for action. . . . To attain perfect clearness in our thoughts of an object, we need only consider what conceivable effects of a practical kind the object may involve—what sensations we are to expect from it, and what reactions we must prepare" (pp. 23–24).

Social psychologists adopted James's (1890/1950) functionalist declaration that thinking is first, and always, for doing. Allport (1954, p. 167) paraphrased this pragmatic view when he stated that "thinking is basically an endeavor to anticipate reality. By thinking we try to foresee consequences and plan actions that will avoid whatever threatens us and will bring our hopes and dreams to pass. There is nothing passive about thinking." Bruner (1957) relied on Peirce's (1878) pragmatic belief that meaning is tied to function; the behavioral consequences of the thing are categorized (e.g., a pencil can write, a diamond is hard). "Let us ask what we mean by calling a thing *hard*. Evidently, that it will not be scratched by many other substances" (Bruner, 1957, p. 126).

Predictive Veridicality

"Predictive veridicality" is a term used by Bruner (1957) to indicate that the truth of an idea is bound up with the extent to which the idea is predictive (i.e., it provides information about the function of the thing categorized). One achievement of categorization is

the *direction it provides for instrumental activity*. To know by virtue of discriminable defining attributes and without need for further direct test that a man is "honest" or that a substance is "poison" is to know in *advance* about appropriate and inappropriate actions to be taken. . . . The moment an object is placed in a category, we have opened up a whole vista of possibilities for "going beyond" the category by virtue of the superordinate and causal relationships linking this category to others. (Bruner et al., 1956, pp. 12–13; emphasis in original)

If an object is classified as an "orange," it not only derives meaning from this classification;

it also allows us to predict what we can do with it—we can eat it.

But there is a danger to arriving at meaning through categorizing, assimilating new data to fit with existing knowledge, and then generalizing from the category to the current experience. The danger is that one's existing categories are not always adequate for explaining the new information. Providing a "satisfactory" explanation, for the sake of preparing appropriate action, can lead either to an incorrect meaning being attained (a miscategorization) or to an incorrect generalization being made (going *too far* beyond the information). James (1907/1991) asserted that defining meaning as that which satisfactorily fits with existing categories is functional because it works most of the time. But he recognized that opponents would view this conception of truth as "a sort of coarse lame second-rate makeshift article of truth. Such truths are not real truth. Such tests are merely subjective. Against this, objective truth must be something non-utilitarian, haughty, refined, remote, august" (p. 32). Bruner (1957) agreed with James that categorization is both functional and ubiquitous, but he also cautioned that attempting to predict appropriate action through the process of categorization produces judgments that are only varyingly veridical:

> The meaning of a thing, thus, is the placement of an object in a network of hypothetical inference concerning its other observable properties, its effects, and so on. . . . All of this suggests, does it not, that veridicality is not so much a matter of representation as it is a matter of what I shall call model building. In learning to perceive, we are learning the relations that exist between the properties of objects and events that we encounter, learning appropriate categories and category systems, learning to predict and to check what goes with what. (p. 126)

In assigning a percept to a category (items with similar features and functions), the veridicality of the inferences that result depends upon the goodness of fit between the thing being categorized and the category to which it has been assigned. Though categorization may be imperfect—"[categories] represent with varying degrees of predictive veridicality the nature of the physical world in which the organism operates" (Bruner, 1957, p. 129)—it typically can provide reliable information about function. Going beyond the information given in this fashion allows one to predict as-yet-untested properties of the person/thing being categorized. As a result, it allows one to prepare appropriate action.

Control

To this point, we have discussed various achievements of categorizing in a manner that is directed by the accessible constructs and wants of the individual. First, this has been described as the process by which meaning and a feeling of "experiencing having truth" are attained. We have described this as being sought because lacking such a state produces an uncomfortable tension that the individual is driven to reduce. The tension has been said to be associated with the fact that survival in the physical and social world is difficult, if not impossible, without being able to predict what others are like.[6] Such prediction affords the individual a menu of appropriate behavior, a guideline for action. However, in addition to this pragmatic function, the ability to predict what can be expected from others also provides a sense of control for the individual over his or her outcomes. Rather than being subjected to the random effects of the social world, the person can control the interactions and situations he or she enters into, and thus can play a role in determining what happens. Heider (1958, p. 71) stated:

> In Lewin's (1936) terms, an unstructured region, that is, a region whose properties are not known to the person, can be considered a barrier which makes action and therefore control difficult if not impossible. Perception helps to structure the region and to remove this barrier.

THE NOTION OF LIMITED CAPACITY AND THE LEAST-EFFORT PRINCIPLE

The Notion of Limited Capacity

Millions of items of the outward order are present to my senses which never properly enter into my experience. Why? Because they have no *interest* for me. *My experience is what I agree to attend to.* Only those items which I *notice* shape my mind—without selective interest, experience is an utter chaos . . . the consciousness of every creature would be a gray, chaotic, indiscriminateness, impossible for us even to conceive.

—JAMES (1890/1950, pp. 402–403; emphasis in original)

We arrive now at the final set of assumptions in the rather functionalistic perspective that characterizes social cognition in general and dual-process models in particular. People construct experience to provide meaning, and they seek meaning to end doubt, to prepare for action, and to gain subjective feelings of control. But why settle for a mere end to doubt? Why cling to past knowledge? Why not seek accuracy and complete verification of each stimulus? If the functional view is maintained, this is deemed not possible for the processing system, because cognitive capacity is bounded and limited. In the quotation above, James characterized the stimulus world as millions of items that bombard the senses, and argued that unless the intake is limited somehow—unless structure is imposed on it from within—experience will be chaotic and meaningless. James (1907/1991) paraphrases Kant's view of experience (*gewühl der erscheinungen, rhapsodie der wahrnehmungen*) as something to be discovered rather than passively labeled—"a motley which we have to unify by our wits" (p. 76). Lippmann (1922) stated that the senses are met by the "great blooming, buzzing confusion of the outer world." He echoed James's notion that experience and interest serve to limit our intake. We handle the confusion of the stimulus world not by scrutinizing each element in it, but by choosing what to attend to—that "which we have picked out in the form stereotyped for us" (p. 55).

Bruner et al. (1956) began their book with this point (p. 1):

> We begin with what seems a paradox. The world of experience of any man is composed of a tremendous array of discriminably different objects, events, people, impressions. There are estimated to be more than 7 million discriminable colors alone . . . [and even subtle differences] we are capable of seeing, for human beings have an exquisite capacity for making distinctions. But were we to utilize fully our capacity for registering the differences in things and to respond to each event encountered as unique, we would soon be overwhelmed by the complexity of our environment. . . . [It] would make us slaves to the particular. . . . [The resolution to this paradox] is achieved by man's capacity to categorize. To categorize is to render discriminably different things equivalent, to group the objects and events and people around us into classes and to respond to them in terms of their class membership.

The phenomenological paradox they propose is that despite being capable of making fine distinctions, we are nonetheless limited in our capacity to do so. The external world is too complex, and attempts to verify and process each stimulus to the fullest degree would render us frozen and inactive, slaves to the details of the environment. Thus, "by categorizing as equivalent discriminably different events, the organism *reduces the complexity of the environment*. It is reasonably clear 'how' this is accomplished. It involves the abstraction and use of defining properties in terms of which groupings can be made" (p. 12; emphasis in original). The eucalyptus and sequoia are discriminably different, but are reacted to similarly; they evoke the same response, "tree." Categorization frees us from being slaves to the particular, reducing the "*necessity of constant learning* . . . we do not have to be taught *de novo* at each encounter that the object before us is or is not a tree. If it exhibits the appropriate defining properties, it 'is' a tree" (p. 12; emphasis in original).

The Principle of Least Effort

The assumption that the capacity for attending to and processing information is limited led researchers interested in attention (e.g., Broadbent, 1958; James, 1890/1950; Kahneman, 1973; Logan, 1980; Treisman & Geffen, 1967) to discuss the metaphor of a preconscious filter that selects what is consciously attended to from the environment. Boring (1932) believed that what an organism picks out is what is important to it for survival and welfare. This metaphor was adopted by social psychologists interested in how people attend to, recall, and judge information about the social world. Kelly (1955) believed that each person's mental constructs can serve as a "scanning pattern which a person continually projects upon his world. As he sweeps back and forth across his perceptual field he picks up blips of meaning" (p. 145). Bruner (1957) assumed that categorization processes serve to simplify the world, leading people to reserve their refined discriminatory skills only for that with which they are specially concerned. Categories are preconsciously used to promote inferences and "the ability to use minimal cues quickly in categorizing the events of the environment is what gives the organism its lead time in adjusting to events. Pause and close inspection inevitably cut down on this precious interval for adjustment" (p. 142). This implies that the information-processing default is to use simplifying strategies "in the service of cognitive and emotional economy" (Jones & Thibaut, 1958, p. 152), but more complex strategies can be called into use when needs and goals are engaged. Similarly, Tajfel (1969) stated that the effort used to pursue meaning "works within the limits imposed by the capacities of the individual" (p. 79), and that "for reasons of cognitive economy [meaning] will tend toward as much simplification as the situation allows for" (p. 92).

Allport (1954) labeled the fact that people seek to maximize outcomes with the least amount of work possible, choosing cognitive economy as a strategy to allow them the ability to maneuver through a complex stimulus environment, as "the principle of least effort." This is a functional account of how people cope with limited resources: They avoid effortful expenditures of cognitive energy by developing simplifying strategies, such as assimilation, stereotype use, and a reliance on heuristics and schemas. This is seen in Kelley's (1973) definition of a "schema" as

> abstract ideas about the operation and interaction of causal factors. These conceptions [enable perceivers to make an] economical and fast attributional analysis, by providing a framework within which bits and pieces of relevant information can be fitted in order to draw reasonably good causal inferences. (p. 115)

We see this assumption reflected in a wide range of dual-process models: Langer's (1978) proposal that processing is often "mindless"; Bargh's (1984) discussion of automatic processing; Fiske and Taylor's (1984) notion of humans as "cognitive misers"; Gilbert and Hixon's (1991) suggestion that stereotype use is ubiquitous because people avoid "the trouble of thinking"; Sedikides and Skowronski's (1991) "law of cognitive structure activation," in which assimilation is said to predominate; Eagly and Chaiken's (1993) description of a "least-effort principle" that promotes a reliance on heuristics; and Uleman et al.'s (1996) discussion of unintended inferences. But the idea of a least-effort principle in psychology can be traced back to James (1890/1950):

> The stream of our thought is like a river. On the whole, easy simple flowing predominates in it, the drift of things is with the pull of gravity, and effortless attention is the rule. But at intervals a log-jam occurs, stops the current, creates an eddy, and makes things temporarily move the other way. If a real river could feel, it would feel these eddies and setbacks as places of effort. (p. 451)

James (1907/1991) named his dual-process theory a "pluralistic monism," with his intent being to characterize two types of individuals—an idealistic, religious, free-willist, theory-driven, monistic type versus a materialistic, fatalistic, data-driven, pluralistic type. But he warned that people are not as uniform as these characterizations suggest; they possess qualities on both sides of the line:

> Most of us have a hankering for the good things on both sides of the line. Facts are good, of course—give us lots of facts. Principles are good—give us plenty of principles. The world is indubitably one if you look at it one way, but as indubitably is it many, if you look at it in another . . . your ordinary philosophic layman never being a radical, never straightening out his system, but living vaguely in one plausible compartment of it or another to suit the temptations of successive hours. (pp. 9–10)

Despite a belief in a default strategy of seeing constancy and relying on prior theories, there is the clear exposition of the idea that the "temptations of successive hours"—that is, fluctuations across time and situations in a person's needs and goals—can lead to a shift from a theory-driven approach to processing the world to a data-driven approach. People are capable of doing more, because they possess an exquisite capacity for making distinctions, but they often choose to do less.

CONCLUSIONS

Evaluation of other persons, important as it is in our existence, is largely automatic, one of the things we do without knowing very much about the "principles" in terms of which we operate. Regardless of the degree of skill which an adult may have in appraising others, he [*sic*] engages in the process most of the time without paying much attention to how he does it.
—TAGIURI (1958, p. ix)

The dual-process models that lean on the set of assumptions concerning limited capacity, least-effort processing, seeking an end to doubt, constructing meaning, and attaining control all describe people as having a default strategy in which "truth" is achieved at the cost of systematic attempts to examine the data. Instead, heuristics, schemas, stereotypes, and expectancies are used to draw conclusions. Bargh (Chapter 18, this volume) tells a fable of how this description of the individual as "cognitive miser" has evolved in recent years to that of a "cognitive monster." The metaphor is used to indicate that perceivers are so adept at effortless processing that much of their social life proceeds automatically— even those aspects of it that are somewhat "ugly" or undesirable. For example, Devine (1989) has concluded that stereotypes are automatically activated, and that only through conscious exertion of the will can people overturn such thoughts and be unprejudiced. Gilbert, Krull, and Malone (1990) state that people automatically believe any assertion put to them, and only subsequently consider its truth or falsity through conscious exertion of the will.

Researchers have rebelled against this extreme position in the 1990s, attempting to "cage" it (thus extending Bargh's "monster" metaphor) by showing the limits to automatic processing. Bargh's point in his thesis is that in attempting to demonstrate that automaticity is indeed limited when discussing social perception, these researchers have attempted too zealously to reassert the role of free will (and to squash the image of humans as mindless automatons), ignoring methodological and interpretive flaws in the findings. This is a point worth noting, for we should opt for rigor over righteousness in science. However, like all monster stories, Bargh's is a bit of a fiction. For the rigor we should exercise when examining attempts to control automaticity should also be exercised when examining the evidence *for* automaticity in social perception. Such examinations would reveal that the monster is not quite what it seems when examined with closer scrutiny (for critiques of the evidence for automaticity, see Gilbert & Hixon, 1991; Lepore & Brown, 1997; Locke, Macleod, & Walker, 1994).

What this discussion reveals is that issues centering around control over cognition are still open to debate and will be moving to the forefront as dual-process models move into the next millennium. Questions concerning the nature of control, and even the possibility of control (given the "cognitive miser/monster" we have described), must be addressed. Dual-process models, to this point, have implicitly conceived of control and exertion of the will as operating via conscious intent— that is, as something effortful. Initial "automatic" responses can be later overturned through cognitive effort, by exerting what Bruner (1957) called a "closer look" at the information. What factors cause people to lack confidence in their judgments and fail to have a sense of closure that will motivate such "close looks"? There have been two general responses to this question (e.g., Chen & Chaiken, Chapter 4, this volume). One has been that this occurs when the information is so inconsistent with prior structures that it challenges the perspective of perceivers and undermines their confidence in judgments arrived at through least-effort processing (for a review, see Moskowitz, 1996). A second response has been that this occurs when "close looks" are willfully chosen. For example, people can desire accuracy (e.g., Tetlock, 1985), thus rendering judgments arrived at through least-effort processing insufficient (see Fiske & Neuberg, 1990). People are not doomed to be cognitive misers, but are "flexible processors" (e.g., Uleman et al., 1996)—capable of elaborate processing when they desire greater certainty in their judgments.

Utilizing "close looks" to control cognition has been shown to be successful at reversing the effects of least-effort processing (see Gollwitzer & Moskowitz, 1996). However, from Bruner (1957) to Bargh (Chapter 18, this volume), reasons have been put forth for us to suspect the utility in everyday life of relying on a regimen of close looking. If control is conceived of as effortful and conscious—capable only of "debiasing" judgment from the effects of automatic responses, rather than *preventing* such responses from ever occurring—then it means that for control to be successful people must be (1) aware of such biases, (2) motivated to "debias," and (3) in possession of cognitive capacity to exert the required effort. But the functional approach we have reviewed in this chapter has suggested that least-effort processing has evolved as a default processing strategy precisely because people typically lack at least one of these elements. The cost of constantly taking "close looks" is too high for organisms that possess only limited capacity. Bruner (1957) stated:

> With enough time and testing of defining cues, "best fit" perceiving can be accomplished for most but not all classes of environmental events with which the person has contact. There are some objects whose cues to identify are sufficiently equivocal so that no such resolution can be achieved, and these are mostly in the sphere of so-called interpersonal perception: perceiving the states of other people, their characteristics, intentions, etc. on the basis of external signs. And since this is the domain where misperception can have the most chronic if not the most acute consequences, it is doubtful whether a therapeutic regimen of "close looking" will aid the misperceiver much in dealing with the more complex cue patterns. But the greatest difficulty rests in the fact that the cost of close looks is generally too high under the conditions of speed, risk, and limited capacity imposed upon organisms by the environment. (pp. 141–142)

Although goals are capable of consciously operating to cause people to initiate closer looks, goals can also preconsciously operate to affect initial categorization. The future for dual-process models must contain an examination of this possibility for preconscious control—one not dependent on "debiasing" or reversals of effects. We have described earlier how preventing least-effort responses from occurring was clearly articulated as possible by Lewin (1936). We conclude this chapter with a discussion of two domains (stereotyping and the truth value of new information) in which motivated control has previously been conceived of as possible only through conscious acts of will, and we instead suggest a role for passive, silently operating, preconscious control.

Preconscious Control and Stereotype Activation

We have noted earlier that Lewin (1936) believed that intentions ("quasi-needs") direct movement in the life space without an individual's being conscious of their impact. Instead, the individual surrenders activation of a motive–plan structure to the environment and the presence of the appropriate cues (those that have valence). Postman et al. (1948) adopted this belief when they asserted that attention is determined by needs and values that preconsciously sensitize the individual to relevant stimuli. Bargh's (1990) "automotives" model directly updates this notion. Bargh suggested that goals are knowledge structures that can be activated, much as any other category can be, and thus are capable of "capturing" relevant stimuli and determining the nature of categorization. Whether a goal is activated upon exposure to a stimulus depends on that goal's having been chronically and habitually paired with the stimulus. Despite the fact that such goal strivings stem from an initial conscious goal intention, the repeated pairing of a goal with a set of situations leads to the eventual movement of goal pursuit from consciousness.

Gollwitzer (1993) similarly applies Lewinian theory to explaining how behavioral control can be willed or intended, yet can still be passive and unconscious. Gollwitzer has defined an "implementation intention" as the process of committing oneself to when, where, and how a goal is to be pursued, as well as what course the subsequent goal pursuit is to take. Such volitional acts connect a goal-directed intention to behave with an anticipated situational context that will allow one to implement the plan of action. The purpose of such intentions is to promote the initiation and efficient execution of goal-directed activity. When relevant cues (occasions or opportunities) are encountered, they prompt the intended behavior. Thus, an initially conscious intent operates to control behavior automatically.

Moskowitz et al. (in press) have adopted this logic and proposed that stereotype activation can be controlled through passively operating goals to be egalitarian (activated by relevant environmental cues). The logic is that both chronically operating goals and temporarily adopted goals (e.g., those adopted through an implementation intention) can interfere with the activation of social stereotypes by promoting the activation of a goal construct instead. In accordance with Allport's (1954) belief that what gets activated by the presence of a member of a stereotyped group is whatever is most dominant in the mind of the perceiver, Moskowitz et al. propose that egalitarian goals can be more dominant than stereotypes, passively capturing the stimulus instead of the stereotype (see also Moskowitz & Salomon, in press).

Fiske (1989) has discussed stereotype control using a similar language—"dominant" (or "easy") choices versus "less dominant" (or "hard") choices. In her analysis, the hard choice is the motive to be egalitarian; the easy choice or dominant goal is the desire to seek simple structure and rely on stereotypes. The point is that both types of motives are "intended," even though the easy choice is a type of intent that gets carried out without awareness or a conscious feeling of having choice from moment to moment. This makes the case that goals promoting stereotyping are intended (and thus an individual performing a goal-relevant behavior is responsible for stereotypic actions), regardless of whether the individual is *aware* of the goal driving the current behavior. At some point even dominant responses have been consciously chosen, and their subsequent routinization does not make action "unintended."[7] Moskowitz et al. (in press) show that egalitarianism can be the dominant rather than the hard choice; preconscious stereotype control can be triggered, rather than preconscious stereotype activation. This means that control can be exercised several ways: (1) if one initiates conscious goals with the intended effect of removing bias, (2) if one initiates conscious goals with the incidental effect of removing bias, and (3) if one develops passively operating goals that prevent the activation of a stereotype and the occurrence of bias.[8]

Preconscious Control in Social Judgment: Metacognition and Correction Processes

The association of mental control with a correction process that requires accuracy, awareness, and effort, and that follow a biased, low-effort, initial judgment, is also common-

place in research on how people "decontaminate" (Wilson & Brekke, 1994) or "correct" (Wegener & Petty, 1995; Strack & Hanover, 1996) their thinking. Gilbert et al. (1990) argued that people represent the truth value of information by accepting information as true automatically, and by correcting this judgment only after expending additional cognitive effort. The logic for this position is drawn from a philosophical debate Gilbert et al. pose between Descartes and Spinoza.

Descartes articulated a position we generally take for granted: First we understand and make sense of information, and then we decide whether it is true or false. For example, Descartes asserted that "I do not see that . . . [Nature] teaches me that for those diverse sense-perceptions we should ever form any conclusion regarding things outside us, without having carefully and maturely examined them beforehand" (1641/1931, p. 97). Gilbert et al. (1990) state that, in contrast to this Cartesian position, Spinoza believed that comprehending information and accepting it as true are two names for the same psychological event. That is, we automatically represent information as true upon comprehension, if only for a fleeting moment. Changing this default "true" response to "false" requires an extra cognitive step that is not automatic. In an experimental test of this debate, Gilbert et al. found that distracting people while they were trying to learn the truth value of information resulted in their mistakenly thinking of false information as "true" more often than wrongly thinking of true information as "false." Since the bias did not emerge without distraction, Gilbert et al. argued that the distraction prevented people from making the effortful change of representation from true to false, leaving them with only the default automatic representation in memory. In other words, our intuitions may tell us we are Cartesian processors, but Gilbert et al.'s evidence suggests that we may be Spinozan processors.

The idea of heuristic responses and systematic corrections has also been invoked to explain a number of phenomena in person perception, such as the correspondence bias (e.g., Gilbert, Pelham, & Krull, 1988) and priming phenomena (e.g., Martin, Seta, & Crelia, 1990). Gilbert et al. (1988) concluded that dispositional inferences occur relatively automatically (see Uleman & Moskowitz,

1994), and that correcting such inferences involves controlled responses that require processing resources. Moskowitz and Skurnik (in press) review the role of correcting for initial inferences in assimilation and contrast effects. In priming studies, participants are exposed to trait-relevant information in such a way as to make the information more accessible in memory. After the priming task, an ostensibly separate judgment task is introduced, in which participants learn about and report their impressions of a "target" person (e.g., Srull & Wyer, 1979; Higgins, Rholes, & Jones, 1977). Generally, participants who have been exposed to primes and participants who have not been primed report different impressions of the target person, despite the fact that the priming task has no logical bearing on resolving the vagueness or ambiguity of the target person. Martin (1986) and Lombardi, Higgins, and Bargh (1987) found that subtle priming produced assimilation effects, but that blatant priming produced contrast effects.

Martin (1986) explained this difference with reference to accuracy motivation (e.g., Thompson et al., 1994). Specifically, when priming is blatant, people become aware of the possible biasing influence of the prime words on their impressions; in the interest of giving a bias-free response, they avoid using the trait construct associated with the prime words when reporting their final impression (resulting in a contrast effect). Martin et al. (1990) found that when participants lacked the motivation or ability to expend cognitive effort, blatant priming led to assimilation effects rather than to contrast effects. Martin et al. (see also Martin & Achee, 1992) reasoned that using a primed construct in impression formation is a relatively low-effort, heuristic response, but that enacting a goal to correct the impression after it has been formed requires cognitive capacity. An expansion of this account of assimilation and contrast effects in priming comes from Wegener and Petty (1995; Petty & Wegener, 1993). These researchers suggest that contrast effects in priming paradigms are the result of participants' using a theory of influence to guide their corrections. That is, if participants believe that the primes will make them assimilate, they will engage corrective processes (when they are able to do so) to counter this perceived influence. If participants believe

that primes will make them contrast their judgments, then correction attempts will lead them to assimilate. In other words, people have an initial judgment that they adjust in light of their theories about the nature of inappropriate influences.

It is important to point out, however, that "theories" or beliefs about the impact of events on mental processing are often employed in initial judgments as well as in later adjustments to judgment. Heuristic cues and theory-based corrections should not be thought of as separate bases for judgment; in fact, a belief about the meaning of heuristic cues is often required in order for them to be employed in judgment. For example, research on the availability heuristic (Tversky & Kahneman, 1973; Schwarz et al., 1991) suggests that when people estimate the frequency or recency of events, they do so in part by considering the ease with which examples of the events come to mind, separately from any aspect of the content of the examples. This habit can lead to error, because many aspects of events that are unconnected with frequency or recency (such as vividness or correspondence with prior expectations) can contribute to ease of recall. Furthermore, it is difficult to tell whether ease of retrieval of an event is the result of the event's frequency, recency, or correspondence with expectations. The availability heuristic can be thought of as a metacognitive misattribution.

What makes a given feature of the context plausible as the source of a reaction is a "theory" or belief about the connections among accessibility, mental processing, and the immediate context. In a sense, such beliefs license the use of heuristic cues as information in judgment processes. In the availability heuristic, ease of recall is diagnostic of frequency or recency. The heuristic would not operate if people did not believe that ease of recall is a sign that the recalled event is a recent or frequent occurrence, and the heuristic would not lead to systematic error if people believed that ease of recall could also be a sign that the recalled event was especially vivid. Indeed, any misattribution effect requires a belief of this general sort. People can employ a theory about the impact that external or internal stimuli have on their thinking, regardless of whether they are processing systematically or heuristically.

This logic can be applied to the Gilbert et al. (1990) research on how people represent the truth value of information. Why would a belief that familiar information is more likely to be true than false develop? People's use of communication rules such as Gricean "conversational norms" leads them to expect information to be truthful (see Schwarz, 1994; and Sperber & Wilson, 1986, for reviews). If most information people encounter is true, then information that is familiar is perforce likely to be true. Hence if familiarity is the only available information when people are judging truth value, the most logical guess is that the information is true. Recall that participants showed a bias to call things "true" if they had seen them before—a bias that did not extend to new information.

A possible alternative explanation to Gilbert et al.'s "Spinozan" model of truth's being inferred automatically is that people have a metacognitive belief about the meaning of familiarity—specifically, that familiarity is more likely to be an indication of truth than of falsehood.[9] Control over this response need not be exerted by effortful correction and conscious theories. Such theories are not automatic and uncontrollable, but subject to change. Thus, preconscious control would be viable if one could change people's metacognitive beliefs about the meaning of familiarity. In several studies, Skurnik and Moskowitz (1997) created contexts where familiar information was more likely to be false than true, and reversed the bias: True items were called "false" more often than false items were called "true" and more often than new items were called "false." People did not automatically label information as true.

Volition versus Effort, Heuristic versus Systematic Processing: Dueling Processes?

In conclusion, we have been discussing the counterintuitive notion that intent, will, and control can operate without awareness. Dual-process models are not inconsistent with this idea of preconscious control. Rather, the models have simply evolved following a set of principles that have shifted the emphasis away from this notion. But there is nothing inherent in the principles underlying these models that rules out the possibility of such control, as evidenced early on by the pioneering research of Lewin, Bruner, Postman, and others. The process-oriented models described in this volume not only do not rule out the possibility of pre-

conscious volitional processes, but are well equipped to address such issues. Examining the interaction of active and passive processes is a fruitful direction for future research; and, despite the placement of such processing strategies at opposing endpoints of a metaphorical continuum in most dual-process models, there is no reason to assume that heuristic and systematic processing cannot operate concurrently (for discussion, see Bohner et al., 1995; Chen & Chaiken, Chapter 4, this volume). These dual processes need not be conceived of as "dueling" processes.

NOTES

1. Bruner's belief that "perceptual experience is necessarily the *end product* of a categorization process" (1957, p. 124; emphasis added) that proceeds unconsciously is most similar to the unconscious inference (*unbewusster schluss*) that Helmholtz (1910) spoke of (in German) decades earlier. The direct translation of *unbewusster schluss* would be "an unconscious ending," and Bruner assumed that the ending Helmholtz referred to is the end product of an inferential process.

2. Similarly, Sherif (1936) emphasized the role that the "ground" plays in shaping the interpretation of the "figure" in social situations. One does not simply respond to figural stimuli such as the face and words of the partner, but regulates one's responses in accordance with the ground as well, such as the setting one is in (e.g., funeral vs. party).

3. This perspective has had a profound impact on modern-day social-cognitive research, as we see it mirrored in the perspective of researchers working in the area known as "person memory." Hamilton (1981, p. 140) stated that "we conceived of impression development as a process of integrating and organizing successively received information about a target person into a coherent cognitive representation of him or her. We assumed that the perceiver seeks coherence and organization in impression and that . . . all items of information characterizing the person should make sense."

4. But meaning was also posited to be produced through the equally simple process of contrast, whereby the event is subjectively interpreted to be opposite to some standard (see Moskowitz & Skurnik, in press, for a review). According to Heider (1944), "Shakespeare makes use of this kind of contrast when he describes Othello as a person to whom jealousy is foreign. If he had introduced Othello as a man inclined to be jealous, his acts of jealousy would have lost much of their dramatic force" (p. 364).

5. As James (1907/1991) informed us, the

very term "pragmatism" (introduced to the philosophical literature by Charles Peirce in 1878) is derived from the Greek word for "action," which is also the source for the English word "practical."

6. Harvey (1963, p. 3) stated:

> One's concepts or system of meaning serves as a transformer through which impinging events are coded and translated into psychological significance. Without some such internal mediating system, the environing world would remain in a state of irrelevance. . . . [Concepts provide] a reliable basis for responding to an otherwise disorganized physical bombardment. Indeed, it is quite probable that without some fairly stable and at least somewhat veridical system of reading and reacting to the situation about him, the individual, both in self structure and biological being, would be doomed to extinction.

7. Ironically, though Fiske frames this argument while making the case for the controllability of stereotype activation, it labels stereotype activation as the "easy choice" and control of that activation as the "hard choice," once again implying that such control is effortful and consciously intended.

8. It is odd that Bargh (1996, p. 172) makes the argument that one needs to be aware a process is occurring to control it: "An individual cannot control a process without awareness that it is occurring. To me, this is an important caveat to any contention that people can make the 'hard choice' and counteract automatic processes from influencing social judgment and behavior." Although it is true that awareness may be required to make the "hard choice," Bargh's "auto-motive" model suggests that a goal can be passively activated, and this can be conceived of as a type of control that does not require awareness—control can become the "easy choice."

9. Gilbert et al.'s (1990) procedure, which involved interrupting participants when they were trying to learn the information, was supposedly preventing the participants from representing the information as false, and was thus demonstrating that the illusion of "truth" was automatic, whereas the assignment of the correct label "false" was effortful. However, this merely could have made it more difficult for the participants to rehearse the information and make associations that would assist recall later. As a result, participants were later forced into an overreliance on familiarity when they were asked to remember truth value, which led them to answer "true."

REFERENCES

Allport, G. (1954). *The nature of prejudice*. Reading, MA: Addison-Wesley.

Aronson, E. (1992). The return of the repressed: Dissonance theory makes a comeback. *Psychological Inquiry, 3*, 303–311.

Asch, S. E. (1946). Forming impressions of personality. *Journal of Abnormal and Social Psychology, 41*, 258–290.

Asch, S. E. (1952). *Social psychology*. New York: Prentice-Hall.

Asch, S. E., & Zukier, H. (1984). Thinking about persons. *Journal of Personality and Social Psychology, 46*, 1230–1240.

Bargh, J. A. (1984). Automatic and conscious processing of social information. In R. S. Wyer & T. K. Srull (Eds.), *Handbook of social cognition* (Vol. 3, pp. 1–44). Hillsdale, NJ: Erlbaum.

Bargh, J. A. (1990). Auto-motives: Preconscious determinants of social interaction. In E. T. Higgins & R. M. Sorrentino (Eds.), *Handbook of motivation and cognition: Foundations of social behavior* (Vol. 2, pp. 93–130). New York: Guilford Press.

Bargh, J. A. (1996). Automaticity in social psychology. In E. T. Higgins & A. W. Kruglanski (Eds.), *Social psychology: Handbook of basic principles* (pp. 169–183). New York: Guilford Press.

Bartlett, F. C. (1932). *Remembering*. Cambridge, England: Cambridge University Press.

Block, J., & Block, J. (1951). An investigation of the relationship between intolerance of ambiguity and ethnocentrism. *Journal of Personality, 19*, 303–311.

Bohner, G., Moskowitz, G. B., & Chaiken, S. (1995). The interplay of heuristic and systematic processing of social information. In W. Stroebe & M. Hewstone (Eds.), *European review of social psychology* (Vol. 6, pp. 33–68). Chichester, England: Wiley.

Boring, E. G. (1932). *The physical dimensions of consciousness* (pp. 194–212). New York: Dover Publications.

Broadbent, D. E. (1958). *Perception and communication*. London, UK: Pergammon Press.

Bruner, J. S. (1957). On perceptual readiness. *Psychological Review, 64*, 123–152.

Bruner, J. S., & Goodman, C. D. (1947). Value and need as organizing factors in perception. *Journal of Abnormal Social Psychology, 42*, 33–44.

Bruner, J. S., Goodnow, J. G., & Austin, G. A. (1956). *A study of thinking*. New York: Wiley.

Descartes, R. (1931). *The philosophical works of Descartes* (E. S. Haldane & G. R. T. Ross, Eds. and Trans.). New York: Cambridge University Press. (Original work published 1641)

Devine, P. G. (1989). Stereotypes and prejudice: Their automatic and controlled components. *Journal of Personality and Social Psychology, 56*, 5–18.

Dewey, J. (1929). *The quest for certainty*. New York: Minton, Balch.

Duncan, B. L. (1976). Differential social perception and attribution of intergroup violence: Testing the lower limits of stereotyping of blacks. *Journal of Personality and Social Psychology, 34*, 590–598.

Eagly, A. H., & Chaiken, S. (1993). *The psychology of attitudes*. Fort Worth, TX: Harcourt Brace Jovanovich.

Festinger, L. (1957). *A theory of cognitive dissonance*. Stanford, CA: Stanford University Press.

Fiske, S. T. (1989). Examining the role of intent: Toward understanding its role in stereotyping and prejudice. In J. S. Uleman & J. A. Bargh (Eds.), *Unintended thought* (pp. 253–283). New York: Guilford Press.

Fiske, S. T., & Neuberg, S. L. (1990). A continuum model of impression formation, from category-based to individuating processes: Influences of information and motivation on attention and interpretation. In M. P. Zanna (Ed.), *Advances in experimental social psychology* (Vol. 23, pp. 1–74). San Diego, CA: Academic Press.

Fiske, S. T., & Taylor, S. (1984). *Social cognition*. NY: McGraw-Hill

Frenkel-Brunswik, E. (1949). Intolerance of ambiguity as an emotional and perceptual personality variable. *Journal of Personality, 18*, 108–143.

Gilbert, D. T., & Hixon, J. G. (1991). The trouble of thinking: Activation and application of stereotypic beliefs. *Journal of Personality and Social Psychology, 60*, 509–517.

Gilbert, D. T., Krull, D. S., & Malone, P. S. (1990). Unbelieving the unbelievable: Some problems in the rejection of false information. *Journal of Personality and Social Psychology, 59*, 601–613.

Gilbert, D. T., Pelham, B. W., & Krull, D. S. (1988). On cognitive busyness: When person perceivers meet persons perceived. *Journal of Personality and Social Psychology, 54*, 733–740.

Gollwitzer, P. M. (1993). Goal achievement: The role of intentions. In W. Stroebe & M. Hewstone (Eds.), *European review of social psychology* (Vol. 4, pp. 141–185). Chichester, England: Wiley.

Gollwitzer, P. M., & Moskowitz, G. B. (1996). Goal effects on thought and behavior. In E. T. Higgins & A. W. Kruglanski (Eds.), *Social psychology: Handbook of basic principles* (pp. 361–399). New York: Guilford Press.

Hamilton, D. L. (1981). Cognitive representations of persons. In E. T. Higgins, C. P. Herman, & M. P. Zanna (Eds.), *Social cognition: Ontario Symposium* (Vol. 1, pp. 135–159). Hillsdale, NJ: Erlbaum.

Harvey, O. J. (1963). *Motivation and social interaction*. New York: Ronald Press.

Heider, F. (1944). Social perception and phenomenal causality. *Psychological Review, 51*, 358–374.

Heider, F. (1958). *The psychology of interpersonal relations*. New York: Wiley.

Helmholtz, H. von. (1866). *Handbuch der physiologischen Optik* (3rd ed.). Leipzig: Voss.

Higgins, E. T. (1996). Knowledge activation: Accessibility, applicability, and salience. In E. T. Higgins & A. W. Kruglanski (Eds.), *Social psychology: Handbook of basic principles* (pp. 133–168). New York: Guilford Press.

Higgins, E. T., King, G. A., & Mavin, G. H. (1982). Individual construct accessibility and subjective impressions and recall. *Journal of Personality and Social Psychology, 43*, 35–47.

Higgins, E. T., Rholes, W. S., & Jones, C. R. (1977). Category accessibility and impression formation. *Journal of Experimental Social Psychology, 13*, 141–154.

Hume, D. (1788). *Essays and treatises on several subjects* (Vol. II). London: Cadell, Elliot, Kay, and Co.

Ichheiser, G. (1943). Misinterpretations of personality in everyday life. *Character and Personality, 11*, 145–160.

James, W. (1950). *The principles of psychology* (Vol. 1). New York: Dover. (Original work published 1890)

James, W. (1991). *Pragmatism*. Buffalo, NY: Prometheus Books. (Original work published 1907)

Jones, E. E. (1979). The rocky road from acts to dispositions. *American Psychologist, 34*, 107–117.

Jones, E. E., & Davis, K. E. (1965). From acts to dispositions: The attribution process in person perception. In L. Berkowitz (Ed.), *Advances in experimental social psychology* (Vol. 2, pp. 219–266). New York: Academic Press.

Jones, E. E., & Thibaut, J. W. (1958). Interaction goals as bases of inference in interpersonal perception. In L. Petrullo & R. Tagiuri (Eds.), *Person perception and interpersonal behavior* (pp. 151–178). Stanford, CA: Stanford University Press.

Kahneman, D. (1973). *Attention and effort*. Englewood Cliffs, NJ: Prentice-Hall.

Kant, I. (1990). *Critique of pure reason*. (J. M. D. Meidlejohn, Trans.). Buffalo, NY: Prometheus Books. (Original work published 1781)

Kelley, H. H. (1973). The processes of causal attribution. *American Psychologist, 28*, 107–128.

Koffka, K. (1922). Perception: An introduction to Gestalt-theorie. *Psychological Bulletin, 19*, 531–585.

Köhler, W. (1930). *Gestalt psychology*. London: Bell.

Langer, E., Blank, A., & Chanowitz, B. (1978). The mindlessness of ostensibly thoughtful action: The role of "placebic" information in interpersonal interaction. *Journal of Personality and Social Psychology, 36*, 635–642.

Lepore, L., & Brown, R. (1997). Category and stereotype activation: Is prejudice inevitable? *Journal of Personality and Social Psychology, 72*, 275–287.

Lewin, K. (1935). Psycho-sociological problems of a minority group. *Character and Personality, 3*, 175–187.

Lewin, K. (1936). *Principles of topological psychology*. New York: McGraw-Hill.

Lippmann, W. (1922). *Public opinion*. New York: Macmillan.

Locke, J. (1844). *An essay concerning human understanding*. Philadelphia: Kay, Jon, and Brother. (Original work published 1690)

Locke, V., MacLeod, C., & Walker, I. (1994). Automatic and controlled activation of stereotypes: Individual differences associated with prejudice. *British Journal of Social Psychology, 33*, 29–46.

Logan, G. D. (1980). Attention and automaticity in Stroop and priming tasks: Theory and data. *Cognitive Psychology, 12*, 523–553.

Lombardi, W. J., Higgins, E. T., & Bargh, J. A. (1987). The role of consciousness in priming effects on categorization. *Personality and Social Psychology Bulletin, 13*, 411–429.

Markus, H. (1977). Self-schemata and processing information about the self. *Journal of Personality and Social Psychology, 35*, 63–78.

Martin, L. L. (1986). Set/reset: Use and disuse of concepts in impression formation. *Journal of Personality and Social Psychology, 51*, 493–504.

Martin, L. L., & Achee, J. W. (1992). Beyond accessibility: The role of processing objectives in judgment. In L. L. Martin & A. Tesser (Eds.), *The construction of social judgments* (pp. 195–216). Hillsdale, NJ: Erlbaum.

Martin, L. L., Seta, J. J., & Crelia, R. A. (1990). Assimilation and contrast as a function of people's willingness and ability to expend effort in forming an impression. *Journal of Personality and Social Psychology, 59*, 27–37.

McArthur, L. Z., & Baron, R. (1983). Toward an ecological theory of social perception. *Psychological Review, 90*, 215–238.

Moskowitz, G. B. (1996). The mediational effects of attributions and information processing in minority social influence. *British Journal of Social Psychology, 35,* 47–66.

Moskowitz, G. B. (in press). On preconscious control: The implicit use of goals. In G. B. Moskowitz (Ed.), *The sovereignty of social cognition.* Mahwah, NJ: Erlbaum.

Moskowitz, G. B., Gollwitzer, P. M., Wasel, W., & Schaal, B. (in press). Preconscious control of stereotype activation through chronic egalitarian goals. *Journal of Personality and Social Psychology.*

Moskowitz, G. B., & Roman, R. J. (1992). Spontaneous trait inferences as self generated primes: Implications for conscious social judgement. *Journal of Personality and Social Psychology, 62,* 728–738.

Moskowitz, G. B., & Salomon, A. (in press). Implicit control of stereotype activation through the preconscious operation of chronic goals. *Social Cognition.*

Moskowitz, G. B., & Skurnik, I. (in press). Contrast effects as determined by the type of prime: Trait versus exemplar primes initiate processing strategies that differ in how accessible constructs are used. *Journal of Personality and Social Psychology.*

Oppenheimer, F. (1922). *System der soziologie.* Jena: Fischer.

Peirce, C. (1877). The fixation of belief. *Popular Science Monthly, 11,*

Peirce, C. (1878). How to make our ideas clear. *Popular Science Monthly, 12,* 286–302.

Petty, R. E., & Wegener, D. T. (1993). Flexible correction processes in social judgment: Correcting for context-induced contrast. *Journal of Experimental Social Psychology, 29,* 137–165.

Postman, L., Bruner, J. S., & McGinnies, E. (1948). Personal values as selective factors in perception. *Journal of Abnormal and Social Psychology, 43,* 142–154.

Schwarz, N. (1994). Judgment in a social context: Biases, shortcomings, and the logic of conversation. In M. P. Zanna (Ed.), *Advances in experimental social psychology* (Vol. 26, pp. 123–162). San Diego, CA: Academic Press.

Schwarz, N., Bless, H., Strack, F., Klummp, G., Rittenauer-Schatka, H., & Simons, A. (1991). Ease of retrieval as information: Another look at the availability heuristic. *Journal of Personality and Social Psychology, 61,* 195–202.

Sedikides, C., & Skowronski, J. J. (1991). The law of cognitive structure activation. *Psychological Inquiry, 2,* 169–184.

Sherif, M. (1936). *The psychology of social norms.* New York: Harper.

Skurnik, I., & Moskowitz, G. B. (1997). *Metacognition and the illusion of truth.* Manuscript submitted for publication.

Smith, E. R., & Mackie, D. M. (1995). *Social psychology.* New York: Worth.

Sperber, D., & Wilson, D. (1986). *Relevance: Communication and cognition.* Cambridge, MA: Harvard University Press.

Srull, T. K., & Wyer, R. S., Jr. (1979). The role of category accessibility in the interpretation of information about persons: Some determinants and implications. *Journal of Personality and Social Psychology, 37,* 1660–1672.

Stangor, C., & Lange, J. E. (1994). Mental representations of social groups: Advances in understanding stereotypes and stereotyping. In M. P. Zanna (Ed.), *Advances in experimental social psychology* (pp. 1357–1416). New York: Academic Press.

Strack, F., & Hanover, B. (1996). Awareness of influence as a precondition for implementing correctional goals. In P. M. Gollwitzer & J. A. Bargh (Eds.), *The psychology of action* (pp. 579–596). New York: Guilford Press.

Tagiuri, R. (1958). Preface. In L. Petrullo & R. Tagiuri (Eds.), *Person perception and interpersonal behavior* (pp. i–xix). Stanford, CA: Stanford University Press.

Tajfel, H. (1969). Cognitive aspects of prejudice. *Journal of Social Issues, 25,* 79–97.

Tetlock, P. E. (1985). Accountability: The neglected social context of judgment and choice. *Research in Organizational Behavior, 7,* 297–332.

Thompson, E. P., Roman, R. J., Moskowitz, G. B., Chaiken, S., & Bargh, J. A. (1994). Accuracy motivation attenuates covert priming effects: The systematic reprocessing of social information. *Journal of Personality and Social Psychology, 66,* 474–489.

Tolman, E. C. (1951). A psychological model. In T. Parsons & E. A. Shils (Eds.), *Toward a general theory of action* (pp. 279–361). Cambridge, MA: Harvard University Press.

Treisman, A., & Geffen, G. (1967). Selective attention: Perception or response? *The Quarterly Journal of Experimental Psychology, 19,* 1–17.

Tversky, A., & Kahneman, D. (1973). Availability: A heuristic for judging frequency and probability. *Cognitive Psychology, 5,* 207–232.

Uleman, J. S., & Moskowitz, G. B. (1994). Unintended effects of goals on unintended inferences. *Journal of Personality and Social Psychology, 66,* 490–501.

Uleman, J. S., Newman, L. S., & Moskowitz, G. B. (1996). Unintended social inference: The case of spontaneous trait inference. In M. P. Zanna (Ed.), *Advances in experimental social psychology* (Vol. 28, pp. 211–279). San Diego, CA: Academic Press.

Wegener, D. T., & Petty, R. E. (1995). Flexible correction processes in social judgment: The role of naive theories in corrections for perceived bias. *Journal of Personality and Social Psychology, 68,* 36–51.

Wilson, T. D., & Brekke, N. (1994). Mental contamination and mental correction: Unwanted influences on judgments and evaluations. *Psychological Bulletin, 116,* 117–142.

Zeigarnik, B. (1927). Das Behalten von erledigten und unerledigten Handlungen. *Psychologische Forschung, 9,* 1–85.

II

Dual-Process Theories in Attitudes
and Social Cognition,
and Single-Process Countermodels

A

Attitudes (and Beyond)

3

The Elaboration Likelihood Model: Current Status and Controversies

RICHARD E. PETTY
DUANE T. WEGENER

It has now been over 20 years since the notion of "two routes to persuasion" was introduced (see Petty, 1977; Petty & Cacioppo, 1981), and over a decade since the elaboration likelihood model (ELM) was translated into a series of formal postulates (Petty & Cacioppo, 1986a, 1986b). The model has garnered some praise (e.g., Ajzen, 1987; Pratkanis, 1989; Sears, 1988), and has guided a large number of basic and applied studies (see Petty & Wegener, 1998, for a recent review), but it has also been misunderstood and criticized on occasion (e.g., Stiff, 1986; Hamilton, Hunter, & Boster, 1993). The goals of this chapter are to provide a brief overview of the model; to discuss some of the major conceptual questions and confusions that have arisen; and to examine the current status of the ELM as a theory of persuasion in particular and of social judgment more generally.

When the idea of two routes to persuasion was first proposed (Petty, 1977), the literature on attitude change was in a state of disarray, to say the least. Seemingly simple variables such as the credibility of the message source or a person's affective state, which were predicted to have relatively straightforward effects on attitude change according to the persuasion theories of the time, instead produced a mystifying diversity of findings. For instance, expert sources, though usually good for persuasion (e.g., Kelman & Hovland, 1953) were not invariably favorable (e.g., Sternthal, Dholakia, & Leavitt, 1978). Similarly, inducing negative affect, though often bad for attitude change (e.g., Zanna, Kiesler, & Pilkonis, 1970), was sometimes associated with more positive influence (e.g., Leventhal, 1970).

The extraordinary complexity of research findings caused some reviewers of the attitude change literature in the late 1970s, both in the United States and abroad, to be quite pessimistic. For example, Jaspers (1978, p. 295) noted that "the most disturbing aspect of these results is their inconsistency." Sherif (1977, p. 370) described the "reigning confusion in the area," and Kiesler and Munson (1975, p. 443) concluded that "attitude change is not the thriving field it once was." Fishbein and Ajzen (1981) characterized the literature as "an accumulation of largely contradictory and inconsistent findings with few (if any) generalizable principles of effective communication" (p. 340). They argued that "a rather serious reconsideration of basic assumptions and thoughtful theoretical reanalyses of problems confronting the field" (Fishbein & Ajzen, 1972, p. 532) were needed. Against this backdrop, the two-routes-to-persuasion notion and the ELM were introduced in order to account for the complicated and perplexing results obtained in the accumulated literature, and to provide an integrative framework with which past research findings could be understood as well as new predictions generated.

OVERVIEW OF THE ELM

In brief, the ELM was formulated as a theory about how the classic source (e.g., expertise), message (e.g., number of arguments), recipient (e.g., mood), and contextual (e.g., distraction) variables have an impact on attitudes toward various objects, issues, and people. More generally, though, the theory can be used to understand how any external or internal variable has an impact on some evaluative (e.g., good–bad) or nonevaluative (e.g., likely–unlikely) judgment. As articulated in more detail shortly, the theory outlines a finite number of ways in which variables can have their impact on judgments; it also specifies when variables take on these roles, as well as the consequences resulting from these different roles. That is, the ELM is a theory about the processes underlying changes in judgments of objects, the variables that induce these processes, and the strength of the judgments resulting from these processes. Because most of the work on the ELM has emphasized evaluative judgments, we focus on evaluations (i.e., attitudes) in this chapter, though similar points can be made for nonevaluative judgments.

The ELM is a dual-route but multiprocess theory (depicted schematically in Figure 3.1). The dual routes—"central" and "peripheral"—refer to attitude changes that are based on different degrees of elaborative information-processing activity. Central-route attitude changes are those that are based on relatively extensive and effortful information-processing activity, aimed at scrutinizing and uncovering the central merits of the issue or advocacy. Peripheral-route attitude changes are based on a variety of attitude change processes that typically require less cognitive effort. As explained further shortly, some low-effort attitude changes are based on processes

that differ primarily in *quantitative* ways from central-route processes, but other peripheral-route changes result from processes that are both less effortful and are *qualitatively* different (Petty, 1997). These low-effort mechanisms are lumped together under the peripheral-route label because of the similarity in the consequences they are postulated to induce (Petty, Wheeler, & Bizer, in press).[1]

Perhaps the most critical construct in the ELM is the elaboration continuum. Points along the elaboration continuum are determined by how motivated and able people are to assess and elaborate upon the central merits of a person, issue, or a position (i.e., the attitude object).[2] As discussed in regard to Postulate 1 shortly, when a person is making an evaluative judgment, the "default" goal is to determine how good or bad the object "really" is; but when a person is judging likelihood, for example, the goal is to determine how likely or unlikely the event "really" is. The more motivated and able people are to assess the central merits of the attitude object (i.e., to determine how good it really is), the more likely they are to effortfully scrutinize all available object-relevant information. This is because effortful scrutiny is usually perceived to be the best way to achieve this goal. Thus, at the high end of the elaboration continuum, people assess object-relevant information in relation to knowledge that they already possess, and arrive at a reasoned (though not necessarily unbiased) attitude that is well articulated and bolstered by supporting information (the "central route" to judgment). At the low end of the elaboration continuum, information scrutiny is reduced. Nevertheless, attitude change can still result from a low-effort scrutiny of the information available (e.g., examining less information than when elaboration is high or examining the same information less carefully); or attitude change can result from a number of less resource-demanding processes, such as classical conditioning (Staats & Staats, 1958), self-perception (Bem, 1972), or the use of heuristics (Chaiken, 1987). Attitudes that are changed with minimal object-relevant thought are postulated to be weaker than attitudes that are changed to the same extent as a result of high object-relevant thought.

The ELM hypothesis of an elaboration continuum comes from recognizing that it is

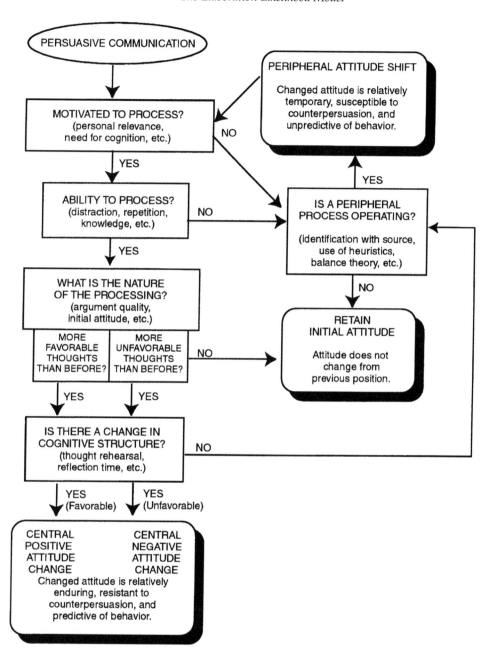

FIGURE 3.1. The elaboration likelihood model of persuasion.

neither adaptive nor possible for people to exert considerable mental effort in thinking about all of the messages and attitude objects to which they are exposed. In order to function in life, people must sometimes act as "cognitive misers" (Taylor, 1981), but at other times it is more adaptive for them to be generous with their cognitive resources. In the remainder of this chapter, we reexamine the formal ELM postulates first presented by Petty and Cacioppo (1986a, 1986b), and address some issues, confusions, and misunderstandings that have been raised since their introduction. We conclude with some discussions of similar dual-process and multiprocess theories that have been developed outside the persuasion domain.

POSTULATE 1: THE CORRECTNESS POSTULATE

People are motivated to hold correct attitudes.

The ELM assumes that at least at a conscious level, people want to hold opinions (and come to judgments) that are correct. That is, in the absence of other competing motives, the correctness motive is presumed to be the default goal. Of course, as Festinger (1954) noted, attitudes cannot be correct in any absolute sense. Rather, the correctness of an attitude is a subjective assessment and can be based on a wide variety of "evidence." Festinger emphasized the extent to which people look to the opinions of others as a means of judging the correctness of their own attitudes. This social comparison process is a relatively simple and easy way of judging correctness. As we will see shortly, the ELM holds open a number of other ways in which a person can achieve a feeling of subjective correctness. For example, people can ignore the opinions of others and effortfully seek out and evaluate all of the relevant information on their own. Or people can consider both the opinions of others and the implications of their personal scrutiny of the object's merits. Or different strategies can be used on different occasions. For example, people who do not enjoy thinking can simply accept what expert and trustworthy sources say, and can thus conserve their cognitive resources. However, if an expert source is untrustworthy, then people who prefer not to think might need to evaluate the message on their own in order to achieve the same feeling of correctness (Priester & Petty, 1995). Finally, the opinions of others might influence the extent or direction of the person's own scrutiny. For example, the greater the number of people who endorse an issue, the more an individual might choose to think about that issue (Burnstein & Vinokur, 1975; Burnstein, Vinokur, & Trope, 1973; Harkins & Petty, 1987). Whatever strategy is used, however,

the ELM assumes that the default goal is to come to a judgment that is subjectively correct.[3]

The assumption that the default motive is to be correct does not imply that people cannot be biased in their assessment of evidence, however (see discussion of Postulate 5). The first postulate of the ELM merely assumes that people are rarely explicitly motivated to be biased. Thus, in situations where people openly acknowledge and rely on a prejudice, they will often think that there is some merit or legitimacy to their view (e.g., a person might be openly biased against women police officers because he or she believes that men can do a better job). That is, people can believe that their bias helps them to be correct! As this implies, sometimes increasing the motive to be correct can actually enhance biased processing. For example, consider a person who is absolutely certain of the validity of a current attitude. In such a situation, the largest threat to correctness comes from the possibility that the person will succumb to influence. Thus, this person's goal will be to defend the attitude from attack, because defending the existing attitude may be the best way of maintaining a subjective sense of correctness. Of course, if a possible bias is made salient and people find this bias to be illegitimate, consistent with Postulate 1, people will often engage in some corrective action (Wegener & Petty, 1997). Additional discussion of bias is postponed until our discussion of Postulate 5.

POSTULATE 2: THE ELABORATION CONTINUUM POSTULATE

Although people want to hold correct attitudes, the amount and nature of issue-relevant elaboration in which they are willing or able to engage to evaluate a message vary with individual and situational factors.

Postulate 2 recognizes that even though people want to be correct, this does not mean that the amount of effort devoted to thinking will be constant across all people and situations. First, consider that the motive to be correct, like other psychological states, can vary with individual and situational factors.

That is, some people probably have a greater desire to be correct than others, and some situations elicit a greater motivation to be correct than others. For example, important issues could elicit a greater desire to be correct than unimportant issues. Therefore, if people think that the best way to form a correct opinion is to effortfully process all of the information provided, then subjectively important issues should elicit more diligent information-processing activity than subjectively unimportant ones (Petty & Cacioppo, 1979b, 1990). A desire to be correct can also motivate consideration of the likelihood that thinking will lead to a correct response. Specifically, although most people presumably believe that the best way to be correct is to effortfully examine all of the information, there may be some people for whom and some situations in which the opposite is the case. For example, if a person knows absolutely nothing about an issue, or has very low confidence in his or her analytic capabilities, the person may feel that the best way to be correct is to eschew effortful thinking and rely on knowledgeable others. For such a person, this tendency should be exacerbated when issue importance (and the need to be correct) is increased (cf. Sorrentino, Bobocel, Gitta, & Olson, 1988). On the other hand, if people who have low confidence in their processing abilities are made to feel that they are capable of effortful analysis, then processing motivation should generally be increased (Bohner, Rank, Reinhard, Einwiller, & Erb, 1998; Evans & Petty, 1998).

Although the desire to be correct and the perception of one's ability to be correct by engaging in effortful thinking are important determinants of the extent of information-processing activity, Postulate 2 explicitly recognizes that a consideration of "correctness" is not the only factor at work in determining the extent of thinking. For example, the hedonic (and other) consequences of thinking can also be important. Thus, putting people in a positive mood gets them to think more about pleasant messages—not because positive moods or pleasant messages increase the desire to be correct (or the need to have greater confidence in one's opinion; Chaiken, Liberman, & Eagly, 1989), but because thinking about a pleasant message is hedonically rewarding, and people in positive moods are

especially attentive to the hedonic consequences of their actions (Wegener & Petty, 1994; Wegener, Petty, & Smith, 1995; cf. Bless & Schwarz, Chapter 21, this volume). In a similar vein, some individuals generally take greater pleasure in thinking than others and thus these individuals (i.e., those high in *need for cognition*; Cacioppo & Petty, 1982) tend to engage in effortful thought because of its intrinsic enjoyment, without regard to the importance of the issue or the need to be correct (see Cacioppo, Petty, Feinstein, & Jarvis, 1996, for a review).

Importantly, Postulate 2 recognizes that motivational variables are not the only factors that influence the extent of thinking. Ability is important as well. Just as motivational variables can stem from the person or the situation, so too can ability. That is, some people are more able to think about issues because of their intelligence or knowledge, but some situations facilitate or impair thinking in most people (e.g., the presence of distraction hinders most people from processing a communication; Petty, Wells, & Brock, 1976). When both motivation and ability are high, people will presumably engage in considerable cognitive effort, and when both are low, effort will be low. If ability is high but motivation is low, people will not engage in much thinking until such time as motivation changes (e.g., following a message, people may learn of its personal relevance). Similarly, if motivation is high but ability is low, people will not process much until such time as they are able. If people continue to be interrupted before they are satisfied that they have achieved a correct opinion (or whatever their salient processing goal is), this can lead to recurrent thought about the object (see Petty, Jarvis, & Evans, 1996, for additional discussion).

Two aspects of Postulate 2 have been misunderstood. The first is that the elaboration likelihood is incorrectly thought to refer to two discrete points rather than a *continuum*. This confusion probably stems in part from the depiction of high- and low-elaboration *endpoints* along the continuum in schematic presentations of the ELM such as that in Figure 3.1, or perhaps from discussion of the two "routes" to change—although such references are meant to describe prototypical points along the continuum. There are a number of important features to this continuum; the most obvious of these is the hypothesis that sometimes attitude change occurs as a result of considerable thinking about and elaboration of the information provided, and at other times attitude change is associated with minimal thinking about and elaboration of the information provided. That is, the elaboration continuum notion implies that the *type* of thought given to object-relevant information can be the same under high- and low-elaboration conditions, but that the *amount* of cognitive activity varies (a "quantitative effect"; see Petty, 1997).

As an example of this quantitative effect, consider a person who is exposed to a message containing eight strong arguments. A high-elaboration processor might think of three or four favorable implications of each of the arguments, whereas a low-elaboration processor might think of only one or two favorable implications (because he or she is not thinking as much). The effect of this is that the high-elaboration processor will probably have more favorable attitudes toward the issue than the low-elaboration processor, because he or she will have generated more favorable implications of the strong arguments presented. An alternative way to bring about this effect is if the low-elaboration processor thinks diligently, but about fewer arguments (e.g., if the person generates three or four favorable thoughts to the first few arguments, but doesn't think at all about the remaining arguments). This is also likely to leave this person with a less favorable attitude than that of the person who has thought carefully about all of the arguments.[4]

The second low-elaboration process—thinking about fewer arguments—can lead to some interesting effects. For example, what if a message contains four strong arguments followed by four weak ones? A high-elaboration processor who thinks about all of the information in a relatively objective manner is likely to have a moderate opinion about the issue, because the arguments are mixed (Friedrich, Fetherstonhaugh, Casey, & Gallagher, 1996; Petty & Cacioppo, 1984a). However, an individual who considers only the early arguments is likely to have a more favorable opinion, because only the strong arguments are given careful consideration. If the message has four weak arguments followed by four strong ones, then the low-elaboration

processor will have a less favorable opinion than the high-elaboration processor who considers all of the arguments objectively.[5] In addition to these quantitative effects, however, the ELM holds that low-elaboration attitude change can be produced by processes that are substantively different from the argument consideration processes just described (a "qualitative effect"; Petty, 1997). Qualitative effects are addressed in more detail later.

A second confusion about the elaboration continuum concerns the nature of the thinking rather than the amount. The term "elaboration" is used to suggest that people add something of their own to the specific information provided in the communication. That is, when elaborating, they go beyond mere verbatim encoding (or learning) of the information provided. As Postulate 2 indicates, the ELM emphasizes *issue*-relevant elaboration (i.e., elaboration of information relevant to the attitude object or advocacy). This issue-relevant (or object-relevant) elaboration is often provoked by message arguments, but can also be sparked if no message is provided, or can be stimulated by nonmessage factors even when a message is presented. As noted by Petty and Cacioppo (1984b), as people approach the high end of the elaboration continuum, they are more likely to "scrutinize *all* available information in the immediate persuasion context . . . in an attempt to evaluate the true merits of the arguments *and position* advocated" (p. 671; emphasis added). Thus, a high elaboration individual might consider factors such as whether the message arguments presented are really cogent and compelling, but might also attempt to evaluate the merits of the position advocated by considering the information value of the source of the message (i.e., "Is the source legitimate to consider and helpful in judging the true merits of the object?"), his or her own currently experienced internal feelings (i.e., "are my feelings legitimate to consider and helpful in judging the true merits of the object?"), and all other factors relevant to judging the merits of the position advocated. Although some reviewers have believed that the ELM identifies central variables or high-effort processing with the message, and peripheral variables or low-effort processing with the source or nonmessage factors (e.g., see Kruglanski & Thompson, in press;

Spiegel, Thompson, & Kruglanski, 1996), this is not the case. In the ELM, content (e.g., source or message variables) and process (e.g., effortful scrutiny, classical conditioning effects, use of heuristics, etc.) are orthogonal. That is, one can engage in effortful scrutiny for merit of source and message factors, and these features of the persuasion context can also be the source of heuristics and other peripheral processes. Although some ELM research has manipulated source versus message variables to *operationalize* high- versus low-elaboration attitude change (e.g., Petty, Cacioppo, & Goldman, 1981), other ELM research has explicitly manipulated only message factors to show their role as peripheral cues in low-elaboration attitude change (e.g., Petty & Cacioppo, 1984a), and some research has manipulated source factors and pointed to their role as arguments in high-elaboration attitude change (Petty & Cacioppo, 1984b).

Research guided by the ELM has shown that just as various message factors (e.g., the mere number of arguments used) can serve as simple cues and can affect judgments when the extent of elaboration is low, various source factors can be relevant to judging the central merits of an object when the extent of elaboration is high. For example, Petty and Cacioppo (1986a) noted that "for teenage smokers . . . the major reason why they smoke may relate to the image of the particular brand. . . . [Thus] . . . the presentation of [various] images might provide important product-relevant information" (p. 17). Similarly, high self-monitors are concerned with the image they project to others (Snyder, 1979), and thus these individuals are likely to think carefully about the image a message source conveys in high-elaboration situations.

There are a number of unexplored implications of the notion that at the extreme high end of the elaboration continuum, people scrutinize all information relevant to judging the position advocated. This means, for example, that people will subject source and message information to more scrutiny under high- than under low-elaboration conditions. Under low-elaboration conditions, people are looking for a simple, quick, and easy way to judge the merits of the position, rather than examining all of the information carefully. Thus, according to the ELM, under these conditions people might base their judgment on the first arguments processed, or on the mere number of arguments presented, or on a cursory analysis of the source (e.g., whether the source seems attractive, likable, expert). However, when people are motivated and able to engage in greater scrutiny, their quick impressions can be modified. That is, later arguments can undermine the implications of early ones, or the large number of arguments may turn out to be specious, or a source who seemed expert on a first glance may turn out to be a fraud upon more careful analysis. Furthermore, as people think about the information more, they may decide that it is inappropriate to use some of the information that they were all too willing to use when they were not thinking very much. For example, when thinking carefully and motivated to be accurate, people might become aware that their mood could be biasing their judgment, and might actively attempt to correct for this influence (see Ottati & Isbell, 1996; Wegener & Petty, 1997). On the other hand, it is possible that with increased scrutiny, people might become even more convinced of the utility of some factor and give it more weight. For example, under high scrutiny people might become more convinced of the expertise, knowledge, and/or informational relevance of the message source, and thus might weight this information even more in their final judgment than when they are not thinking carefully (e.g., Kirmani & Shiv, 1998).

The point is that when a person's goal in scrutinizing all of the information is to determine the true merits of the proposal, the person will use whatever information seems useful in reaching that goal. Thus, if providing a message recipient with extensive information about the credibility of the source convinces the person more of the validity of the position when the source information is scrutinized, the impact of credibility can be even higher under high- than under low-elaboration conditions. Conversely, if providing extensive information about the attractiveness of the source (e.g., number of beauty pageants won, etc.) does not convince the person of the validity of the position when this information is scrutinized (e.g., if this information is viewed as irrelevant to the advocacy), the impact of the attractiveness manipulation can be lower under high- than under low-elaboration conditions. Treating the same information differently under different levels of elaboration is at the heart of the next ELM postulate.

POSTULATE 3: THE MULTIPLE-ROLES POSTULATE

Variables can affect the amount and direction of attitude change by (a) serving as persuasive arguments, (b) serving as peripheral cues, and/or (c) affecting the extent or direction of issue and argument elaboration.

Postulate 3 is perhaps the most misunderstood of all of the ELM postulates. This postulate does a number of things, but we focus on two here. First, it makes a distinction between the processes by which variables have an impact on persuasion. Second, it suggests that any one variable can have an impact on attitude change by more than one mechanism. We discuss each of these notions in turn.

Central versus Peripheral Processes of Attitude Change

One of the important things that Postulate 3 is intended to do is to make a distinction between treating information as an "argument" or as a "cue." Postulate 2 introduced the elaboration continuum, and we have seen that a number of interesting effects can be predicted simply by considering the extent to which people process each of the items of information presented as arguments. That is, the items of information available in the persuasion situation (whether stemming from the source, the message, the context, or one's own mind or body) can be subjected to scrutiny and examined for relevance in determining the merit of the position advocated. As noted in discussing Postulate 2, this scrutiny of the information as arguments falls along a continuum and thus can be maximal, moderate, or minimal. In addition to this quantitative variation in the treatment of information as arguments, however, Postulate 3 notes that some information can be treated as a peripheral cue. The aim here is to make a *qualitative* distinction, to complement the *quantitative* variation encompassed by the elaboration continuum outlined in Postulate 2. If the only differences involved in persuasion were quan-

titative ones, then one might simply speak of one persuasion process that operated in varying degrees. In fact, some social psychologists have argued that there is just one persuasion process. Fishbein and Middlestadt (1995), for example, explicitly reject current multiprocess models such as the ELM and the heuristic–systematic model (HSM; Chaiken et al., 1989), arguing that all attitude change is "cognitive" and can be captured by changes in the composite created by combining the perceived desirability of an object's attributes and the perceived likelihood of the object's possessing those attributes. Similarly, Kruglanski's lay epistemic theory (LET; see Kruglanski, 1989; Kruglanski, Thompson, & Spiegel, Chapter 14, this volume) rejects the need for multiprocess frameworks, preferring to lump all proposed mechanisms of persuasion into one process of "hypothesis testing." Of course, if one process were sufficient to account for persuasion, then the LET and other one-process models would be more parsimonious than and thus superior to multiprocess models.

While acknowledging the importance of quantitative variations in the extent of elaboration in Postulate 2, the ELM holds that no single process or mechanism is sufficient to account for the complexity of judgment phenomena. Rather, the ELM holds that various peripheral mechanisms of attitude change, which do not involve much (if any) thought about the substantive merits of the information presented, occur when the elaboration likelihood is low. For example, when presented with a lengthy list of arguments, the low-elaboration processor might not just process the first few arguments and quit (quantitative effect), but might instead simply count the arguments and reason that "if there are 20 reasons to favor it, it must be worthwhile" (see Petty & Cacioppo, 1984a). Note that this process of attitude change, on some dimensions at least, is qualitatively different from the argument elaboration process: This mechanism does not involve consideration of the merits of *any* of the arguments, but instead involves reliance on a rule of thumb or heuristic that the person generates or retrieves from memory (see Chaiken, 1987, and Chen & Chaiken, Chapter 4, this volume, for more on heuristic processing). Other relatively low-effort mechanisms that are capable of producing attitude change without processing the substantive merits of the information presented include classical conditioning (Staats & Staats, 1958; Cacioppo, Marshall-Goodell, Tassinary, & Petty, 1992), identification with the source of the message (Kelman, 1958), misattribution of affect to the message (Petty & Cacioppo, 1983; Schwarz & Clore, 1983), and mere-exposure effects (Bornstein, 1989; Zajonc, 1968). When one of these peripheral processes has a substantial influence on attitudes, this typically indicates that either motivation or ability is rather low in that persuasion setting and that the resulting attitudes are likely to be rather weak. We discuss the consequences of different attitude change processes further in connection with Postulate 7.[6]

Distinguishing Qualitative from Quantitative Effects along the Elaboration Continuum

At the conceptual level, it is relatively easy (we think) to distinguish between qualitatively different argument (central) and cue (peripheral) processes of persuasion. At the empirical level, however, it might sometimes be difficult to discern whether any given low-elaboration effect differs from a high-elaboration effect, because of the qualitative or the quantitative mechanism specified by the ELM. For example, consider a study reported by Petty and Cacioppo (1984b) in which the attractiveness of the message source in an advertisement for a beauty product was manipulated. In this study, the attractiveness of the source had an impact under both high- and low-involvement conditions (designed to manipulate the elaboration likelihood), but the manipulation of the quality of the verbal arguments had an impact only under high-involvement conditions. Stated differently, only source attractiveness had an impact under low-involvement (low-elaboration) conditions, but both source attractiveness and argument quality had an impact under high-involvement (high-elaboration) conditions. A clear conclusion from this study, consistent with the ELM, is that low-involvement participants engaged in less effortful information processing activity than high-involvement individuals because they considered a smaller quantity of information than high-involvement participants. But is this explana-

tion, based on the ELM prediction of quantitative variation along the elaboration continuum, sufficient to account for the results? Or did the processing of low-involvement individuals differ from that of high-involvement individuals in its quality as well as its quantity? Petty and Cacioppo (1984b) argued that the high-involvement individuals considered all information—including source attractiveness—and determined that the attractiveness of a person using a beauty product was a relevant consideration in judging the merit of the product; thus source attractiveness, when processed as an argument, added to the impact of the other (verbal) arguments presented for the product. Petty and Cacioppo further argued that in the low-involvement conditions, however, source attractiveness had an impact because of its function as a peripheral cue.

To summarize, one account for the different effects under high- and low-involvement conditions is simply a quantitative one. That is, low-involvement individuals could have processed the source attractiveness information in the same way as high-involvement individuals (i.e., they could have judged its relevance for the merit of the product), but they did not process the other information because the verbal arguments were less salient, more difficult to process, were introduced later in the communication, and so forth. Thus, this interpretation of the study, consistent with the ELM, says that involvement induced differences in the extent of information-processing activity, with high-involvement individuals engaging in greater information processing than low-involvement individuals (i.e., they processed more information as arguments). However, the ELM allows for another interpretation as well. Specifically, the low-involvement participants might have processed the source information in a qualitatively different way than high-involvement participants. For example, the attractive source could have produced positive affect that generalized to the product, as specified by classical conditioning models of attitude change (Staats & Staats, 1958). Or the positive regard for the attractive source could have led people to evaluate the product by means of a retrieved heuristic (e.g., "I agree with people I like"; Chaiken, 1987). In this study it was not possible to determine whether a quantitative or a qualitative difference along the elaboration continuum was responsible for the differences observed under conditions of high and low involvement. However, it is possible to design a study that could tease these apart. For example, one could vary the relevance of the product to source attractiveness.

Consider a study that varies the elaboration likelihood (via involvement, distraction, etc.), the quality of the verbal arguments in the message, and the relevance of source attractiveness for the attitude object. Thus, some people might receive an ad for a beauty product as in the Petty and Cacioppo (1984b) study (high relevance of attractiveness), but others would receive an ad for a roofing contractor (low relevance of attractiveness). Both the quantitative and qualitative interpretations would suggest that the manipulation of verbal argument quality would have a greater impact under high- than under low-elaboration conditions. However, the quantitative and qualitative interpretations make different predictions for the low-relevance (low-elaboration) conditions.

Both frameworks agree that under high-elaboration conditions, people would process the source attractiveness information as an argument, leading to rejection of attractiveness in the ad for the roofing contractor but acceptance of it for the beauty product. Because processing the argument value of the source would lead to rejection of the source for the roofing ad (i.e., little or no impact of the attractive source), the quantitative explanation suggests that the attractive source would also have no effect for the roofing contractor under low-elaboration conditions (for the same reason that it would have no effect under high-elaboration conditions). However, the qualitative explanation suggests that the attractive source could have an impact for both the beauty product and the roofing ads under low-elaboration conditions, because the information could presumably be having an impact on judgment by a different mechanism (e.g., classical conditioning, invocation of a heuristic, etc.) that would be applicable regardless of the relevance of attractiveness to the product.

As we have just noted, both the quantitative and the qualitative possibilities are consistent with the ELM, so perhaps the key question is whether the qualitative feature of the ELM is *ever* needed to account for results. If all results can be accommodated by the quantitative aspect of the ELM, then there would be no need to postulate a separate category of peripheral attitude change mechanisms (classical conditioning, use of heuristics, etc.). In our view, the empirical evidence to date clearly suggests that quantitative variations in elaboration alone are insufficient to account for the obtained results.

For example, in one relevant study, Miniard, Bhatla, Lord, Dickson, and Unnava (1991) varied motivation to think about an advertisement, as well as whether the pictures featured in the advertisement were relevant to judging the merits of the featured product or not (e.g., a picture of a fluffy kitten could suggest "softness" for a facial tissue, but a picture of an equally positive sunset would be irrelevant for this product). Miniard et al. found that the relevance of a picture to a product did not matter under low-elaboration conditions. That is, as long as the picture was rated positively, equally favorable attitudes toward the product were induced. Under high-elaboration conditions, however, the relevance of the picture was consequential. Specifically, the high-relevance picture was associated with more liking of the product than was the equally positive low-relevance picture. This finding is consistent with the idea that the pictures were processed in a qualitatively different manner under high- and low-elaboration conditions (i.e., as arguments and as peripheral cues, respectively).

In another study, mentioned earlier, Petty and Cacioppo (1984a) varied involvement, the quality of verbal arguments, and the number of verbal arguments in a message. Under low-involvement conditions, people reported agreeing with the message more when it contained more arguments, regardless of whether the arguments were cogent or specious. In contrast, under high-involvement conditions, more arguments led to more persuasion when the arguments were compelling, but to less persuasion when the arguments were specious (i.e., argument quality was more important than the mere number of arguments). It is not clear how a framework allowing only quantitative variations in processing could account for this pattern of results. That is, counting arguments seems to be a qualitatively different mechanism for producing attitude change than evaluating arguments for merit.[7]

In sum, although a number of interesting predictions can be made from consideration of the amount of elaboration alone (quantitative variation), additional interesting and unique predictions can be made from consideration of qualitatively different peripheral-route processes. As just noted, these qualitative predictions have been supported in some research, suggesting that one-process models may be overly limited (for discussions of unimodal versus multimode models of persuasion, see Haugtvedt, 1997; Priester & Fleming, 1997; Schwartz, 1997; Wegener & Claypool, in press).

Multiple Roles for Variables along the Elaboration Continuum

A second important feature of Postulate 3 is that it introduces the notion of multiple roles for persuasion variables. That is, the ELM notes that a variable can influence attitudes in four ways: (1) by serving as an argument, (2) by serving as a cue, (3) by determining the extent of elaboration, and (4) by producing a bias in elaboration. Importantly, the postulate is meant to suggest that variables (such as source attractiveness) need not serve in only one of the roles specified. At the time the postulate was originally presented, no research had been conducted demonstrating that any one variable could serve in *all* of the postulated roles, though Petty and Cacioppo (1986a) reviewed some studies showing that any one variable could serve in at least two different roles in different situations, and provided speculation about when and how any one variable could serve in all of the roles (see pp. 204–215).

In essence, the multiple-roles notion is that any given variable can influence attitudes by different processes, and Petty and Cacioppo (1986a, 1986b) noted that variables can take on different roles at different points along the elaboration continuum. In brief, variables serve as cues (or work via peripheral mechanisms) at the low end of the elaboration continuum. Variables serve as arguments or bias information processing at the high end of the elaboration continuum. Variables are most likely to affect the amount of thinking when the elaboration likelihood is not constrained by other variables to be high or low (e.g., at about the middle of the continuum). The fact that variables can take on

different roles at different points along the elaboration continuum implies that the *impact* of any given variable that serves as a peripheral cue under low-elaboration conditions can be enhanced, can be reduced, can be reversed, or can remain the same as the elaboration likelihood is increased (Petty, 1994).

For example, consider whether a manipulation of "beautiful scenery" in an advertisement for a vacation location should increase or decrease in impact as the elaboration likelihood is increased. If a person is not thinking about the ad very much, then the beautiful scenery might have a positive impact simply because of its mere association with the target location, much as it might have a similar positive impact on evaluations of a new car that is located in the scenery. However, as the elaboration likelihood is increased and the scenery is processed for its merits with respect to the product, then the impact of the scenery on attitudes might be increased in the ad for the vacation location because of its perceived relevance and merit (or might have the same impact but for a different reason than under low elaboration), but might show decreased impact in the ad for the car because of its perceived irrelevance for this product when processed as an argument. The positive impact of beautiful scenery can also be reversed if the scenery makes the ad seem more interesting (and thus people think about the ad more) when the ad contains only weak arguments for the vacation location.

As noted previously, one misunderstanding of the ELM is the mistaken belief that the model holds that source (and other nonmessage) variables are peripheral but message variables are central. Because of this misunderstanding, some have interpreted the ELM to say that source factors must invariably decrease in impact as the elaboration likelihood is increased (e.g., Kruglanski & Thompson, in press; Spiegel et al., 1996). Yet, as we have explained, there are multiple ways in which source (and other nonmessage) variables can *increase* in impact as a person moves up the elaboration continuum. For example, as the source information is scrutinized more carefully along with all other information, confidence in the validity of the message position might be increased (i.e., when the source is processed as an argument, confidence in the correctness of the position espoused might be increased, decreased, or show no change). Second, the source impact can increase because the source biases information-processing activity. Thus an expert source might bias processing of the verbal arguments presented (Chaiken & Maheswaran, 1994), or might lead to the self-generation of arguments consistent with the position the source is advocating (see Burnstein & Vinokur, 1975). Of course, if a potential cue (e.g., an attractive source) is scrutinized and found lacking (e.g., "Attractiveness is not a good reason to favor this" or "It is biasing to go along just because he or she is attractive"), then the presumably positive cue can actually reduce persuasion (e.g., if an overcorrection for the perceived bias occurs; Petty, Wegener, & White, 1998). If the cue is deemed relevant and informative when scrutinized, however, then it will add to the impact of the other information. Note that in the ELM, the additive impact under high-elaboration conditions is not a result of a low-effort heuristic adding to the impact of high-effort central/systematic processing (see Maheswaran & Chaiken, 1991), but is due to the fact that the cue/heuristic is effortfully scrutinized as a potential argument supporting the advocacy of the message.[8]

In general, misunderstanding of the multiple-roles postulate shows up whenever scholars assume that the ELM holds that variables can take on only *one* of the postulated roles. Thus, some critics of the model (e.g., Allen & Reynolds, 1993) have (inappropriately) asked for a list of what variables work via the "central route" and what variables work via the "peripheral route." In a similar vein, scholars who review the effects of certain variables have sometimes struggled to determine whether a variable is a "central" or a "peripheral" one, rather than recognizing the multiple roles for variables. For example, in reviewing the effects of group membership on persuasion, McGarty, Haslam, Hutchinson, and Turner (1994) stated that "in the elaboration likelihood model (ELM) of Petty and Cacioppo (1986[b]), group memberships are persuasive by the peripheral route" (p. 269). Although this is a possibility, the multiple-roles postulate for variables outlined by Petty and Cacioppo (1986b) applies to group membership as much as it does to other variables. That is, in some circumstances persuasive influence of group membership might be a pe-

ripheral-cue effect, but at other times group membership might serve as an argument, might bias processing, or might influence how much people scrutinize arguments (see Fleming & Petty, in press, for additional discussion of multiple roles for group membership in persuasion).

In addition, when some investigators find that some seemingly "peripheral" variables can affect the amount of information processing, this is seen as a surprising revelation rather than as a result consistent with the ELM. For example, when Soldat, Sinclair, and Mark (1997) found that the color of the paper on which a task was printed influenced the extent of information processing, they noted that "it appears to be the case that cues that are traditionally seen as peripheral (e.g., color . . .) can affect whether people engage in elaboration" (p. 69). As noted previously, even early research guided by the ELM multiple-roles notion showed that a variety of seemingly peripheral variables, such as source expertise (e.g., Heesacker, Petty, & Cacioppo, 1983) and source attractiveness (e.g., Puckett, Petty, Cacioppo, & Fisher, 1983), could influence the extent of information processing (see Petty & Cacioppo, 1986a, for a review, see also DeBono & Harnish, 1988).

In general, whenever researchers postulate or document just one role for a variable, the ELM multiple-roles postulate suggests that this variable might operate by different mechanisms in different situations. For example, in a recent study (Ottati, Terkildsen, & Hubbard, 1997), a speaker's facial expressions were shown to influence the extent of processing of the speaker's message (i.e., happy facial expressions elicited less elaboration than neutral expressions). The ELM suggests that a speaker's facial expressions should be capable of influencing attitudes by other mechanisms as well (e.g., by serving as a peripheral cue if the elaboration likelihood is constrained to be low).

POSTULATE 4: THE OBJECTIVE-PROCESSING POSTULATE

Variables affecting motivation and/or ability to process a message in a relatively objective manner can do so by either enhancing or reducing argument scrutiny.

Postulate 4 has been relatively uncontroversial. It simply notes that some variables influence the extent of information scrutiny in a relatively objective manner by invoking various motivational factors (encompassing a person's intentions and goals) and ability factors (encompassing a person's capabilities and opportunities). Persuasion researchers have identified a number of ways to assess the extent to which persuasion is based on effortful consideration of information. Perhaps the most popular procedure has followed Petty et al. (1976) and has varied the quality of the arguments contained in a message, in order to gauge the extent of message processing by the size of the argument quality effects on attitudes. Greater argument quality effects suggest greater argument scrutiny. Although the purpose of argument quality manipulation in ELM studies is sometimes misunderstood (see O'Keefe, 1990), such manipulation is simply a methodological tool for examining the impact of some other variable on thinking (for further discussion, see Petty & Cacioppo, 1986b; Petty, Wegener, Priester, Fabrigar, & Cacioppo, 1993).

Other procedures for assessing the extent of mental effort include assessment of the number and profile of issue-relevant thoughts generated (Petty, Ostrom, & Brock, 1981). High-elaboration conditions are sometimes associated with more thoughts (e.g., Burnkrant & Howard, 1984), and even if the total number of thoughts does not vary, under high-elaboration conditions the thoughts better reflect the quality of the issue-relevant information presented (e.g., Harkins & Petty, 1981). For example, low elaborators might generate an average of two favorable and three unfavorable thoughts following a message, reflecting their initially unfavorable attitudes regardless of the quality of the arguments presented. However, high elaborators might generate three favorable and two unfavorable thoughts following the presentation of strong arguments, and one favorable and four unfavorable thoughts following the presentation of weak arguments. Note that in this example, the total number of thoughts does not vary across elaboration conditions, but the thoughts better reflect the fact that the individuals have considered the substantive message information presented. Also, correlations between message-relevant thoughts and

postmessage attitudes tend to be greater when argument scrutiny is high (e.g., Chaiken, 1980; Petty & Cacioppo, 1979b), and high message elaboration can produce longer reading or exposure times than more cursory analyses (e.g., Mackie & Worth, 1989; see Wegener, Downing, Krosnick, & Petty, 1995, for a discussion of measures of elaboration).

The notion in Postulate 4 that variables can influence persuasion by enhancing or reducing information processing is a key hypothesis in helping to explain how the same variable can both increase and decrease persuasion. For example, because distraction reduces information processing, it inhibits whatever thoughts a person normally would be thinking in the absence of distraction. Thus, if a person would normally be generating many unfavorable thoughts because a message is highly counterattitudinal or contains specious arguments, distraction will reduce these unfavorable thoughts and will thereby increase persuasion. On the other hand, if the person would normally be generating many favorable thoughts because the message takes a highly desirable position or contains compelling arguments, distraction will reduce these favorable thoughts, and persuasion will be reduced as well (Petty et al., 1976).

Following the distraction studies (Petty et al., 1976), numerous investigations have manipulated some variable of interest (such as source expertise), along with some other variable (usually the cogency of the message arguments) that normally makes the profile of thoughts generated very favorable or very unfavorable when people think about the message. If source expertise influences thinking in a relatively objective manner, then one of the two patterns of results presented in Figure 3.2 can be expected. The top panel depicts the case in which a high-expertise source has led to greater differentiation of strong from weak arguments, suggesting that a high-expertise source produces more message processing than a low-expertise source. The bottom panel depicts the opposite result: A low-expertise source produces more message processing than a high-expertise source. Note that whichever processing outcome is produced, such results move understanding of the variable beyond the first-generation persuasion conclusion (i.e., that the variable either enhances or reduces persuasion) to the second-generation conclusion (i.e., that the variable can both enhance and reduce persuasion because of its effect on information processing; see Petty, 1997, for additional discussion of the generations of persuasion research).

In the first wave of research examining the impact of some variable on message processing, it was typically assumed that variables either enhance or reduce information processing. Many such variables have been examined in this regard. For example, just as distraction was shown to reduce ability to process a message, repeating a message was shown to increase ability to process (Cacioppo & Petty, 1989). Also, just as some variables were shown to increase motivation to process (e.g., enhancing personal relevance; Petty & Cacioppo, 1979b, 1990), other variables were shown to decrease motivation to

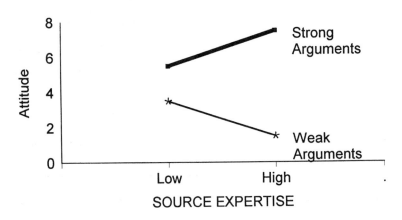

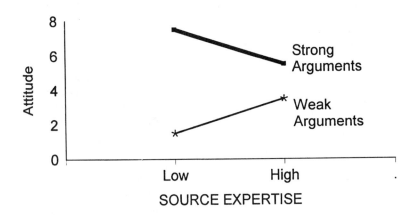

FIGURE 3.2. Two patterns of results that can be expected if source expertise influences thinking in a relatively objective manner: (Top) A high-expertise source leads to greater differentiation of strong from weak arguments. (Bottom) A low-expertise source leads to greater differentiation of strong from weak arguments.

process (e.g., making the person part of a group responsible for evaluating the message; Petty, Harkins, & Williams, 1980). Some variables (such as distraction and repetition) were part of the persuasion context, but other variables influencing processing stemmed from the message itself (e.g., overly complex messages tend to receive less processing than simple messages; Hafer, Reynolds, & Obertynski, 1996), or the source (e.g., knowledgeable sources who are untrustworthy induce more processing than knowledgeable sources who are trustworthy; Priester & Petty, 1995), or the recipient of the message (e.g., those high in need for cognition engage in greater message processing than those low in need for cognition; Cacioppo, Petty, & Morris, 1983). The number of variables that have been crossed with argument quality to examine the effect of the variables on information processing is now quite large; in addition to those just mentioned, these variables include mood (Worth & Mackie, 1987; Bless, Bohner, Schwarz, & Strack, 1990; see Bless & Schwarz, Chapter 21, this volume), recipient posture (Petty, Wells, Heesacker, Brock, & Cacioppo, 1983), deprivation of control (Pittman, 1993), expectation of discussion with another (Chaiken, 1980; Leippe & Elkin, 1987), number of message sources (e.g., Harkins & Petty, 1987; Moore & Reardon, 1987), ambivalence about the message topic (Maio, Bell, & Esses, 1996), speed of speech (Smith & Shaffer, 1991), physiological arousal (Sanbonmatsu & Kardes, 1988), time pressure (e.g., Ratneshwar & Chaiken, 1991), knowledge about the issue (Wood, Rhodes, & Biek, 1995), and others.

Thus, a number of studies have supported the second-generation conclusion that many variables can increase or decrease persuasion by increasing or decreasing information processing. More recently, however, a number of studies have addressed the third-generation possibility that the same variable can increase processing in some situations, but decrease it in others. The first such study examined the effect of rhetorical questions on persuasion and found that summarizing arguments as rhetorical questions (e.g., "Wouldn't increasing tuition lead to an improvement in the library?") rather than as statements (e.g., "Increasing tuition would lead to an improvement in the library") led to increased message

processing when the issue was of low personal relevance and people ordinarily would not be thinking about the message, but to reduced message processing when the issue was of high personal relevance and people ordinarily would be thinking about the message (Petty, Cacioppo, & Heesacker, 1981). The latter effect presumably occurred because people who were already engaged in thinking about the message were distracted from their natural chain of thoughts by the rhetorical questions.

Since the rhetorical-questions study, several variables have been shown both to increase and to decrease message processing in different situations. For example, endorsement of an advocacy by a majority of one's peers leads to more message processing than minority endorsement when the message topic is counterattitudinal, but majority endorsement leads to less message processing than majority endorsement when the message topic is proattitudinal (Baker & Petty, 1994). Framing the message arguments in a positive way (e.g., "If you stop smoking you will live longer") leads to more processing than negative framing (e.g., "If you don't stop smoking you will die sooner") when people expect negatively framed arguments, but positive framing leads to less processing than negative framing when people expect positively framed arguments (Smith & Petty, 1996). Happy mood leads to less message processing than sad mood when the message topic is expected to be unpleasant, but happy mood leads to more processing when the message topic is expected to be pleasant (Wegener, Petty, & Smith, 1995).

These patterns of data are very complex when one attempts to describe the impact of a variable on persuasion. For example, majority endorsement increases persuasion over minority endorsement when the topic is counterattitudinal and the arguments are strong (because in this case majority endorsement increases processing of the strong arguments over minority endorsement), or when the topic is proattitudinal and the arguments are weak (because in this case majority endorsement reduces processing of the weak arguments over minority endorsement). However, at the conceptual level the findings can be understood quite readily. For example, both the research on majority–minority endorsement and the research on positive–negative framing can be understood by the simple principle that "surprise leads to more message processing" (e.g., it is surprising for people to find that a majority disagrees with them or a minority agrees). Similarly, the mood results can be understood through application of mood management motives (i.e., people in a positive mood process the pleasant message more because they are more sensitive to the hedonic consequences of their actions; Wegener & Petty, 1994). We suspect that a relatively small number of processing principles will ultimately integrate these third-generation studies.

POSTULATE 5: THE BIASED-PROCESSING POSTULATE

Variables affecting message processing in a relatively biased manner can produce either a positive (favorable) or negative (unfavorable) motivational and/or ability bias to the issue-relevant thoughts attempted.

Whereas Postulate 4 notes that some variables have an impact on thinking (elaboration) by influencing thinking in a relatively objective manner, Postulate 5 recognizes that thinking can also be biased. The variables just discussed, such as distraction or need for cognition, tend to influence information-processing activity in a relatively objective manner. That is, all else being equal, distraction tends to disrupt whatever thoughts a person is thinking (Petty et al., 1976). The distraction per se does not specifically target one type of thought (e.g., favorable or unfavorable) to impede. Similarly, individuals with high need for cognition are more motivated to think in general than are people low in need for cognition (Cacioppo et al., 1983). They are not more motivated to think certain kinds of thoughts over others. Some variables, however, are selective in their effects on thinking.

Motivational and Ability Factors in Bias

Just as motivational and ability factors contribute to relatively objective information processing, Postulate 5 notes that both motivational and ability factors contribute to biased processing. Regarding motivation, the ELM holds that motivation is relatively objective when no *a priori* judgment is preferred and a person's implicit or explicit goal is to "seek the truth wherever it might lead" (Petty & Cacioppo, 1986b, p. 19). In contrast, a motivated bias can occur whenever people implicitly or explicitly prefer one judgment or conclusion over another. Petty and Cacioppo (1986b) noted that the distinction between objective and biased processing has much in common with an earlier cognitive distinction between "bottom-up" and "top-down" processing (cf. Bobrow & Norman, 1975). Whereas objective processing tends to be data-driven (i.e., drawing whatever conclusions the data imply), biased processing is directed in such a way as to favor an existing attitude schema or current goal. Biased processing also has much in common with a subsequent distinction made by Kruglanski (1990) between the need for "specific closure" and the need for "nonspecific closure." When a person is seeking nonspecific closure, *any* answer will do, and thus processing can be relatively objective; however, when a person is seeking specific closure, some answers are preferred over others, and thus processing is more likely to be biased.

In the ELM, a wide variety of motivations can determine which particular judgment is preferred in any given situation. For example, if the reactance motive (Brehm, 1966) is aroused, people will prefer to hold whatever judgment is forbidden or restricted and to resist whatever opinion is pressured. If balance motives (Heider, 1958) are operating, people will prefer to adopt the position of a liked source but to distance themselves from a disliked source. If impression management motives (Tedeschi, Schlenker, & Bonoma, 1971) are in ascendance, people will prefer to hold whatever position they think will be ingratiating and to avoid those that will make them look bad. If self-affirmation motives (Steele, 1988) are high, people will prefer the position that will make them feel best about themselves, and so forth. Importantly, many of these biasing motives can influence judgments by either the central or the peripheral route. That is, biasing motives can have their impact on judgments by effortful or noneffortful means. For example, invocation of reactance can lead to simple rejection of the forbidden position without much thought (i.e., based on the reactance motive alone), or the reactance motive can lead to a more effortful rejection by motivating intense counterarguing of the position. Whether the motive produces a biased outcome by relatively effortful or noneffortful means will depend on other variables such as whether the person is motivated (e.g., high vs. low personal relevance) or able (e.g., high vs. low distraction) to think carefully about object-relevant information (Petty & Cacioppo, 1979, 1990). Finally, it is worth noting that if the overall elaboration likelihood is high, motivated biases will presumably lead to a biased assessment of *all* information in the persuasion environment. In such circumstances, people might "allow" certain peripheral cues consistent with their motivational goals to influence their judgments, whereas in the absence of these motives they will discount or correct for these cues (see "Bias Correction," below). If the overall elaboration likelihood is low, however, then motivated biases will either have a direct impact on judgment, or lead to a biased assessment of a more limited set of information (e.g., only the most salient peripheral cues).

The ELM holds that biased processing can occur even if no specific judgment is preferred (i.e., if motivational factors alone will promote relatively objective processing). This is because ability factors can also introduce a bias in the information-processing activity. For example, in some circumstances, knowledge stored in memory is simply imbalanced (and thus favors some conclusions over others). In other circumstances, variables in the persuasion setting can bias retrieval of information even if what is stored in memory is completely balanced and no motivational biases are operating (see Petty, Priester, & Wegener, 1994, for additional discussion). For example, a positive mood might increase access to positive material in memory (e.g., Bower, 1981; see Bless & Schwarz, Chapter 21, this volume). The result could be that favorable heuristics are more likely to be retrieved and used than unfavorable ones when the elaboration likelihood is low, and that favorable interpretations of arguments are generated and applied when the elaboration likelihood is high (Petty, Schumann, Richman, &

Strathman, 1993). In general, biases in processing a persuasive message are fostered when the message contains information that is ambiguous or mixed rather than clearly strong or weak (Chaiken & Maheswaran, 1994).

Bias can occur because of what people choose to process, how they choose to process it, and/or how they integrate the results of their information-processing efforts. Furthermore, these processes can be driven by motivational factors, by ability factors, or by both. Consider the well-known study by Lord, Ross, and Lepper (1979) in which people received information both favoring and opposing capital punishment information. Following the message, people reported their own side to be more compelling than the other side. This could have occurred for a number of reasons. Assume for the moment that in some objective sense, the arguments presented on both sides were equally compelling. Why would people have found their own side to be more persuasive? According to the ELM, there are a number of possibilities. First, people might have engaged in relatively little processing of either side, but simply demonstrated an "ownness bias" (Perloff & Brock, 1980) and reasoned that "my side is better" (i.e., using their initial attitude as a peripheral cue to validity; Petty, Cacioppo, & Haugtvedt, 1992). Second, the biased outcome could have come about as a result of various more effortful message-processing biases. For example, people could have engaged in greater thinking about their own side of the issue over the other side. Even if this processing was objective, this difference in amount of thought could have led them to find their own side to be more compelling. Alternatively, people could have engaged in biased processing of one or the other side—selectively arguing in favor of their own side and/or counterarguing the other side. Finally, even if people processed both sides objectively and to an equal extent, generating a balanced set of thoughts, the thoughts favoring their own side (and/or opposing the other side) might have been given greater weight in forming a final judgment than the thoughts favoring the other side (and/or opposing their own side; Anderson, 1981). It is important to note that these processes could have been mostly attributable either to ability or to motivational factors. For example, people might have selectively processed their own side mostly because it would be uncomfortable if their side did not "come out on top" (motivational factor), or mostly because they were more capable of thinking about the side that fit with their existing attitude schema (ability factor).

Consideration of both motivational and ability variables in bias can lead to some rather complex outcomes (see Biek, Wood, & Chaiken, 1996). For example, consider how a person's knowledge about an attitude issue can influence persuasion. Knowledge (i.e., information about the attitude object) can vary in both its nature and its amount, and can have an impact by both motivational and ability means. In most prior studies on knowledge, the amount of knowledge is measured (see Wood et al., 1995, for a review) rather than manipulated. Because people are likely to have knowledge that is consistent with or supportive of their attitudes, people who are categorized as especially high in knowledge are likely to be those who are also especially high in *attitude-congruent* knowledge. In general, the greater one's attitude-congruent knowledge, the more able one will be to defend one's position from attack. Thus, it might not be surprising that the typical effect reported in the literature between amount of knowledge and persuasion is that increased knowledge increases resistance to persuasion (e.g., Wood, Kallgren, & Priesler, 1985).

If a person has relatively objective or balanced knowledge about an issue, however, there is unlikely to be a bias due to ability factors (unless, of course, one type of knowledge is more easily activated than the other). Rather, as the extent of a person's balanced knowledge about the issue increases, the individual might be more able to see the merits (or faults) of either side of the issue to an equal degree, compared to a person with little knowledge about the issue. This might especially be the case if the message is rather complex and requires some prior knowledge to understand. If the message is relatively simple and does not require much in the way of background to understand, increasing one's balanced knowledge might not confer much ability benefit on processing (but might still affect motivation). Thus, in terms of ability factors, a biased knowledge base enables a person to see the merits of his or her own side

and to counterargue opposing sides, but relatively balanced knowledge is less likely to confer this ability bias. The nature of one's knowledge is considered an ability bias, because even if people are trying as hard as possible to be objective, it will be more difficult for them to do so the more they have a biased store of previous knowledge on the topic.

However, it is also important to recognize that increasing knowledge about a topic, whether that knowledge is balanced or not, can have various motivational consequences as well. For example, if the message topic is a relatively unimportant one, a person might use the perceived amount of knowledge on a topic as a cue to reject the message. That is, the person might reason that he or she is likely to have more expertise than the message source, and thus that there is no need to change. In addition, however, a person's knowledge can be used as an indication of whether or not to process the message. For example, the person might reason, "I'm uninformed, so I need to learn more," or "I know enough, so I don't need to process," or maybe even "I have some knowledge, so this must be worth thinking about." These postulated motivational effects are really effects of *perceived* knowledge rather than actual knowledge, since, for example, a person with objectively little knowledge might still perceive himself or herself as an expert! Of course, when the message topic is also important, thinking oneself to be more expert than the source can also lead to extensive counterarguing of what the source has to say on the topic.

Bias Correction

The mere fact that some motivational or ability factor encourages biased processing does not mean that a biased outcome will inevitably result. One reason for this is that people sometimes attempt to correct for factors they believe might unduly influence (or might have unduly influenced) their evaluations (e.g., Strack, 1992; Petty & Wegener, 1993; Wilson & Brekke, 1994). According to the flexible-correction model (FCM; Wegener & Petty, 1995, 1997), corrections for bias can proceed in different directions, depending on recipients' theories of how the biasing event or stimulus (e.g., an attractive source) is likely to influence their views. The FCM posits that in order for corrections to occur, people should (1) be motivated and able to identify potentially biasing factors, (2) possess or generate a naive theory about the magnitude and direction of the bias, and (3) be motivated and able to make the theory-based correction. In some cases, integrative processing of the information (e.g., Schul & Burnstein, 1985) can make it difficult for people to correct for the biasing effect of an individual piece of information that contributes to an overall evaluation. That is, even if motivated to correct, people might not have the ability to do so, or to do so accurately.

When people are motivated and able to correct, theory-based corrections can actually result in reversals of typical persuasion effects (e.g., if people believe that the persuasion factor has had a greater impact than it actually has). For example, in one study, when people were made aware of possible biases due to source likability, an overcorrection led a disliked source to be more persuasive than a liked source (Petty et al., 1998).

POSTULATE 6: THE TRADEOFF POSTULATE

As motivation and/or ability to process arguments is decreased, peripheral cues become relatively more important determinants of persuasion. Conversely, as argument scrutiny is increased, peripheral cues become relatively less important determinants of persuasion.

Postulate 6 says that as one moves along the elaboration continuum, the impact of peripheral-cue processes on attitudes varies. That is, at low levels of information scrutiny, relatively low-elaboration judgment strategies (such as going with the early information or relying on heuristics) and low-elaboration judgment mechanisms and processes (such as identification with the source or classical conditioning) have a greater impact on attitudes than they do at high levels of scrutiny. In essence, Postulate 6 articulates a tradeoff between the impact of central and peripheral mechanisms on judgments along the elaboration likelihood continuum. That is, as the impact of central-route processes on judgments increases, the impact of peripheral-route

mechanisms on judgments decreases. One aspect of this postulate that has been misunderstood is that the postulated tradeoff is not in the *occurrence* of central and peripheral processes, but in the impact of these processes on attitudes and judgments. For example, the presence of one's friend might invoke the heuristic "I agree with people I like" (Chaiken, 1980) under both high- and low-elaboration conditions, because the heuristic is so well practiced that it is automatically accessed. Under high-elaboration conditions, however, when this heuristic enters consciousness it will be subjected to careful scrutiny, just as the other information in the persuasion context is subjected to scrutiny (Petty & Cacioppo, 1986a; Petty, 1994). That is, the retrieved heuristic, like all other available information in one's consciousness, will be evaluated as an argument. If the heuristic is found to lack merit as an argument for supporting the advocated view, then it will have little impact on one's overall judgment. On the other hand, if the heuristic is deemed cogent, then it will have an impact. This scrutiny of the heuristic for merit is less likely under low-elaboration conditions, where the mere invocation of the heuristic could be sufficient for persuasion.[9]

It is important to note that the ELM tradeoff hypothesis implies a number of things. First, at most points along the continuum, central and peripheral processes will co-occur and jointly influence judgments (Petty, Kasmer, Haugtvedt, & Cacioppo, 1987). Second, however, movement in either direction along the continuum will tend to enhance the *relative* impact of one or the other *process* (e.g., effortful scrutiny for merit vs. reliance on a heuristic) on judgments. It is important to note that changing the relative impact of one *process* over another on attitudes does not imply that the impact of any given *variable* (e.g., source expertise, mood) on judgments must increase or decrease as one moves along the continuum. This is because of the multiple-roles postulate discussed previously. Recall that the multiple-roles notion is that any given variable can influence attitudes by different processes at different points along the elaboration continuum (Petty & Cacioppo, 1986a). In fact, as noted previously, the ELM holds that the impact of variables serving as cues under low-elaboration conditions can be reduced, unchanged, enhanced, or even reversed as the elaboration likelihood is increased! In sum, the tradeoff hypothesis basically means that a variable is less likely to have its impact on attitudes via a peripheral process as the elaboration likelihood is increased.[10]

Reduced-Impact Effects

The earliest research on the ELM (and HSM) focused on the reduced impact of variables serving as cues as the elaboration likelihood was increased. For example, Petty, Cacioppo, and Goldman (1981) found that a manipulation of source expertise (i.e., whether the message on an educational issue came from a Princeton University professor or a local high school student) had a smaller impact on attitudes when the personal relevance of the communication was increased (and that a manipulation of argument quality had an increased impact). Similarly, as noted previously, Petty and Cacioppo (1984a) found that the mere number of arguments in a message had a smaller impact on attitudes as the personal relevance of the message was increased (but that argument quality had a larger effect).

Petty (1994) outlined a number of possible explanations for these reduced-impact effects. For example, features of a message that serve as peripheral cues when the elaboration likelihood is low (e.g., source attractiveness, message length) might initially be effective under high-elaboration conditions as well (leading to a tentatively favorable attitude), but might subsequently be drowned out or undermined by the more substantive arguments (see also Chaiken et al., 1989). Or these features might simply be less salient than other substantive features of the message when elaboration is high, and thus might be viewed as less extreme, weighted less, or ignored. Or people might process the feature intently (i.e., as an argument), but might find that it is not useful or relevant to evaluating the central merits of the issue. People might even explicitly attempt to discount or correct for the impact of these features if they are seen as biasing.

Unchanged-, Enhanced-, and Reversed-Impact Effects

As just noted, according to the ELM, variables such as source attractiveness can have a favorable impact on attitudes for different reasons along the elaboration continuum. For example, attractiveness can influence attitudes by some peripheral mechanism under low-elaboration conditions (e.g., if people are distracted), but can serve to influence the amount of thinking if the elaboration likelihood is a bit higher (e.g., if people are unsure whether or not cognitive effort is merited). Under even higher-elaboration conditions, attractiveness can serve as an argument if it provides information central to the merits of the attitude object, can bias the processing of whatever issue-relevant information is presented, or both. Furthermore, as noted previously, the biased processing can result from either motivational or ability factors. For example, an attractive source, like a positive mood, might make it more likely that positive associations and ideas will come to mind. Or, to the extent that self-affirmation motives or impression management motives are present in the situation, people might wish to agree with an attractive source for purposes of enhancing esteem in their own eyes or the eyes of others. The key point here is that depending on the *outcome* of these different processes, a variable that serves as a peripheral cue under low-elaboration conditions can lose the impact it had under low-elaboration conditions, can have an unchanged impact, can have an enhanced impact, or can even have a reversed impact on attitudes as the elaboration likelihood is increased.

For example, consider a study by Petty, Wegener, and White (1997, raw data; cited in Petty et al., 1998) in which a manipulation of liking for a source had an increased impact as the elaboration likelihood increased. In this study, students at Ohio State University were given a message from a person who either praised them in comparison to the students at the University of Michigan or derogated them. Part of the study was conducted prior to and part was conducted shortly after the University of Michigan football team defeated Ohio State for the second year in a row—once again ruining what would have been a perfect season and a chance at a national championship. For data collected prior to the game, the typical source effect emerged (with the likable source being more persuasive than the dislikable source to a greater extent under low- than under high-processing conditions; Chaiken, 1980; Petty,

Cacioppo, & Schumann, 1983). Shortly after the second-season ending loss to Michigan, however, the reverse was obtained. Following the loss, students reported that they didn't care about being highly biased against Michigan supporters. Thus, one would expect that the disliked source would lead to counterarguing when the topic was important. If the counterarguing of the disliked source was especially intense, it could lead to the observed result that the source manipulation had a greater impact in the high- than in the low-elaboration conditions. That is, the negative impact of counterarguing of the disliked source on attitudes could be greater than the negative impact of the disliked source's serving as a cue.

POSTULATE 7: THE ATTITUDE STRENGTH POSTULATE

Attitude changes that result mostly from processing issue-relevant arguments (central route) will show greater temporal persistence, greater prediction of behavior, and greater resistance to counterpersuasion than attitude changes that result mostly from peripheral cues.

Postulate 7 suggests that basing one's attitude on considerable issue-relevant thinking (high elaboration) leads to stronger attitudes than basing one's attitude on little issue- relevant thinking (low elaboration), such as occurs when attitudes change by the peripheral route. As Petty and Cacioppo (1986b) explained, this postulate is based on the notion that high-effort, central-route processes generally require greater cognitive effort than peripheral-route processes, and that issue-relevant cognitive effort is related to the various indicators of attitude strength (e.g., resistance to counterpersuasion). Thus, carefully processing three message arguments will lead to stronger attitudes than carefully processing just one argument (quantitative effect), and carefully processing just one argument will lead to stronger attitudes than less effortfully basing one's attitude on one salient heuristic retrieved from memory, or on one inference (e.g., self-perception) generated on-line (qualitative effect). Because the latter prediction assumes that processing one argument requires greater object-relevant cognitive effort than

using one heuristic or inference, this comparison involves both a qualitative and a quantitative difference.

Several features of Postulate 7 have been misunderstood. First, it is important to consider that the postulate applies to a comparison between attitudes changed to the same degree by high and low amounts of elaboration. Thus, it would not be appropriate to compare, for example, the persistence of a very small change produced by high elaboration with a very large change produced by low elaboration. At a subsequent point in time, the absolute amount of change could well be larger for the low-elaboration change than for the high-elaboration change, given the very different starting points.

Second, in generating predictions from the postulate, it is important to understand why high amounts of elaboration are thought to produce the postulated strength consequences. That is, Petty and Cacioppo (1986b) noted that several mediating mechanisms are likely to be responsible for the effects of elaboration on attitude strength. They noted, for example, that high amounts of thinking about an object can render the attitude more accessible than low amounts of thinking, and that increased accessibility will make it more likely that the same attitude will be reported at two points in time and be available to guide behavior. Also, increased object-relevant thinking will make it more likely that the object-relevant information linked to the attitude will be more salient and thus can be used to defend one's attitude at a later point in time. Similarly, thinking might enhance confidence in one's attitude, making it more likely that one will be willing to act on the attitude (see also Petty, Haugtvedt, & Smith, 1995). It is also possible that elaboration will enhance the consistency of the attitude with one's underlying beliefs, making it easier to resist counter-communications (see Chaiken, Pomerantz, & Giner-Sorolla, 1995). In any case, it is important to consider that object-relevant elaboration should produce strength consequences only to the extent that it is associated with the postulated mediating mechanisms. To the extent that elaboration does not result in the presumed mediating processes, it should not be associated with the strength consequences. Thus, for example, if increased thinking results in greater uncertainty about one's attitude rather than in greater confidence, thinking should not necessarily result in greater strength than not thinking.

Furthermore, consideration of the presumed mediating mechanisms suggests that low-effort processes can also produce one or more of the strength consequences. Petty and Cacioppo (1986a) noted, for example, that increased repetition of one or more peripheral cues (e.g., Johnson & Watkins, 1971; Weber, 1972) can enhance the accessibility of the attitude and the memorability of the cue(s), resulting in relatively persistent attitudes. In fact, Zanna, Fazio, and Ross (1994) reported that merely having people rehearse their attitudes (presumably enhancing accessibility without encouraging any additional thinking) was sufficient to increase attitude persistence. Similarly, increasing the memorability or accessibility of a cue, by increasing its relevance to the attitude object, can also enhance persistence (Sengupta, Goodstein, & Boninger, 1997).

Another area of confusion is whether the various postulated strength consequences invariably co-occur, given that each results from elaboration. The ELM holds that the strength consequences can be independent. For example, Petty and Cacioppo (1986a) noted that "the resistance of an attitude to attack is conceptually distinct from the temporal persistence of the attitudes. Thus, some attitudes may be highly persistent, but only if they are not challenged. Likewise, it is possible for some attitudes to be very resistant to change, but only in the short term" (p. 190; see also McGuire, 1964). As one instance of independence, Petty and Cacioppo noted that repeatedly pairing peripheral cues with an attitude object can produce an accessible attitude that is relatively persistent. However, individuals with these peripherally based persistent attitudes are still likely to be susceptible to counterpersuasion, because they will presumably have difficulty mounting a defense of their attitudes if they are attacked with strong arguments.

In an empirical demonstration of the independence of attitude persistence and resistance, Haugtvedt, Schumann, Schneier, and Warren (1994) presented one group of participants with an advertising campaign for a consumer product in which the substantive arguments for the campaign were varied across multiple exposures of the ads. Another group of participants was presented with a campaign in which the ads were varied cosmetically (e.g., different endorser cues in each ad), but the ads did not vary in the substantive arguments they presented. That is, the substantive variation strategy involved keeping the peripheral cues constant across exposures, but presenting different substantive information in each ad. The cosmetic-variation strategy involved keeping the substantive information the same across ad exposures, but varying the positive cues contained in the advertisements. Substantive variation strategies would be expected to encourage attitude formation by high-effort evaluation of the substantive arguments, but cosmetic variations would encourage attitude formation by low-effort processes, such as reliance on source heuristics (see Schumann, Petty, & Clemons, 1990).

Previous research comparing high- and low-effort attitude changes has typically involved a single exposure to a message containing multiple pieces of substantive information (arguments) but just one salient cue. Haugtvedt et al. (1994) noted that such research might have provided central-route participants with mnemonic advantages (e.g., multiple retrieval cues) over peripheral-route participants. However, if recipients were presented with multiple peripheral cues (cosmetic-variation strategy), or if a single cue was repeated multiple times, attitude persistence might be greater than that obtained in the typical low-effort condition, in which there was just one exposure to an ad containing a peripheral cue. Consistent with this hypothesis, Haugtvedt et al. (1994) found that people receiving three exposures to the substantively varied ads, to the cosmetically varied ads, or to a single ad showed greater (and equivalent) persistence in attitude change over a 1-week period, compared to people who received just one exposure. That is, by the persistence criterion, each of the repetition conditions produced equivalently more favorable attitudes than the single-exposure control 1 week after message presentation.

What about resistance? To assess this, after completing the delayed attitude measure, recipients were presented with a message that weakly attacked the product presented in the critical advertisements. On the attitude measure taken after the attacking message, people who had received the substantively varied ads showed greater resistance than people in any of the other groups. Thus, even though the repetition strategies were all more effective in enhancing persistence over 1 week than the single-exposure control condition was, the different repetition strategies were not all more effective in inducing resistance. Specifically, the attitudes based on exposure to substantively varied ads were more resistant in the face of attack than were the attitudes resulting from the other repetition strategy. That is, repetition and variation of peripheral cues were useful for increasing persistence, but were ineffective in increasing resistance. This can be understood by consideration of the presumed mediating mechanisms outlined above. That is, for example, both substantively and cosmetically varied ads could have increased the accessibility or memorability of the attitude to an equivalent extent, but only effortful processing of the substantive ads led people to have sufficient information to be able to defend their attitudes when attacked.

In sum, the key to Postulate 7 is understanding the impact of elaboration on the mechanisms mediating the strength consequences. Thus, if a message recipient elaborates a source factor and thinks about its relevance to validity, this should enhance strength over use of the same source factor as a cue (e.g., acceptance as a result of a heuristic) if the former process results in an attitude that is more accessible, associated with greater confidence, and so forth.

What happens when a strong (e.g., relatively persistent and accessible) attitude is changed as a result of the provision of new information? Is the old attitude simply replaced with the new one? This is a question with numerous conceptual and practical implications. For example, in the field of health education, people's initially strong attitudes in favor of smoking or high-fat foods can be changed by new information to be less favorable toward these objects. Yet, a common anecdotal occurrence is that when confronted with the attitude object (cigarettes, ice cream), the "old," highly favorable attitude can come to mind prior to the "new," less favorable one and guide behavior. Petty, Baker, and Gleicher (1991) suggested that this phenomenon should be especially likely when people are

under some cognitive load and are therefore unable to reflect upon their new attitude and/ or to discount their old one (see also Petty, Gleicher, & Jarvis, 1993). Importantly, our discussion of Postulate 7 above implies that it isn't only old attitudes based on the central route that might continue to have some influence even after they are ostensibly changed. Consider an initial attitude based on classical conditioning—a peripheral attitude change mechanism that doesn't rely on effortful, issue-relevant thinking. However, this procedure pairs the attitude object with positive (or negative) affective cues over many trials. Because of this, an "old" conditioned attitude is likely to remain highly accessible and might continue to influence behavior even if the person supposedly adopts a "new" attitude—especially if the newly changed attitude is not as accessible as the old one, and the behavioral opportunity is one that does not allow time for contemplation (see Jarvis, Tormala, & Petty, 1998; Petty & Jarvis, 1998). This phenomenon suggests the possibility that people can simultaneously possess two (or more) evaluative predispositions (attitudes) toward a given attitude object (perhaps residing in separate memory systems; e.g., McClelland, McNaughton, & O'Reilly, 1995; see Smith & DeCoster, Chapter 16, this volume). Which attitude is activated and guiding can depend on the contextual conditions, such as whether some minimal time for reflection and discounting of the prior opinion is provided or not (see also Dovidio, Kawakami, Johnson, Johnson, & Howard, 1997; Gilbert, 1991; Wilson & Schooler, 1998). The ELM strength postulate has been examined largely under conditions that allow at least some minimal time for deliberation. As just suggested, the consequences of attitudes examined under cognitive load or time pressure (or on implicit measures) might vary markedly from those observed when some reflection is permitted.

THE ELM AND SOCIAL JUDGMENT

Thus far in this chapter, we have reviewed the formal postulates of the ELM, and addressed some areas of confusion that have appeared in the literature. Because most of the work on the ELM has been conducted in a persuasion context, our review and examples have focused on this context as well. In this section of the chapter, we briefly compare the ELM to other multiprocess models that have been developed outside of the persuasion context (for comparisons of the ELM with the HSM, see Chaiken, Wood, & Eagly, 1996; Eagly & Chaiken, 1993; Petty, 1994; Petty & Wegener, 1998). As noted in introducing the ELM, the basic tenets of the model can be used to understand both evaluative and nonevaluative judgments in a variety of domains (see also Petty et al., 1994), and in some cases basic elements of the ELM approach have been incorporated into these nonpersuasion models. In some cases, we believe that a more direct application of the ELM principles might provide a more complete framework for understanding the phenomena of interest.

Person Perception

One of the most influential models of person perception is Fiske's (Fiske & Neuberg, 1990; Fiske & Pavelchak, 1986; see Fiske, Lin, & Neuberg, Chapter 11, this volume) continuum model of impression formation (for another prominent model in this area that shares some features with the continuum model, see Brewer, 1988, and Brewer & Harasty, Chapter 12, this volume). The continuum model distinguishes between category-based impressions and impressions based on individuating information. In brief, this model holds that when one encounters a new person, an attempt is made to fit the person into some preexisting category for which one already possesses an evaluation (e.g., the person is a "schizophrenic" or an "athlete"). Category-based evaluation is assumed to be a relatively efficient and effortless way to engage in evaluation. On the other hand, if categorization fails, one is "forced" to engage in an attribute-by-attribute assessment of the new person in order to form an evaluation. This "piecemeal" processing is less efficient and requires greater cognitive effort. Thus, this models shares with the ELM the basic assumption that sometimes evaluation is relatively thoughtful and effortful, but sometimes it is not. Fiske's model also highlights a particular low-effort evaluation process—reliance on a preexisting category. This mechanism seems most similar to Chaiken's (1980) em-

phasis on preexisting evaluative heuristics that are retrieved from memory. In any case, the ELM therefore predicts that impressions formed of new individuals on the basis of previously stored categories will be less strong (on some dimensions at least) than impressions formed by an effortful analysis of the traits and behaviors that the new person displays.

One potentially important difference between the Fiske model and the ELM is that the Fiske model implies a two-step process. That is, the high-effort evaluation is only postulated to occur to the extent that category processing fails. In the ELM, this two-step process provides a reasonable account of what happens in some circumstances (e.g., individuals low in need for cognition might rely on source trustworthiness cues if these are present, but if not, they might be "forced" to process the message; Priester & Petty, 1995). On the other hand, the ELM holds that there are a variety of situations in which people are highly motivated to think, and thus are not "forced" to think by a failure of peripheral cues to fit the target. In such situations, the ELM holds that people will engage in what Fiske has called "piecemeal" processing, and any category accessed will be evaluated along with all of the other person-relevant information, or the category might bias processing of the other information. Of course, the ELM also incorporates a variety of additional low-effort means of evaluating a person (beyond a stored assessment of the person's "category").

Attitude–Behavior Consistency

Fazio (1990) has proposed a two-route model of behavioral choice (the "motivation and opportunity as determinants" [MODE] model; see Fazio & Towles-Schwen, Chapter 5, this volume). That is, sometimes people's behavior is thought to be determined largely by the accessibility of their existing attitudes, but at other times behavior is thought to be determined largely by people's effortful scrutiny of all of the available information in the behavioral context. Although the latter, more reasoned process has much in common with the high-effort, central-route process of attitude formation, the accessibility process does not necessarily map well onto the peripheral route. This is because the ELM holds that an accessible attitude (like other variables) can influence behavioral judgments (like other judgments) in both effortful and noneffortful ways. Thus, a person's highly accessible attitude might come to mind and guide behavior rather automatically without much thought (e.g., "I like you, so I'll give you money"); or an accessible attitude might increase scrutiny of the information available in the behavioral situation in a rather objective way (see Fabrigar, Priester, Petty, & Wegener, 1998); or the attitude might bias processing of the information available (as emphasized by Fazio, 1995; e.g., liking the person makes the cause seem more worthy, leading to a greater monetary donation).

Affect and Judgment

Forgas (1992, 1995) has recently proposed a multiroute model of the impact of affect on judgment (the affect infusion model, or AIM). In the AIM, several information-processing modes are described. Two of the modes address when affect has an impact on judgment, and two address when affect does not have an impact. Specifically, Forgas notes that affect can have an impact on judgment in two ways. In what Forgas calls "heuristic processing," affect influences judgment because people "use their affect as a short cut to infer their evaluative reactions to the target." In what he calls "substantive processing," affect influences judgment "through its selective influence on attention, encoding, retrieval, and associative processes" (Forgas, 1995, p. 40). In essence, these two processing modes map nicely onto the ELM notion that affect can influence judgment under low-elaboration conditions by serving as a peripheral cue, and under high-elaboration conditions by biasing thinking (see Petty, Schumann, et al., 1993, for evidence). Forgas further notes that affect will not have an impact on judgment if a person has a strong prior attitude that is retrieved directly "direct access"). This mode points to one prior cue (i.e., a person's own attitude) that can be more salient than the cue effect produced by mood. The ELM argues that under low-elaboration conditions, a variety of cues might compete with mood—not just one's prior attitude. Thus, a salient dislikable message source might be used as a cue under low-elaboration conditions, rather

than one's mood. That is, in the ELM, one's prior attitude is not be the only cue that can override the impact of mood as a cue or can be used instead of mood. Finally, Forgas notes that affect will not have an impact on judgment under high-elaboration conditions if some strong motivational bias is at work ("motivated processing"). Stated in ELM terms, processing can be biased by a number of motivational factors when the elaboration likelihood is high, and some of these can undermine the impact of mood. For example, if a person is placed in a positive mood, but reactance is induced by the speaker, the desire to reject the message might overwhelm any favorable impact that normally would be produced by the positive mood. In sum, Forgas's four strategies map well onto a 2 (high elaboration, low elaboration) × 2 (no other bias present, other bias present) matrix, where under low elaboration the other bias is supplied by nonmood variables that can serve as cues (e.g., source likability), and under high elaboration the other bias is supplied by other motivational (e.g., reactance) or ability (e.g., prior knowledge) variables that compete with the mood bias.

There are also a number of crucial differences between the ELM and the AIM. For example, Forgas (1992, 1995) posits that stored judgments of the target are only used when the target (or judgment) is unimportant to the judge, whereas a person's stored attitude or judgment can serve in multiple roles within the ELM (see discussion of the MODE model, above). The models also diverge in their treatment of effects of mood. For example, in the AIM, both heuristic use of mood and effects of mood on information scrutiny occur only if the judgment is important (if the judgment is unimportant, direct access of a prior judgment is used). Within the ELM, heuristic and other "direct" influences of mood (e.g., classical conditioning) are more likely under low- rather than high-elaboration conditions (i.e., low rather than high importance of the attitude object or judgment), and effects of mood on amount of information scrutiny are most likely when elaboration likelihood is not constrained to be either high or low. Whereas the AIM (Forgas, 1992, 1995) hypothesizes decreased processing in happy moods, research guided by the ELM has shown that happy moods can either increase or decrease processing of judgment-relevant information (see Wegener, Petty, & Smith, 1995). Finally, in addition to Forgas's heuristic-processing mode (based on a "How do I feel about it?" heuristic; Schwarz, 1990) and substantive-processing mode, the ELM postulates that affect can serve as an argument relevant to the central merits of a judgment target. Although the AIM might lump such an effect under the heuristic mode, we believe that there would be different consequences of using affect in these different ways.

Survey Responding

Krosnick (1991) has presented a conceptual analysis of people's responses to survey questions. Two strategies are distinguished: "satisficing" and "optimizing." When satisficing, people do not engage in effortful thought about the survey question, and thus give answers that are based on salient cues in the environment or on more simplistic strategies (e.g., selecting the first plausible answer, or always saying "yes"). When optimizing, people engage in the effortful scrutiny of the questions and think carefully before answering. Thus, Krosnick notes that optimizing is more likely when people are both motivated and able to think about the survey questions, but that satisficing is more likely when either motivation or ability are low. Thus, consistent with the ELM, Krosnick postulates thoughtful and nonthoughtful routes to survey responding, which are moderated by motivational and ability factors. One important difference between the ELM analysis of survey responding and Krosnick's satisficing–optimizing analysis, however, is that Krosnick assumes that optimizing (i.e., high-effort processes) results in less biased judgments than satisficing (low-effort processes). In contrast, according to the ELM, bias can result from either low- or high-effort processes. For example, recall how mood can bias judgment by high-effort and low-effort processes (Petty, Schumann, et al., 1993). Thus, in the ELM, high effort is no guarantee that survey responses will be any more accurate than low-effort responses. In fact, in some cases, giving quick, highly accessible responses can result in greater accuracy than highly thoughtful but biased responses (cf. Wilson, Kraft, & Dunn, 1989; see Petty & Jarvis, 1996, for more on high- and low-effort processes in survey responding).

CONCLUSIONS

Although it is sometimes misunderstood, the ELM has proven to be a useful framework for studying attitude change and persuasion. Incorporation of many ELM principles in models outside the persuasion domain suggests that the ELM might prove equally beneficial in a variety of related areas. Although existing non-persuasion-related models have incorporated some aspects of the ELM, we believe that many of these models have lost some of the complexities and flexibilities (e.g., the notion of multiple roles) that might make the ELM especially useful in those domains. It is our hope that the present discussion of some misunderstood aspects of the ELM will clarify aspects of the model and encourage interpretations true to the conceptualization intended.

NOTES

1. That is, as articulated shortly, the peripheral route to persuasion refers to attitude changes that result from low-effort central route processes (i.e., putting minimal effort into elaborating issue-relevant information) as well as peripheral processes (e.g., use of heuristics, identification with the source) since these mechanisms tend to produce similarly weak attitudes.

2. We refer to the elaboration *likelihood* continuum when assessing in advance of a message or judgment how *likely* it is that a person will think about it. For example, if there are many distractions in the situation, the likelihood of elaboration is low. The actual placement of an individual along the continuum, of course, cannot be known until after the message or attitude object has been processed.

3. Following Festinger (1954), the ELM talks about achieving subjective correctness; however, similar points can be made about achieving *confidence* in one's opinion (see Chaiken, Liberman, & Eagly, 1989), since confidence is presumably based mostly on a feeling that one's opinion is correct.

4. This effect is expected whether the cognitive responses to the arguments are added or averaged, as long as the person's initial opinion (either toward the particular object or the class of objects to which this object belongs) is added/averaged along with the new cognitive responses (see Anderson, 1981).

5. If the high-elaboration processor does not consider all of the information objectively, then the attitudinal outcomes might be the same as for the low-elaboration processor, but for different reasons. For example, if a high-elaboration processor encounters strong arguments first and becomes convinced of the merit of the position, the subsequent weak arguments might be actively reconceptualized so as to appear strong (i.e., belief in the position can lead to biased processing of the weak arguments). That is, primacy effects can occur for both effortful and noneffortful reasons (Haugtvedt & Wegener, 1994; Hawkins, Petty, & Wegener, 1996).

6. Of course, on some level, the issue of whether to lump all processes of persuasion together or to split them into two or more categories depends on the utility of the distinctions involved, as well as on how one defines what is qualitatively different from something else (Petty et al., in press). At the most general level, truly uniprocess models postulate something akin to "People think." Although true enough, such a view is relatively incapable of predicting when a given variable is likely to influence persuasion in a simple way (e.g., when mood is used as a heuristic; Petty & Cacioppo, 1983; Schwarz, 1990) as opposed to a more complex way (e.g., when mood influences interpretations of object-relevant information; Petty, Schumann, Richman, & Strathman, 1993; Wegener, Petty, & Klein, 1994).

7. Interestingly, what variables have the potential to serve as cues versus arguments can vary with situational and individual factors. For example, in a study conducted with Chinese students in Hong Kong (Aaker & Maheswaran, 1997), the mere number of arguments in a message became a less influential determinant of attitudes as task importance (i.e., elaboration likelihood) increased, whereas argument quality became more important, duplicating the data just described for U.S. college students (Petty & Cacioppo, 1984b). This cross-cultural replication suggest that Chinese students treat the mere number of arguments as a peripheral cue that is unrelated to the true merit of the advocacy when they are carefully processing a message, just as U.S. college students do. In another study, however, Chinese students were still influenced by a manipulation of the number of people who favored a product under high-elaboration conditions, whereas U.S. students were not (Maheswaran & Chaiken, 1991). The latter finding is consistent with the idea that the number of people who endorse something is viewed as more closely related to the central merits of an advocacy in a collectivist than in an individualistic culture.

8. This is not to imply that heuristics cannot add to the impact of argument processing, but rather that the same additive outcome can occur if the variable that invokes a heuristic and/or the heuristic itself are processed for merit under high-elaboration conditions (we postpone discussion of the co-occurrence of central and peripheral processes until Postulate 6).

9. We do not mean to imply that all peripheral processes are subjected to scrutiny under high-elaboration conditions. Rather, people scrutinize both the external and internal information that is available. Thus, people might have conscious access to some peripheral information, such as retrieved heuristics (even if the retrieval process itself is automatic), but are not likely to have conscious access to other peripheral mechanisms, such as mere association (as in classical conditioning). Because of this, the output of some peripheral mechanisms can be subjected to scrutiny, whereas the output of other peripheral mechanisms cannot. Attitudinal effects of the latter mechanisms might be detected with implicit measures.

10. Different peripheral-route processes require different *minimal* motivation and ability levels to have an impact on attitudes (e.g., a self-perception process presumably requires that people have greater motivation and ability to evaluate a message than does classical conditioning or mere exposure). Thus, when one is going from extremely low levels of elaboration likelihood to moderately low levels, the impact of some peripheral processes (such as self-perception and other attributional inferences) might be increased. Once one is past the minimal point on the continuum necessary to invoke the process, however, moving higher along the continuum should reduce the impact of the process on attitudes. That is, as the elaboration likelihood is increased further, the peripheral process should account for less variance in the overall attitude.

REFERENCES

Aaker, J. L., & Maheswaran, D. (1997). The effect of cultural orientation on persuasion. *Journal of Consumer Research*, 24, 315–328.

Ajzen, I. (1987). A new paradigm in the psychology of persuasion. *Contemporary Psychology*, 32, 1009–1010.

Allen, M., & Reynolds, R. (1993). The elaboration likelihood model and the sleeper effect: An assessment of attitude change over time. *Communication Theory*, 3, 73–82.

Anderson, N. (1981). Integration theory applied to cognitive responses and attitudes. In R. Petty, T. Ostrom, & T. Brock (Eds.), *Cognitive responses in persuasion* (pp. 361–397). Hillsdale, NJ: Erlbaum.

Bem, D. J. (1972). Self-perception theory. In L. Berkowitz (Ed.), *Advances in experimental social psychology* (Vol. 6, pp. 1–62). New York: Academic Press.

Baker, S. M., & Petty, R. E. (1994). Majority and minority influence: Source–position imbalance as a determinant of message scrutiny. *Journal of Personality and Social Psychology, 67*, 5–19.

Biek, M., Wood, W., & Chaiken, S. (1996). Working knowledge and cognitive processing: On the determinants of bias. *Personality and Social Psychology Bulletin, 22*, 547–556.

Bless, H., Bohner, G., Schwarz, N., & Strack, F. (1990). Mood and persuasion: A cognitive response analysis. *Personality and Social Psychology Bulletin, 16*, 331–345.

Bobrow, D. G., & Norman, D. A. (1975). Some principles of memory schemata. In D. G. Bobrow & A. G. Collins (Eds.), *Representation and understanding: Studies in cognitive science* (pp. 131–150). New York: Academic Press.

Bohner, G., Rank, S., Reinhard, M., Einwiller, S., & Erb, H. (1998). Motivational determinants of systematic processing: Expectancy moderates effects of desired confidence on processing effort. *European Journal of Social Psychology, 28*, 185–206.

Bornstein, R. F. (1989). Exposure and affect: Overview and meta-analysis of research, 1968–1987. *Psychological Bulletin, 106*, 265–289.

Bower, G. H. (1981). Mood and memory. *American Psychologist, 36*, 129–148.

Brehm, J. W. (1966). *A theory of psychological reactance.* New York: Academic Press.

Brewer, M. B. (1988). A dual process model of impression formation. In T. K. Srull & R. S. Wyer (Eds.), *Advances in social cognition* (Vol. 1, pp. 177–183). Hillsdale, NJ: Erlbaum.

Burnkrant, R. E., & Howard, D. J. (1984). Effects of the use of introductory rhetorical questions versus statements on information processing. *Journal of Personality and Social Psychology, 47*, 1218–1230.

Burnstein, E., & Vinokur, A. (1975). What a person thinks upon learning he has chosen differently from others: Nice evidence for the persuasive-arguments explanation of choice shifts. *Journal of Experimental Social Psychology, 11*, 412–426.

Burnstein, E., Vinokur, A., & Trope, Y. (1973). Interpersonal comparison versus persuasive argumentation: A more direct test of alternative explanations for group induced shifts in individual choice. *Journal of Experimental Social Psychology, 9*, 236–245.

Cacioppo, J. T., Marshall-Goodell, B. S., Tassinary, L. G., & Petty, R. E. (1992). Rudimentary determinants of attitudes: Classical conditioning is more effective when prior knowledge about the attitude stimulus is low than high. *Journal of Experimental Social Psychology, 28*, 207–233.

Cacioppo, J. T., & Petty, R. E. (1982). The need for cognition. *Journal of Personality and Social Psychology, 42*, 116–131.

Cacioppo, J. T., & Petty, R. E. (1989). Effects of message repetition on argument processing, recall, and persuasion. *Basic and Applied Social Psychology, 10*, 3–12.

Cacioppo, J. T., Petty, R. E., Feinstein, J., & Jarvis, W. B. G. (1996). Dispositional differences in cognitive motivation: The life and times of individuals varying in need for cognition. *Psychological Bulletin, 119*, 197–253.

Cacioppo, J. T., Petty, R. E., & Morris, K. J. (1983). Effects of need for cognition on message evaluation, recall, and persuasion. *Journal of Personality and Social Psychology, 45*, 805–818.

Chaiken, S. (1980). Heuristic versus systematic information processing in the use of source versus message cues in persuasion. *Journal of Personality and Social Psychology, 39*, 752–766.

Chaiken, S. (1987). The heuristic model of persuasion. In M. P. Zanna, J. M. Olson, & C. P. Herman (Ed.), *Social influence: The Ontario Symposium* (Vol. 5, pp. 3–39). Hillsdale, NJ: Erlbaum.

Chaiken, S., Liberman, A., & Eagly, A. H. (1989). Heuristic and systematic information processing within and beyond the persuasion context. In J. S. Uleman & J. A. Bargh (Ed.), *Unintended thought* (pp. 212–252). New York: Guilford Press.

Chaiken, S., & Maheswaran, D. (1994). Heuristic processing can bias systematic processing: Effects of source credibility, argument ambiguity, and task importance on attitude judgment. *Journal of Personality and Social Psychology, 66*, 460–473.

Chaiken, S., Pomerantz, E. M., & Giner-Sorolla, R. (1995). Structural consistency and attitude strength. In R. E. Petty & J. A. Krosnick (Eds.), *Attitude strength: Antecedents and consequences* (pp. 387–412). Mahwah, NJ: Erlbaum.

Chaiken, S., Wood, W., & Eagly, A. H. (1996). Principles of persuasion. In E. T. Higgins & A. W. Kruglanski (Eds.), *Social psychology: Handbook of basic principles* (pp. 702–742). New York: Guilford Press.

DeBono, K. G., & Harnish, R. J. (1988). Source expertise, source attractiveness, and the processing of persuasive information: A functional approach. *Journal of Personality and Social Psychology, 55*, 541–546.

Dovidio, J. F., Kawakami, K., Johnson, C., Johnson, B., & Howard, A. (1997). On the nature of prejudice: Automatic and controlled processes. *Journal of Experimental Social Psychology, 33*, 510–540.

Eagly, A. H., & Chaiken, S. (1993). *The psychology of attitudes.* Fort Worth, TX: Harcourt Brace Jovanovich.

Evans, L. M., & Petty, R. E. (1998, May). *The effect of expectations on knowledge use.* Presented at the annual meeting of the Midwestern Psychological Association, Chicago, IL.

Fabrigar, L. R., Priester, J. R., Petty, R. E., & Wegener, D. T. (1998). The impact of attitude accessibility on cognitive elaboration of persuasive messages. *Personality and Social Psychology Bulletin, 24*, 339–352.

Fazio, R. H. (1990). Multiple processes by which attitudes guide behavior: The MODE model as an integrative framework. In M. P. Zanna (Ed.), *Advances in experimental social psychology* (Vol. 23, pp. 75–109). San Diego, CA: Academic Press.

Fazio, R. H. (1995). Attitudes as object–evaluation associations: Determinants, consequences, and correlates of attitude accessibility. In R. E. Petty & J. A. Krosnick (Eds.), *Attitude strength: Antecedents and consequences* (pp. 247–282). Mahwah, NJ: Erlbaum.

Festinger, L. (1954). A theory of social comparison processes. *Human Relations, 7*, 117–140.

Fishbein, M., & Ajzen, I. (1972). Attitudes and opinions. *Annual Review of Psychology, 23*, 487–544.

Fishbein, M., & Ajzen, I. (1981). Acceptance, yielding and impact: Cognitive processes in persuasion. In R. E. Petty, T. M. Ostrom, & T. C. Brock (Eds.), *Cognitive responses in persuasion* (pp. 339–359). Hillsdale, NJ: Erlbaum.

Fishbein, M., & Middlestadt, S. (1995). Noncognitive effects on attitude formation and change: Fact or artifact? *Journal of Consumer Psychology, 2,* 181–202.

Fiske, S. T., & Neuberg, S. L. (1990). A continuum of impression formation, from category-based to individuating processes: Influences of information and motivation on attention and interpretation. In M. P. Zanna (Ed.), *Advances in experimental social psychology* (Vol. 23, pp. 1–74). San Diego, CA: Academic Press.

Fiske, S. T., & Pavelchak, M. A. (1986). Category-based versus piecemeal-based affective responses: Developments in schema-triggered affect. In R. M. Sorrentino, & E. T. Higgins (Eds.), *Handbook of motivation and cognition: Foundations of social behavior* (Vol. 1, pp. 167–203). New York: Guilford Press.

Fleming, M. A., & Petty, R. E. (in press). Identity and persuasion: An elaboration likelihood approach. In D. Terry & M. Hogg (Eds.), *Attitudes, behavior, and social context: The role of norms and group membership.* Mahwah, NJ: Erlbaum.

Forgas, J. P. (1992). Affect in social judgments and decisions: A multi-process model. In M. P. Zanna (Ed.), *Advances in experimental social psychology* (Vol. 25, pp. 227–275). San Diego, CA: Academic Press.

Forgas, J. P. (1995). Mood and judgment: The affect-infusion model (AIM). *Psychological Bulletin, 117,* 39–66.

Friedrich, J., Fetherstonhaugh, D., Casey, S., & Gallagher, D. (1996). Argument integration and attitude change: Suppression effects in the integration of one-sided arguments that vary in persuasiveness. *Personality and Social Psychology Bulletin, 22,* 179–191.

Gilbert, D. T. (1991). How mental systems believe. *American Psychologist, 46,* 107–119.

Hafer, C. L., Reynolds, K., & Obertynski, M. A. (1996). Message comprehensibility and persuasion: Effects of complex language in counterattitudinal appeals to laypeople. *Social Cognition, 14,* 317–337.

Hamilton, M. A., Hunter, J. E., & Boster, F. J. (1993). The elaboration likelihood model as a theory of attitude formation: A mathematical analysis. *Communication Theory, 3,* 50–65.

Harkins, S. G., & Petty, R. E. (1981). Effects of source magnification of cognitive effort on attitudes: An information processing view. *Journal of Personality and Social Psychology, 40,* 401–413.

Harkins, S. G., & Petty, R. E. (1987). Information utility and the multiple source effect. *Journal of Personality and Social Psychology, 52,* 260–268.

Haugtvedt, C. P. (1997). Beyond fact or artifact: An assessment of Fishbein and Middlestadt's perspectives on attitude change processes. *Journal of Consumer Psychology, 6,* 99–106.

Haugtvedt, C. P., Schumann, D. W., Schneier, W. L., & Warren, W. L. (1994). Advertising repetition and variation strategies: Implications for understanding attitude strength. *Journal of Consumer Research, 21,* 176–189.

Haugtvedt, C. P., & Wegener, D. T. (1994). Message order effects in persuasion: An attitude strength perspective. *Journal of Consumer Research, 21,* 205–218.

Hawkins, C., Petty, R. E., & Wegener, D. T. (1996, May). *Need for cognition and primacy/recency: Understanding when each occurs.* Paper presented at the annual meeting of the Midwestern Psychological Association, Chicago.

Heider, F. (1958). *The psychology of interpersonal relations.* New York: Wiley.

Heesacker, M. H., Petty, R. E., & Cacioppo, J. T. (1983). Field dependence and attitude change: Source credibility can alter persuasion by affecting message-relevant thinking. *Journal of Personality, 51,* 653–666.

Jarvis, W. B. G., Tormala, Z., & Petty, R. E. (1998, May). *Do attitudes really change?* Paper presented at the annual meeting of the American Psychological Society, Washington, DC.

Jaspers, J. M. G. (1978). Determinants of attitude and attitude change. In H. Tajfel & C. Fraser (Eds.), *Introducing social psychology* (pp. 277–301). Harmondsworth, England: Penguin.

Johnson, H. H., & Watkins, T. A. (1971). The effects of message repetition on immediate and delayed attitude change. *Psychonomic Science, 22,* 101–103.

Kelman, H. C. (1958). Compliance, identification, and internalization: Three processes of attitude change. *Journal of Conflict Resolution, 2,* 51–60.

Kelman, H. C., & Hovland, C. I. (1953). "Reinstatement" of the communicator in delayed measurement of opinion change. *Journal of Abnormal and Social Psychology, 48,* 327–335.

Kiesler, C. A., & Munson, P. A. (1975). Attitudes and opinions. *Annual Review of Psychology, 26,* 415–456.

Kirmani, A., & Shiv, B. (1998). Effects of source congruity on brand attitudes and beliefs: The moderating role of issue-relevant elaboration. *Journal of Consumer Psychology, 7,* 25–47.

Krosnick, J. A. (1991). Response strategies for coping with the cognitive demands of attitude measures in surveys. *Applied Cognitive Psychology, 5,* 213–236.

Kruglanski, A. W. (1989). *Lay epistemics and human knowledge.* New York: Plenum Press.

Kruglanski, A. W. (1990). Lay epistemic theory in social-cognitive psychology. *Psychological Inquiry, 1,* 181–197.

Kruglanski, A. W., & Thompson, E. P. (in press). Persuasion by a single route: A view from the unimodel. *Psychological Inquiry.*

Leippe, M. R., & Elkin, R. A. (1987). When motives clash: Issue involvement and response involvement as determinants of persuasion. *Journal of Personality and Social Psychology, 52,* 269–278.

Leventhal, H. (1970). Findings and theory in the study of fear communications. In L. Berkowitz (Ed.), *Advances in experimental social psychology* (Vol. 5, pp. 119–186). New York: Academic Press.

Lord, C. G., Ross, L., & Lepper, M. R . (1979). Biased assimilation and attitude polarization: The effects of prior theories on subsequently considered evidence. *Journal of Personality and Social Psychology, 37,* 2098–2109.

Mackie, D. M., & Worth, L. T. (1989). Processing deficits and the mediation of positive affect in persuasion. *Journal of Personality and Social Psychology, 57,* 27–40.

Mahesharan, D., & Chaiken, S. (1991). Promoting systematic processing in low-motivation settings: Effect of incongruent information on processing and judgment. *Journal of Personality and Social Psychology, 61,* 13–33.

Maio, G. R., Bell, D. W., & Esses, V. M. (1996). Ambivalence and persuasion: The processing of messages about immigrant groups. *Journal of Experimental Social Psychology, 32*, 513–536.

McClelland, J. L., McNaughton, B. L., & O'Reilly, R. C. (1995). Why are there complementary learning systems in the hippocampus and neocortex?: Insights from the successes and failures of connectionist models of learning and memory. *Psychological Review, 102*, 419–457.

McGarty, C., Haslam, S. A., Hutchinson, K. J., & Turner, J. C. (1994). The effects of salient group memberships on persuasion. *Small Group Research, 25*, 267–293.

McGuire, W. J. (1964). Inducing resistance to persuasion: Some contemporary approaches. In L. Berkowitz (Ed.), *Advances in experimental social psychology* (Vol. 1, pp. 191–229). New York: Academic Press.

Miniard, P. W., Bhatla, S., Lord, K. R., Dickson, P. R., & Unnava, H. R. (1991). Picture-based persuasion processes and the moderating role of involvement. *Journal of Consumer Research, 18*, 92–107.

Moore, D. L., & Reardon, R. (1987). Source magnification: The role of multiple sources in the processing of advertising appeals. *Journal of Marketing Research, 24*, 412–417.

O'Keefe, D. J. (1990). *Persuasion: Theory and research.* Newbury Park, CA: Sage.

Ottati, V. C., & Isbell, L. M. (1996). Effects on mood during exposure to target information on subsequently reported judgments: An on-line model of misattribution and correction. *Journal of Personality and Social Psychology, 71*, 39–53.

Ottati, V., Terkildsen, N., & Hubbard, C. (1997). Happy faces elicit heuristic processing in a televised impression formation task: A cognitive tuning account. *Personality and Social Psychology Bulletin, 23*, 1144–1156.

Perloff, R. M., & Brock, T. C. (1980). And thinking makes it so: Cognitive responses to persuasion. In M. Roloff & G. Miller (Eds.), *Persuasion: New directions in theory and research* (pp. 67–100). Beverly Hills, CA: Sage.

Petty, R . E. (1977). *A cognitive response analysis of the temporal persistence of attitude changes induced by persuasive communications.* Unpublished doctoral dissertation, Ohio State University.

Petty, R. E. (1994). Two routes to persuasion: State of the art. In G. d'Ydewalle, P. Eelen, & P. Bertelson (Eds.), *International perspectives on psychological science* (Vol. 2, pp. 229–247). Hillsdale, NJ: Erlbaum.

Petty, R. E. (1997). The evolution of theory and research in social psychology: From single to multiple effect and process models of persuasion. In C. McGarty & S. A. Haslam (Eds.), *The message of social psychology: Perspectives on mind in society* (pp. 268–290). Oxford: Blackwell.

Petty, R. E., Baker, S., & Gleicher, F. (1991). Attitudes and drug abuse prevention: Implications of the elaboration likelihood model of persuasion. In L. Donohew, H. E. Sypher, & W. J. Bukoski (Eds.), *Persuasive communication and drug abuse prevention* (pp. 71–90). Hillsdale, NJ: Erlbaum.

Petty, R. E., & Cacioppo, J. T. (1979a). Effects of forewarning of persuasive intent and involvement on cognitive responses and persuasion. *Personality and Social Psychology Bulletin, 5*, 173–176.

Petty, R. E., & Cacioppo, J. T. (1979b). Issue-involvement can increase or decrease persuasion by enhancing message-relevant cognitive responses. *Journal of Personality and Social Psychology, 37*, 1915–1926.

Petty, R. E., & Cacioppo, J. T. (1981). *Attitudes and persuasion: Classic and contemporary approaches.* Dubuque, IA: William C. Brown.

Petty, R. E., & Cacioppo, J. T. (1983). The role of bodily responses in attitude measurement and change. In J. T. Cacioppo & R. E . Petty (Eds.), *Social psychophysiology: A sourcebook* (pp. 51–101). New York: Guilford Press.

Petty, R. E., & Cacioppo, J. T. (1984a). The effects of involvement on response to argument quantity and quality: Central and peripheral routes to persuasion. *Journal of Personality and Social Psychology, 46*, 69–81.

Petty, R. E., & Cacioppo, J. T. (1984b). Source factors and the elaboration likelihood model of persuasion. *Advances in Consumer Research, 11*, 668–672.

Petty, R. E., & Cacioppo, J. T. (1986a). *Communication and persuasion: Central and peripheral routes to attitude change.* New York: Springer-Verlag.

Petty, R. E., & Cacioppo, J. T. (1986b). The elaboration likelihood model of persuasion. In L. Berkowitz (Ed.), *Advances in experimental social psychology* (Vol. 19, pp. 123–205). New York: Academic Press.

Petty, R. E., & Cacioppo, J. T. (1990). Involvement and persuasion: Tradition versus integration. *Psychological Bulletin, 107*, 367–374.

Petty, R. E., Cacioppo, J. T., & Goldman, R. (1981). Personal involvement as a determinant of argument-based persuasion. *Journal of Personality and Social Psychology, 41*, 847–855.

Petty, R. E., Cacioppo, J. T., & Haugtvedt, C. (1992). Involvement and persuasion: An appreciative look at the Sherifs' contribution to the study of self-relevance and attitude change. In D. Granberg & G. Sarup (Ed.), *Social judgment and intergroup relations: Essays in honor of Muzifer Sherif* (pp. 147–175). New York: Springer-Verlag.

Petty, R. E., Cacioppo, J. T., & Heesacker, M. (1981). Effects of rhetorical questions on persuasion: A cognitive response analysis. *Journal of Personality and Social Psychology, 40*, 432–440.

Petty, R. E., Cacioppo, J. T., & Schumann, D. (1983). Central and peripheral routes to advertising effectiveness: The moderating role of involvement. *Journal of Consumer Research, 10*, 135–146.

Petty, R. E., Gleicher, F. H., & Jarvis, B. (1993). Persuasion theory and AIDS prevention. In J. B. Pryor & G. Reeder (Eds.), *The social psychology of HIV infection* (pp. 155–182). Hillsdale, NJ: Erlbaum.

Petty, R. E., Harkins, S. G., & Williams, K. D. (1980). The effects of group diffusion of cognitive effort on attitudes: An information processing view. *Journal of Personality and Social Psychology, 38*, 81–92.

Petty, R. E., Haugtvedt, C., & Smith, S. M. (1995). Elaboration as a determinant of attitude strength: Creating attitudes that are persistent, resistant, and predictive of behavior. In R. E. Petty & J. A. Krosnick (Eds.), *Attitude strength: Antecedents and consequences* (pp. 93–130). Mahwah, NJ: Erlbaum.

Petty, R. E., & Jarvis, W. B. G. (1996). An individual differences perspective on assessing cognitive processes. In N. Schwarz & S. Sudman (Eds.), *Answering questions: Methodology for determining cognitive and communicative processes in survey research* (pp. 221–257). San Francisco: Jossey-Bass.

Petty, R. E., & Jarvis, W. B. G. (1998). *What happens to*

the "old" attitude when attitudes change? Presented at the annual meeting of the Society of Experimental Social Psychology, Lexington, KY.

Petty, R. E., Jarvis, W. B. G., & Evans, L. M. (1996). Recurrent thought: Implications for attitudes and persuasion. In R. S. Wyer (Ed.), *Advances in social cognition* (Vol. 9, pp. 145–164). Mahwah, NJ: Erlbaum.

Petty, R. E., Kasmer, J. A., Haugtvedt, C. P., & Cacioppo, J. T. (1987). Source and message factors in persuasion: A reply to Stiff's critique of the elaboration likelihood model. *Communication Monographs, 54,* 233–249.

Petty, R. E., Ostrom, T. M., & Brock, T. C. (Eds.). (1981). *Cognitive responses in persuasion.* Hillsdale, NJ: Erlbaum.

Petty, R. E., Priester, J. R., & Wegener, D. T. (1994). Cognitive processes in attitude change. In R. S. Wyer & T. K. Srull (Eds.), *Handbook of social cognition* (2nd ed., Vol. 2, pp. 69–142). Hillsdale, NJ: Erlbaum.

Petty, R. E., Schumann, D. W., Richman, S. A., & Strathman, A. J. (1993). Positive mood and persuasion: Different roles for affect under high- and low-elaboration conditions. *Journal of Personality and Social Psychology, 64,* 5–20.

Petty, R. E., & Wegener, D. T. (1993). Flexible correction processes in social judgment: Correcting for context induced contrast. *Journal of Experimental Social Psychology, 29,* 137–165.

Petty, R. E., & Wegener, D. T. (1998). Attitude change: Multiple roles for persuasion variables. In D. Gilbert, S. Fiske, & G. Lindzey (Eds.), *Handbook of social psychology* (4th ed., pp. 323–390). New York: McGraw-Hill.

Petty, R. E., Wegener, D. T., Fabrigar, L. R., Priester, J. R., & Cacioppo, J. T. (1993). Conceptual and methodological issues in the elaboration likelihood model of persuasion: A reply to the Michigan State critics. *Communication Theory, 3,* 336–363.

Petty, R. E., Wegener, D. T., & White, P. (1998). Flexible correction processes in persuasion. *Social Cognition, 16,* 93–113.

Petty, R. E., Wells, G. L., & Brock, T. C. (1976). Distraction can enhance or reduce yielding to propaganda: Thought disruption versus effort justification. *Journal of Personality and Social Psychology, 34,* 874–884.

Petty, R. E., Wells, G. L., Heesacker, M., Brock, T. C., & Cacioppo, J. T. (1983). The effects of recipient posture on persuasion: A cognitive response analysis. *Personality and Social Psychology Bulletin, 9,* 209–222.

Petty, R. E., Wheeler, C. S., & Bizer, G. Y. (in press). Is there one persuasion process or more?: Lumping versus splitting in attitude change theories. *Psychological Inquiry.*

Pittman, T. S. (1993). Control motivation and attitude change. In G. Weary, F. Gleicher, & K. Marsh (Eds.), *Control motivation and social cognition* (pp. 157–175). New York: Springer-Verlag.

Pratkanis, A. R. (1989). Advances in social psychology during the postcrisis era. *Contemporary Psychology, 34,* 547–548.

Priester, J. R., & Fleming, M. A. (1997). Artifact or meaningful theoretical constructs?: Examining evidence for nonbelief- and belief-based attitude change processes. *Journal of Consumer Psychology, 6,* 67–76.

Priester, J. R., & Petty, R. E. (1995). Source attributions and persuasion: Perceived honesty as a determinant of message scrutiny. *Personality and Social Psychology Bulletin, 21,* 637–654.

Puckett, J. M., Petty, R. E., Cacioppo, J. T., & Fisher, D. L. (1983). The relative impact of age and attractiveness stereotypes on persuasion. *Journal of Gerontology, 38,* 340–343.

Ratneshwar, S., & Chaiken, S. (1991). Comprehension's role in persuasion: The case of its moderating effect on the persuasive impact of source cues. *Journal of Consumer Psychology, 18,* 52–62.

Sanbonmatsu, D. M., & Kardes, F. R. (1988). The effects of physiological arousal on information processing and persuasion. *Journal of Consumer Research, 15,* 379–385.

Schul, Y., & Burnstein, E. (1985). When discounting fails: Conditions under which individuals use discredited information in making a judgment. *Journal of Personality and Social Psychology, 49,* 894–903.

Schumann, D., Petty, R. E., & Clemons, S. (1990). Predicting the effectiveness of different strategies of advertising variation: A test of the repetition–variation hypotheses. *Journal of Consumer Research, 17,* 192–202.

Schwarz, N. (1990). Feelings as information: Informational and motivational functions of affective states. In E. T. Higgins & R. M. Sorrentino (Eds.), *Handbook of motivation and cognition: Foundations of social behavior* (Vol. 2, pp. 527–561). New York: Guilford Press.

Schwarz, N. (1997). Moods and attitude judgments: A comment on Fishbein and Middlestadt. *Journal of Consumer Psychology, 6,* 93–98.

Schwarz, N., & Clore, G. L. (1983). Mood, misattribution, and judgments of well-being: Informative and directive functions of affective states. *Journal of Personality and Social Psychology, 45,* 513–523.

Sears, D. O. (1988). [Review of *Communication and persuasion: Central and peripheral routes to attitude change*]. *Public Opinion Quarterly, 52,* 262–265.

Sengupta, J., Goodstein, R. C., & Boninger, D. S. (1997). All cues are not created equal: Obtaining attitude persistence under low-involvement conditions. *Journal of Consumer Research, 23,* 351–361.

Sherif, M. (1977). Crisis in social psychology: Some remarks towards breaking through the crisis. *Personality and Social Psychology Bulletin, 3,* 368–383.

Smith, S. M., & Petty, R. E. (1996). Message framing and persuasion: A message processing analysis. *Personality and Social Psychology Bulletin, 22,* 257–268.

Smith, S. M., & Shaffer, D. R. (1991). Celerity and cajolery: Rapid speech may promote or inhibit persuasion through its impact on message elaboration. *Personality and Social Psychology Bulletin, 17,* 663–669.

Snyder, M. (1979). Self-monitoring processes. In L. Berkowitz (Ed), *Advances in experimental social psychology* (Vol. 12, pp. 86–128). New York: Academic Press.

Soldat, A. S., Sinclair, R. C., & Mark, M. M. (1997). Color as an environmental processing cue: External affective cues can directly affect processing strategy without affecting mood. *Social Cognition, 15,* 55–71.

Sorrentino, R. M., Bobocel, D. R., Gitta, M. Z., & Olson, J. M. (1988). Uncertainty orientation and persuasion: Individual differences in the effects of personal relevance on social judgments. *Journal of Personality and Social Psychology, 55,* 357–371.

Spiegel, S., Thompson, E. P., & Kruglanski, A. (1996, July). *Toward a unimodal theory of persuasion: On the effortful processing of "heuristic" information.* Paper presented at the annual meeting of the American Psychological Society, Washington, DC.

Staats, A. W., & Staats, C. K. (1958). Attitudes established by classical conditioning. *Journal of Abnormal and Social Psychology, 57,* 37–40.

Steele, C. M. (1988). The psychology of self-affirmation: Sustaining the integrity of the self. In L. Berkowitz (Ed.), *Advances in experimental social psychology* (Vol. 21, pp. 261–302). New York: Academic Press.

Sternthal, B., Dholakia, R., & Leavitt, C. (1978). The persuasive effect of source credibility: A test of cognitive response analysis. *Journal of Consumer Research, 4,* 252–260.

Strack, F. (1992). The different routes to social judgments: Experiential versus informational based strategies. In L. L. Martin & A. Tesser (Eds.), *The construction of social judgments* (pp. 249–275). Hillsdale, NJ: Erlbaum.

Stiff, J. B. (1986). Cognitive processing of persuasive message cues: A meta-analytic review of the effects of supporting information on attitudes. *Communication Monographs, 53,* 75–89.

Taylor, S. E. (1981). The interface of cognitive and social psychology. In J. H. Harvey (Ed.), *Cognition, social behavior, and the environment* (pp. 189–211). Hillsdale, NJ: Erlbaum.

Tedeschi, J. T., Schlenker, B. R., & Bonoma, T. V. (1971). Cognitive dissonance: Private ratiocination or public spectacle? *American Psychologist, 26,* 685–695.

Weber, S. J. (1972). *Opinion change is a function of the associative learning of content and source factors.* Unpublished doctoral dissertation, Northwestern University.

Wegener, D. T., & Claypool, H. M. (in press). The elaboration continuum by any other name does not smell as sweet. *Psychological inquiry.*

Wegener, D. T., Downing, J., Krosnick, J. A., & Petty, R. E. (1995). Measures and manipulations of strength related properties of attitudes: Current practice and future directions. In R. E. Petty & J. A. Krosnick (Eds.), *Attitude strength: Antecedents and consequences* (pp. 455–488). Mahwah, NJ: Erlbaum.

Wegener, D. T., & Petty, R. E. (1994). Mood management across affective states: The hedonic contingency hypothesis. *Journal of Personality and Social Psychology, 66,* 1034–1048.

Wegener, D. T., & Petty, R. E. (1995). Flexible correction processes in social judgment: The role of naive theories in corrections for perceived bias. *Journal of Personality and Social Psychology, 68,* 36–51.

Wegener, D. T., & Petty, R. E. (1997). The flexible correction model: The role of naive theories of bias in bias correction. In M. P. Zanna (Ed.), *Advances in experimental social psychology* (Vol. 29, pp. 141–208). San Diego, CA: Academic Press.

Wegener, D. T., Petty, R. E., & Klein, D. J. (1994). Effects of mood on high elaboration attitude change: The mediating role of likelihood judgments. *European Journal of Social Psychology, 24,* 25–43.

Wegener, D. T., Petty, R. E., & Smith, S. M. (1995). Positive mood can increase or decrease message scrutiny: The hedonic contingency view of mood and message processing. *Journal of Personality and Social Psychology, 69,* 5–15.

Wilson, T. D., & Brekke, N. (1994). Mental contamination and mental correction: Unwanted influences on judgments and evaluations. *Psychological Bulletin, 116,* 117–142.

Wilson, T. D., Kraft, D., & Dunn, D. S. (1989). The disruptive effects of explaining attitudes: The moderating effect of knowledge about the attitude object. *Journal of Experimental Social Psychology, 25,* 379–400.

Wilson, T. D., & Schooler, T. (1998). *Dual attitudes.* Unpublished manuscript, University of Virginia.

Wood, W., Kallgren, C. A., & Preisler, R. M. (1985). Access to attitude-relevant information in memory as a determinant of persuasion: The role of message attributes. *Journal of Experimental Social Psychology, 21,* 73–85.

Wood, W., Rhodes, N., & Biek, M. (1995). Working knowledge and attitude strength: An information processing analysis. In R. E. Petty & J. A. Krosnick (Ed.), *Attitude strength: Antecedents and consequences* (pp. 283–313). Mahwah, NJ: Erlbaum.

Worth, L. T., & Mackie, D. M. (1987). Cognitive mediation of positive affect in persuasion. *Social Cognition, 5,* 76–94.

Zajonc, R. B. (1968). Attitudinal effects of mere exposure. *Journal of Personality and Social Psychology Monograph Supplements, 9,* 1–27.

Zanna, M. P., Fazio, R. H., & Ross, M. (1994). The persistence of persuasion. In R. C. Schank & E. Langer (Eds.), *Beliefs, reasoning, and decision-making: Psychologic in honor of Bob Abelson* (pp. 347–362). Hillsdale, NJ: Erlbaum.

Zanna, M. P., Kiesler, C. A., & Pilkonis, P. A. (1970). Positive and negative attitudinal affect established by classical conditioning. *Journal of Personality and Social Psychology, 14,* 321–328.

4

The Heuristic–Systematic Model in Its Broader Context

SERENA CHEN
SHELLY CHAIKEN

In the spirit of the current volume, this chapter articulates new, and expands on old, conceptual links between the heuristic–systematic model (e.g., Chaiken, 1980, 1987; Chaiken, Liberman, & Eagly, 1989) and related concepts in the social-cognitive literature on alternative modes of information processing. Our hope is to demonstrate the utility of applying the heuristic–systematic model to a diverse range of judgmental domains. To lay the groundwork, we first present the basic heuristic–systematic model in its multiple-motive formulation (Chaiken, Giner-Sorolla, & Chen, 1996), and then briefly discuss how our dual-process theory relates to various other models of social judgment.

To place the model in its broader context, we begin by considering heuristic and systematic modes of processing, along with the social-cognitive principles thought to govern the activation and use of stored knowledge. Consistent with the growing emphasis on the role of applicability in determining when stored knowledge will be activated and used in social judgment (see Higgins, 1996), we discuss this principle in particular detail. From there we turn to the increasingly critical distinction between conscious and unconscious processes (e.g., Bargh, 1989, 1994),

and discuss how it relates to our distinction between heuristic and systematic processing. Having considered both conscious and unconscious aspects of each processing mode, we then focus on unconscious forms of heuristic processing. Specifically, we examine the impact of subjective experiences on judgment, and argue that this reflects the unconscious activation and application of stored heuristics that pertain distinctly to these experiences. Finally, we discuss some of the implications of our conceptualization of subjective experiences for heuristic and systematic processing more broadly.

In drawing connections between the heuristic–systematic model and related concepts in the social-cognitive literature, our primary aim is to highlight the novel ramifications of these connections for heuristic and systematic modes of processing. As such, this chapter focuses more on extending the heuristic–systematic model than on recapitulating earlier discussions of it, and more on suggesting new avenues of empirical inquiry than on reviewing past research. For aspects of heuristic and systematic processing on which this chapter may fall short, prior discussions of the model and relevant empirical evidence can be consulted (Bohner, Moskowitz, & Chaiken,

1995; Chaiken, 1980, 1987; Chaiken, Giner-Sorolla, & Chen, 1996; Chaiken et al., 1989; Chaiken, Wood, & Eagly, 1996; see also Eagly & Chaiken, 1993).

THE HEURISTIC–SYSTEMATIC MODEL

Heuristic and Systematic Modes of Information Processing

Within any given judgmental context, the heuristic–systematic model delineates two basic modes by which perceivers may determine their attitudes and other social judgments. *Systematic processing* entails a relatively analytic and comprehensive treatment of judgment-relevant information. Judgments formed on the basis of systematic processing are thus responsive to the actual content of this information. Given its nature, systematic processing requires both cognitive ability and capacity. Hence, for example, systematic forms of processing in a given judgmental domain are less likely to be seen among perceivers who possess little knowledge in the domain, or among individuals who are processing with time constraints.

The other basic mode, *heuristic processing*, entails the activation and application of judgmental rules or "heuristics" that, like other knowledge structures, are presumed to be learned and stored in memory (e.g., "Experts' statements can be trusted," "Length implies strength," "Consensus opinions are correct"). Judgments formed on the basis of heuristic processing reflect easily processed judgment-relevant cues (e.g., message length; Wood, Kallgren, & Preisler, 1985), rather than individualistic or particularistic judgment-relevant information.[1] Relative to systematic processing, heuristic processing makes minimal cognitive demands on the perceiver. The heuristic mode is constrained, however, by social-cognitive principles of knowledge activation and use—namely, availability, accessibility, and applicability (e.g., Higgins, 1996). Specifically, in heuristic processing, judgment-relevant heuristics must be stored in memory (i.e., available), and that within a given judgmental setting they must be somehow retrieved from memory and thus ready to be used (i.e., accessible). Beyond this, an available and accessible heuristic must also

be applicable—that is, somehow relevant to the judgmental task at hand. We return to a more detailed discussion of these principles in a later section.

The Sufficiency Principle

Reflecting widespread notions of perceivers as limited in cognitive resources (e.g., Shiffrin & Schneider, 1977) and thus as "economy-minded" information processors (e.g., Chaiken, 1980, 1987; Fiske & Taylor, 1991), the heuristic–systematic model assumes that perceivers are guided in part by a "principle of least effort." That is, in the interest of economy, heuristic processing often predominates over relatively more effortful systematic processing. Information processing, however, is often guided by motivational concerns beyond economy. Recognizing this, the heuristic–systematic model incorporates least-effort notions into its *sufficiency principle*, which maintains that perceivers attempt to strike a balance between minimizing cognitive effort on the one hand and satisfying their current motivational concerns on the other (Chaiken, Giner-Sorolla, & Chen, 1996; Chaiken et al., 1989; see also Simon, 1976). Thus, for example, perceivers who are motivated to determine accurate judgments will exert as much cognitive effort as is necessary (and possible) to reach a sufficient degree of confidence that their judgments will satisfy their accuracy goals.

For any given judgment, the sufficiency principle proposes a continuum of judgmental confidence, along which two critical points lie: one designating perceivers' level of *actual* confidence, and the other designating their level of *desired* confidence, or *sufficiency threshold*. Perceivers will exert cognitive effort until their level of actual confidence reaches (if it can) their sufficiency threshold, thereby closing the gap between actual and desired levels of confidence. When low-effort heuristic processing fails to confer sufficient judgmental confidence (or cannot occur due to, for example, the absence of any judgment-relevant heuristic-cue information), perceivers are likely to engage in systematic processing in an attempt to close the confidence gap.[2]

Processing predictions follow directly from the sufficiency principle. Systematic processing is likely to emerge when the gap between actual and desired judgmental confidence is widened as a result of either an increase in one's sufficiency threshold (e.g., when the importance of the judgment task is enhanced; Darke et al., in press) or a decrease in one's level of actual confidence (e.g., when judgment-relevant information contradicts the judgmental implications of previously encountered heuristic-cue information; Maheswaran & Chaiken, 1991). Underlying this prediction is the assumption that perceivers generally believe that more processing will provide them with more confident judgments (Chaiken et al., 1989; Tordesillas & Chaiken, in press). When this self-efficacy expectation is not held, increasing the gap between actual and desired confidence will not necessarily instigate systematic processing (Bohner, Rank, Reinhard, Einwiller, & Erb, 1998).

It is important to keep in mind that the sufficiency principle is based on a judgmental *continuum*, which implies that varying degrees of heuristic and systematic processing may occur, corresponding to variations in the width of the confidence gap. And of course, as discussed above, heuristic and systematic processing depend not only on one's motivational concerns, but also on the availability, accessibility, and applicability of judgment-relevant heuristics, and on the availability of adequate cognitive resources, respectively.

Co-Occurrence of Heuristic and Systematic Processing

Although either processing mode may occur alone, our theory delineates specific and predictable ways in which heuristic and systematic processing may co-occur (Chaiken et al., 1989; cf. Petty & Cacioppo, 1986). Below we describe several different patterns of co-occurrence and point out situational, cognitive, and motivational factors that render one pattern more or less likely than another.

According to the heuristic–systematic model's *additivity hypothesis*, heuristic and systematic processing may exert independent and judgmentally consistent effects. Such additivity was shown in one study, in which participants were asked to make evaluations of a consumer product. When the judgmental implication of a "brand-name heuristic" was congruent with the judgmental implication of

attribute information about the product, participants who were led to believe that their product evaluations would be highly consequential based these evaluations on both their heuristic and systematic processing of the product information (Maheswaran, Mackie, & Chaiken, 1992; see also Chaiken & Maheswaran, 1994; Darke et al., in press; Maheswaran & Chaiken, 1991).

The model's *bias hypothesis* refers to the notion that the judgmental implications of heuristic cue information may establish expectancies about subsequently encountered judgment-relevant information, which may then bias the nature of more effortful systematic processing of this information. Such bias is most likely to occur in judgmental settings in which individuating judgment-relevant information is ambiguous and hence amenable to differential interpretation, or when no such information is provided but perceivers generate judgment-relevant cognitions of their own. Considerable support for the bias hypothesis exists (e.g., Chaiken & Maheswaran, 1994; Chen, Shechter, & Chaiken, 1996; Darke et al., in press; Erb, Bohner, Schmäelzle, & Rank, in press). For example, in one study, exposure to heuristic-cue information (i.e., source credibility) led participants who were told that their judgments would be highly consequential to systematically process ambiguous individuating information about the object of judgment in ways congruent with the judgmental implications of the source credibility information (Chaiken & Maheswaran, 1994). More specifically, participants exposed to the *high*-credibility heuristic cue elaborated upon the ambiguous information in more favorable ways than did those exposed to the *low*-credibility cue, presumably because high source credibility engendered favorable expectancies about the ambiguous individuating information. In turn, participants' biased systematic processing of this ambiguous information predicted their judgments about the object. In another study, which examined the impact of consensus information in the absence of persuasive arguments, college students for whom the issue (requiring comprehensive exams) was personally important generated thoughts that were favorable (vs. unfavorable) toward the issue when a sizable majority of their peers favored (vs. opposed) the issue, and these biased cognitions mediated their issue attitudes; in contrast, consensus information exerted a direct heuristic impact on the issue attitudes of participants for whom the issue was not personally relevant (Darke et al., in press).

Heuristic and systematic processing may also work in opposition—a proposition embodied in the model's *attenuation hypothesis*. For example, the judgmental implications derived from systematic processing may contradict and thus attenuate the judgmental impact of heuristic processing. Support for such a pattern of co-occurrence has been found in several studies (Chaiken & Maheswaran, 1994; Maheswaran & Chaiken, 1991; Maheswaran et al., 1992). For example, high-motivation participants in one study were presented with consensus-cue information that was either congruent or incongruent with the valence of individuating information about the object of judgment. When the judgmental implication derived from their heuristic processing of consensus-cue information was *in*congruent with that of their systematic processing of the individuating information, these highly motivated participants relied solely on their more effortful cognitions to determine their judgments (Maheswaran & Chaiken, 1991).

Our discussion of different patterns of co-occurrence is not exhaustive (for further discussion, including contrast/correction effects, see Bohner et al., 1995; Ruder, Bohner, & Erb, 1997; Ruder, Erb, & Bohner, 1996). Through the examples we have given, our intention has been to illustrate the *predictability* of the co-occurrence of heuristic and systematic processing. That is, just as knowledge of the characteristics of the perceiver and of the current judgmental setting permits predictions of when each processing mode is likely to occur alone, knowledge of these same parameters enables predictions regarding the co-occurrence of heuristic and systematic processing and its particular form. So, for example, situational factors such as the presence of heuristic-cue information—as well as its congruence with other available, judgment-relevant information—may largely determine the nature of perceivers' heuristic and systematic processing. Specifically, assuming adequate cognitive resources and relatively high levels of motivation, if the judgmental implication of heuristic-cue information is congruent with

that of other available judgment-relevant information, perceivers may well engage in heuristic *and* systematic processing in additive ways. In contrast, if the judgmental implication of the heuristic-cue information is incongruent with other available judgment-relevant information, perceivers' systematic processing is likely to attenuate the judgmental impact of the heuristic cue (but see Bohner et al., 1995). Alternatively, if perceivers have neither the cognitive resources nor the motivation to process systematically, whether heuristic-cue information is congruent or incongruent with other available judgment-relevant information will exert little if any impact on the nature of information processing. In both cases, perceivers are likely simply to engage in heuristic processing, resulting in judgments that directly reflect the judgmental implications of the heuristic-cue information.

The Multiple-Motive Framework

In discussing the motivational underpinnings of our model, we have focused so far on the implications of variations in the *level* or *amount* of motivation on heuristic and systematic processing. We have argued that higher levels of motivation correspond to larger discrepancies between actual and desired judgmental confidence (via higher sufficiency thresholds, reduced actual confidence, or both), and thus to an enhanced willingness to engage in systematic processing in the effort to reach these thresholds (however, see Note 2). What we have not yet addressed are variations in the *types* of motives that perceivers may have and the distinct impact that different motivations are likely to exert on information processing. Below we consider three broad motivations and the heuristic and systematic ways in which perceivers process information to satisfy each.

Accuracy Motivation

In developing the heuristic–systematic model, we (Chaiken, 1980, 1987; Chaiken, Giner-Sorolla, & Chen, 1996) originally assumed that perceivers are motivated to hold accurate attitudes and beliefs. Thus initial research on heuristic and systematic processing focused on judgmental contexts in which *accuracy motivation* was paramount. The hallmark of accuracy-motivated processing is a relatively open-minded and evenhanded treatment of judgment-relevant information.[3] When motivation is low, judgment-relevant information is scarce, or cognitive capacity is constrained, accuracy-motivated perceivers may simply base their attitudes on the heuristic-cue information that is seen as best suited for achieving their accuracy goals (e.g., "Length implies strength"). Given higher levels of motivation and sufficient cognitive resources, however, they may also engage in systematic forms of processing in the effort to reach their (often) heightened accuracy sufficiency thresholds. Considerable research conducted both within and beyond the heuristic–systematic framework supports the notion that accuracy motives can be satisfied by either more or less effortful cognition, or both (see Chaiken, Giner-Sorolla, & Chen, 1996; Chaiken et al., 1989; Chaiken, Wood, & Eagly, 1996; Chaiken & Stangor, 1987; Eagly & Chaiken, 1993; see also Petty & Wegener, 1998).

Recognizing that in many situations other motives may coexist with or even supplant accuracy goals, the heuristic–systematic model presently acknowledges two other broad motivations—namely, defense and impression motives (Chaiken, Giner-Sorolla, & Chen, 1996; see also Chaiken et al., 1989). Together, accuracy, defense, and impression motivations comprise the multiple-motive framework of the model. Although conceptually analogous motives have long existed in the literature (e.g., Festinger, 1957; Jones, 1990; Kunda, 1990; Smith, Bruner, & White, 1956; Tetlock, 1992), the heuristic–systematic model is distinct in its joint consideration of multiple motives on the one hand and multiple modes of processing on the other. In the same way that accuracy goals may be satisfied by either or both processing modes, the heuristic–systematic model suggests ways in which heuristic processing, systematic processing, or both can serve both defense and impression concerns.

Defense Motivation

Defense motivation refers to the desire to hold attitudes and beliefs that are congruent with one's perceived material interests or existing self-definitional attitudes and beliefs (Chaiken, Giner-Sorolla, & Chen, 1996). Self-definitional attitudes and beliefs are those closely tied to the self—for example, those involving one's values (e.g., equality), social identities (e.g., occupation), or personal attributes (e.g., intelligence). The defense-motivated perceiver aims to preserve the self-concept and associated world views, and thus processes information selectively—that is, in a way that best satisfies such defense concerns.

Defense motives may be addressed heuristically by the selective application of heuristics. For example, heuristics with judgmental implications that are congenial to the defense-motivated perceiver's existing attitudes and beliefs are particularly likely to be applied, while uncongenial heuristics are less likely to be invoked; indeed, they may be disparaged or entirely ignored. Thus defense-motivated perceivers can and do use the same heuristics that accuracy-motivated perceivers use, but they do so in a biased way. To illustrate, in one study, participants with and without a vested interest in the target issue were exposed to consensus heuristic-cue information in the form of poll results stating that the majority of students were opposed or in favor of the issue (Giner-Sorolla & Chaiken, 1997). Participants rated the poll as significantly more reliable, and criticized it significantly less, if its results supported their vested interest. Indeed, in the effort to protect their vested interests, these participants determined their attitudes on the issue primarily on the basis of their heuristic processing of the congenial consensus-cue information.

When defense motivation is high and cognitive resources are available, defense-motivated systematic processing is likely to emerge, characterized by effortful but biased scrutiny and evaluation of judgment-relevant information. Information that is congruent with one's existing attitudes and beliefs, such as research supporting one's position on abortion, will be judged more favorably than incongruent information will be (e.g., Lord, Ross, & Lepper, 1979; Pomerantz, Chaiken, & Tordesillas, 1995; Pyszczynski & Greenberg, 1987). In fact, incongruent information may be subjected to great scrutiny in a defense-motivated effort to derogate its validity (e.g., Ditto & Lopez, 1992; Giner-Sorolla & Chaiken, 1997; Liberman & Chaiken, 1992).

For example, participants in a study by Ditto and Lopez (1992) were told that a self-administered saliva test indicated either the presence or absence of an undesirable medical condition. Those who were diagnosed as having the condition were not only more likely to rate the test as less accurate and the condition as less serious, but were also more likely to spontaneously administer the test again, subjecting the threatening information to further inspection.

As with accuracy motivation, predictions for defense-motivated processing follow the sufficiency principle. However, unlike accuracy sufficiency thresholds, defensive sufficiency thresholds are determined not by whether processing yields a judgment that is accurate, but rather by whether processing yields a judgment that reinforces one's self-definitional attitudes and beliefs. Thus, whether defense motives engender heuristic processing, systematic processing, or some combination of the two depends on factors that influence perceivers' actual and desired levels of confidence that their judgments will address their defense concerns. For example, encountering heuristic-cue information that is incongenial to one's vested interests or cherished opinions may undermine the level of one's actual defensive confidence, triggering defense-motivated systematic processing in the effort to close a widened defensive confidence gap (assuming requisite cognitive resources). Congenial heuristic-cue information, on the other hand, can boost actual defensive confidence, narrowing the confidence gap and thus rendering effortful processing less likely (Giner-Sorolla & Chaiken, 1997).

Beyond the congeniality of judgment-relevant heuristic-cue information, the extent and nature of defense-motivated processing will reflect motivational factors, such as the centrality of one's threatened attitudes; situational factors, such as the presence of heuristic-cue information that pertains to defense goals; and cognitive factors, such as knowledge about the given judgmental domain, the possession of which may facilitate the derogation of threatening information (for further discussion of defense-motivated processing, see Chaiken, Giner-Sorolla, & Chen, 1996; Chaiken, Wood, & Eagly, 1996; Giner-Sorolla & Chaiken, 1997).

Impression Motivation

Impression motivation refers to the desire to hold attitudes and beliefs that will satisfy current social goals. Thus impression motives elicit a consideration of the interpersonal consequences of expressing a particular judgment in a given social context. Like defense-motivated processing, impression-motivated processing is marked by a selective bias. However, the selectivity of heuristic and systematic processing in the service of impression motivation is specifically aimed at satisfying immediate social goals, rather than at preserving existing self-definitional attitudes and beliefs (Chaiken, Giner-Sorolla, & Chen, 1996).

Impression-motivated heuristic processing entails the selective application of heuristics. For instance, the heuristic "Moderate opinions minimize disagreement" may be applied to serve the goal of having a smooth interaction with a person of unknown views. On the other hand, when others' opinions are known, the heuristic "Go along to get along" may be used to serve the same goal. With sufficient cognitive resources and higher levels of impression motivation, individuals may also process in more effortful but similarly selective ways. For example, an interviewee who is motivated not only to be well liked by his or her interviewer, but also to appear forceful, may systematically process information on an issue so as to be prepared to counterargue views in opposition to those of the interviewer.

As with accuracy and defense motivation, processing predictions for impression motivation are guided by the sufficiency principle. The impression sufficiency threshold is that point of processing at which perceivers feel sufficiently confident that their judgments will satisfy their interpersonal goals. Heuristic processing should confer sufficient judgmental confidence in situations that elicit minimal impression motivation, given correspondingly low impression sufficiency thresholds. When impression motivation is higher and sufficient cognitive ability and capacity exist, perceivers, in the effort to reach their heightened impression sufficiency thresholds, are likely to engage in systematic forms of processing that are biased toward achieving their social goals. Beyond factors that directly affect perceivers' actual and/or desired levels of confidence that their judgments will address their interpersonal concerns, the extent and nature of impression-motivated processing will of course depend on cognitive factors, such as perceivers' current cognitive capacity, as well as on situational factors, such as the presence of judgment-relevant heuristic-cue information.

Considerable evidence for impression-motivated heuristic and systematic processing exists (for a review, see Chaiken, Giner-Sorolla, & Chen, 1996). In one study, for example, participants anticipated a discussion about a social issue with an alleged partner who they were told held either a favorable or an unfavorable opinion on the discussion issue (Chen et al., 1996, Experiment 2). In an initial task that was ostensibly unrelated to the upcoming discussion, participants engaged in a task that primed either accuracy motivation or impression motivation. It was reasoned that either the accuracy goal to determine a valid attitude on the issue or the impression goal to get along with the partner was potentially relevant in the experimental discussion setting. The partner attitude information represented information that could be used as a basis for invoking an impression-motivated "Go along to get along" heuristic. After the priming task, participants were given an evaluatively balanced essay to read about the discussion issue so as to prepare for the upcoming discussion, and were then asked to list their thoughts while reading the essay and to indicate their attitudes on the issue.

Consistent with their validity concerns, accuracy-motivated participants based their attitudes on their evenhanded, systematic processing of the issue information—that is, processing that was unbiased by the partner attitude heuristic-cue information. In contrast, impression-motivated participants' systematic processing of the essay information was biased in a direction that was judgmentally consistent with the attitudes of their alleged partners, resulting in attitudes that were similarly biased. To serve the social goal of getting along with others, impression-motivated participants appeared to have selectively applied the "Go along to get along" heuristic on the basis of the partner attitude information, and the judgmental implications of this information biased the evaluative nature of their more

effortful systematic processing of issue-relevant information.

Multiple Motives

Although we have thus far discussed the multiple-motive framework of the heuristic–systematic model as if different motives operate in isolation from one another, we do not mean to preclude the possibility that more than one motive may be relevant in a given setting, or the possibility that at times perceivers may in fact be multiply motivated (e.g., Leippe & Elkin, 1987). Indeed, it is probably the case that in most everyday judgmental contexts, perceivers are *primarily* rather than *solely* accuracy-, defense-, or impression-motivated. Thus, we recognize that perceivers may at times engage in hybrid forms of motivated processing in their efforts to satisfy multiple goals. Greater attention needs to be directed at assessing the nature of heuristic and systematic processing in such ecologically meaningful settings in which several motives are potentially relevant, as well as the factors that may lead perceivers to engage in one form of motivated processing over another.

In the latter vein, recent research indicates that perceivers' transitory mood states may influence which motive is pursued in contexts in which multiple motives are potentially operative (Zuckerman & Chaiken, 1997). This work is noteworthy in several respects. First, it explicitly addresses the possibility that multiple motives may be relevant in a given judgmental context. Second, this work importantly extends the literature on mood's effects on information processing. Specifically, whereas most prior research on mood and information processing has simply focused on the impact of mood on the *amount* of cognitive processing that perceivers engage in (e.g., Mackie & Worth, 1989; Bless & Schwarz, Chapter 21, this volume), this research examines the impact of mood on *type* of processing—namely, type of *motivated* processing.

In one study in this research program, positive-mood and neutral-mood participants anticipated a discussion about a social issue with an alleged partner who they were led to believe held either a favorable or unfavorable opinion on the discussion issue (Zuckerman

& Chaiken, 1997, Experiment 2). As in prior work using this experimental paradigm, described above (Chen et al., 1996), it was reasoned that both accuracy motivation and impression motivation were possibly relevant in the discussion context set up in this paradigm. Unlike most research on mood's effects on information processing, this research did not simply focus on the impact of mood on the amount of processing of judgment-relevant information. Rather, the central hypothesis of this study was that mood would influence whether impression or accuracy motives would be primarily operative, and thus whether participants would primarily engage in impression- or accuracy-motivated processing.

Evidence consistent with this hypothesis was in fact found. Neutral-mood participants in this study processed information in a way suggesting that they were primarily impression-motivated—namely, concerned with getting along with their discussion partner. Specifically, they appear to have invoked the "Go along to get along" heuristic on the basis of the partner attitude information, resulting in attitudes that directly reflected their anticipated partner's opinion on the issue. Positive-mood participants, on the other hand, were relatively more accuracy-motivated, in that their attitudes were unaffected by the partner attitude information. These individuals based their attitudes solely on the thoughts that they generated in response to an essay containing issue-relevant information. Presumably, positive mood instilled these participants with the interpersonal confidence necessary to focus less on determining an attitude that would facilitate getting along with the anticipated discussion partner, and more on determining an attitude that would be backed by a fairly systematic assessment of issue-relevant information (Zuckerman & Chaiken, 1997).

To summarize, we have used the multiple-motive framework of our model to examine the heuristic and systematic ways that perceivers process judgment-relevant information in an effort to satisfy their current goals. We and others have found this framework to be useful within as well as beyond the validity-seeking persuasion context in which the heuristic–systematic model was originally conceived (e.g., Bodenhausen, Macrae, & Sherman, Chapter 13, this vol-

ume; Smith, 1994; Thompson, Roman, Moskowitz, Chaiken, & Bargh, 1994; for a recent review, see Chaiken, Giner-Sorolla, & Chen, 1996). Before we conclude our discussion of this framework, it is important to note that although we view heuristic and systematic processing as directed toward satisfying particular goals, we do not mean to imply that perceivers are necessarily aware of their motives, or of the biases that they might exert on their information processing. In fact, recent trends in the literature on attitudes and social cognition are leading to an increased appreciation of the power of motives to guide thought and behavior without perceivers' conscious knowledge of such influences (e.g., Bargh, Chapter 18, this volume; Bargh & Barndollar, 1996). We return to the issue of the conscious versus unconscious nature of motivated heuristic and systematic processing in a later section.

Relations to Other Models of Social Judgment

As evidenced by the contributions to this book, the heuristic–systematic model is one of a growing family of dual-process theories in the literature on attitudes and social cognition (e.g., Fiske, Lin, & Neuberg, Chapter 11, this volume; Petty & Wegener, Chapter 3, this volume; Brewer & Harasty, Chapter 12, this volume) as well as in other areas of psychology (e.g., Epstein & Pacini, Chapter 23, this volume; Sloman, 1996; Smith & DeCoster, Chapter 16, this volume). As such, it is worthwhile to briefly point out some of the similarities and differences between our formulation and some of these other models (see also Chaiken, Wood, & Eagly, 1996; Eagly & Chaiken, 1993; Smith & DeCoster, Chapter 16, this volume).

Dual-process theories vary in how widely they have been applied, although they often focus on a single domain such as persuasion (e.g., Petty & Cacioppo, 1986) or impression formation (e.g., Fiske & Neuberg, 1990; see also Bodenhausen et al., Chapter 13, this volume). Despite these variations, dual-process models converge in the recognition that social judgments are not always formed on the basis of relatively effortful processing of judgment-relevant information; rather, judgments may also be formed on the basis of relatively low-effort processing of more peripheral forms of information (e.g., heuristic-cue information). Furthermore, the hallmark of any dual-process approach is the attempt to specify cognitive and motivational factors that determine when judgments are likely to be mediated by each of these processing modes. At this level of specification, predictions across dual-process theories are often quite similar.

Among these approaches, the heuristic–systematic model is perhaps most closely allied with the elaboration likelihood model (ELM; Petty & Cacioppo, 1981, 1986; Petty & Wegener, Chapter 3, this volume). To touch briefly on some of the similarities between the two models, we point out that both maintain that "central" or "systematic" processing requires capacity and motivation, whereas "peripheral" or "heuristic" processing may occur with little of either. Both make least-effort assumptions; that is, they assume that perceivers tend to process information minimally unless they are motivated to do otherwise. Both acknowledge the potential influence of motivational factors (e.g., personal relevance) and of cognitive factors (e.g., time constraints). Nonetheless, the models diverge in several important respects, among them the degree to which the two processing modes are thought to be exclusive, and the ways in which motivational influences on processing are thought to operate. The ELM assumes that as motivation, ability for argument scrutiny, or both increase, peripheral mechanisms become less important determinants of attitude judgment. In contrast, the heuristic–systematic model explicitly assumes that its two modes may co-occur and that both heuristic and systematic processing can have an impact on judgment when motivation and ability for argument scrutiny are high. In terms of motivational biases, the ELM makes the overarching assumption that perceivers are accuracy-motivated and that the level of this motivation may vary, resulting in corresponding levels of elaboration likelihood. Motives other than accuracy are discussed in the model, however, and can exert a biasing effect on judgment via either peripheral-route or central-route mechanisms. For example, impression-motivated concerns may make social cues in the environment more salient, triggering reliance on some relevant peripheral mechanism as a basis for one's judgment (see

Chaiken, Wood, & Eagly, 1996; Petty & Wegener, Chapter 3, this volume). In contrast, as discussed earlier, our recent multiple-motive formulation of the heuristic–systematic model makes no overriding motivational assumptions; moreover, it treats motive type and processing mode as orthogonal dimensions. As such, we assume that any given motive can influence heuristic processing, systematic processing, or both. More extensive discussions of the similarities and differences of these two models appear elsewhere (see Eagly & Chaiken, 1993; Chaiken, Wood, & Eagly, 1996).

Our model also has much in common with dual-process approaches such as Fiske's (Fiske et al., Chapter 11, this volume), Brewer's (Brewer & Harasty, Chapter 12, this volume), and Bodenhausen's (Bodenhausen et al., Chapter 13, this volume)—all of which focus on the domain of person perception, especially the important issue of stereotyping. Category-based processing in these models, for example, involves making a simple inference about a particular target person's character, based on his or her group category membership. Such processing can easily be seen as an example of heuristic processing. For example, when a female target is regarded as "unassertive" simply on the basis of her womanhood (i.e., without scrutiny of individuating information), perceivers are essentially employing the heuristic or stereotype "Women are unassertive." Similarly, what these models refer to as "individuated" processing is essentially the same as our model's notion of systematic processing. Indeed, we have elsewhere argued for the applicability of the heuristic–systematic model to impression formation and other domains outside the persuasion area in which it was originally developed (e.g., decision making—Tordesillas & Chaiken, in press; see also Smith & DeCoster, Chapter 16, this volume).

On the whole, dual-process approaches have had a large impact on theory and research in the domain of attitudes and social cognition, as evidenced not only by the large number of models grounded in dual-process logic, but also by the considerable degree of compatibility among them. We briefly acknowledge, however, that a single-process alternative to our dual-process approach has been offered (Kruglanski, Thompson, &

Spiegel, Chapter 14, this volume; see also Kunda, Chapter 15, this volume). This "unimodel" perspective contends that forming a judgment on the basis of either heuristic or systematic processing reflects the same underlying process. Specifically, it argues that both processing modes involve linking evidence with a particular conclusion in an "if–then" fashion. Certainly we agree that heuristic processing involves "if–then" associations; indeed, a heuristic may be defined *as* an "if–then" linkage. We do not, however, view systematic processing solely in "if–then" terms. Although we would agree that systematic processing may involve recognizing "if–then" linkages between pieces of evidence and the conclusions they allow, none of these conclusions in and of itself constitutes the overriding judgment toward which a perceiver is processing. Forming a judgment on the basis of systematic processing, then, may involve integrating multiple "if–then" associations with other available judgment-relevant information. Although we have yet to specify the precise nature of such integration processes, we believe that conceptualizing heuristic and systematic processing in terms as abstract as "if–then" associations obscures fundamental differences in the nature of the two processing modes. Given the current state of evidence, the distinctions that dual-process theories draw between processing modes allow a level of predictive specificity whose value seems to outweigh that of the presumed parsimony offered by a single-process approach (see also Bodenhausen et al., Chapter 13, and Smith & DeCoster, Chapter 16, this volume).

THE AVAILABILITY, ACCESSIBILITY, AND APPLICABILITY OF HEURISTICS

"Heuristics" have been defined as learned, declarative or procedural knowledge structures stored in memory (e.g., Chaiken et al., 1989). To begin examining the heuristic–systematic model in its broader context, we elaborate on this definition by considering how the heuristic mode of processing relates to social-cognitive work on the principles that underlie the activation and use of stored knowledge. We first briefly discuss availability and accessibility principles, both of which have been previously discussed vis-à-vis heuristic pro-

cessing (see Chaiken et al., 1989). We then consider applicability in particular detail, given the relatively little attention that has been given to this principle in earlier work both within and beyond the heuristic–systematic model.

The Role of Availability and Accessibility in Heuristic Processing

A heuristic's "availability" refers to whether or not the knowledge structure is stored in memory. Heuristic processing can only occur if judgment-relevant heuristics are available in memory for retrieval and use. In existing research in which the judgmental impact of heuristic processing has been assessed, it has been widely assumed that all participants have the focal heuristic stored in memory. The availability of a judgment-relevant heuristic, however, does not guarantee its use in a given judgmental context; an available heuristic must also be "accessible." "Accessibility" refers to the activation potential of stored knowledge (e.g., Higgins, 1989). In order for stored knowledge to exert an impact on processing and judgment, its activation potential must exceed a certain threshold level, above which the knowledge is ready for use. As with any other knowledge structure, the activation potential of a heuristic will vary as a function of factors that can be internal and/or external to the perceiver (e.g., Higgins, King, & Mavin, 1982; Higgins, Rholes, & Jones, 1977). For example, frequent use of a heuristic is likely to result in the chronic accessibility of the heuristic, or the chronic readiness of the heuristic to be used. Such chronic accessibility is an internal source of activation potential. Salient cues in the current judgmental context that are relevant to a stored heuristic are potential external sources of the accessibility of the heuristic (see Chaiken, Axsom, Liberman & Wilson, 1992; Eagly & Chaiken, 1993, Ch. 7).

Accessibility's role in instigating the heuristic mode of processing is of particular interest, in part because it may carry some important implications for the likelihood of *systematic* forms of processing. Specifically, the accessibility of a heuristic may not simply correspond to the likelihood of its use, but may also affect the confidence with which a judgment determined on the basis of the heuristic is held. In turn, of course, judgmental confidence affects the likelihood of systematic processing, such that increasing confidence generally decreases perceivers' motivation to engage in more effortful forms of cognition—a prediction that follows directly from the heuristic–systematic model's sufficiency principle, discussed earlier. In other words, the ease with which a heuristic comes to mind may heighten a perceiver's confidence in the judgment implied by the heuristic, lowering the need to process further to attain a sufficient level of judgmental confidence (see also Giner-Sorolla & Chaiken, 1997).

Linking the accessibility of heuristics to judgmental confidence also implies that different heuristics may confer differential amounts of judgmental confidence, leaving room for differences both within and between perceivers. Thus, for example, the differential ease with which a domain-relevant heuristic is accessed by experts versus novices in the domain may correspond to differences not only in the likelihood that the heuristic will be used, but also in the confidence with which the judgment implied by the heuristic is held. Overall, these possibilities imply that a heuristic may exert a judgmental impact in at least two ways: the first having to do with the judgmental implication of the heuristic, and the second having to do with the judgmental confidence that the heuristic may confer by virtue of the ease with which it is accessed from memory. Indeed, the judgmental impact of ease in retrieving a heuristic may itself reflect the activation and application of a stored heuristic rule delineating the judgmental implications of such ease-of-retrieval experiences—a possibility we explore in subsequent sections.

The Role of Applicability in Heuristic Processing

Beyond availability and accessibility, a heuristic will only exert a judgmental impact to the extent that it is applicable to the current judgmental task or domain. "Applicability" refers to the relevance or appropriateness of stored knowledge to a given judgmental task, and it exists at both nonconscious and conscious levels (e.g., Hardin & Rothman, 1997; Higgins, 1989, 1996). In nonconscious form, applicability refers to the activation arising from "matches," or overlap, between a stimulus event and some stored knowledge construct; the activation level of the stored construct (e.g., a trait concept, a heuristic) increases to the extent that there is greater overlap between features of the construct and features of the stimuli at hand. In its more conscious form, perceived applicability, or "judged usability" (Higgins, 1996), refers to the conscious process of perceivers' deciding whether it is appropriate to use activated mental constructs as guides to judgment. Although applicability has been much less thoroughly examined than either availability or accessibility principles, recognition of its importance is on the rise (e.g., Bargh, 1997; Hardin & Rothman, 1997; Higgins, 1996; Leyens, Yzerbyt, & Corneille, 1996; Smith, 1990). Indeed, research has demonstrated that stored knowledge may be differentially applicable across judgmental tasks, although this work has focused mainly on the applicability of stored trait constructs (e.g., Higgins & Brendl, 1995; Higgins et al., 1977).

What determines the applicability of a stored heuristic? The applicability of a heuristic to a judgmental task is based in part on the degree to which the heuristic somehow "matches" features of the task (e.g., Higgins, 1989, 1996). For instance, the applicability of the heuristic "Experts' statements can be trusted" to the task of expressing one's attitude on capital punishment on the basis of a highly reputable newspaper article on the issue is relatively high, given the "match" between the heuristic and the article's source expertise features. In comparison, the applicability of the heuristic "Consensus opinions are correct" to the same task is likely to be considerably lower.

Beyond the amount of "match" between a heuristic and aspects of a judgmental task, the degree to which a heuristic is applicable to a task is also determined by the extent to which it has been activated and used for the particular task in the past. Specifically, the applicability of a heuristic to a task should increase with its repeated activation and use for that task. This implies an increase in the likelihood and speed with which the heuristic will be brought to bear on the same task in the future. Such facilitation in processing has been referred to as a "specific-practice effect," and

reflects the formation of a mental linkage between the heuristic and the particular task
(e.g., Smith, 1990, 1994; see also Anderson,
1983, 1987; Higgins, 1989, 1996; Wyer &
Srull, 1986). Unlike a "general-practice effect," which refers simply to an across-the-
board increase in the accessibility of a heuristic with increasing use, a specific-practice effect refers to an increase in the likelihood of
heuristic processing specifically for the task in
which the heuristic was previously "practiced" (i.e., activated and used).

Finally, over and above degree of match
and degree of previous usage in a particular
task, whether a heuristic is applied to a judgment task depends also on its judged usability
in the task. In previous work, we have used the
term "perceived reliability" to refer to this
more conscious type of applicability (e.g.,
Darke et al., in press). We have argued, for example, that some heuristics (e.g., "Experts'
statements can be trusted") may be generally
perceived as more reliable or more valid guides
to judgment than other heuristics (e.g., "Likable people say agreeable things"). Moreover,
situational factors may affect the perceived reliability of heuristics, and perceivers may differ
chronically in the degree of reliability they attribute to different heuristics (see Chaiken et
al., 1989; Darke et al., in press; Eagly &
Chaiken, 1993, Ch. 7). Overall, applicability
principles are clearly relevant to understanding
how the heuristic mode operates, in that the
likelihood of heuristic processing is in part determined by the nature and strength of associations between particular heuristics and particular judgmental tasks or domains.

*Applicability-Based Predictions Regarding
Heuristic Processing*

Only a few studies have explicitly recognized
the potential role of such stored linkages between particular heuristics and particular
tasks or domains (e.g., Chaiken et al., 1992;
Darke et al., in press; Roskos-Ewoldsen &
Fazio, 1992; Rothman & Hardin, 1997). For
example, Chaiken et al. (1992) examined individual differences in the perceived reliability
of the "Length equals strength" heuristic, and
found that high-reliability participants applied this rule in evaluating a (long vs. short)
persuasive message, if this rule had been made
temporarily accessible (via a prior priming

task). Regardless of its temporary accessibility, however, the length–strength rule had no
impact on judgments made by participants
who regarded this rule as low in reliability or
judged usability. More recently, Darke et al.
(in press) found that participants for whom
an issue was low in personal relevance (i.e.,
who were unmotivated for systematic processing) used the "Consensus implies correctness" heuristic in forming their issue attitudes, even when the sample size upon which
consensus information was based (a poll of
student peers) was very small (vs. very large).
More interestingly, high-personal-relevance
participants also used the consensus heuristic,
but only when sample size was large; presumably, these participants doubted the reliability
of consensus information when it was based
on only a small number of observations.

In most previous work, however, the
heuristics that have been examined have typically been ones that researchers assumed to be
fairly comparable across research participants
in terms of their availability, accessibility, and
applicability (although see Chaiken et al.,
1992; Roskos-Ewoldsen & Fazio, 1992). For
example, research on the heuristic "Experts'
statements can be trusted" has generally made
the assumption that most individuals have
this heuristic available in memory, and that
neither the accessibility nor the applicability
of the heuristic varies substantially across individuals (e.g., Chaiken & Maheswaran,
1994). Thus variations in the likelihood of
heuristic processing that are attributable to
characteristics of the heuristics and their relation to the particular judgmental task in question have not been widely considered. Yet, as
implied above, one way to conceptualize the
impact of different variables on the likelihood
of heuristic processing is in terms of differences in the stored associations that exist in
memory between particular heuristics and
particular judgmental tasks or domains.
Heuristics may be differentially applicable for
different tasks and for different individuals,
depending on the nature and extent of prior
processing in these tasks and among these individuals, respectively. What this implies is
that knowing which associations are likely to
be most accessible and applicable in a given
judgmental context, and for whom this is
more and less likely to be the case, may substantially enhance the predictability of heuristic processing.

To illustrate, the impact that knowledge-ability about an attitudinal issue may have on processing and judgment may not simply reflect differences in the issue-relevant knowledge that high- versus low-knowledge individuals possess (e.g., Biek, Wood, & Chaiken, 1996; Wood, Rhodes, & Biek, 1995). This impact may also reflect differences in the nature and strength of the heuristics that high-versus low-knowledge individuals typically perceive as appropriate to use in domains in which personal views on the attitudinal issue are relevant. In other words, individuals high versus low in knowledge about an issue may differ not only in the number and types of heuristics they are likely to have available and accessible, but also in the applicability of these heuristics—that is, in the heuristics that they are most likely to bring to bear on similar judgmental tasks involving the attitudinal issue. Thus, for example, the applicability of the heuristic "Consensus opinions are correct" to the task of expressing a judgment on recent policies on affirmative action may be substantially higher among individuals who do not possess very much knowledge about this issue than among those who are highly knowledgeable about it.

Applicability's Role in Motivated Heuristic Processing

The idea that associations may exist between particular heuristics and particular judgmental tasks also has direct implications for *motivated* forms of heuristic processing. For example, each time a Republican is asked for his or her opinion regarding allegedly questionable Republican campaign finance practices, defense motives may be triggered that then bias his or her processing of judgment-relevant information. As discussed earlier, such motives are likely to produce selectivity in the heuristics that the Republican chooses to invoke; judgment-relevant heuristics that support his or her existing beliefs and attitudes are more likely to be applied than heuristics that threaten these beliefs and attitudes. Repeated, motivated use of these heuristics in similar judgment tasks should result in an across-the-board increase in the likelihood and speed of such motivated heuristic processing, as well as an increase that is specific to future judgmental tasks involving

such campaign finance issues. On a more conscious level, people may judge a particular heuristic as a more reliable or less reliable guide to judgment, depending on whether its judgmental implications are congenial or incongenial to their overarching defense or impression goals (Giner-Sorolla & Chaiken, 1997).

The applicability concept is thus readily incorporated into the multiple-motive heuristic–systematic model. In fact, integrating this concept may offer a novel way to conceptualize classic functional theories of attitudes (e.g., Katz, 1960; Smith et al., 1956; for a recent review, see Eagly & Chaiken, 1998), by which our model's multiple-motive framework was in part inspired. Functional approaches contend that attitudes serve specific functions or motives. For instance, a person's proabortion attitude may serve a value-expressive function, insofar as it reflects his or her value-laden belief that people should have the right to choose. Although some contemporary work has addressed the information-processing implications of attitude functions (e.g., DeBono, 1987; Snyder & DeBono, 1987), explicit consideration of applicability in conjunction with the motivated use of heuristics helps to forge clearer connections. That is, particular forms of motivated heuristic processing may be part of what constitutes and what maintains the functional underpinnings of an attitude. Interestingly, this may be especially true in judgment settings in which perceivers are not particularly motivated or are in some way capacity-constrained. For example, an attitude that serves a value-expressive function may be one that is backed not simply by a value-expressive goal, but also by stored attitude-specific heuristics that are distinctly aimed at preserving consistency between one's attitude and one's cherished values (see also Giner-Sorolla & Chaiken, 1997).

CONSCIOUS VERSUS UNCONSCIOUS HEURISTIC AND SYSTEMATIC PROCESSING

So far, we have considered how the heuristic–systematic model relates to social-cognitive work on the principles that determine when stored knowledge will be activated and used. We now examine how heuristic and systematic modes of processing relate to another rapidly growing area of social-cognitive inquiry—namely, theorizing and research on conscious versus unconscious processes (e.g., Bargh, 1989, 1994, and Chapter 18, this volume; Greenwald & Banaji, 1995; Uleman & Bargh, 1989).

In previous work, we have generally assumed that systematic processing involves conscious processes, whereas heuristic processing, given its less resource-demanding nature, involves either conscious or unconscious processes (Chaiken et al., 1989). We continue to make these assumptions, but we try here to specify more clearly what is meant by the conscious versus unconscious nature of each processing mode. We then focus on the idea that heuristics may be unconsciously activated and used by examining how the heuristic mode of processing is related to research on the judgmental impact of subjective experiences (for a recent review, see Schwarz & Clore, 1996). Specifically, we argue that the judgmental impact of subjective experiences reflects the activation and application of stored heuristics that pertain distinctly to these experiences, and contend that such forms of heuristic processing are especially likely to occur unconsciously. Throughout, we consider some of the broader implications of our view of subjective experiences.

Conscious and Unconscious Systematic Processing

Systematic processing is resource-demanding by definition, as it requires cognitive effort and capacity, and entails intentionally and controllably attending to judgment-relevant information. In these senses, systematic processing is appropriately characterized as conscious (see Bargh, 1994). However, awareness is another dimension along which a mental process can be judged as conscious or unconscious. Although perceivers are clearly aware when they are systematically processing information, they are by no means necessarily aware of the precise form of this processing, or of the factors that may influence it. For instance, perceivers may seldom be aware of the potential biasing impact of heuristic processing on their systematic processing. Beyond this, perceivers may also frequently lack awareness of the motivational biases that color the evaluative nature of their systematic

processing. Take, for example, the defense-motivated perceiver. Such persons are unlikely to be aware of their selectivity in processing threatening self-relevant information, experiencing instead an "illusion of objectivity" (Taylor, 1991; see also Chaiken, Giner-Sorolla, & Chen, 1996). Indeed, in many cases, processing biases are likely to be ones that perceivers would exert effort to counteract if they were aware of them.

Conscious and Unconscious Heuristic Processing

So far, theory and research on heuristic processing have focused on examining the judgmental impact of heuristics that are presumably activated by the heuristic-cue information available in a given judgmental setting. For instance, research participants may be presented with consensus-cue information, along with other judgment-relevant information, and their use of the heuristic "Consensus opinions are correct" in the judgmental task is then assessed. Although the processing of such heuristic cues is typically less resource-demanding than systematic processing, such forms of heuristic processing nonetheless involve perceivers' awareness of the heuristic-cue information. To the extent that perceivers attend to and are cognizant of the judgmental implications of heuristic-cue information, and judge the information as relevant to the judgmental task at hand, heuristic processing should be characterized as conscious. Indeed, heuristic-cue information (e.g., information about source credibility) may at times be attended to precisely because a perceiver consciously judges it as not only appropriate, but also highly informative, to use in the current judgmental task (e.g., Darke et al., in press).

As with systematic processing, however, there are various dimensions along which heuristic processing can be considered conscious or unconscious. We focus again on the awareness dimension. Although heuristic processing entails, minimally, an awareness of a heuristic cue in the environment, this does not imply that perceivers are necessarily aware of the activation of a corresponding heuristic that occurs as a result of encountering this information, or of their application of this rule to their current judgmental task. The distinction between awareness of heuristic-cue information and awareness of its role in triggering the use of a relevant heuristic stored in memory is analogous to the distinction drawn in the priming literature between awareness of a priming stimulus and awareness of its potential judgmental influence (e.g., Bargh, 1992). To the extent that perceivers are unaware of the ways in which stimulus information of which they are aware influences their processing, heuristic processing may be deemed unconscious.

Indeed, often the nature of heuristic-cue information would be judged irrelevant, if not inappropriate, for use if perceivers *were* aware of its potential judgmental impact. For example, perceivers may at times be vigilant and weary of the potential judgmental influence of stereotype-based heuristic-cue information. In this regard, contrast effects have been discussed within the framework of the heuristic–systematic model (e.g., Bohner et al., 1995; Ruder et al., 1997). Within the model, the "contrast hypothesis" refers to the possibility that the judgmental implications of heuristic-cue information may at times lead to contrasting, or precisely opposite, judgmental effects. This may occur when perceivers are aware of both the heuristic-cue information *and* its potential judgmental impact, and are motivated and have the capacity to "correct" for this biasing effect (see also Lombardi, Higgins, & Bargh, 1987; Martin, Seta, & Crelia, 1990; for reviews of contrast phenomena, see Higgins, 1996; Strack & Hannover, 1996).[4] The idea that avoiding the judgmental influence of heuristic-cue information requires effort and an awareness of the nature of the influence is consistent with the possibility that perceivers may at times use heuristic-cue information in judgmentally consistent ways, in the absence of an awareness of having done so.

Although heuristic processing often occurs on the basis of the heuristic-cue information that is available in a given judgmental context, heuristic processing may also be triggered by *internal* sources of information, such as one's own attitudes (e.g., Giner-Sorolla, Lutz, & Chaiken, 1998)—and, of particular interest here, perceivers' subjective experiences. For example, current mood states or the fluency with which information is processed may serve as heuristic-cue information.

Relative to external sources of heuristic-cue information, such internal sources may be more likely to trigger heuristic processing that is unconscious in nature. In other words, perceivers may be especially likely to be unaware of their subjective experiences as a source of judgment-relevant information, and thus to be unaware of the nature of the influence of these experiences on their processing and judgments.

Conceptualizing the Judgmental Impact of Subjective Experiences as Heuristic Processing

In our view, in order for a subjective experience to exert a judgmental impact, perceivers must possess some knowledge or a "theory" about what the experience implies judgmentally. That is, they must have previously learned judgment rules or heuristics stored in memory that link specific subjective experiences with specific judgmental implications. Although this assumption has been made, implicitly or explicitly, in prior work on subjective experiences (see Schwarz & Clore, 1996), its implications have not been extensively considered.

Schwarz and Clore (1996) have distinguished subjective experiences associated with affective states from those associated with cognitive states. We focus on cognitive states, or subjective experiences that pertain to perceivers' current state of knowledge (see also Clore & Parrott, 1991). Relative to work on affective states, such as those associated with moods and emotions, less work has addressed the idea that the judgmental impact of "cognitive feelings" may reflect the activation and use of heuristics that specify the judgmental implications of such subjective experiences of knowing. Indeed, considerable research conducted both within and beyond the framework of the heuristic–systematic model has conceptualized mood states in heuristic terms (see Bless & Schwarz, Chapter 21, this volume; Bohner et al., 1995; Chaiken, Wood, & Eagly, 1996; Schwarz, 1990; Schwarz & Clore, 1996). To flesh out our view of subjective experiences as reflecting heuristic processing, we focus on two cognitive experiences: the experienced ease of retrieving knowledge from memory, and the familiarity experienced upon encountering previously seen stimulus information.

Ease-of-Retrieval Experiences

Research examining the judgmental impact of perceivers' ease-of-retrieval experiences has grown steadily (e.g., Schwarz et al., 1991; Rothman & Hardin, 1997; Rothman & Schwarz, 1998; Wanke, Bless, & Biller, 1996; Zimmerman & Chaiken, 1994). In this work, research participants are typically induced to experience either ease or difficulty in retrieving knowledge required for an experimental task, and the degree to which participants (mis)attribute their subjective experience of ease of retrieval to an object of judgment rather than to the task serves as the primary dependent measure. For example, in the Schwarz et al. (1991) studies, participants were asked to recall either 6 or 12 examples of their own past assertive or unassertive behaviors, and were then asked to make self-assessments of assertiveness or unassertiveness. The self-assessments of those who were asked to recall 6 such behaviors were higher than of those who were asked to recall 12 behaviors. These findings were interpreted as reflecting participants' misattribution of their experienced ease in retrieving 6 versus 12 examples of assertive or unassertive behaviors to their degree of assertiveness or unassertiveness. Other researchers have produced conceptually analogous effects, demonstrating, for example, the misattribution of the experienced ease of retrieving arguments in favor of or against a social issue to the favorability or unfavorability of one's attitude on the issue (Wanke et al., 1996; Zimmerman & Chaiken, 1994).

Familiarity Experiences

Considerable social-psychological research examining the judgmental impact of familiarity experiences also exists (see Schwarz & Clore, 1996). In this work, familiarity experiences are typically induced by exposing participants to judgment-relevant stimulus information that they have previously seen. The extent to which participants misattribute such familiarity experiences to some aspect of the object of judgment is the primary focus of this research. In one study, for example, participants who had been exposed to a list consisting entirely of nonfamous names misattributed the familiarity they experienced upon seeing the names again 24 hours later to their fame (Jacoby, Kelley, Brown, & Jasechko, 1989). The same "famous-name" paradigm has also been used in research on implicit gender stereotyping (Banaji & Greenwald, 1995). In this work, a gender bias was found in the tendency for participants to misattribute their familiarity experiences upon encountering previously seen nonfamous names to fame. Specifically, previously seen, nonfamous male names were more likely to be judged famous than were similarly familiar, nonfamous female names.

Familiarity effects have also been discussed in other domains. For instance, mere-exposure effects have been interpreted in terms of the misattribution of familiarity experiences (e.g., Bornstein & D'Agostino, 1994; Chaiken, Wood, & Eagly, 1996). Specifically, mere exposure to an attitude object may result in enhanced liking of the object, due to perceivers' misattribution of the familiarity they experience upon reencountering the object to their liking of it. As another example, research on the effects of prior exposure to trivia information on perceivers' perceptions of the validity of this information can similarly be construed in terms of the judgmental impact of familiarity experiences. This research has demonstrated that earlier exposure to trivia statements enhances perceptions of the validity of these statements upon reexposure (e.g., Arkes, Boehm, & Xu, 1991; Begg, Armour, & Kerr, 1985; Hasher, Goldstein, & Toppino, 1977). In our view, the results of this research can be readily interpreted in terms of the misattribution of familiarity experiences to statement validity.

Subjective Experiences as Heuristic-Cue Information

What is common to each of the ease-of-retrieval and familiarity effects discussed above is the need to make the assumption that participants somehow associated their subjective experiences with specific judgmental implications. In the Schwarz et al. (1991) research, participants must have linked their ease of retrieving behavioral exemplars of assertiveness or unassertiveness with the degree to which they were assertive or unassertive.

For example, they may have invoked the "theory" that the ease of coming up with instances of assertive behavior implied that there were many such instances, and therefore that they were relatively assertive persons. In the Jacoby et al. (1989) work, participants must have somehow associated familiarity with fame, perhaps by calling upon the explanation that the familiarity of the names was a product of their fame. Thus, as argued earlier, each of these demonstrations of the judgmental impact of a subjective experience implies the existence of a "theory"—essentially, a heuristic—that delineates the judgmental implications of the experience. In our view, then, subjective experiences may serve as heuristic-cue information. So, just as externally provided information (e.g., consensus information, gender information) may trigger the retrieval and use of a heuristic stored in memory (e.g., "Consensus implies correctness," "Women are unassertive"), so too may subjective experiences trigger the activation and application of relevant stored heuristics.

Implications of Viewing the Judgmental Impact of Subjective Experiences as Heuristic Processing

Conceptualizing the impact of subjective experiences on judgment in terms of the activation and use of stored "theories" or heuristics carries implications for several aspects of heuristic and systematic modes of processing. We consider some of these here. Specifically, we discuss the implications for the conscious versus unconscious nature of heuristic and systematic processing, for the predictability of heuristic processing based on subjective experiences, and for perceivers' judgmental confidence.

Conscious and Unconscious Heuristic and Systematic Processing Revisited

As should be apparent from the examples given above, existing demonstrations of the judgmental impact of subjective experiences have generally relied on a misattribution logic: Research participants are experimentally induced to have a particular subjective experience, and are then expected to (incorrectly) attribute the experience to some feature of the object of judgment, rather than to the features of the experimental setting that

actually produced it (e.g., Schwarz et al., 1991; Jacoby et al., 1989). At times, however, the correct attribution for the subjective experience is made salient to participants (Schwarz & Clore, 1983), or the informativeness of the subjective experience is called into question (e.g., Schwarz et al., 1991), producing an absence or reversal of the judgmental impact of the subjective experience. The underlying logic of such paradigms implies, then, that to the extent that perceivers (mis)attribute their subjective experiences to aspects of the object of judgment, it is likely that such experiences exert their judgmental impact outside of awareness. It is in this way that interpreting such effects in terms of the use of stored heuristics supports the notion that particular forms of heuristic processing often occur unconsciously—namely, those triggered by subjective experiences.

We note, however, that existing demonstrations of the judgmental impact of subjective experiences vary in terms of the degree to which they represent solid evidence for the unconscious nature of these effects. In research based on the Jacoby et al. (1989) paradigm, the judgmental impact of familiarity is properly deemed unconscious, in that in this paradigm the judgmental influence of conscious processes opposes that of unconscious processes (see also Jacoby, Toth, Lindsay, & Debner, 1992). Thus, to the extent that the effects of the predicted unconscious process emerge—despite the opposing conscious process—one can be fairly certain that the intended unconscious influence did in fact occur unconsciously. For example, in Jacoby et al.'s (1989) famous-name studies, participants were told that if they could consciously recall having seen a name earlier, they could be sure that the name was part of the list of nonfamous names to which they had been previously exposed. In direct opposition to the influence of conscious recollection on participants' fame judgments was the impact of the familiarity experienced upon encountering previously seen nonfamous names—namely, inferring fame from familiarity. The oppositional nature of this paradigm substantiates the claim that the impact of the subjective experience of familiarity on participants' fame judgments occurred unconsciously.

Research on mere-exposure effects also suggests that the impact of familiarity experiences may occur unconsciously, in that the impact of prior stimulus exposure on liking judgments for the stimuli has been shown to occur even (indeed, particularly) when the initial stimulus exposure is subliminal in nature (e.g., Bornstein, 1989; Bornstein & D'Agostino, 1992; see Chaiken, Wood, & Eagly, 1996, for a related discussion). In comparison, however, research on ease-of-retrieval experiences speaks less definitively to the unconscious–conscious distinction. In this work, the judgmental implications of conscious versus unconscious processes are not typically placed in direct opposition to each other (e.g., Rothman & Hardin, 1998; Schwarz et al., 1991; Zimmerman & Chaiken, 1994). Nonetheless, we argue that unlike heuristic-cue information existing in the environment, heuristic-cue information based on subjective experiences is more likely to lead to heuristic processing of which perceivers are unaware.

In our view, internal sources of heuristic-cue information are less likely to be the focus of conscious attention, thereby decreasing the likelihood that perceivers apply the heuristics that link this information with specific judgmental implications consciously. This distinction we have drawn between external and internal sources of heuristic-cue information—together with the parallel we have made to conscious and unconscious forms of heuristic processing, respectively—is consistent with Polanyi's (1958) distinction between "tools" and "objects." Whereas external sources of heuristic-cue information are likely to be "objects" of attention, and thus consciously attended to and used, we suggest that internal sources of heuristic-cue information, such as subjective experiences, are more likely to be used as "tools" in the course of information processing (see also Jacoby & Kelley, 1987). That is, perceivers are less likely to be consciously aware of heuristic-cue information that emanates from within them, rendering them particularly unlikely to be aware of the activation and use of the heuristic "tools" that are triggered by such internal information.

Finally, it is important to point out that although we have interpreted the judgmental impact of subjective experiences in terms of heuristic processing, we believe that these experiences may also exert an influence on the systematic mode of processing, which may co-occur with the heuristic mode in various ways (see earlier discussion). Thus, for example,

when heuristic processing based on subjective experiences does in fact occur unconsciously, systematic processing that is biased by this processing may also be considered unconscious. Indeed, consistent with our view that heuristic processing triggered by subjective experiences is particularly likely to occur outside of perceivers' awareness, we suggest that perceivers are especially likely to be unaware of processing biases in their systematic processing that are attributable to the activation and application of heuristics pertaining distinctively to their subjective experiences.

Predicting the Judgmental Impact of Subjective Experiences

Beyond the question of the conscious versus unconscious nature of heuristic and systematic processing, conceptualizing the judgmental impact of subjective experiences in heuristic terms allows for greater precision in predicting how, when, and for whom subjective experiences are likely to exert an impact. Specifically, acknowledging the existence of heuristic rules that designate the judgmental implications of particular subjective experiences permits predictions to be made on the basis of the same social-cognitive principles of knowledge activation and use discussed earlier. We focus again on applicability, and suggest that a considerable amount of existing evidence on the judgmental impact of subjective experiences can be interpreted in terms of the differential applicability of stored heuristics (for a related discussion, see Hardin & Rothman, 1997).

As mentioned earlier, in the effort to demonstrate that the judgmental impact of subjective experiences reflects misattribution processes, past research has often included experimental conditions in which the correct attribution for the subjective experience is made salient to participants, or the informativeness of the subjective experience is called into question (e.g., (Schwarz & Clore, 1983; Schwarz et al., 1991). In these conditions, the absence or reversal of the judgmental impact of the subjective experience is predicted and typically found. In our view, these findings are readily interpretable in terms of the differential applicability of the heuristic that presumably underlies the impact of the particular subjective experience. It is likely that participants for whom the subjective experience was made salient, or for whom the informativeness of the experience was cast into doubt, were able to appropriately judge the applicability of such a heuristic to the judgmental task at hand as low.

Several empirical examples illustrating how the applicability concept fits with our view of the judgmental impact of subjective experiences now exist. In research on the impact of familiarity on judgments of the fame of male and female names (Banaji & Greenwald, 1995), it was found that only male names "became famous overnight." This finding is readily explained in terms of the differential application of the theory or heuristic "Familiarity implies fame" to the task of judging male versus female names. That is, the applicability of this heuristic to the task of judging the fame of *male* names was presumably higher than its applicability to the task of judging the fame of *female* names. In other words, it is likely that participants in this study had had more practice inferring fame from familiarity for male names than for female names, rendering the appropriateness of applying the "Familiarity implies fame" heuristic to the task of judging the fame of male names particularly high.

Evidence for the differential impact of the experienced ease of retrieving behavioral exemplars on judgments of the extent to which ingroup versus outgroup members possess the trait implied by the behaviors has explicitly been considered in terms of the differential applicability of a stored heuristic (Rothman & Hardin, 1998). For example, in this research, the judgmental impact of the subjective experience of ease in retrieving behavioral exemplars emerged only for judgments of outgroup members (Experiment 1). Rothman and Hardin discuss this finding in terms of the differential applicability of an availability heuristic to ingroup versus outgroup judgments—a difference that they argue reflects corresponding differences in prior use of this heuristic for judgments of ingroup versus outgroup members. That is, they argue that their results reflect the fact that people are typically more likely to invoke the use of an availability heuristic when judging outgroup members. Thus Rothman and Hardin's interpretation of their findings is entirely consistent with our view that the judgmental impact of subjective experiences re-

flects heuristic processing, and that as such, the concept of applicability can be used to predict the likelihood of such processing.

Also consistent with our view of subjective experiences is research demonstrating the differential attitudinal impact of the ease of retrieving persuasive arguments about a social issue among individuals high versus low in their commitment to their attitudinal position on the issue (Zimmerman & Chaiken, 1994). In this work, low-commitment participants expressed more favorable (unfavorable) attitudes toward the target issue after coming up with three versus nine arguments in favor of (against) the issue. Presumably, these participants invoked the use of a heuristic that specifically links the experienced ease of retrieving attitude-relevant arguments to the favorability of one's position on the issue (i.e., ease in coming up with arguments in favor of an issue implies that a favorable position on the issue is well substantiated). The ease of retrieving arguments did not trigger the activation and application of such a heuristic among high-commitment participants. These participants expressed more favorable (unfavorable) attitudes after coming up with nine versus three arguments in favor of (against) the issue. The differential attitudinal impact of the ease of retrieving attitude-relevant arguments for high- versus low-commitment participants can be interpreted in terms of the differential applicability of the stored heuristic linking this subjective experience with specific attitudinal implications. When asked for their opinion on the target issue, highly committed individuals were probably far less likely than less committed individuals to rely on ease-of-retrieval experiences as a basis for determining their issue opinion, and far more likely to rely on information that was more directly relevant to the attitude in question. As a result, the applicability of an ease-of-retrieval heuristic to the task of expressing one's attitude on the target issue was likely to be relatively lower among these individuals.

Similar results have recently been found in research on risk perception (Rothman & Schwarz, 1998). In this work, analogous to the moderating effect of high versus low attitudinal commitment (see above), high versus low perceived self-relevance moderated the impact of ease-of-retrieval experiences on participants' perceptions of their risk of heart disease. Specifically, individuals low in perceived self-relevance relied on experienced ease in recalling risk-relevant behaviors when making judgments of their vulnerability to heart disease, whereas individuals high in perceived self-relevance relied on the content of what they recalled. Here again, the differential use of an ease-of-retrieval heuristic among participants high versus low in perceived self-relevance can be interpreted as reflecting the differential applicability of this judgment rule to the task of assessing one's vulnerability to heart disease.

Also interpretable in terms of the differential applicability of a heuristic linking a specific subjective experience with particular judgmental implications are preliminary data suggesting the differential effects of prior exposure to persuasive arguments on judgments of the validity of these arguments among individuals high versus low in knowledge on the issue (Chen & Chaiken, 1997). In this research, low-knowledge individuals misattributed the familiarity they experienced upon encountering previously seen persuasive arguments to the validity of these arguments. In heuristic terms, they appear to have applied the heuristic "Familiarity implies validity" to the tasks of making validity judgments. The validity-enhancing effects of familiarity were not seen among high-knowledge individuals. For low-knowledge individuals, the applicability of such heuristics may have been particularly high because they lacked the informational resources needed to use a relatively more analytic basis to judge validity. For high-knowledge individuals, who had the informational resources that enabled them to rely on relatively more analytic bases to make validity judgments (e.g., the arguments themselves), these same heuristics were presumably not applicable to the judgmental tasks at hand.

The Potential Impact of Subjective Experiences on Judgmental Confidence

Finally, as alluded to earlier, the impact of a heuristic may stem not only from its judgmental implication, but also from the ease with which it is retrieved from memory. That is, the ease of retrieving a heuristic may itself serve as heuristic-cue information, triggering the activation and application of a heuristic delineating the judgmental implications of

such ease. The precise nature of these implications depends, of course, on the nature of perceivers' heuristics or "theories" regarding the subjective experience. One possibility, however, is that perceivers may attribute the ease of retrieving a heuristic to the applicability of the heuristic to the judgmental task at hand (e.g., "Judgmental rules that come to mind easily must be appropriate for use"). Alternatively, perceivers may attribute such ease to the validity or even infallibility of the heuristic (e.g., "Judgmental rules that come to mind easily must be accurate"). Importantly, in both cases, the subjective experience is likely to increase the confidence with which perceivers hold the judgment implied by the heuristic (cf. Downing, Judd, & Brauer, 1992). In turn, this increase in judgmental confidence is likely to dampen the likelihood that perceivers will engage in additional, more effortful systematic forms of processing—to the extent that their judgmental-confidence needs have been satisfied.

To summarize, we argue that, as with heuristic-cue information that is available in the external environment, subjective experiences may serve as heuristic-cue information, triggering the activation and use of stored heuristics that pertain distinctly to them. As such, we interpret the impact that subjective experiences may have on judgment as reflecting heuristic processing, recognizing that stored "theories" that link particular subjective experiences with specific judgmental implications must exist in memory if such experiences are to exert any impact at all.

CONCLUDING COMMENTS

In this chapter, our main goal has been to place the heuristic–systematic model in its broader context. We have laid the groundwork by reviewing the basic postulates of our model and its multiple-motive framework, and by highlighting some recent data that support our assumptions. We have then examined how social-cognitive theory on the principles underlying the activation and use of stored knowledge pertains to the heuristic mode of processing. Here we have paid special attention to the concept of applicability, viewing its role in the heuristic mode of processing as especially promising in terms of suggesting new research directions. Next we have articulated largely implicit connections between our heuristic–systematic distinction and the distinction drawn between conscious and unconscious processes. In this domain, we have focused on the impact of subjective experiences on processing and judgment, and have argued that often this impact reflects the unconscious activation and application of stored heuristics or "theories" that designate the particular judgmental implications of such experiences.

By drawing connections between the heuristic–systematic model and related concepts in the literature on attitudes and social cognition, and by discussing some of their implications, we hope to help spur new directions for theorizing and research on the mediation of social judgment. Reflecting the mission of this volume, we believe that the time is ripe for considering dual-process approaches in the context of other constructs and models that similarly speak to the processes that underlie our judgments and behaviors. By considering the heuristic–systematic model more broadly, we have certainly enriched our own understanding of the role of heuristic and systematic modes of processing in everyday social judgment, and we hope to have demonstrated the potential utility of applying the model in domains within as well as beyond the attitudes and persuasion arena in which it originally developed.

ACKNOWLEDGMENTS

We thank Gerd Bohner, Peter Darke, Roger Giner-Sorolla, Richard Petty, and Yaacov Trope for their comments on an earlier draft of this chapter.

NOTES

1. In most persuasion research examining heuristic processing, heuristic-cue information is presented prior to and separately from persuasive argumentation (see Eagly & Chaiken, 1993). For example, participants may be exposed to consensus-cue information in the form of poll results that appear prior to and separately from a persuasive message containing judgment-relevant persuasive arguments (e.g., Giner-Sorolla & Chaiken, 1997). Nonetheless, we do not assume that heuristic-cue information is by definition processed prior to and separate from persuasive argumentation—although we submit that this may often be the case (for a re-

lated point, see Bodenhausen, Macrae, & Sherman, Chapter 13, this volume). Heuristic-cue information may exist in many forms and appear in various places beyond those examined in the modal persuasion study. For example, heuristic-cue information may be embedded in the context of a persuasive appeal and discovered only in the course of systematically processing persuasive arguments. More distinctly, as argued later in this chapter, internal affective and cognitive states may also serve as heuristic-cue information, triggering heuristics that specify their judgmental implications.

2. Although we contend that systematic processing is generally more effective in decreasing the gap between actual and desired confidence, we note that engaging in systematic processing does not guarantee that the gap will be closed. Moreover, we also recognize the possibility that there may be particular instances in which heuristic processing contributes as much as or even more than systematic processing to decreasing the gap between actual and desired confidence—although this possibility has yet to be examined empirically.

3. Although the goal of accuracy-motivated individuals by definition is to seek the truth, this does not imply that their processing is necessarily unbiased. Cognitive factors, such as bias in one's knowledge base, may color the evaluative nature of processing. For instance, a person's greater knowledge of arguments on one side of an issue may result in stronger counterarguing information supporting the other side of the issue (for further discussion of knowledge-based biases in information processing, see Wood, Rhodes, & Biek, 1995).

4. Contrast effects may not always result from perceivers' attempts to correct for potential unwanted judgmental influences of available heuristic-cue information. At times, perceivers may treat the judgmental implications derived from heuristic-cue information as a standard against which to evaluate other judgment-relevant information, leading to similarly contrasted judgments (for a recent discussion of the underlying nature of contrast effects, see Higgins, 1996).

REFERENCES

Anderson, J. R. (1983). *The architecture of cognition.* Cambridge, MA: Harvard University Press.

Anderson, J. R. (1987). Skill acquisition: Compilation of weak-method problem solutions. *Psychological Review, 84,* 192–210.

Arkes, H. R., Boehm, L. E., & Xu, G. (1991). Determinants of judged validity. *Journal of Experimental Social Psychology, 27,* 576–605.

Banaji, M. R., & Greenwald, A. G. (1995). Implicit gender stereotyping in judgments of fame. *Journal of Personality and Social Psychology, 68,* 181–198.

Bargh, J. A. (1989). Conditional automaticity: Varieties of automatic influence in social perception and cognition. In J. S. Uleman & J. A. Bargh (Eds.), *Unintended thought* (pp. 3–51). New York: Guilford Press.

Bargh, J. A. (1992). The ecology of automaticity: Toward establishing the conditions needed to produce automatic processing effects. *American Journal of Psychology, 105*, 181–199.

Bargh, J. A. (1994). The four horsemen of automaticity: Awareness, intention, efficiency, and control in social cognition. In R. S. Wyer & T. K. Srull (Eds.), *Handbook of social cognition* (2nd ed., pp. 1–40). Hillsdale, NJ: Erlbaum.

Bargh, J. A. (1997). The automaticity of everyday life. In R. S. Wyer, Jr. (Ed.), *Advances in social cognition* (Vol. 10, pp. 1–61). Mahwah, NJ: Erlbaum.

Bargh, J. A., & Barndollar, K. (1996). Automaticity in action: The unconscious as repository of chronic goals and motives. In P. M. Gollwitzer & J. A. Bargh (Eds.), *The psychology of action: Linking cognition and motivation to behavior* (pp. 457–481). New York: Guilford Press.

Begg, I., Armour, V., & Kerr, T. (1985). On believing what we remember. *Canadian Journal of Behavioural Science, 17*, 199–214.

Biek, M., Wood, W., & Chaiken, S. (1996). Working knowledge, cognitive processing, and attitudes: On the determinants of bias. *Personality and Social Psychology Bulletin, 22*, 547–556.

Bohner, G., Moskowitz, G. B., & Chaiken, S. (1995). The interplay of heuristic and systematic processing of social information. In W. Stroebe & M. Hewstone (Eds.), *European review of social psychology* (Vol. 6, pp. 33–68). New York: Wiley.

Bohner, G., Rank, S., Reinhard, M.-A., Einwiller, S., & Erb, H.-P. (1998). Motivational determinants of systematic processing: Expectancy moderates effects of desired confidence on processing effort. *European Journal of Social Psychology, 28*, 185–206.

Bornstein, R. F. (1989). Exposure and affect: Overview and meta-analysis of research, 1968–1987. *Psychological Bulletin, 106*, 265–289.

Bornstein, R. F., & D'Agostino, P. R. (1992). Stimulus recognition and the mere exposure effect. *Journal of Personality and Social Psychology, 63*, 545–552.

Bornstein, R. F., & D'Agostino, P. R. (1994). The attribution and discounting of perceptual fluency: Preliminary tests of a perceptual fluency/attributional model of the mere exposure effect. *Social Cognition, 12*, 103–128.

Chaiken, S. (1980). Heuristic versus systematic information processing and the use of source versus message cues in persuasion. *Journal of Personality and Social Psychology, 39*, 752–766.

Chaiken, S. (1987). The heuristic model of persuasion. In M. P. Zanna, J. M. Olson, & C. P. Herman (Eds.), *Social influence: The Ontario Symposium* (Vol. 5, pp. 3–39). Hillsdale, NJ: Erlbaum.

Chaiken, S., Axsom, D., Liberman, A., & Wilson, D. (1992). *Heuristic processing of persuasive messages: Chronic and temporary sources of rule accessibility.* Unpublished manuscript, New York University.

Chaiken, S., Giner-Sorolla, R., & Chen, S. (1996). Beyond accuracy: Defense and impression motives in heuristic and systematic information processing. In P. M. Gollwitzer & J. A. Bargh (Eds.), *The psychology of action: Linking cognition and motivation to behavior* (pp. 553–578). New York: Guilford Press.

Chaiken, S., Liberman, A., & Eagly, A. H. (1989). Heu-

ristic and systematic processing within and beyond the persuasion context. In J. S. Uleman & J. A. Bargh (Eds.), *Unintended thought* (pp. 212–252). New York: Guilford Press.

Chaiken, S., & Maheswaran, D. (1994). Heuristic processing can bias systematic processing: Effects of source credibility, argument ambiguity, and task importance on attitude judgment. *Journal of Personality and Social Psychology, 66*, 460–473.

Chaiken, S., & Stangor, C. (1987). Attitudes and attitude change. *Annual Review of Psychology, 38*, 575–630.

Chaiken, S., Wood, W., & Eagly, A. H. (1996). Principles of persuasion. In E. T. Higgins & A. W. Kruglanski (Eds.), *Social psychology: Handbook of basic principles* (pp. 702–742). New York: Guilford Press.

Chen, S., & Chaiken, S. (1997, May). *Unconscious influences of the past: Misattributing familiarity to validity and to agreement.* Paper presented at the annual meeting of the American Psychological Society, Washington, DC.

Chen, S., Shechter, D., & Chaiken, S. (1996). Getting at the truth or getting along: Accuracy- vs. impression-motivated heuristic and systematic information processing. *Journal of Personality and Social Psychology, 71*, 262–275.

Clore, G. L., & Parrott, W. G. (1991). Moods and their vicissitudes: Thoughts and feelings as information. In J. Forgas (Ed.), *Emotion and social judgment* (pp. 107–123). Oxford: Pergamon Press.

Darke, P. R., Chaiken, S., Bohner, G., Einwiller, S., Erb, H.-P., & Hazelwood, J. D. (in press). Accuracy motivation, consensus information, and the law of large numbers: Effects on attitude judgment in the absence of argumentation. *Personality and Social Psychology Bulletin, 24*, 1205–1215.

DeBono, K. G. (1987). Investigating the social-adjustive and value-expressive functions of attitudes: Implications for persuasion processes. *Journal of Personality and Social Psychology, 52*, 279–287.

Ditto, P. H., & Lopez, D. F. (1992). Motivated skepticism: Use of differential decision criteria for preferred and nonpreferred conclusions. *Journal of Personality and Social Psychology, 63*, 568–584.

Downing, J. W., Judd, C. M., & Brauer, M. (1992). Effects of repeated expression on attitude extremity. *Journal of Personality and Social Psychology, 63*, 17–29.

Eagly, A. H., & Chaiken, S. (1993). *The psychology of attitudes.* Fort Worth, TX: Harcourt Brace Jovanovich.

Eagly, A. H., & Chaiken, S. (1998). Attitude structure and function. In D. T. Gilbert, S. T. Fiske, & G. Lindzey (Eds.), *The handbook of social psychology* (Vol. 2, 4th ed., pp. 269–322). New York: McGraw-Hill.

Erb, H.-P., Bohner, G., Schmälzle, K., & Rank, S. (1998). Beyond conflict and discrepancy: Cognitive bias in minority and majority influence. *Personality and Social Psychology Bulletin, 24*, 620–633.

Festinger, L. (1957). *A theory of cognitive dissonance.* Evanston, IL: Row, Peterson.

Fiske, S. T., & Neuberg, S. L. (1990). A continuum of impression formation, from category-based to individuating processes: Influences of information and motivation on attention and interpretation. In M. P. Zanna (Ed.), *Advances in experimental social psychology* (Vol. 23, pp. 1–74). San Diego, CA: Academic Press.

Fiske, S. T., & Taylor, S. E. (1991). *Social cognition* (2nd ed.). New York: McGraw-Hill.

Giner-Sorolla, R., & Chaiken, S. (1997). Selective use of heuristic and systematic processing under defense motivation. *Personality and Social Psychology Bulletin*, 23, 84–97.

Giner-Sorolla, R., Lutz, S., & Chaiken, S. (1998). *Attitudes and issue beliefs as heuristics in a simulated judicial decision.* Manuscript submitted for publication.

Greenwald, A. G., & Banaji, M. R. (1995). Implicit social cognition: Attitudes, self-esteem, and stereotypes. *Psychological Review*, 102, 4–27.

Hardin, C. D., & Rothman, A. J. (1997). Rendering accessible information relevant: The applicability of everyday life. In R. S. Wyer (Ed.), *Advances in social cognition* (Vol. 10, pp. 143–156). Mahwah, NJ: Erlbaum.

Hasher, L., Goldstein, D., & Toppino, T. (1977). Frequency and the conference of referential validity. *Journal of Verbal Learning and Verbal Behavior*, 16, 107–112.

Higgins, E. T. (1989). Knowledge accessibility and activation: Subjectivity and suffering from unconscious sources. In J. S. Uleman & J. A. Bargh (Eds.), *Unintended thought* (pp. 75–123). New York: Guilford Press.

Higgins, E. T. (1996). Knowledge activation: Accessibility, applicability, and salience. In E. T. Higgins & A. W. Kruglanski (Eds.), *Social psychology: Handbook of basic principles* (pp. 133–168). New York: Guilford Press.

Higgins, E. T., & Brendl, C. M. (1995). Accessibility and applicability: Some "activation rules" influencing judgment. *Journal of Experimental and Social Psychology*, 31, 218–243.

Higgins, E. T., King, G. A., & Mavin, G. H. (1982). Individual construct accessibility and subjective impressions and recall. *Journal of Personality and Social Psychology*, 43, 35–47.

Higgins, E. T., Rholes, W. S., & Jones, C. R. (1977). Category accessibility and impression formation. *Journal of Experimental Social Psychology*, 13, 141–154.

Jacoby, L. L., & Kelley, C. M. (1987). Unconscious influences of memory for a prior event. *Personality and Social Psychology Bulletin*, 13, 314–336.

Jacoby, L. L., Kelley, C. M., Brown, J., & Jasechko, J. (1989). Becoming famous overnight: Limits on the ability to avoid the unconscious influences of the past. *Journal of Personality and Social Psychology*, 56, 326–338.

Jacoby, L. L., Toth, J. P., Lindsay, D. S., & Debner, J. A. (1992). Lectures for a layperson: Methods for revealing unconscious processes. In R. F. Bornstein & T. S. Pittman (Eds.), *Perception without awareness* (pp. 81–120). New York: Guilford Press.

Jones, E. E. (1990). *Interpersonal perception.* New York: Freeman.

Katz, I. (1960). The functional approach to the study of attitudes. *Public Opinion Quarterly*, 24, 163–204.

Kunda, Z. (1990). The case for motivated reasoning. *Psychological Bulletin*, 108, 480–498.

Leippe, M. R., & Elkin, R. A. (1987). When motives clash: Issue involvement and response involvement as determinants of persuasion. *Journal of Personality and Social Psychology*, 52, 269–278.

Leyens, J., Yzerbyt, V., & Corneille, O. (1996). The role of applicability in the emergence of the overattribution bias. *Journal of Personality and Social Psychology*, 70, 219–229.

Liberman, A., & Chaiken, S. (1992). Defensive processing of personally relevant health messages. *Personality and Social Psychology Bulletin*, 18, 669–679.

Lombardi, W. J., Higgins, E. T., & Bargh, J. A. (1987). The role of consciousness in priming effects on categorization: Assimilation versus contrast as a function of awareness of the priming task. *Personality and Social Psychology Bulletin*, 13, 411–429.

Lord, C. G., Ross, L., & Lepper, M. R. (1979). Biased assimilation and attitude polarization: The effects of prior theories on subsequently considered evidence. *Journal of Personality and Social Psychology*, 37, 2098–2109.

Mackie, D. M., & Worth, L. T. (1989). Cognitive deficits and the mediation of positive affect in persuasion. *Journal of Personality and Social Psychology*, 57, 27–40.

Maheswaran, D., & Chaiken, S. (1991). Promoting systematic processing in low-motivation settings: Effect of incongruent information on processing and judgment. *Journal of Personality and Social Psychology*, 61, 13–25.

Maheswaran, D., Mackie, D. M., & Chaiken, S. (1992). Brand name as a heuristic cue: The effects of task importance and expectancy confirmation on consumer judgments. *Journal of Consumer Psychology*, 1, 317–336.

Martin, L. L., Seta, J. J., & Crelia, R. A. (1990). Assimilation and contrast as a function of people's willingness and ability to expend effort in forming an impression. *Journal of Personality and Social Psychology*, 59, 27–37.

Petty, R. E., & Cacioppo, J. A. (1981). *Attitudes and persuasion: Classic and contemporary approaches.* Dubuque, IA: William C. Brown.

Petty, R. E., & Cacioppo, J. A. (1986). The elaboration likelihood model of persuasion. In L. Berkowitz (Ed.), *Advances in experimental social psychology* (Vol. 19, pp. 123–205). New York: Academic Press.

Petty, R. E., & Wegener, D. T. (1998). Attitude change: Multiple roles for persuasion variables. In D. T. Gilbert, S. T. Fiske, & G. Lindsey (Eds.), *The handbook of social psychology* (Vol. 1, 4th ed., pp. 323–390). Boston: McGraw-Hill.

Polanyi, M. (1958). *Personal knowledge: Towards a post-critical philosophy.* Chicago: University of Chicago Press.

Pomerantz, E. M., Chaiken, S., & Tordesillas, R. S. (1995). Attitude strength and resistance processes. *Journal of Personality and Social Psychology*, 69, 408–419.

Pyszczynski, T., & Greenberg, J. (1987). Toward an integration of cognitive and motivational perspectives on social inference: A biased hypothesis-testing model. In L. Berkowitz (Ed.), *Advances in experimental social psychology* (Vol. 20, pp. 297–340). New York: Academic Press.

Roskos-Ewoldsen, D. R., & Fazio, R. H. (1992). The accessibility of source likability as a determinant of persuasion. *Personality and Social Psychology Bulletin*, 18, 19–25.

Rothman, A. J., & Hardin, C. D. (1997). Differential use of the availability heuristic in social judgment. *Personality and Social Psychology Bulletin*, 23, 123–138.

Rothman, A. J., & Schwarz, N. (1998). Constructing perceptions of vulnerability: Personal relevance and the use of experiential information in health judgments. *Personality and Social Psychology Bulletin, 24,* 1053–1064.

Ruder, M., Bohner, G., & Erb, H.-P. (1997, June). *Die Kontrasthypothese: Paradoxe Effekte heuristischer Cues bei Erwartungsverletzung* [The contrast hypothesis: Paradoxical effects of heuristic cues under expectancy violation]. Paper presented at the 6th Tagung der Fachgruppe Sozialpsychologie, Konstanz, Germany.

Ruder, M., Erb, H.-P., & Bohner, G. (1996). Wenn hoher Sachverstand zu Ablehnung fuhrt: Der Professor mit den fadenscheinigen Argumenten [When expertise fails: The professor who presents specious arguments]. In A. Schorr (Ed.), *Experimentelle psychologie: Beitrage zur 38. Tagung experimentell arbeitender Psychologen/Beitrage zur DGMF–Tagung Medienpsychologie–Medienwirkungsforschung* (pp. 270–271). Lengerich, Germany: Pabst.

Schwarz, N. (1990). Feelings as information: Informational and motivational functions of affective states. In E. T. Higgins & R. Sorrentino (Eds.), *Handbook of motivation and cognition: Foundations of social behavior* (Vol. 2, pp. 527–561). New York: Guilford Press.

Schwarz, N., Bless, H., Strack, F., Klumpp, G., Rittenauer-Schatka, H., & Simons, A. (1991). Ease of retrieval as information: Another look at the availability heuristic. *Journal of Personality and Social Psychology, 61,* 195–202.

Schwarz, N., & Clore, G. L. (1983). Mood, misattribution, and judgments of well-being: Informative and directive functions of affective states. *Journal of Personality and Social Psychology, 45,* 513–523.

Schwarz, N., & Clore, G. L. (1996). Feelings and phenomenal experiences. In E. T. Higgins & A. W. Kruglanski (Eds.), *Social psychology: Handbook of basic principles* (pp. 433–465). New York: Guilford Press.

Shiffrin, R. M., & Schneider, W. (1977). Controlled and automatic human information processing: II. Perceptual learning, automatic attending, and general theory. *Psychological Review, 84,* 127–190.

Simon, H. A. (1976). *Administrative behavior* (3rd ed.). New York: Free Press.

Sloman, S. A. (1996). The empirical case for two systems of reasoning. *Psychological Bulletin, 119,* 3–22.

Smith, E. R. (1990). Content and process specificity in the effects of prior experiences. In R. S. Wyer & T. K. Srull (Eds.), *Advances in social cognition* (Vol. 3, pp. 1–59). Hillsdale, NJ: Erlbaum.

Smith, E. R. (1994). Procedural knowledge and processing strategies in social cognition. In R. S. Wyer & T. K. Srull (Eds.), *Handbook of social cognition* (2nd ed., pp. 99–152). Hillsdale, NJ: Erlbaum.

Smith, M. B., Bruner, J. S., & White, R. W. (1956). *Opinions and personality.* New York: Wiley.

Snyder, M., & DeBono, K. G. (1987). A functional approach to attitudes and persuasion. In M. P. Zanna, J. M. Olson, & C. P. Herman (Eds.), *Social influence: The Ontario Symposium* (Vol. 5, pp. 107–125). Hillsdale, NJ: Erlbaum.

Strack, F., & Hannover, B. (1996). Awareness of influence as a precondition for implementing correctional goals. In P. M. Gollwitzer & J. A. Bargh (Eds.), *The psychology of action: Linking motivation and cognition to behavior* (pp. 579–596). New York: Guilford Press.

Taylor, S. E. (1991). Asymmetrical effects of positive and negative events: The mobilization-minimization hypothesis. *Psychological Bulletin, 110,* 67–85.

Tetlock, P. E. (1992). The impact of accountability of judgment and choice: Toward a social contingency model. In M. P. Zanna (Ed.), *Advances in experimental social psychology* (Vol. 25, pp. 331–376). San Diego, CA: Academic Press.

Thompson, E. P., Roman, R. J., Moskowitz, G. B., Chaiken, S., & Bargh, J. A. (1994). Accuracy motivation and the reprocessing of social information. *Journal of Personality and Social Psychology, 66,* 474–489.

Tordesillas, R. S., & Chaiken, S. (in press). Thinking too much, or thinking too little: The effects of introspection on the decision-making process. *Personality and Social Psychology Bulletin.*

Uleman, J. S., & Bargh, J. A. (Eds.). (1989). *Unintended thought.* New York: Guilford Press.

Wanke, M., Bless, H., & Biller, B. (1996). Subjective experience versus content of information in the construction of attitude judgments. *Personality and Social Psychology Bulletin, 22,* 1105–1113.

Wood, W., Kallgren, C. A., & Preisler, R. M. (1985). Access to attitude-relevant information in memory as a determinant of persuasion: The role of message attributes. *Journal of Experimental Social Psychology, 21,* 73–85.

Wood, W., Rhodes, N., & Biek, M. (1995). Working knowledge and attitude strength: An information-processing analysis. In R. E. Petty & J. A. Krosnick (Eds.), *Attitude strength: Antecedents and consequences* (pp. 283–313). Mahwah, NJ: Erlbaum.

Wyer, R. S., & Srull, T. K. (1986). Human cognition in its social context. *Psychological Review, 93,* 322–359.

Zimmerman, J., & Chaiken, S. (1994, July). *Subjective experiences influence attitudes: Ease of retrieval.* Paper presented at the annual meeting of the American Psychological Society, Washington, DC.

Zuckerman, A., & Chaiken, S. (1997, May). *Mood influences persuasion in an interpersonal setting.* Paper presented at the annual meeting of the American Psychological Society, Washington, DC.

5

The MODE Model
of Attitude–Behavior Processes

RUSSELL H. FAZIO
TAMARA TOWLES-SCHWEN

Like other chapters in this volume, this chapter focuses on a dual-process model. In our case, the specific issue of concern is the question of how attitudes guide behavior. That is, by what processes do attitudes exert their influence on behavior? We review the MODE model of attitude–behavior processes (Fazio, 1990) that aims to address this question, as well as research that has been conducted to test the model.

TWO CLASSES OF
ATTITUDE–BEHAVIOR PROCESSES

The MODE model to be described in this chapter distinguishes between two classes of attitude–behavior processes. The basic difference between the two types centers on the extent to which deciding on a particular course of action involves conscious deliberation regarding the alternatives or a spontaneous reaction to one's perception of the immediate situation. An individual may analyze the costs and benefits of a particular behavior, and in so doing may deliberately reflect upon the attitudes relevant to the behavioral decision. These attitudes may serve as one of the possibly many dimensions that are considered in

arriving at a behavior plan, which then may be enacted. Alternatively, attitudes may guide an individual's behavior in a more spontaneous manner, without the individual's having actively considered the relevant attitudes and without his or her necessarily being aware of the attitudes' influence. Instead, the attitudes may influence how the person interprets the event that is occurring, and thus may affect the person's behavioral response in that way. In either case, attitudes are having an effect upon behavior, but the process by which they are doing so differs markedly.

Spontaneous Processing

Let's turn first to the spontaneous processing alternative. In the mid 1980s, Fazio and his colleagues proposed a model of attitude–behavior processes that focused upon the accessibility of attitudes from memory and the influence that attitudes can have upon perceptions of the object in the immediate situation (Fazio, Powell, & Herr, 1983; Fazio, 1986). The spontaneous process that was outlined begins with the presence of an environmental trigger. A behavioral opportunity presents itself. The individual encounters the attitude object, and the immediate situation requires some response—either because the individual is interacting with the object (as in the case of a social interaction with another person), or because a request for a certain action is made. The model postulates that behavior is largely a function of the individual's perceptions in this immediate situation.

Beginning with the "New Look" movement (e.g., Bruner, 1957), which so heavily emphasized the constructive nature of perception, psychology has recognized that such perceptions are affected by the knowledge structures, affect, values, and expectations that the individual brings to the situation. Advances in the area of social cognition make it evident that such constructs in memory can have an influence through a passive, automatic process. That is, the individual need not consciously reflect upon a construct and its applicability to the current information for the construct to affect interpretations. Instead, the priming of a construct from memory is sufficient for that construct to influence interpretations.

Obviously, the individual's attitude toward the object is such a construct—one that can guide perceptions of the attitude object in the immediate situation in which it is encountered. A considerable amount of evidence consistent with this proposition has accrued over the decades of research concerning the biasing influence of attitudes (see Fazio, Roskos-Ewoldsen, & Powell, 1994, for a general discussion of this issue). For example, documenting a phenomenon well known to any sports fan, Hastorf and Cantril (1954) observed varying perceptions of possible infractions committed during the course of a football game as a function of team allegiance. Regan, Straus, and Fazio (1974) found that attitudes toward a confederate influenced attributions regarding the confederate's behavior, such that attitudinally inconsistent behavior was attributed to external forces and attitudinally consistent behavior was attributed to internal causes. Carretta and Moreland (1982) found that Nixon supporters (as identified by earlier voting behavior) were more likely than McGovern supporters to evaluate Nixon's involvement with Watergate as within legal limits and to maintain their positive attitudes toward Nixon through the course of the Watergate hearings. Research by Lord, Ross, and Lepper (1979) revealed that judgments of the quality of two

purported scientific studies concerning the deterrent efficacy of capital punishment varied as a function of the participants' own attitudes toward the death penalty.

By influencing perceptions in this way, attitudes may have an impact on eventual behavior, even without the individual's reflecting upon the attitudes. An attitude that is highly accessible from memory, and hence likely to be activated automatically upon the individual's encountering the attitude object, is apt to result in immediate perceptions that are congruent with the attitude. A positive attitude that has been activated is likely to lead the individual to notice, attend to, and process primarily the positive qualities that the object is exhibiting in the immediate situation. Likewise, a negative attitude will direct attention to negative qualities of the object. Thus, selective processing produces perceptions of the object in the immediate situation that are consistent with the attitude. These immediate perceptions of the object, as well as any constructs regarding the situation itself that might be activated (e.g., norms), will influence the individual's definition of the event that is occurring. Approach behaviors are prompted by a definition of the event that consists primarily of positive perceptions of the attitude object in the immediate situation. Avoidance behaviors follow from a negative definition of the event.

This entire sequence need not involve any deliberate reflection or reasoning. Instead, behavior simply follows from a definition of the event that has itself been influenced by the automatically activated attitude. Neither the activation of the attitude from memory nor the selective-perception component requires conscious effort, intent, or control on the part of the individual. Indeed, it is within an entirely automatic sequence that attitude activation and selective processing take on a necessary role if the attitude is to exert any influence upon the behavior. If the attitude is not activated from memory, immediate perceptions are likely to be based upon momentarily salient, and potentially unrepresentative, features of the attitude object—ones that are not necessarily congruent with the attitude. As a result, greater attitude–behavior consistency is observed when attitudes are highly accessible from memory than when attitudes are relatively less accessible.

In a variety of laboratory and field investigations concerning the attitude–behavior relation, Fazio and his colleagues have obtained evidence of such a moderating role of attitude accessibility (Fazio, Chen, McDonel, & Sherman, 1982; Fazio, Powell, & Williams, 1989; Fazio & Williams, 1986; see Fazio, 1995, for a review). For example, individuals with more accessible attitudes toward the candidates at the beginning of the 1984 presidential election were more likely, months later, to vote consistently with those attitudes (Fazio & Williams, 1986). Evidence also indicates that the extent of biased processing of information related to the attitude object varies as a function of attitude accessibility (Fazio & Williams, 1986; Houston & Fazio, 1989; Schuette & Fazio, 1995). For example, the investigation of the 1984 presidential election revealed a relation between attitudes toward the candidates and judgments of the quality of the candidates' performance during the nationally televised debates—a relation that, once again, increased as attitude accessibility increased.

A Deliberative Attitude-to-Behavior Process

The spontaneous-process model focuses upon preexisting attitudes and their accessibility from memory. This can be contrasted with a much more deliberative process in which the individual focuses not upon any preexisting attitude, but upon the raw data (i.e., the attributes of the behavioral alternative).

Beyond question, some social behavior is planned and deliberate. Indeed, people sometimes decide how they *intend* to behave and then follow through on that intention when they enter the situation. This deliberative processing is characterized by considerable cognitive work. It involves the scrutiny of available information and an analysis of positive and negative features, of costs and benefits. The specific attributes of the attitude object and the potential consequences of engaging in a particular course of action may be considered and weighed. Such reflection forms the basis for deciding upon a behavioral intention and, ultimately, upon behavior.

Unquestionably, the most familiar model of this sort is the Ajzen and Fishbein (1980) theory of reasoned action, and its descendant,

Ajzen's (1991) theory of planned behavior (see Ajzen & Sexton, Chapter 6, this volume). Because the Ajzen and Fishbein model is so well known and so well specified, we focus upon it here as an excellent illustration of deliberative processing. However, it should be kept in mind that any specific model that involves individuals' engaging in an effortful analysis of attributes can be considered within the class of deliberative-processing models of the attitude–behavior relation. In the judgment and decision-making literature, these models are often said to involve a focus upon an analysis of the attributes via weighted averaging, the application of lexicographic rules, or elimination by aspects (see Abelson & Levi, 1985; Einhorn & Hogarth, 1981).

The Ajzen and Fishbein model is clearly based upon deliberative processing. "Generally speaking, the theory is based on the assumption that human beings are usually quite rational and make systematic use of the information available to them. . . . We argue that people consider the implications of their actions before they decide to engage or not engage in a given behavior" (Ajzen & Fishbein, 1980, p. 5). According to the theory of reasoned action, behavior stems from a behavioral intention, which is itself the consequence of the individual's considering and weighing his or her attitude toward the behavior and subjective norms. "Subjective norms" refer to the person's beliefs that significant others think that he or she should or should not perform the behavior, as well as the person's motivation to comply with these specific referents. It is important to note that within this model the attitude under consideration is not a general attitude toward the object in question, but an attitude toward performing the specific behavior in question. According to the model, attitude toward the behavior is itself a function of the person's beliefs concerning the outcomes that are likely to result from performing the behavior and the person's evaluations of those outcomes. Thus, individuals are assumed to systematically weigh the available information, including the likely consequences of their engaging in the behavior under consideration.

The critical distinction between the spontaneous-process and deliberative-process models centers upon the extent to which the behavioral decision involves effortful reasoning as opposed to flowing spontaneously from individuals' appraisals in the immediate situation. The deliberative process can be viewed as relatively "data-driven"; it involves consideration of the specific attributes of the attitude object and of the potential consequences of engaging in a particular behavior. In contrast, focusing as it does upon attitude toward the object and upon the activation of this attitude from memory, the spontaneous process can be viewed as more "theory-driven."

MOTIVATION AND OPPORTUNITY AS DETERMINANTS: THE MODE MODEL

The obvious question that arises concerns the conditions under which a spontaneous attitude–behavior process versus a deliberative one might operate. The MODE model addresses this question. MODE is an acronym for "Motivation and Opportunity as DEterminants." Given the effortful reflection that is required by the deliberative-processing alternative, it would appear that some motivating force is necessary to induce individuals to engage in the reasoning. A fruitful way of conceptualizing the sort of situations that may foster the deliberative attitude–behavior process is provided by Kruglanski's theory of lay epistemics (Kruglanski, 1989; Kruglanski & Freund, 1983; Kruglanski & Webster, 1996; see also Kruglanski, Thompson, & Spiegel, Chapter 14, this volume). Kruglanski attempts to delineate the general processes and motivating variables relevant to the acquisition of knowledge. In so doing, he discusses the importance of the motivation to avoid reaching an invalid conclusion—motivation that stems from the perceived costliness of a judgmental mistake. The theory suggests that high "fear of invalidity" motivates careful reflection; it induces individuals to undergo the effortful reflection and reasoning involved in a deliberative attitude–behavior process. Without such inducement, individuals have little reason to deliberate. Instead of considering and weighing the potential consequences of the behavior, individuals can allow themselves the effortless luxury of being "theory-driven." That is, any attitudinal evaluation that has been activated from memory can guide individuals'

definitions of the event and, ultimately, their behavior.

Much like other dual-process models, then, the MODE model tends to focus on a broad motivation to be accurate (see, e.g, Chen & Chaiken, Chapter 4, this volume; Fiske, Lin, & Neuberg, Chapter 11, this volume; Petty & Wegener, Chapter 3, this volume). However, as shall be evident later in this chapter, we do recognize that the motivation to deliberate can also stem from more specific goals regarding the standards that individuals maintain for their behavior in a given domain or the manner in which they wish to present themselves in that domain. Later, we will be concerned with the extent to which individuals are motivated to avoid acting in a prejudiced manner. In such a case, the perceived costliness of a judgmental error centers not on inaccuracy per se, but on the possibility that the judgment or behavior may be a sign of prejudice. Generally speaking, the motivating perception of potential costliness stems from any indication that specific judgments vary markedly in the extent to which they are likely to produce positive or negative consequences for the individual. Negative consequences can result from a given judgment's deviation from reality and/or from its discordance with internally or externally imposed standards for behavior. In any case, it is the perception of a potential for costs that motivates more careful deliberation.

Of course, the motivation to engage in the deliberative process is not in and of itself sufficient. The time and the resources to deliberate—what the MODE model refers to as "opportunity"—also must exist. Situations that require one to make a behavioral response quickly can deny one the opportunity to undertake the sort of reflection and reasoning that may be desired. Likewise, competing task demands may interfere with one's ability to deliberate. Moreover, some kinds of behaviors (e.g., nonverbal behavior) may limit opportunity because they are inherently less amenable to direct, conscious control. In such cases, individuals may have no alternative to the "theory-driven" mode characterized by the spontaneous-processing model.

Several tests of each component of the MODE model have been conducted, and research supporting the validity of each component is discussed next.

THE ROLE OF MOTIVATION

Two tests of the MODE model have explicitly examined the role of motivation in the attitude-to-behavior process. Sanbonmatsu and Fazio (1990) presented participants with attributes of two department stores. The information provided about the camera departments of the two stores was inconsistent with participants' overall evaluations of the stores. Participants were given generally positive information about Brown's department store, but the statements about the camera department were negative. The reverse was true for the second department store, Smith's. After participants had finished reading about both stores and had formed general attitudes about them, they were asked to decide where they would choose to buy a camera. Obviously, participants could base their decisions on their overall evaluations of each store or on their memory of the specific attributes of each store. Given the configuration of the stimuli, their choice of store provided information regarding the basis for their decisions. If participants chose Smith's (the generally more positive store with the inferior camera department), they were likely to have relied on their overall evaluations and would appear to have been using a relatively noneffortful, spontaneous process to arrive at their decisions. If they chose Brown's, which received generally negative reviews but had the superior camera department, they were likely to have engaged in the effortful process of retrieving specific attribute information about each store from memory.

Motivation to reach a valid decision was manipulated by enhancing fear of invalidity for half the participants (Kruglanski & Freund, 1983). These participants were told that their store selections would be compared to those of the other students participating in the session, and that they would have to explain their decisions to the experimenter and the other participants. The other half of the participants did not receive such instructions. Opportunity to deliberate was also manipulated, by inducing time pressure. Some participants were instructed that they would have only 15 seconds to reach a decision. Thus, motivation and opportunity were manipulated in a 2 × 2 factorial design.

In this and related experiments, Sanbonmatsu and Fazio found that more participants in the high-fear-of-invalidity (i.e., high-motivation) and low-time-pressure (i.e., high-opportunity) conditions chose the store indicative of attribute-based decision making than in any of the other conditions. Thus, motivated individuals who were not under time pressure appeared to have reached their decisions via the deliberative process delineated earlier. Apparently, unless participants had both sufficient motivation and opportunity, they failed to retrieve the specific attribute information and instead relied only on their overall attitudes toward the stores. Both motivation and opportunity were necessary for individuals to engage in the more effortful process of retrieving and evaluating their beliefs about the camera departments of the two stores, just as predicted by the MODE model. The implication is that the reasoned-action process upon which Ajzen and Fishbein (1980) focus—one that involves individuals' "computation" of attitudes toward the act by integrating their evaluations of relevant beliefs—occurs only when people are properly motivated and have the opportunity to pursue such effortful reflection.

In another test of the MODE model, Schuette and Fazio (1995) extended the findings of Sanbonmatsu and Fazio (1990) to situations involving on-line, as opposed to memory-based, judgments. In the Sanbonmatsu and Fazio (1990) work, participants' use of a deliberative process required them to expend effort by searching their memories for the relevant attribute information. Moreover, the specific attributes describing each store were unambiguously desirable or undesirable. Motivation and opportunity served to induce and permit the effort expenditure necessary to retrieve the attributes of the camera departments from memory. In contrast, the Schuette and Fazio (1995) study attempted to understand the role of motivation in a deliberative process that required participants to expend more effort considering the information that was *currently* available to them. In addition, the information that participants were to judge was ambiguous; it was open to varied interpretations. Therefore, instead of exploring the MODE model in tasks requiring retrieval of previously stored facts, the Schuette and Fazio study tested the MODE model in a context requiring more careful examination of the facts that were being presented at that time. The critical question was whether more properly motivated individuals would engage in the cognitive effort of considering alternative possibilities, instead of readily accepting the interpretation implied by their attitudes. If so, they should show less evidence of having processed the stimulus information in an attitudinally biased manner.

In the Schuette and Fazio (1995) study, participants were asked to judge the quality of two studies concerning the effectiveness of capital punishment at deterring crime (see Lord et al., 1979). One study reached a "pro" conclusion about the death penalty, and the other reached a "con" conclusion. Judgments of the quality of the two studies were examined as a function of two experimentally manipulated variables. Attitude accessibility was manipulated in the same manner as in an earlier study, which found the accessibility of subjects' attitudes toward the death penalty to moderate the influence of these attitudes on their judgments of the two studies' quality (Houston & Fazio, 1989). Participants were asked to complete attitude surveys that required them to express their attitudes regarding the death penalty just once or several times. Motivation was manipulated via a fear-of-invalidity technique similar to that used by Kruglanski and Freund (1983) and by Sanbonmatsu and Fazio (1990). Participants were told that their judgments would be compared to that reached by a "blue-ribbon panel" of social scientists, and that they would discuss their decisions later with the experimenter and their fellow participants.

The relation between participants' attitudes toward the death penalty and their judgments of the studies' quality was found to vary jointly as a function of the accessibility of attitudes and motivation. Those with accessible attitudes and low motivation to reach "valid" conclusions were more likely to judge the quality of the studies in a manner that was consistent with their attitudes toward the death penalty. That is, attitudinally biased processing was most apparent in the high-attitude-accessibility/low-motivation condition. The effect of attitude accessibility within the low-motivation condition replicated the findings of the study by Houston and Fazio (1989): The more accessible an attitude, the more likely it was that the attitude would in-

fluence an individual's interpretation of ambiguous information. However, the findings also indicated that individuals could overcome the potential biasing influences of even a relatively accessible attitude when they were properly motivated. Under these circumstances, individuals apparently attended to the attributes of the studies that were presented in a relatively objective fashion, instead of readily accepting the interpretation implied by their attitudes.

THE ROLE OF OPPORTUNITY

The importance of opportunity as a prerequisite for deliberative processing is demonstrated by the Sanbonmatsu and Fazio (1990) study described earlier. Additional evidence to support this notion is available in the literature. For example, Kruglanski and Freund (1983) demonstrated that when time pressure was applied to participants who were asked to compare essays written by children from two different ethnic backgrounds, they were more likely to make judgments about quality that corresponded to their stereotypes about the ethnic groups. Further support is provided by Jamieson and Zanna (1989). Jamieson and Zanna measured participants' attitudes about affirmative action and then asked them to make a judgment about an ambiguous court case involving a charge of sex discrimination. When participants' time to read about the case and make a decision was limited, Jamieson and Zanna found that low self-monitors, who were assumed to possess more accessible attitudes, were more likely to be influenced by their personal attitudes than either the high self-monitors or those in the no-time-pressure condition. Thus, there is ample evidence that the opportunity to consider the available information carefully is necessary for a deliberative process to occur.

MIXED PROCESSES

In addition to delineating two distinct classes of attitude–behavior processes, the MODE model explicitly postulates the possibility of processes that are neither purely spontaneous nor purely deliberative, but instead are "mixed" processes involving a combination of automatic and controlled components. An attitude-to-behavior process that is essentially deliberative in nature may still involve some components that are influenced by automatically activated attitudes. For example, an accessible attitude may serve as a retrieval cue that enhances the likelihood that the individual will retrieve and consider attribute information that is evaluatively congruent with the attitude. An individual may be sufficiently motivated to analyze attribute information, but not sufficiently so to consider the possibility that the sample of evidence being considered may itself be biased.

Likewise, an essentially spontaneous process may sometimes involve some components that are controlled. A particularly striking instance is a situation in which the activation of knowledge regarding normative requirements induces an individual to define the event as one in which he or she needs to control and monitor impulsive behavior carefully. People often experience situations in which they feel that they need to "bite their tongues." This sort of active control over one's responses is particularly likely when normative constraints intervene and prevent one from behaving in accordance with perceptions of the attitude object in the immediate situation. However, any such controlled component within a mixed sequence requires, yet again, that one be both *motivated* to engage in the necessary cognitive effort and have the *opportunity* to do so—just as is true of a purely deliberative process.

In fact, the Schuette and Fazio (1995) study described earlier may illustrate such a mixed process. Recall that participants characterized by more accessible attitudes displayed greater attitudinally biased processing than those with less accessible attitudes, unless their motivation to avoid an invalid conclusion had been enhanced. Presumably, the attitudes of the high-attitude-accessibility/high-motivation participants were activated automatically while they were reading the stimulus information, but their enhanced motivation induced them to consider the information in a more objective fashion. In effect, this was an instance of an automatic process (attitude activation) followed by a controlled process aimed at ensuring a more objective consideration.

If the individual is aware of the potential biasing influence of an automatically activated attitude, then such a motivated process may involve an attempt to "correct" for the influence of the attitude. This particular form of a mixed process, then, parallels the manner in which recent theoretical models have discussed trait inference processes (e.g., Gilbert, Pelham, & Krull, 1988; Trope, 1986). These models hypothesize a sequence of processes in which an initial characterization of a target person's behavior may be followed by a more demanding, effortful stage of reasoning that corrects for the influence of situational constraints on the target's behavior. In a similar manner, individuals sometimes may be motivated to correct for the influence of an automatically activated attitude.

Alternatively, enhanced motivation may simply ensure a more careful, two-sided examination of the available information—scrutiny that has the consequence of attenuating the impact of the automatically activated attitude. In such a case, the attitude may foster a particular interpretation of a given piece of information, but the motivation may induce the individual to consider the information from multiple perspectives (see Lord, Lepper, & Preston's, 1984, discussion of a "consider-the-opposite" strategy). This more balanced consideration will attenuate the influence of the individual's own attitude (see Chen & Chaiken, Chapter 4, this volume, for a discussion of such attenuation processes in the persuasion domain).

IMPLICATIONS FOR RACIAL ATTITUDES, JUDGMENTS, AND BEHAVIOR

One domain in which such mixed attitude-to-behavior processes may commonly occur involves racial attitudes and prejudice. This is one of the few attitudinal domains in which it is obvious that both automatic and controlled processes can operate simultaneously. Some people for whom negativity is automatically activated in response to African Americans are disturbed by such negativity and are motivated to control their prejudiced reactions. In fact, this thesis forms the core of Devine's theoretical and empirical work on racial prejudice (Devine, 1989a, 1989b). Much like our MODE model of attitude–behavior processes, her model focuses upon automatic and controlled components. Devine maintains that as a result of common socialization histories, people are all equally knowledgeable about cultural stereotypes. She argues that the automatic process involved in prejudice against blakc people consists of this socially shared cultural stereotype, which is predominantly negative, being automatically activated in the presence of a black target person. What distinguishes prejudiced and unprejudiced individuals, according to Devine's model, is not this automatic component, but the controlled component. The nonprejudiced are motivated to inhibit the influences of the automatically activated cultural stereotype.

Although concurring with Devine about the potential importance of controlled processes for race-related judgments and behavior, the MODE model offers a different perspective regarding the role of automatic processes. The MODE model assumes that variability exists in the automatic component, as well as the controlled component. That is, the model does not postulate that the predominantly negative cultural stereotype possesses any necessary advantage over personal evaluations in terms of their likelihood of being activated automatically upon an individual's encountering a black person. Instead, the MODE model suggests that there will be meaningful variability in the nature of the evaluations that are activated from memory automatically. For some people, blacks will be strongly associated with negativity; for others, however, they will not, or they may even be strongly associated with a positive evaluation. In other words, what is automatically activated from memory is not necessarily some socially shared cultural stereotype, but personal evaluations—attitudes.

In any case, the notion that both automatic and controlled processes may operate when it comes to racial attitudes and behavior makes race an ideal domain for testing the MODE model. In particular, the mixed processes that the MODE model proposes can be fruitfully investigated in the domain of race-related judgments and behavior. The MODE model offers predictions regarding three general classes of individuals. First, we can consider individuals who are characterized by automatically activated negative attitudes toward blacks, but who at the same time are motivated to control prejudiced reactions. The prediction for such persons is that whether they will express negative judgments will depend upon whether they have sufficient opportunity to counter the influence of their automatically activated negativity. If so, their judgments should not be negative. In contrast, a second class of individuals—those for whom negativity is automatically activated, but who lack any motivation to control those reactions—are predicted to exhibit negative judgments and behavior. Such people simply have no qualms about experiencing and expressing negativity toward blacks. Finally, and as noted earlier, the MODE model posits the existence of individuals for whom negativity is not activated in response to black targets or for whom positive evaluations are automatically activated. These individuals should not, of course, show any evidence of negative judgments or behavior.

Motivated by this reasoning, we have conducted a number of experiments concerning racial attitudes. It is to these empirical tests of the MODE model in the context of race-related judgments and behavior that we now turn.

TESTS OF THE MODE MODEL IN THE DOMAIN OF RACIAL ATTITUDES AND PREJUDICE

All the experiments that have been conducted involve the direct assessment of the evaluations that are automatically activated in response to black target persons. The assessment procedure, which has been termed the "bona fide pipeline" technique (Fazio, Jackson, Dunton, & Williams, 1995), involves a priming paradigm that was first developed in the mid-1980s (Fazio, Sanbonmatsu, Powell, & Kardes, 1986) and has since been used widely to study automatic attitude activation (e.g., Bargh, Chaiken, Govender, & Pratto, 1992; Greenwald, Klinger, & Liu, 1989; Hermans, De Houwer, & Eelen, 1994). The participants' task on each trial is to indicate the connotation of an evaluative adjective as quickly as possible. They are to determine whether the adjective means "good" or "bad." The latency with which this judgment is made, and how it is affected by the prior presentation of a prime, constitute the core of the technique.

In our laboratory's very first report regarding automatic activation (Fazio et al., 1986), the possibility was raised that the procedure might have utility as an unobtrusive measure of attitude. Essentially, the pattern of facilitation that is exhibited on positive versus negative adjectives can provide an indication of an individual's attitude toward the primed object. Relatively more facilitation on positive adjectives should be indicative of a more positive attitude, and relatively more facilitation on negative adjectives should be indicative of a negative attitude. Furthermore, these estimates are obtained in a situation in which the individual is not aware that his or her attitude is being assessed. During the priming task, the participant is not asked to consider his or her attitude toward the object. Yet it is possible to ascertain from the facilitation data the degree to which positive or negative evaluations are activated when the attitude object is presented.

This is the methodology that Fazio and his colleagues have adapted to the measurement of automatically activated racial attitudes. Because some individuals may be reluctant to admit, to themselves or others, that they have negative reactions to blacks, their self-reported attitudes may be suspect. By attempting to "get inside the head" of a respondent, the bona fide pipeline technique provides an unobtrusive estimate of attitude that avoids the problems inherent to self-report measures.

Details regarding the procedure are available in Fazio et al. (1995). For the present purposes, a brief sketch of the procedure should suffice. The participants are told that the experiment involves word meaning as an automatic skill, and that a variety of different tasks will be performed during the experiment. The procedure actually consists of several phases, the fourth phase being the actual priming task.

The purpose of the first task is to obtain baseline data. On each trial, the participant is presented with an adjective and asked to indicate as quickly as possible whether the adjective meant "good" or "bad." Some examples are "attractive," "likable," "wonderful," "annoying," "disgusting," and "offensive." The next two phases of the experiment are in-

tended to prepare participants for the priming task, which involves the presentation of faces as primes and adjectives as targets. The second phase is presented to the participants as involving the ability to learn faces. They simply attend to the faces presented on the computer screen. The third phase involves a recognition test. Participants are presented with a face and asked to indicate whether the face was one that they have or have not seen in the previous task.

Next, the actual priming task of interest occurs. Participants are told that the previous tasks will now be combined. They are told that the researchers' interest is in determining the degree to which judging word meaning is an automatic skill. The experimenter indicates that if it truly is an automatic skill, individuals should be able to perform just as well as in the very first phase of the experiment, even if they have to do something else at the same time. In this case, the task to be performed simultaneously is learning faces. Thus participants are led to believe that this phase of the experiment involves both the learning of the faces and the judgment of adjective connotation. On the target trials, color photographs of white and black undergraduates serve as the primes. All photographs are head shots taken against a common background and are digitized as 256-color, 640 × 480 resolution images.

This procedure yields a multitude of observations for each participant. Fazio and colleagues have routinely reduced the data that are obtained from any given respondent to a single index that serves as the estimate of the individual's attitude toward blacks. To do so, average facilitation scores are computed for each person on positive and negative adjectives for each face that is presented. This preliminary step yields mean facilitation scores for each of the multiple white and black faces. Thus, it is possible to examine the interaction between race of photo and valence of adjective for every participant. The effect size of this interaction is computed and serves as the estimate of the individual's attitude. Given this computational procedure, more negative scores reflect a pattern of facilitation indicating greater negativity toward blacks. That is, negative scores involve relatively more facilitation on negative adjectives when they are preceded by a black face than a white face, and relatively less facilitation on positive adjectives when they are preceded by a black face. The opposite pattern produces a positive score.

Validity of the Attitude Estimates

The initial study employing the bona fide pipeline procedure (Fazio et al., 1995, Experiment 1) was aimed at assessing the validity of the attitude estimates obtained. The first indication that the technique has some validity stemmed from the finding that the 45 white participants and 8 black participants in the sample displayed very different patterns of facilitation. On the average, the white participants displayed more negative attitudes toward blacks than did the black participants. However, considerable variability existed among the white participants. Some were characterized by relatively extreme negative attitudes. However, some of them were not; in fact, some displayed data similar to those displayed by some of the black participants. The obvious question is whether this variability was simply noise, or whether it was meaningful in the sense that it proved predictive of some of the other data that were collected.

One such measure is especially relevant to the present purposes. It involved the participants' interacting with a black female. Participants were introduced to this person after completing the computer tasks and interacted with her for about 10 minutes in the context of her providing a "bogus debriefing." Based on this interaction, the black experimenter rated each individual in terms of the friendliness and interest that he or she exhibited. She paid particular attention to such factors as amount of smiling, eye contact, spatial distance, and body language. The sum of her two ratings served as the measure of the quality of the interaction. The unobtrusive estimates of the white participants' attitudes toward blacks correlated significantly with this measure.

Thus, the unobtrusive measure does appear to have some validity. Not only did the attitude estimates for black and white participants differ markedly, but the variability that existed among white participants proved to have predictive value. The variability that existed in the nature of the evaluations that were automatically activated from memory was predictive of subsequent behavior during an interaction with a black person.

Evidence Regarding Spontaneous Attitude–Behavior Processes

This latter finding is especially important for the MODE model, and in particular for its postulate regarding a spontaneous attitude-to-behavior process—one in which behavior is a direct function of the attitudes that are automatically activated from memory when the attitude object is encountered. As noted earlier, many correlational and experimental studies on attitude–behavior consistency have compared people whose attitudes were highly accessible (and hence capable of automatic activation) to those with less accessible attitudes. Greater consistency between attitudes and behavior has been observed within the group with more accessible attitudes. In other words, the work has demonstrated the moderating role of attitude accessibility. In contrast, this study directly assessed of any evaluation that was automatically activated from memory upon exposure to black stimulus persons, and then used that information as an individual-difference measure for predicting subsequent behavior. In that sense, the finding provides more direct support for the MODE model's depiction of a spontaneous attitude–behavior process than has been available previously.

A recent study by Jackson (1997) leads to a similar conclusion. After an initial session in which the bona fide pipeline procedure was employed to assess automatically activated attitudes toward blacks, the participants returned for a session that included their judging the quality of an essay presumably written by a black male undergraduate. Ostensibly, the essay had been submitted as an entry in a competition intended to select a description of the student's university for publication in a guide to colleges and universities. Participants were provided a folder that included a brief biography and photo of the author, as well as the essay. After answering a few questions regarding their impressions of the described university, participants rated the quality of the essay. A composite measure was created from responses to questions regarding how informative, persuasive, and well written the essay was, and from a rating of the extent to which the essay deserved to win the competition. This measure of the quality of the essay correlated significantly with the attitude estimates provided by the unobtrusive measure of racial attitudes. Thus, judgments of a black target person's work were evidently affected by the evaluations that were automatically activated in response to the author's race.

Recent research by Dovidio, Kawakami, Johnson, Johnson, and Howard (1997) also provides support for the MODE model's postulate regarding a spontaneous attitude–behavior process. These researchers developed a measure of automatically activated racial attitudes conceptually similar to the technique employed by Fazio et al. (1995). The latency with which participants responded to positive versus negative words that had been preceded by the subliminal presentation of a police-like sketch of a white or a black face provided the basis for computing an estimate of attitude toward blacks. In a later part of the experiment, the participants were videotaped while interacting with a black and a white interviewer. Significant correlations were observed between the attitude estimates obtained in the first part of the experiment and the participants' nonverbal behavior toward the black interviewer. The more participants' response latencies during the priming task reflected automatically activated negativity toward blacks, the more frequently they blinked and the less eye contact they maintained with the black relative to the white interviewer.

Evidence Regarding Mixed Attitude–Behavior Processes

The findings summarized above indicate that assessments of the extent to which negativity is automatically activated in response to black targets can be predictive of race-related judgments and behavior. However, correlations with such assessments have not always been observed. It has not been possible to predict some race-related judgments from attitude estimates based on automatically activated evaluations (see Fazio et al., 1995). According to the MODE model, such null-effect cases are likely to have involved a judgment that evoked a motivation to control seemingly prejudiced reactions and a context that provided the opportunity to exert such control successfully. The findings noted above regard-

ing actual interactions with a black target person (Dovidio et al., 1997; Fazio et al., 1995) focused upon nonverbal behaviors, which are known to be difficult to control consciously (DePaulo, Stone, & Lassiter, 1985; Zuckerman, DePaulo, & Rosenthal, 1981). Thus, even though some individuals may have been motivated to counter the influence of any automatically activated negativity that they experienced in the presence of the black target person, the opportunity to do so may have been lacking. As a result, automatically activated attitudes may have directly influenced the nonverbal behaviors that were emitted. Presumably, any such motivations were not engaged by Jackson's (1997) essay judgment task. Apparently, rating the essay's quality in the context of a competition did not lead individuals to construe the situation and the requested responses as related to their racial attitudes. If no motivation to control seemingly prejudiced reactions is aroused, then the MODE model again predicts that automatically activated attitudes should directly influence the judgments. However, as noted in our earlier discussion of mixed attitude–behavior processes, the MODE model does maintain that the influence of any automatically activated negativity toward blacks can be attenuated if *both* the motivation and the opportunity to do so exist.

In order to examine such mixed processes, Dunton and Fazio (1997) developed a 17-item scale assessing motivation to control seemingly prejudiced reactions. The scale includes such statements as "In today's society, it's important that one not be perceived as prejudiced in any manner," "It's never acceptable to express one's prejudices," and "I feel guilty when I have a negative thought or feeling about a Black person." By administering this scale, as well as having participants undergo the bona fide pipeline procedure, investigators can examine the joint influence of automatic and controlled processes on race-related judgments.[1] Recent research has followed this strategy as a means of testing the MODE model's predictions regarding mixed processes.

The first study to do so (Fazio et al., 1995, Experiment 4) focused on responses to the Modern Racism Scale (McConahay, 1986)—a measure for which earlier studies indeed had failed to observe any correlation with automatically activated racial attitudes (Fazio et al., 1995, Experiments 1 and 2). The scale, which includes such items as "Over the past few years, Blacks have gotten more economically than they deserve," "Discrimination against Blacks is no longer a problem in the United States," and "Blacks are getting too demanding in their push for equal rights," appeared likely to engage a motivation to control prejudiced reactions. Moreover, experimental research (Fazio et al., 1995, Experiment 3) revealed that the Modern Racism Scale is quite reactive, despite claims to the contrary (McConahay, Hardee, & Batts, 1981). Participants presented themselves as less prejudiced when they completed the scale for a black experimenter than when they did so for a white experimenter. This reactivity

suggests that at least some individuals experience some motivation to control prejudiced reactions when responding to the items of the Modern Racism Scale.

Scores on the Motivation to Control Prejudiced Reactions Scale (Dunton & Fazio, 1997), along with estimates of participants' racial attitudes derived from the unobtrusive priming procedure, were used to predict Modern Racism Scale scores. The interaction between the unobtrusive estimates and motivation to control prejudice was significant and is plotted in Figure 5.1, which displays the regression lines predicting Modern Racism Scale scores from attitude estimates for high and low Motivation to Control Prejudiced Reactions Scale scores. As motivation to control prejudice decreased, the relation be-

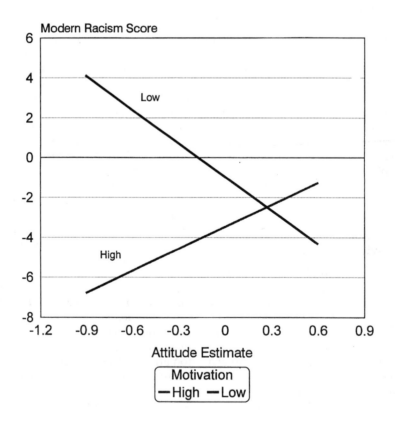

FIGURE 5.1. Regression lines predicting scores on the Modern Racism Scale as a function of the unobtrusive attitude estimates and motivation to control prejudice. Higher scores reflect more prejudice. From Fazio, Jackson, Dunton, and Williams (1995). Copyright 1995 by the American Psychological Association. Reprinted by permission.

tween the unobtrusive attitude estimates and Modern Racism Scale scores grew stronger, such that more negative automatically activated attitudes were associated with more prejudiced Modern Racism scores. Motivation to control prejudice mattered little among those for whom little or no negativity was automatically activated in response to black faces. However, motivation to control prejudice exerted a strong influence among those individuals for whom negativity was automatically activated. Those with little such motivation felt free to respond to the Modern Racism Scale items in a manner that was indicative of prejudice, whereas the more motivated described themselves as far less prejudiced.

A similar interaction between automatic and controlled components of racial prejudice has been obtained in subsequent work (Dunton & Fazio, 1997). In this research, two direct self-report measures of evaluation of blacks were examined. One measure asked respondents to list feelings that came to mind when they thought about the "typical Black male undergraduate" (see Haddock, Zanna, & Esses, 1993). The participants then scored their listed feelings by rating each of the feelings on a scale of –2 (extremely negative) to +2 (extremely positive). These ratings were averaged to arrive at a final feeling score for each respondent. The second measure involved a simple thermometer rating (from 0 to 100) of favorability toward black male undergraduates. Given that these two ratings were highly correlated, they were standardized and then combined into a single composite score reflecting each participant's self-reported attitude toward blacks.

Approximately 1 month after providing their self-reports, these individuals participated in a two-session experiment. The first session was devoted to the bona fide pipeline procedure. Participants completed the Motivation to Control Prejudiced Reactions Scale in a second session 1 week later, while participating in an ostensibly unrelated experiment. A regression analysis predicting the self-reports regarding black male college students revealed a significant interaction between estimates of automatically activated attitudes and motivation to control prejudice. As shown in Figure 5.2, when subjects were not motivated to control prejudiced reactions, their self-

reported evaluations tended to be consistent with their automatically activated evaluations. For example, low-motivation students who were estimated to have negative attitudes by the unobtrusive measure also reported negative attitudes when questioned directly. Highly motivated participants, on the other hand, being motivated to inhibit racial prejudice, tended to report positive evaluations even when negativity was automatically activated. Thus, this work provides additional evidence regarding the interplay of automatic and controlled processes in race-related judgments and behavior.

Both the findings with respect to the Modern Racism Scale and those concerning the direct self-reports indicate that some individuals for whom negativity was automatically activated in response to blacks were motivated to counter the effects of that negativity. In fact, among individuals highly motivated to control prejudiced reactions, the relations between the attitude estimates and both the Modern Racism Scale and the direct evaluation measure were in a direction opposite to that of the relations for individuals characterized by low motivation. As motivation increased, the slope of the regression lines changed from negative to positive in the case of the Modern Racism Scale (for which higher numbers reflect more prejudice) and from positive to negative in the case of the evaluation measure (for which higher numbers reflect more positive evaluations). It certainly would have been reasonable to expect no relation (i.e., a flat regression line) between unobtrusive attitude estimates and self-reports to emerge among motivated respondents. However, the findings consistently revealed a relation. It appeared that individuals characterized by automatically activated negativity and relatively strong motivation to control prejudiced reactions tended to overcompensate for their negativity. Their high motivation to control prejudiced reactions led to the expression of judgments that were even more positive than the responses of individuals for whom positivity was activated.

This overcompensation can be interpreted in terms of Petty and Wegener's (1993; Wegener & Petty, 1995) flexible-correction model. This model postulates that judgmental corrections are a function of individuals' naive theories regarding the influence of a force

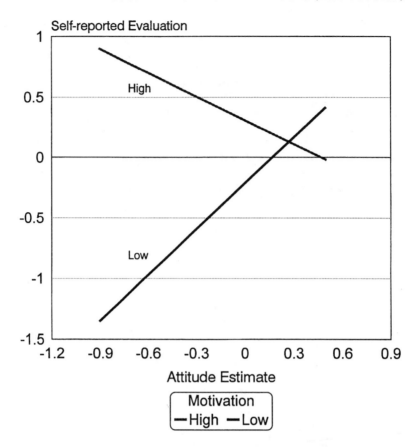

FIGURE 5.2. Regression lines predicting self-reported evaluations as a function of unobtrusive attitude estimates and motivation to control prejudice. Higher evaluation scores reflect a more positive evaluation. From Dunton and Fazio (1997). Copyright 1997 by Sage Publications, Inc. Reprinted by permission.

that they believe to be biasing their judgments. Apparently, individuals who experience automatically activated negativity toward blacks, yet are highly motivated to control prejudiced reactions, believe that this negativity exerts a large biasing impact on their judgmental processes. As a result, they display a relatively large correction in order to eliminate the presumed biasing effects of their automatically activated negativity toward blacks.

Categorization by Race

Additional support for the MODE model is provided by a recent study that examined the automatic and controlled processes involved in the categorization of stimulus persons (Fazio & Dunton, 1997). Given that people can typically be thought of as members of multiple categories, it is valuable to consider the processes involved in categorization by race. What factors determine whether stimulus persons will be categorized by race, as opposed to the multiple other possibilities that exist? Fazio and Dunton reasoned that both automatically activated attitudes and motivation to control prejudiced reactions should influence categorization by race. The prediction regarding motivation was very straightforward: The more motivated an individual is to avoid a seemingly prejudiced reaction, the more the individual should search for means of construing the stimulus persons other than race.

The reasoning regarding the role of automatic attitude activation was more complex; it was based largely upon research findings concerning the role of attitude accessibility in visual attention. Roskos-Ewoldsen and Fazio (1992) found that when subjects were visually presented with an array of line drawings of objects, their attention was inescapably and automatically attracted to those objects that were attitude-evoking (i.e., objects toward which they had accessible attitudes). For example, these attitude-evoking objects were more likely to be noticed after very brief exposures of display, and more likely to be noticed incidentally during a task in which attending to these items was neither required nor optimal. On the basis of these findings, Roskos-Ewoldsen and Fazio suggested that an attitude toward an object in the visual field may be activated from memory at an early stage in the processing of visual information. Such activation then may direct further attention to the visual stimulus, so that ultimately the stimulus receives sufficient processing for it to be consciously noticed and reported.

Models of categorization—for example, those of Medin and Schaffer (1978), Nosofsky (1986), and Smith and Zarate (1992)—posit a pivotal role for such attentional mechanisms. These models suggest that categorization follows from the allocation of attention to particular dimensions of the stimulus. Greater attention to a given attribute increases the likelihood that the stimulus person will be categorized accordingly. Therefore, it appears that possessing highly accessible attitudes toward a given attribute of a stimulus person may lead to greater attention's being drawn to this specific attitude-evoking characteristic of the stimulus person. In turn, this greater attention increases the likelihood that the target will be categorized according to the dimension toward which subjects hold accessible attitudes.[2]

On the basis of this reasoning, Fazio and Dunton (1997) hypothesized that the more attitude-evoking race is for a given individual, the more likely it is that the individual will attend to the target's race and categorize by race. The bona fide pipeline procedure provides an indication of how attitude-evoking race is for a given individual, because it is based upon evaluations that are automatically activated from memory. For some people, blacks automatically evoke positivity; for others, blacks automatically evoke negativity; for still others, neither occurs. Thus, a curvilinear,

U-shaped relation between this measure and categorization by race was predicted.

In order to assess categorization by race, a similarity rating procedure and multidimensional scaling were employed. The participants returned for a second, ostensibly unrelated session 1 week after having participated in the bona fide pipeline procedure. They were met by a different experimenter, who instructed them that they would be presented with pairs of photos on the computer screen. Their task was to rate the similarity of the individuals in each pair. The photos varied in race, gender, and occupation (e.g., a black female cashier). Each photo presented cues as to the occupation of the individual in the photo; therefore, the photos could be categorized in any number of ways. These similarity ratings were subjected to a multidimensional scaling procedure, INDSCAL. A four-dimensional solution emerged, with one of the dimensions readily identifiable as race. An advantage of INDSCAL is that it yields not only this multidimensional space, but also a set of weights for each individual, showing the extent to which the individual weighted each dimension in making his or her similarity ratings. When squared, these weights indicate the proportion of variance in the similarity ratings that is accounted for by each dimension.

Obviously, the weights for the race dimension were of primary interest. A multiple regression predicting these weights from the estimate of automatically activated attitudes and from the squared values of these attitude estimates revealed the predicted curvilinear relation to be significant. Those participants for whom negativity was automatically activated in response to blacks had weights indicating that they used the race dimension heavily in making their similarity ratings. The same was true of those participants for whom positive attitudes were automatically activated. It was those individuals for whom little or no attitude activation occurred automatically who tended not to use the race dimension much.

When scores on the Motivation to Control Prejudiced Reactions Scale were added to the regression equation predicting use of the race dimension, a significant main effect was observed. Individuals who described themselves as being highly motivated to control seemingly prejudiced reactions did not use the race dimension as heavily when judging similarity as did those individuals with lower motivation scores.

The findings suggest that upon the presentation of a black target, attitudes toward blacks were automatically activated at a very early stage of processing for some individuals. As a result, their attention was automatically drawn to the race information. Greater attention to the race information led the participants to weigh race more heavily in judging similarity. However, some participants apparently did not appreciate having their attention drawn to race in this way. Those who were motivated to control prejudiced reactions exerted some effort to counter this influence, and hence used the race dimension less.

Corroborating evidence for this particular account was provided by analyses of the latencies with which the participants made the similarity judgments. At least in the first third of the 276 trials (prior to the participants' having developed much efficiency at this rather lengthy task), those individuals for whom race was attitude-evoking were relatively faster to respond on trials involving a black stimulus person than were those for whom race was more neutral. Apparently the attention of the former individuals was automatically drawn to race, providing them with an easy basis for judging similarity, and hence allowing them to respond relatively quickly. The analysis also revealed that those participants who were relatively motivated to control prejudiced reactions were significantly slower to respond. Thus, they apparently found it necessary to exert some time-consuming effort to counter having their attention drawn to race. This finding suggests that the motivation to control seemingly prejudiced reactions prompted a controlled process involving a search for alternative bases for judging similarity.

This study illustrates the importance of both automatic and controlled processes for attention and categorization. When they encounter a target person who is categorizable in multiple ways, people do not necessarily "see" the same person. People for whom race is attitude-evoking are the ones who most readily notice that the target is black, and are most likely to categorize the target as black.

What does this imply for an actual interaction with a black target? Someone characterized by automatically activated positivity is very likely to categorize the target as black, but the outcome should be relatively benign, because judgment and behavior will be influenced by a positive attitude. The same cannot be said about an individual for whom negativity is automatically activated. Such an individual is also relatively likely to categorize the target as black, as opposed to relying on other potentially relevant categories (e.g., "female" or "cashier"). However, in such a case, perceptions of the target person in this immediate situation and ultimately, behavior toward the target will be influenced by the automatically activated negativity.

Implications Regarding Racial Prejudice

The application of the MODE model to the domain of racial attitudes has proven quite fruitful. The empirical research has confirmed that both automatic and controlled processes can be involved in race-related judgments and behavior. Individuals vary both with respect to the attitudes that are automatically activated in response to a black person and with respect to their motivation to control seemingly prejudiced reactions. It is this variability across two different components of racial prejudice that has formed the basis for our earlier discussion of the MODE model's consideration of three classes of individuals—a discussion to which it is now useful to return. Some people, who might be labeled as truly nonprejudiced, do not experience any automatically activated negativity when they encounter a black person, or may even experience activation of a positive evaluation relative to what occurs when they encounter a white target. Others, who might be labeled as truly prejudiced, do experience automatically activated negativity and are not motivated to control its influence.

Finally, and just as hypothesized by Devine (1989a, 1989b; see also Devine & Monteith, Chapter 17, this volume), there is a class of individuals who are motivated to correct for the influence of the automatically activated negativity that they experience. This motivation may stem from a sincere distaste for the negative reaction that has been automatically activated, from a simple desire to avoid dispute, or from a more strategic self-presentational desire to comply with the perceived social norms in a given situation. In any case, judgments and behavior may be monitored carefully so as to avoid what might be construed as a prejudiced response. The more these controlled efforts stem from a sincere displeasure with an individual's having experienced automatically activated negativity, the more the individual appears to be moving toward a truly nonprejudiced stand. The importance of such self-dissatisfaction has been documented by recent research concerned with the process of prejudice reduction (Devine, Monteith, Zuwerink, & Elliot, 1991; Monteith, 1993; Monteith, Devine, & Zuwerink, 1993). The obvious hope is that with sufficient practice at controlling prejudiced reactions, the negative associations with blacks that are stored in memory will eventually lose strength or even be replaced by positive associations, so that ultimately the automatic activation of negativity will no longer occur.

The MODE model and the empirical investigations conducted to date emphasize the importance of both motivation and opportunity. As noted earlier, whether a motivation to control seemingly prejudiced reactions is engaged in any given situation will depend on individuals' construals of the situation and the judgmental or behavioral response that they have been requested to provide. Construals that note the relevance of racial attitudes to the situation and the requested response appear to be necessary to evoke such motivation among any individuals who are so disposed. The findings concerning the Modern Racism Scale and self-reported favorability toward blacks indicate that requests for verbal evaluations of blacks as a group are construed as related to racial attitudes and do evoke motivational concerns. Likewise, requests to judge the similarity of stimulus persons who vary in race, gender, and occupation seem sufficient to engage a motivation to avoid seemingly prejudiced responses. It appears that at least some of the participants in the categorization study viewed the use of race as an inappropriate dimension by which to judge similarity and believed that doing so would be indicative of a negative racial attitude. However, Jackson's (1997) finding regarding judgments of the quality of an essay submitted to a competition by a black author suggests that

motivational concerns are not inevitably evoked for all judgments and behavior concerning a black target. In this study, the judgments of quality varied as a function of automatically activated attitudes, but did not vary with scores on the Motivation to Control Prejudiced Reactions Scale. Apparently, the participants did not construe the task of judging the quality of an essay produced by a black student for a competition as being related to racial attitudes.

Assuming that a situation is construed as relevant to racial attitudes, and that motivational concerns are evoked for people who seek to avoid responses that might be indicative of prejudice, the MODE model maintains that the opportunity factor will be the key determinant of whether any such motivated efforts are successful. Motivation is not sufficient; the opportunity to monitor one's responses is also necessary. Motivated persons need the time and the cognitive resources to deliberate about their responses if they are to correct for the influence of any automatically activated negativity. As noted earlier, some behaviors may be more easily monitored and controlled than others. Nonverbal behaviors, in particular, may be subject to "leakage" of the negativity that has been automatically activated, despite any efforts an individual may be making to behave in a nonprejudiced manner. In addition, some situations may provide a greater opportunity for the motivated individual to engage in correction processes than other situations do. The research discussed earlier concerning time pressure suggests that situations that demand an immediate response may decrease the opportunity to inhibit the influence of automatically activated negativity. Likewise, when cognitive resources are limited or taxed by the need to attend to multiple demands, the opportunity to engage in controlled processing may be limited (see Sanbonmatsu & Kardes, 1988).

Judgments and behaviors that provide the opportunity for controlling one's response should be predictable from the joint influence of automatically activated attitudes and motivation to control prejudice—just as was observed for the Modern Racism Scale, the self-reports of favorability toward blacks, and the similarity judgments. However, as opportunity decreases, either because the behavior itself is not easily controllable or because the situation limits the opportunity, the behavior should be less influenced by motivational concerns and more directly and singly influenced by any automatically activated evaluations.

CONCLUSION

The MODE model appears to provide a useful framework for considering the multiple processes by which attitudes may guide judgments and behavior. Attitudes that are automatically activated from memory upon an individual's encountering the attitude object can influence perceptions of the attitude object in the immediate situation and, ultimately, behavior (a relatively spontaneous process). However, given sufficient motivation for accuracy and sufficient opportunity, individuals can consider the attitude object in terms of the attributes that it is known to possess, instead of relying on their previously stored summary evaluations of the object (a relatively deliberative process). In addition, automatic and controlled processes may sometimes both be involved in judgments and behavior. Such mixed processes can assume any number of forms, but one especially interesting form is illustrated by the research concerning racial prejudice. In this case, a motivation to achieve the specific goal of behaving in a nonprejudiced manner may prompt efforts that have the effect of mitigating the influence of an automatically activated attitude. The MODE model suggests that race-related judgments and behavior will depend upon automatically activated evaluations; upon any motivation that the individual may experience to respond without prejudice; and, finally, upon the extent to which the behavior in question and the situation provide an opportunity for such a motivated process to succeed.

ACKNOWLEDGMENT

Preparation of this chapter, as well as much of the research summarized within it, was supported by Research Scientist Development Award No. MH00452 and Grant No. MH38832 from the National Institute of Mental Health.

NOTES

1. Factor analyses have revealed that the scale consists of two distinct factors: (1) a concern with acting prejudiced, which involves a personal commitment to avoid reactions that others and oneself might consider prejudiced, as well as a sincere distaste for any violations of this personal standard that one may exhibit; and (2) restraint to avoid dispute, which involves a willingness to inhibit the expression of one's own thoughts and feelings in the interest of avoiding dispute with or about blacks. Although the two factors have been found to bear somewhat different relations to self-reports regarding blacks, we will, for the sake of simplicity, limit the present discussion to a consideration of the total scale scores. The interested reader is referred to Dunton and Fazio (1997) for corresponding analyses involving each of the two factors.

2. A recent series of experiments yielded evidence supporting the hypothesis that attitude accessibility does influence categorization (Smith, Fazio, & Cejka, 1996). These experiments focused upon attitude objects that can be categorized in multiple ways. For example, yogurt can be viewed as a health food or as a dairy product. When the accessibility of attitudes toward health food was experimentally enhanced, yogurt was more likely to cue "health food"; when attitudes toward dairy products were rehearsed, yogurt was more likely to cue "dairy products." Thus, the potential category toward which the individual had the more accessible attitude was more likely to dominate the categorization process. The Fazio and Dunton (1997) study examined this same general hypothesis, but with photos of people as the stimuli of interest.

REFERENCES

Abelson, R. P., & Levi, A. (1985). Decision making and decision theory. In G. Lindzey & E. Aronson (Eds.), *Handbook of social psychology* (3rd ed., Vol. 2, pp. 231–310). New York: Random House.

Ajzen, I. (1991). The theory of planned behavior. *Organizational Behavior and Human Decision Processes, 50,* 179–211.

Ajzen, I., & Fishbein, M. (1980). *Understanding attitudes and predicting social behavior.* Englewood Cliffs, NJ: Prentice-Hall.

Bargh, J. A., Chaiken, S., Govender, R., & Pratto, F. (1992). The generality of the automatic activation effect. *Journal of Personality and Social Psychology, 62,* 893–912.

Bruner, J. S. (1957). On perceptual readiness. *Psychological Review, 64,* 123–152.

Carretta, T. R., & Moreland, R. L. (1982). Nixon and Watergate: A field demonstration of belief perseverance. *Personality and Social Psychology Bulletin, 8,* 446–453.

DePaulo, B. M., Stone, J. I., & Lassiter, G. D. (1985). Deceiving and detecting deceit. In B. R. Schlenker (Ed.), *The self and social life* (pp. 323–370). New York: McGraw-Hill.

Devine, P. G. (1989a). Stereotypes and prejudice: Their automatic and controlled components. *Journal of Personality and Social Psychology, 56,* 5–18.

Devine, P. G. (1989b). Automatic and controlled processes in prejudice: The role of stereotypes and personal beliefs. In A. R. Pratkanis, S. J. Breckler, & A. G. Greenwald (Eds.), *Attitude structure and function* (pp. 181–212). Hillsdale, NJ: Erlbaum.

Devine, P. G., Monteith, M. J., Zuwerink, J. R., & Elliot, A. J. (1991). Prejudice with and without compunction. *Journal of Personality and Social Psychology, 60,* 817–830.

Dovidio, J. F., Kawakami, K., Johnson, C., Johnson, B., & Howard, A. (1997). On the nature of prejudice: Automatic and controlled processes. *Journal of Experimental Social Psychology, 33,* 510–540.

Dunton, B. C., & Fazio, R. H. (1997). An individual difference measure of motivation to control prejudiced reactions. *Personality and Social Psychology Bulletin, 23,* 316–326.

Einhorn, H. J., & Hogarth, R. M. (1981). Behavioral decision theory: Processes of judgment and choice. *Annual Review of Psychology, 32,* 52–88.

Fazio, R. H. (1986). How do attitudes guide behavior? In R. M. Sorrentino & E. T. Higgins (Eds.), *Handbook of motivation and cognition: Foundations of social behavior* (Vol. 1, pp. 204–243). New York: Guilford Press.

Fazio, R. H. (1990). Multiple processes by which attitudes guide behavior: The MODE model as an integrative framework. In M. P. Zanna (Ed.), *Advances in experimental social psychology* (Vol. 23, pp. 75–109). San Diego, CA: Academic Press.

Fazio, R. H. (1995). Attitudes as object–evaluation associations: Determinants, consequences, and correlates of attitude accessibility. In R. E. Petty & J. A. Krosnick (Eds.), *Attitude strength: Antecedents and consequences* (pp. 247–282). Mahwah, NJ: Erlbaum.

Fazio, R. H., Chen, J., McDonel, E. C., & Sherman, S. J. (1982). Attitude accessibility, attitude–behavior consistency, and the strength of the object–evaluation association. *Journal of Experimental Social Psychology, 18,* 339–357.

Fazio, R. H., & Dunton, B. C. (1997). Categorization by race: The impact of automatic and controlled components of racial prejudice. *Journal of Experimental Social Psychology, 33,* 451–470.

Fazio, R. H., Jackson, J. R., Dunton, B. C., & Williams, C. J. (1995). Variability in automatic activation as an unobtrusive measure of racial attitudes: A bona fide pipeline? *Journal of Personality and Social Psychology, 69,* 1013–1027.

Fazio, R. H., Powell, M. C., & Herr, P. M. (1983). Toward a process model of the attitude–behavior relation: Accessing one's attitude upon mere observation of the attitude object. *Journal of Personality and Social Psychology, 44,* 723–735.

Fazio, R. H., Powell, M. C., & Williams, C. J. (1989). The role of attitude accessibility in the attitude-to-behavior process. *Journal of Consumer Research, 16,* 280–288.

Fazio, R. H., Roskos-Ewoldsen, D. R., & Powell, M. C. (1994). Attitudes, perception, and attention. In P. M. Niedenthal & S. Kitayama (Eds.), *The heart's eye: Emotional influences in perception and attention* (pp. 197–216). San Diego: Academic Press.

Fazio, R. H., Sanbonmatsu, D. M., Powell, M. C., & Kardes, F. R. (1986). On the automatic activation of attitudes. *Journal of Personality and Social Psychology, 50,* 229–238.

Fazio, R. H., & Williams, C. J. (1986). Attitude accessibility as a moderator of the attitude–perception and attitude–behavior relations: An investigation of the 1984 presidential election. *Journal of Personality and Social Psychology, 51,* 505–514.

Gilbert, D. T., Pelham, B. W., & Krull, D. S. (1988). On cognitive busyness: When person perceivers meet persons perceived. *Journal of Personality and Social Psychology, 54,* 733–740.

Greenwald, A. G., Klinger, M. R., & Liu, T. J. (1989). Unconscious processing of dichoptically masked words. *Memory and Cognition, 17,* 35-47.

Haddock, G., Zanna, M. P., & Esses, V. M. (1993). Assessing the structure of prejudicial attitudes: The case of attitudes toward homosexuals. *Journal of Personality and Social Psychology, 65,* 1105–1118.

Hastorf, A. H., & Cantril, H. (1954). They saw a game: A case study. *Journal of Abnormal and Social Psychology, 49,* 129–134.

Hermans, D., De Houwer, J., & Eelen, P. (1994). The affective priming effect: Automatic activation of evaluative information in memory. *Cognition and Emotion, 8,* 515–533.

Houston, D. A., & Fazio, R. H. (1989). Biased processing as a function of attitude accessibility: Making objective judgments subjectively. *Social Cognition, 7,* 51–66.

Jackson, J. R. (1997). *Automatically activated racial attitudes.* Unpublished doctoral dissertation, Indiana University.

Jamieson, D. W., & Zanna, M. P. (1989). Need for structure in attitude formation and expression. In A. R. Pratkanis, S. J. Breckler, & A. G. Greenwald (Eds.), *Attitude structure and function* (pp. 383–406). Hillsdale, NJ: Erlbaum.

Kruglanski, A. W. (1989). *Lay epistemics and human knowledge: Cognitive and motivational bases.* New York: Plenum Press.

Kruglanski, A. W., & Freund, T. (1983). The freezing and unfreezing of lay-inferences: Effects on impressional primacy, ethnic stereotyping, and numerical anchoring. *Journal of Experimental Social Psychology, 19,* 448–468.

Kruglanski, A. W., & Webster, D. M. (1996). Motivated closing of the mind: "Seizing" and "freezing." *Psychological Review, 103,* 263–283.

Lord, C. G., Lepper, M. R., & Preston, E. (1984). Considering the opposite: A corrective strategy for social judgment. *Journal of Personality and Social Psychology, 47,* 1231–1243.

Lord, C. G., Ross, L., & Lepper, M. R. (1979). Biased assimilation and attitude polarization: The effects of prior theories on subsequently considered evidence. *Journal of Personality and Social Psychology, 37,* 2098–2109.

McConahay, J. B. (1986). Modern racism, ambivalence, and the Modern Racism Scale. In J. F. Dovidio & S. L. Gaertner (Eds.), *Prejudice, discrimination, and racism* (pp. 91–125). Orlando, FL: Academic Press.

McConahay, J. B., Hardee, B. B., & Batts, V. (1981). Has racism declined in America?: It depends on who is asking and what is asked. *Journal of Conflict Resolution, 25,* 563–579.

Medin, D. L., & Schaffer, M. M. (1978). Context theory of classification learning. *Psychological Review, 85,* 207–238.

Monteith, M. J. (1993). Self-regulation of prejudiced responses: Implications for progress in prejudice-reduction efforts. *Journal of Personality and Social Psychology, 65,* 469–485.

Monteith, M. J., Devine, P. G., & Zuwerink, J. R. (1993). Self-directed versus other-directed affect as a consequence of prejudice-related discrepancies. *Journal of Personality and Social Psychology, 64,* 198–210.

Nosofsky, R. M. (1986). Attention, similarity, and the identification–categorization relationship. *Journal of Experimental Psychology: General, 115,* 39–57.

Petty, R. E., & Wegener, D. T. (1993). Flexible correction processes in social judgment: Correcting for context-induced contrast. *Journal of Experimental Social Psychology, 29,* 137–165.

Regan, D. T., Straus, E., & Fazio, R. H. (1974). Liking and the attribution process. *Journal of Experimental Social Psychology, 10,* 385–397.

Roskos-Ewoldsen, D. R., & Fazio, R. H. (1992). On the orienting value of attitudes: Attitude accessibility as a determinant of an object's attraction of visual attention. *Journal of Personality and Social Psychology, 63,* 198–211.

Sanbonmatsu, D. M., & Fazio, R. H. (1990). The role of attitudes in memory-based decision making. *Journal of Personality and Social Psychology, 59,* 614–622.

Sanbonmatsu, D. M., & Kardes, F. R. (1988). The effects of arousal on information processing and persuasion. *Journal of Consumer Research, 15,* 379–385.

Schuette, R. A., & Fazio, R. H. (1995). Attitude accessibility and motivation as determinants of biased processing: A test of the MODE model. *Personality and Social Psychology Bulletin, 21,* 704–710.

Smith, E. R., Fazio, R. H., & Cejka, M. A. (1996). Accessible attitudes influence categorization of multiply categorizable objects. *Journal of Personality and Social Psychology, 71,* 888–898.

Smith, E. R., & Zarate, M. A. (1992). Exemplar-based model of social judgment. *Psychological Review, 99,* 3–21.

Trope, Y. (1986). Identification and inferential processes in dispositional attribution. *Psychological Review, 93,* 239–257.

Wegener, D. T., & Petty, R. E. (1995). Flexible correction processes in social judgment: The role of naive theories in corrections for perceived bias. *Journal of Personality and Social Psychology, 68,* 36–51.

Zuckerman, M., DePaulo, B. M., & Rosenthal, R. (1981). Verbal and nonverbal communication of deception. In L. Berkowitz (Ed.), *Advances in experimental social psychology* (Vol. 14, pp. 1–59). New York: Academic Press.

6

Depth of Processing, Belief Congruence, and Attitude–Behavior Correspondence

ICEK AJZEN
JAMES SEXTON

Evaluation is an essential aspect of all human judgment. Work on the semantic differential (Osgood, Suci, & Tannenbaum, 1957) has shown that objects, people, and events are assessed first and foremost along an evaluative dimension. Evaluative reactions of good or bad, desirable or undesirable, confer on the judged concept a large measure of its connotative meaning. Additional evidence for the importance of evaluative reactions comes from research on the automatic activation of attitudes. Not only do evaluative judgments account for a large proportion of variance in our considered responses to various stimuli; it is now known that immediate, initial evaluations are ubiquitous and virtually inevitable. Automatic evaluative or affective reactions occur prior to any focused deliberations and are often outside of conscious awareness (Bargh, 1997; Bargh, Chaiken, Govender, & Pratto, 1992; Bargh, Chaiken, Raymond, & Hymes, 1996; Murphy, Monahan, & Zajonc, 1995; Murphy & Zajonc, 1993). In fact, it has been suggested that positive versus negative reactions constitute a basic dimension by which the brain deals with information (Lang, Bradley, & Cuthbert, 1990), and that these evaluative responses are part of what makes us uniquely human (Kagan, 1996).

The pervasiveness and prominence of evaluative reactions to stimuli are not incidental. It was recognized long ago that evaluative responses, or attitudes, are preparatory to behavior; they predispose individuals to decisions and actions consistent with the valence of the attitude (e.g., Allport, 1935; Lewin, 1935). Positive attitudes are thus expected to produce an approach tendency, and negative attitudes to produce an avoidance tendency. Despite occasional doubts and many blind alleys (e.g., Blumer, 1955; Festinger, 1964; Wicker, 1969), this article of faith has been affirmed in a large number of studies on the relation between attitudes and behavior (see Ajzen & Fishbein, 1977; Eagly & Chaiken, 1993; Kraus, 1995).

The present chapter explores some of the cognitive processes that may be responsible for correspondence or lack of correspondence between attitudes and behavior. We first examine the role of belief accessibility in the framework of the expectancy–value model of attitudes, followed by a discussion of the different ways in which attitudes can be activated. We briefly address automatic affective and evaluative responses, but our focus is on considered judgments that are based on varying amounts of deliberation. We try to show that effortful activation of attitudes can be biased by various personal and contextual factors, thus influencing the type and number of considerations on which an evaluative reaction is based. Attitude–behavior correspondence can then be explained by comparing the considerations that are accessible when attitudes are expressed and when behavior is performed. A general principle of belief congruence is proposed, according to which attitude–behavior correspondence is strong when the considerations match, but weak when they don't match. The belief congruence principle is used to explain how various personal and situational factors moderate the attitude–behavior relation, and to propose directions for future research.

ATTITUDE RETRIEVAL VERSUS CONSTRUCTION

We begin by exploring some of the cognitive processes that underlie evaluative responses in a given context. A basic understanding of these processes is required as a starting point for our analysis of the attitude–behavior relation.

Subjectively, most cognitive processes appear to be immediate and unitary experiences. We humans perceive situations and events with little cognitive effort, and our memories for people and events seem to be stored intact and retrieved with relative ease. Yet cognitive research has shown otherwise: Only certain features of our experiences are stored in long-term memory, and the retrieval of information, though guided by the contents stored in memory, is an active process that involves inferences and reconstruction of the experiences in question (see Neisser, 1976). Even when initially stored more or less intact, memory traces are subject to retroactive interference by later events, so that the original information can only be retrieved with difficulty if at all (Waugh & Norman, 1965). Moreover, memories are stored not in isolation, but in relation to other mental constructs. They are grouped with similar ideas and organized under superordinate categories. Exposure to new information can change this structure, and the resulting reorganization can modify the meaning of the stored memories. In fact, memory for past events appears to be quite

fragile. It can be altered by the context in which it is retrieved (e.g., Loftus & Palmer, 1974), and entirely imaginary scenarios can be induced by providing suggestions and misinformation that interact with existing memories and expectations (Loftus, Feldman, & Dashiell, 1995).

Attitude Formation: The Expectancy–Value Model

These conclusions regarding perception and memory have important parallels in the formation of attitudes, their storage, and their retrieval. The most widely accepted theory of attitude formation relies on an expectancy–value model (see Feather, 1982). One of the first and most complete statements of the expectancy–value model can be found in Fishbein's (1963, 1967) summation theory of attitude, although somewhat narrower versions were proposed earlier by Peak (1955), Carlson (1956), and Rosenberg (1956). In Fishbein's theory, people's evaluations of, or attitudes toward, an object are determined by their salient beliefs about the object; a "belief" is defined as the subjective probability that the object has a certain attribute (Fishbein & Ajzen, 1975). The terms "object" and "attribute" are used in the generic sense, and they refer to any discriminable aspect of an individual's world.

Each belief associates the object with a certain attribute. According to the expectancy–value model, a person's overall attitude toward an object is determined by the subjective values or evaluations of the attributes associated with the object, as well as by the strength of these associations. Specifically, the evaluation of each attribute ontributes to the attitude in direct proportion to the person's subjective probability that the object possesses the attribute in question. The basic structure of the model is shown in the following equation (Fishbein & Ajzen, 1975; Feather, 1959):

$$A \propto \sum_{f=1}^{n} b_i e_i$$

In this equation, A is the attitude toward the object; b_i is the strength of the belief (the subjective probability) that the object has attribute *i*; e_i is the evaluation of attribute *i*; and *n* is the number of salient attributes (see Fishbein & Ajzen, 1975).

Accessibility of Beliefs

One important implication of the expectancy–value model of attitude formation is that attitudes toward an object are acquired automatically and inevitably as people form beliefs about the object's attributes, and as the subjective values of these attributes become linked to the object (Fishbein, 1967). People can, of course, form many different beliefs, but it is assumed that they can attend to only a relatively small number at any given moment. It is these *salient* beliefs that are considered to be the prevailing determinants of a person's attitude. Some correlational evidence is available to support the importance of belief salience. The subjective probability associated with a given belief (i.e., its strength) correlates with the frequency with which the belief is emitted in a sample of respondents (i.e., with its salience) (Fishbein, 1963), as well as with order of belief emission (Kaplan & Fishbein, 1969). In addition, salient beliefs tend to correlate more highly with an independent measure of attitude than do nonsalient beliefs (Petkova, Ajzen, & Driver, 1995; van der Pligt & Eiser, 1984). The likelihood that a given belief will be emitted in a free-response format is also found to correspond to its *accessibility*, as measured by response latency (Ajzen, Driver, & Nichols, 1995). Because "accessibility" is the currently preferred term, we will use it in the remainder of this chapter.

Domain of Accessible Beliefs

From an expectancy–value perspective, attitudes have an emergent quality. They develop in the course of acquiring information about the attitude object, and they keep evolving as existing beliefs change and new beliefs are formed. It follows that the evaluative reaction to an attitude object depends on the particular beliefs that are accessible at the time of observation. Attitudes should vary with the *number* of accessible beliefs, with their *strength* (i.e., the subjective probabilities of the object–attribute associations), and with

their *evaluative implications* (i.e., the subjective values of the associated attributes).

As a general rule, individuals with different accessible beliefs regarding a given object, behavior, or event also hold different attitudes toward the issue in question. Similarly, situations that make different beliefs accessible tend to produce different attitudes. These observation must be qualified, however, because in the expectancy–value model the attitude toward an object is given by the aggregated evaluation inherent in the *total set* of accessible beliefs, regardless of the number and kind of beliefs involved. Theoretically, therefore, two very different sets of accessible beliefs could result in the same or very similar overall attitudes.

Attitude Storage

We have little direct information about the ways in which attitudes are stored in memory, but some insight can be gained by examining work in social cognition. Relevant to the question of attitude storage, research has provided evidence for the relative independence of memory for general evaluative judgments (e.g., overall impressions of another person) and memory for specific items of information on which the evaluations are based (Dreben, Fiske, & Hastie, 1979; Fiske & Pavelchak, 1986). These findings parallel the distinction between "semantic memory" and "episodic memory" (Tulving, 1983). Semantic memory is procedural in nature and relatively abstract; it involves skills and habits, as well as cognitive schemas and relations among schemas. Overall evaluations would seem to fall into this category and, like other aspects of semantic memory, should be available without much cognitive effort. In contrast, contextual and concrete information about people and events that stems from personal experience is stored in episodic memory. Recall of such information is more deliberate, requiring greater cognitive effort. Beliefs about an attitude object that are based on a small sample of data probably reside in episodic memory. However, as the number of relevant episodic memories increases, a semantic memory is typically formed. Because beliefs and evaluations are stored and retrieved in different ways, they may become divorced from each other. As new information becomes available, existing beliefs may change and new beliefs may be formed, without necessarily having an immediate impact on the relevant attitudes. However, in a fashion similar to the "Socratic effect" shown by McGuire (1960) with respect to probabilistic judgments, thinking about one's beliefs and attitudes in the same context is likely to produce pressures toward consistency.

Attitude Activation

It stands to reason that attitudes must somehow be activated before they can be reported and before they can exert an effect on behavior. Several chapters in the present volume present a variety of perspectives on dual-mode processing. Although differing in detail, these perspectives compare a relatively automatic, effortless processing mode with a more deliberate, systematic mode (e.g., Chen & Chaiken, Chapter 4; Epstein & Pacini, Chapter 23; Fazio & Towles-Schwen, Chapter 5; and Petty & Wegener, Chapter 3, this volume). Our conception of attitude activation and retrieval follows similar lines.

Effortless Attitude Activation

Automatic Affective Responses. We have thus far drawn no clear distinction between "affect" and "evaluation." There is now general agreement that "attitude" is best defined as an overall evaluative response that takes account of various reactions to the object of the attitude, and that affect or feelings concerning the object are a relatively independent class of responses that may be one of the factors influencing the attitude (Eagly & Chaiken, 1993). Consistent with this view, research has shown that although affective and evaluative responses are correlated, they can be empirically distinguished (e.g., Ajzen & Driver, 1991; Breckler, 1984; Sparks, Guthrie, & Shepherd, 1997).

Stimuli can elicit positive or negative feelings in an immediate and spontaneous fashion, even if a person has had no prior exposure to them. The strongest evidence for automatic activation of affect comes from work on the affective-primacy hypothesis (Murphy & Zajonc, 1993; Zajonc, 1980). This work has demonstrated that stimuli can elicit affective reactions outside of awareness, and that these reactions tend to be quite diffuse, generalizing easily to novel stimuli in the situation.

Evidence for automatic activation of affect is consistent with Epstein's (1990) cognitive–experiential self-theory (see also Epstein & Pacini, Chapter 23, this volume). This theory postulates two parallel, interactive systems: a rational system and an experiential system. The rational system is assumed to operate at the conscious level; processing in this system is intentional, analytical, primarily verbal, and relatively free of affect. In contrast, processing in the experiential system is said to be automatic, preconscious, holistic, primarily nonverbal, and closely linked to affect. Automatic affective reactions outside of conscious awareness thus have to be handled by the experiential system.

Direct Retrieval of Evaluative Responses. Direct retrieval of evaluative reactions presupposes that an overall evaluation was formed in the past, has been stored in memory, and is now available for relatively effortless retrieval. It must be recalled, however, that stored information is subject to interference and reconstruction, and that the evaluation retrieved even in this relatively direct mode of activation may differ from the evaluation that was originally stored in memory.

As a general rule, the likelihood of direct attitude retrieval should be a function of the attitude's accessibility in memory. Research has shown that an attitude's accessibility, as measured by response latency, increases with the frequency of prior retrievals (Powell & Fazio, 1984). Perhaps not surprisingly, responses to attitudinal inquiries are faster following recent expressions of the same or a similar attitude. Of greater substantive interest is that response latencies are also lower for attitudes formed by direct experience than for attitudes based on secondhand information (Fazio & Zanna, 1981; Regan & Fazio, 1977). Explanations of these effects assume that repeated expressions and direct experience tend to strengthen the attitude, thus resulting in a faster evaluative response. Moreover, Fazio and his associates (Fazio, Sanbonmatsu, Powell, & Kardes, 1986) have argued that only strong attitudes (with relatively low response latencies) are activated automatically. When a strong bond has been formed between an object and an evaluative response, the actual or symbolic presence of the object is assumed to activate the attitude toward the object in a spontaneous and effortless manner. In contrast, weaker attitudes are said to be retrievable only by means of a conscious effort.

This view of automatic attitude activation is challenged by recent priming research, which has shown that all attitudes, whether strong or weak, can be automatically activated (Bargh et al., 1992). Whatever the advantages of strong over weak attitudes, therefore, these advantages may have little to do with their automatic or deliberate activation. We will return to this issue below in our discussion of attitude–behavior correspondence.

Effortful Attitude Activation:
Derivation and Construction

What characterizes the automatic and retrieval-from-memory modes of attitude activation is that they occur without added processing of relevant information. This contrasts with the remaining modes, which assume an active, though not necessarily thorough, activation of the evaluative response. One effortful mode involves the *derivation* of an attitude from existing information or beliefs about the attitude object. Attitude derivation in real time is likely to occur when relevant information is available but no overall evaluation has been stored in memory, or when that evaluation cannot be easily retrieved (for whatever reason). In the most effortful mode of activation, an attitude is *formed* on-line as new information about an object or issue becomes available. We discuss some implications of these alternative modes of attitude activation below.

Initial, preconscious processing of an affective nature, with only minimal stimulus input, will usually be followed by a more careful, conscious assessment before a general evaluative reaction is expressed. Moreover, on many occasions a person cannot simply retrieve an attitude from memory, but must instead arrive at an evaluative judgment on the basis of available information. The information may be stored in memory and may be retrieved in the form of beliefs about the attitude object. In this case, attitudes are activated in real time by deriving an evaluative response consistent with the accessible beliefs. Many people have given little or no thought to their attitudes toward such issues as term limits for elected officials, protection of endangered species, the desirability of space exploration, or support for English as the official language of the United States. Yet they possess information and beliefs relevant to these issues. When they are asked to express their attitudes in the course of an attitude survey, they can derive an evaluation in real time on the basis of the existing and accessible beliefs.

Alternatively or in addition, new information may become available, and this new information may be used to form an attitude on-line (Hastie & Park, 1986). This process is perhaps best illustrated by research on impression formation. In the typical impression formation paradigm, individuals are exposed to concrete items of information about another person (usually in the form of trait adjectives), and are asked how much they would like or dislike the person thus described. Research has shown that respondents tend not merely to base their attitudes on the information provided, but instead to draw wide-ranging inferences about the other person that go beyond the information given (see Ajzen, 1977; Schneider, 1973).

Heuristic Processing. Real-time derivation of evaluations on the basis of existing information, as well as construction of attitudes on-line by integrating incoming information, involves relatively controlled, effortful processes. This is not to say, however, that a logical and in-depth review of all relevant considerations must necessarily take place. On the contrary, it is generally assumed that the default processing mode keeps cognitive effort to the required minimum, especially when motivation is low or opportunities for extensive deliberation are limited (Chaiken, 1980; Petty & Cacioppo, 1986; Taylor, 1981).

One way to bypass excessively effortful considerations of an issue's pros and cons is to rely on cognitive heuristics or rules of thumb to arrive at an evaluative judgment. Although it is not conceptualized in this manner, the self-attribution account of dissonance phenomena implies use of cognitive heuristics. People are said to arrive at their attitudes not by deliberating the positive and negative aspects of a given issue, but by inferring the attitude from their own behavior and from the circumstances under which it occurred (Bem, 1965).

The most explicit assumption of heuristic processing as a basis for attitude formation can be found in Chaiken's (1980) heuristic–systematic model of persuasion. Under conditions of low motivation or limited cognitive capacity, receivers of a persuasive communication are said to rely on relatively simple cognitive heuristics to form their opinions. Consistent with this view, it has been found that under the conditions specified to favor heuristic processing, receivers tend to rely on such relatively superficial cues as the communicator's attractiveness or the number of arguments contained in the message (for a review, see Eagly & Chaiken, 1993). However, the actual cognitive heuristics used in such situations have not been systematically investigated. It is assumed that receivers use simple and apparently reasonable rules of inference, such as "If an expert source makes this claim, it must be valid." Although the data are consistent with this account, it would be useful to have more direct information about the actual heuristics used by receivers exposed to a persuasive communication.

Research on stereotyping has also implicated heuristic processing as a possible underlying mechanism. When making stereotypic judgments, people are said to rely not on a "piecemeal" analysis of characteristics possessed by another person, but rather on perceived features of the group to which the person belongs (Fiske & Neuberg, 1990; Fiske & Pavelchak, 1986; see also Fiske, Lin, & Neuberg, Chapter 11, this volume). Categorical, stereotypic judgments of this kind are likely to be made by individuals in positions of power and under conditions of competition for rewards (Fiske & Dépret, 1996; Ruscher & Fiske, 1990).

Systematic Processing. Although people are said to prefer the relatively effortless heuristic mode of processing, it is recognized that attitudinal judgments can be based on systematic deliberations of an issue's pros and cons. In fact, the expectancy–value model described earlier assumes some degree of systematic processing by postulating that attitudes are based on accessible beliefs about the attitude object. Systematic processing is especially likely to occur in new situations, with previously unencountered issues, when circumstances have changed, or when attitudes are challenged. However, there is widespread agreement among theorists that this effortful central processing of information requires the ability and motivation to devote cognitive resources to the task (Chaiken, 1980; Fazio, 1990; Petty & Cacioppo, 1986). Thus, with sufficient ability and motivation, attitudes are likely to be based on a systematic consideration of relevant beliefs about the attitude object.

Although the proposition that systematic processing requires ability and motivation is noncontroversial, it is less clear how *much* processing will occur in the systematic mode. The expectancy–value model fails to address this issue; it simply stipulates that attitudes are determined by the prevailing accessible beliefs. The various models of dual-mode processing, however, would suggest that degree of processing increases with cognitive ability and with motivation to process. In other words, these models imply a continuum that ranges from little to intense systematic processing of relevant information.

Note that the distinction between shallow and deep processing is independent of the distinction between heuristic and systematic processing, or between automatic and deliberate processing. Although heuristic processing is considered to be relatively shallow, systematic, issue-relevant processing can be either shallow or deep. Similarly, whereas automatic responding involves little or no conscious activity, deliberate processing can vary in depth. The depth-of-processing continuum is located in only one mode—namely, deliberate processing of information that is of substantive relevance to the issue under consideration. However, this continuum ranges from low to high.

The depth-of-processing dimension is of importance for our purposes because it speaks to the domain of beliefs that become accessible in a given context. Clearly, the number of accessible beliefs is likely to increase with processing depth, and the strength and evaluative implications of accessible beliefs may also change as a result of continued deliberation. To understand systematic activation of attitudes, it is thus important to explore the factors that influence depth of processing.

It is easy to see that competing cognitive demands, distractions, and lack of requisite skills or information may interfere with a person's ability to perform an in-depth analysis of a given attitudinal issue. Perhaps less obvious are the factors that influence motivation to process attitudinally relevant information. Kruglanski's (1980, 1989) theory of lay epistemics posits two complementary motivational factors: the need for structure, which discourages continued deliberation so that a judgment or decision can be made; and the fear of invalidity, which prolongs information processing when the cost of making a mistake looms large.

Within these general motives to cut off or continue deliberation, we can identify more specific factors that may influence depth of processing. Especially in the context of persuasive communication, the *personal relevance* of the issue being considered can greatly influence motivation to process issue-relevant information. Using a thought-listing task to elicit cognitive responses to a message, research on the elaboration likelihood model (Petty & Cacioppo, 1986) has shown that the number of cognitive responses increases with the personal relevance of the issue to the receiver (e.g., Leippe & Elkin, 1987; Petty & Cacioppo, 1979).

The Action Context

Our focus up to this point has been on evaluative judgments, and in particular on the ways in which attitudes are retrieved, derived, or constructed with varying degrees of cognitive effort. These considerations regarding attitude activation have distinct parallels in the behavioral context. Like attitudes, behavioral decisions may be made in a relatively automatic fashion; action sequences stored in memory may be retrieved and performed without a great deal of cognitive effort. Alternatively, decisions may be based on more or less extensive deliberations of the pros and cons of available alternatives. When deliberations occur, decisions may be made in real time on the basis of existing information about the available alternatives, or they may

be made on-line as new information becomes available.

Automaticity in Behavior

Behaviors of interest to social psychologists rarely occur in a completely automatic fashion, without any conscious deliberation whatsoever. Nevertheless, several lines of theory and research suggest that even relatively complex social behaviors can become routinized to the point of being performed without much cognitive effort. On the basis of past experience, people are assumed to have stored in memory a behavioral script (Abelson, 1976) or to have formed a habit (Triandis, 1980), and the appropriate context is thought to elicit the learned course of action in a more or less automatic or "mindless" fashion (Langer, 1975).

Deliberate Decision Making

In contrast to automatic responding, the most popular model of decision making— the subjective expected utility model—assumes at least some degree of deliberation. This model is very similar in structure, even if not in all its underlying assumptions, to the expectancy–value model of attitudes (see Ajzen, 1996a, for a comparison). As in the expectancy–value model, individuals are assumed to evaluate each available course of action in terms of the likelihood that the action will produce various outcomes and the subjective value or utility of these outcomes. Subjective probabilities and values are then multiplied, and the products are summed over all outcomes. It is expected that the alternative with the highest subjective expected utility is the preferred course of action (see Edwards, 1954).

However, just as attitude theorists had to allow for simplifying modes of attitude activation, decision theorists soon recognized that the subjective expected utility model may overstate the degree to which people engage in systematic information processing. Simon (1955, 1956) proposed that actual decision-making behavior can better be described as a process of "bounded rationality." The strategy of a person who operates under bounded rationality is to reach a satisfactory level of outcomes, not necessarily the best possible level. The principle of utility maximization, and statistical models of probability, are now seen as ideals that prescribe how judgments and decisions should be made, but it is recognized that they provide only limited information about the actual processes that underlie judgments and decisions.

Conclusions

Our discussion up to this point can be summarized as follows. Evaluative reactions provide a primary basis for acting, either verbally or behaviorally, in relation to social objects. These evaluative reactions, especially reactions of an affective nature, may be relatively automatic and preconscious, but more often they involve some degree of deliberation. Deliberate processing can be quite shallow, or, given sufficient motivation and cognitive capacity, can go into considerable depth. In either case, people derive their attitudes from existing and currently accessible beliefs, or they construct an attitude on the basis of new incoming information. The ultimate evaluative judgments and overt behaviors are the results of these cognitive processes.

BIASING FACTORS

Processing of information in the attitudinal and behavioral contexts need not involve a disinterested, objective survey of an issue's or action's pros and cons. On the contrary, the deliberations are often characterized by considerable biases, which may be inherent in the person or induced by the context. Of particular interest for our understanding of the attitude–behavior relation are any biases that favor either the positive or the negative side of the evaluative continuum. Biases of this kind will tend to influence overall evaluations in the attitudinal context and behavioral dispositions in the action context. When personal or contextual factors make positive beliefs more accessible, attitudes and behaviors will shift in a favorable direction; when the biases make negative beliefs more accessible, attitudes and behaviors will shift in the opposite direction.

Many lines of research document the operation of cognitive biases that may influence the kinds of beliefs that are accessible in attitudinal and behavioral contexts. We review here the major types of biases that have the potential for affecting evaluative judgments and behavioral decisions.

Existing Attitudes

The idea that information processing is biased by a person's attitudes has had a pervasive impact on social-psychological theorizing. As a general rule, it is assumed that people are more likely to attend to information consistent with their attitudes, to evaluate ambiguous events in line with their attitudes, and to remember attitude-consistent information better. Initial research failed to provide clear-cut support for these biases, and it is now recognized that their operation is contingent on a variety of conditions and that they may be overshadowed by other motivating factors, such as the utility of the information for the individual's goals (for a review, see Eagly & Chaiken, 1993, pp. 589–604).

Biased processing of information in line with existing attitudes can influence the evaluative reactions elicited in attitudinal and behavioral contexts. In a series of experiments, Tesser and his associates (e.g., Tesser & Conlee, 1975; Tesser & Leone, 1977; see Tesser, 1978) have shown that thinking about an attitude object tends to polarize evaluative responses to it, such that initially positive attitudes become more favorable and initially negative attitudes become more unfavorable. It thus appears that merely thinking about an object can strengthen existing beliefs or make new attitude-consistent beliefs accessible.[2]

It has also been shown that attitudes can influence the direction of cognitive and behavioral responses. Strongly held attitudes, as indicated by fast response latencies, were found to influence evaluations of the performance of political candidates in a debate (Fazio & Williams, 1986) and evaluations of the quality of empirical research (Houston & Fazio, 1989). Although not directly proving the point, these findings have been taken as evidence that existing attitudes bias perception of the behavioral context in such a manner as to induce attitude-consistent behavior (see Fazio, 1990).

Biased Samples of Past Behavior

If attitudes are often not simply retrieved from memory, but are instead derived in real time or constructed on-line, then any personal or contextual factors that bias accessible information in a favorable or unfavorable direction will tend to affect the attitude produced. As noted earlier, one type of information that may be important in attitude derivation or construction is people's knowledge of their own past behavior. People may proceed to derive an attitude by reviewing behaviors they have performed in the past with respect to the attitude object. To the extent that the context focuses attention on behaviors favorable to the object, people will tend to infer a positive attitude, but if it focuses attention on negative behaviors, the attitude inferred will tend to be negative.

Salancik and Conway (1975) demonstrated this possibility experimentally by means of a linguistic manipulation that biased perception of past behavior in a positive or a negative direction. In one of their studies, respondents were asked to indicate which of a series of behaviors relevant for religiosity they performed "on occasion" or "frequently." Because they were more likely to agree that they performed a behavior on occasion, this manipulation tended to bias perception of past behavior in a positive direction when proreligion items incorporated the adverb "on occasion" and antireligion items used the adverb "frequently." Conversely, the opposite use of the two adverbs biased perception of past behavior in a negative direction. Attitudes toward religion expressed after the behavior check-list were consistent with this manipulation: They were significantly more favorable in the positive-bias than in the negative-bias condition.

Priming

Memory for ideas and concepts is said to be organized in an associative network (e.g., Hastie, 1988; Srull & Wyer, 1989). Activation of one node in the network spreads to associated nodes; once made accessible, the network of ideas remains active for a while and can influence subsequent information processing (see Collins & Loftus, 1975). This phenomenon is known as "priming." Activation of a dimension or construct—the "priming event"—can bias judgments in the direction consistent with the activated idea. Thus, an ambiguous behavior can be interpreted in a favorable or an unfavorable light, depending on the nature of the priming event; it has also been shown that this effect can occur outside of conscious awareness (e.g., Bargh & Pietromonaco, 1982; Higgins, Rholes, & Jones, 1977).

The possibility of priming effects suggests that when people construct an attitude or try to reach a decision, immediately preceding events can direct their thinking in either a positive or a negative direction. Evidence for the priming of evaluative judgments can be found in a number of experiments that have used existing positive and negative attitudinal stimuli as priming events (e.g., Bargh et al., 1992; Fazio, Sanbonmatsu, Powell, & Kardes, 1986). Presented at subliminal exposure times, these primes are found to influence the speed at which subsequent target adjectives are judged to be good or bad. Judgments are faster when the valence of the target adjective matches the valence of the prime.

The essential function of a priming event is that it can serve as a reference point or anchor for the retrieval of information from memory and for the construction of an attitudinal judgment. The effect of priming tends to be rather brief, however—limited to a short period immediately following activation of a construct (Fiske & Taylor, 1991). Nevertheless, recent activation makes the primed dimension more readily accessible and causes more attention to be given to that dimension (Higgins, 1989; Higgins, Bargh, & Lombardi, 1985). As a result, priming is likely to influence the set of beliefs accessible in a given situation, and thus the nature of the attitude that is derived or constructed. In addition, priming can direct thinking toward use of one cognitive heuristic as opposed to another, and can in this fashion influence the final attitudinal judgment (Chaiken, Axsom, Liberman, & Wilson, 1992).

Although it can occur outside of awareness, priming of positive or negative reactions can affect evaluations of considerable personal relevance. For example, when questions about general life satisfaction are preceded by a question about marital satisfaction, either assimilation or contrast effects can be observed, depending on the linguistic context in which the questions are asked (see Schwarz, Strack, & Mai, 1991). Life in general may be contrasted with one's marriage, resulting in a less favorable judgment if marital satisfaction is high and a more favorable judgment if marital satisfaction is low. Such a contrast effect is likely when respondents implicitly or explicitly exclude marital satisfaction from their judgments of satisfaction with life in general. Alternatively, general life satisfaction can be assimilated, appearing more favorable if marital satisfaction is high and less favorable if marital satisfaction is low. This is likely to occur when respondents implicitly or explicitly include the specific domain in their judgment of general life satisfaction (see Schwarz & Bless, 1992).

In a similar fashion, priming of certain dimensions can influence people's attitudes toward important social issues. For example, drawing attention to the fact that Senator Edward Kennedy is a liberal or a catholic has been shown to influence expressed attitudes toward abortion (Granberg, 1985).

Mood

A considerable body of research has documented the effects of positive and negative moods on information processing. Much of this work has focused on mood congruity in memory and judgment. Interpretation of ambiguous material can be biased, such that it is viewed more favorably when a person is happy rather than sad (Robles, Smith, Carver, & Wellens, 1987; Schaller & Cialdini, 1990). Mood also influences retrieval, with favorable information more likely to be retrieved during a positive mood and negative information more likely to be retrieved during negative mood (Blaney, 1986; Bower, 1981; Erber & Erber, 1984; Isen, 1987; Mayer, McCormick, & Strong, 1995). And, in a similar manner, mood tends to bias the perceived likelihood of events. Negative events appear more probable during a bad mood than during a good mood (Johnson & Tversky, 1983); positive events are perceived as more likely under conditions of good mood, especially when the event is personally relevant (Forgas, Bower, & Krantz, 1984), but sometimes even when it is not (Mayer, Gaschke, Braverman, & Evans, 1992).

In addition to their tendency to recall and judge information in a mood-congruent manner, people may rely on mood to infer their own attitudes. To the extent that they consider their mood to be relevant to the attitude, or to be the result of thinking about the attitude object, they tend to use their mood as a cue and express more favorable attitudes when in a positive mood and more unfavorable attitudes when in a negative mood (Schwarz, 1990; Schwarz & Clore, 1988).

Directed Thinking

Perhaps the simplest way to bias people's accessible beliefs in a positive or a negative direction is to ask them to think about positive or negative aspects of the attitude object. In a series of experiments, McGuire and McGuire (1996) showed that this procedure can have an effect even on such a fundamental aspect of personality as self-esteem. College students asked to list desirable characteristics they possess or undesirable characteristics they do not possess express more favorable attitudes toward the self than do students who are asked to list undesirable characteristics they possess or desirable characteristics they do not possess.

Processing Goals

A person's goals or motivation can influence the evaluative direction of information processing. It is often assumed that processing prior to making a judgment or reaching a decision is a relatively unbiased and open-minded analysis of information designed to produce the best possible decision (Festinger, 1964). More recent theorizing has drawn attention to alternative potential processing goals, such as defensive motivation (which seeks to confirm the validity of a preferred attitude position and to disconfirm the validity of contrary positions) and impression motivation (which biases evaluative reactions in the direction of socially acceptable positions) (Chaiken, Liberman, & Eagly, 1989). Personal as well as situational factors may activate one processing goal rather than another, resulting in biases that produce either a more favorable or a more unfavorable reaction.

Framing

The way in which a decision problem is structured or framed can greatly affect the judgments and choices that are made (Tversky & Kahneman, 1981). For example, most people prefer the prospect of winning $3,000 with certainty to the prospect of winning $4,000 with a probability of .80, even though the second prospect has a greater expected value (Kahneman & Tversky, 1979). This "certainty effect" is reversed, however, when the gains are replaced by losses. Thus, most people prefer the prospect of losing $4,000 with a probability of .80 to the prospect of losing $3,000 with certainty. This reversal implies risk aversion in the case of gains and risk proneness in the case of losses. Framing can affect other evaluative judgments by making salient likely consequences of a positive or negative nature. According to Tversky and Kahneman's prospect theory, the particular frame adopted depends on the way the problem is formulated, on individual differences in perspective, and on problem-solving style.

Time Perspective

Attitudes and decisions regarding complex issues almost inevitably involve a mixture of positive and negative beliefs, of attractive and repulsive forces. In his influential analysis of conflict and conflict resolution, Lewin (1935, 1938) visualized a potential course of action as an activity region in a person's life space, and its positive and negative attributes as force fields that create approach and avoidance tendencies. Lewin argued that as the individual approaches the activity region (i.e., comes closer to making a decision), the region's positive and negative valences grow in strength, and he postulated that the avoidance gradient is steeper than the approach gradient. Figure 6.1 depicts a typical approach–avoidance conflict in which neither tendency is completely dominant. In a conflict of this kind, the individual is predicted at first to approach the decision point, because the attractive force generated by the positive valence dominates the avoidance force generated by the negative valence. However, as the psychological distance from the decision grows smaller, the avoidance tendency overcomes the approach tendency, and the individual retreats to the point of equilibrium.

The assumption that the slope of the avoidance gradient is steeper than the slope of the approach gradient implies a biasing effect of time perspective. When people are considering a course of action in the distant future,

positive consequences are more readily accessible or are given more weight than negative consequences. Attitudes toward the behavior are therefore relatively favorable. When the time of action approaches, however, the negative consequences loom large in people's minds, and their attitudes toward the contemplated course of action become correspondingly unfavorable. Commitments that are accepted readily well ahead of a scheduled event take on a burdensome quality as the time of the event draws near.

A related conclusion regarding the effect of time perspective is reached on the basis of temporal-construal theory (Liberman & Trope, 1998). According to this theory, different aspects of an event can be construed at relatively abstract or relatively concrete levels. With regard to goal-directed activities, the goal's desirability is represented at an abstract level, whereas the likelihood that the goal will be attained is construed on a more concrete level. Furthermore, the value of the abstract aspects of the goal (the goal's desirability) increases with temporal distance from the goal, whereas the value of the concrete aspects (i.e., its probability) decreases with temporal distance. In a series of experiments, Liberman and Trope obtained support for their theory. Of greatest relevance for our purposes, they found that people give weight to a goal's positive aspects (its desirability) when making decisions for the long term, and to the goal's negative aspects (its difficulty) when making decisions for the short term. These findings imply that positive beliefs about the goal are more readily accessible in long-term decisions, whereas negative beliefs predominate in short-term decisions.

Conclusions

Clearly, a large number of personal and contextual factors can bias the kinds of considerations that are accessed prior to the activation of evaluative reactions and behavioral decisions. Priming cues, mood, problem framing, time perspective, and many other factors produce either a more favorable or a more unfavorable set of accessible beliefs in any given context. The implications of these biases for the attitude–behavior relation are discussed in the following section.

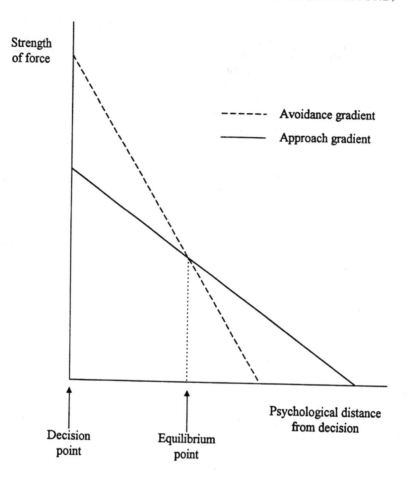

FIGURE 6.1. A typical approach–avoidance conflict.

ATTITUDES AND BEHAVIOR

The Principle of Belief Congruence

We are now ready to consider the relation between attitudes and behavior in light of the ways in which attitudes are activated and decisions are made. Our focus in this discussion is on situations that involve at least some degree of active deliberation, rather than on completely automatic retrieval of attitudes or behavioral scripts. The starting point for our analysis is the recognition that in situations of this kind, attitudes as well as behaviors are guided by the considerations that occur at the time. Whether these considerations are the result of simple cognitive heuristics or of a more complex and systematic review of relevant information, they provide the basis for an evaluative reaction in the attitudinal context and for a behavioral decision in the action context. The crucial question for the attitude–behavior relation is the degree of congruence between the considerations or beliefs available in the attitudinal and behavioral contexts. Only when belief congruence is high should we expect a strong relation between attitudes and behavior. Under conditions of low belief congruence, the considerations that produce the evaluative attitudinal response differ from those that precede a behavioral decision. As a result, attitudes and behavior may show little consistency.[3]

In view of the potential biases reviewed above, it is clear that many factors can influence the types of beliefs or considerations that become accessible as a basis for expressed attitudes and behavioral decisions. However, these processes need not have a detrimental effect on the attitude–behavior relation, so long as the biasing factors in the attitudinal and in the behavioral contexts produce congruent sets of beliefs. The relation between attitudes and behavior is likely to deteriorate only when the biases are such that the beliefs made accessible in the attitudinal context differ in their overall evaluative implications from the beliefs made accessible in the behavioral context. The fact that verbal attitudes are often found to have little or no relation to overt behavior (Ajzen & Fishbein, 1977; Wicker, 1969) suggests that low belief congruence may be quite common. Any factor or combination of factors that produces different sets of accessible beliefs in the attitudinal context and in the behavioral context will tend to reduce observed correspondence between attitudes and behavior. Only when access to beliefs is completely unbiased in both contexts, or when circumstances produce the same biases, can we expect to obtain strong attitude–behavior correlations. It is thus the potential for *differential* bias that is of greatest concern when we are trying to predict overt behavior from verbal expressions of attitude.

Cognition versus Affect

We sometimes observe a divergence between evaluative reactions of a cognitive or instrumental kind and reactions of an affective kind. This divergence is evident in the context of health behavior. Individuals tend to hold favorable beliefs about the consequences of engaging in exercise or maintaining a prescribed medical regimen; yet when it comes to carrying out the required course of action, negative affect may predominate and lead to procrastination or lack of compliance. Although more general in its application, the belief congruence principle, first formulated by Ajzen (1996b), is consistent with the hypothesis of affective–cognitive mismatch (Millar & Tesser, 1986, 1992). According to this hypothesis, individuals may focus on either affective or cognitive aspects when expressing their attitudes and when performing a behavior. Attitudes are expected to be poor predictors of behavior when there is a mismatch be-

tween the attitudinal focus and the behavioral focus (i.e., when attitudes are expressed under an affective focus but behavior is performed under a cognitive focus, or vice versa). In support of this prediction, Millar and Tesser (1986) showed that correlations between attitudes toward different intellectual puzzles and time spent solving those puzzles were stronger when attention in the attitudinal and behavioral contexts was focused on the same type of considerations (instrumental or affective) than when it was focused on different types of considerations.

Social Category Exemplars

The belief congruence principle is also consistent with theorizing concerning the accessibility of social category exemplars (Sia, Lord, Lepper, Blessum, & Ratcliff, 1997). Evaluative as well as behavioral responses with respect to a social category are likely to be influenced by the exemplars of the category that come to mind at the time the response is made. Attitudes and behaviors are therefore expected to vary with changes in the accessibility of category exemplars across situations. In a series of experiments, Sia et al. showed that congruence of category exemplars across time and contexts increased stability of attitudes over time and improved prediction of behavior from attitudes.

Attribute Salience

Perhaps most similar to the principle of belief congruence is the suggestion made by Shavitt and Fazio (1991) that any attribute dimension relevant to an evaluative judgment may vary in salience as a function of the judgmental context. Shavitt and Fazio theorized that for any given attitude object, certain dimensions are naturally salient, and are therefore the prime determinants of behavior with respect to the object. It follows that attitudes should predict behavior best when the dimensions that are salient at the time of attitude assessment are those that are naturally salient at the time of the behavior. This hypothesis was confirmed in two laboratory experiments that first manipulated the accessibility of a selected dimension prior to attitude assessment, and then used the expressed attitudes to predict behavioral intentions with respect to objects whose naturally salient attributes either did or did not match the attributes that had been made accessible in the attitudinal context.

Depth of Processing

As noted earlier, belief congruence is independent of processing mode, but depth of processing can have important implications for congruence. In comparison to shallow processing, deep processing is likely to result in a greater number of accessible beliefs. The research on mere thought reviewed earlier suggests that these beliefs tend to be evaluatively biased in the direction of the original attitude. If processing depth varies from attitudinal to behavioral context, therefore, there is the potential for differential bias in accessible beliefs. It is not clear, however, that processing mode or depth differs systematically from the attitudinal context to the behavioral context. Requiring a commitment to action, the behavioral context may induce greater motivation to process than the attitudinal context. On the other hand, time limitations or other external pressures may afford less ability to process information in the behavioral context.

Attitude–Behavior Correspondence

We now take another look at past research and theorizing regarding the attitude–behavior relation in light of belief congruence. Although beliefs in attitudinal and behavioral contexts have not been directly assessed, we will try to show that different lines of research have produced results consistent with the belief congruence principle.

The Principle of Compatibility

Perhaps the most frequently cited explanation for differences in observed attitude–behavior relations is the principle of correspondence (Ajzen & Fishbein, 1977; Fishbein & Ajzen, 1974) or compatibility (Ajzen, 1988). According to this principle, verbal (attitudinal) and nonverbal (overt behavioral) responses to an attitude object can be expected to correlate to the extent that these responses reflect the same underlying evaluative disposition (i.e.,

the same attitude). It is argued that this is likely to be the case only when the measure of attitude is compatible with the measure of behavior in terms of four elements: the action specified, if any; the target at which the action is directed; the context in which the action occurs; and the time of its occurrence. As a general rule, it is expected that specific actions in particular contexts can be predicted only from equally specific attitudes toward those actions, and that general attitudes toward social issues or objects correlate only with equally broad, aggregated measures of behavior relevant to the issue or object in question. Many empirical studies have supported this idea by reporting greater attitude–behavior correspondence under conditions of high as opposed to low compatibility (for reviews, see Eagly & Chaiken, 1993, pp. 162–168; Kraus, 1995).

Although the principle of compatibility is quite effective in accounting for differences in observed attitude–behavior relations, it was formulated without much attention to the underlying psychological mechanisms. We now suggest that its function can be explained in terms of belief congruence. Under conditions of high compatibility, the measure of attitude is concerned with exactly the same issue or action as the measure of behavior. For example, if applying to the police academy is the behavioral criterion, attitudes toward applying to the academy should be assessed. The considerations or beliefs that are accessed in the attitudinal and behavioral contexts are likely to be about the same. In contrast, under conditions of low compatibility, different issues or actions are the focus of attention in the two contexts. Thus, expressing attitudes toward the police may bring to mind very different beliefs than considering the possibility of joining the police academy does. The resulting lack of belief congruence will tend to produce low attitude–behavior correlations.

This discussion also suggests, however, that compatibility between measures of verbal and nonverbal responses does not necessarily ensure a strong relation. Even if the two measures involve exactly the same action, target, context, and time elements, differential biases in the attitudinal and behavioral contexts may well reduce belief congruence, resulting in behavior that is inconsistent with the verbally expressed attitude.

"Symbolic" versus "Authentic" Responses

An example illustrating this state of affairs can be found in research on racial attitudes and behavior. It is often maintained that attitudinal responses are "symbolic" in nature and differ in principle from realistic or "authentic" nonverbal behavior, and that this is the reason why attitudes often fail to predict behavior (e.g., Blumer, 1955; Deutscher, 1966). Among other things, symbolic attitudes are said to lack validity because they are subject to social desirability responding, acquiescence tendencies, strategic considerations, and other response biases. By way of contrast, overt behaviors are considered real and thus inherently valid indicators of a person's response tendencies.

Although we agree that there are important differences between responses observed in the attitudinal and the behavioral contexts, we argue that these differences may have little to do with response biases or other issues related to measurement validity. After all, observed actions may also be biased to create favorable impressions, to avoid conflict, or to gain an advantage by means of ingratiation. Observations of nonverbal behavior thus have, in terms of validity, no inherent advantage over verbal responses (see Merton, 1940). From our perspective, the question of greater interest is the extent to which "symbolic" expressions of attitude derive from the same beliefs as the performance of "authentic" behavior. A strong attitude–behavior relation depends on a high degree of belief congruence.

In an experiment dealing with racial attitudes and behavior, Linn (1965) observed considerable inconsistency, despite the fact that his measures were strictly compatible in terms of action, target, context, and time elements. White female students were asked to indicate their willingness to pose for a photograph with a black male. The photo was to be used for seven different purposes of an increasingly public nature; the proposed uses ranged from psychological research to a racial integration campaign conducted by the National Association for the Advancement of Colored People. The behavior observed in this study was the actual signing or refusal to sign releases of a photograph to be taken with a black male—one release for each of the seven

purposes. The number of releases signed served as the dependent variable.

Postexperimental interviews conducted by the experimenter showed that for many participants, the beliefs about releasing the photos that were prominent at the time of attitude assessment differed greatly from the beliefs that were accessible when behavioral commitment was requested. As one participant put it, "At that time [time of the questionnaire] I was thinking of what I *should* do, but when confronted with the situation, I thought more deeply about participating. I was worried about other people and what they would think" (quoted in Linn, 1965, p. 362). Consistent with the lack of belief congruence, a large proportion of participants displayed inconsistencies between their verbally expressed intentions and their actual signing behavior.

Direct Experience

Individuals who have had direct experience in a behavioral domain are likely to form beliefs about the behavior's consequences and constraints that are more realistic than the beliefs of individuals who have only received secondhand information about the behavior (see Doll & Ajzen, 1992). Direct experience is therefore likely to promote congruence between beliefs that are accessible at the time of attitude measurement and beliefs that become available during behavioral performance. And indeed, attitudes are consistently found to predict behavior better under conditions of direct experience (see Fazio & Zanna, 1981). Also consistent with the belief congruence notion, attitudes based on secondhand information tend to change as new information becoming available in the behavioral context influences the domain of accessible beliefs (Doll & Ajzen, 1992).

Issue Involvement versus Vested Interest

As a general rule, involvement or interest in an attitudinal issue will tend to increase motivation to attend to and process information regarding that issue. Because of greater processing depth, attitudinal responses should be based on a relatively large set of accessible beliefs. This should be true in the attitudinal as well as in the behavioral context, because issue involvement is a relatively stable feature that is likely to exert its influence across time and situations. Individuals involved in an issue can be expected to have a great deal of information readily available to form their attitudes and to aid them in deciding on a course of action. In comparison to uninvolved individuals, therefore, they should exhibit a high degree of belief congruence and a strong relation between their attitudes and their behavior. Findings consistent with this idea were reported by Fazio and Zanna (1978), who used latitude of rejection to operationalize involvement in the issue of psychological research. Readiness to participate as a subject in psychological experiments was predicted with greater precision from attitudes toward psychological research for individuals with high as opposed to low involvement in this issue.

Whereas issue involvement is expected to produce congruent beliefs in the attitudinal and behavior contexts, vested interest in a particular attitudinal position or behavior may have a more complex pattern of effects. When vested interest is present in both the attitudinal and the behavioral contexts, it should, like issue involvement, increase processing depth, produce a high degree of belief congruence, and result in a strong attitude–behavior correlation. Evidence for such effects due to vested interest was provided by Sivacek and Crano (1982).

However, the personal relevance of an issue may be more evident in one context than in another. For example, it is possible to measure students' attitudes toward a tuition increase in general, and the personal relevance of this issue may not be readily apparent. But when students are asked to sign a petition in opposition to a tuition increase, they may become aware that an increase is to take place very soon, thus arousing their vested interests. In this case, the beliefs accessible in the behavioral context may differ from the beliefs that have been considered in the attitudinal context, and this should tend to lower the observed attitude–behavior correlation.

Explaining One's Attitude

We saw earlier that thinking about an attitude object tends to polarize the evaluative reac-

tion to it (see Tesser, 1978). This systematic bias in the direction of the original attitude stands in contrast to the effect of asking individuals to analyze the reasons for their attitudes, which tends to be a disruptive effect (see Wilson, Dunn, Kraft, & Lisle, 1989; Wilson & Hodges, 1992). Consistent with the position taken in the present chapter, Wilson and his associates have argued that attitudes are often temporary constructions that depend on the considerations accessible in a given context. Because various factors can bias the reasons that come to mind for adopting a certain position on an issue, attitudes expressed immediately after reviewing one's reasons tend to shift temporarily in the direction implied by the accessible considerations. These effects can wear off quickly, resulting in low congruence between the beliefs that are accessible in the attitudinal context and the beliefs that become accessible in a later behavioral context. It follows that asking respondents to think about the reasons for their attitudes prior to expressing them can have a detrimental effect on the prediction of later behavior. Support for this expectation can be found in a series of experiments by Wilson, Dunn, Bybee, Hyman, and Rotondo (1984).

Conclusions

Several lines of thought converge on the idea that attitude–behavior correspondence depends on the extent to which the considerations that arise in the attitudinal context are comparable to the considerations that arise in the behavioral context. According to the mismatch hypothesis, attitude–behavior correlations will suffer if affective considerations are prominent in one context and cognitive or instrumental considerations are prominent in the other. Similarly, for strong attitude–behavior correlations to be observed, the exemplars of a social category that come to mind when an evaluative judgment is made must be the same or similar to the exemplars that are evoked when a category-relevant behavior is performed. The principle of belief congruence is a more general application of these ideas; it goes beyond affective–cognitive mismatch and category exemplars to deal with any factors that influence correspondence between accessible beliefs. Using this principle, we are able to explain the operation of various factors that have been found to affect the relation between attitude and behavior, including measurement compatibility, direct experience, and issue involvement.

EXTENSIONS AND IMPLICATIONS

In the preceding section, we have tried to show that the belief congruence principle can account for many findings regarding the relation between attitudes and behavior. The present section examines some further extensions and implications.

Attitude Stability

Underlying the principle of belief congruence is the assumption that attitudes are no more stable than the cognitive and affective considerations on which they are based. Belief congruence thus implies stable attitudes, and stable attitudes are better predictors of behavior (Doll & Ajzen, 1992). This idea also suggests, however, that like attitude stability, belief congruence should vary as a function of attitude strength. Beliefs and attitudes held with a great deal of conviction are less likely to change with context than are relatively indifferent attitudes. The research mentioned earlier regarding the effects of involvement on the attitude–behavior relation is consistent with this idea. Similarly, the finding that highly accessible attitudes tend to predict behavior better than less accessible attitudes (see Fazio, 1990) can also be attributed to their greater stability. In an experiment testing this interpretation, Doll and Ajzen (1992) showed that, as had been found in previous research (Fazio & Williams, 1986), attitudes based on direct experience had lower response latencies, were thus more readily accessible in memory, and predicted behavior better than attitudes based on secondhand information. In addition, this study revealed that the effect of information type on the attitude–behavior relation was mediated by the greater stability of attitudes under direct-experience conditions.

Prospects for Future Research

Beyond helping to account for the results of past investigations on the attitude–behavior relation, the principle of belief congruence has intriguing implications for future research. Of greatest interest in this regard are effects of the various potential biasing factors discussed earlier. Each of these factors can influence belief congruence by producing different sets of considerations in the attitudinal and behavioral contexts, and hence each biasing factor can affect the prediction of behavior from attitudes. We will here consider only a few biasing factors whose implications for the attitude–behavior relation have received little attention.

Depth of Processing

As noted earlier, processing can be relatively shallow or deep in the attitudinal context as well as in the behavioral context. Because the domain of accessible beliefs will tend to increase with processing depth, belief congruence is likely to obtain when depth of processing is about the same in the two contexts. Of course, even with equivalent degrees of deliberation, the nature of the beliefs accessed in the two contexts can vary. To ensure attitude–behavior correspondence, therefore, respondents can be encouraged to consider all positive and negative beliefs prior to expressing their attitudes and prior to deciding on a course of action.

Time Perspective

We have noted earlier that according to Lewin's (1935) analysis of approach–avoidance conflicts, positive considerations predominate at some distance from the goal, but negative considerations predominate at close range. This hypothesis itself has yet to be directly tested, but if we assume that it will be confirmed, we can derive several predictions regarding the attitude–behavior relation. As a general rule, and of only minor interest, we expect that the predictive validity of attitudes will increase with proximity to the goal behavior. The reason for this expectation is that attitudes assessed immediately prior to the behavior will reflect the same relative prominence of negative and positive considerations as the behavioral decision. Behavioral prediction of practical significance, however, requires that attitudes be assessed some time prior to performance of the behavior. The conflict model implies that in situations involving relatively complex decisions, differential bias may be operative, such that positive beliefs are more readily accessible in the attitudinal context and negative beliefs in the behavioral context. The result will be lack of correspondence between attitudes and behavior. To improve prediction, we can try to increase the accessibility of negative considerations at the time of attitude measurement, try to raise awareness of positive features prior to performance of the behavior, or use a combination of these approaches.

Framing

If framing of the situation can influence attitudes as well as actions, it also has the potential for affecting the attitude–behavior relation. Specifically, belief congruence will depend on equivalent framing of the issue in the attitudinal and the behavioral contexts. When framed differently, attitudes may be based on one set of accessible beliefs, while behaviors may be based on a somewhat different set of beliefs. For instance, studies may examine beliefs and attitudes with respect to smoking or drug use, and the behavioral criterion is quitting or reduced consumption. The cognitive frame in the attitudinal context tends to focus attention on the harmful consequences of *continued* use of cigarettes or drugs, while in the behavioral context, the focus tends to be on the steps required to *stop* using cigarettes or drugs. Clearly, these two different frames of reference may make accessible very different types of beliefs, resulting in a lack of belief congruence and relatively low attitude–behavior correspondence. To secure optimal prediction, framing of the behavioral context should be as similar as possible to framing of the attitudinal context.

Mood and Affect

The mood congruence effects discussed earlier suggest that attitude–behavior correspondence may be enhanced by ensuring that, to the extent possible, the attitudinal context creates moods or affective states similar to those likely to be encountered in the behavioral context. When affect in the behavioral context is similar to the affect that is present at the time of attitude measurement, the same or similar kinds of beliefs are likely to be accessed, resulting in greater belief congruence. Conversely, if, for example, a respondent is in a positive mood while filling out an attitude survey, but in a negative mood when making a behavioral decision, different beliefs may become accessible in the two contexts, resulting in a weak attitude–behavior correlation.

SUMMARY AND GENERAL CONCLUSIONS

In this chapter, we have proposed to take seriously and quite literally the notion that attitudes are based on beliefs that are salient or accessible in a given situation. Generally speaking, attitudes can be viewed as composed of a relatively stable core as well as a more variable component. The strength of the stable part, relative to the unstable component, is likely to differ from situation to situation and from one individual to another. Although attitudes based on strongly held convictions are unlikely to vary with the context in which they are assessed, research has shown that many attitudes of considerable importance are greatly influenced by contextual factors. Existing attitudes, biased scanning of past behavior, priming, mood, and framing can all influence the nature of the beliefs that are accessible when an attitude is brought to mind, or when a behavioral decision is made. In addition, the scope and nature of accessible beliefs can also be affected by processing mode and depth of processing. A heuristic mode of processing relies on different kinds of beliefs than does a systematic mode, and shallow processing will usually bring to mind fewer and perhaps different beliefs than will deep processing.

The belief congruence principle serves as a link between contextual bias and the attitude–behavior relation. It helps explain why attitudes often fail to predict behavior, and it suggests ways to improve the prediction of behavior from attitudes. According to this principle, attitudes often fail to predict behavior because they are based on a set of accessible beliefs that differs from the set of beliefs providing the basis for the behavior. This is likely to happen when attitudes are assessed in a context that biases accessible beliefs in one direction (positive or negative), while the behavioral context biases accessible beliefs in the opposite direction. The resulting lack of congruence between accessible beliefs produces behavior that is inconsistent with expressed attitudes. A strong attitude–behavior relation can be obtained only when the attitudinal and behavioral contexts afford a high degree of belief congruence.

ACKNOWLEDGMENT

We would like to thank Wolfgang Stroebe and Yaacov Trope for their helpful comments on an earlier draft of this chapter.

NOTES

1. Existing attitudes can, of course, influence the nature of the new beliefs that are formed, but this possibility is not part of the expectancy value perspective.

2. Attitude polarization, however, is not the only possible effect of thinking about an object. We will consider other possibilities below.

3. Because automatic affective responses and retrieval of stored evaluations do not require systematic deliberations, belief congruence is largely irrelevant for these modes of attitude activation. However, issues of congruence can arise if one mode is employed in the attitudinal context and the other mode in the behavioral context. An attitude retrieved from memory, for example, will be based on a set of considerations that predominated at the time the attitude was formed, but if the behavioral context encourages deliberation, new and different kinds of considerations may determine the action taken.

REFERENCES

Abelson, R. P. (1976). Script processing in attitude formation and decision-making. In J. S. Caroll & J. W. Payne (Eds.), *Cognition and social behavior* (pp. 33–45). Hillsdale, NJ: Erlbaum.

Ajzen, I. (1977). Information processing approaches to interpersonal attraction. In S. Duck (Eds.), *Theory and practice in interpersonal attraction* (pp. 51–77). London: Academic Press.

Ajzen, I. (1988). *Attitudes, personality, and behavior.* Homewood, IL: Dorsey Press.

Ajzen, I. (1996a). The social psychology of decision making. In E. T. Higgins & A. W. Kruglanski (Eds.), *Social psychology: Handbook of basic principles* (pp. 297–325). New York: Guilford Press.

Ajzen, I. (1996b). The directive influence of attitudes on behavior. In P. M. Gollwitzer & J. A. Bargh (Eds.), *The psychology of action: Linking motivation and cognition to behavior* (pp. 385–403). New York: Guilford Press.

Ajzen, I., & Driver, B. L. (1991). Prediction of leisure participation from behavioral, normative, and control beliefs: An application of the theory of planned behavior. *Leisure Sciences, 13,* 185–204.

Ajzen, I., Driver, B. L., & Nichols, A. J., III. (1995). Identifying salient beliefs about leisure activities: Frequency of elicitation versus response latency. *Journal of Applied Social Psychology, 25,* 1391–1410.

Ajzen, I., & Fishbein, M. (1977). Attitude behavior relations: A theoretical analysis and review of empirical research. *Psychological Bulletin, 84,* 888–918.

Allport, G. W. (1935). Attitudes. In C. Murchinson (Ed.), *A handbook of social psychology* (pp. 798–844). Worcester, MA: Clark University Press.

Bargh, J. A. (1997). The automaticity of everyday life. In R. S. Wyer (Ed.), *Advances in social cognition* (Vol. 10, pp. 1–61). Mahwah, NJ: Erlbaum.

Bargh, J. A., Chaiken, S., Govender, R., & Pratto, F. (1992). The generality of the automatic attitude activation effect. *Journal of Personality and Social Psychology, 62,* 893–912.

Bargh, J. A., Chaiken, S., Raymond, P., & Hymes, C. (1996). The automatic evaluation effect: Unconditionally automatic attitude activation with a pronunciation task. *Journal of Experimental Social Psychology, 32,* 104–128.

Bargh, J. A., & Pietromonaco, P. (1982). Automatic information processing and social perception: The influence of trait information presented outside of conscious awareness on impression formation. *Journal of Personality and Social Psychology, 43,* 437–449.

Bem, D. J. (1965). An experimental analysis of self persuasion. *Journal of Experimental Social Psychology, 1,* 199–218.

Blaney, P. H. (1986). Affect and memory: A review. *Psychological Bulletin, 99,* 229–246.

Blumer, H. (1955). Attitudes and the social act. *Social Problems, 3,* 59–65.

Bower, G. H. (1981). Mood and memory. *American Psychologist, 36,* 129–148.

Breckler, S. J. (1984). Empirical validation of affect, behavior, and cognition as distinct components of attitude. *Journal of Personality and Social Psychology, 47,* 1191–1205.

Carlson, E. R. (1956). Attitude change through modification of attitude structure. *Journal of Abnormal and Social Psychology, 52,* 256–261.

Chaiken, S. (1980). Heuristic versus systematic information processing and the use of source versus message cues in persuasion. *Journal of Personality and Social Psychology, 39,* 752–766.

Chaiken, S., Axsom, D., Liberman, A., & Wilson, D. (1992). *Heuristic processing of persuasive messages: Chronic and temporary sources of rule accessibility.* Unpublished manuscript, New York University.

Chaiken, S., Liberman, A., & Eagly, A. H. (1989). Heuristic and systematic information processing within and beyond the persuasion process. In J. S. Uleman & J. A. Bargh (Eds.), *Unintended thought* (pp. 212–252). New York: Guilford Press.

Collins, A. M., & Loftus, E. F. (1975). A spreading-activation theory of semantic processing. *Psychological Review, 82,* 407–428.

Deutscher, I. (1966). Words and deeds. *Social Problems,* 13, 235–254.

Doll, J., & Ajzen, I. (1992). Accessibility and stability of predictors in the theory of planned behavior. *Journal of Personality and Social Psychology,* 63, 754–765.

Dreben, E. K., Fiske, S. T., & Hastie, R. (1979). The independence of evaluative and item information: Impression and recall order effects in behavior-based impression formation. *Journal of Personality and Social Psychology,* 37, 1758–1768.

Eagly, A. H., & Chaiken, S. (1993). *The psychology of attitudes.* Fort Worth, TX: Harcourt Brace Jovanovich.

Edwards, W. (1954). The theory of decision making. *Psychological Bulletin,* 51, 380–417.

Epstein, S. (1990). Cognitive–experiential self-theory. In L. A. Pervin (Ed.), *Handbook of personality: Theory and research* (pp. 165–192). New York: Guilford Press.

Erber, R., & Erber, M. W. (1994). Beyond mood and social judgment: Mood incongruent recall and mood regulation. *European Journal of Social Psychology,* 24, 79–88.

Fazio, R. H. (1990). Multiple processes by which attitudes guide behavior: The MODE model as an integrative framework. In M. P. Zanna (Ed.), *Advances in experimental social psychology* (Vol. 23, pp. 75–109). San Diego, CA: Academic Press.

Fazio, R. H., Sanbonmatsu, D. M., Powell, M. C., & Kardes, F. R. (1986). On the automatic activation of attitudes. *Journal of Personality and Social Psychology,* 50, 229–238.

Fazio, R. H., & Williams, C. J. (1986). Attitude accessibility as a moderator of the attitude–perception and attitude–behavior relations: An investigation of the 1984 presidential election. *Journal of Personality and Social Psychology,* 51, 505–514.

Fazio, R. H., & Zanna, M. (1978). Attitudinal qualities relating to the strength of the attitude–behavior relationship. *Journal of Experimental Social Psychology,* 14, 398–408.

Fazio, R. H., & Zanna, M. P. (1981). Direct experience and attitude–behavior consistency. In L. Berkowitz (Ed.), *Advances in experimental social psychology* (Vol. 14, pp. 161–202). New York: Academic Press.

Feather, N. T. (1959). Subjective probability and decision under uncertainty. *Psychological Review,* 66, 150–164.

Feather, N. T. (Ed.). (1982). *Expectations and actions: Expectancy–value models in psychology.* Hillsdale, NJ: Erlbaum.

Festinger, L. (1964). *Conflict, decision, and dissonance.* Stanford, CA: Stanford University Press.

Fishbein, M. (1963). An investigation of the relationships between beliefs about an object and the attitude toward that object. *Human Relations,* 16, 233–240.

Fishbein, M. (Ed.). (1967). *Readings in attitude theory and measurement.* New York: Wiley.

Fishbein, M., & Ajzen, I. (1974). Attitudes toward objects as predictors of single and multiple behavioral criteria. *Psychological Review,* 81, 59–74.

Fishbein, M., & Ajzen, I. (1975). *Belief, attitude, intention, and behavior: An introduction to theory and research.* Reading, MA: Addison-Wesley.

Fiske, S. T., & Dépret, E. (1996). Control, interdependence and power: Understanding social cognition in its social context. In W. Stroebe & M. Hewstone (Eds.), *European review of social psychology* (Vol. 7, pp. 31–61). New York: Wiley.

Fiske, S. T., & Neuberg, S. L. (1990). A continuum of impression formation, from category-based to individuating processes: Influences of information and motivation on attention and interpretation. In M. P. Zanna (Ed.), *Advances in experimental social psychology* (Vol. 23, pp. 1–74). San Diego, CA: Academic Press.

Fiske, S. T., & Pavelchak, M. A. (1986). Category-based versus piecemeal-based affective responses: Developments in schema-triggered affect. In R. M. Sorrentino & E. T. Higgins (Eds.), *Handbook of motivation and cognition: Foundations of social behavior* (Vol. 1, pp. 167–203). New York: Guilford Press.

Fiske, S. T., & Taylor, S. E. (1991). *Social cognition* (2nd ed.). New York: McGraw-Hill.

Forgas, J. P., Bower, G. H., & Krantz, S. (1984). The influence of mood on perceptions of social interactions. *Journal of Experimental Social Psychology,* 20, 497–513.

Granberg, D. (1985). An anomaly in political perception. *Public Opinion Quarterly,* 49, 504–516.

Hastie, R. (1988). A computer simulation model of person memory. *Journal of Experimental Social Psychology,* 24, 423–447.

Hastie, R., & Park, B. (1986). The relationship between memory and judgment depends on whether the judgment task is memory-based or on-line. *Psychological Review,* 93, 258–268.

Higgins, E. T. (1989). Knowledge accessibility and activation: Subjectivity and suffering from unconscious sources. In J. S. Uleman & J. A. Bargh (Eds.), *Unintended thought* (pp. 75–123). New York: Guilford Press.

Higgins, E. T., Bargh, J. A., & Lombardi, W. (1985). The nature of priming effects on categorization. *Journal of Experimental Psychology: Learning, Memory, and Cognition,* 11, 59–69.

Higgins, E. T., Rholes, W. W., & Jones, C. R. (1977). Category accessibility and impression formation. *Journal of Experimental Social Psychology,* 13, 141–154.

Houston, D. A., & Fazio, R. H. (1989). Biased processing as a function of attitude accessibility: Making objective judgments subjectively. *Social Cognition,* 7, 51–66.

Isen, A. M. (1987). Positive affect, cognitive processes and social behavior. In L. Berkowitz (Ed.), *Advances in experimental social psychology* (Vol. 20, pp. 203–253). San Diego, CA: Academic Press.

Johnson, E. J., & Tversky, A. (1983). Affect, generalization, and the perception of risk. *Journal of Personality and Social Psychology,* 45, 20–31.

Kagan, J. (1996). Three pleasing ideas. *American Psychologist,* 51, 901–908.

Kahneman, D., & Tversky, A. (1979). Prospect theory: An analysis of decision under risk. *Econometrica,* 47, 263–291.

Kaplan, K. J., & Fishbein, M. (1969). The source of beliefs, their saliency, and prediction of attitude. *Journal of Social Psychology,* 78, 63–74.

Kraus, S. J. (1995). Attitudes and the prediction of behavior: A meta-analysis of the empirical literature. *Personality and Social Psychology Bulletin,* 21, 58–75.

Kruglanski, A. W. (1980). Lay epistemo-logic—process

and content: Another look at attribution theory. *Psychological Review, 87,* 70–87.

Kruglanski, A. W. (1989). *Lay epistemics and human knowledge.* New York: Plenum Press.

Lang, P. J., Bradley, M. M., & Cuthbert, B. N. (1990). Emotion, attention, and the startle reflex. *Psychological Review, 97,* 377–395.

Langer, E. J. (1975). The illusion of control. *Journal of Personality and Social Psychology, 32,* 311–328.

Leippe, M. R., & Elkin, R. A. (1987). When motives clash: Issue involvement and response involvement as determinants of persuasion. *Journal of Personality and Social Psychology, 52,* 269–278.

Lewin, K. (1935). *A dynamic theory of personality.* New York: McGraw-Hill.

Lewin, K. (1938). The conceptual representation and measurement of psychological forces. *Contributions to Psychological Theory, 1*(4).

Liberman, N., & Trope, Y. (1998). The role of feasibility and desirability considerations in near and distant future decisions: A test of temporal construal theory. *Journal of Personality and Social Psychology, 75,* 5–18.

Linn, L. S. (1965). Verbal attitudes and overt behavior: A study of racial discrimination. *Social Forces, 43,* 353–364.

Loftus, E. F., Feldman, J., & Dashiell, R. (1995). The reality of illusory memories. In D. L. Schacter (Ed.), *Memory distortion: How minds, brains, and societies reconstruct the past* (pp. 47–68). Cambridge, MA: Harvard University Press.

Loftus, E. F., & Palmer, J. C. (1974). Reconstruction of automobile destruction: An example of the interaction between language and memory. *Journal of Verbal Learning and Verbal Behavior, 13,* 585–589.

Mayer, J. D., Gaschke, Y. N., Braverman, D. L., & Evans, T. W. (1992). Mood congruent judgement is a general effect. *Journal of Personality and Social Psychology, 63,* 119–132.

Mayer, J. D., McCormick, L. J., & Strong, S. A. (1995). Mood-congruent memory and natural mood: New evidence. *Personality and Social Psychology Bulletin, 21,* 736–746.

McGuire, W. J. (1960). A syllogistic analysis of cognitive relationships. In C. I. Hovland & M. J. Rosenberg (Eds.), *Attitude organization and change* (pp. 65–111). New Haven, CT: Yale University Press.

McGuire, W. J., & McGuire, C. V. (1996). Enhancing self-esteem by directed-thinking tasks: Cognitive and affective positivity asymmetries. *Journal of Personality and Social Psychology, 70,* 1117–1125.

Merton, R. K. (1940). Fact and factitiousness in ethnic opinionnaires. *American Sociological Review, 5,* 13–27.

Millar, M. G., & Tesser, A. (1986). Effects of affective and cognitive focus on the attitude–behavior relation. *Journal of Personality and Social Psychology, 51,* 270–276.

Millar, M. G., & Tesser, A. (1992). The role of beliefs and feelings in guiding behavior: The mismatch model. In L. L. Martin & A. Tesser (Eds), *The construction of social judgments* (pp. 277–300). Hillsdale, NJ: Erlbaum.

Murphy, S. T., Monahan, J. L., & Zajonc, R. B. (1995). Additivity of nonconscious affect: Combined effects of priming and exposure. *Journal of Personality and Social Psychology, 69,* 589–602.

Murphy, S. T., & Zajonc, R. B. (1993). Affect, cognition, and awareness: Affective priming with optimal and suboptimal stimulus exposures. *Journal of Personality and Social Psychology, 64,* 723–739.

Neisser, U. (1976). *Cognition and reality: Principles and implications of cognitive psychology.* San Francisco: Freeman.

Osgood, C. E., Suci, G. J., & Tannenbaum, P. H. (1957). *The measurement of meaning.* Urbana: University of Illinois Press.

Peak, H. (1955). Attitude and motivation. In M. R. Jones (Ed.), *Nebraska Symposium on Motivation* (Vol. 3, pp. 149–188). Lincoln: University of Nebraska Press.

Petkova, K. G., Ajzen, I., & Driver, B. L. (1995). Salience of anti-abortion beliefs and commitment to an attitudinal position: On the strength, structure, and predictive validity of anti-abortion attitudes. *Journal of Applied Social Psychology, 25,* 463–483.

Petty, R. E., & Cacioppo, J. T. (1979). Issue involvement can increase or decrease persuasion by enhancing message-relevant cognitive responses. *Journal of Personality and Social Psychology, 37,* 1915–1926.

Petty, R. E., & Cacioppo, J. T. (1986). *Communication and persuasion.* New York: Springer-Verlag.

Powell, M. C., & Fazio, R. H. (1984). Attitude accessibility as a function of repeated attitudinal expression. *Personality and Social Psychology Bulletin, 10,* 139–148.

Regan, D. T., & Fazio, R. H. (1977). On the consistency between attitudes and behavior: Look to the method of attitude formation. *Journal of Experimental Social Psychology, 13,* 38–45.

Robles, R., Smith, R., Carver, C. S., & Wellens, A. R. (1987). Influence of subliminal visual images on the experience of anxiety. *Personality and Social Psychology Bulletin, 13,* 399–410.

Rosenberg, M. J. (1956). Cognitive structure and attitudinal affect. *Journal of Abnormal and Social Psychology, 53,* 367–372.

Ruscher, J. B., & Fiske, S. T. (1990). Interpersonal competition can cause individuating impression formation. *Journal of Personality and Social Psychology, 58,* 832–842.

Salancik, G. R., & Conway, M. (1975). Attitude inferences from salient and relevant cognitive content about behavior. *Journal of Personality and Social Psychology, 32,* 829–840.

Schaller, M., & Cialdini, R. B. (1990). Happiness, sadness, and helping: A motivational integration. In E. T. Higgins & R. M. Sorrentino (Eds.), *Handbook of motivation and cognition: Foundations of social behavior* (Vol. 2, pp. 265–296). New York: Guilford Press.

Schneider, D. J. (1973). Implicit personality theory: A review. *Psychological Bulletin, 79,* 294–309.

Schwarz, N. (1990). Feelings as information: Informational and motivational functions of affective states. In E. T. Higgins & R. M. Sorrentino (Eds.), *Handbook of motivation and cognition: Foundations of social behavior* (Vol. 2, pp. 527–561). New York: Guilford Press.

Schwarz, N., & Bless, H. (1992). Constructing reality and its alternatives: An inclusion/exclusion model of assimilation and contrast effects in social judgment. In L. L. Martin & A. Tesser (Eds.), *The construction of* social judgments (pp. 217–245). Hillsdale, NJ: Erlbaum.

Schwarz, N., & Clore, G. L. (1988). How do I feel about it? The informative function of affective states. In K. Fielder & J. P. Forgas (Eds.), Affect, cognition and social behavior (pp. 44–62). Toronto: Hogrefe.

Schwarz, N., Strack, F., & Mai, H. (1991). Assimilation and contrast effects in part–whole question sequences: A conversational logic analysis. Public Opinion Quarterly, 55, 3–23.

Shavitt, S., & Fazio, R. H. (1991). Effects of attribute salience on the consistency between attitudes and behavioral predictions. Personality and Social Psychology Bulletin, 17, 507–516.

Sia, T. L., Lord, C. G., Lepper, M. R., Blessum, K. A., & Ratcliff, C. S. (1997). Is a rose always a rose?: The role of social category exemplar change in attitude stability and attitude–behavior consistency. Journal of Personality and Social Psychology, 72, 501–514.

Simon, H. A. (1955). A behavioral model of rational choice. Quarterly Journal of Economics, 69, 99–118.

Simon, H. A. (1956). Rational choice and the structure of the environment. Psychological Review, 63, 129–138.

Sivacek, J., & Crano, W. D. (1982). Vested interest as a moderator of attitude–behavior consistency. Journal of Personality and Social Psychology, 43, 210–221.

Sparks, P., Guthrie, C. A., & Shepherd, R. (1997). The dimensional structure of the "perceived behavioral control" construct. Journal of Applied Social Psychology, 27, 418–438.

Srull, T. K., & Wyer, R. S., Jr. (1989). Person memory and judgment. Psychological Review, 96, 58–83.

Taylor, S. E. (1981). A categorization approach to stereotyping. In D. L. Hamilton (Ed.), Cognitive processes in stereotyping and intergroup behavior (pp. 88–114). Hillsdale, NJ: Erlbaum.

Tesser, A. (1978). Self-generated attitude change. In L. Berkowitz (Ed.), Advances in experimental social psychology (Vol. 11, pp. 289–338). New York: Academic Press.

Tesser, A., & Conlee, M. C. (1975). Some effects of time

and thought on attitude polarization. Journal of Personality and Social Psychology, 31, 262–270.

Tesser, A., & Leone, C. (1977). Cognitive schemas and thought as determinants of attitude change. Journal of Experimental Social Psychology, 13, 340–356.

Triandis, H. C. (1980). Values, attitudes, and interpersonal behavior. In H. E. Howe, Jr., & M. M. Page (Eds.), Nebraska Symposium on Motivation (Vol. 27, pp. 195–259). Lincoln: University of Nebraska Press.

Tulving, E. (1983). Elements of episodic memory. Oxford: Clarendon Press.

Tversky, A., & Kahneman, D. (1981). The framing of decisions and the psychology of choice. Science, 211, 435–458.

van der Pligt, J., & Eiser, J. R. (1984). Dimensional salience, judgment, and attitudes. In J. R. Eiser (Ed.), Attitudinal judgment (pp. 161–177). New York: Springer-Verlag.

Waugh, N., & Norman, D. (1965). Primary memory. Psychological Review, 72, 89–104.

Wicker, A. W. (1969). Attitudes versus actions: The relationship of verbal and overt behavioral responses to attitude objects. Journal of Social Issues, 25, 41–78.

Wilson, T. D., Dunn, D. S., Bybee, J. A., Hyman, D. B., & Rotondo, J. A. (1984). Effects of analyzing reasons on attitude–behavior consistency. Journal of Personality and Social Psychology, 47, 5–16.

Wilson, T. D., Dunn, D. S., Kraft, D., & Lisle, D. J. (1989). Introspection, attitude change, and attitude–behavior consistency: The disruptive effects of explaining why we feel the way we do. In L. Berkowitz (Ed.), Advances in experimental social psychology (Vol. 19, pp. 123–205). San Diego, CA: Academic Press.

Wilson, T. D., & Hodges, S. D. (1992). Attitudes as temporary constructions. In L. L. Martin & A. Tesser (Eds.), The construction of social judgments (pp. 37–65). Hillsdale, NJ: Erlbaum.

Zajonc, R. B. (1980). Feeling and thinking: Preferences need no inferences. American Psychologist, 35, 151–175.

B

Person Perception

7

Spontaneous versus Intentional Inferences in Impression Formation

JAMES S. ULEMAN

> Psychology also attempts to conceptualize what it is doing. . . . How do we do that?
> Mostly, so it seems to me, by the construction of oppositions—usually binary ones. We
> worry about nature versus nurture, about central versus peripheral, about serial versus
> parallel, and so on . . . far from providing the rungs of a ladder by which psychology
> gradually climbs to clarity, this form of conceptual structure leads rather to an ever
> increasing pile of issues, which we weary of or become diverted from, but never really
> settle.
>
> —NEWELL (1973, pp. 287, 289)

This chapter takes a look at yet another binary opposition: how spontaneous inferences seem to differ from intentional ones when we form impressions of other people. The literature on intentional inferences in impression formation is huge (e.g., Gilbert, 1997; Kenny, 1994), and no attempt is made to summarize it here. But our picture of impression formation processes would be incomplete if it were restricted to intentional processes. Impressions are formed spontaneously (unintentionally) as well. So at the risk of adding yet another dichotomy to Newell's pile of oppositions, and with a promissory note to move beyond mere dichotomies in future work, this chapter examines the newer and more limited spontaneous-inference literature for clues about how impressions formed spontaneously may differ from those formed intentionally. Spontaneous processes are engaged by mere attention to others, whereas intentional processes are engaged by intend-ing to form an impression or make a decision about others. These two sets of processes may interact, but this possibility will not be developed here because there is no relevant research evidence.

I begin this chapter with a cautionary sketch of some properties of dualities, so that we do not assume that every duality is a good one, or mistake all dichotomies for latent dual-process theories. I then consider the criteria traditionally used to distinguish between strategic and automatic processes, and conclude that the distinction between intentional and unintentional (spontaneous) processes is the most defensible duality. A brief discussion of some complexities inherent in the notions of "intentional" and "unintentional" follows.

To illustrate the idea of unintentional (or spontaneous) inferences in general, three are described for which there is some research evidence: logical, predicting, and counterfactual. Then the major portion of the chapter describes the ways in which spontaneous inferences seem to differ from intentional inferences in impression formation. These are summarized in a table. In addition, I offer a metaphor to capture these differences and perhaps to suggest others. Finally, the spontaneous–intentional duality is compared with some other prominent dual-process models. This produces several suggestions for future research that may help transform this "pile of issues" into the "rungs of a ladder" we can climb to gain a clearer view of their relations to one another.

FALSE AND TRUE DUALITIES

A duality may be false for many reasons. The underlying reality may actually be continuous (e.g., as posited in Kruglanski's unimodel; see Kruglanski, Thompson, & Spiegel, Chapter 14, this volume). The duality may implicitly deny additional categories (e.g., "heterosexual men" and "women" as "natural" categories). It may imply mutually exclusivity when that is inaccurate (e.g., the duality "straight" and "gay/lesbian" denies bisexuality). Or it may represent only one level of a hierarchical taxonomy (e.g., biological taxonomies).

Dual-process theories should be based on coherent dichotomies. One popular dichotomy in psychology has been that between automatic and controlled (or automatic and strategic) processes. But the current consensus is that automatic processes have several properties that do not always co-occur, and that some of these properties are continuous. Bargh (1994) has discussed four properties of automaticity: efficiency, lack of awareness, lack of control, and lack of intention. Three of these are arguably continuous. Smith's (1994) work on the proceduralization of social judgments clearly demonstrates that the efficiency of cognitive processes varies continuously.

Awareness is also a matter of degree, but in several senses. First, people can be "aware" of varying amounts of any cognitive process and outcome. The literature is replete with discussions of what that amount may be in particular instances (e.g., Ericsson & Simon, 1993; Nisbett & Wilson, 1977; Smith & Miller, 1978), but there seems to be no dispute that a potentially continuous "amount"

is involved. Second, because awareness of what happened is necessarily assessed after the fact, retrospective certainty of what one was aware of at the time (rather than what one surmised afterward) can vary continuously. So both the extent of what one is aware of, and one's certainty that such awareness does not reflect retrospective reconstruction, can vary continuously.

Control is also a matter of degree in at least two senses. One concerns how closely the outcome can be made to match some standard or goal. One's backhand in tennis may not perfectly match one's ideal, but it may still evidence some degree of control. The second sense concerns the proportion of constituent subprocesses that are controlled or actively guided *during* their execution. When a skill is highly practiced, more of the subroutines are chained and executed automatically, so that conscious guidance serves only to disrupt the performance (e.g., "the Zen of" archery, typing, or tennis). However this proportion may be measured, it is clear that the acquisition of such expertise is a matter of degree.

Thus, among Bargh's "four horsemen of automaticity," intention may be the clearest candidate for a dichotomy on which to base a dual-process theory. Either you intend to do something, or you don't. Intentions are *a priori*, so they don't have the ambiguity of awareness assessed post hoc. (Note that post hoc reconstructions of intentions, which can vary in certainty and are subject to all kinds of self-justifying biases, are not included here.) Of course, intentions may have continuous features. The specificity of your plan for implementing your intention can vary. Your determination to carry out your intention may be strong or weak. Your success at doing so may also vary continuously. But the intention itself either exists or it does not. Some sort of mental Rubicon is crossed when you go from thinking about what to do to adopting a particular intention (see Gollwitzer, 1990). Operationally, participants in studies can be instructed to (have the intention to) form impressions of others, or to attend to information about them for some unrelated purpose.

This suggests that a dual-process theory may attempt to account for whatever differences occur when a cognitive process occurs *intentionally versus unintentionally*. The prerequisite for this is that the intentional process also occurs, in some sense, unintentionally. Fortunately, many cognitive processes do. Evidence of their occurrence can be obtained from patterns of cued recall, recognition probe reaction times (RTs), lexical-decision RTs, word stem completions, and savings in relearning tasks. Some of these are considered in detail below.

This chapter describes emerging evidence on differences between intentional and unintentional inferences in impression formation. It focuses particularly on spontaneous trait inferences (STIs), because these have been defined from the outset (Winter & Uleman, 1984) as unintentional. STIs have typically been demonstrated by having participants read descriptions of trait-implying behaviors, in the absence of intentions to infer traits or form impressions, and then obtaining evidence that trait inferences occurred. For example, "The reporter steps on his girlfriend's feet during the tango" implies "clumsy." "The secretary solved the mystery halfway through the book" implies "clever." The research evidence indicates that reading such sentences with a goal that does not involve impression formation—such as memorizing them, reading them as distractors, or familiarizing oneself with them—is enough to prompt trait inferences. Participants are not instructed to form trait inferences, and typically deny that they have done so. Yet evidence from a variety of paradigms provides evidence of STIs. (See Uleman, Newman, & Moskowitz, 1996, for a recent review of this evidence.)

There is also research suggesting that people make spontaneous emotion inferences. Gernsbacher, Goldsmith, and Robertson (1992, Study 3) had participants read stories, some of which implied emotions. For example:

Joe worked at the local 7-11, to get spending money while in school. One night, his best friend, Tom, came in to buy a soda. Joe needed to go back to the storage room for a second. While he was away, Tom noticed the cash register was open. From the open drawer Tom quickly took a ten dollar bill. Later that week, Tom learned that Joe had been fired from the 7-11 because his cash had been low one night. (p. 105)

The stories appeared on a computer screen, one sentence at a time. Some stories were followed by a probe word (e.g., "guilt"), 150 milliseconds (ms) after the last sentence, which the participants were to pronounce as quickly as possible. When the emotion matched the one implied by the story, pronunciation times were reliably faster (by 50 ms), suggesting that the emotion concept had been activated by the story.

Neither this research nor most research on STIs has contrasted intentional and unintentional conditions directly. Instead, stimulus materials have been selected on the basis of their trait implications under impression formation instructions, and then used in unintentional (spontaneous) conditions to seek evidence of trait inferences. Recently, however, some research has emerged that directly compares intentional and unintentional conditions (e.g., Carlston & Skowronski, 1994; Stapel, Koomen, & van der Pligt, 1996; Zelli, Cervone, & Huesmann, 1996). This chapter focuses on this and related research as a source of suggestions and speculations about possible differences between intentional and unintentional inferences in impression formation. So the chapter is part review, part elaboration and speculation, and part program for future research.

SOME COMPLEXITIES OF INTENTIONS

As noted above, intentions have properties more complex than their simple dichotomous presence or absence. A brief reminder of some of these may prevent conceptual confusion later on.

First, a different dichotomy is possible. People may intend to do X, or *intend to not do X*. This is different from *not intending to do X*: The first involves an intention not to do something, whereas the second involves the absence of an intention. Processes occurring in the absence of an intention are what I have called "spontaneous." Intentions to not do something are central to Jacoby's (1991) process dissociation procedures. These contrast results obtained when participants are instructed to do X (the "inclusion" condition) versus instructed to not do X (the "exclusion" condition). Such a contrast makes it possible to assess how much cognitive control is possible (when various additional assumptions are met), but it is not the present contrast. I return to Jacoby's procedures at the end of this chapter. (See also Wegner & Wenzlaff, 1996, for a different approach to the issue of control.)

Second, "the absence of an intention to do X" is an ill-defined condition; it may include anything from intentions to do A through Z (except X) to being asleep. Clearly, this is too broad. So to be more precise, the absence of the intention must occur within a task that requires attention to the stimulus information under some other intention, Y. Furthermore, intention Y must not necessarily entail intention X. Thus, people may be asked to memorize the information (Y) because this requires attention to the information without requiring that they infer traits (X). The complication here is that one does not always know what is entailed by a particular intention, because this requires detailed knowledge of the processes used to carry it out. Deciding whether a stimulus person resembles your mother may involve inferring traits ("Let's see, my mother is warm but demanding. Is this person warm but demanding?"), but it may not ("My mother is female and 5'2". This guy is not"). So doing Y may turn out to entail X for some people and not others (because there are many ways to do Y), or may entail X for everyone (because that is the only way to do Y). At the very least, Y must not necessarily entail X. (See Uleman & Moskowitz, 1994, for more on the effects of other goals on STIs.)

One cannot assume that people can accurately report on what processes, or intermediate outcomes, an intention entails. Nisbett and Wilson's (1977) classic demonstrations make this point, even with their limitations (Smith & Miller, 1978) and important exceptions (e.g. Ericsson & Simon, 1993). Research on the role of intuition in discovery (e.g., Bowers, Regehr, Balthazard, & Parker, 1990) also illustrates this point. Thus, although post hoc reports that Y was done without doing X may be desirable, they cannot be decisive for the issue of what an intentional process entails.

Third, the present discussion excludes unconscious goals and intentions. Global unconscious goals may be essential in the development of spontaneous processes (Uleman, Newman, & Moskowitz, 1996). But the current operation and psychological reality of unconscious goals are difficult to verify empirically (Uleman, 1996; cf. Bargh, Chen, & Burrows, 1996). In addition, unconscious intentions do not entail the kind of deliberate monitoring and corrective processes that characterize conscious intentions (see below). So in this chapter, "intention" means conscious intention.

EXAMPLES OF OTHER SPONTANEOUS INFERENCES

Spontaneous inferences are not limited to the STI literature. A brief look at some other types of spontaneous inferences may sharpen the spontaneous–intentional distinction.

Spontaneous Logical Inferences

Many inferences are made in the course of text comprehension. For example, to understand "Linda finally decided to be daring and to get a dye job done on her hair," one must infer that "her" refers to Linda. On the other hand, not all possible inferences are made; one doesn't imagine all the colors that Linda could choose or everything that might have prompted her decision. Inferences that are necessarily entailed by comprehension are those required to maintain the coherence of what has been read, such as the anaphoric inference above and bridging inferences that link widely separated clauses (Graesser, Singer, & Trabasso, 1994; Kintsch, 1988; McKoon & Ratcliff, 1992). The number of potential inferences is infinite, and most are not necessary for comprehension and textual coherence.

Lea (1995b) has shown that some types of simple logical inferences, which are not required for text coherence, are nevertheless made during text comprehension. One series of stories permitted "or-elimination" inferences. For instance, the Linda story (see above) continued, "According to her hairdresser, Linda's complexion would look good with either a dark shade or a red shade. She let her hairdresser, Yvette, make the final decision. 'Well,' said Yvette, 'I'm sure you want to look different from everybody else this year, so we're not going to dye your hair red.'" Participants spontaneously inferred "dark" after reading this last sentence. In two studies, they were faster to make lexical decisions about associates of the inferences (e.g., "light") than they were when the last sentence did not permit the inference (e.g., "Linda flipped through a few hairstyle magazines and saw a lot of people with red hair"). In another study, pronunciation times for the inferences themselves (e.g., "dark,") were faster.

Another pair of studies provides lexical-decision evidence for the spontaneous use of *modus ponens* ("If *P*, then *Q*; *P*; therefore *Q*"). In these, participants read stories such as, "Fred, the forest ranger, was trying to decide which National Park to work for. He knew that if he decided on the one in Alaska, then he would be working to protect the eagles. . . . After much consideration, Fred decided to work for the park in Alaska." Reading about this decision facilitated a lexical decision about "bird," but reading that "Fred wondered whether the park in Alaska would be too cold for his liking" did not. Note that comprehending neither text requires the activation of "eagles," and that both texts mention Alaska toward the end. But only the first enables (but does not require) the spontaneous logical inference of "eagles."

Spontaneous Predicting Inferences

Most inferences that are necessary to establish textual coherence are "backward" inferences, relating material currently in working memory to previous material. McKoon and Ratcliff (1986) showed that another kind of "forward" inference, not required for textual coherence, occurs spontaneously. "Predicting inferences" represent predictions about what will follow. For example, reading "After locating the cavity, the dentist told John to open his mouth" may prompt the prediction "drill," but it does not require it. In three studies, McKoon and Ratcliff found that participants responded to recognition probes such as "drill" either more slowly, or with more errors, than after control stories that did not imply the predictions (e.g., "John opened his mouth for the dentist, but there were no cavities"). They interpreted this as evidence that "drill" was activated by the first but not by the second story, so that it was harder to say it had not appeared in the story. A fourth study showed that these predicting inferences were more effective recall cues for the predicting stories than for the control stories.

The emotions implied in the Gernsbacher et al. (1992) study described above could also be thought of as predicting inferences, in that they followed the events in the stories. However, to encourage comprehension, their participants expected to write continuations of some of the stories. So it might be argued that inferring the future implications of each story was entailed in their task, and therefore not spontaneous.

Thus, at least two kinds of forward inferences occur spontaneously during text comprehension: predicting and simple logical inferences. Neither is necessary for textual coherence. They may depend on intending to comprehend the text (the *Y* intention that doesn't entail the *X* intention to infer, described above). In Lea's (1995b) studies, participants answered a comprehension question after each story to ensure comprehension. McKoon and Ratcliff's (1986) participants rated how interesting each sentence was before they got the unexpected cued-recall test. However, in their recognition probe RT studies, there was no instruction to ensure comprehension; in fact, comprehension worked against optimal performance, because predicting inferences that were implied but absent slowed responses and produced more errors. Nevertheless, participants seemed to employ their usual comprehension procedures anyway (at least on initial trials; see Uleman, Hon, Roman, & Moskowitz, 1996).

Spontaneous Counterfactual Inferences

Counterfactual inferences may come to mind spontaneously under some circumstances. Roese and Olson (1997, pp. 21–23) report evidence that negative but not unexpected or novel events prompt counterfactual thinking. They measured RTs to counterfactual probes (e.g., "yes" or "no" to "My score could have been much different") following feedback on an anagram task. RTs were shorter following failure, and negative affect (but neither unexpectedness nor controllability) significantly mediated this effect.

Roese and Olson obtained similar results from nondirective thought listings. Although such measures can be informative, and have been central in earlier research on "spontaneous" inferences (e.g., Weiner, 1985), there is always the danger that the instruction to list thoughts prompts thinking that would not have otherwise occurred. The RT results are much more relevant and convincing.

Spontaneous Inferences versus Simpler Unintended Processes

As these examples illustrate, "inferring" refers to relatively complex symbolic processing of information in which several meanings are combined to produce an emergent meaning that is not present in any of the constituent meanings. Thus an inference (trait, logical, predicting, or counterfactual) goes well beyond the simple activation of concepts that is found in repetition or semantic priming. These simpler processes differ from spontaneous inferences in that priming activates concepts rather directly, whereas inferring invokes more extensive knowledge structures and more complex processes than simple associations and lexical access.

The trait, logical, predicting, and counterfactual inferences described above illustrate this difference. Well-designed studies always contain control stimuli in which associations that might activate the target concept can operate (e.g., "dentist" and "cavities" can activate "drill"), but these stimuli do *not* produce the target inference (e.g., "John opened his mouth for the dentist, but there were no cavities") to the same extent as the concept-implying stimulus. Although STIs themselves can act as primes once they occur (Moskowitz & Roman, 1992), they depend on more complex cognitive processes than semantic priming or association. Of course, priming and stereotype category activation play important roles in unintended-impression formation. But they are beyond the scope of this chapter.[1]

SPONTANEOUS VERSUS INTENTIONAL IMPRESSIONS

Spontaneous impressions occur when one is attending to other people without an impression formation goal in mind. "Uneventful people watching" provides a prototypical case. "Uneventful" is important, because negative or surprising observations may initiate questions and epistemic goals: "What's going on? What caused that? What kind of person would do something like that?" When such questions occur, the inferred answers are not spontaneous. "Watching" is also important, because spontaneous inferences can only occur if the information is attended to. By contrast, intentional impressions occur when one is attending to, and even interacting with others with an impression formation goal in mind. Getting acquainted at a party and unstructured job interviews illustrate such situations, where the perceiver is actively engaged in information search and hypothesis testing in order to form an impression. Sometimes the impression formation goal is content-specific (e.g., "Is she a good candidate for the statistician job?" or "Does he have my sense of humor?"). Such content-specific goals activate relevant knowledge structures, which influence how any new information is encoded. Reflecting on these examples suggests several possible differences between spontaneous and intentional impressions, which are summarized in Table 7.1.

1. Spontaneous impressions are guided more by chronically accessible constructs, whereas intentional impressions are guided more by temporarily activated goal-relevant constructs and procedures, and by implicit theories (about the meanings of actions, relationships of traits to each other, the properties of an adequate impression, etc.). If you are engaging in uneventful people watching at the annual picnic, and are chronically concerned with other people's sense of humor or with how they treat children, your observations should be spontaneously encoded in terms of these particular concerns. On the other hand, if you have the goal of deciding who would work well in your lab, that should temporarily activate such constructs as intelligence and conscientiousness and your theories about good scientists, should prompt competing interpretations of whatever you observe, and should engage a host of hypothesis-testing processes. All of this may obscure individual differences in chronic accessibility.

2. Spontaneous impressions are less focused, more wide-ranging, and more promiscuous, whereas intentional impressions are focused; goal-irrelevant inferences are inhibited in the latter. A chronic concern with funniness, sexiness, a sense of social injustice, or the like should produce spontaneous inferences about any of these that are applicable.

TABLE 7.1. Possible Differences between Spontaneous and Intentional Inferences in Impression Formation

Spontaneous	Intentional
1. Inferences are guided by chronically accessible constructs and procedures.	1. Inferences are guided by temporary goal-relevant constructs and deliberative processes.
2. Multiple unrelated inferences occur and persist.	2. Goal- and context-irrelevant inferences are inhibited.
3. Prior construct activation affects impressions, but subsequent information is less likely to.	3. Both prior and subsequent information is integrated into coherent impressions.
4. Trait inferences are implicitly linked to actors by association, appropriately or not.	4. Trait inferences are explicitly linked to the actors about whom one intends to form impressions.

Multiple spontaneous inferences may occur in parallel. Intentional impressions are more focused and limited by serial processes that check for goal relevance, consistency, etc.

3. Spontaneous impressions arise in the course of comprehending events (or text). Rather than being revised when inconsistent or qualifying information is encountered, they are simply replaced by the new information's implications. This differs from intentional-impression formation in that the additional information is not used to revise and reinterpret prior information, which has to be retrieved from long-term memory. Instead, it simply forms an overlay and replaces prior impressions. Prior information may affect spontaneous impressions by priming relevant constructs. But little or no effort is made to revise prior inferences in light of subsequent information, partly because there is no awareness that they have been made.

4. Spontaneous impressions are linked to actors by mere association (if they are linked at all), whereas intentional impressions are correctly linked to the logically appropriate actor. Trait concepts activated spontaneously by one actor's behavior may become associated with another person in that setting, or may not even be associated with any particular person. Thus you may remember that someone (or something) was pretty funny at the annual picnic without remembering who it was, or you may even be mistaken about who it was. Such errors are less likely for intentional impressions, because one has the

question in mind ("What's John really like when he lets his hair down?") before the answer is generated.

In short, relative to intentional impressions, spontaneous impressions reflect the perceiver more than the target (i.e., the perceiver's chronically activated constructs and a wider range of such constructs); are relatively unfocused; reflect little or no integration of inconsistent information; and may be associated with salient others who did not give rise to the impression, or may not be associated with anyone at all. This is a list of hypotheses, not a list of well-established research findings. Nevertheless, each was suggested by research evidence. I turn to that next, to describe the evidence, elaborate on these ideas, and examine the limits of the support that already exists for them.

Chronically Accessible Constructs versus Goal-Activated Constructs

Goals select and activate goal-relevant constructs and processes. For example, deciding whether someone is suitable for a particular job activates relevant constructs and hypothesis-testing processes (see Gollwitzer & Moskowitz, 1996; Trope & Liberman, 1996). Without such goals, the effects of chronic concerns and chronically accessible constructs should be more evident. In addition, the simple goal of being thorough in forming an impression may generate multiple inferences—

inferences that would not occur spontaneously, or with a specific but superficial processing goal in mind.

Zelli and his colleagues (Zelli et al., 1996; Zelli, Huesmann, & Cervone, 1995) conducted two studies that contrasted spontaneous inferences with those made by participants who were asked to "think about the reasons *why* the persons described in the statement did what they did. Think about what caused the outcome described" (Zelli et al., 1996, p. 174). All participants read a group of sentences with the goal of memorizing them for a subsequent recall test; the "deliberate-inference" participants also thought about reasons for the actors' behaviors. Participants in each study were in the extreme quartiles on a self-report measure of the frequency of engaging in aggression (e.g., "threatened, or actually cut with a knife, or shot with a gun") in the past year. On this basis, they could be assumed to be high or low in the chronic activation of hostility-related constructs.

Some of the sentences participants read had both hostile and nonhostile interpretations. For example, "The electrician looks at his younger brother and starts laughing" can imply "ridicule" or "playful." "The man in the second row starts screaming when the athlete runs by" can imply "insulting" or "excited." The prediction was that more aggressive participants would spontaneously encode these sentences in hostile ways, but that this difference would disappear under deliberative conditions because all participants would generate both interpretations. That is, extensive deliberations should lead to multiple interpretations, not just to those occurring spontaneously on the basis of chronically accessible constructs.

This prediction was supported in both studies. Zelli et al. (1995) compared recall cued by hostile cues with that cued by semantic cues ("wires" and "audience," respectively, for the sentences above). Under spontaneous processing, hostile cues were relatively more effective for aggressive participants; under intentional processing, there were no differences. Zelli et al. (1996) compared the effectiveness of hostile and nonhostile trait cues, to control for the possibility that participants might differ in their tendency to make trait inferences of any kind. Under spontane-

ous processing, hostile cues were more effective for aggressive participants, but not for nonaggressive participants. Under deliberative processing, the pattern was reversed, but the difference was not significant.

These results suggest that spontaneous impressions are more sensitive to the influence of chronically accessible constructs than the "traditional deliberate processing paradigms, which have yielded relatively small aggressive/nonaggressive differences [Dodge, 1993]" (Zelli et al., 1995, p. 415). They are also consistent with findings on the assessment of social problem-solving skills. Rabiner, Lenhart, and Lockman (1990) examined such skills among three groups of fourth- and fifth-graders: nonrejected, rejected–aggressive, and rejected–nonaggressive. These children responded to six short conflict vignettes either (1) immediately, with the first thought that came to mind; or (2) after 20 seconds of reflection about alternative responses. In the immediate condition, both groups of rejected boys gave more "conflict escalation" and fewer nonaggressive "verbal assertion" solutions, consistent with their behavior in the rough-and-tumble round of daily social interactions. In the reflective condition, however, the only difference was that rejected–aggressive boys gave fewer verbal assertion solutions (suggesting that such solutions were not only inaccessible but unavailable to these boys). Although these immediate solutions were not "spontaneous" in precisely the unprompted sense used here, they were clearly less reflective and thus more revealing of differences in chronic accessibility.

There is a large body of evidence indicating that differences in the chronic accessibility of constructs *do* affect intentional-impression formation (see Higgins, 1996, pp. 139–141, for a recent review). Why, then, was this not the case in these studies? Note that these participants were asked to think about the reasons for and causes of the actions. Although this faithfully replicated traditional procedures in research on the cognitive mediators of aggressive behavior, it called for more extensive processing than the instruction to simply "form an impression." This more extensive thought may have activated most of the applicable available constructs in all the participants, swamping differences in chronic accessibility. That is, traditional impression formation studies may have prompted less extensive processing than could easily have occurred, thereby allowing chronically accessible constructs to have a larger impact. The results of impression formation studies may not be particularly representative of the impression formation processes engaged in during social interaction, where more extensive thought may lead to multiple competing inferences (hypotheses to be examined), and where multiple goals may activate more goal-relevant constructs. Daily social interaction, especially where future interaction is anticipated, may engage more complex impression formation than those engaged by traditional "impression formation" instructions and settings. Research is needed to test this idea directly.

Although the studies by Zelli et al. (1995, 1996) are the only ones that directly compare spontaneous with intentional impressions, additional research also suggests the importance of chronic accessibility in STIs. My colleagues and I (Uleman, Winborne, Winter, & Shechter, 1986) examined whether a personality trait that predicts differences in impressions of others would also predict differences in STI. Our participants were high or low in authoritarianism. Sentence stimuli had clear intentional trait implications for one of these two groups but not the other. For example, "The architect loved the excitement of military parades" implied "patriotic" to those who were high on authoritarianism; among low-authoritarianism participants, there was much less consensus about its implications. On the other hand, when low-authoritarianism participants read "The reporter slapped his daughter several times whenever she left her clothes on the floor," they inferred that the reporter was "harsh" or "abusive," whereas high-authoritarianism participants did not. When these sentences were read "for a memory study," the most effective trait cues for participants low in authoritarianism (e.g., "harsh") were not effective for those high in authoritarianism. This was interpreted as support for the idea that differences in authoritarianism reflect (among other things) differences in chronically accessible constructs, which affect spontaneous impressions.

Newman (1993) reported two studies suggesting individual differences in the chronic accessibility of trait constructs in general. People in individualistic cultures use traits in their open-ended self-descriptions more than people from collectivistic cultures do (e.g., Rhee, Uleman, Lee, & Roman, 1995). This suggests that individual differences in individualism (or, more accurately, idiocentrism; Triandis, Bontempo, Villareal, Asai, & Lucca, 1988) may in part reflect differences in the chronic accessibility of trait constructs generally. In Study 1, participants read trait-implying sentences for a subsequent memory test. Analyses of cued-recall evidence for STIs revealed more STIs among idiocentric men (but not women). In Study 2, participants read trait-implying sentences and responded to trait and nontrait recognition probes. As predicted, there was more evidence of STI among participants (both men and women) who were higher in idiocentrism.

More recently, Duff and Newman (1997) found that idiocentric participants made more STIs and fewer spontaneous situational inferences. Participants read 12 sentences (e.g., "On her lunch break, the receptionist steps in front of another person in line," "The photographer complains about the service in the new restaurant") for a subsequent memory test. Each sentence had both a trait interpretation (e.g., "rude" and "picky," respectively) and a situational interpretation (e.g., "in a hurry" and "slow," respectively). Half the sentences were cued with trait cues, and half with situational cues. Idiocentrism correlated (1) positively with trait-cued sentence recall (but only among men, again), and (2) negatively with situation-cued recall.

An unpublished study supports the importance of individualism and collectivism in STIs. Zárate and Uleman (1994) found that on a lexical decision task, Anglo and Chicano students differed as predicted (Latino cultures are more collectivistic). Participants read sentences on a computer screen, and then their recall was tested, to simulate "an exam" taken after "study with distraction." During the sentences, the subjects were "distracted" unpredictably by lexical decisions. Among Anglos, RTs to trait words were shorter following trait-implying sentences than following control sentences, indicating STIs. But there was absolutely no evidence of STIs among Chicanos, even though there were almost two and a half times as many Chicanos as Anglos, and the intentional inferences of Anglo and Chicano students did not differ.

Moskowitz (1993) reported an individual difference in STIs that reflected differences in chronic goals rather than in chronically accessible constructs. Using a cued-recall paradigm, he found that participants who were high in "personal need for structure" were more likely to engage in STIs. Personal need for structure is a desire for certainty and clarity, and a corresponding aversion to ambiguity. Those with the chronic goal of obtaining structure are thought to be more practiced at and more interested in inferring traits from behavior. They prefer not to suspend judgment, and tend to avoid more complex impressions that include situational contingencies. Therefore, they are more likely to interpret trait-implying sentences spontaneously in simple trait terms.

Thus there is considerable evidence consistent with the hypothesis that differences in chronically accessible constructs and goals are reflected in spontaneous impressions, and some evidence that extensive intentional thought about the same information obscures these effects (Zelli et al., 1995, 1996; Zárate & Uleman, 1994). But two kinds of studies are needed to provide clearer support for this hypothesis. The first kind is studies that include more direct measures of chronic construct accessibility, and that distinguish this from construct availability. The second is studies that compare the results of spontaneous, "traditional intentional" (the usual impression formation condition), and "deliberative" (Zelli et al., 1996) processes of impression formation. If my speculation is correct, spontaneous impressions should be most affected by chronically accessible constructs, and deliberative impressions should be least affected. Traditional intentional impressions should fall somewhere in between.

Multiple Unrelated Inferences versus Goal-Relevant Inferences

Goals not only activate constructs, but also inhibit them. In negative priming, stimuli that are to be ignored on one trial take longer to respond to on the next trial than when they had not been ignored. Such inhibition does not simply reduce overall attention to a stimulus; it selects which of several aspects of a stimulus to ignore. "The behavioral goals of the task, whether semantic identification or manual reaching, determine what representations of a stimulus will be accessed and inhibited by attention" (Tipper, 1992, p. 108).

Inhibition is important in comprehension. The classic demonstrations have been carried out with ambiguous words (see Simpson, 1994, for a recent review). If participants read, "The man was not surprised when he found several spiders, roaches, and other bugs," and then immediately make a lexical decision about "ant" or "spy" or "sew", *both* "ant" and "spy" are facilitated because they are related to the meanings of "bug." If the lexical decision is delayed by just four more syllables (200 ms), decisions for "ant" are still facilitated, but those for "spy" are not. That is, all of the meanings of homonyms are initially activated in parallel, but the context-irrelevant ones are quickly inhibited (Swinney, 1979).

Gernsbacher (1991) gives a prominent role to suppression processes in her "structure-building framework" of comprehension. Suppression dampens activation through inhibitory signals transmitted to context-irrelevant cognitive nodes. It plays an important role in lexical access (as in Swinney, 1979), in anaphoric inference, in cataphoric access (maintaining greater activation for marked referents), and in the loss of surface information while retaining the meaning of text. Relative to good comprehenders, poor comprehenders are less efficient suppressers when understanding stories in written, in spoken, and even in pictorial form (Gernsbacher & Faust, 1991a). Thus the inhibition of context-irrelevant meanings is an important general mechanism in comprehending events.

What happens when comprehension goals or context do not require the inhibition of multiple meanings? For example, "Pam was annoyed by a quack" does not provide any basis for deciding whether the "quack" was a doctor or a sound from a duck, whereas "Pam was diagnosed by a quack" and "Pam heard a sound like a quack" do. Gernsbacher and Faust (1991b) used a lexical-decision task with probes such as "doctor" and "duck." They showed that both concepts were active immediately after unambiguous sentences, but that the context-irrelevant meanings were suppressed 500 ms later. Following ambiguous sentences, however, both concepts remained just as active in the delay condition as appropriate concepts were after unambiguous sentences. Thus multiple contradictory meanings can remain active in the absence of disambiguating contexts.

Spontaneous inferences about others are more likely to resemble the associates of ambiguous sentences than those of unambiguous ones. No content-specific goals are operating to inhibit irrelevant meanings. No general goal of forming a coherent impression—one that takes other information about the person into account—is operating. So factors that might select the most relevant from among several meanings and suppress the rest are absent, permitting the persistence of multiple inferences.

Unfortunately, there is no direct research evidence on this possibility. But we (Uleman & Moskowitz, 1994) used a cued-recll paradigm to examine the co-occurrence of trait inferences and inferences of "behavioral gists." Behavioral gists describe behavior in ways that are not directly relevant to traits. "The child tells his mother that he ate the chocolates" implies "honest," but the behavior can also be characterized as "confessing." We expected STIs and spontaneous gist inferences to compete for limited processing capacity or procedures, and therefore to be mutually exclusive. But instead of finding that traits' and gists' effectiveness as cues were negatively correlated, we found that they were positively correlated. These correlations reached significance in some conditions but not others (with Ns about 35); however, they were always positive. Thus, STIs and spontaneous gist inferences tend to co-occur rather than to be mutually exclusive. Whether or not multiple and even mutually inconsistent trait inferences co-occur in spontaneous impressions remains to be examined in future research.

Forward versus Backward Information Integration

Because spontaneous impressions are unintended and often unnoticed (unconscious), inconsistencies with subsequent information are unnoticed too. The usual processes of resolving inconsistencies when forming impressions of others are thus neglected. This does not mean that some sort of information integration doesn't occur. But, at least for STIs, it is more likely for information that precedes rather than follows the trait-implying information. Three studies have demonstrated the effect of preceding information on STIs, and others have demonstrated the failure of subsequent information to affect STIs.

We (Newman & Uleman, 1990) primed trait concepts in an "unrelated-study" paradigm, before trait-implying sentences were read for a subsequent memory test. Either the positive or the negative pole of four trait constructs was primed. The trait-implying sentences were ambiguous, in the sense that they could imply either the positive or negative pole of one of the traits (e.g., "Molly would not take no for an answer" could imply that she was "determined" or "pushy.") Trait-cued recall of the sentences was followed by an unexpected recall test for the primes from the "first study."

Previous research had found that when primes were recalled, contrast effects occurred on a subsequent intentional-impression formation task, whereas assimilation occurred when they were not recalled. Apparently primes that could be remembered served as standards against which to compare subsequent information, resulting in a contrast or overcorrection effect. If they could not be recalled, subsequent information was simply assimilated to the primed construct. We obtained parallel findings for STIs. When participants recalled the prime (e.g., "persistent" or "stubborn"), the cue with the opposite valence ("pushy" and "determined," respectively) was most effective—a contrast effect. When participants did not recall the prime, the cue synonymous with the prime was most effective—an assimilation effect. Thus the activation of relevant trait concepts prior to forming spontaneous impressions affects the inferences from ambiguous behaviors.

In view of the earlier discussion of inhibition above, it is interesting to note that we found that, relative to a no-prime condition, the primes inhibited the effectiveness of the other cue (whether contrasting or synonymous) rather than enhancing the effectiveness of the target cue. "This pattern of results thus seems to indicate that, without priming, more than one interpretation of an observed ambiguous behavior is encoded spontaneously . . . and the primed construct predominates only by inhibiting alternative ones" (Newman & Uleman, 1990, p. 237).

Lupfer, Clark, and Hutcherson (1990) examined whether the preceding narrative context would affect STIs. Instead of reading paragraphs of context and trait-implying behavior for a subsequent memory test, participants read them as distractors from what they believed was their focal task, memorizing digits. One example of such a distractor, "The businessman steps on his girlfriend's feet during the foxtrot" (which implies "clumsy") was preceded by either "The businessman and his girlfriend plan a 'night on the town.' He spills a drink on her dress," or "The businessman and his girlfriend are trying to dance on a very crowded dance floor. Everyone is bumping into others." The first context supports a trait inference, whereas the second does not. On each trial, participants read a string of digits to remember, then read the distractor information, then repeated the final trait-implying sentence aloud from memory, and finally recalled the digits. Relative to reading only the trait-implying sentence as a distractor, STIs were more likely with a preceding context that supported a trait inference.

Lea (1995a) asked participants to read brief stories and make lexical decisions after each one. The critical stories ended with trait-implying sentences. Some stories supported the trait implication and some did not. For example, "The minister gets his poem published in *The New Yorker*" (which implies "talented") was the last sentence in either the story "An Unusual Hobby" or "The Printing Errors." The first story included the following: "Last year a published book of his poems won a prize. This year he has written, he thinks, his best poem." The second story began, "The minister writes a poem for the church newsletter. A couple of printing errors occur. His poem becomes something so hilarious that the national press is alerted." Lexical decisions were faster to trait words (e.g., "talented") when the context supported the trait implication than when it did not, replicating the findings of Lupfer et al. (1990).

Note that both of these studies used narrative contexts that also implied the relevant traits. The clumsy businessman with big feet

also spills a drink on his companion; the talented minister has already won a prize. So these studies may simply show that two trait activations are better than one, or that the preceding context is integrated in more complex ways. In either case, it makes STIs more likely.

What happens when trait-relevant information clearly follows the trait-implying sentences? Lupfer, Clark, Church, DePaola, and McDonald (1995) examined effects of covariation information. They developed focal sentences that were either (1) trait-implying; (2) ambiguous, with traits and situations equally likely explanations; or (3) situation-implying. For some participants, these were followed by covariation information supporting trait inferences; for others, information supporting situational inferences. In both Studies 2 and 3, the resulting three-sentence paragraphs were presented as distractors from a focal task of digit memory (as in Lupfer et al., 1990). In Study 2, STIs were detected with a recognition probe task, with four probes following each paragraph: the trait implication, the situation implication, and two words that actually were presented. Error rates for trait probes showed that STIs were most likely following trait-implying focal sentences, as expected, but were unaffected by the covariation information. In Study 3, STIs were detected with a lexical-decision task. Error rates and latencies for traits again showed that STIs were more likely following trait-implying focal sentences, as expected, but were again unaffected by the covariation information. Thus both studies found that covariation information did not affect spontaneous impressions when it followed the trait-implying information, even though it did have the predicted effects on intentional impressions that were generated in Study 1.

On the basis of work by Moskowitz and Roman (1992), Stapel et al. (1996) used spontaneous- and intentional-impression formation tasks as primes in two studies of assimilation and contrast effects. In Study 1, participants in an "impersonal" condition read simple trait-implying sentences (e.g., "He knew he could handle most problems that would come up"), for the purpose of either forming an impression of the actor (intentional inference) or preparing for a subsequent memory test (STI). The sentences' trait implications were either positive ("confident" and "persistent"), negative ("conceited" and "stubborn"), or irrelevant to the second task. Then in a subsequent "unrelated" task, participants formed an impression of "Erik," modeled after the ambiguous "Donald" in Higgins, Rholes, and Jones (1977). STIs on the first task produced assimilation effects on the second task, whereas intentional impressions produced contrast effects. This was consistent with their theory that activated "abstract" trait concepts ("in the background," not linked to particular actors) would produce assimilation, whereas "concrete" concepts (linked to an actor) would produce contrast.

More to the present point, in Study 2 participants read these same trait-implying sentences under memory (STI) or impression formation instructions, and the sentences were followed by covariation information implying either situational or personal causality. Then participants formed impressions of Erik. Stapel et al. predicted that the situational information would make the activated trait concepts abstract; that the personal information would render them concrete; and that subsequent impressions of Erik would show assimilation or contrast effects, respectively. This was what occurred, regardless of whether the sentences were read under memory or impression instructions.

In other words (and contrary to Lupfer et al., 1995), the covariation information *did* have reliable effects in the STI condition, even though it followed the trait-implying sentences. Why this discrepancy? Although comparisons across studies are hazardous when there are so many differences between them (number and nature of sentences, dependent variables, etc.), recall that Lupfer et al.'s participants read the sentences as distractors rather than for a memory test, giving them less opportunity or incentive for the kind of elaborative processing that could alter inferences from the initial focal behaviors. Although both studies presented covariation information after the trait-implying information, the task demands in Stapel et al. (1996) called for more thorough processing than did those in Lupfer et al. (1995). Thus, whether subsequent information that could modify an intentional impression is processed for a

spontaneous impression depends on the processing demands of the other task (the "Y" task discussed earlier in this chapter). Reading information as a momentary distractor requires less processing than reading for a subsequent memory test, which apparently calls for the construction of a more coherent "text base" (Kintsch, 1988) or "structure" (Gernsbacher, 1991) when several related sentences are involved.

This evidence is consistent with the hypothesis that, like intentional impressions, STIs are affected by preceding information that activates relevant constructs. But STIs are less likely to be revised by subsequent information than intentional impressions are. If new information suggests a new spontaneous impression, it is more likely to replace a prior impression than to be integrated with it. In short, forward integration (based on simple construct activation) occurs for both kinds of impressions, but backward integration is less likely with spontaneous impressions.

Spontaneous versus Intentional Associations with Actors

When you ask yourself (or are asked) a question (e.g., "What kind of a person is Rashid?"), and then an answer to that question occurs to you, you know what question is being answered. Unlike Carnac the Magnificent on the old *The Tonight Show with Johnny Carson* (who would guess at the question when given an answer), you don't have to guess at the question. So if the trait concept "clever" occurs to you as you're wondering about Rashid, your initial inference will be that Rashid is clever.

Krull (1993) demonstrated as much when he showed that the stages in forming impressions of a situation parallel those of forming impressions of a person. His participants were asked to watch a silent videotape of a woman responding nervously to unknown interview questions, and to form an impression of either the person or the situation. Half of each group was under cognitive load, which interferes with the "correction" stage of Gilbert's well-known model of intentional person inferences (in which "categorization" and "correction" are more efficient than the final correction stage; Gilbert, Pelham, & Krull, 1988; see also Gilbert, 1997).

Consistent with the model, participants under cognitive load who were asked to form an impression of the woman saw her as more anxious than those under no load did. More interestingly, those under load who were asked to form an impression of the situation saw it as more anxiety-provoking than those under no load did. That is, without the more deliberative correction stage, participants attributed more anxiety to whatever they had a question about: either the person or the situation.

What happens when you don't have a question in mind—when your inference is spontaneous? The answer seems to be that if you attach the inferred concept to anything, it will be linked to the most salient feature(s) in the situation.

There are several ways to define and assess links between actors and trait inferences, and not all of them produce the same results. Explicit memory links between trait inferences and actors seem to be relatively rare and to require particular conditions (see Uleman, Newman, & Moskowitz, 1996, on "manifest reference"). However, a relearning paradigm provides strong evidence of implicit memory links between actors and STIs. In relearning, participants memorize stimuli on one occasion and then memorize them again later. It takes less time or fewer trials to reach the same performance criterion on the second occasion, or the old material is learned more thoroughly in the same amount of time than new material on the second occasion. This savings is usually unrelated to whether participants recognize the old material on the second session. Thus savings on relearning provides a measure of implicit memory.

Carlston and Skowronski (1994; Carlston, Skowronski, & Sparks, 1995) have studied STI with a relearning paradigm. In a typical study, participants viewed a series of photos of people paired with self-descriptive statements that implied traits. (For example, "I hate animals. Today I was walking to the pool hall and I saw this puppy. So I kicked it out of my way" implies "cruel.") They were asked either to form impressions of the people or simply to "familiarize [yourself] with materials to be used later in the experiment." Then they attempted to learn photo–trait pairs on a later occasion. Some photos were paired with traits implied by the previous self-descriptive

behaviors, and some were not. The difference in memory for "old" and "new" pairs provided a measure of savings. Large savings effects were found in nine studies, and, remarkably, they did not differ by condition. Thus, mere familiarization led to (spontaneous) trait inferences as much as intentional-impression formation did.

In Study 4, Carlston et al. (1995) told participants that the descriptions were given by the people in the photos, but that they were about *other people*. To emphasize that these were not self-descriptions, the photos and descriptions had different genders. Some participants familiarized themselves with the materials (as in previous studies), whereas others formed intentional impressions of either the person in the photo or the person being described. Savings occurred under familiarization (where it revealed an erroneous implicit association between photo and trait), but not reliably under either impression formation condition. That is, the trait inference was reliably associated with the (salient) photo only in spontaneous impressions. This suggests that when people intentionally form impressions, potentially misleading associative links can be prevented or inhibited.

Skowronski, Carlston, Mae, and Crawford (1998) have dubbed this effect "spontaneous trait transference" (STT). In a series of four studies, they documented how robust it is. Study 1 used the relearning paradigm to show that it persists over a 2-day delay. (It also found some evidence of STT in the intentional-impression condition with no delay, but this disappeared after the 2-day delay.) Studies 2–4 used an explicit trait-rating task instead of relearning, after initial familiarization. In Study 2, 2 days after participants had simply familiarized themselves with the communicators' (in photos) descriptions of cross-gender acquaintances, they erroneously attributed the traits implied by those descriptions to the communicators. Study 3 showed that even when participants were explicitly told that the photos of the "communicators" and "their descriptions" were randomly paired, and that they should simply study them for a subsequent test of their memory for the pairings, their trait ratings of the photos 2 days later reflected traits implied by the descriptions. Study 4 demonstrated STT with videotaped interviews rather than printed stimuli. Interviewees described either themselves or others. Some participants intentionally formed trait impressions of those described; others familiarized themselves with the interview format; and still others judged whether the taped vignettes were staged or authentic. Trait ratings of interviewees 2 days later showed STT of equal magnitude for all goal conditions. And, replicating a finding from Study 2, explicit memory for whether the interview had been about self or other did not mediate STT.

These results suggest that STT is based on simple associations between activated trait concepts and communicators. It is reminiscent of the "innuendo" effect reported by Wegner, Wenzlaff, Kerker, and Beattie (1981). And it provides a sharp contrast with intentional-impression formation processes, in which intentions link trait concepts firmly to the intentional object of inquiry. Spontaneous impressions are implicitly associated with salient people, even if they are not the people the impression should be about.

A METAPHOR, NOT A MODEL

Table 7.1 summarizes the four differences described above, but omits the reasons for suggesting them and the reliability of that evidence. This evidence may suggest other differences to the reader (or may suggest that some suggestions should not be taken very seriously without further research). Because many of these ideas are speculative, a metaphorical summary is more appropriate than a more formal model. Here's mine.

Spontaneous-impression formation processes are part of an underground stream of unconscious thought—guided by long-established constructs and procedures, flowing in multiple unrelated directions, carrying prior inferences forward to color the current stream, but never circling back or flowing uphill to change the source. (New inferences supplant old ones, but are not integrated with them in complex ways.) They attach themselves promiscuously to any plausible target in their path. Intentional-impression formation processes are an above-ground aqueduct system—flexibly channeled to destinations consistent with current needs, protected from leaks and contaminants by inhibitory pro-

cesses, integrated with other complex processing systems, and accompanied by a record-keeping and control system for self-corrective feedback. The underground stream and the aqueduct system may interact, but in ways as yet unfathomed.

SOME RELATIONSHIPS WITH OTHER DUAL-PROCESS THEORIES

Dual-process theories often identify distinct kinds of processing, and then describe the unique instigators and consequences of each. Thus one often starts with a clear conception of the processes' characteristics and then investigates the conditions that give rise to them, as well as their unique consequences (e.g., Sloman, 1996). My approach has been different. I have begun with a dichotomous instigating condition—the presence or absence of intentions to form an impression—and asked whether there is any empirical evidence that different processes flow from each. Recent evidence suggests that they do. These differences, summarized in Table 7.1, have some interesting similarities to and differences from other dual-process formulations.

Greenwald and Banaji's (1995) distinction between implicit and explicit social cognitions rests on whether the person is aware of them and their influence on behavior. (This is a feature of the outcome, rather than an instigating condition or a feature of the process.) They make a strong case for using measures of attitudes, self-esteem, and stereotypes that do not depend on accurate introspective self-reports, because these often fail to reflect the effects of past experience that mediate valenced responses toward others (attitudes), toward the self (self-esteem), and toward members of social categories (stereotypes). By their broad criterion, a spontaneous inference is an implicit social cognition—that is, "the introspectively unidentified (or inaccurately identified) trace of past experience that mediates" responses (p. 5). As noted above, these responses include explicit recall of behaviors, lexical decisions, recognition RTs, savings in relearning, and explicit impressions (see Uleman, Newman, & Moskowitz, 1996, for more details). All of these are implicit measures, in that none requires awareness either of making an inference or of its effect on the response. In fact, participants usually deny that they have inferred anything, and these inferences interfere with some response tasks. So spontaneous impressions are usually implicit social cognitions. Thus the research on STIs extends the domain of responses that depend on implicit cognition beyond the highly valenced ones considered by Greenwald and Banaji, to include the more specific effects of activating particular constructs.

Epstein's experiential system (see Epstein & Pacini, Chapter 23, this volume) has some suggestive similarities to spontaneous inference processes, although it is described as noncognitive, and it attempts to account for a different and broader range of phenomena. Perhaps spontaneous inferences are one kind of input that goes primarily to the experiential system.

Trope's dual-process model of impression formation distinguishes between identification and inference processes (see Trope & Gaunt, Chapter 8, this volume). All of the relevant research has been done under intentional impression formation instructions, so possible roles for spontaneous inferences are as yet unexamined. However, two lines of evidence suggest that identification (at least) may occur spontaneously as well as intentionally. First, some kinds of prior information can affect STIs (point 3, Table 7.1). Thus, prior situational information that could disambiguate the identification of behavior may facilitate STIs, as it does intentional identification. Second, identification and STIs are relatively unaffected by concurrent cognitive load. The possibility of spontaneous identification remains to be tested directly. Spontaneous "inferences" (in Trope's more specific sense) are probably less likely than spontaneous identifications because intentional "inferences" require substantial cognitive capacity, and the discounting of trait causes may involve a more complex, coherent cognitive sequence than spontaneous processing can sustain. In addition, Trope's trait "inference" process produces a clear causal attribution to the actor, whereas STIs are merely associated with the actor. Their status as "real explanations" or "causes" is unclear, and they are probably best regarded as potential hypotheses, at least until a question is posed and an answer is sought intentionally.

Neither the heuristic–systematic distinction (Chen & Chaiken, Chapter 4, this vol-

ume) nor the central–peripheral distinction (Petty & Wegener, Chapter 3, this volume) seems to map very well onto the spontaneous–intentional dichotomy, because both describe intentional processes of attitude change. That is, both distinguish between ways of intentionally processing persuasive messages. And both have been studied almost exclusively within situations of intentional attitude change. Heuristic and peripheral processing seem to have more in common with spontaneous processing, because neither produces complex integration of all the relevant message content (point 3, Table 7.1). And systematic and central processing are clearly intentional. However, heuristic and peripheral processing can also be intentional, whereas spontaneous processing cannot, by definition.

It may be interesting to see whether spontaneous processing of persuasive messages, accompanied by heuristic cues, will favor the use of heuristic cues when heuristic cues (e.g., source expertise) and systematic cues (e.g., argument strength) are equated for ease of encoding. It seems more likely that attitudes will be determined by other features of the presentation. One possibility, given the associationistic nature of spontaneous processes (point 4, Table 7.1), is that attitudes will be determined by the relative frequency of positive and negative associations with the attitude object, regardless of whether the associations have heuristic or systematic value. Another possibility, given spontaneous inferences' failure to integrate subsequent information (point 3, Table 7.1) and the idea that new associations simply supplant old ones, is that attitudes will be determined by the last information presented (a recency effect), regardless of its heuristic or systematic relevance. Neither possibility accords heuristic cues any special role in spontaneously processing persuasive messages.

Mapping Sloman's (1996) "two systems of reasoning" onto the spontaneous–intentional dichotomy is also difficult, because Sloman's work is exclusively based on studies where reasoning, whether associative or rule-based, was intentional. People tried to solve problems, apply theories, or arrive at conclusions intentionally. Although his "associative system" seems to share some features with spontaneous inferences (e.g., both are more associative, and both may contribute more to intuition, fantasy, and creativity), his associative reasoning is intentional. Just because spontaneous inferences are associative, and associative reasoning can occur intentionally, spontaneous inferences need not be the same as intentional associative reasoning. For example, people are aware "of the result of the computation" (p. 6) in associative reasoning (although not of the process). This is usually not true of spontaneous inferences. Finally, unlike the case of spontaneously processing persuasive messages, it is difficult to imagine what it could mean to spontaneously reason or attempt to solve problems.

Jacoby, Kelley, and McElree (Chapter 19, this volume) argue persuasively that there are no "process-pure" tasks, and that all cognitive tasks are performed through some combination of controllable and uncontrollable processes. Their process dissociation procedures and models yield estimates of the relative effect of each in any task where these two operate independently. How can these models be applied to STIs? It is useful to distinguish between (1) making STIs in the first place, or encoding; and (2) STIs' effects on subsequent impression formation or other processes (i.e., those involving retrieval). Speed–accuracy tradeoff procedures should be useful for tracking the time courses and relative importance of controllable and uncontrollable processes in producing STIs under a variety of encoding conditions, such as variations in goals (Uleman & Moskowitz, 1994), in concurrent cognitive load (Uleman, Newman, & Winter, 1992), in prior trait priming (Newman & Uleman, 1990), and in the linguistic structure of the stimulus materials (the focus of most of the literature on text comprehension). There is evidence that people can gain control of STI encoding processes over the course of many trials with feedback, when STI interferes with the primary task (Uleman, Hon, et al., 1996). Encoding processes that are initially uncontrolled seem to come under control. Speed–accuracy tradeoff analyses over the course of multiple trials may provide insight into how this occurs.

The process dissociation procedures familiar to most social psychologists through Jacoby's false-fame effect (e.g., Jacoby, Kelley, Brown, & Jasechko, 1989) can be used to estimate the relative contribution of controllable and uncontrollable processes to STIs' effects on retrieval tasks, such as savings in relearning (e.g., Carlston stem completion (e.g., W Zingmark, 1992), or any both controlled retrieval st matic "habits" or familiari (e.g., Moskowitz & Romar ...uper et al., 1996).

For example, Skowronski et al. (1998) have shown that when participants "familiarize" themselves with pairs of photos and trait-implying descriptions, the resulting STIs affect subsequent trait ratings of the people in the photos 2 days later. This effect occurs even when it is clear to participants that those in the photos were describing someone else, and it does not depend on subsequent confusion about this issue. Thus one might set up "inclusion" versus "exclusion" trait-rating conditions, in which participants are invited to "use whatever comes to mind for your trait ratings, including the material you familiarized yourself with earlier" or to "be sure to avoid being influenced by the erroneous material you familiarized yourself with earlier," respectively. The relative effect of controlled retrieval processes could be varied by varying the delay between familiarization and ratings. The automatic effects of familiarity might be varied by manipulating relevant encoding conditions. Such a program of research could determine the relative importance of controllable and uncontrollable processes in both the encoding of STIs and their subsequent effects on a variety of impression formation tasks.

As I hope this section begins to indicate, one way to avoid the "pile of issues" Newell (1973) decried in the quotation that opens this chapter is to look for ways in which these dichotomies may duplicate, extend, cross-cut, or complement one another. The fact that these comparisons generate several clear suggestions for future research supports the heuristic value of "dual-process theories" after all.

ACKNOWLEDGMENT

Preparation of this chapter was supported by National Science Foundation Grant No. SBR-9319611. I would like to thank Frank Van Overwalle, Len Newman, Yaacov Trope, and Arnaldo Zelli for their thoughtful comments and suggestions on an earlier draft.

_ES

1. The clarity of this intuitive distinction between complex inferences and simple semantic priming and associations depends upon what models of inference processes, priming, and associations are adopted. Explicating and defending a model for inferences are well beyond the scope of this chapter, although I suspect it would resemble the recent proposals by Kunda and Thagard (1996), modified perhaps to handle the telling criticisms of Bodenhausen, Macrae, and Sherman (Chapter 13, this volume). Their models are clearly symbolic, in that the nodes symbolize something. If one adopts a mixed symbolic–connectionist model of information processing—a course supported by several compelling arguments (e.g., Marcus, 1997; Smolensky, 1988)—this distinction may become less clear. Nevertheless, it seems useful for present purposes.

REFERENCES

Bargh, J. A. (1994). The four horsemen of automaticity: Awareness, intention, efficiency, and control in social cognition. In R. S. Wyer, Jr., & T. K. Srull (Eds.), *Handbook of social cognition* (2nd ed.): *Vol. 1. Basic processes* (pp. 1–40). Hillsdale, NJ: Erlbaum.

Bargh, J. A., Chen, M., & Burrows, L. (1996). Automaticity of social behavior: Direct effects of trait construct and stereotype activation on action. *Journal of Personality and Social Psychology, 71,* 230–244.

Bowers, K. S., Regehr, G., Balthazard, C., & Parker, K. (1990). Intuition in the context of discovery. *Cognitive Psychology, 22,* 72–110.

Carlston, D. E., & Skowronski, J. J. (1994). Savings in the relearning of trait information as evidence for spontaneous inference generation. *Journal of Personality and Social Psychology, 66,* 840–856.

Carlston, D. E., Skowronski, J. J., & Sparks, C. (1995). Savings in relearning: II. On the formation of behavior-based trait associations and inferences. *Journal of Personality and Social Psychology, 69,* 420–436.

Dodge, K. A. (1993). Social-cognitive mechanisms in the development of conduct disorder and depression. *Annual Review of Psychology, 44,* 559–584.

Duff, K. J., & Newman, L. S. (1997). Individual differences in the spontaneous construal of behavior: Idiocentrism and the automatization of the trait inference process. *Social Cognition, 15,* 217–241.

Ericsson, K. A., & Simon, H. A. (1993). *Protocol analysis: Verbal reports as data* (rev. ed.). Cambridge, MA: MIT Press.

Gernsbacher, M. A. (1991). Cognitive processes and mechanisms in language comprehension: The structure building framework. In G. H. Bower (Ed.), *The psychology of learning and motivation* (Vol. 27, pp. 217–263). San Diego: Academic Press.

Gernsbacher, M. A., & Faust, M. E. (1991a). The mechanism of suppression: A component of general comprehension skill. *Journal of Experimental Psychology: Learning, Memory, and Cognition, 17,* 245–262.

Gernsbacher, M. A., & Faust, M. E. (1991b). The role of suppression in sentence comprehension. In G. B. Simpson (Ed.), *Understanding word and sentence* (pp. 97–128). Amsterdam: North-Holland.

Gernsbacher, M. A., Goldsmith, H. H., & Robertson, R. R. W. (1992). Do readers mentally represent characters' emotional states? *Cognition and Emotion, 6,* 89–111.

Gilbert, D. T. (1997). Ordinary personology. In D. T. Gilbert, S. T. Fiske, & G. Lindzey (Eds.), *Handbook of social psychology* (4th ed., Vol. II, pp. 89–150). New York: McGraw-Hill.

Gilbert, D. T., Pelham, B. W., & Krull, D. S. (1988). On cognitive busyness: When person perceivers meet persons perceived. *Journal of Personality and Social Psychology, 54,* 733–740.

Gollwitzer, P. M. (1990). Action phases and mind-sets. In E. T. Higgins & R. M. Sorrentino (Eds.), *Handbook of motivation and cognition* (Vol. 2, pp. 53–92). New York: Guilford Press.

Gollwitzer, P. M., & Moskowitz, G. B. (1996). Goal effects on action and cognition. In E. T. Higgins & A. W. Kruglanski (Eds.), *Social psychology: Handbook of basic principles* (pp. 361–399). New York: Guilford Press.

Graesser, A. C., Singer, M., & Trabasso, T. (1994). Constructing inferences during narrative text comprehension. *Psychological Review, 101,* 371–395.

Greenwald, A. G., & Banaji, M. R. (1995). Implicit social cognition: Attitudes, self-esteem, and stereotypes. *Psychological Review, 102,* 4–27.

Higgins, E. T. (1996). Knowledge activation: Accessibility, applicability, and salience. In E. T. Higgins & A. W. Kruglanski (Eds.), *Social psychology: Handbook of basic principles* (pp. 133–168). New York: Guilford Press.

Higgins, E. T., Rholes, W. S., & Jones, C. R. (1977). Category accessibility and impression formation. *Journal of Experimental Social Psychology, 13,* 141–154.

Jacoby, L. L. (1991). A process dissociation framework: Separating automatic from intentional uses of memory. *Journal of Memory and Language, 30,* 513–541.

Jacoby, L. L., Kelley, C. M., Brown, J., & Jasechko, J. (1989). Becoming famous overnight: Limits on the ability to avoid unconscious influences of the past. *Journal of Personality and Social Psychology, 56,* 326–338.

Kenny, D.A. (1994). *Interpersonal perception: A social relations analysis.* New York: Guilford Press.

Kintsch, W. (1988). The role of knowledge in discourse comprehension: A construction–integration model. *Psychological Review, 95,* 163–182.

Krull, D. S. (1993). Does the grist change the mill?: The effect of the perceiver's inferential goal on the process of social inference. *Personality and Social Psychology Bulletin, 19,* 340–348.

Kunda, Z., & Thagard, P. (1996). Forming impressions from stereotypes, traits, and behaviors: A parallel-constraint-satisfaction theory. *Psychological Review, 103,* 284–308.

Lea, R. B. (1995a). [Lexical decision evidence for spontaneous trait inference]. Unpublished raw data.

Lea, R. B. (1995b). On-line evidence for elaborative logical inferences in text. *Journal of Experimental Psychology: Learning, Memory and Cognition, 21,* 1469–1482.

Lupfer, M. B., Clark, L. F., Church, M., DePaola, S. J., & McDonald, C. D. (1995). *Do people make situational as well as trait inferences spontaneously?* Unpublished manuscript, University of Memphis.

Lupfer, M. B., Clark, L. F., & Hutcherson, H. W. (1990). Impact of context on spontaneous trait and situational attributions. *Journal of Personality and Social Psychology, 58,* 239–249.

Marcus, G. F. (in press). Rethinking eliminative connectionism. *Cognitive Psychology, 37.*

McKoon, G., & Ratcliff, R. (1986). Inferences about predictable events. *Journal of Experimental Psychology: Learning, Memory, and Cognition, 12,* 82–91.

McKoon, G., & Ratcliff, R. (1992). Inference during reading. *Psychological Review, 99,* 440–466.

Moskowitz, G. B. (1993). Individual differences in social categorization: The effects of personal need for structure on spontaneous trait inferences. *Journal of Personality and Social Psychology, 65,* 132–142.

Moskowitz, G. B., & Roman, R. J. (1992). Spontaneous trait inferences as self-generated primes: Implications for conscious social judgment. *Journal of Personality and Social Psychology, 62,* 728–738.

Newell, A. (1973). You can't play 20 Questions with nature and win. In W. G. Chase (Ed.), *Visual information processing* (pp. 283–308). New York: Academic Press.

Newman, L. S. (1993). How individualists interpret behavior: Idiocentrism and spontaneous trait inference. *Social Cognition, 11,* 243–269.

Newman, L. S., & Uleman, J. S. (1990). Assimilation and contrast effects in spontaneous trait inferences. *Personality and Social Psychology Bulletin, 16,* 224–240.

Nisbett, R. E., & Wilson, T. D. (1977). Telling more than we can know: Verbal reports on mental processes. *Psychological Review, 84,* 231–259.

Rabiner, D. L., Lenhart, L., & Lockman, J. E. (1990). Automatic versus reflective social problem solving in relation to children's sociometric status. *Developmental Psychology, 26,* 1010–1016.

Rhee, E., Uleman, J. S., Lee, H. K., & Roman, R. J. (1995). Spontaneous self-concepts and ethnic identities in individualistic and collectivistic cultures. *Journal of Personality and Social Psychology, 69,* 142–152.

Roese, N. J., & Olson, J. M. (1997). Counterfactual thinking: The intersection of affect and function. In M. P. Zanna (Ed.), *Advances in experimental social psychology* (Vol. 29, pp. 1–59). San Diego, CA: Academic Press.

Simpson, G. (1994). Context and the processing of ambiguous words. In M. A. Gernsbacher (Ed.), *Handbook of psycholinguistics* (pp. 359–374). San Diego, CA: Academic Press.

Skowronski, J. J., Carlston, D. E., Mae, L., & Crawford, M. T. (1998). Spontaneous trait transference: Communicators take on the qualities they describe in others. *Journal of Personality and Social Psychology, 74,* 837–848.

Sloman, S. A. (1996). The empirical case for two systems of reasoning. *Psychological Bulletin, 119,* 3–22.

Smith, E. R. (1994). Procedural knowledge and processing strategies in social cognition. In R. S. Wyer, Jr., & T. K. Srull (Eds.), *Handbook of social cognition* (2nd ed.) *Vol. 1. Basic processes* (pp. 99–152). Hillsdale, NJ: Erlbaum.

Smith, E. R., & Miller, F. D. (1978). Limits on perception of cognitive processes: A reply to Nisbett and Wilson. *Psychological Review, 85,* 355–362.

Smolensky, P. (1988). On the proper treatment of connectionism. *Behavioral and Brain Sciences, 11,* 1–23.

Stapel, D. A., Koomen, W., & van der Pligt, J. (1996). The referents of trait inferences: Impact of trait concepts versus actor–trait links on subsequent judgments. *Journal of Personality and Social Psychology, 70,* 437–450.

Swinney, D. A. (1979). Lexical access during sentence comprehension: (Re)consideration of context effects. *Journal of Verbal Learning and Verbal Behavior, 18,* 645–659.

Tipper, S. P. (1992). Selection for action: The role of inhibitory mechanism. *Current Directions in Psychological Science, 1,* 105–109.

Triandis, H. C., Bontempo, R., Villareal, M. J., Asai, M., & Lucca, N. (1988). Individualism and collectivism: Cross-cultural perspectives on self–ingroup relationships. *Journal of Personality and Social Psychology, 54,* 323–338.

Trope, Y., & Liberman, A. (1996). Social hypothesis testing: Cognitive and motivational mechanisms. In E. T. Higgins & A. W. Kruglanski (Eds.), *Social psychology: Handbook of basic principles* (pp. 239–270). New York: Guilford Press.

Uleman, J. S. (1996). When do unconscious goals cloud our minds? [a commentary on Martin & Tesser's target chapter, Ruminative thoughts]. In R. S. Wyer, Jr. (Ed.), *Advances in social cognition* (Vol. 9, pp. 165–176). Mahwah, NJ: Erlbaum.

Uleman, J. S., Hon, A., Roman, R., & Moskowitz, G. B. (1996). On-line evidence for spontaneous trait inferences at encoding. *Personality and Social Psychology Bulletin, 22,* 377–394.

Uleman, J. S., & Moskowitz, G. B. (1994). Unintended effects of goals on unintended inferences. *Journal of Personality and Social Psychology, 66,* 490–501.

Uleman, J. S., Newman, L. S., & Moskowitz, G. B. (1996). People as flexible interpreters: Evidence and issues from spontaneous trait inference. In M. P. Zanna (Ed.), *Advances in experimental social psychology* (Vol. 28, pp. 211–279). San Diego, CA: Academic Press.

Uleman, J. S., Newman, L., & Winter, L. (1992). Can personality traits be inferred automatically? Spontaneous inferences require cognitive capacity at encoding. *Consciousness and Cognition, 1,* 77–90.

Uleman, J. S., Winborne, W. C., Winter, L., & Shechter, D. (1986). Personality differences in spontaneous personality inferences at encoding. *Journal of Personality and Social Psychology, 51,* 396–403.

Wegner, D. M., & Wenzlaff, R. M. (1996). Mental control. In E. T. Higgins & A. W. Kruglanski (Eds.), *Social psychology: Handbook of basic principles* (pp. 466–492). New York: Guilford Press.

Wegner, D. M., Wenzlaff, R., Kerker, R. M., & Beattie, A. E. (1981). Incrimination through innuendo: Can media questions become public answers? *Journal of Personality and Social Psychology, 40,* 822–832.

Weiner, B. (1985). "Spontaneous" causal thinking. *Psychological Bulletin, 97,* 74–84.

Whitney, P., Waring, D. A., & Zingmark, B. (1992). Task effects on the spontaneous activation of trait concepts. *Social Cognition, 10,* 377–396.

Winter, L., & Uleman, J. S. (1984). When are social judgments made? Evidence for the spontaneousness of trait inferences. *Journal of Personality and Social Psychology, 47,* 237–252.

Zárate, M. A., & Uleman, J. S. (1994). *Lexical decision evidence that Anglos do, and Chicanos do not make spontaneous trait inferences.* Unpublished manuscript, University of Texas–El Paso.

Zelli, A., Cervone, D., & Huesmann, R. L. (1996). Behavioral experience and social inference: Individual differences in aggressive experience and spontaneous versus deliberate trait inference. *Social Cognition, 14,* 165–190.

Zelli, A., Huesmann, L. R., & Cervone, D. (1995). Social inference and individual differences in aggression: Evidence for spontaneous judgments of hostility. *Aggressive Behavior, 21,* 405–417.

8

A Dual-Process Model of Overconfident Attributional Inferences

YAACOV TROPE
RUTH GAUNT

The present chapter is concerned with the role of deliberate, resource-dependent processes and implicit, resource-independent processes in attributional judgments. We use the distinction between these two types of processes to examine how attribution of behavior to some focal factor is affected by the presence of other factors (called "contextual inducements") that might also produce the behavior. According to the "discounting principle" (Kelley, 1972), attribution of behavior to any given cause should be attenuated in the presence of other potential causes of behavior. However, a considerable amount of research has found that perceivers often violate this principle (see, e.g., Jones, 1979; Ross, 1977). For example, research on dispositional inferences has found that perceivers often attribute behavior to the corresponding disposition even in the presence of strong situational inducements to perform the behavior (see reviews by Gilbert & Malone, 1995; Jones, 1990; Trope & Higgins, 1993). As a result, perceivers often draw overconfident attributional inferences. The question we address, then, is this: What are the cognitive processes that underlie such overconfident attributional inferences?

On the basis of Trope's (1986) attribu-

tion model, it is proposed that contextual inducements affect attribution via two different processes. First, contextual inducements determine how behavioral input is identified. Here, context activates a behavior category or interpretive frame in terms of which the input is represented. Second, contextual inducements suggest an alternative explanation for the identified behavior, which in turn acts to attenuate attribution of behavior to the focal property. For example, seeing someone being teased or insulted may lead perceivers to identify the actor's response as angry, but may also attenuate perceivers' certainty that the angry response is attributable to the actor's dispositional aggressiveness.

We view the first process as an implicit process of assimilating behavioral input into a contextually activated category. This process presumably requires little conscious attention and few processing resources. The second process of using contextual inducements as an alternative explanation of the identified behavior presumably reflects a diagnostic strategy of evaluating an attributional hypothesis. Diagnostic evaluation is a deliberate and relatively effortful process. Under suboptimal processing conditions, perceivers are therefore likely to rely on a simpler heuristic method, called "pseudodiagnostic evaluation," which is relatively insensitive to contextual inducements.

According to this analysis, then, overconfident attributions result from context-produced misidentification of behavior and from failure to perform a diagnostic evaluation of a related attributional hypothesis. For example, perceivers will misattribute an actor's reaction to dispositional aggressiveness if situational provocation leads perceivers to misidentify the reaction as angry, without attenuating its diagnostic value regarding the actor's dispositional aggressiveness.

In the following sections, we develop the present dual-process model of context effects in attributional judgments, and we present research bearing on the model. First, we describe in more detail the use of contextual inducements for identifying behavior and for explaining it, and we apply the distinction to dispositional attributions. Next, we present recent research testing our assumption that the use of contextual inducements for behavior identification is an implicit, resource-independent process, whereas the use of contextual inducements for explaining behavior is a deliberate, resource-dependent process. We then relate the present dual-process model to Gilbert's three-stage correction model (Gilbert & Malone, 1995). According to Gilbert's model, situational inducements are used in a separate correction stage—one that follows categorization of behavior and attribution of the behavior to the correspondent disposition. This section presents new research designed to test these models. Finally, we presents a summary of general conclusions about the present dual-process approach to social attributions.

ATTRIBUTIONAL-HYPOTHESIS EVALUATION

Attributional judgment is viewed here as a product of a hypothesis evaluation process. An "attributional hypothesis" refers to a personal or situational property that serves to explain one's own or another person's behavior. In some cases, perceivers may test hypotheses about personality traits, skills, and attitudes; in other cases, they may test hypotheses about characteristics of tasks, role requirements,

and social norms. For example, one is likely to use a student's reaction to a class for evaluating hypotheses about the student's personality traits when one's goal is to form an impression of that student, but the same reaction will be used to test hypotheses about the quality of the class when one needs to decide whether to take that class (see Krull, 1993).

Attributional-hypothesis evaluation presumably proceeds in two stages. In the first stage, behavioral input is identified in terms of an attribution-relevant category (e.g., "John acted nervously"). In the second stage, an attributional hypothesis regarding the identified behavior is evaluated (e.g., "Is John a nervous person?"). Information about contextual inducements (e.g., "John is about to receive the results of an important health examination") may affect both stages. That is, this information may provide both (1) a frame for behavior identification and (2) an alternative explanation of the identified behavior. Both the use of contextual inducements as an identification frame and their use as an alternative explanation presumably depend on the same general knowledge activation and utilization factors, such as salience, accessibility, and applicability (see Higgins, 1996; Higgins & King, 1981; Ginossar & Trope, 1987). That is, contextual inducements are likely to be used to the extent that they are perceptually salient, cognitively accessible, and applicable to the behavior. We argue, however, that beyond these general factors the use of contextual inducements as an alternative explanation depends on perceivers' hypothesis evaluation strategy, whereas the use of contextual inducements as an identification frame is independent of the hypothesis evaluation strategy and instead depends on the nature of contextual and behavioral information. Below, we first describe the use of contextual inducements as an alternative explanation, and then we describe the use of contextual inducements as an identification frames.

The Use of Contextual Inducements as an Alternative Explanation

We distinguish between two hypothesis evaluation strategies, "diagnostic" and "pseudo-diagnostic." Diagnostic evaluation represents an orderly and systematic method for assessing the validity of an attributional hypothesis. It takes into account base rate probabilities of the attributional hypothesis, the reliability with which the immediate behavior was identified, and its diagnostic value regarding the attributional hypothesis. The diagnostic value of behavior is assessed on the basis of perceivers' models of the determinants of behavior. These models are causal theories that link behavior to personal and situational factors in specific domains, such as aggressiveness, friendliness, and helpfulness (see, e.g., Dweck, Hong, & Chiu, 1993; Reeder, 1993; Shoda & Mischel, 1993; Trope & Liberman, 1993). Behavior is diagnostic to the extent that it is probable, given that the hypothesized property is true, and improbable, given that the hypothesized property is false. Diagnostic evaluation thus takes into account not only the extent to which the hypothesized property is *sufficient* to produce the behavior, but also the extent to which the hypothesized property is *necessary* to produce the behavior.

Contextual inducements make the behavior seem probable, whether the attributional hypothesis is true or false. The hypothesized property remains sufficient to produce the behavior, but it becomes unnecessary. As a result, contextual inducements attenuate the diagnostic value of behavior regarding the attributional hypothesis. For example, the fact that a target person is waiting for an important job interview may render his or her nervous reaction nondiagnostic of the target's dispositional nervousness to the extent that a nervous reaction becomes probable, whether or not the target is dispositionally nervous.

Diagnostic evaluation is a systematic but effortful process. People may engage in diagnostic evaluation when alternative hypotheses are salient, when motivation to reach an accurate conclusion is high, and when attentional resources are unimpaired by competing tasks (see Ginossar & Trope, 1987; Harkness, Debono, & Borgida, 1985; Kruglanski & Mayseless, 1988; Trope, 1997). However, under less optimal conditions, perceivers are likely to resort to less systematic but simpler heuristic rules (see Chaiken & Stangor, 1987; Kahneman & Tversky, 1973; Sherman & Corty, 1984). A number of hypothesis evaluation heuristics have been proposed, including the representativeness heuristic (Kahneman & Tversky, 1973), hypothesis matching (Evans

& Lynch, 1973; Higgins & Bargh, 1987), and positive testing (Klayman & Ha, 1987). These heuristics focus on the consistency of the evidence with the current hypothesis and do not place enough emphasis on the consistency of the evidence with alternative hypotheses. The general tendency to use evidence according to its consistency with one's hypothesis has been called "pseudodiagnostic evaluation" (see Doherty, Mynatt, Tweeney, & Schiavo, 1979; Fischhoff & Beyth-Marom, 1983; Trope & Liberman, 1996). Diagnostic hypothesis evaluation requires one to generate alternative hypotheses and to assess both the sufficiency of the focal hypothesis (i.e., the probability of the evidence, given that the hypothesis is true) and its necessity (i.e., the probability of the evidence, given that the hypothesis is false). In contrast, pseudodiagnostic evaluation is primarily based on the sufficiency of the focal hypothesis. That is, the perceived validity of a hypothesis in light of identified evidence is mainly a function of the perceived likelihood of the evidence, given the hypothesis. Thus, pseudodiagnostic inferences are made as if evidence consistent with the hypothesis is inconsistent with its alternatives, and vice versa.

Pseudodiagnostic strategy embodies the speed–accuracy tradeoff of judgmental heuristics (Chaiken, Liberman, & Eagly, 1989; Fiske, 1993; Sherman & Corty, 1984). On the one hand, pseudodiagnostic evaluation is simple, fast, and relatively uneffortful. Inferences are primarily based on the relationship between the evidence and the hypothesis. In the extreme case, alternative hypotheses are not generated, and their evidential implications are not assessed. Pseudodiagnostic evaluation may thus require little mental effort. On the other hand, pseudodiagnostic evaluation may produce unwarranted judgments. Such evaluation assumes that base rates are uninformative (see Kahneman & Tversky, 1973), that the evidence is perfectly reliable (see Trope, 1978), and that what is consistent with the hypothesis is inconsistent with its alternatives. When these default assumptions apply, pseudodiagnostic evaluation will provide reasonable approximations to diagnostic judgments. However, when these assumptions do not apply, pseudodiagnostic and diagnostic inferences may be uncorrelated.

In the evaluation of attributional hypotheses, contextual inducements reduce the necessity of the focal property for producing the behavior. However, because pseudodiagnostic evaluation focuses on the sufficiency of the focal property rather than on its necessity, contextual inducements are likely to have little effect on judgment. For example, the fact that a target person is waiting for an important job interview is unlikely to attenuate attributions of the target's nervous reaction to his or her dispositional anxiety, because pseudodiagnostic evaluation gives little weight to the possibility that most persons (not only dispositionally nervous persons) would behave anxiously in this situation. The same holds true for pseudodiagnostic evaluation of situational hypotheses. For example, attribution of a target's anxious behavior to the nature of the job interview is unlikely to be attenuated by prior knowledge that the target is an anxious person. In general, pseudodiagnostic evaluation leads to overconfident attribution of behavior to any personal or situational property that perceivers test.

According to the present analysis, then, the use of contextual inducements as an alternative explanation requires diagnostic evaluation of attributional hypotheses. Because diagnostic evaluation is an effortful process, it is likely to depend on perceivers' motivation to draw accurate conclusions and processing resources. Perceivers are therefore more likely to make overconfident attributions under unfavorable processing conditions—that is, when their attentional resources are limited (see Gilbert & Krull, 1988; Gilbert & Osborne, 1989; Gilbert, Pelham, & Krull, 1988) or when their motivation to reach an accurate conclusion is low (see Tetlock, 1985). It should be pointed out, however, that diagnostic evaluation and pseudodiagnostic evaluation represent the endpoints of a continuum, rather than a dichotomy. Under highly favorable conditions, perceivers may engage in extensive generation, assessment, and integration of alternative explanations of the behavioral evidence. Under less favorable conditions, perceivers may generate fewer alternatives and process them less extensively. Motivational and cognitive resources thus determine the weight of contextual inducements in attributional judgment.

The Use of Contextual Inducements as an Identification Frame

Contextual inducements may determine not only how behavior is explained, but also how it is identified. Contextual inducements activate an associated behavior category that may be used to represent the behavioral input. In this way, contextual inducements may produce an assimilative bias in the identification of behavior. For example, knowing that a target person is waiting for an important job interview may activate the associated category of anxious behavior and lead to the identification of the target's behavior as anxious, even when it is not. Similarly, knowing that the target is an anxious person may bias perceivers toward identifying the target's behavior as anxious (see Trope, 1986; Trope & Alfieri, 1997; Trope, Cohen, & Maoz, 1988; Trope, Cohen, & Alfieri, 1991).

The behavioral input may constrain the assimilative effects of contextual inducements. However, a considerable amount of research has shown that when input is ambiguous—namely, associated with different categories—its representation will depend on the context in which it is processed (see Higgins & King, 1981; Higgins & Stangor, 1988; Wyer & Srull, 1981). Context presumably determines which one of the alternative categorizations of the input will be sufficiently activated to reach conscious awareness, thus resolving the ambiguity of behavioral input. Perceivers may be unaware of the alternative meanings of the behavioral input and the fact that contextual inducements have determined which one is selected. As a result, perceivers may treat their identifications as *independent* behavioral evidence rather than as *context-produced*. For example, in conflict situations, direct eye contact, close physical proximity, silence, and even a smile are likely to be perceived as hostile responses. Benevolent identifications of these same responses as sympathetic or cooperative are unlikely to be consciously considered. As a result, the identification of these responses as hostile is likely to be used as evidence for the target's dispositional hostility.

Context-produced behavior identifications may thus be misattributed to the hypothesized causal property and contribute to overconfidence in its validity. Diagnostic evaluation is unlikely to prevent this effect of assimilative behavior identification. Perceivers may attempt to avoid identification error. However, because disambiguation may be unconscious, perceivers may be unaware of alternative identifications of the behavioral input and may rely on their identifications as perceptual givens.

In sum, contextual inducements may affect attribution via two different processes. One process, called "diagnostic inference," uses contextual inducements as an alternative explanation for an identified behavior. Contextual inducements render the behavior probable, whether the attributional hypothesis is true or false, thus attenuating the diagnostic value of behavior. The other process, called "assimilative identification," uses contextual inducements as an identification frame. Here contextual inducements activate an associated behavior category into which the behavioral input is assimilated.

Diagnostic inference is presumably a controlled and resource-dependent process. It requires deliberate and critical evaluation of one's attributional hypothesis against alternative hypotheses. The process is optional, in that it depends on incentives for drawing accurate conclusions and on one's beliefs about the contextual inducements. In contrast, assimilative identification is an implicit process that requires few processing resources. Perceivers may be aware of contextual inducements, but not of the process whereby they disambiguate the behavioral input. The process is inflexible, in that it is independent of accuracy incentives and one's beliefs about the contextual inducements. Instead, assimilative identification depends on the ambiguity of the behavioral input and whether this input is preceded by information about contextual inducements.

The Combined Effect of Contextual Inducements as an Identification Frame and as an Alternative Explanation

According to the present dual-process analysis, contextual inducements produce two opposite effects on attributional judgments. As an alternative explanation, contextual inducements attenuate confidence in attributional hypotheses via diagnostic inference. In contrast, as an identification frame, contextual inducements enhance confidence in attributional hypotheses via assimilative identification. Thus, via diagnostic inference, contextual inducements act to produce discounting effects; via assimilative identification, contextual inducements act to reverse discounting effects. The observed effect of contextual inducements on attribution should be a result of these two mediating processes. Four types of

	Inference	
	Diagnostic	**Pseudodiagnostic**
Nonassimilative	**A** Discounting effect	**B** Null
Assimilative	**C** Null	**D** Discounting reversal

(Identification)

FIGURE 8.1. The combined effect of contextual inducements as an identification frame and as an alternative explanation.

observed effects are therefore possible (see Figure 8.1). One type of effect is a discounting effect (see Quadrant A). This effect requires perceivers to use contextual inducements for diagnostic inference, but not for behavior identification. Theoretically, these requirements are likely to be met when (1) the behavioral input is sufficiently unambiguous to prevent context from biasing identification of the input, and (2) perceivers possess sufficient cognitive and motivational resources to adjust the diagnostic value of behavior for the influence of contextual inducements.

Failure to meet either one of these two requirements should result in null effects of contextual inducements on attribution. One type of null effect results from failure to perform diagnostic inference (Quadrant B). In this case, perceivers presumably fail to use contextual inducements as an alternative explanation of behavior because of suboptimal processing conditions. The other type of null effect results from context-produced biases in behavior identification (Quadrant C). Here contextually produced behavior identifications are used as independent evidence for the hypothesized property, thus offsetting the use of contextual inducements as an alternative explanation. For example, knowing that a target person is responding to an anxiety-provoking situation is unlikely to attenuate attributions of dispositional anxiety to that person if this situation leads perceivers to identify the target's response as anxious, when it is in fact not anxious.

Finally, the fourth type of effect that contextual inducements may produce on attributional judgment is an extreme form of discounting failure—namely, discounting reversal (see Quadrant D). Here, the presence of contextual inducements increases rather than decreases confidence in one's attributional hypotheses. Reverse discounting effects presumably occur when perceivers use contextual inducements to identify behavior, but not to adjust the diagnostic value of the identified behavior. Context is used here as an identification frame, but not as an alternative explanation of the identified behavior. For example, the fact that a target person responds to an anxiety-provoking situation will enhance attribution of dispositional anxiety to the target if (1) the situation leads perceivers to misidentify the target's response as anxious, and (2) the situation is ignored as an alternative explanation of the anxious response.

Summary

According to the present dual-process analysis, discounting failures result from identification errors and inferential errors. Identification errors lead perceivers to misidentify behavior as consistent with the focal hypothesis, whereas inferential errors lead perceivers to give little weight to the consistency of the behavior with alternative hypotheses. Both types of errors contribute to overconfident attributions. Inferential errors contribute to overconfidence because perceivers underweight the influence of contextual inducements on the actor's behavior. Identification errors contribute to overconfidence because perceivers underweight the influence of contextual inducements on their own representation of the actor's behavior. Inferential errors result from failure to engage in deliberate and effortful testing of diagnostic attributions; they should therefore depend on perceivers' motivational and attentional resources. Identification errors result from implicit assimilative encoding of the behavioral input; they should therefore depend on ambiguity of the behavior and on whether its processing is preceded by processing of contextual information.

RESEARCH ON DETERMINANTS OF OVERCONFIDENT ATTRIBUTIONS

We now turn to research bearing on the predictions of the present dual-process analysis (see Figure 8.1). This research has been concerned with discounting effects of situational inducements on attribution of behavior to personal dispositions, such as attitudes and personality traits. A general finding in this area is that perceivers often show what has been termed "correspondence bias"—that is, a tendency to overattribute behavior to personality dispositions (see reviews by Gilbert & Malone, 1995; Jones, 1979, 1990; Trope & Higgins, 1993). From the present perspective, this bias is a manifestation of overconfidence in an attributional hypothesis, the hypothesis in this case being a behavior-correspondent disposition. Below, we first briefly summarize research that relates overconfident dispositional attributions either to the use of situational inducements as a behavior identification frame or to the use of situational inducements as an alternative explanation. We then describe more recent research that relates overconfident dispositional attributions to both types of processes.

Determinants of the Use of Situational Inducements as an Alternative Explanation

A number of attribution theorists have viewed low perceptual salience of situational inducements as a major cause of dispositional bias and actor–observer differences (Heider, 1958; Jones & Nisbett, 1971). Perceivers presumably focus on others' behavior because it is seen as figure against the situational background. A considerable amount of research has supported this proposal (see, e.g., Taylor & Fiske, 1975). From the present hypothesis evaluation perspective, perceptual salience of the situation increases diagnostic inference, because it alerts perceivers to an alternative to their dispositional hypothesis—namely, the possibility that the behavior will occur without the target's necessarily possessing the corresponding disposition.

A number of studies have investigated how cognitive and motivational resources influence dispositional attributions. These studies manipulated situational constraints on the actor and assessed perceivers' attributions of a target person's unambiguous behavior to his or her attitudes, traits, or abilities. From the present perspective, the manipulation of cognitive and motivational resources determines whether dispositional inferences will be adjusted for the influence of the situation, as required by diagnostic hypothesis evaluation. That is, because this research used unambiguous behavior, this research compared Quadrant A of Figure 8.1 (where discounting effects should be observed) and Quadrant B (where null effects should be observed).

Gilbert and his colleagues (see Gilbert & Krull, 1988; Gilbert et al., 1988) studied the effect of cognitive resources by comparing a condition where perceivers were free to devote their full attention to the inference problem (no-load condition) and a condition where participants were distracted by a secondary task, such as keeping in memory an eight-digit number (load condition). Perceivers saw an interviewee responding nervously to questions that were either anxiety-provoking or neutral. These researchers found that anxiety-provoking questions produced discounting effects—that is, these questions attenuated attributions of targets' nervous reactions to their dispositional nervousness—in the no-load condition, but not in the load condition.

Tetlock (1985) investigated the impact of making perceivers accountable for their judgments on discounting effects of situational inducements. This research concerned the role of the motivation to make accurate attributions. As expected, Tetlock found that accountability attenuated perceivers' tendency to infer a writer's attitude from his or her essay. Accountable perceivers showed greater sensitivity to situational constraints on a writer's behavior—specifically, whether or not the writer had a choice of what position to advocate. Together, these findings are consistent with the assumption that suboptimal cognitive and motivational resources lead perceivers to evaluate dispositional hypotheses pseudodiagnostically rather than diagnostically, which in turn results in failure to use situational inducements as an alternative explanation of the target's behavior (see Quadrant B of Figure 8.1).

Determinants of the Use of Situational Inducements as an Identification Frame

Ambiguity of Behavior and Order of Presentation

Research on the use of situational inducements as a behavior identification frame has examined how ambiguity of behavior and the order of behavioral and situational information influence discounting effects of situational inducements (for a review, see Trope & Liberman, 1993). Theoretically, situational information is more likely to produce assimilative identification when behavior is ambiguous and preceded by situational information than when behavior is unambiguous or followed by situational information. Because there was no distraction or time pressure in this research, participants could draw diagnostic inferences. That is, this research compared Quadrants A and C in Figure 8.1. For example, in a study by Trope et al. (1991), participants heard an evaluator present an ambiguous or an unambiguously positive evaluation of another person, under demands to present either a positive or a negative evaluation. Participants then judged both the favorability of the evaluation (behavior identification) and the evaluator's true attitude toward the evaluatee (dispositional judgment).

The discounting effects of situational demands on attitude attributions were consistent with Figure 8.1's predictions. Specifically, situational demands to present a positive evaluation attenuated attribution of a positive attitude to the evaluator when the evaluation was unambiguous or followed by situational demands (Quadrant A), but not when the evaluation was ambiguous and preceded by situational demands (Quadrant C). A mediation analysis of attitude attributions, with perceived favorability of the evaluation as a mediator, tested the present dual-process analysis of these attitude attributions. This analysis decomposed the overall effect of situational demands on attitude attribution into an indirect effect, via assimilative identification of the evaluation, and a direct effect, reflecting diagnostic inference. This analysis showed that the ambiguity of the evaluation and the order of presentation of situational and behavioral information affected the use of situational demands in assimilative identification, but did not affect the use of situational demands in diagnostic inference.

More specifically, when the evaluation was unambiguous or followed by situational demands, the latter affected attitude attributions via diagnostic inference, but not via assimilative identification. Here perceivers apparently used situational information as an alternative explanation of the identified behavior, but not as a behavior identification frame. In contrast, when behavior was ambiguous and preceded by situational demands, the latter affected attitude attributions both via assimilative identification and via diagnostic inference. In this condition, perceivers used situational demands both as an identification frame and as an alternative explanation. Because these two uses of situational demands produce opposite effects on dispositional

judgment, they canceled each other out, as evidenced by the null effect of situational demands on attribution of the ambiguous evaluation. Consistent with the present analysis, then, behavior ambiguity and order of presentation determined the use of situational inducements for behavior identification, but not for diagnostic inference.

Awareness of the Alternative
Meanings of Behavior

How does ambiguity facilitate assimilative identification? We assume that ambiguity allows perceivers to identify the behavior by using a situationally activated category, without being aware of alternative meanings of the behavior. This implies that activation of the alternative meanings of an ambiguous behavior should reduce assimilative identification.

Trope and Sikron (1992) tested this hypothesis using Trope el al.'s (1991) attitude attribution paradigm, in which participants hear an evaluator present an evaluation of another person. The alternative meanings of behavior were activated in two ways. The first method was to prime both the positive and negative meanings of the ambiguous evaluation (e.g., superficial and efficient) before participants heard the evaluation, as part of a purportedly unrelated experiment. The second method used mixed evaluations. Specifically, whereas the ambiguous evaluation consisted of statements that each had both a positive and a negative meaning, the mixed evaluation consisted of some statements that had a positive meaning and others that had a negative meaning.

Priming produced the predicted effects, both on behavior identification and on dispositional inferences. Specifically, when the alternative meanings of the ambiguous evaluation were primed, situational inducements no longer affected perception of the ambiguous evaluation, but continued to be used in adjusting inferences regarding the evaluator's attitude. That is, priming of alternatives led subjects to treat ambiguous evaluations as unambiguous, which resulted in strong discounting effects of situational inducements on attitude attributions (see Quadrant A). Mixed evaluations yielded similar results: Situational inducements produced weak assimilative effects on identification of the content of the evaluation and strong discounting effects on attitude attributions.

In sum, this research suggests that situational inducements affects dispositional attribution via assimilative identification when perceivers are unaware of any alternative meaning of the behavior. Under these circumstances, context-produced identification is used as evidence for the target's dispositions. However, when an alternative meaning of a behavior is strongly activated, situational inducements are unlikely to affect identification, and their effect on dispositional attributions will reflect only their use as an alternative explanation of the behavior.

The Combined Effect of the Two Types of Determinants

The research reviewed above manipulated either determinants of the use of situational inducements as an alternative explanation (e.g., Gilbert et al., 1988) or determinants of the use of situational inducements as an identification frame (e.g., Trope et al., 1991). In terms of Figure 8.1, the former studies compared Quadrants A and B, whereas the latter studies compared Quadrants A and C. Recently, Trope and Alfieri (1997) conducted two studies that compared all four quadrants. One study focused on the effortfulness of using situational inducements for identification and for diagnostic inference; the other focused on the flexibility of theses two uses of situational inducements.

Effortfulness

Trope and Alfieri's first study varied both behavior ambiguity (and thus the use of situational inducements as an identification frame) and cognitive load (and thus the use of situational inducements as an alternative explanation). Subjects heard an evaluator describing another person, John, to a boss who either liked or disliked John. The boss' opinion about John created a situational demand on the evaluator to present a positive or negative evaluation of John. The evaluation was either ambiguous or unambiguous, and the information was presented under cognitive load (keeping in memory an eight-digit number) or

no cognitive load. Participants judged the favorability of the evaluation (behavior identification) and the evaluator's true attitude toward John (attitude attribution).

A mediation analysis of the attitude attributions was carried out, using behavior identifications as a mediator (see Figure 8.2). This analysis decomposed the effect of situational demands on attitude attribution into an indirect effect, via assimilative identification of the evaluation, and a direct effect, via diagnostic inference. As expected, the indirect effect of situational demands via assimilative identification increased with behavioral ambiguity. Moreover, this effect was independent of cognitive load; that is, situational demands affected behavior identification even when subjects were under cognitive load. In contrast, the direct effect of situational demands on attitude attribution via diagnostic inference depended on cognitive load and was independent of behavioral ambiguity. Specifically, the direct effect was significant under no load and negligible under load. Thus, ambiguity determined whether situational demands were used to identify the content of the evaluation, whereas cognitive load determined whether demands were used as an alternative explanation of the evaluation.

Reflecting these results, the overall effects of situational demands on attitude attribution were consistent with Figure 8.1. First, situational demands produced a discounting effect only when subjects were under no load and behavior was unambiguous (Quadrant A). In this condition, subjects used the situation as an alternative explanation but not as an identification frame. They committed neither an identification error nor an inferential error. Second, situational demands failed to produce discounting effects when either subjects were under load or the behavior was ambiguous (Quadrants B and C). Specifically, when subjects were under cognitive load, discounting failure was due to an inferential error—namely, failure to use the situation as an alternative explanation (Quadrant B). When the behavior was ambiguous, discounting failure was due to an identification error—namely, the use of the situation as an identification frame (Quadrant C). Finally, situational demands produced reverse discounting effects, enhancing rather than attenuating attitude attributions, when subjects were under

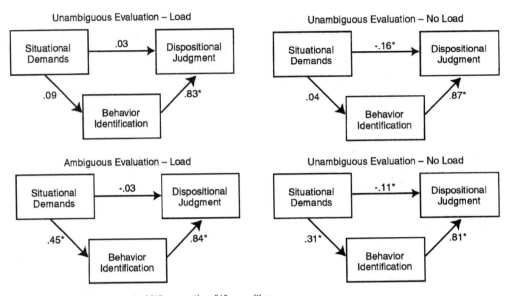

FIGURE 8.2. Direct and indirect effects of situational demands on dispositional judgment as a function of behavior ambiguity and cognitive load. *$\beta \neq 0$, $p < .05$. From Trope and Alfieri (1997). Copyright 1997 by the American Psychological Association. Reprinted by permission.

load and the behavior was ambiguous (Quadrant D). Here participants used the situation as an identification frame and did not use it as an alternative explanation. These participants committed both an identification error and an inferential error.

This study thus obtained all three possible effects of situational inducements—discounting effects, null effects, and reverse discounting effects—in accordance with the predictions presented in Figure 8.1. This required taking into account factors that determined both the use of the situation as an identification frame and its use as an alternative interpretation of the identified behavior. Because past research is focused on one set of factors, it can account for some but not all types of effects of situational inducements on dispositional attribution. For example, cognitive and motivational resources may enable perceivers to use the situation as an alternative explanation, but these resources may not prevent the more implicit use of the situation as an identification frame. As a result, when behavior is unambiguous, ample cognitive and motivational resources may eliminate overconfident dispositional attributions (Quadrant A), as Gilbert and his colleagues

have shown. However, when behavior is ambiguous, assimilative identification may produce overconfident dispositional attributions, regardless of cognitive and motivational resources (Quadrant C).

The Reversibility of Situational Effects

Suppose perceivers initially think that an evaluator is expected to present a positive evaluation, but then learn that the evaluator is unaware of these demands. The question is whether perceivers with ample cognitive and motivational resources can undo the judgmental effects of their invalid assumptions about the situation. From the present dual-processing viewpoint, the use of the situation as an identification frame and as an alternative explanation should differ in this respect. Specifically, the use of the situation as an alternative explanation is presumably a deliberate process and should therefore be reversible. The use of the situation as an identification frame, on the other hand, is presumably a largely implicit process and hence should be irreversible. Perceivers may see their initial behavior identifications as perceptual givens rather than as context-derived, and may therefore fail to change them when the original situational information is invalidated.

Trope and Alfieri's (1997) second experiment tested this analysis. Subjects heard an evaluator describing another person, John, to a supervisor who either liked or disliked John. The description strongly implied, but did not actually state, that the evaluator knew the supervisor's opinion about John and thus was under demand to present a positive or negative evaluation. Before making their judgments, some of the subjects were told that this assumption was valid (validation condition), whereas others were told that this assumption was invalid—that the evaluator was actually unaware of the supervisor's opinions about John (invalidation condition). As before, the evaluation was either unambiguously positive or ambiguous, and subjects judged the favorability of the evaluation (behavior identification) and the evaluator's true attitude toward John (attitude attribution).

Mediation analysis decomposed the observed effect of situational demands on attitude attribution into an indirect effect via identification of the evaluation, reflecting the use of the situation as an identification frame, and a direct effect, reflecting the use of the situation as an alternative explanation (see Figure 8.3). This analysis yielded two main results. First, the indirect effect of situational demands via behavior identification depended on the ambiguity of the behavior, not on the validity of situational demands. That is, situational demands continued to affect identification of the ambiguous evaluation even when the demands were invalidated. Second, the direct effect of situational demands on attitude attributions (reflecting the use of the situation as an alternative explanation) depended on the validity of situational demands, not on ambiguity of the behavior. The direct effect was significant when situational demands were validated, but it was negligible when these demands were invalidated.

The overall effects of situational demands on attitude attribution reflected these findings. First, when behavior was unambiguous and the demands were validated, a discounting effect was obtained. This reflected the fact that in this condition situational demands were used only as an alternative explanation of the evaluation, thus discounting at-

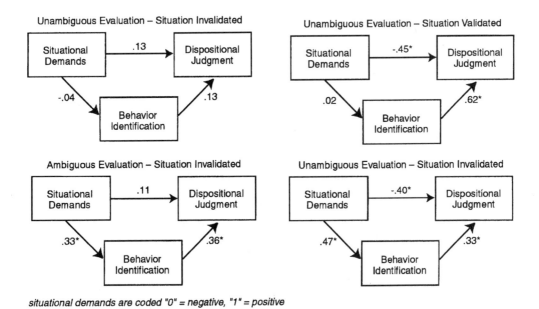

situational demands are coded "0" = negative, "1" = positive

FIGURE 8.3. Direct and indirect effects of situational demands on dispositional judgment as a function of behavior ambiguity and situational validation. *$\beta \neq 0$, $p < .05$. From Trope and Alfieri (1997). Copyright 1997 by the American Psychological Association. Reprinted by permission.

titude attributions. Second, the overall effect was nullified when either the behavior was ambiguous or situational demands were invalidated. Specifically, when behavior was ambiguous, situational demands produced a null effect because situational demands produced two opposite effects on attributions—one reflecting the use of situational demands as an identification frame, and the other reflecting the use of situational demands as an alternative explanation of the evaluation. When situational demands were invalidated, the null effect simply reflected the fact that participants undid their initial use of the situation as an alternative explanation of the evaluation. Finally, situational demands produced a reverse discounting effect on attitude attribution when the behavior was ambiguous and the demands were invalidated. Here participants undid their initial use of situational demands as an alternative explanation, but not the biasing influence of these demands on behavior identification.

The results of this study are consistent with the assumption that the use of the situation to identify behavior is less reversible than the use of the situation to draw inferences regarding the target's dispositions. Perceiver who learn that their assumptions about the situation are false can reverse their use of the situation as an alternative explanation of behavior, but not their use of the situation as a frame for identifying the meaning of the behavior.

Conclusions

Together, the results of the studies by Trope and Alfieri (1997) support the present distinction between the use of situational inducements as an identification frame and as an alternative explanation of behavior. The use of situational inducements as an alternative explanation depends on attentional resources and the validity of information about the situation. Thus, this use of situational inducements seems a deliberate and effortful process—a process that presumably requires diagnostic assessment of a dispositional hypothesis against situational alternatives. In contrast, the use of the situation as an identification frame is independent of attentional resources and the validity of the information

about the situation. Instead, this use of the situation depends on the ambiguity of the behavior, awareness of the alternative meanings of the ambiguous behavior, and the order in which situational and behavioral information is presented. Thus, the use of situational inducements for behavior identification seems to be an unintentional and uneffortful process of representing behavioral input in terms of the situationally activated category.

THE USE OF SITUATIONAL INFORMATION: CORRECTION OR INTEGRATION?

In this section, we relate the present dual-process model to Gilbert's three-stage model, wherein perceivers initially make a dispositional attribution and then use situational inducements to correct this attribution. We then describe recent research designed to subject these models to empirical test.

Gilbert has suggested that attributional inferences proceed in three stages (see Gilbert et al., 1988; Gilbert, 1989, 1995). In the first, called "categorization," perceivers identify what the target does; in the second, called "characterization," they infer that the target possesses the corresponding disposition; and in the third, called "correction," they correct this inference for situational inducements. The first two stages presumably require few processing resources, whereas the third is effortful. Thus, Gilbert's three-stage model assumes that situational information is used in a separate correction stage—one that depends on cognitive resources, and that comes after identifying behavior and inferring that the target possesses the behavior-correspondent disposition.

The present dual-process model and Gilbert's model agree in distinguishing between categorizing or identifying behavior and drawing inferences regarding its cause. The models also agree that discounting effects are resource-dependent. However, the models differ in two respects. First, whereas Gilbert's model focuses on the use of the contextual inducements in explaining behavior, the present model emphasizes that under specifiable conditions contextual inducements are used in the earlier stage of categorizing or identifying behavior (see Trope, 1986; Trope et al., 1988,

1991). Furthermore, the present model emphasizes that the use of contextual inducements for behavior identification, unlike its use for explanation, is resource-independent (see Trope & Alfieri, 1997).

Second, the models make different assumptions regarding the use of situational inducements in explaining behavior—namely, the inferential processes following behavior identification. This section discusses these assumptions and describes new research designed to test the two models.

At What Stage Are Situational Inducements Utilized?

Gilbert proposes a "correction model" for the use of situational inducements. That is, perceivers first attribute behavior to the corresponding personal disposition, and only then use situational inducements to correct this attribution. Unlike the initial dispositional attribution, the correction for situational inducements is presumably effortful. According to Gilbert, cognitive load therefore eliminates the correction stage, but not the preceding dispositional-attribution stage.

According to the present model, the use of situational inducements is an integral part of diagnostic evaluation of a dispositional hypothesis, rather than a separate correction process that follows dispositional attribution of behavior. Such evaluations integrate information about the target's immediate behavior with information about situational inducements and prior information about the target. The integration of these sources of information does not necessarily follow a fixed temporal sequence (see Trope, 1986). The relative weight of situational information may be low, but this does not necessarily mean that situational information is processed only after a dispositional attribution of behavior is made. In this "integration model," cognitive load (as well as a variety of other factors) may diminish the weight of situational information, rather than eliminate a separate situational correction stage.

Thus, although the correction and integration models make different assumptions regarding underlying process, they make similar predictions regarding the effect of cognitive load on the use of situational information in dispositional judgment. The question, then,

is how the two models can be empirically distinguished. One possibility has to do with the role of general utilization knowledge factors—namely, the salience, accessibility, and applicability of situational information. Consider, for example, the role of salience of situational inducements. Physical properties of situational information (loudness, brightness, movement, contrast, etc.) may render this same information more or less perceptually salient (see Taylor & Fiske, 1975). Gilbert's correction model assumes that situational inducements are considered at the final correction stage. In this model, then, salience of situational inducements cannot influence judgment unless perceivers perform the correction stage. If, as Gilbert assumes, cognitive load eliminates this stage, then perceptual salience of situational inducements cannot affect the use of these inducements by cognitively loaded perceivers. In short, under cognitive load situational discounting effects should be eliminated, regardless of the perceptual salience of situational inducements.

The present integration model makes different predictions regarding the effect of perceptual salience as a function of cognitive load. In this model, load impairs perceivers' ability to fully integrate alternative informational factors into judgment. The perceptual salience of an informational factor, whether dispositional or situational, is therefore likely to be a strong determinant of its weight in judgment. This model predicts, then, that perceptually salient situational inducements should produce strong discounting effects even when perceivers are under load. Thus, whereas Gilbert's correction model predicts that the influence of perceptual salience of situational inducements should be eliminated or at least drastically reduced under cognitive load, the present integration model predicts that the influence of perceptual salience should be no smaller or even greater under cognitive load than under no cognitive load.

The same logic applies to the effect of other determinants of knowledge utilization—namely, the accessibility and applicability of information (see Higgins, 1996; Ginossar & Trope, 1987). For example, Ginossar and Trope found that base rates are likely to be utilized (1) when base rate information is perceptually salient, (2) when the base rate rule is made cognitively accessible by initial priming, and (3) when the perceived applicability of the base rate rule is enhanced by creating a match between the rule and properties of the immediate inference problem. In an analogous manner, situational information may become momentarily more accessible as a result of priming situational causes prior to the current inference task. Furthermore, situational inducement may seem more applicable to the current inference task to the extent that they are specifically relevant to the target person under consideration.

According to Gilbert's correction model, accessibility and applicability of situational information cannot affect the utilization of this information unless perceivers reach the situational correction stage. Assuming that cognitive load prevents them from reaching this stage, it follows that under load situational information will fail to produce discounting effects, regardless of its accessibility and applicability. In contrast, the present integration model predicts that accessibility and applicability of situational information should increase discounting effects to the same or even to a greater extent when perceivers are under cognitive load than when they are under no cognitive load.

The Role of Salience, Accessibility, and Applicability of Situational Information: An Empirical Test

We conducted a series of three studies to investigate the joint influence of cognitive load and situational activation factors (salience, accessibility, and applicability) on the utilization of situational information in dispositional inferences (Trope & Gaunt, 1998). The results of these studies are described below.

Perceptual Salience of Situational Information

Using an attitude attribution paradigm, the first study varied situational inducements, salience of situational inducements, and cognitive load. Participants read an essay favoring the legalization of marijuana, allegedly written by another student under free-choice or no-choice conditions. In the control, low-situational-salience condition, participants read the choice or no-choice instructions to the essay writer in a booklet. This procedure

was similar to that used in most attitude attribution studies (see reviews by Gilbert & Malone, 1995; Jones, 1990; Trope & Higgins, 1993). In the high-situational-salience condition, participants heard an audio recording of the same instructions. The information was presented under cognitive load (memorizing an eight-digit number) or no cognitive load. The main dependent variable was participants' ratings of the essay writer's true attitude regarding legalization of marijuana.

The results of the low-situational-salience condition replicated Gilbert's findings. Attitude attributions showed a significant situational discounting effect on attitude attribution in the no-load condition, but no discounting effect in the load condition. Consistent with Gilbert's findings, participants remembered the content of the instructions, but the manipulation of cognitive load was sufficiently effective to eliminate any discounting effects in the low-situational-salience condition. A different pattern of results was obtained, however, in the high-situational-salience condition. Here, inconsistent with Gilbert's correction model's predictions, cognitive load did not eliminate situational discounting effects. On the contrary, attitude attributions under load showed a strong and significant situational discounting effect, similar in magnitude to the discounting effect obtained for attitude attributions under no load. Thus, as predicted by the present integration model, cognitive load increased rather than decreased the influence of situational salience on discounting effects.

Accessibility of Situational Information

The second study examined the role of accessibility of situational information, using the same attitude attribution paradigm that was used in the study of perceptual salience study. Accessibility was manipulated by priming situational explanations of behavior before the attitude attribution task. Specifically, as part of a supposedly unrelated experiment, participants read and answered questions concerning a set of four proverbs. In the situational-priming condition, the proverbs concerned influences of situational forces on people's behavior (e.g., "When in Rome, do as the

Romans do"). In the neutral-priming condition, the proverbs were unrelated to situational influences on behavior (e.g., "When life gives you lemons make lemonade"). Participants then read an essay favoring the legalization of marijuana, allegedly written by a student under choice or no-choice conditions. The information was presented either under cognitive load or no cognitive load, as in the study of perceptual salience.

The results of this study were analogous to those obtained in our earlier study. Following neutral priming, situational inducements produced a discounting effect on attitude attribution in the no-load condition, but not in the load condition. Like the earlier study, these results replicated earlier findings by Gilbert regarding the effect of cognitive load under neutral conditions. However, following situational priming, attitude attribution showed strong and significant discounting effects in both the load and no-load conditions. Again, these results are consistent with the integration model, but not with the correction model. As predicted by the integration model, the influence of situational accessibility on discounting effects was greater rather than smaller under cognitive load than under no cognitive load.

Perceived Applicability of Situational Information

In the third study, participants read about a teaching assistant who, under situational pressure, gave low grades in a statistics exam. The applicability of the situational pressure varied according to conditions. In high-applicability condition, the situational pressure was specifically applicable to the teaching assistant and statistics exam under consideration. Specifically, participants were told that the professor instructed the teaching assistant to use strict criteria in grading this particular exam. In the low-applicability condition, participants were informed about university-wide guidelines encouraging the use of strict grading criteria. The information was presented either under cognitive load (memorizing an eight-digit number) or no cognitive load. The primary dependent variable was participants' ratings of the teaching assistant as dispositionally strict or lenient.

The findings of this third study were also quite clear. When applicability was low, situational pressure to use strict grading criteria produced discounting effects on attribution of dispositional strictness by participants who were under no load, but not by participants who were not under load. However, when applicability was high, situational pressures produced significant and strong discounting effects both under load and under no load. Again supporting the integration model, the results of this study show, then, that cognitive load does not eliminate and actually increases the effect of situational applicability on the use of situational information.

Conclusions

Together, the results of the three studies seem to have clear theoretical implications regarding the correction and integration models. The correction model assumes that situational inducements are used if and only if inferences proceed to a correction stage following a dispositional attribution of behavior. If cognitive load prevents perceivers from reaching this stage, as Gilbert assumes, then under load situational information should not affect attributional judgment, regardless of the properties of this information—namely, its perceptual salience, accessibility, and applicability. Our findings have disconfirmed this prediction, showing that when situational information is salient, accessible, or applicable, it produces strong discounting effects even when perceivers are under cognitive load. In fact, the effect of these properties of situational information on dispositional attribution is more pronounced when perceivers are under load than when they are under no load.

The present findings are thus consistent with an integration model of dispositional attribution. This model assumes that situational information is integrated with other information sources to form a dispositional judgment. The integration of these information sources does not necessarily follow a fixed temporal sequence. Cognitive load may impair perceivers' ability to fully integrate the various information sources. Therefore, under load the weight of any factor, whether situational or dispositional, is likely to be highly dependent on its activation level. Because the activation level of situational information is often low, cognitive load is likely to eliminate the use of this information, as Gilbert's and our own studies show. However, when situational information is highly salient, accessible, and applicable, it is likely to have a relatively strong impact on dispositional attributions even under cognitive load, as our studies show.

SUMMARY AND GENERAL CONCLUSIONS

This chapter has presented a dual-process model of the use of contextual inducements in attributional judgment. According to this model, contextual inducements are initially used as a frame for behavior identification and then as an alternative explanation for the identified behavior. As an identification frame, contextual inducements influence the representation of behavior through an assimilation process. This is presumably an implicit and uneffortful process, and therefore irreversible and independent of perceivers' cognitive and motivational resources. Instead, it depends on properties of the behavioral episode, such as the ambiguity of the behavior and the order of behavioral information and contextual information. As an alternative explanation of the identified behavior, contextual inducements affect attribution through diagnostic evaluation of one's attributional hypothesis against alternative hypotheses. The evaluation of alternative explanations is presumably a deliberate and effortful process, and therefore reversible and dependent on perceivers' cognitive and motivational resources. Under suboptimal processing conditions, perceivers presumably resort to pseudodiagnostic hypothesis evaluation. This is a short-cut heuristic that focuses on the consistency of the behavior with the focal attributional hypothesis and gives less weight to the consistency of the behavior with alternative attributional hypotheses. In pseudodiagnostic hypothesis evaluation, contextual inducements have a relatively small effect on attribution.

Research has tested some of these assumptions (Trope et al., 1988, 1991; Trope & Alfieri, 1997). Supporting the present distinction between the two uses of contextual inducements, this research has found that the use of contextual inducements for behavior identification depends on behavior ambiguity and the order of contextual and behavioral information, but not on cognitive load and the validity of information about contextual inducements. In contrast, the use of contextual inducements as an alternative explanation has been found to depend on cognitive load and the validity of information about contextual inducements, but not on the ambiguity of behavior and order of presentation.

According to the present analysis, discounting failures and the resulting overconfident attributions stem from two types of errors: biased identification of behavior, and failure to consider alternative explanations of the identified behavior. For example, conflict situations will fail to attenuate and may even enhance attribution of dispositional hostility to an actor when conflict (1) initially leads perceivers to misidentify the actor's reaction as angry and (2) is subsequently ignored as an alternative explanation of the actor's hostile reaction. The first type of error contributes to overconfidence because perceivers underweight the influence of contextual inducements on their representation of behavior. The second type of error contributes to overconfidence because perceivers underweight the influence of contextual inducements on the actor's behavior. Overconfident attributions thus result from misattributing to a focal property the effects of contextual inducements (1) on the actor's behavior (inferential error) and (2) on the perceiver's identification of the actor's behavior (identification error). Errors of inferences from identified behavior are presumably more controllable and dependent on perceivers' motivation and attentional resources than errors of behavior identification are.

The present analysis is applicable to any kind of attributional hypothesis. In many cases, perceivers will use behavior or performance to evaluate a hypothesis about the actor's traits or abilities. This is often the case in person perception experiments where participants are encouraged to find out something about the actor's personal characteristics. Situational forces will then serve as contextual inducements for the behavior. In some cases, however, perceivers may use behavior to test a hypothesis about the situation. In explaining their own behavior, for example, perceivers are more likely to evaluate situational hypotheses. Here the actor's personal characteristics may serve as contextual inducements. In all of these cases, perceivers are likely to make overconfident attributions (personal or situational) to the extent that they use contextual inducements as a frame for identifying behavior, but not as an an alternative explanation of the identified behavior.

Finally, this chapter has related the present dual-process model to Gilbert's three-stage attribution model (see Gilbert & Malone, 1995). Unlike Gilbert's model, the present model emphasizes the use of situational information in identifying or categorizing behavioral input. Moreover, the models make different assumptions about the use of situational information following behavior identification. According to Gilbert, situational inducements are used in a separate correction stage—one that follows attribution of behavior to the corresponding disposition. This model assumes (1) that perceivers do not use situational inducements unless inferences reach the final correction stage, and (2) that cognitive load prevents perceivers from reaching this stage. This model predicts, then, that situational information will fail to affect attributions under cognitive load, regardless of how strongly this information is activated.

A recent series of studies we conducted (Trope & Gaunt, 1998) found that cognitive load indeed eliminated the use of situational information when activation level of this information was relatively low, thus replicating earlier research by Gilbert. However, inconsistent with Gilbert's model, our studies also found that when situational information was made perceptually salient, accessible, and applicable, it strongly influenced dispositional attributions even when perceivers were under cognitive load. These findings were interpreted as consistent with the assumptions of the present model that situational information is integrated with other information sources to form a dispositional judgment, and that the integration of these information sources does not necessarily follow a fixed temporal sequence.

REFERENCES

Chaiken, S., Liberman, A., & Eagly, A. H. (1989). Heuristic and systematic information processing within and beyond the persuasion context. In J. S. Uleman & J. A. Bargh (Eds.), *Unintended thought* (pp. 212–252). New York: Guilford Press.

Chaiken, S., & Stangor, C. (1987). Attitude and attitude change. *Annual Review of Psychology, 38,* 575–630.

Doherty, M. E., Mynatt, C. R., Tweeney, R. D., & Schiavo, M. D. (1979). Pseudodiagnosticity. *Acta Psychologica, 43,* 111–121.

Dweck, C. S., Hong, Y., & Chiu, C. (1993). Implicit theories: Individual differences in the likelihood and meaning of dispositional inference. *Personality and Social Psychology Bulletin, 19,* 633–643.

Evans, J. S. B. T., & Lynch, J. S. (1973). Matching bias in the selection task. *British Journal of Psychology, 64,* 391–397.

Fischhoff, B., & Beyth-Marom, R. (1983). Hypothesis evaluation from a Bayesian perspective. *Psychological Review, 90,* 239–260.

Fiske, S. T. (1993). Social cognition and social perception. *Annual Review of Psychology, 44,* 155–194.

Gilbert, D. T. (1989). Thinking lightly about others: Automatic components of the social inference process. In J. S. Uleman & J. A. Bargh (Eds.), *Unintended thought* (pp. 189–211). New York: Guilford Press.

Gilbert, D. T. (1997). Ordinary personology. In D. T. Gilbert, S. T. Fiske, & G. Lindzey (Eds.), *Handbook of social psychology* (4th ed.). New York: McGraw-Hill.

Gilbert, D. T., & Krull, D. S. (1988). Seeing less and knowing more: The benefits of perceptual ignorance. *Journal of Personality and Social Psychology, 54,* 93–102.

Gilbert, D. T., & Malone, P. S. (1995). The correspondence bias: The what, when, how and why of unwarranted dispositional inference. *Psychological Bulletin, 117,* 21–38.

Gilbert, D. T., & Osborne, R. E. (1989). Thinking backward: Some curable and incurable consequences of cognitive busyness. *Journal of Personality and Social Psychology, 57,* 940–949.

Gilbert, D. T., Pelham, B. W., & Krull, D. S. (1988). On cognitive busyness: When person perceivers meet persons perceived. *Journal of Personality and Social Psychology, 54,* 733–740.

Ginossar, Z., & Trope, Y. (1987). Problem solving in judgment under uncertainty. *Journal of Personality and Social Psychology, 52,* 464–476.

Harkness, A. R., DeBono, K. G., & Borgida, E. (1985). Personal involvement and strategies for making contingency judgments: A stake in the dating game makes a difference. *Journal of Personality and Social Psychology, 49,* 22–32.

Heider, F. (1958). *The psychology of interpersonal relations.* New York: Wiley.

Higgins, E. T. (1998). Knowledge activation: Accessibility, applicability, and salience. In E. T. Higgins & A. W. Kruglanski (Eds.), *Social psychology: Handbook of basic principles* (pp. 133–168). New York: Guilford Press.

Higgins, E. T., & Bargh, J. A. (1987). Social cognition and person perception. *Annual Review of Psychology, 38,* 369–425.

Higgins, E. T., & King, G. (1981). Accessibility of social constructs: Information-processing consequences of individual and contextual variability. In N. Cantor & J. F. Kihlstrom (Eds.), *Personality, cognition and social interaction* (pp. 69–121). Hillsdale, NJ: Erlbaum.

Higgins, E. T., & Stangor, C. (1988). Context-driven social judgment and memory: When "behavior engulfs the field" in reconstructive memory. In D. Bar-Tal & A. Kruglanski (Eds.), *Social psychology of knowledge* (pp. 262–298). Cambridge, England: Cambridge University Press.

Jones, E. E. (1979). The rocky road from acts to dispositions. *American Psychologist, 34,* 107–117.

Jones, E. E. (1990). *Interpersonal perception.* New York: Macmillan.

Jones, E. E., & Nisbett, R. E. (1971). *The actor and the observer: Divergent perception of the causes of behavior.* Morristown, NJ: General Learning Press.

Kahneman, D., & Tversky, A. (1973). On the psychology of prediction. *Psychological Review, 80,* 237–251.

Kelley, H. H. (1972). Causal schemata and the attribution process. In E. E. Jones, D. E. Kanouse, H. H. Kelley, R. E. Nisbett, S. Valins, & B. Weiner (Eds.), *Attribution: Perceiving the causes of behavior* (pp. 151–174). Morristown, NJ: General Learning Press.

Klayman, J., & Ha, Y.-W. (1987). Confirmation, disconfirmation, and information in hypothesis-testing. *Psychological Review, 94,* 211–228.

Kruglanski, A. W., & Mayseless, O. (1988). Contextual effects in hypothesis testing: The role of competing alternatives and epistemic motivations. *Social Cognition, 6,* 1–20.

Krull, D. S. (1993). Does the grist change the mill?: The effect of the perceiver's inferential goal on the process of social inference. *Personality and Social Psychology Bulletin, 19,* 340–348.

Kunda, Z. (1990). The case for motivated reasoning. *Psychological Bulletin, 108,* 480–498.

Reeder, G. D. (1993). Trait–behavior relations and dispositional inference. *Personality and Social Psychology Bulletin, 19,* 586–593.

Ross, L. (1977). The intuitive psychologist and his shortcomings: Distortion in the attribution process. In L. Berkowitz (Ed.), *Advances in experimental social psychology* (Vol. 10, pp. 174–221). New York: Academic Press.

Sherman, J. S., & Corty, E. (1984). Cognitive heuristics. In R. S. Wyer, Jr., & T. K. Srull (Eds.), *Handbook of social cognition* (Vol. 1, pp. 189–286). Hillsdale, NJ: Erlbaum.

Shoda, Y., & Mischel, W. (1993). Cognitive social approach to dispositional inferences: What if the perceiver is a cognitive social theorist? *Personality and Social Psychology Bulletin, 19,* 574–595.

Taylor, S. E., & Fiske, S. T. (1975). Point-of-view and perceptions of causality. *Journal of Personality and Social Psychology, 32,* 439–445.

Tetlock, P. E. (1985). Accountability: A social check on the fundamental attribution error. *Social Psychology Quarterly, 48,* 227–236.

Trope, Y. (1978). Inferences of personal characteristics on the basis of information retrieved from one's memory. *Journal of Personality and Social Psychology, 36,* 93–106.

Trope, Y. (1986). Identification and inferential processes in dispositional attribution. *Psychological Review, 93,* 239–257.

Trope, Y., & Alfieri, T. (1997). Effortfulness and flexibility of dispositional inference processes. *Journal of Personality and Social Psychology, 73,* 662–675.

Trope, Y., Cohen, O., & Alfieri, T. (1991). Behavior identification as a mediator of dispositional inference. *Journal of Personality and Social Psychology, 61,* 873–883.

Trope, Y., Cohen, O., & Maoz, Y. (1988). The perceptual and inferential effects of situational inducements on dispositional attributions. *Journal of Personality and Social Psychology, 55,* 165–177.

Trope, Y., & Gaunt, R. (1998). *The use of situational information in dispositional inferences: Correction or integration?* Unpublished manuscript, New York University.

Trope, Y., & Higgins, E. T. (1993). The what, how, and when of dispositional inference: New questions and answers. *Personality and Social Psychology Bulletin, 19,* 493–500.

Trope, Y., & Liberman, A. (1993). Trait conceptions in identification of behavior and inferences about persons. *Personality and Social Psychology Bulletin, 19,* 553–562.

Trope, Y., & Liberman, A. (1996). Social hypothesis testing: Cognitive and motivational mechanisms. In E. T. Higgins & A. W. Kruglanski (Eds.), *Social psychology: Handbook of basic principles* (pp. 239–270). New York: Guilford Press.

Trope, Y., & Sikron, F. (1992). *Perceptual and inferential mechanism underlying trait attributions.* Paper presented at the joint Society for Experimental Social Psychology–European Association for Experimental Social Psychology meeting, Louvain, Belgium.

Wyer, R. S., & Srull, T. K. (1981). Category accessibility: Some theoretical and empirical issues concerning the processing of social stimulus information. In E. T. Higgins, C. P. Herman, & M. P. Zanna (Eds.), *Social cognition: The Ontario Symposium* (Vol. 1, pp. 161–197). Hillsdale, NJ: Erlbaum.

9

Modes of Social Thought

IMPLICIT THEORIES AND SOCIAL UNDERSTANDING

SHERI R. LEVY
JASON E. PLAKS
CAROL S. DWECK

Early social psychologists (e.g., Heider, 1958; Kelly, 1955) recognized that people's lay theories about personality play a pivotal role in their social understanding (see also Dweck & Leggett, 1988; Epstein, 1989; Murphy & Medin, 1985; Ross, 1989; Sternberg, 1985). Such "implicit" theories, although generally unconscious and unarticulated, contain key assumptions that can underlie different patterns of social information processing. For example, imagine a relatively static social reality in which people have fixed qualities, and a more dynamic reality where personal qualities are malleable. Such fundamentally different perspectives on human nature are likely to spawn very different mental models about how humans function, and therefore very different beliefs about what information is needed in order to understand and predict their behavior.

The idea of static versus dynamic implicit theories has a precedent in the work of the philosopher Alfred North Whitehead, who compared a static world view to a dynamic one (Whitehead, 1929, 1938; see also Johnson, Gerner, Efran, & Overton, 1988). He proposed that one metaphysical system, the

static world view, leads naturally to the desire to measure enduring properties and to create taxonomies based on them, whereas the other system, the dynamic world view, leads to the desire to analyze, understand, and influence the processes underlying these dynamic systems. He proposed that this distinction applies to scientists seeking to know the world that they study, as well as to laypeople seeking to know the world in which they live. Our research has focused on the information-processing consequences of these contrasting views, or theories, as people seek to know their social world.

In this chapter, we present research that compares individuals who believe in a more static social reality to those who believe in a more dynamic one, and we demonstrate how these two groups of people exhibit two different modes of social thought. One mode is organized around traits: seeking trait information, viewing traits as causes of behavior, drawing trait-centered inferences, and categorizing people by traits. The other mode is organized around more dynamic psychological mediators (e.g., people's goals, needs, states of mind); as we shall see, people who operate in

179

this mode tend to analyze and understand people in terms of these processes.

We then integrate the findings from the research, showing how these two implicit theories generate distinct, coherent, mental models that result in distinct patterns of social information processing and social judgment. In the final section, we then turn to existing models of social information processing and social inference, and describe how considering people's implicit theories can illuminate these models—or, in some cases, lead us to rethink them entirely.[1]

SOCIAL JUDGMENT

Earlier work in our laboratory, which examined the impact of fixed ("entity") versus malleable ("incremental") theories on people's self-judgments, led to the question of whether implicit theories would also play a role in predicting people's judgments of others (see Legett & Dweck, 1988; Levy & Dweck, 1998). The earlier work showed that individuals holding entity theories of personal attributes (intelligence or personality) tended to blame or condemn their attributes when they failed, whereas those holding incremental theories tended to focus instead on mediating processes (such as effort or strategies) when they encountered setbacks (Erdley, Cain, Loomis, Dumas-Hines, & Dweck, 1997; Henderson & Dweck, 1990). Would the same pattern emerge when people's implicit theories were applied to the judgments of others? Would entity theorists make stronger trait judgments based on minimal information about others and see underlying traits as the causes of others' behaviors? Would incremental theorists focus on more dynamic explanations for others' behavior, such as psychological mediators within the person (e.g., emotion states, needs, goals)?

A number of studies have now addressed these questions. In this section, we first describe studies that address differences in extremity of trait judgments of novel individuals (Chiu, Hong, & Dweck, 1997; Erdley & Dweck, 1993), of unfamiliar groups (Levy, Stroessner, & Dweck, 1998; Levy & Dweck, in press), and of familiar groups (Levy et al., 1998). Second, we describe other ways in which entity and incremental theorists' trait judgments differ—namely, in how inflexible they are (Erdley & Dweck, 1993) and in how valid individuals expect them to be over time (Erdley & Dweck, 1993) and across situations (Chiu, Hong, & Dweck, 1997). Third, we discuss studies revealing differences in nontrait person inferences. Here, we show how incremental theorists, in judging individuals and explaining their behavior, put more emphasis than entity theorists on psychological processes within a person (e.g., goals or needs; Hong, 1994) and on situational or environmental factors impinging on the person (Hong, 1994; Levy & Dweck, in press; Levy et al., in press). Finally, we describe the consequences of entity and incremental theorists' differing social judgments for how they believe people should be treated and for how they would behave toward them (Chiu, Dweck, Tong, & Fu, 1997; Erdley & Dweck, 1993; Freitas, Levy, & Dweck, 1997; Gervey, Chiu, Hong, & Dweck, in press; Levy & Dweck, in press).

Differences in Extremity of Trait Judgments

Unfamiliar Persons

People are often faced with making rapid trait judgments based on minimal behavioral information—for example, when relevant contextual information is not available. In order to assess how readily people form trait judgments, researchers have presented participants with just this kind of information (e.g., "Stephanie donated money to a charity") (Hastie & Kumar, 1979; Uleman, Newman, & Moskowitz, 1996). We have also presented participants with sparse behavioral information, but with the goal of examining individual differences in readiness to form strong trait judgments.

In one such study, Chiu, Hong, and Dweck (1997, Study 3) presented college students with 35 statements depicting a range of behaviors from mildly positive (e.g., "making one's bed in the morning") to clearly positive (e.g., "risking one's life for another"), and from mildly negative (e.g., "interrupting someone who is speaking") to clearly negative (e.g., "stealing a car"). Participants were asked to judge how indicative each behavior would be of a person's moral goodness or badness—in other words, to indicate how sweeping a trait judgment they would draw from the behavior. It was found that entity theorists rated both positive and negative behaviors, even those that were mildly valenced, as significantly more indicative of the target's moral traits than did incremental theorists. This finding of the relation between implicit theories and trait judgments also held for students in a more collectivistic culture (Hong Kong), indicating that these implicit theories are not simply culture-specific constructs, but may transcend variations in culture (Chiu, Hong, & Dweck, 1997, Study 4).

Would entity theorists more readily and strongly draw trait inferences about others even if their attention were drawn to the situational and psychological-process information surrounding a target's behavior? Or would the differences be eliminated if such contextual details were provided? To explore this, Erdley and Dweck (1993) provided late-grade school children with some negative behavioral information about a "new boy at school" (e.g., he lied about his background, copied from a classmate's paper, and appropriated a classmate's leftover art materials), as well as situational information (the boy had moved in the middle of the school year to the new school) and information relevant to possible psychological mediators (the boy was very nervous about making a good impression). On the basis of all this information, children were asked to evaluate the boy on a number of attributes. Results indicated that entity theorists rated the target significantly more negatively than did incremental theorists on global moral traits (e.g., "bad," "mean," "nasty").

In a study with college students, Sorich and Dweck (1996) corroborated these findings. Participants read scenarios about a person performing undesirable actions (peeking at a copy of an upcoming exam). Information about the target's psychological state (distraught about performing poorly) and the situational pressures (came across a copy of the exam) was also included. When asked to rate the causes of the target's action, entity theorists, relative to incremental theorists, endorsed negative traits (e.g., dishonesty or selfishness) as significantly more important causes of the target's actions.

These findings suggest that making situational and psychological-process state information about a target salient does not eliminate the tendency of entity theorists to draw stronger trait inferences.

Unfamiliar Groups

Do entity theorists draw stronger trait inferences when the behavioral information describes an unfamiliar group, as they do when the information describes an unfamiliar target person? A recent series of studies has answered this question (Levy & Dweck, in press; Levy et al., 1998, Study 3).

In one of their studies, Levy et al. (1998) provided college students with behavioral information about a novel group, ostensibly a student group at another university (cf. Ford & Stangor, 1992; Hastie & Kumar, 1979). The group was characterized either by 12 positive and 6 neutral behaviors (e.g., "ran after a person who left a package," "bought a magazine from a newsstand"), or by 12 negative and 6 neutral behaviors (e.g., "pushed to the front of the line at a movie theater," "went to the post office to buy some stamps"). Each behavior was attributed to a different group member. After receiving the information, participants were given 2 minutes to provide an open-ended description of the group as a whole. Although traits made up much of the open-ended descriptions, entity theorists generated significantly more traits and, in addition, tagged the traits with more extreme qualifiers (e.g., "very, " "extremely") than did incremental theorists.

Participants were also asked to evaluate the group as a whole on a set list of traits. Entity theorists, relative to incremental theorists, made significantly more extreme attribute ratings in both the positive group condition (attributes such as "virtuous," "good," "moral") and the negative-group condition (attributes such as "evil," "mean," and "rude"). In addition, they were more extreme in their judgments of the group's homogeneity, rating the group members as being more similar to one another on these attributes than incremental theorists.

The speed with which participants made the trait ratings was also assessed via computer, as another measure of readiness to associate strong trait labels with groups. Entity theorists were found to make significantly more rapid trait judgments than incremental theorists. This finding suggests that entity theorists not only make more extreme judgments of a group's attributes, but also access those judgments more readily.

In two studies of stereotype formation with late-grade school students, a similar pattern of differences emerged (Levy & Dweck, in press). In one study, children learned about and judged a mostly negatively behaving school; in a second study, they judged two groups in relation to one another (a negatively behaving and a positively behaving school). Across the studies, Levy and Dweck found that children with an entity theory, compared with those children with an incremental theory, made more extreme group judgments—both in their ratings of each group's traits and in their perception of greater within group homogeneity on these traits. Moreover, entity theorists' impressions generalized to a completely unknown member of the negative group (a student who was described as absent the day the observer visited the school). Specifically, entity theorists expected the unknown student to be "bad" and "mean" whereas incremental theorists reported a neutral expectation of the unknown student.

It is important to note that although entity theorists, compared to incremental theorists, tend to attach stronger trait labels both to individuals and to groups on the basis of limited behavioral information, entity theorists do not make more extreme judgments in general. That is, when entity and incremental theorists are asked simply to rate the behaviors, their ratings are virtually identical (Chiu, Hong, & Dweck, 1997; Levy & Dweck, in press; Levy et al., 1998). This suggests that entity theorists' stronger trait inferences do not stem from their evaluating the behaviors themselves differently or from a generalized tendency to make more extreme judgments.

Sufficiency of Information for Judging Unfamiliar Others

The findings reviewed thus far suggest that entity theorists view even limited behavioral information as more sufficient for making strong trait inferences of individuals and

groups than do incremental theorists. To examine directly whether entity theorists indeed believe more firmly than incremental theorists that people's behavior easily and reliably reveals their underlying traits, Sorich and Dweck (1996) asked entity and incremental theorists to evaluate a series of statements about the relation between behaviors and underlying traits. They found that entity theorists agreed with, and agreed significantly more than incremental theorists with, the following statements: "Each person has a basic character, and you can tell what kind of person someone is even by details of their behavior or appearance," "A single act often tells you a lot about a person's fundamental character," and "It's fairly easy to tell what kind of a person someone is by observing them on one or two occasions." In contrast, incremental theorists' mean response to these statements fell on the "disagree" side of the rating scale.

If a single act provides sufficient information for entity theorists to know the kind of person someone is, then do they also believe that limited information is sufficient for forming an impression of a group of people? In the study of novel groups with college students, participants were asked how sufficient the amount of information given was for forming an impression of the larger group (i.e., 18 behaviors—12 positive or negative and 6 neutral—performed by different group members; Levy et al., 1998, Study 3). The results indicated that entity theorists, significantly more than incremental theorists, believed that the information provided about a subset of group members (in both the positive and negative conditions) was sufficient for forming an impression of the entire group.

Thus, entity theorists tend to believe that strong inferences are more warranted from limited information.

Familiar Groups

If entity theorists *form* impressions of others more readily than do incremental theorists, do they also place more stock in their existing beliefs about others? In several studies, Levy et al. (1998) explored the extremity of college students' beliefs about ethnic and occupational stereotypes. In the first study, stereotypical beliefs were assessed by having participants list all the stereotypes they knew of African Americans, Asians, Latinos, Jews, and Caucasians (cf. Devine, 1989; Eagly, Mladinic, & Otto, 1994). Participants were then asked to review the stereotypes they had listed, and to evaluate how true they thought each one was. The findings showed that although both theory groups were equally knowledgeable about societal stereotypes, entity theorists endorsed both the positive and negative stereotypes they listed for each of the five groups significantly more strongly than did incremental theorists—examples included "lazy" for African Americans; "hard-working" for Asians, "criminal" for Latinos, "cheap" for Jews, and "racist" for Caucasians.

In follow-up studies, participants rated a specified set of stereotypes of three of the ethnic groups (African Americans, Asians, Latinos) and four occupational groups (doctors, lawyers, politicians, teachers) (Levy et al., 1998, Studies 2 and 5). Consistent and significant differences in endorsement of positive and negative stereotypes of these groups were again found.

To summarize, entity theorists, compared to incremental theorists, tend to attach stronger trait labels to novel groups and individuals; they also show a greater tendency to endorse stereotypes of existing groups.

Differences in Types of Trait Judgments: Dispositional versus Descriptive

Besides differing in extremity, entity and incremental theorists' trait inferences differ in other important ways. In a study reviewed earlier in which children formed impressions of a new boy at school who performed a series of transgressions, Erdley and Dweck (1993) also explored the extent to which the children would incorporate new, contradictory information into their initial impression. Toward this end, they provided half of the participants with an "inconsistent" ending to the story, in which the boy exhibited positive behaviors. Consistent with their belief that traits cannot be changed, entity theorists did not revise their trait judgments of the target (as a liar, a thief, or a cheat) in light of the new information. In contrast, incremental theorists significantly revised their judgments in response to the inconsistent information.

Do entity theorists expect the traits they infer to be more stable over time and across situations (key inferential practices of "lay dispositionism"—see Kunda & Nisbett, 1986; cf. Wright & Mischel, 1987)? Erdley and Dweck found that entity theorists expected their trait inferences to remain valid over time; they rated the boy as significantly more likely to act negatively in both the short-term future (a few weeks later) and the long-term future (several years later) than did incremental theorists.

Chiu, Hong, and Dweck (1997, Study 1) assessed college students' expectations that trait-relevant behavior would be consistent across different situations. They used a measure designed by Kunda and Nisbett (1986), which assessed participants' behavioral predictions for targets who had performed positive or negative social and intellectual behaviors. For example, participants were asked to "suppose . . . you observed Jack and Joe in one particular situation and found that Jack was more friendly than Joe." They were then asked to estimate the probability that in a completely different situation the relative behavior would be consistent. Chiu et al. found that entity theorists predicted far greater behavioral consistency than did incremental theorists (who, in fact, expected *Joe* to be the friendly one in a completely different situation).

In short, entity theorists' trait judgments are qualitatively different from those of incremental theorists. Not only do entity theorists, relative to incremental theorists, infer traits more readily and more strongly from limited social information (Chiu, Hong, & Dweck, 1997; Levy & Dweck, in press; Levy et al., 1998); they also (1) are less apt to revise their trait judgments in the face of counterinformation (Erdley & Dweck, 1993; see also Plaks & Dweck, 1997) and (2) are more likely to expect their trait judgments to remain valid over time and across situations (Chiu, Hong, & Dweck 1997; Erdley & Dweck, 1993). Incremental theorists' trait judgments thus seem to be more provisional. Their judgments are seen as valid only for the present (Erdley & Dweck, 1993), and are readily revised when new, discrepant information is presented to them (Erdley & Dweck, 1993; Plaks & Dweck, 1997).

These findings suggest that entity and incremental theorists' trait attributions are invested with different meanings. For entity theorists, traits seem to reflect enduring dispositional labels, whereas for incremental theorists, traits seem to reflect more temporary, descriptive labels (for discussions of different meanings of traits, see Bassili, 1989; Uleman et al., 1996).

Differences in Nontrait Judgments

Internal versus External (Situational) Attributions

Thus far, we have reviewed evidence that entity theorists focus more on traits as a way to understand others' actions than do incremental theorists. In this section, we review studies showing what incremental theorists tend to focus on as they seek to understand people's behavior and outcomes. As one would expect, incremental theorists, relative to entity theorists, focus more on explanations for behavior that are themselves dynamic—such as situational or environmental factors that affect a person, or psychological processes within a person (e.g., a person's goals, emotion states, needs).

Let us look first at group differences in situational explanations. As an initial exploration of whether incremental theorists would provide more situational explanations for behavior, Hong (1994) provided college students with 24 statements to evaluate in an open-ended manner. The statements depicted either a positive or negative action ("Arthur brought his colleagues some souvenirs from a trip") or a positive or negative outcome ("Lee's last two relationships ended badly"). Participants were asked to provide brief causal explanations for each of the 24 episodes by completing this stem: "This probably occurred because . . ." Hong found that although both groups provided far more internal than external explanations, incremental theorists made significantly more external, situational attributions for people's behaviors and outcomes than did entity theorists.

Internal versus external explanations were also explored in a study described earlier. In this study (Levy & Dweck, in press, Study 1), late-grade school children were asked to judge a novel school based on the behaviors of a subset of the students from the

school, and then were asked to explain why they thought the "kids from the school" acted the way they did. In line with Hong's (1994) findings, children holding incremental theories reported significantly more external explanations (such as situational and environmental/learning factors—e.g., "The picture was ugly," "Their friends taught them how to be bad") than did entity theorists. Also, as might be expected, entity theorists provided significantly more internal, trait explanations (e.g., "They are mean") than did incremental theorists.

To summarize, incremental theorists tend to think more in terms of situational influences on behavior than do entity theorists. Entity theorists, more often than incremental theorists, locate the causes of behavior inside a person—most often in a person's traits. Both groups, however, ascribe much of behavior to internal factors, yet there is a critical difference in the internal factors they favor.

Different Internal Attributions: Trait versus Process Explanations

Hong (1994), for example, found that within the internal attributions that were made for positive and negative behaviors, entity theorists made significantly more trait attributions (e.g., "Arthur is good-hearted"), whereas incremental theorists made significantly more process-centered attributions—attributions that portrayed the behavior as resulting from psychological processes, such as the person's goals, needs, beliefs, emotions, and so on (e.g., "Arthur wanted to please his colleagues"). In fact, incremental theorists offered significantly more process attributions than trait attributions, whereas entity theorists made more trait attributions than process attributions. Thus, when invoking internal causes of behavior (both positive and negative ones), entity theorists seem to focus relatively more on traits, and incremental theorists seem to focus more on mediating psychological processes (see also Levy, 1998, for a similar finding with fifth- and sixth-graders).

This differential emphasis on traits versus psychological processes was observed in a study (Chiu, 1994, Study 2) in which college students were given both trait-relevant and goal-relevant information about a number of individuals, and then were asked to judge the similarity–dissimilarity of the individuals. Chiu found that incremental theorists categorized the targets (saw them as similar–dissimilar) on the basis of their goals, whereas entity theorists categorized the targets on the basis of their traits. Therefore, whether they are judging the causes of behavior or judging the similarity of individuals, entity and incremental theorists focus on different internal psychological qualities—underlying traits *vs.* more specific and dynamic psychological processes.

Implications of Differences in Trait and Nontrait Judgments

Our findings on trait versus nontrait (situational and psychological process) explanations have implications for social perception research. For instance, our findings may shed light on the "fundamental attribution error," the general tendency to overestimate the role of people's traits (dispositions) and to underestimate situational factors in explaining their behaviors, even when situational factors are made salient (e.g., Jones & Davis, 1965; for a review, see Ross & Nisbett, 1991). Our findings suggest that incremental theorists may not be falling prey to the fundamental attribution error to the same extent as entity theorists. For one thing, incremental theorists give somewhat more situational explanations and fewer trait explanations than entity theorists (Hong, 1994; Levy & Dweck, in press). In addition, incremental theorists have been shown to give more process explanations than entity theorists (Hong, 1994; Levy, 1998). Attributions that invoke the target's mediating psychological processes (such as goals, emotional reactions, or states of mind) can be viewed as placing the person in a situational context more than do trait attributions, which tend to refer to context-free personal attributes. For example, if one believes that a person acted aggressively because he or she felt threatened, this explanation assumes the impact of the situation. In sum, because of their greater recognition of situational factors, as well as of the psychological impact of these factors, incremental theorists may be less prone to the fundamental attribution error.

The differences that have emerged within internal attributions are important to highlight further. Social judgment research has tended *not* to emphasize the distinction between different types of internal attributions (for notable exceptions, see Trope, 1989, and Trope & Liberman, 1993; see also Weiner, 1993, and Graham & Weiner, 1991), concentrating instead on the distinction between internal (dispositional) attributions and external (situational) attributions (e.g., Fiedler, Semin, & Bolten, 1989; Jones & Davis, 1965). Yet, as we have seen, trait and process attributions, although they are both internal attributions, may have very different meanings and ramifications.

Consequences of Differing Social Judgments

Besides predicting differences in judgments and attributions, implicit theories also predict differences in the course of actions people generate, the decisions they make, and the behavior they display toward other people.

First, several studies (Chiu, Dweck, et al., 1997; Erdley & Dweck, 1993; Gervey et al., in press) have found that entity theorists, having rendered a negative judgment, are significantly more likely to recommend punishment or are likely to recommend a significantly greater degree of punishment. By contrast, incremental theorists, focusing more on malleable processes, are significantly more likely to recommend education or rehabilitation for wrongdoers.

Recently, Gervey et al. (in press) showed that entity theorists were not only more willing to render a negative judgment on the basis of personal information, but were also more willing to base a guilty–innocent verdict on the information. Participants (college students) were asked to imagine that they were jurors and had to decide the guilt or innocence of a defendant accused of murder. Specifically, they were given a summary transcript of the trial, which in some cases described the defendant's appearance the day of the crime—as either characteristic of "respectable" individuals (he was wearing a business suit and tie) or characteristic of somewhat "less respectable" individuals (he was wearing blue jeans, a black leather jacket with many zippers, and a black T-shirt). Regardless of the strength of the evidence provided, entity theorists rated the less respectably dressed defendant as less moral and more likely to be guilty than did incremental theorists. Incremental theorists, by contrast, disregarded the clothing information and focused on the strength of the evidence in rendering their judgments. However, when no information about the defendant's social category was available, entity and incremental theorists made equivalent judgments based on the strength of the evidence, showing that the "category" information was the key determinant of differences in their jury decisions.

The study reviewed earlier on children's judgments of a novel group of students also revealed differences in desired interaction with group members (Levy & Dweck, in press, Study 1). Children in the study were asked to report the extent to which they were willing to socialize with the students from the "negatively behaving" school (e.g., to go to a party, to be a friend, to be a best friend). Although both entity and incremental theorists indicated that they did not want to socialize much with the students from the school, entity theorists wanted to do so significantly less than did incremental theorists.

In a study with college students, Freitas et al. (1997) examined whether entity theorists would be more likely than incremental theorists to act on existing stereotypes when interacting with members of stereotyped groups. Participants were led to believe that they were playing a two-person Prisoner's Dilemma game (Schelling, 1960) against either a "law student" or a control opponent. Entity and incremental theorists played equally competitively against the unidentified opponent. However, whereas entity theorists played more competitively against the "law student," incremental theorists did not, indicating that entity but not incremental theorists acted on the societal stereotype of law students.

Thus, implicit theories appear to have consequences not just for how people will be judged, but also for how they are likely to be treated.

INFORMATION-PROCESSING SYSTEMS

Much of the research we have described has focused on "later" processes, such as judgment of and decisions about targets. Yet, if

implicit theories do indeed underlie truly distinct processing frameworks, then entity and incremental theorists may differ not only in how they interpret a given set of target information, but also in how they capture information from the environment in the first place. In other words, just as judgment and interpretation processes seem to be strongly influenced by implicit theories, attention and encoding strategies may be similarly influenced. Accordingly, we have recently begun to focus on "earlier" processes by addressing whether there are differences in how entity and incremental theorists attend to, encode, and organize incoming social information.

Attention and Encoding

The fact that entity and incremental theorists often reach very different judgments on the basis of the same input raises the question: "Do entity and incremental theorists gather social information in the same manner and then *apply* it differently, or do they actually gather incoming information in different manners?"

Prior research has suggested that structures such as beliefs, expectancies, values, and attitudes can lead to people to devote greater attention to particular aspects of incoming information (e.g., Bruner, 1957; Derryberry & Tucker, 1994; Erber & Fiske, 1984; Fazio, Roskos-Ewoldsen, & Powell, 1994; Hilton, Klein, & von Hippel, 1991; Moray, 1959; Newtson, 1976; Treisman, 1964). In light of this research, it is plausible that entity and incremental theorists, given their different beliefs about human qualities, might focus their attention on different aspects of incoming social information.

What function might such different attention strategies serve? Strategic attention allocation might be employed in order to facilitate the formation of trait judgments (for entity theorists) or situational/process-oriented judgments (for incremental theorists). For example, consider a case in which entity and incremental theorists are faced with inconsistent information about a target (e.g., when a target behaves at first in an immoral manner and then in a moral manner, as in Erdley & Dweck, 1993). Our model predicts that because incremental theorists are not heavily invested in trait labels, they should be relatively attentive to inconsistent information about a target. Entity theorists, on the other hand, because they tend to think of others mainly in terms of (fixed) traits, should prefer a set of incoming data that is consistent with a single global trait (either "good" or "bad"), and therefore should selectively attend in a manner that facilitates such a trait judgment.

Plaks and Dweck (1997) tested differences in selective attention to inconsistent target information. Following a previously established attention allocation paradigm (Sherman, Lee, Bessenoff, & Frost, 1998; Hastroudi, Mutter, Cole, & Green, 1984), Plaks and Dweck provided participants with a target label implying that the target was morally good (a priest) or morally bad (a neo-Nazi skinhead). Then participants read 30 sentences about the target, one at a time, on a computer screen. In 10 of the sentences, the target behaved in a morally exemplary fashion; in 10 of the sentences, the target behaved in a morally negative fashion; and the remaining 10 sentences contained information about the target that was irrelevant to the morality dimension. To assess how much attention participants were paying to each of the three kinds of sentences, a concurrent-task reaction time paradigm was used. For 9 of the sentences (3 of each type, randomized), a tone was emitted by the computer; participants were to press a key as quickly as possible, with the computer measuring reaction time. Presumably, the more attention being paid to the sentence currently on the screen, the more interference there would be with the concurrent task of pressing a key, and thus the slower the response time. Less attention to the sentence currently on the screen would presumably lead to less interference with the concurrent task of pressing a key, and in turn to a faster response time.

Plaks and Dweck found that entity theorists responded significantly more quickly (reflecting less attention) than incremental theorists to *inconsistent* target information. Moreover, it was found that entity theorists responded more slowly (reflecting more attention) than incremental theorists to *consistent* target information. This suggests that entity theorists pay less attention than incremental theorists to target information that might dilute or confuse their impression of the target

and instead focus on information that supports a single, clear, trait-based impression. In contrast, incremental theorists appear to pay more attention than entity theorists to inconsistent information (presumably because it might provide a more comprehensive picture of the target) and less attention to consistent information (presumably because it appears redundant). In other words, these data suggest that incremental theorists find inconsistent information more engaging, whereas entity theorists consider consistent information more attention-worthy.

These findings raise the possibility that entity–incremental differences in the extent to which an initial impression guides later judgment may be at least partially mediated by differential allocation of attentional resources. Entity theorists appear to "hold on tighter" to an impression in the face of contradictory information (Erdley & Dweck, 1993). It may be that this is accomplished in part by employing strategic selective-attention processes. Perhaps at an early, less conscious stage, information that violates entity theorists' expectancies serves as a signal to initiate strategically selective processing. Incremental theorists, on the other hand, seem less put off by counter-expectant information, perhaps even relishing it for its diagnostic value.

Thus, we raise the possibility that implicit theories about the mutability of human attributes constitute an important predictor of who will pay more attention to inconsistent target information and who will pay more attention to consistent target information. This approach may shed light on the long-standing question in person perception of when people will embrace inconsistent information (Brewer, Dull, & Lui, 1981; Hastie & Kumar, 1979; Taylor & Fiske, 1978) and when they will selectively focus on confirmatory information (see Erber & Fiske, 1984, and Stangor & Ruble, 1989).

Encoding

A second early social-cognitive processing stage at which entity and incremental theorists may diverge is the encoding stage. It is possible that just as they appear to use selective attention to facilitate trait judgments, entity theorists may also *encode* incoming information in ways that facilitate trait judgments.

For example, entity theorists may tag incoming information in a more evaluative manner than do incremental theorists. The act of tagging each incoming piece of information as positive or negative could presumably allow each individual piece to fit more readily into a subsequently recalled set of "evidence" used in later trait judgments. That is, if entity theorists are inclined to judge someone as morally good or bad, it is easier to amass evidence of goodness or badness from memory if each piece of information is clearly tagged as "good" or "bad" than if each piece of information is not clearly tagged in this way.

To test differences in evaluative encoding of incoming person information, Hong, Chiu, Dweck, and Sacks (1997) used a variation of an established procedure for examining the extent to which an attitude object activates an evaluation (see Bargh, Chaiken, Govender, & Pratto, 1992; Fazio, Sanbonmatsu, Powell, & Kardes, 1986). In this paradigm, if an attitude object (e.g., snakes) activates a negative evaluation, then a participants' response time to a subsequently presented negative word (e.g., "disgusting") will be facilitated, and their response to a positive word (e.g., "lovely") will be retarded.

Hong et al. (1997) first presented college students with information about the performance of a pilot trainee on 20 subscales of an aptitude test. (Some scores were high, some low, some average.) These scores were subsequently presented as primes, one at a time, on a computer screen. Each prime was followed by either a positive or negative adjective (e.g., "lovely" or "gruesome"), and participants were asked to decide as quickly as possible whether the adjective was positive or negative. If the pilot's scores were encoded in evaluative terms (positive vs. negative), then responses to adjectives congruent in valence (positive or negative ones) would be facilitated. As predicted, Hong et al. found that high and low test scores significantly facilitated entity theorists' responses to subsequent adjectives that were congruent in valence. That is, entity theorists responded more quickly to positive target adjectives when the primes were high test scores than when the primes were low test scores, and more quickly to negative target adjectives when the primes were low test scores than when the primes were high test scores. In contrast, incremental

theorists' responses to the adjectives were not influenced by the primes. This finding suggests that entity theorists encoded the test scores in a more evaluative manner than did incremental theorists, and thus in a way that might facilitate later trait inferences.

Organization of Information in Memory

If entity theorists seek to make trait judgments, and if they encode person information with evaluative tags, do they also organize information in memory based on the valence of evaluative tags (see Asch & Zukier, 1984)? In other words, if entity theorists do seek to make evaluative trait judgments (e.g., good or bad, intelligent or unintelligent), segregating the information into information that supports a positive judgment versus information that supports a negative judgment may facilitate subsequent decisions.

As part of the study on evaluative encoding described earlier, Hong et al. (1997) assessed whether the entity and incremental theorists differed in the extent to which they segregated information in memory based on valence. They reasoned that if, relative to incremental theorists, entity theorists tended to segregate valenced information, then they would be more susceptible to biased retrieval (if, e.g., a question oriented them toward the positive or the negative information store) (Asch & Zukier, 1984; Wyer & Carlston, 1994). To test this, participants, after exposure to the pilot's positive and negative test scores, were randomly assigned to a positive-, negative-, or neutral-framing condition. The positive or negative frames were introduced in the instructions as follows: "You have to estimate how likely it is that he would do well [poorly] in the pilot training course and pass [fail] the licensing examination when he leaves the training school . . ." The neutral frame was introduced as follows: "You will have to estimate how he would perform in the pilot training course and on the licensing examination when he leaves the training school . . ." When asked to recall the trainee's scores, entity theorists' mean recalled score was significantly affected by the framing manipulation: Their mean recalled score was highest in the positive condition, lower in the neutral condition, and even lower in the negative condition. In contrast, incremental theorists' mean recalled score was not systematically affected by the framing conditions. These findings provided preliminary support for the idea that entity theorists are more likely than incremental theorists to separate person information by valence, and that incremental theorists, not seeking as much to make trait judgments, may be more likely to integrate positive and negative information in forming an impression.

How else might entity and incremental theorists' representations in memory differ? Chiu (1994, Study 2), in a study discussed earlier, tested whether entity theorists, in line with their trait focus, would categorize people in terms of similarities in their traits, and incremental theorists, in line with their process focus, would categorize people more in terms of similarities in their goals. Chiu presented participants with both goal and trait information about a number of targets, and asked them to judge the similarity and dissimilarity of the targets. More specifically, the targets were fictitious team leaders at a summer camp who were described in terms of both goal information (e.g., a target reported that he was working at the camp to "fulfill a school requirement") and trait information (e.g., a reference letter described a target as "a kind and generous person"). By providing both kinds of information about each target, Chiu (1994) could assess the relative weight entity and incremental theorists gave to trait versus goal information in judging the similarity. Results provided clear evidence that incremental theorists were more goal-focused in their categorization of the targets, whereas entity theorists were more trait-focused.

In short, there is mounting empirical evidence that entity and incremental theorists tend to encode and organize new information in ways that facilitate and reflect their trait-versus process-centered social judgments.

CAUSAL RELATION BETWEEN IMPLICIT THEORIES AND INFERENCES

Implicit theories appear to be knowledge constructs that can be either chronically accessible or situationally induced. Because our model portrays the link between people's implicit theories and their allied inference processes as a causal link, it is important to find direct support for that link—for example, by showing that situationally induced implicit theories have the predicted impact on subsequent processes. Research in our laboratory (Bergen, 1991; Chiu, Hong, & Dweck, 1997; Dweck, Tenney, & Dinces, 1982, reported in Dweck & Leggett, 1988; Levy, 1998; Levy et al., 1998) has now shown that the link between people's implicit theories and allied processes in various domains is indeed a causal one.

Dweck et al. (1982, reported in Dweck & Leggett, 1988) experimentally manipulated children's theories of intelligence by presenting a compelling passage that portrayed the intelligence of notable individuals (e.g., Albert Einstein) as either fixed or malleable. The results showed that, as predicted, the induction affected children's goal choice on an upcoming task: Children in the entity theory condition showed relatively greater concern with how their intelligence would be judged, and children in the incremental theory condition showed greater concern with developing their ability. In another study, Bergen (1991) persuaded college students to adopt either an entity or an incremental view through the use of compelling "scientific" articles (*Psychology Today*-type articles)—ones that vividly described and quoted extensive (fictitious) research attesting to each view. Results from this study showed that those who read the entity-oriented article reacted to failure feedback in the way predicted by an entity theory (i.e., with a more "helpless" reaction). In both of these studies, great care was taken to ensure that the theory manipulation in no way suggested particular goals or reactions.

More recently, Chiu, Hong, and Dweck (1997, Study 5) successfully manipulated college students' implicit theories of personality and provided initial evidence for the causal relation between implicit theories and the inference patterns we have been addressing. Participants in the study read versions of short scientific article modeled on the ones used by Bergen (1991). The entity and incremental versions of the article each cited evidence from several sources—case studies of individuals (including famous people), longitudinal studies conducted over several decades, and large-scale intervention programs. These induction articles, although quite thoroughly addressing the entity and incremental beliefs, in no way were related to the specific dependent measures used. Some time after reading the article, participants completed two measures that assessed trait inferences (drawn from Kunda & Nisbett, 1986): a trait judgment questionnaire (e.g., "If Jack hits John in a particular situation, to what extent can it be concluded with confidence that Jack is an aggressive person?") and a questionnaire about behavioral consistency (e.g., "Henry is more aggressive than Edward on average. What do you suppose is the probability that Henry would act more aggressively than Edward in a particular situation?"). Results indicated that those who were led to adopt an entity theory scored higher on both questionnaires, indicating that they made stronger trait judgments and predicted greater cross-situational consistency than those who were led to believe in an incremental theory.

Levy et al. (1998, Study 4) have also obtained preliminary results suggesting that the relation between implicit theories and endorsement of group stereotypes is a causal one. Participants in this research were led to adopt an entity or an incremental view (with the articles used in Chiu, Hong, & Dweck, 1997), and then were asked to complete a stereotype measure that was presented as part of another study. Specifically, participants were asked to evaluate occupational groups (lawyers, doctors, teachers, and politicians) and ethnic groups (African Americans, Asians, and Latinos) on 17 attributes (e.g., "intelligent," "hard-working," "competitive," "untrustworthy," and "dishonest"). It was found that those who were led to adopt the entity view agreed significantly more with stereotypes relevant to these groups than did those who were led to adopt the incremental view (see also Levy, 1998, for a similar finding with fifth-graders).

In summary, these findings indicate that theories can be successfully manipulated in the intelligence and personality domains. In addition to providing evidence for the causal role of theories, these findings suggest that these theories do not belong to different types of people but rather are different belief systems that impact social perception when salient.

THEORIES, MENTAL MODELS, AND PROCESSING CONSEQUENCES

The consistently distinct patterns displayed by entity and incremental theorists across a variety of tasks and across numerous studies suggest that these implicit theories may lay the foundation for distinct mental models of human personality and behavior. In other words, our findings lead us to conclude that an entity theory and an incremental theory probably do not "act alone"; instead, each theory is one important component of an organized network of beliefs and causal schemas, the sum of which constitutes a coherent mental model.

We have presented findings that fill in many of the "nodes" of the entity and incremental mental models with particular beliefs and causal schemas. In this section we highlight the most important of these beliefs, schemas, and associated processing strategies. Figure 9.1 displays the suggested components of each mental model.

The Entity Mental Model

The entity mental model is built around the core implicit theory that people's qualities are fixed and cannot be changed. In Figure 9.1, we have illustrated this implicit theory with one of the items from our questionnaire on which participants must indicate their extent of agreement or disagreement: "Everyone is a certain kind of person, and there is not much that can be done to really change that."

What exactly do entity theorists mean when they indicate that personality is not changeable? Overall, this line of research suggests that they tend to believe that personal attributes are largely immune to a person's efforts or motivation to change (e.g., Mueller & Dweck, 1998). Furthermore, different situations play little role in shaping personality. Thus, when entity theorists indicate that personality is fixed, this implies that personal qualities are resistant to change over time and are stable across situations.

The entity mental model seems to contain the assumption that not only are traits fixed, but in an important sense, they are what personality is composed of (as opposed to being composed of such psychological con-

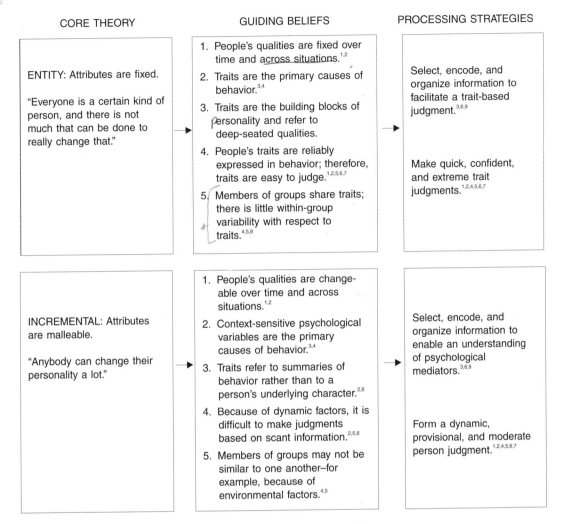

FIGURE 9.1. Proposed mental models of entity and incremental theorists. [1]Chiu, Hong, and Dweck (1997); [2]Erdley and Dweck (1993); [3]Hong (1994); [4]Levy and Dweck (1998b) [5]Levy et al. (1998); [6]Plaks and Dweck (1997); [7]Sorich and Dweck (1996); [8]Gervey et al. (In press); [9]Chiu (1994).

structs as goals, values, ideals, competencies, etc.). According to this view, traits are the building blocks of personality, and any meaningful appraisal of someone must address his or her underlying traits. Moreover, this belief in fixed traits as the building blocks of personality fits with the view that traits are the primary cause of behavior.

Within the entity mental model, not only does personality consist of fixed traits that cause trait-consistent behavior over time and across situations, but these traits are reliably displayed in behavior. That is, rather independently of the particular point in time or the particular situation, traits frequently and reliably generate trait-consistent behavior. This means that a given behavior can be taken as representing an underlying trait and that only a few instances of behavior are needed to judge a person's personality. "After all," the implicit logic appears to be saying, "this person is not going to be very different in another situation or in the future, so why waste time and cognitive resources assembling a pool of redundant information?"

If entity theorists focus on traits as the

primary "stuff" of personality and as the primary cause of behavior, what is their view of other factors, such as psychological processes? Even though we have little direct evidence on this point, the findings we do have lead us to suggest that while entity theorists may acknowledge that people experience various psychological processes and that they are subject to situational presses, entity theorists may view these variables as mere epiphenomena of the person's underlying trait. That is, a given trait leads not only to behavior, but to specified goals, specified feelings, and so on, as well as tendencies to enter specified situations. However, although these goals, feelings, and situations may often accompany the behavior, they are seen as correlates, not causes. These psychological and situational factors may be seen as only adding "noise" to the system and are ultimately reducible to the person's underlying trait.

Finally, our findings on entity theorists' tendency to stereotype more than incremental theorists suggest that just as they perceive low variability of behavior within a single person, they also perceive low variability of behavior or traits within a group of people. Thus the behavior of a few group members is indicative of the traits of the entire group (Levy & Dweck, in press; Levy et al., 1998), and knowing a person's group membership allows you to predict how an individual will act (Gervey et al., in press). This belief in low within-group variability with respect to traits may be partly due to a belief that traits are inherent. Levy et al. (1998) asked participants to provide explanations for differences that exist between groups. Entity theorists were more likely than incremental theorists to ascribe the differences to innate differences in group members' traits, whereas incremental theorists were more likely than entity theorists to ascribe the differences to environmental or experiential factors. The belief that members of a group share key traits from the start may foster the view that group members are basically interchangeable.

To date, we have identified two main processing strategies that seem to emanate from the entity mental model. In terms of decisions and judgments about the target, entity theorists seem inclined to pursue relatively quick, confident, and extreme judgments about the target's trait characteristics. In terms of selection, organization, and encoding strategies, entity theorists seem to process in a manner that facilitates and simplifies the task of making a trait-based judgment. For example, entity theorists tend to selectively favor information that confirms an initial, trait-based appraisal of the target over information that disconfirms the initial appraisal.

To summarize, the entity mental model is built around the core belief that people's qualities are fixed—over time and across situations. This model then guides what information will be attended to and how it will be encoded and organized, which in turn influences the judgments that are based on this information.

The Incremental Mental Model

The incremental mental model is built around the core theory that people's qualities are malleable and are susceptible to change due to such factors as effort and motivation. In Figure 9.1, we have illustrated the incremental theory with an item taken from our questionnaire: "Anybody can change their personality a lot." Our research has shown that incremental theorists also appear to believe not only that people can change over time, but also that their behavior can vary meaningfully with the situation or context.

A central belief that accompanies the incremental theory is that if people are susceptible to change over time and across situations, then more dynamic processes (e.g., such context-sensitive psychological variables as needs, goals, emotions, competencies, etc.) are the primary building blocks of personality and the causes of behavior. Several of our studies have indicated that incremental theorists, although they can invoke traits, nevertheless tend to cite psychological and situational processes as explanations for systematic variation in someone's behavior much more often than do entity theorists.

Despite the fact that incremental theorists do employ trait terms, our research suggests that when they do so, they are often (1) referring to a summary of the observed behaviors rather than the actor's underlying character, and (2) using the terms in a provisional manner that may be revised readily in the face of new information.

Because behavior is dependent on context-sensitive psychological processes, what someone is like is not easy to diagnose from a small number of behaviors. Instead, it is likely that to gain an understanding of the systematic, coherent aspects of an individual's personality, observation of behavior over time and across situations is necessary (Shoda & Mischel, 1993).

Finally, just as incremental theorists consider an individual to be variable with respect to his or her behavior, they consider a group to be variable with respect to the personalities and behavior of its constituent members. Therefore, incremental theorists are more likely than entity theorists to believe that observing how a few individuals act indicates little about the group as a whole.

These beliefs have been found to manifest themselves in at least two processing strategies. First, incremental theorists' initial judgments often seem to display a more cautious and less extreme pattern than those of entity theorists. Second, incremental theorists' selection, encoding, and organizational processes are not focused on supporting a trait-based judgment of the target. Non-trait-related information, such as psychological states or situational presses, is accorded at least equal (if not greater) weight in the encoding process. In addition, incremental theorists devote more attention than entity theorists to information that contradicts a trait-based expectancy (e.g., information describing the immoral actions of a supposedly moral person).

In sum, the incremental mental model is built around the core belief that people's attributes are changeable—over time and across situations. The mental model then orients information processing toward more dynamic variables and flexible judgments.

This "mental-model" approach provides a fuller account of entity and incremental theorists' differences. By identifying the networks of beliefs and processing strategies that emanate from each theory, we can begin to explain how the underlying theory leads to certain deductive practices. It should be noted that according to our mental-models account, the differences in processing exhibited by entity and incremental theorists are not due to differences in general processing sophistication or overall motivation to be accurate. Instead, these differences appear to be mediated

by the different emphases that grow out of the two mental models with their different underlying assumptions about human nature. Furthermore, people may possess both mental models, but for some the entity mental model may be more accessible, whereas for others the incremental model may be more accessible.

In the remainder of this chapter, we apply this "implicit-theories/mental-models" approach to thorny questions in the field of person perception, and describe how this approach may provide new insights.

APPLICATION OF IMPLICIT THEORIES AND MENTAL MODELS APPROACH

Relation to Models of Dispositional Inference

Historically, researchers have proposed that making a dispositional inference on the basis of observed behavior is a relatively automatic act that requires less effort than taking into account the influence of the situation on the behavior (Heider, 1958; Jones & Davis, 1965). Jones (1990) described an actor and his or her act as "a natural, fundamental Gestalt," whereas situations are referred to as "contextual shapers" and "part of the background" (p. 147). That is, people are more attention-grabbing than situations, which leads perceivers to think about actors more often than situations. This in turn leads perceivers to trace causal attribution to the most accessible source—that is, the actor (Jones & Harris, 1967; Ross, 1977).

In this literature, "actor" has come to mean "the presumed trait(s) of the actor." Our research, however, suggests that although perceivers do tend to trace causal attribution to actors more than to situations, for some perceivers "actor" does not necessarily refer to the actor's traits. It appears that for incremental theorists, "actor" often refers to the actor's more temporary psychological processes or states. Earlier we illustrated how this distinction may shed light on the fundamental attribution error. In what follows, we describe how this distinction may illuminate other dispositional inference processes as well.

In the past decade, a number of prominent approaches to dispositional inference (e.g., Gilbert, Pelham, & Krull, 1988; Hilton, Fein, & Miller, 1993; Krull & Erickson, 1995; Reeder, 1993; Trope, 1986, 1989; Uleman et al., 1996) have identified processes and variables that further specify the path from observed behavior to inferred dispositional trait. In particular, these models have tended to interpose additional processing steps on the road from the observation of behavior to the inference of a disposition.

In this section, we propose that although a number of these recent models of dispositional inference have contributed valuable insights, they may not tell the entire story. They assume that people in general follow only one route (be it simple or multistaged) that starts with the observation and identification of behavior and is aimed toward attributing this behavior to the target's underlying trait disposition. Our findings, however, lead us to suggest that different people may have different goals or endpoints when they process social information.

Trait versus Nontrait Orientation:
Implications for Information Processing

More concretely, our findings suggest that not all people are equally oriented toward traits. We have demonstrated that upon observing a target's behavior, entity theorists make trait inferences more readily than incremental theorists, and incremental theorists often show a preponderance of psychological-process-related inferences.

These distinctions are critical because they may suggest that incremental theorists follow a route of processing that is markedly different not only from that of entity theorists, but also from the routes of processing outlined by most existing models of dispositional inference. Because incremental theorists are less trait-oriented, it appears that their processing has an alternate "destination" and, therefore, an alternate "route." Thus, existing models may be inherently "entity" models, in that they assume that people are trait-focused. That is, they may fail to account for a possible processing route that is not inevitably oriented toward reaching a trait-based characterization of the target (see Shoda & Mischel, 1993, for a notable exception).

Moreover, it is possible that these models describe *neither* theory group with great accuracy. In other words, combining entity and incremental theorists together obscures their important differences and creates an artificial mean that, in the end, describes neither group fully. Not only may incremental theorists be less trait-oriented, but entity theorists may be even *more* trait-oriented than these models imply.

Different Meanings of Traits:
Implications for Automatic Trait Inferences

The implications of different groups' being differentially oriented toward traits can be further seen in the issue of whether people make automatic trait inferences. Uleman and colleagues (Uleman et al., 1996; Winter & Uleman, 1984) presented evidence that people automatically infer traits from observed behavior. After reading about an actor's behavior, participants exhibited facilitation in their response times to relevant trait terms. Uleman et al. initially concluded that people automatically link the target's behavior to an associated trait label. These findings were subsequently reinterpreted, however, by several researchers (including Uleman and colleagues) who distinguished between traits as labels of behavior versus labels of people (Bassili, 1989; Claeys, 1990; Higgins & Bargh, 1987; Uleman et al., 1996). It was argued that at least some of the participants in the original Uleman et al. studies, when responding to a trait term (e.g., "aggressive"), may have affixed trait-type labels to behaviors (e.g., "an aggressive act"), but did not necessarily draw the link between the trait term and the actor's underlying disposition (e.g., "an aggressive person").

We raise the possibility that both explanations are correct, in that each applies to a different subset of theorists. As noted, our research indicates that there appear to be components of the entity mental model that draw an immediate and direct causal link between a behavior, a trait term, and the actor's underlying disposition. The incremental mental model, by contrast, appears to contain the belief stating that traits describe patterns of behavior, but are not necessarily underlying disositions or causes of behavior. The spontaneous trait inferences of entity theorists may thus be truly *dispositional*, in that they refer to the underlying properties of the actor, whereas the spontaneous trait inferences generated by incremental theorists may be a shorthand way of referring to the behavior only.

Implications for Revision of Dispositional Inferences

These critical differences in how entity and incremental theorists approach and process social information may be associated with yet another difference in dispositional-inference processing. Entity and incremental theorists may differ in their readiness to revise an initial dispositional appraisal of a target once it has been activated. (A possible revision stage is proposed by several multistage models of person perception [e.g., Devine, 1989; Gilbert et al., 1988]; cf. Jones, 1979; Quattrone, 1982.) One means of accomplishing this revision is to make more extensive use of psychological or situational information about the target. Inasmuch as this multistage, serial approach is valid, the components of the entity and incremental mental model may precipitate different strategies toward an already activated dispositional inference (see Read & Miller, 1993, for an interesting alternative model based on parallel processes; see also Trope & Gaunt, Chapter 8, this volume). Entity theorists, with their belief that dispositional traits are reliably reflected in a person's behavior, may be more likely to consider a dispositional characterization of a target as satisfactory, and consequently may be less likely to initiate a "revision" stage. In contrast, incremental theorists' belief in dynamic attributes and mediating processes may lead them to view an initial disposition-based characterization as merely provisional and open to change. Therefore, incremental theorists may be more likely to overturn an already activated dispositional inference on the basis of new information.

Recent findings in our laboratory (Plaks & Dweck, 1997) suggest that this is indeed the case. In one study, participants were provided with strong expectancies about a target's intellectual ability, and then half of the participants witnessed the target performing in a highly counterexpectant manner on an exam. Entity theorists were less likely than incremental theorists to revise their initial appraisal of a target in the face of information that contradicted their original trait diagnosis. Entity and incremental theorists, then, may differ not only in the meaning of their spontaneous trait inferences, but in their readiness to revise a trait inference once it has been activated. Existing models do not adequately account for the possibility of different perceivers' having differing approaches to revision, based on differing beliefs and assumptions about personality.

It is important to stress that we are not claiming that entity theorists are invariably or necessarily less complex social information processors than incremental theorists are. Consider, for instance, Krull and Erickson's (1995) reinterpretation of the classical notion that situational information is harder than dispositional information to integrate into an impression. Contrary to Heider's and Jones's assumption that actors offer more compelling causal explanations than situations, Krull and Erickson have suggested that the real difficulty for perceivers may be in generating and thinking about alternatives. When the typical dispositional-inference paradigm is reversed (i.e., participants are asked to make judgments about a situation rather than an actor), these researchers showed that it requires effort for perceivers to incorporate dispositional information about the *actor* into their judgment of the *situation*. For example, imagine that Bob tells a perceiver that a class is boring and hard. Imagine also that Bob happens to be a lazy student. It requires effort for people to incorporate the fact that Bob is lazy into their appraisal of the class. Thus, under conditions of cognitive load, people tend to take Bob's description of the class at face value; without cognitive load, people factor in Bob's disposition and take his description of the class with a grain of salt, given his "slacker" nature. Although Krull and Erickson did not pit situational inferences against dispositional inferences to see which are ultimately more influential, these data are instructive in suggesting that the very process of considering alternative explanations—regardless of whether the alternative is situational or dispositional in nature—is an effortful one.

In such a case, when dispositional and situational information are reversed so that dispositional information might modify situational judgments, one intriguing possibility is that incremental theorists may actually use the moderating dispositional information *less* than entity theorists do. If so, incremental theorists would be the less effortful processors in this case. Because an entity mental model places such emphasis on the actor's static, underlying disposition, this type of information may be more readily integrated than situational information by entity theorists. Because an incremental mental model emphasizes the dynamic nature of personality, using static, dispositional information may actually require considerable effort for incremental theorists. Then, in the case of judging situations like the one concerning Bob, entity theorists may be the ones who process information in a more optimal, integrative manner.

In sum, we propose that consideration of the perceiver's implicit theory, in conjunction with the mental model of personality that emanates from this core theory, may contribute to a more developed understanding of what exactly it is that people infer from observed behavior and how they go about doing it. Specifically, we suggest that different theories and mental models lead to different foci in processing—one on traits and one on context-sensitive psychological mediators—which in turn lead to notably different processing patterns. The fact that different people seem to have different aims and to follow different routes of person perception suggests that future models of social inference should not assume that everyone follows the same route to the same destination.

As we have seen from the Krull and Erickson (1995) example, underlying the various processes involved in dispositional inference is the notion that some of these processes require more effort than others. In the next section, we discuss implicit theories, mental models, and their implications for a perceiver's level of cognitive effort exertion in the context of prominent dual-process models of social cognition.

Relation to More General Dual-Process Models of Social Judgment

Both the models of dispositional inference just described and more general dual-process models of social cognition (e.g., Brewer, 1988; Chaiken, Liberman, & Eagly, 1989; Fiske & Neuberg, 1990; Petty & Cacioppo, 1986) rest on a proposed tension between less elaborative and more elaborative modes of processing. The claim in this section is that just as entity and incremental mental models are sufficient to drive distinct modes of processing when it comes to dispositional inference, entity and incremental mental models are sufficient to drive the different modes of processing found in more general dual-process models.

What is the nature of these distinct processing patterns? We propose that the trait-focused assumptions and beliefs of the entity mental model underlie entity theorists' tendency to think about people in a manner that is often less complex and effortful, compared to that of incremental theorists. In contrast, the incremental mental model tends to focus on ways of describing people involving mediating psychological states or situational presses. This tendency, we propose, often (but not invariably) expresses itself in more complex, more effortful social information processing on the part of incremental theorists.

For example, although the processing strategies elaborated in the heuristic–systematic model (Chaiken, 1980) as well as in the elaboration likelihood model (Petty & Cacioppo, 1986) are typically used to characterize two routes of persuasion, they seem particularly applicable to characterizing how entity and incremental theorists' social judgments might be formed (see Chaiken et al., 1989, for a discussion of how their model is applicable to the domain of social judgment). Systematic processing (or central-route processing) is characterized by thorough, effortful processing of available information. In contrast, heuristic processing (or peripheral-route processing) is characterized by more superficial, rapid, and cognitively untaxing processing. When behavioral information is provided, it seems likely that entity theorists may engage in a form of heuristic processing. For instance, many of the "nodes" of the entity mental model may be formulated as heuristics for social understanding (e.g., "Fixed traits cause people's behavior," "A small set of behaviors reliably reflects a person's underlying traits"; see Sorich & Dweck, 1996). Given their focus on mediating processes in social judgment, it seems likely that incremental theorists generally find such heuristics to be inadequate. Instead, they seem to engage in more elaborative processing of behavioral information, because their social understanding may involve the interplay of multiple variables—both variables that are external to the person (the situation) and ones that are internal to the person (goals, needs, beliefs) (see Erdley & Dweck, 1993; Hong, 1994; Levy & Dweck, in press; Sorich & Dweck, 1996).

In fact, it may be that the distinction between systematic and heuristic processing is more typically applicable to incremental theorists than to entity theorists. Limited resources or motivation may lead incremental theorists to restrict their focus to a trait diagnosis and to devote less effort to variables that may moderate that trait diagnosis (e.g., contextual information or psychological-process information). Entity theorists, on the other hand, appear to prefer trait diagnoses under most capacity conditions. After all, if entity theorists consider contextual or psychological-process information to be relatively uninformative compared to the actor's trait in explaining the actor's behavior, then we should expect them to prefer the trait explanation even when capacity or motivational conditions allow for the consideration of alternative explanations. Thus, incremental theorists may engage in systematic versus heuristic processing, depending on available cognitive resources; however, but given their mental model focused on fixed traits, entity theorists may often engage in heuristic processing independently of their current processing capacity.

Furthermore, consideration of perceivers' theory-based mental models may add refinement to the distinctions proposed in models of impression formation (e.g., the dual-process model of Brewer, 1988, or the continuum model of Fiske & Neuberg, 1990). In these models, two modes of processing are contrasted—category-based and individuating (or attribute-based) processing. Category-based processing is characterized by immediate categorization of information into meaningful social categories (e.g., roles, occupations, demographic categories). In contrast, when information about a target cannot be easily categorized (e.g., a secretary who is Black, Danish, and qualitatively oriented and who believes in the genetic determination of

intelligence; Fiske & Neuberg, 1990), then individuating processing is proposed to occur. In other words, single attributes of a target are integrated into an impression one at a time in a piecemeal manner (see Anderson, 1974).

Even though both theory groups may utilize both modes of processing, our findings suggest that when the task involves determining what the target is "like," entity theorists may be more inclined than incremental theorists to seek and utilize category information. This is especially true if the social category in question has implications for the target's traits. Incremental theorists' judgments, by contrast, seem to reflect more consideration of individuating information (e.g., psychological-process and situational information; Erdley & Dweck, 1993; Sorich & Dweck, 1996) and less consideration of trait-related categorical information (Gervey et al., in press). In a study we reviewed earlier, in which category information about a defendant was provided in some conditions, Gervey et al. (in press) found that only entity theorists made category-based judgments. Despite the fact that incremental theorists, like most social perceivers, took note of the category information (e.g., Brewer, 1988; Devine, 1989; Fiske & Neuberg, 1990), Gervey et al.'s results suggest that incremental theorists' final judgment of the defendant did not reflect initial category information, but rather reflected the particular evidence presented in the transcript of the case.

The Impact of Prior Beliefs and Assumptions on Motivation

Although researchers have identified a host of motivational variables that predict when people will pursue the "quick and easy" mode and when they will pursue the "complex and effortful" mode—for example, need for closure (Webster & Kruglanski, 1994), need for cognition (Cacioppo & Petty, 1982), task importance (Maheswaran & Chaiken, 1991), accountability for one's judgments (Tetlock, 1983), positive mood (Mackie & Worth, 1989), and anxiety (Jepson & Chaiken, 1990) (for a review, see Petty & Cacioppo (1986)—none of these variables refer to perceivers' underlying assumptions and beliefs about others. Yet people do enter social situations with important assumptions and beliefs (either chronic or recently primed) about what people are typically like and what is the best way to gain an understanding of other people. These assumptions and beliefs can lead to differences in processing that are largely conceptually independent of the motivational variables listed above.

This is not to deny the importance of motivational variables when one is considering dual-process models. In fact, much work in our laboratory has focused on the relationship between implicit theories and the goals that are allied with each type of implicit theory. We do wish to argue, however, that the study of motivational and individual-difference variables that affect the extent of processing can be enriched by placing it in the context of implicit theories and mental models.

"Entitativity" as a General Principle of Social Perception

Throughout this chapter, we have described how distinct implicit theories about the mutability of human attributes drive differences in social processing. In this section, we draw links between our research and other research that has focused on a related dimension.

Prior research has shown that in general, perceivers display differences in processing of information about individuals versus groups. Weisz and Jones (1993) found that impressions of individuals tend to be more stable (i.e., more resistant to counterexpectant information) than impressions of groups. Similarly, Stern, Mars, Millar, and Cole (1984), and Wyer, Bodenhausen, and Srull (1984) found that perceivers focus on different kinds of information when the target is an individual compared to when the target is a group.

What is it about individuals compared to groups that accounts for these differences in processing? Hamilton, Sherman, and colleagues (Hamilton & Sherman, 1996; McConnell, Sherman, & Hamilton, 1997) have proposed that a perceiver's implicit belief about the internal consistency (the "entitativity") of a target is a crucial predictor of these differences in processing. Specifically, Hamilton and Sherman (1996) have noted that perceivers typically consider individuals to possess greater entitativity than groups, and it is this difference in perceived enti-

tativity that underlies such findings as perceivers' tendency to make more spontaneous trait inferences about individuals than about groups. Indeed, when asked to make a judgment about a highly entitative group (such as a college fraternity, which presumably self-selects members with high similarity to one another), perceivers treat the group like an individual and are more willing to make trait judgments. Conversely, when an individual is presented as having low entitativity (e.g., a mentally unstable person), then perceivers are more reluctant to come to quick trait judgments (see Hamilton, Sherman, & Maddox, Chapter 30, this volume).

In other words, Hamilton et al.'s research indicates that the differential processing of information about individuals versus groups is not attributable to differences between individuals and groups per se. Rather, differences in how consistent, monolithic, or "entitative" a target is perceived to be (whether it is an individual or a group) seems to be what primarily drives these effects.

Our approach employs a related dimension, but instead underscores the often neglected notion that people can differ in their implicit theories about the "entitativity" of individuals or a given group. Whereas Hamilton et al. (Chapter 30, this volume) focus on the differences in inherent entitativity of different classes of targets, we focus on perceivers and their personal proclivity for believing that individuals are entitative or not. The convergent findings from both laboratories suggest that the entitativity dimension may underlie many social perception phenomena.

CONCLUSION

In this chapter, we have portrayed two modes of social thought—one organized around rather global evaluative traits, and the other organized around more dynamic psychological processes (see Figure 9.1). In the former, trait-relevant information is sought; incoming information is encoded in ways that support future trait inferences; and available information is readily converted to traits. Traits appear to be the unit of analysis for organizing, describing, and explaining social phenomena.

In the latter mode, human behavior is viewed more as the product of a chain of psychological processes: People have beliefs, values, goals, hopes, and fears that lead them to act as they do. These processes, then, are the units that are used to understand people and to organize information about them.

Each mode of thought is linked to a different implicit person theory, and it is through the study of these implicit theories that we may come to understand how people can construct disparate social worlds for themselves—each world being entirely logical and internally consistent within the framework set up by its implicit theory.

We have also found that these different modes of social thought engender different modes of reaction. Entity theorists, observing a negative behavior and rendering a global evaluative judgment, wish to punish the wrongdoer, whereas incremental theorists, observing the same behavior and identifying a mediating process, wish to educate the wrongdoer (see Dweck, 1996; Dweck et al., 1995). Thus, the implicit theories may set up not only meaning systems, but also meaning–action systems (Chiu, Dweck, et al., 1997).

Over 60 years ago, Whitehead (1929, 1938) proposed two modes of thought stemming from beliefs in a static versus dynamic physical reality. We have applied a similar analysis to the social world, and by doing so, we hope, have illuminated some basic phenomena of social perception and cognition.

NOTES

1. It should be noted that in the studies reported in this chapter, domain-general implicit person theories were typically assessed rather than more domain-specific theories (e.g., theory of intelligence, theory of moral character). This is because the social behaviors examined in these studies cut across different person attributes. Implicit theories can be domain-specific. For example, some people can believe that intelligence is fixed, but personality is malleable, or vice versa. Thus, when the behavior in question falls clearly into one domain, it is preferable to use the domain-specific measure. Moreover, our assessment of implicit theories assumes that although these theories are usually not clearly articulated, people are nonetheless able to judge whether they agree or disagree with the simple straightforward beliefs presented in our measures. Categorization of participants as entity or incremental theorists is based on an index of agreement or disagreement with items such as this: "Everyone is a certain kind of person, and there is not much that can be done to really change that." Across studies, approximately 85% of the respondents are categorized clearly (and fairly equally) into entity and incremental theorists while the remaining 15%, who show no clear pattern of agreement or disagreement, are excluded (for validity and reliability information, see Dweck, Chiu, & Hong, 1995; Levy et al., 1998).

There are a growing number of individual-difference variables that predict differences in social information processing and judgment (e.g., need for closure—Webster & Kruglanski, 1994; need for cognition—Cacioppo & Petty, 1982; personal need for structure—Neuberg & Newsom, 1993). Our measure is not only largely conceptually distinct from other individual-difference variables, in that it represents a core belief rather than a need or motive, but it also appears to be largely statistically distinct (see Levy et al., 1998, Study 5).

REFERENCES

Anderson, N. H. (1974). Information integration: A brief survey. In D. H. Krantz, R. C. Atkinson, R. D. Luce, & P. Suppes (Eds.), *Contemporary developments in mathematical psychology* (pp. 236–305). San Francisco: Freeman.

Asch, S. E., & Zukier, H. (1984). Thinking about persons. *Journal of Personality and Social Psychology, 46,* 1230–1240.

Bargh, J. A., Chaiken, S., Govender, R., & Pratto, F. (1992). The generality of the automatic attitude activation effect. *Journal of Personality and Social Psychology, 62,* 893–912.

Bassili, J. N. (1989). Traits as action categories versus traits as person attributes in social cognition. In J.N. Bassili (Ed.), *On-line condition in person perception* (pp. 61–89). Hillsdale, NJ: Erlbaum.

Bergen, R. (1991). *Beliefs about intelligence and achievement-related behaviors.* Unpublished doctoral dissertation, University of Illinois.

Brewer, M. B. (1988). A dual process model of impression formation. In T. K. Srull & R. S. Wyer, Jr. (Eds.), *Advances in social cognition* (Vol. 1, pp. 1–36). Hillsdale, NJ: Erlbaum.

Brewer, M. B., Dull, V., & Lui, L. (1981). Perceptions of the elderly: Stereotypes as prototypes. *Journal of Personality and Social Psychology, 41,* 656–670.

Bruner, J. S. (1957). On perceptual readiness. *Psychological Review, 64,* 123–152.

Cacioppo, J. T., & Petty, R. E. (1982). The need for cognition. *Journal of Personality and Social Psychology, 42,* 116–131.

Chaiken, S. (1980). Heuristic versus systematic information processing and the use of source message cues in persuasion. *Journal of Personality and Social Psychology, 39,* 752–766.

Chaiken, S., Liberman, A., & Eagly, A. E. (1989). Heuristic and systematic information processing within and beyond the persuasion context. In J. S. Uleman & J. A. Bargh (Eds.), *Unintended thought* (pp. 212–252). New York: Guilford Press.

Chiu, C. (1994). *Bases of categorization and person cognition.* Unpublished doctoral dissertation, Columbia University.

Chiu, C., Dweck, C. S., Tong, Y. Y., & Fu, H. Y. (1997). Implicit theories and conceptions of morality. *Journal of Personality and Social Psychology, 73,* 923–940.

Chiu, C., Hong, Y., & Dweck, C. S. (1997). Lay dispositionism, culture and implicit theories of personality. *Journal of Personality and Social Psychology, 73,* 19–30.

Claeys, W. (1990). On the spontaneity of behavior categorization and its implications for personality measurement. *European Journal of Personality, 4,* 173–186.

Derryberry, D., & Tucker, D. (1994). Motivating the focus of attention. In P. Niedenthal & S. Kitayama (Eds.), *The heart's eye: Emotional influences in perception and attention* (pp. 167–196). San Diego, CA: Academic Press.

Devine, P. G. (1989). Stereotypes and prejudice: Their automatic and controlled components. *Journal of Personality and Social Psychology, 56,* 5–18.

Dweck, C. S. (1996). Implicit theories as organizers of goals and behavior. In P. M. Gollwitzer & J. A. Bargh (Eds.), *The psychology of action* (pp. 69–90). New York: Guilford Press.

Dweck, C. S., Chiu, C., & Hong, Y. (1995). Implicit theories and their role in judgments and reactions: A world from two perspectives. *Psychological Inquiry, 6,* 267–285.

Dweck, C. S., & Leggett, E. L. (1988). A social-cognitive approach to motivation and personality. *Psychological Review, 25,* 109–116.

Eagly, A. H., Mladinic, A., & Otto, S. (1994). Cognitive and affective bases of attitudes toward social groups and social policies. *Journal of Experimental Social Psychology, 30,* 113–137.

Epstein, S. (1989). Values from the perspective of cognitive–experiential self-theory. In N. Eisenberg, J. Reykowski, & E. Staub (Eds.), *Social and moral values: Individual and social perspectives* (pp. 3–61). Hillsdale, NJ: Erlbaum.

Erber, R., & Fiske, S. T. (1984). Outcome dependency and attention to inconsistent information. *Journal of Personality and Social Psychology, 47,* 709–726.

Erdley, C. A., Cain, K. M., Loomis, C. C., Dumas-Hines, F., & Dweck, C. S. (1997). The relations among children's social goals, implicit personality theories, and responses to social failure. *Developmental Psychology, 33,* 283–272.

Erdley, C. A., & Dweck, C. S. (1993). Children's implicit personality theories as predictors of their social judgments. *Child Development, 64,* 863–878.

Fazio, R. H., Roskos-Ewoldsen, D. R., & Powell, M. C. (1994). Attitudes, perception, and attention. In P. Niedenthal & S. Kitayama, (Eds.), *The heart's eye: Emotional influences in perception and attention* (pp. 197–216). San Diego, CA: Academic Press.

Fazio, R. H., Sanbonmatsu, D. M., Powell, M. C., & Kardes, F. R. (1986). On the automatic activation of attitudes. *Journal of Personality and Social Psychology, 50,* 229–238.

Fiedler, K., Semin, G. R., & Bolten, S. (1989). Language

use and reification of social information: Top-down and bottom-up processing in person cognition. *European Journal of Social Psychology, 19,* 271–295.

Fiske, S. T., & Neuberg, S. L. (1990). A continuum of impression formation, from category based to individuating processes: Influences of information and motivation on attention and interpretation. In M. P. Zanna (Ed.), *Advances in experimental social psychology,* (Vol. 23, pp. 1–74). San Diego, CA: Academic Press.

Ford, T. E., & Stangor, C. (1992). The role of diagnosticity in stereotype formation: Perceiving group means and variances. *Journal of Personality and Social Personality, 63,* 356–67.

Freitas, A. L., Levy, S. R., & Dweck, C. S. (1997, May). *Implicit theories predict behavioral stereotyping in a Prisoner's Dilemma game.* Paper presented at the Eighth Annual Convention of the American Psychological Society, Washington, DC.

Gervey, B. M., Chiu, C., Hong, Y., & Dweck, C. S. (in press). The use of personality information in decision making: The role of implicit theories. *Personality and Social Psychology Bulletin.*

Gilbert, D. T., Pelham, B. W., & Krull, D. S. (1988). On cognitive business: When person perceivers meet person perceived. *Journal of Personality and Social Psychology, 54,* 733–740.

Graham, S., & Weiner, B. (1991). Testing judgments about attribution–emotion–action linkages: A lifespan approach. *Social Cognition, 9,* 254–276.

Hamilton, D. L., & Sherman, S. J. (1996). Perceiving persons and groups. *Psychological Review, 103,* 336–355.

Hastie, R., & Kumar, R. (1979). Person memory: Personality traits as organizing principles in memory for behaviors. *Journal of Personality and Social Psychology, 37,* 25–38.

Hashtroudi, S., Mutter, S. A., Cole, E. A., & Green, S. K. (1984). Schema-consistent and schema inconsistent information: Processing demands. *Personality and Social Psychology Bulletin, 10,* 269–278.

Heider, F. (1958). *The psychology of interpersonal relations.* New York: Wiley.

Henderson, V. L., & Dweck, C. S. (1990). Motivation and achievement. In S. S. Feldman & G. R. Elliott (Eds.), *At the threshold: The developing adolescent* (pp. 308–329). Cambridge, MA: Harvard University Press.

Higgins, E. T., & Bargh, J. A. (1987). Social cognition and social perception. In M. R. Rosenzweig & L. W. Porter (Eds.), *Annual review of psychology* (Vol. 38, pp. 369–425). Palo Alto, CA: Annual Reviews.

Hilton, J. L., Fein, S., & Miller, D. T. (1993). Suspicion and dispositional inference. *Personality and Social Psychology Bulletin, 19,* 501–512.

Hilton, J. L., Klein, J. G., & von Hippel, W. (1991). Attention allocation and impression formation. *Personality and Social Psychology Bulletin, 17,* 548–559.

Hong, Y. Y. (1994). *Predicting trait versus process inferences: The role of implicit theories.* Unpublished doctoral dissertation, Columbia University.

Hong, Y. Y., Chiu, C., Dweck, C. S., & Sacks, R. (1997). Implicit theories and evaluative processes in person cognition. *Journal of Experimental Social Psychology, 33,* 296–323.

Jepson, D., & Chaiken, S. (1990). Chronic issue-specific fear inhibits systematic processing of persuasive communications. *Journal of Social Behavior and Personality*, 5, 61–84.

Johnson, J. A., Gerner, C. K., Efran, J. S., & Overton, W. F. (1988). Personality as a basis for theoretical predilections. *Journal of Personality and Social Psychology*, 55, 824–835.

Jones, E. E. (1979). The rocky road from acts to dispositions. *American Psychologist*, 34, 107–117.

Jones, E. E. (1990). *Interpersonal perception*. New York: Freeman.

Jones, E. E., & Davis, K. E. (1965). From acts to dispositions: The attribution process in person perception. In L. Berkowitz (Ed.), *Advances in experimental social psychology*, (Vol. 2, pp. 219–266). New York: Academic Press.

Jones, E. E., & Harris, V. A. (1967). The attribution of attitudes. *Journal of Experimental Social Psychology*, 3, 1–24.

Kahneman, D., & Tversky, A. (1973). On the psychology of prediction. *Psychology Review*, 80, 237–251.

Kelley, H. H. (1973). The processes of causal attribution. *American Psychologist*, 28, 107–128.

Kelly, G. A. (1955). *The psychology of personal constructs*. New York: Norton.

Klein, S. B., & Loftus, J. (1990). Rethinking the role of organization in person memory: An independent trace storage model. *Journal of Personality and Social Psychology*, 59, 400–410.

Kruglanski, A. W., & Freund, T. (1983). The freezing and unfreezing of lay inferences: Effects on impressional primacy, ethnic stereotyping, and numerical anchoring. *Journal of Experimental Social Psychology*, 19, 448–468.

Kruglanski, A. W., & Webster, D. M. (1996). Motivated closing of the mind: "Seizing" and "freezing." *Psychological Review*, 103, 263–283.

Krull, D. S., & Erickson, D. J. (1995). Judging situations: On the effortful process of taking dispositional information into account. *Social Cognition*, 13, 417–438.

Kunda, Z., & Nisbett, R. E. (1986). The psychometrics of everyday life. *Cognitive Psychology*, 18, 195–224.

Levy, S. R. (1998). *Children's static vs. dynamic conceptions of people: Their impact on intergroup attitudes*. Unpublished doctoral dissertation, Columbia University.

Levy, S. R., & Dweck, C. S. (1998). Trait- vs. process-centered social judgment. *Social Cognition*, 16, 151–172.

Levy, S. R., & Dweck, C. S. (in press). The impact of children's static vs. dynamic conceptions of people on stereotype formation. *Child Development*.

Levy, S. R., Stroessner, S. J., & Dweck, C. S (1998). Stereotype formation and endorsement: The role of implicit theories. *Journal of Personality and Social Psychology*, 74, 1421–1436.

Mackie, D. M., & Worth, L. T. (1989). Processing deficits and the mediation of positive affect in persuasion. *Journal of Personality and Social Psychology*, 57, 27–40.

Maheswaran, D., & Chaiken, S. (1991). Promoting systematic processing in low-motivation settings: Effect of incongruent information on processing and judgment. *Journal of Personality and Social Psychology*, 61, 13–25.

McConnell, A., Sherman, J. W., & Hamilton, D. L. (1997). Target entitativity: Implications for information processing about individual and group targets. *Journal of Personality and Social Psychology*, 72, 750–762.

Moray, N. (1959). Attention in dichotic listening: Affective cues and the influence of instructions. *Quarterly Journal of Experimental Psychology*, 11, 56–60.

Mueller, C., & Dweck, C. S. (1998). Praise for intelligence can undermine children's motivation and performance. *Journal of Personality and Social Psychology*, 75, 33–52.

Murphy, G. L., & Medin, D. L. (1985). The role of theories in conceptual coherence. *Psychological Review*, 92, 289–316.

Neuberg, S. L., & Newsom, J. T. (1993). Personal need for structure: Individual differences in the desire for simple structure. *Journal of Personality and Social Psychology*, 65, 113–131.

Newtson, D. (1976). Foundations of attribution: The perception of ongoing behavior. In J. H. Harvey, W. J. Ickes, & R. F. Kidd (Eds.), *New directions in attribution research* (pp. 223–247). Hillsdate, NJ: Erlbaum.

Petty, R. E., & Cacioppo, J. T. (1986). The elaboration likelihood model of persuasion. In L. Berkowitz (Ed.), *Advances in experimental social psychology* (Vol. 19, pp. 123–205). San Diego, CA: Academic Press.

Plaks, J., & Dweck, C. S. (1997, May). *Implicit person theories and attention to counterexpectant social information*. Paper presented at the Eighth Annual Convention of the American Psychological Society, Washington, DC.

Quattrone, G. A. (1982). Overattribution and unit formation: When behavior engulfs the person. *Journal of Personality and Social Psychology*, 42, 593–607.

Read, S. J., & Miller, L. C. (1993). Rapist or "regular guy": Explanatory coherence in the construction of mental models of others. *Personality and Social Psychology Bulletin*, 19, 526–540.

Reeder, G. D. (1993). Trait-behavior relations and dispositional inference. *Personality and Social Psychology Bulletin*, 19, 586–593.

Ross, L. (1977). The intuitive psychologist and his shortcomings: Distortion in the attribution process. In L. Berkowitz (Ed.) *Advances in experimental social psychology* (Vol. 10, pp. 174–221). New York: Academic Press.

Ross, L., & Nisbett, R. E. (1991). *The person and the situation*. New York: McGraw-Hill.

Ross, M. (1989). Relation of implicit theories to the construction of personal histories. *Psychological Review*, 96, 341–357.

Schelling, T. C. (1960). *The strategy of conflict*. Cambridge, MA: Harvard University Press.

Sherman, J. W., Lee, A. Y., Bessenoff, G. R., & Frost, L. A. (1998). Stereotype efficiency reconsidered: Encoding flexibility under cognitive load. *Journal of Personality and Social Psychology*, 75, 589–606.

Shoda, Y., & Mischel, W. (1993). Cognitive social approach to dispositional inferences: What if the perceiver is a cognitive social theorist? *Personality and Social Psychology Bulletin*, 19, 574–585.

Sorich, L., & Dweck, C. S. (1996). [Implicit theories as predictors of attributions for and response to wrongdoing]. Unpublished raw data, Columbia University.

Stangor, C., & Ruble, D. (1989). Strength of expectancies and memory for social information: What we remember depends on how much we know. *Journal of Experimental Social Psychology, 25,* 18–35.

Stern, L. D., Marrs, S., Millar, M. G., & Cole, E. (1984). Processing time and recall of inconsistent and consistent behavior of individuals and groups. *Journal of Personality and Social Psychology, 47,* 253–263.

Sternberg, R. J. (1985). Implicit theories of intelligence, creativity, and wisdom. *Journal of Personality and Social Psychology, 49,* 607–627.

Taylor, S. E., & Fiske, S. (1978). Salience, attention, and attribution: Top of the head phenomena. In L. Berkowitz (Ed.) Advances in experimental social psychology (Vol. 11, pp. 249–268). New York: Academic Press.

Tetlock, P. (1983). Accountability and the perseverance of first impressions. *Social Psychology Quarterly, 46,* 285–292.

Treisman, A. M. (1964). Selective attention in man. *British Medical Bulletin, 20,* 12–16.

Trope, Y. (1986). Identification and inferential processes in dispositional attribution. *Psychological Review, 93,* 239–257.

Trope, Y. (1989). Levels of inference in dispositional judgment. *Social Cognition, 7,* 296–314.

Trope, Y., & Liberman, A. (1993). The use of trait conceptions to identify other people's behavior and to draw inferences about their personalities. *Personality and Social Psychology Bulletin, 19,* 553–562.

Uleman, J. S., Newman, L. S., & Moskowitz, G. B. (1996). People as flexible interpreters: Evidence and issues from spontaneous trait inference. In M. P. Zanna (Ed.), *Advances in experimental social psychology* (Vol. 28, pp. 211–279). San Diego, CA: Academic Press.

Webster, D. M., & Kruglanski, A. W. (1994). Individual-differences in need for cognitive closure. *Journal of Personality and Social Psychology, 67,* 1069–1062.

Weiner, B. (1993). On sin versus sickness: A theory of perceived responsibility and social motivation. *American Psychologist, 48,* 957–965.

Weisz, C., & Jones, E. E. (1993). Expectancy disconfirmation and dispositional inference: Latent strength of target-based and category-based expectations. *Personality and Social Psychology Bulletin, 19,* 563–573.

Whitehead, A. N. (1929). *Process and reality.* New York: Free Press.

Whitehead, A. N. (1938). *Modes of thought.* New York: Free Press.

Winter, L., & Uleman, J.L. (1984). When are social inferences made?: Evidence for the spontaneousness of trait inferences. *Journal of Personality and Social Psychology, 47,* 237–252.

Wright, J. C., & Mischel, W. (1987). A conditional approach to dispositional constructs: The local predictability of social behavior. *Journal of Personality and Social Psychology, 53,* 1159–1177.

Wyer, R. S., Bodenhausen, G. V., & Srull, T. K. (1984). The cognitive representation of persons and groups and its effect on recall and recognition memory. *Journal of Experimental Social Psychology, 20,* 445–469.

Wyer, R. S., & Carlston, D. E. (1994). The cognitive representation of persons and events. In R. S. Wyer, Jr. & T. K. Srull (Eds.), *Handbook of social cognition: Basic processes* (pp. 41–98). Hillsdale, NJ: Erlbaum.

10

Dual-Processing Accounts of Inconsistencies in Responses to General versus Specific Cases

STEVEN J. SHERMAN
DENISE R. BEIKE
KENNETH R. RYALLS

Walking through the Anne Frank House in Amsterdam is a chilling experience. Here is the room where Anne Frank slept. Here is where she wrote in her diary every day. Here is the very wall on which she pasted pictures of movie stars. Here is the window out of which she looked longingly at the trees in bloom in the spring, wishing she could leave her prison of a house. And here is where she was dragged off to a concentration camp and to her death.

Walking through the Anne Frank House is also a curious experience. One little girl and her simple diary—and so much human impact. One story out of so many broad descriptions of the Holocaust—and so much interest. Hundreds of other books have been written about the atrocities of the Nazi occupation, about the concentration camps, and about the horrible medical experiments and techniques of torture. And yet this one book by one girl has been translated into virtually every language and has sold more copies than all the historical documentations of the Nazi occupation combined. More people, in fact, visit this one house than any other site in Amsterdam, a city of countless museums and of much history.

It is observations such as this that led to the thinking that has gone into this chapter—observations in which specific instances seem to have quite different impacts and effects on thoughts, feelings, judgments, and behaviors than do general or abstract cases. Specific instances and general cases are different in the ways in which they touch both the mind and the heart. Before we begin to delve into a discussion of the processes that may underlie such differences, we might do well to document some of the other observations that have served to stimulate and direct our thinking. What these observations seem to share is that all of them reflect a difference in the way individuals make judgments of or responses to specific or particular occurrences and instances, as opposed to more general, global, or holistic instances. Even when the general case is simply a collection of a number of known and identifiable specific instances, there seem to be some important specifiable differences in how people think about and deal with these different levels of specificity and generality.[1]

1. *Bush loses to "the Democratic nominee," but defeats each and every viable specific candidate.* In the spring of 1992, it was clear that George Bush would be the Republican nominee for U.S. President. The Democratic convention had not yet taken place, and it was still very unclear who the Democratic nominee would be. A clear and finite number of candidates had been identified—Clinton, Kerry, Gephardt, Harkin, Brown, and Tsongas. At this time, several political polls were taken. In one type of poll, voters were asked to choose between Bush and "the Democratic nominee" (whoever that might be) if the election were held today. This general, unspecified, abstract Democratic nominee beat Bush consistently. Other polls asked the same question of voters, but pitted Bush against some specific potential nominee. Bush consistently beat each and every specifically identified Democratic opponent.

2. *"Not in my back yard."* As a city council representative, one of us is struck time and again by the great difference in the way that constituents consider a general community principle and the way that they make judgments about a specific proposal that instantiates that principle. For example, most citizens endorse the idea of mixed zoning rather than total separation and isolation of residential, commercial, industrial, and business zones. And yet when any specific plan emerges to bring a neighborhood commercial development into a particular residential setting, the inhabitants line up at meetings in droves to protest about how such a development would interfere with their property rights and their quality of life. This "not in my back yard" (NIMBY) philosophy shows very dramatically the disjunctures in judgment that occur between general policy principles and specific plans.

3. *The girl in the well.* It is typically difficult to convince people to donate money to charities or causes that will deliver global assistance to an abstractly identified general population, such as "the starving children of the world." And yet every so often a case of a specific needy child comes to the attention of the mass media. For example, several

years ago a little girl from Texas fell into a well and was stuck there for quite a long time. For specific cases such as this, people send millions of dollars in cash and gifts, even when such giving is unsolicited. This phenomenon is not limited to cases of human need. People will donate large amounts of money to help rescue a specific few whales that are pictured in the media and are stranded near a beach (even though these whales are likely to die in any case), and yet will not donate a dime to a general "save the whales" cause.

4. *Mr. Butts.* In the *Doonesbury* cartoon depicted in Figure 10.1, Garry Trudeau illustrates the difference in the way we think about individual, idiosyncratic cases as opposed to general principles or abstract statistical averages. This particular demonstration—focusing on the general principle that cigarette smoking is harmful to health, as opposed to the likelihood that any specific smoker may be adversely affected—has been verified in research that shows differences between smokers' general beliefs about the risks of smoking and their risk assessments of their own health (Matthews & Piper, 1974). It is, of course, quite rational to differentiate a judgment of a specific case from an average general principle when there is diagnostic information about the specific case. However, as we know from years of research on the underutilization of base rates (Bar-Hillel, 1990; Kahneman & Tversky, 1973), people seem to ignore general principles and general information in the judgment of specific cases, even when the information about these individual cases is quite undiagnostic.

5. *Failure rates versus specific instances of failure.* In the achievement realm, where outcomes can be classified as successes or failures, there appears to be a substantial difference in the way that people respond emotionally to general or global levels of outcome as opposed to specific instances of success or failure. For example, surgeons may be quite willing to accept a general failure rate of 10% for a difficult operation. Yet they may also respond to any specific failure of this operation with feelings of frustration, anger, or guilt. Similarly, a college basketball coach may gladly accept a preseason offer of a turnover rate of 7 per game. Yet even when the specific circumstances of any game or season are well

Doonesbury

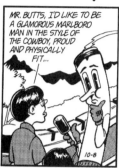
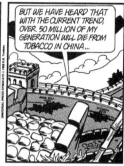
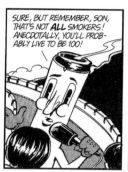
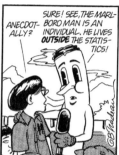

FIGURE 10.1. Mr. Butts, a recurring character in Garry Trudeau's *Doonesbury*, demonstrates a focus on the individual case rather than on the statistics. *Doonesbury* © G. B. Trudeau. Reprinted with permission of Universal Press Syndicate. All rights reserved.

within these acceptable limits, this coach will react quite negatively to specific errors and turnovers. He or she may scream, grimace, and even throw chairs when errors or bad outcomes occur, and may punish players for these errors. The players themselves will also experience regret, dissatisfaction, and guilt for errors, turnovers, or missed free throws. In other words, people express a variety of negative emotions following specific failure experiences, despite their understanding, that at a general level some such failures are inevitable.

6. *Overconfidence in judgments, but only for specific items.* It is a well-documented fact that the probabilities of correctness that people assign to questions of general knowledge are too high by a substantial amount (Lichtenstein, Fischhoff, & Phillips, 1982). For example, Sniezek, Paese, and Switzer (1990) reported a mean subjective probability for specific items of general knowledge in the range of .67. Yet subjects were correct on only 41% of the items. On the other hand, when subjects were asked not about individual items but about their general overall success across an entire array of items (an aggregate performance estimate), not only did they fail to show overconfidence, but they were in fact quite a bit underconfident (Sniezek et al., 1990). In addition, the correlation between subjective probabilities for individual items and a global assessment of performance was essentially zero. In other words, people seem to have low confidence in their assessment of general ability in a task, but high confidence about each and every item that makes up the task—another instance of a disjunction in the way that people think about general versus specific instances.

From this set of observations, it should be apparent that responses to specific cases can often be quite different from, and incompatible with, responses to global or abstract cases. Moreover, these incompatibilities seem to exist across a number of different response measures. The examples of Bush versus the Democrats and the NIMBY principle show that *attitudes* toward general versus specific cases can be quite different. The Mr. Butts cartoon and the overconfident responses for specific items, but not for general estimates, demonstrate discrepancies for *nonevaluative judgments*. The reactions to general failure rates versus specific instances of failure, as well as the observations of the impact of Anne Frank, the girl in the well, and the stranded whales, dramatically demonstrate the differences in *emotional reactions* to specific as opposed to general instances of negative outcomes. In addition, all of the examples imply that different *behavioral consequences* can be expected for specific versus general cases, based on the differences in attitudinal, judgmental, and emotional responses.

Beginning with these examples, and recognizing that in one way or another they all illustrate an inconsistency in responses to general versus specific cases, we now begin to pursue the possible mechanisms underlying such inconsistencies. Two of these possibilities are discussed only briefly and superficially. The third, a dual-process approach, is most relevant to this text, and it is put forth in much greater detail.

INTEGRATION–DEGRADATION

One class of explanations for inconsistencies in responses to general versus specific instances involves processes of "integration" and "degradation"—how people put parts together to form a whole, and how they dissect a whole into its component parts. According to this class of explanation, if integration and degradation strategies were complete, rational, and unbiased, no discrepancies would exist between the judgments of the whole and the judgments of its parts. However, we know that there are numerous biases and a lack of completeness in both kinds of strategies. In the area of integration strategies (Anderson, 1965, 1981, 1988), it is clear that averaging and weighted-averaging strategies can lead to a judgment of the whole that does not closely resemble the judgment of any of the component parts. In addition, judges may combine pieces of information according to a faulty integration strategy. For example, Lichtenstein, Earle, and Slovic (1975) reported that subjects generally used an averaging rule for combining items of diagnostic information, rather than a normatively appropriate rule that involved the multiplication of likelihood ratios. This led to global judgments that were far too conservative. Troutman and Shanteau (1977) found that subjects often used irrelevant specific cues to arrive at a global or general judgment. Such dilution effects occur only when the implications of the nondiagnostic information are less extreme than the implications of the diagnostic information (Zukier & Jennings, 1983–1984), and this may have been the case for several of the examples presented earlier. Finally, Higgins and Rholes (1976) discuss overassimilation effects, in which the judgment of the whole can be more extreme than the judgment of any of its parts.

With regard to degradation strategies, several recent models address the process by which wholes are decomposed into their parts, and demonstrate how inconsistencies between judgments of general cases and specific instances may occur. Fiedler and Armbruster (1994) report that estimates of the frequency of a whole category are substantially less than estimates of the frequencies of the parts composing the whole. For example, subjects who are asked to estimate the number of Japanese cars in the United States will give a significantly lower estimate than subjects who are asked to estimate the number of Nissans, Toyotas, Hondas, and so forth (and then to sum these estimates). Fiedler and Armbruster (1994) use an information loss approach that depends on random error in recall plus the tendency of frequency estimates to regress to the mean, in order to account for the significantly larger estimates for the parts than for the global whole. Tversky and Koehler (1994) are also concerned with the degradation of wholes into their component parts. They suggest that incomplete "unpacking" of the whole into its parts can lead to discrepancies in judgments. When subjects fail to completely unpack a global set when making judgments of the whole, the frequency of the whole will be less than the sum of the frequencies of the parts. Incomplete unpacking can explain several of the observations presented at the beginning of this chapter. For example, subjects may have unpacked the "Democratic nominee" into only their first and second favorites, leaving all subjects with a very attractive "Democratic candidate." But each specific candidate may have been objectionable to a large proportion of the subjects who were polled.

In short, the processes by which perceivers integrate specifics into a global judgment, or decompose global entities into their component parts, can lead in predictable ways to incompatible judgmental responses to general cases versus specific instances. These processes can result in a whole that is either more or less extreme than the parts of which it is composed.

REPRESENTATION

A second class of explanations for general–specific mismatches is that of differential cognitive representation. The cognitive traces of general and specific items may be different in any number of the ways in which memory representations differ from one another. These differences may include differing amounts of detail in the representation, the closeness of association between this representation and other traces, the presence or absence of certain features (e.g., affective tags), representation in different types of systems, and so on. To the extent that general entities are represented cognitively in a qualitatively (not just quantitatively) different way from specific entities, responses based on these retrieved traces are likely to be inconsistent with one another.

One basic way in which specific versus general information is represented differently is in terms of the abstract versus concrete nature of the representation. There is much support for the idea that abstract and concrete information is represented and handled in different ways by the human cognitive system, leading to differential accessibility and different subjective experiences of the two types of information. These differences can serve as the basis for the inconsistencies of responses that we attempt to explain in this chapter. For example, stereotypes appear to apply more readily to abstract than to concrete representations (Nisbett, Zukier, & Lemley, 1981). Similarly, base rate information is more likely to be applied to social targets that are represented abstractly as opposed to concretely (Tversky & Kahneman, 1982). Concrete and specific entities inspire more flexible, context-dependent judgments than abstract, general entities, which are easier to judge via context-insensitive precomputed expectancies. In addition, more affect, imagery, and self-relevance seem to be tied to the representation of concrete information (Nisbett & Ross, 1980), again leading to differences in responses toward these entities as opposed to abstract instances.

Tulving's (1983) distinction between "episodic" and "semantic" representations is also relevant. Episodic memories are engaged for specific instances, and these memories are experiential, self-referenced, contextual, and affective. They are retrieved more deliberately and are experienced as information "remembered." Semantic memories are engaged for generalities, and these are symbolic, universe-referenced, context-free, and affectless. They

are retrieved automatically and are experienced as information "known." Thus, knowledge about the plight of poor children is stored in semantic memory, whereas an encounter with a specific unfortunate child is stored in episodic memory. Because episodic memory involves self-relevance and has close ties with autobiographical memory (Brewer, 1986), episodic representations are more likely to inspire action, especially action that is not filtered through rational contemplation.

Another cognitive-representational approach to explaining general–specific incongruities is found in the literature on hierarchical representation (Collins & Quillian, 1967; Rosch, 1978). Representations of concepts at the basic level are easier to access and to use, as well as being more informative in terms of amount of featural information. We suggest that specific instances are more likely to be represented at the basic level, whereas generalities more often are represented at the superordinate level. Thus, accessing a generality requires "moving up" a level of abstraction and thereby losing featural information. The features must be actively retrieved, which takes processing time and effort. As the basic level is the more common one for perception and categorization, it is also the level at which attitudes toward the objects are most likely to be automatized. The "motivation and opportunity as determinants" (MODE) model (Fazio, 1990) suggests that the strength of an attitude is determined by the strength of association in long-term memory between the object and its corresponding evaluation. Objects at the basic level, because their representations are more frequently accessed, should be more frequently associated with their attitudes, and thus attitudes to specific cases are more likely to be automatically activated. This further implies that attitudes associated with specific objects are more likely to guide behavior than are attitudes associated with general-level objects.

Finally, Gelman and Markman (1987) distinguish between "natural kinds" and "artificial kinds." Natural kinds have an essential nature that affords fast and confident inferences about other category members. We believe that specific cases are more likely to be perceived and represented as natural kinds than general cases are. This would imply that greater predictability for the future can be made for specific instances and that a greater number of inferences will be made for such instances.

In sum, specifics tend to have a richer and more complex representation, whereas generalities tend to be represented more vaguely and are one step removed from the basic level of operation. This abstract, semantic, and superordinate representation results in a phenomenal experience of difficult retrieval, little information on which to base inferences, difficult mapping to actions, and personal irrelevance. Specifics, on the other hand, are more associated with the self and have more affect associated with the representation. These representational differences can lead to strikingly different response outputs for general items in contrast to specific cases.

DUAL PROCESSING

The third class of explanations that can help us to understand why different and sometimes inconsistent responses are made for general as opposed to specific cases involves differences in the ways that general and specific types of information are processed. Here we consider the idea that two different types of information processing are involved—one for general or abstract information and another for specific instances. None of the currently prevalent dual-process models directly addresses the issue of alternative systems for processing general as opposed to specific information, and none explicitly claims that information of a general nature is processed by one of the two modes of the particular model, whereas information of a more specific nature is processed by the other mode. However, we believe that there is a relationship between the degree of generality of information and the likelihood that this information will be processed by one mode or another, and we believe that several dual-process models can be fruitfully applied to this issue.

If indeed different modes of processing are engaged for general versus specific cases, then it should not be surprising that attitudes, judgments, and emotions toward these two types of cases may be quite different and seemingly inconsistent. In considering each potentially applicable dual-process model (many of which are considered in greater detail in other chapters of this volume), we shall try to indicate which mode of processing is likely to be engaged by specific instances and which mode by general, abstract instances. Furthermore, we shall try to indicate what implications this should have for the kinds of responses given to specific versus general cases. Finally, we shall attempt to apply these analyses in order to understand some of the observations of disjunctures in responses to specific and general cases with which we have begun this chapter.

The Use of Comparison Cases: Prior Expectancies versus Postevent Constructions

When people try to understand, judge, or provide causal explanations for events, they often must depend on a comparison case or cases in order to provide a standard or a context for judgment. Which comparison case is adopted will very much affect the judgment or interpretation of the target event, as well as the evaluative, affective, and behavioral responses to the event. Several approaches have suggested that the usual, prototypic, or expected case is often chosen as the comparison or background case (Hesslow, 1983; Hilton & Slugoski, 1986). Evaluative or causal judgments will then depend on the ways in which and the degree to which the target case deviates from the expected case.

Kahneman and Miller (1986) suggest an alternative approach to the development and selection of a comparison case. According to their norm theory, each episode suggests and recruits its own idiosyncratic comparison case. This comparison case is constructed in an ad hoc manner after the event rather than in advance, and does not preexist as an expectation. Each event brings its own comparison standard into being. This postevent comparison case will share certain features with the target case and will differ on other features. It will differ from the target case according to the features of the target that appear most mutable (nonessential) to the perceiver. Thus, the rules that govern mutability are what guide the construction of the comparison case. And, again, as with the use of preexisting expectancies, different comparison cases will lead to different judgments and interpretations of the target case.

In applying Kahneman and Miller's (1986) norm theory to causal explanations, McGill (1989, 1993) demonstrated that individuals who are confronted with the same target event but who utilize different comparison cases (through experimental manipulation, individual differences, or situational constraints) come to quite different explanations of the event. For example, actors tend to compare their own behavior to another instance of their own behavior in some other situation. On the other hand, observers tend to compare the behavior of an actor with the behavior of some other actor in the same situation (McGill, 1989). This difference in the construction of a comparison context can explain the classic attributional differences between actors and observers (Jones & Nisbett, 1971). When McGill (1989) controlled for the comparison case that was employed, actor–observer differences disappeared.

Thus, which comparison case is used for understanding an event and whether that comparison case preexists as an expectancy or is computed after the fact as it is recruited by the episode will very much affect the interpretation of and the responses to the event. The use of preexisting expectancies and the computation of postevent comparison cases can be considered as alternative (or dual) processes that are employed in the understanding and explanation of events. The former involves a straightforward memory process in which the trace of an expectancy for the current situation is activated. This trace has been stored on the basis of prior experience and should capture the usual or typical circumstances or outcomes that occur. The development of such expectancies should be similar to the processes involved in the development and storage of any schema, script, or prototype.

For the computation of postevent comparison cases, the process depends less on memory and more on active construction. There are no stored abstract representations to consider, as each event is different in suggesting its own idiosyncratic comparison case. The process involves the mutation of certain features of the event, so that a novel comparison event is generated, depending on which of the features are most easily psychologically altered.

The use of preexisting expectancies should be quite rapid, efficient, and stable. As an abstracted, expected case, the same comparison alternative should be generated for a rather large variety of generally similar events. On the other hand, the computation of postevent comparison cases is likely to involve a slower and less stable process. Here the generation of a comparison case will be unique to the event itself, and will depend on the perceived mutability of the features of the event, as well as on the accessibility of features based on chronic individual differences or on the recent priming of features.

Once a comparison case has been generated (through either the process of expectancy retrieval or "on-the-fly" computation), the comparison process itself is likely to be similar in the two cases. Deviations of the target episode from the comparison case will be noted, and these deviations will determine one's satisfaction with, affect toward, and causal interpretation of the target episode.

How might this process distinction be relevant for our understanding of responses to general versus specific cases? We argue that specific instances with their identifiable and unique features afford comparison cases constructed after the event, such as Kahneman and Miller (1986) discuss. The unusual or salient features of the specific target event will be mutated to yield alternative possible events. These events will serve as comparison cases for the target episode. On the other hand, general cases have fewer particular or unique features that can be mutated. In this case, it is more likely that preexisting, preevent expectancies will be used as comparison standards. The processing difference therefore involves a differential reliance on exemplars versus prototypes. In norm theory, an event evokes its own comparison exemplars, based on similarity, salience, or accessibility, and these exemplars are integrated to construct a norm for the various attributes of the target event. This norm in turn serves as a standard for judging the abnormality and inevitability of the event. An exemplar model of this type involves on-line computation and context sensitivity. The event acts as a memory probe, which serves as a reminder of similar experiences from the past. However, it is likely that similar exemplars and experiences can be activated and recruited only when the target event has specific characteristics and features. In the absence of such specific features, a generalized instance will establish no postevent comparison case, and it is more likely that (the prototype) category knowledge will be used as a standard for judging the target event.

What are the implications of using preexisting expectancies for general cases but postevent computations of specific comparison standards for specific cases? The key is that the postevent alternatives that are generated according to the processes specified by norm theory often involve the construction of counterfactual alternatives to real experience, in relation to which the target event is judged. These counterfactual alternatives to reality indicate to a perceiver what could have been, what might have been, and what should have been. Judgments of real events and affective reactions toward these events are very much affected by this mutation of conditions. For example, counterfactual alternatives are easier to generate following actions as opposed to inactions. Thus, those who experience negative outcomes based on an action will feel greater regret than will those who experience the same negative outcomes based on an inaction (Kahneman & Miller, 1986; Landman, 1988). This is due to the ease of generating or retrieving the counterfactual world afforded by a specific action event. Without a counterfactual world constructed after an event, affective reactions to the event will not be as extreme, and judgments will not be based on considerations of "what could have been" or "what should have been." This is likely to be the case for general or abstract events, where salient or mutable features are difficult to find.

The idea that counterfactual generation is likely to occur for specific cases but not for general cases can help us understand some of the important differences in responses to general versus specific cases. Consider the example of the acceptance of a 10% overall failure rate, but the lack of acceptance of any specific failure. In basketball, when a 90% free-throw shooter hits 9 shots and misses the 10th, coaches, fans, and shooter alike will be disappointed with the miss. We argue that this acceptance of general levels of failure and lack of acceptance of specific failure experiences is due to the difference in the ease with which counterfactual alternatives can be generated

as contrast comparison cases. General cases and global achievement outcomes do not easily afford counterfactual alternatives, which require the mutation of specific circumstances, behaviors, or choices. The notion of a 10% failure rate or a turnover average of 7 per game do not allow for the development of a counterfactual comparison case. The comparison case here is likely to be the general rate based on one's prior expectancies, and judgments of acceptability or satisfaction will depend only on the direction and extent of deviation of the outcome from this preexisting expectation. However, for any specific negative experience, a mutation that would have undone some particular feature or circumstance is often easy to generate. For example, for a specific error in baseball or softball, an infielder may have failed to keep his or her head down, to set his or her feet before throwing, or to be in position to make the right play. That is, the contrast case is a perfect play rather than a 95% perfect record. The ease of mutating specific features of the play causes the specific error to appear unnecessary and avoidable, and this in turn leads to affective reactions such as frustration, anger, or embarrassment.

Thus, the counterfactual generations that follow specific failures are likely to be one reason why specific negative occurrences are more difficult to accept and are reacted to more strongly than are global levels of failure. Unfortunately, as people generate counterfactual alternatives following specific negative experiences, and as they imagine how these negative outcomes need not have occurred, they further assume that what *need* not have occurred *should* not have occurred. This confusion of what might have been with what should have been has been termed the "counterfactual fallacy" by Miller and Turnbull (1990). Such a tendency will cause people to judge the quality of thinking and the competence of the decision maker solely by the outcome of the specific decision, rather than on the basis of the antecedent conditions or of the generally expected outcome (Baron & Hershey, 1988). This inability to recognize that bad outcomes can follow good decision strategies can lead people to change good strategies into bad ones. Thus, the tendency to respond to specific failures with counterfactual alternatives can lead both to heightened negative emotions and to poor subsequent decisions.

In fact, people may actually feel better and function more effectively if they can simply accept specific negative outcomes and failures (especially if these failures are within an acceptable general level of occurrence) as inevitable and unavoidable, and move on to the next decision. Those decision makers who can avoid the counterfactual alternatives to specific failures may be in the best position, both cognitively and emotionally, to render good subsequent decisions. For example, Tony LaRussa, the very successful manager of the Oakland A's and now of the St. Louis Cardinals, seems to be one of those rare managers who does not cringe or scream or bang his fists when a relief pitcher is hammered or a defensive replacement makes an error. It is possible that a decision maker's lack of reactivity to each and every specific negative outcome, and the tendency not to generate counterfactual alternatives to such specific outcomes, are related to subsequent success rate.

In short, specific as opposed to abstract or general events recruit similar prior events and experiences that serve as comparison standards. These standards are experienced as counterfactual alternatives to reality—as worlds that could have or should have happened. In turn, the presence of counterfactual alternatives where outcomes have been changed is a key component to the level of affect or emotion that an event evokes. In fact, many theories of emotion (Abelson, 1983; Kahneman & Miller, 1986; Niedenthal, Tangney, & Gavanski, 1994) maintain that alternatives to reality determine the type and degree of emotion experienced, and stress the role of counterfactual alternatives in affective experience. Because generalized events do not readily evoke counterfactual alternatives, both the judgments of these events and the emotional experiences surrounding the event will differ from the judgments of and reactions to more specific events.

The type of difference in the processing of general versus specific information based on the generation of different comparison cases is similar in many respects to the process distinction employed by Sniezek and Buckley (1991) to account for why people are overconfident about the accuracy of their judgments for specific items, but are not overconfident for judgments of their general ability across an entire set of items. For example, in estimations of answers to specific problems (e.g., the total current value of the university's land), subjects set 90% confidence intervals for each item, whereas only 22.5%(!) of these contained the actual value of the estimated variable. However, subjects' mean global confidence about their accuracy across all items showed significantly less overconfidence, and the mean of the confidence ratings for specific items was significantly higher than the global confidence rating.

Sniezek and Buckley (1991) argue that the assessments of judgment quality for specific events and for global performance are fundamentally different and involve unique psychological processes. For single, specific items (e.g., "Is absinthe a jewel or an alcoholic drink?"), confidence is determined by the amount of item-specific evidence that one can gather in support of an answer. And for any item, a memory search (perhaps a biased search) can bring to mind facts that would support one or another answer (e.g., "I think that I remember a bar in New Orleans called The Olde Absinthe Bar," "Absinthe contains the word 'sin,' and so probably applies to liquor"). As we know from work on hypothesis confirmation biases and positive-test strategies (Klayman & Ha, 1987), people generally generate support in favor of whatever hypothesis is being entertained. Koriat, Lichtenstein, and Fischhoff (1980) suggest that when subjects are working on a specific knowledge problem to solve, they begin with a random search for information, find an initial cue that one of the alternatives is correct, set up that alternative as the focal hypothesis, engage in a biased information search for supportive evidence, ignore the alternative answers, and end up very confident that their answer is correct.

Such a process is not possible for global judgments, where specific supporting evidence elicited by a particular item cannot be part of the process. Rather, one must make the assessment by depending more on general expectations for and memories of one's global attributes and skills in the area, task difficulty, luck, and so on. These general expectations are stored as abstract representations based on one's past experiences and past performances, and they include global notions about self-relevant traits and tendencies. This difference in processes has much in common with the two different ways in which comparison cases can be generated for the assessment of an event (prior expectancies vs. postevent computations), and it clearly indicates how one can have low confidence in one's global performance on a task and yet high confidence for each and every item that makes up the task.

Assimilation versus Contrast, and Construal Processes

The preceding discussion about comparison cases indicates that different comparison alternatives are used in dealing with general instances as opposed to specific events. Prior expectancies are more likely to be employed as comparison cases for general events, whereas postevent counterfactual worlds are more likely to be constructed for the purpose of comparison with specific cases. We now shall consider the situation where researchers control for and provide exactly the same comparison alternative for a general and for a specific case. Interestingly, we believe that other processing differences may play a role, so that reactions to general versus specific events will still differ, given the identical comparison case. Consider a study by Schwarz and Bless (1992a), who primed subjects with examples of sleazy and scandalous politicians. Having been thus primed, subjects then evaluated the trustworthiness of politicians in general or the trustworthiness of three specific politicians. The priming of scandalous politicians decreased the evaluations of trustworthiness of politicians in general, but increased the perceived trustworthiness of specific individual politicians.

According to Schwarz and Bless, the primed sleazy political figures served as a standard for subsequent judgments. For the judgment of the general category of politicians, this standard became a salient part of the identity and definition of the term "politician," and the general case was assimilated to this target. In this case, the task of the subjects was to identify and characterize this term—to find its meaning as a category (Herr, 1986; Herr, Sherman, & Fazio, 1983). The fact that the general case of politicians was

ambiguous and open to several different definitions and interpretations allowed this definition to change, depending on recent and frequent activation of category attributes such as sleaziness or activation of specific sleazy exemplars, and assimilation to these activated attributes or exemplars was the outcome. For the judgments of specific and unambiguously defined cases, on the other hand, the primed examples served as anchors against which the specific cases were judged. The outcome of this process was contrast away from the anchor (Schwarz & Bless, 1992b). Compared to these sleazy politicians, the current specific cases seemed quite positive and trustworthy by contrast.

The processes of assimilation and contrast have indeed been characterized as dual processes, rather than as differential judgment outcomes that occur as a consequence of a single underlying process (Herr, 1986; Martin, 1986; Wedell, Parducci, & Geiselman, 1987). For example, according to Martin (1986), assimilation results from using a primed concept for categorization, which usually occurs spontaneously. Contrast results from an attempt to refrain from using a primed concept, which usually requires more attention and effort. Others have proposed that contrast may occur more spontaneously than assimilation (Petty & Wegener, 1993). In either set of circumstances, however, assimilation and contrast operate as separate processes, with one process engaged as a correction for the other.

Interestingly, not only does the priming of an identical event lead to the differential processes and outcomes of assimilation and contrast for general versus specific instances; the priming of a general event leads to the assimilation of a subsequently presented target stimulus, whereas the priming of a specific instance leads to the contrasting of that very same subsequently presented target stimulus (Stapel, Koomen, & van der Pligt, 1996). Thus, general instances compel assimilation, whereas specific cases compel contrast, regardless of whether the general and specific cases are the primes or the targets to be judged. As indicated, these effects are consistent with models of social judgment (e.g., Herr et al., 1983) that predict assimilation effects for ambiguous stimuli (such as general cases) where identification is necessary and construal plays a role, but that predict contrast effects for unambiguous stimuli (specific cases) based on a different process that involves anchoring effects.

This difference in the social judgment process for general versus specific cases can lead to situations where the evaluation of each and every specific case is quite positive (or quite negative), and yet the evaluation of the general case is negative (or positive). In other words, the differential operation of the processes involved in contrast and assimilation can lead to very different and even opposite evaluations of specific and general cases. For example, consider the case where George Bush lost to "the Democratic candidate" in the polls, but beat each and every specific candidate. If we assume that past positive political heroes are often invoked during an election year, it is likely that voters were primed with well-respected party members prior to the polls. According to Schwarz and Bless (1992a), this would have led to a positive evaluation of a party in general due to assimilation effects (and thus Bush lost to the general Democratic nominee), but would have led to a negative evaluation of any specific party member due to contrast effects (and thus Bush beat specific nominees).

These findings with regard to assimilation and contrast processes raise the broader point that general cases are typically more ambiguous than specific instances, and require categorization and identification. General cases are thus open to a rather wide variety of definitions and interpretations, whereas specific cases are usually well defined. The terms "Democratic nominee" and "athlete" may be interpreted in very different ways by different individuals, or even by the same individual at different points in time. On the other hand, "Bill Clinton" and "Pete Rose" are not easily open to a variety of definitions or interpretations. The consideration of differential susceptibility to multiple construals can help to account for certain differences in responses to general and specific cases.

Let us consider a series of studies reported by Gilovich (1990). Gilovich was interested in explaining the "false-consensus effect"—the tendency for people to believe that their opinions, preferences, values, and attributes are rather widely shared throughout the population. Thus, individuals who themselves prefer vacations in Europe to vacations in South America believe that more people in the general population also prefer vacations in Europe (compared to estimates by those individuals who prefer vacations in South America). Similarly, individuals who prefer the music of the 1960s to the music of the 1980s give higher estimates of the percentage of 1960s preferrers than do individuals who prefer the music of the 1980s. Gilovich accounted for this finding by noting that a false-consensus effect usually occurs only for estimates of general kinds of preferences or beliefs (e.g., European vacations, music of the 1960s). He found that different individuals construed these general terms in very different ways. For example, subjects who preferred 1960s music construed 1960s music to consist of talented groups such as The Beatles, whereas subjects who preferred 1980s music construed 1960s music to consist of less talented groups such as The Monkees. When general terms such as "1960s music" were used in these experiments, large false-consensus effects were observed. However, when Gilovich presented subjects with very specific exemplars, the size of the false-consensus effect diminished markedly. Thus, an important difference in the way that general versus specific items are responded to in terms of frequency estimations across a large number of respondents may be due to the fact that general cases are construed in a large variety of ways, whereas specific cases are construed very similarly across the whole population.

The process of identifying, construing, or categorizing an object is an important part of the determination of an emotional, evaluative, or judgmental response toward that object. Specific items are usually easily and quickly identified. This process is likely to be automatic and effortless, and will result in the same categorization across a wide range of respondents. For abstract and general instances, on the other hand, with the large degree of ambiguity involved, the process of identification and construal is likely to be rather slow and effortful. As we have pointed out earlier, automatically activated evaluative responses or categorizations are less likely to develop for general cases than for specific instances. In addition, there are likely to be differences in the construal of the same general item, and thus far more variability in the identification of and in responses to general items than specific instances.

What is likely to determine the particular construal that will be applied to a general object or concept? First, there are important cognitive aspects to construal, and these operate for both general and specific instances. These aspects involve the degree to which the object matches various category representations that are in one's head. In general, there will be a larger variety of "good" or "acceptable" matches for general than for specific cases, and thus greater differential construal for general instances. In addition, the recent and frequent activation or priming of certain categories and exemplars will affect the identification of both general and specific objects. Thus, a round yellow blob is more likely to be identified as a lemon than as a tennis ball if the match between the blob and one's representation of a lemon is better and/or if there has been recent activation of other fruits as opposed to sports objects. If the construal of objects (both general and specific objects) depended only on these kinds of cognitive factors, then one might well argue that there are not alternative processing systems involved. These processes of categorization and construal would seem like differential outcomes involving only a single underlying process.

However, because of the ambiguity of general cases, there is also the opportunity for motivational factors to enter into the construal process. Motivated distortions, categorizations, and construals are far less likely to occur in the case of unambiguous specific instances. We would thus argue that the inclusion of motivated reasoning in the disambiguation of general cases renders it quite a different process from the one involved in the unmotivated reasoning that characterizes the categorization of specific instances.

Recall again the finding that Bush lost in the polls to "the Democratic nominee" but beat every specific opponent. Specific opponents were not open to differential motivated construals of identity: Bill Clinton is Bill Clinton, and Jerry Brown is Jerry Brown. However, "the Democratic nominee" was ambiguous as to identity. It is possible that most subjects construed "the Democratic nominee" to be their favorite Democratic candidate,

based on their preferences and motivations. If the respondents in the polls differed greatly in their preferred Democratic candidate, and if each respondent preferred only one (or two) Democratic candidates to Bush but preferred Bush to all the other Democratic candidates, the seeming inconsistency in the polls for general versus specific cases makes sense. The motivated-construal processes involved in the identification of a general term are what allow for the differential reactions to general and specific instances.

In a similar way, many findings in the stereotype literature demonstrate very different responses to the general case (e.g., blacks, businesswomen), as opposed to responses to a specific black person or a specific businesswoman. Many years ago, LaPiere (1934) demonstrated a seeming inconsistency in responses to an Asian couple. When LaPiere telephoned a number of hotels and restaurants, told the managers that he was traveling in their city with an Asian couple, and asked whether this couple would be accommodated, many respondents said "no." On the other hand, when LaPiere simply showed up at these very same restaurants and hotels with the actual Asian couple, the couple was given accommodations nearly 100% of the time. Why was a specific Asian couple treated differently from the general category of Asian couples? One likely answer lies in the processes of construal. It is possible that the hotel and restaurant managers' construal of the ambiguous term "Asian couple" was a poorly dressed, uneducated, sneaky pair of people. The specific couple that accompanied LaPiere and showed up at the hotel or restaurant was not subject to construal on the basis of abstract, stereotypic information, but was categorized on the basis of the specific facts at hand. The two people were well dressed, educated, and friendly. In other words, base rate information is used for the construal or categorization of general instances, whereas individuated information is used more for specific instances (Krueger & Rothbart, 1988). Thus, the managers were not responding to the same stimulus when they considered the general concept over the telephone as opposed to the specific case that showed up in person. It is not clear whether the differences in the LaPiere experiment were based on motivational processes that operated only in the general case (over the telephone) or on purely cognitive processes, but in any case there is certainly sufficient evidence for the role of motivation in construal and judgment, and for the position that such motivated distortions represent quite different psychological processes from those involved in cognitively based distortions (Kunda, 1990).

Another area where differential processes of construal can account for disjunctures between reactions to general and specific cases involves the difficulty that people have in predicting their own future behavior. Sherman (1980) has shown that subjects are quite inaccurate in predicting behaviors such as future willingness to devote time to a charity or to participate in a psychology experiment. In responding to the hypothetical general case, no doubt subjects are motivated to think of themselves and to present themselves in the most positive light. Thus, they predict that in general they will be helpful. The actual situation, however, will usually occur at a time when such motivations are overridden by the specific factors surrounding the request. Thus, subjects actually agree to very little help in the specific case. In addition to these differences in the operation of social desirability motives, the construal of the general hypothetical situation where "someone calls and asks you to devote an afternoon's time to collecting money for charity" is likely to be quite different (strictly in terms of cognitive-representational factors) from the actual specific situation that arises when someone actually calls and asks for a specific commitment. In a similar way, most people (wrongly) predict that they would never keep shocking the learner in a Milgram-type study. However, due to both cognitive and motivational factors, their construal of the general situation is often not at all like the actual situation. Subjects omit from their construals such things as the experimenter's air of authority and the pressures to help in a scientific experiment. Thus, people can mispredict their own future behavior because their interpretation and construal of the hypothetical, general future possible case are quite different from what the actual specific situation in the future will actually be like. The incompatibility in response to general and specific cases may thus not be a difference in response to the same stimulus event at different levels of generality, but

rather a difference based on the fact that the stimulus event being responded to is quite different in its perceived characteristics at the ambiguous general level as opposed to the precise specific level.

On-Line versus Memory-Based Processing

Consider the disjuncture between citizens' attitudes toward Congress as a whole (which are quite negative) and their attitudes toward their own representatives (which are very positive and which result in a large advantage for incumbents, despite a general dislike and mistrust of Congress). This is an example of inconsistency between the evaluation of a general group and the evaluations of the specific individuals who constitute the group. Sears (1983) has discussed this phenomenon and labeled it the "person positivity bias." This bias refers to the fact that attitude objects that resemble individual human beings are evaluated more favorably than less person-like attitude objects, such as inanimate objects or aggregates of individuals. Thus individual people are evaluated both more positively than the traits that they possess, and more positively than the groups to which they belong. According to this reasoning, individual members of Congress are evaluated far more positively than is the Congress as a whole.

Sears explains this phenomenon by the degree of personhood or humanness that is inherent in an attitude object. Objects high in personhood are viewed as similar to ourselves, and this similarity promotes liking (Byrne, 1971). Groups or aggregates of individuals have less personhood than specific individual members, and will thus be viewed as less similar to the self and will be more negatively evaluated. Although Sears's (1983) explanation is viable, and he presents evidence that supports his predictions of person positivity bias, we feel that more recent evidence involving differences in processing information about individuals and groups provides a more compelling explanation for the differences observed in the evaluations of individual and group social targets.

Hamilton and Sherman (1996) have considered similarities and differences in the ways in which social perceivers form impressions of individuals as opposed to groups on the basis of behavioral information about those social targets. They delineate important differences in perceivers' assumptions and expectations about individual and group targets. Differences in processing information about these targets ensue, and these can result in inconsistent judgments of groups versus individuals.

According to Hamilton and Sherman (1996), a perceiver confronted with an individual target (as opposed to a group as a target) assumes that the specific individual target person's underlying dispositions are stable and can be discerned from the target's behavior. Furthermore, the perceiver assumes that the specific individual target is consistently behaving in ways that support the underlying disposition of that person. Third, the perceiver assumes an organization in the inherent dispositions of the target, such that one disposition deduced by the perceiver ought to fit with other behaviors and dispositions already observed in that target individual by the perceiver, forming a coherent whole. The three components of stability, consistency, and coherence guide information processing with regard to individuals in meaningful ways.

Because the perceiver expects to find a stable personality in almost every individual, he or she spontaneously attends to that target's behavior with the goal of identifying the dispositions (Anderson, 1981; Carlston & Skowronski, 1994; Uleman, 1987). The formation of a coherent impression and the abstraction of personality traits will allow the perceiver to achieve a degree of predictability and control in interactions with the individual target.

Spontaneous impression formation implies that information about a specific individual is processed on-line (Hastie & Park, 1986), as it is being received, in order to enable the perceiver to form an accurate and immediate impression of the individual target. On-line processing of information, however, is costly. It is often effortful, requiring the commitment of many of the available cognitive resources in order to integrate incoming information as it is received. The cost of engaging in on-line processing is offset by the benefit of apprehending the individual's presumed stable disposition up front and allowing for greater predictability in the future.

Hamilton and Sherman (1996) argue that the assumptions of stability, consistency, and coherence are not held as strongly when

perceivers are dealing with general groups as targets. Because groups are assumed not to be as high in unity, and thus not to possess stable dispositions, a perceiver does not waste time and cognitive energy trying to discern dispositional traits of the group on-line. Instead, the perceiver will wait until it is necessary to make a judgment of the group, and at that point will integrate the behavioral information received earlier into a summary evaluation. Thus, at the time of judgment, the perceiver must attempt to access from memory as much of the previously received behavioral information as possible, and to integrate this available information into an overall judgment or impression. Because of their reliance on the content of recall of previously received information, these judgments of group targets are termed "memory-based judgments" (Hastie & Park, 1986). Of course, the behavioral information that happens to be most salient and accessible at the time of judgment will carry the most weight in such a memory-based judgment. In addition, when judgments are memory-based, there will be a strong relationship between the valence of what is remembered and the valence of the judgment. This is not necessarily the case for on-line judgments, where subsequent memory for information may not correlate with the previously formed impressions.

In short, Hamilton and Sherman (1996) propose on-line impression formation for individuals as targets, and memory-based impressions for groups. Quickly creating an impression of a specific individual who is assumed to have a stable, enduring disposition will facilitate the encoding of incoming information in the future, leading to more efficient processing, and will allow for predictable interactions with the individual. However, creating an on-line impression of a general group is not usually advantageous, as groups are not expected to have underlying general dispositions. Any impression will tend to be formed later, if necessary, from information available in memory at the time of judgment. These ideas can be used to make sense of the findings of empirical work looking into the processing of information about individual as opposed to group social targets. These findings focus on differences in recall for individuals and groups, differences in the extent of illusory-correlation formation for individuals and groups, and differences in judgments of individual and group social targets. These results are summarized in Hamilton and Sherman (1996) and are elaborated further and discussed in terms of dual-process implications in a different chapter in this volume (Hamilton, Sherman, & Maddox, Chapter 30).

Thus, different processing strategies for information about individuals (specific social entities) and groups (general social entities) can account for differences in various judgments of these two types of entities. The process of impression formation involves on-line judgments for individual targets and memory-based judgments for group targets. On-line judgments are characterized by integrative processing as the relevant information is received. This kind of processing includes organization of the information into a coherent structure, evaluation of the target, and the attribution of traits and abilities. Memory-based judgments entail retrieval of whatever information is accessible at the time of judgment, and thus these judgments do not use all the original information. Processes involving forgetting and accessibility play a major role in memory-based judgments. When the preponderance of behaviors about the social target is positive (as is usually the case for perceivers' interactions with people), evaluations based on on-line information integration will generally be very positive. Such evaluations are usually extremitized in the direction of the prevailing information, and thus evaluations of individual social targets are likely to be positive. On the other hand, when evaluations of the social target are memory-based (as is the case for group targets), these evaluations may well be more negative, because negative and distinctive information is often highly accessible, is more memorable, and will carry great weight in the judgment. This difference in processes, then, predicts that individuals will be evaluated more positively than the groups to which they belong, which is precisely what Sears (1983) reported.

Let us thus apply this processing distinction to an analysis of why Congress in general is evaluated so much more negatively than are specific members of Congress. According to our analysis, people process information about the two types of social targets in very different ways. Judgment of specific members

of Congress are in all likelihood created on-line, perhaps during a political debate or while perceivers are listening to speeches. Integrative processing about the individual Congressperson is done on-line as relevant information is received, with an evaluative impression likely to be formed as behaviors and political positions are observed. Because the Congressperson is likely to be good at public relations and at gearing comments to the target audience at hand, the majority of information is likely to be positive, and the on-line manner of judgment will ensure quite a positive evaluation. Whenever voters are asked about any specific Congressperson, they need only retrieve this predetermined evaluation and report that they feel quite positively. Congress, on the other hand, is a diffuse and general group, perhaps perceived as somewhat high in unity, but probably not unified enough for the average perceiver to assume underlying stable group traits. Instead, when confronted with a need to evaluate Congress in general, the perceiver makes a memory-based judgment, attempting to recall information relevant to the judgment currently being made. Negative behaviors will be more accessible, especially the salient negative behaviors popularly reported in the press, such as scandal and wasted taxes. The resulting judgment of Congress is negative, even though the individuals making up the group are looked upon favorably. The memory-based judgment of the general group thus differs in its outcome from the on-line judgments for the individual members of the group.

Central versus Peripheral Processing

The persuasion literature offers us two models that posit dual-processing systems for dealing with information received in a persuasive communication: Petty and Cacioppo's (1981, 1986) elaboration likelihood model (with central and peripheral processing routes), and Chaiken's (1980) heuristic–systematic model. Although there are certain fundamental differences between the two models, they are similar enough that, for the level of our discussion, we will use the terminology employed in Petty and Cacioppo's (1986) model to refer to ideas found in both. These models of persuasion offer evidence of two different types of processing of persuasive arguments, depending on the perceiver's involvement in the topic of the message, as well as the perceiver's ability and capacity to process the message.

Perceivers who are highly involved in the message topic and who have the resources and ability to process the message carefully will be motivated to engage in central-route processing. This involves analyzing the contents of the message deliberatively and thinking about the merits of the arguments rationally and critically. In this case, the strength of the persuasive arguments will determine the amount of persuasion. Central-route processing requires a large degree of cognitive effort, because the facts contained in the message are evaluated for their merits, and the message is analyzed rationally and carefully (Petty & Cacioppo, 1981, 1986).

Peripheral-route processing, on the other hand, involves handling incoming information in a more global fashion, using simplifying heuristics and salient cues in the message to determine the validity of the message. This kind of processing is engaged when one is uninvolved in the topic of the message and/or is unable or unwilling to devote the resources necessary for careful processing of the message content. Peripheral-route processing is done on a more holistic level and relies on the "feel" of the message or on shortcuts that facilitate message processing. The validity of the message content is judged by heuristic principles such as the length of the message or the credibility of the communicator.

There can be significant differences in the judgments and evaluations of a persuasive message, depending on whether central or peripheral processing is engaged. For example, let us consider the case of a persuasive message consisting of a few weak arguments that is delivered by a highly credible source. If this message is processed centrally, its content will be judged as invalid because of the weak arguments, and it will be an ineffective persuasion tool. On the other hand, if the message is processed peripherally, the content will be judged as valid because of the use of source credibility as a heuristic cue. The message will now be an effective persuasion tool. Through similar reasoning, a set of strong arguments presented by a noncredible source will be effective under central processing but ineffective under peripheral processing (Axsom, Yates, & Chaiken, 1987).

This central–peripheral dual-processing model can be used to help understand inconsistencies in responses to general and specific cases. Our assumption from a careful reading of Petty and Cacioppo (1986) is that as a rule, general cases will engage peripheral processing, whereas specific cases will engage central processing. We base this assumption on an application of the differences between general and specific information to several of the important mediating variables in the central–peripheral model. The first mediating variable is affective involvement. We have argued that specific cases usually inspire higher affective involvement with the decision at hand. For instance, it is easy to identify with the suffering of an individual child, but difficult to identify with the global problem of world hunger. Therefore, a decision based on information about a specific starving child will be more personally and affectively involving, and more likely to engage central processing.

The second mediating variable is confidence or certainty. The feeling of certainty or being done with a decision determines the thoroughness of processing, with lower certainty leading to central processing (Chaiken, Liberman, & Eagly, 1989; Trope & Lieberman, 1996). Dealing with general versus specific cases may alter one's confidence threshold for an accurate answer in one of two ways. One, arousal of affect may lower one's certainty, depending upon the framing of the decision (Martin, Ward, & Achee, 1993). As specific cases arouse greater affect, they may also tend to raise the threshold for feeling that a decision is accurate. This will necessitate more careful processing.

Two, we have argued that precomputed rules or heuristics for making a decision are more likely to exist for general cases. It is simply easier to find an appropriate rule for general cases than for specific cases. The very difficulty of finding an appropriate rule for specific cases may decrease one's certainty and thereby engage central processing. In our example of "the Democratic candidate" versus individual Democrats, a readily available decision rule about Democrats being preferable to Republicans may have already been formed and stored, and could have been arrived at through simple cueing by the framing of the survey question. A rule about Tsongas, Brown, or Clinton versus George Bush may never have been computed, and the preexisting rule about Democrats being preferred to Republicans may not have been as applicable to these specific cases. This candidate-specific framing of the survey question would increase uncertainty for the specific instances about how to approach the decision; therefore more extensive, central processing would be required. Thus, the difference between general cases and instances in the use of central versus peripheral processing may lie not only in the level of affective involvement, but also in the availability of preexisting strategies, rules, and solutions. Consistent with this possibility, it has been noted that abstract entities are easier to judge by stereotypes, whereas concrete and specific entities inspire context-dependent judgments that require piecemeal processing (Fiske & Neuberg, 1990).

Given the potential for differences in judgments and evaluations when central as opposed to peripheral processing is engaged, and given the likelihood that specific and general cases are likely to engage central and peripheral processing, respectively, it follows that one reason for differences in responses to general and specific cases is the differential use of central and peripheral processing that they entail. Although this dual-processing distinction has not been applied to the domain of the generality–specificity of the information under consideration, we can speculate about what some of the implications might be. With specific cases (the Anne Frank story, the particular little girl who was trapped in the well, any specific possible opponent of George Bush), central processing will be the rule. This will entail thorough and careful consideration of the information presented. It will lead to judgments and attitudes that are stable, resistant to change, and ultimately are held with great confidence (Petty & Cacioppo, 1986). The central processing of specific cases should lead to high levels of commitment for any decision that is made, and the high levels of self-involvement should ensure affective responsivity.

For general or abstract instances (the needy children of the world, Bush's "Democratic opponent," the principle of mixed zoning for a community), peripheral processing will ensure that the facts are not carefully or thoroughly considered. Judgments and attitudes that follow from the processing should be held with less ultimate confidence and should be subject to change on the basis of new information. There should be low levels of commitment to any decision about general issues, and a minimum of attachment or affective response.

As an example, peripheral processing about what to do for all the needy children of the world may lead to the "quick and dirty" conclusion that one cannot save all the world by a donation, that one cannot give to every single cause, and that one should not get involved in other people's problems. On the other hand, the central processing engaged by the specific case of the girl in the well may have led to a careful consideration of her particular plight. The combination of high affective involvement and the careful consideration that what one does can clearly have an effect on a single occurrence may have ensured that the likelihood of trying to help in this case would be high. Perhaps this is why many charities that involve help to needy and starving children assign a specific identified child to each donor, rather than having all contributions go into a general fund. Indeed, Miller (1977) reports that subjects, especially high believers in a just world, offered more help to a specified isolated individual with a need than to a situation where there were many unidentified victims in need. The logic of this discussion is most clearly demonstrated by an actual television ad for one such charity. "This isn't some abstract concept like millions of starving children," the spokesperson explains. "This is a *real* child."

Cognitive–Experiential Self-Theory

The last two dual-processing models that we have considered—on-line versus memory-based processing, and central versus peripheral processing—suggest that specific instances are more involving to the perceiver, and that specific cases are thus more likely to get more integrative processing, more cognitive attention, and deeper, rational consideration (in the form of on-line or central processing). Abstract cases, on the other hand, are less emotionally involving, and judgments of them are more likely to be made on the basis of peripheral or heuristic cues and in a memory-based manner.

We now consider a different process model that can be applied to the processing of specific and general cases: Epstein's cognitive–experiential self-theory (CEST; Epstein, 1983, 1985; Epstein, Lipson, Holstein, & Huh, 1992). Like the two models just discussed, CEST posits two major systems for processing incoming information—in this case, the experiential system and the rational system. However, these two processing modes handle information in a manner strikingly different from that of the models discussed previously. In Epstein's view, it is the *less* rational system that handles specific cases.

According to Epstein (1985), the experiential system processes information rapidly, providing people with the speed and cognitive ability necessary to get through everyday judgments without bogging down in each individual decision. The experiential system utilizes a quick and simple approach when processing information, relying on the information's "feel" in order to make judgments. This system operates in an automatic, associationistic, and holistic manner and is associated with affective experience. In Epstein's view, the more emotionally engaging the situation, the more likely it is that the perceiver will use the experiential system rather than utilize rational, deliberative processing to arrive at a decision. The experiential system can be viewed as the domain of the perceiver's personal reality, where beliefs are established on experiences rather than on logical deduction or induction. Validity is not ascertained through systematic logic; rather, according to Epstein, "experiencing is believing" (Epstein et al., 1992, p. 329). Because specific instances are usually more emotionally engaging and personally relevant, CEST predicts that decision makers will actually be *less* apt to analyze specific instances in a plodding, rational, logical, or careful way. Instead, decision makers will follow their gut reactions for specific cases.

In contrast, the rational system is a slow, plodding system, employing rules governed by logical processes to arrive at the decision. It is a deliberative, verbally mediated, conscious, and analytical system that relies on logical rules of evidence for its judgments. The rational system, because it is comparatively slow, is better suited for tasks that need not be completed immediately. It demands much of the cognitive energy and attention available to the decision maker, and thus it is not employed as often as is the experiential system when making decisions. The less involving the situation is emotionally, the more likely it is that the rational system will be employed. Therefore, abstract instances, with their lack of self-involvement and their emotional distance, are more likely to be processed rationally. It is difficult to have a gut feeling about vague, abstract ideas to which one has paid little or no attention in the past.

A consideration of the judgments represented in Garry Trudeau's *Doonesbury* cartoon about Mr. Butts (see Figure 10.1, above) provides an excellent example of the differences between the experiential and rational systems. Often one is presented with many abstract statistics concerning the dangers of smoking, all at a very uninvolving, general level. Indeed, the young potential smoker in the cartoon is well aware of the statistical information associated with smoking. A consideration of smokers as a general class thus causes concern when the young man thinks about taking up smoking. He has heard the negative information and knows that smoking is a health hazard in general, or statistically.

Mr. Butts, however, seems to be encouraging the young man to develop a more experientially based approach to the analysis, and to consider his own case as a specific instance. Anecdotes provide wonderful evidence for those concerned only with outcome, not with logic. Smokers can continue to justify smoking, in spite of all the statistical evidence against them, by relying on specific anecdotes and their own feelings of invulnerability to keep them outside of the statistics. The judgment of the diminished harm of smoking rests on such feelings and on experiential evidence possessed by a smoker, such as "My Uncle Mike lived to be 95 years old, smoking three packs a day." What appears to be rationalization or cognitive-dissonance reduction may be, according to CEST, simply a different type of processing of the available information. Logic takes a back seat, and gut feelings take over.

This difference in judgments arrived at through rational versus experiential processing has recently been demonstrated by Denes-Raj and Epstein (1994) in the domain of probability judgments. Subjects could judge general probability levels correctly, but when confronted with specific choices, their gut feelings took over and their decisions were quite different. For example, subjects knew logically that they were more likely to draw a red bean from a bowl that had 1 red bean out of 10 total beans as opposed to 7 red beans out of 100 total beans. Yet, when faced with a self-relevant choice (i.e., drawing a red bean was rewarding), they often elected to draw from the bowl with 7 out of 100 red beans, because the greater frequency of winning opportunities made them *feel* more likely to win. Thus, judgments made by the experiential system are likely to differ from judgments made by the rational system, and these systems may be differentially engaged by specific and general instances.

The CEST approach suggests, then, that specific cases (one pick from the bowl of beans, the particular little girl in the well) will be responded to from the heart, on the basis of emotional responses and gut feelings. These affective responses to specific cases are likely to be quite different from the conclusions of the head in the case of abstract instances (the overall probability of choosing a red bean, all the needy children of the world), which depend on careful consideration and the logic of a cost–benefit analysis. That the heart and the head may lead us in separate directions is, of course, not a novel idea. Psychologists, as well as authors, songwriters, and poets, have made similar observations for many years. What is interesting about the CEST model is how it seems to differ from another dual-processing model that we have considered, the central–peripheral model. We have inferred that specific cases engage both central processing and the experiential system, whereas general cases engage both peripheral processing and the rational system. At first blush, our inferences seem to conflict with each other. Central processing is more thorough than peripheral processing, but the rational system would seem to be more careful than the experiential system. How can specific information engage both central and experiential processing?

One way to resolve the apparent conflict between CEST and the central–peripheral model is to consider the degree to which the various systems involve extensive processing.

The central–peripheral model assumes that more extensive processing occurs when the information is processed centrally. Although CEST makes a distinction between automatic and controlled processing, the question of whether the experiential or rational system entails more extensive processing is open. It may take a good deal of processing, albeit low-level and automatic processing, to reach an experiential conclusion. If experiential processing is usually more extensive than rational processing, no conflict between the two models remains.

This possibility can be explored by again considering the presence and the role of preexisting rules for these different systems. Petty and Cacioppo (1986) suggest that preexisting solutions and heuristics are employed by the peripheral system, which we have identified with the processing of general cases. CEST suggests that there may be preexisting rules for specific cases as well; these rules are simply generalized from different data sets and by different procedures. Rules that are stored in and applied by the rational system, which is more applicable to the processing of general cases, are likely to be acquired through formal education—for example, "The volume of a gas is proportional to temperature and pressure." Rules that are stored in and applied by the experiential system, which is more applicable to the processing of specific cases, are likely to be acquired from one's own experience—for example, "My tires always look flat in the winter." Although these rules may sometimes agree, as in the preceding examples, decades of psychological research on people's ability to induce appropriate rules from experience shows that these rules may often conflict, with the experiential rules more likely to be in error (e.g., McCloskey, 1983). Because the preexisting rules that are learned for specific cases may be more difficult to apply than the heuristic principles applied to general cases, the experiential system may require more extensive processing for its handling of specific cases than the rational system requires for its processing of general cases. Thus, CEST and the central–peripheral model may be similar in suggesting more extensive processing for specific cases.

The suggestion by CEST of separate rules for the rational and experiential systems helps to explain the dilemma of how smokers can recognize the health risks of smoking, yet continue to light up cigarette after cigarette. The rational system's rule says that smoking is bad for health, and yet the experiential system of most smokers develops a conflicting rule. The average smoker has engaged in this behavior time and again, but has not (so far) become sick from doing so. The experiential system therefore develops the equally valid rule that smoking leads to no ill consequences for the self. These conflicting rules continue to coexist, as each is applied to different situations. In fact, one reason a smoker may continue to smoke is that the decision to smoke each individual cigarette is usually framed in specific rather than general terms. The usual framing, "Should I have a cigarette?", cues knowledge of the person's own experiences with smoking, whereas "Should I remain a smoker?" cues the person's competing knowledge about smokers in general. For this reason, the experiential system's rule is more likely to be cued each time the smoker lights up, and the behavior continues despite the rational system's rule.

A final distinction between CEST and the central–peripheral model should be noted. Petty and Cacioppo (1986) are clear about the outcomes of these two processing systems. Central processing, with its high affective involvement and careful consideration, leads to judgments that are firmly held and resistant to change. It is not as clear what the CEST model implies in this regard. Does the experiential or the rational system lead to attitudes and judgments that are more strongly and confidently held and are more resistant to change? Does the heart or the head get a person more committed to a cause or to a judgment?

In summary, we interpret both CEST and the central–peripheral model as suggesting more extensive processing for specific cases. This processing is necessitated by the greater affective involvement in some cases, by the stronger feeling that the decision must involve thorough processing in some cases, and/or by the lesser availability of rules in some cases. It should be noted, however, that extensive processing may not always result in more accurate decisions. Motivated processing, even when extensive, may result in a biased outcome. In addition, the use of the experiential system's rules may also lead to biases, as may the use of heuristic principles such as availability and representativeness by the rational system.

CONCLUSION

We have proposed that there are numerous instances of choice, evaluation, or decision making where the judgments of specific or particular occurrences are somehow inconsistent or discordant with judgments of the more general or abstract cases that these specific occurrences combine to form. Moreover, we have suggested several possibilities for the psychological processes and mechanisms that may be responsible for such inconsistencies in judgment. We have briefly outlined processes that involve strategies of integration and degradation, as well as the role of cognitive representations. The main discussion has concerned dual-processing models that assume the engagement of one of the two systems for specific instances and the other system for the processing of general cases.

It is likely the case that no one of these processes is responsible for all of the examples and seeming inconsistencies that we have considered throughout this chapter. Nor is it even likely that any one of the inconsistencies is determined by only one such process. No doubt this phenomenon involves multiple determination, and we offer the process accounts as only a first step toward a full account of why responses to specific versus general cases show some inconsistency. It will take further refinement in conceptualization and a dedicated program of empirical research to tease out which processes operate, and the conditions under which different processes may operate or combine with other processes, in order to produce the kinds of effects that we have described.

Thus, we suggest that our different dual-process accounts all operate to some extent, and that which mechanism predominates will depend on certain limiting conditions. Some of these conditions are likely to involve factors about the decision maker. We have discussed throughout the chapter factors involving the self-relevance of the judgment, the degree to which the decision maker is cognitively busy, and the extent to which the person has the motivation and the ability to process the information at hand carefully.

Many of our accounts have depended on a distinction between careful and systematic processing versus heuristic or simplified processing. In addition to person factors, there are likely to be situational factors that determine which mechanism is most likely to operate. Factors concerning the kind of information involved in the judgment should be most important in this regard. We have discussed the importance of the following aspects of the information base: completeness, ambiguity, salience, extremity, and variability. In short, both factors about the judge and aspects of the information being judged will determine whether or not we observe inconsistencies in the judgment of general and specific cases, the degree to which such inconsistencies will emerge, and the processes responsible for the inconsistencies.

It is also important to recognize that we have treated the application of the dual-processing models to the general–specific distinction in an all-or-none fashion. That is, we have proposed that one of the two dual-processing modes (e.g., on-line, central, experiential) will be engaged for specific cases, and that the other (e.g., memory-based, peripheral, rational) will be engaged for general or abstract cases. Although such an assumption may be a reasonable starting point for analysis and discussion, it is no doubt oversimplified in several important ways. First, the very distinction between a specific and a general case is not always clear. Some specific cases are more specific than others, and general cases vary in their degree of abstractness. It is perhaps more fruitful to think of a continuum of cases from the very specific to the very general, and to propose that a different probability of applying one processing mode or the other exists for different points along the continuum.

Second, we have implied that for the application of dual-processing models to our questions of interest, it is reasonable to assume that either one or the other processing mode will be engaged at any point in time. It is unlikely that thinking can be characterized as involving one system or the other in a serial fashion. Rather, it makes more sense to suggest that the processing of social information almost always involves a combination of the two modes of processing in parallel. This issue of simultaneous versus sequential dual-processing systems has been addressed by several social-psychological models. With regard to models of persuasion, the central–peripheral model of Petty and Cacioppo (1986) proposes that these two processes of persuasion are mutually exclusive and operate sequentially in an all-or-none fashion. On the other hand, Chaiken (1980) suggests that the heuristic and systematic routes to persuasion can operate simultaneously and in a complementary fashion. With regard to CEST, as we have seen, individual cases and concrete exemplars tend to strongly engage the experiential system. However, they may also engage the rational system at the same time if they are presented in a context recognized as appropriate for logical solution, and if there is strong motivation to engage in such processing. Thus, for vivid and emotional cases, either experiential or rational processing or both (or central or peripheral processing or both) may be engaged, depending on the motivations and resources available and on the extent to which the operation of one system may interfere with the operation of the other. When both systems operate simultaneously, each may lead to its own output. At times like this, people realize that they must choose between what their hearts are pulling them toward and what their heads are telling them to do logically.

If the dual-processing systems for general versus specific information that we have discussed do indeed operate in parallel, and if each system leads to its own independent judgment or output, the question arises as to what is done when these two outputs are incompatible. For example, the processing of general-level information may indicate that the error rate is fine and that the system needs no fixing, whereas the simultaneous processing of specific-case information may indicate that there are serious performance problems that need addressing. In cases such as this, it is possible, as Chaiken (1980) suggests, that the outputs of the two processes will be integrated and that any conflict will be resolved. On the other hand, recent models of Sloman (1996) and Abelson (1994) suggest that the incompatible judgments derived from parallel processing systems might both remain strongly represented at the same time and that one or the other judgment could be used depending upon the context or the requirements of the situation. A more in-depth discussion of this issue of parallel processing by dual systems is provided in Chapter 30 of this volume by Hamilton et al.

Interestingly, the idea of differential processing mechanisms for general versus specific items at the conceptual level is mirrored by processing differences at the perceptual level. Perception of the whole appears to be automatic and unavoidable, whereas perception of the parts composing that whole takes time and effort (Navon, 1977). That is, perceivers can process information at the global level of organization without being affected by information at the local level of organization. On the other hand, as global information is automatically attended to, the local information cannot be perceived without the global information's getting through as well. It is possible that in processing general versus specific cases at the conceptual level, there may be a similar dominance of the general level over the specific level. Judgments of the general case may not be influenced by the judgments of its specific components (just as perceptions of the general case are not influenced by perceptions of specific components), whereas judgments of specific cases may always be affected by one's judgment of the general entity. That is, one may be able to consider Democrats without necessarily being influenced by one's attitude toward Bill Clinton, but one's judgment of Bill Clinton may always be affected by one's attitude toward Democrats.

It is also interesting to consider the differences between the general and the specific from a linguistic point of view. Languages have ways of grammatically marking the extent to which nouns are generic or specific (Givon, 1989). However, the English language can be quite unclear about whether a referent is general or specific. For example, "The person who killed Smith is insane" may be referring to a specific identified individual who killed Smith and who is known to be insane. It may also indicate that an unknown person killed Smith, but that whoever it is must be insane. Other languages—for example, Spanish—more carefully mark the gradation in the generality and specificity of referents (definite, semidefinite, and nonreferential). Because language can affect thinking and judgment, it may be useful to compare the degree of disjuncture in responses to general and specific cases with the extent to which the language

that is spoken codes patently for this difference.

Finally, we should consider why our observations and analyses may be important from the point of view of researchers of human judgment. In the first place, we believe that we have identified a generally important source of errorful judgments. Some of these errorful judgments are based on quite rational processes, and some involve irrational judgment strategies. Some of these errorful judgments are based on motivational factors, and some are more purely cognitive in nature. In any case, the focus on these errors and inconsistencies of judgment can certainly help us to understand such errors, to develop ways to reduce them, and to improve our judgmental processes. Second, our focus on a variety of mechanisms that are involved in the consideration of general and specific instances can enlighten us about the various processes involved in decision making. We have considered processing possibilities that have not received a lot of attention in the judgment literature. For example, we feel that more attention should be given to the roles of comparison and construal in the judgment process.

It is apparent that the observations we have made have important applied implications. The examples and analyses that we have considered have touched on political judgments, charity donations, legal decision making, and sports judgments. In addition, the distinctions that we have made have been discussed in terms of their implications for differences in the effectiveness of various compliance techniques or persuasive messages. In a broad way, the consideration of a judgment as a general case or as a collection of specific instances is an example of the importance of framing in decision making. All of the ways in which framing has been demonstrated to influence applied decision making should apply to our distinction.

Although we believe that there is something important and useful in the issues that we have raised, and although we have enjoyed putting our thoughts together, we realize that this chapter provides more speculation than resolution. In short, we may be guilty of raising more questions than we have answered. However, our goal is to titillate and motivate the readers of this chapter to move from theoretical speculation to empirical undertakings. We hope we have succeeded in generating interest in a more programmatic examination of these preliminary ideas.

ACKNOWLEDGMENT

Work on this chapter was supported by Grant No. MH40058 from the National Institute of Mental Health to Steven J. Sherman.

NOTE

1. It should be noted that these observations, anecdotal in nature, are meant to serve as a useful background (and, we hope, a compelling background) to indicate interesting instances in which naturalistic responses to general and specific cases differ greatly, often with important and serious consequences. We shall not attempt to identify the process operating in each observation. Nor do we claim that the differences in response to general versus specific instances are necessarily inconsistent. In some cases, "reasonable" differences in self-interest for general versus specific instances, or "understandable" differences in the properties of general as opposed to specific cases, render the differences comprehensible and even sensible. Yet, in each case, the differential response to the two levels of abstraction leaves one with the feeling or perception that one or the other response ought to change.

REFERENCES

Abelson, R. P. (1983). Whatever became of consistency theory? *Personality and Social Psychology Bulletin, 9,* 37–54.

Abelson, R. P. (1994). A personal perspective on social cognition. In P. G. Devine, D. L. Hamilton, & T. M. Ostrom (Eds.), *Social cognition: Impact on social psychology* (pp. 15–37). San Diego, CA: Academic Press.

Anderson, N. H. (1965). Averaging versus adding as a stimulus-combination rule in impression formation. *Journal of Experimental Psychology, 70,* 394–400.

Anderson, N. H. (1981). *Foundations of information integration theory.* New York: Academic Press.

Anderson, N. H. (1988). A functional approach to person cognition. In T. K. Srull & R. S. Wyer, Jr. (Eds.), *Advances in social cognition* (Vol. 1, pp. 37–51). Hillsdale, NJ: Erlbaum.

Axsom, D., Yates, S., & Chaiken, S. (1987). Audience response as a heuristic cue in persuasion. *Journal of Personality and Social Psychology, 53,* 30–40.

Bar-Hillel, M. (1990). Back to base rates. In R. M. Hogarth (Ed.), *Insights in decision making: A tribute to Hillel J. Einhorn.* Chicago: University of Chicago Press.

Baron, J., & Hershey, J. C. (1988). Outcome bias in deci-

sion evaluation. *Journal of Personality and Social Psychology, 54,* 569–579.

Brewer, W. F. (1986). What is autobiographical memory? In D. C. Rubin (Ed.), *Autobiographical memory* (pp. 25–49). Cambridge, England: Cambridge University Press.

Byrne, D. (1971). *The attraction paradigm.* New York: Academic Press.

Carlston, D. E., & Skowronski, J. J. (1994). Savings in the relearning of trait information as evidence for spontaneous inference generation. *Journal of Personality and Social Psychology, 66,* 840–856.

Chaiken, S. (1980). Heuristic versus systematic information processing and the use of source versus message cues in persuasion. *Journal of Personality and Social Psychology, 39,* 752–766.

Chaiken, S., Liberman, A., & Eagly, A. E. (1989). Heuristic and systematic information processing within and beyond the persuasion context. In J. S. Uleman & J. A. Bargh (Eds.), *Unintended thought* (pp. 212–252). New York: Guilford Press.

Collins, A. M., & Quillian, M. R. (1969). Retrieval time from semantic memory. *Journal of Verbal Learning and Verbal Behavior, 8,* 240–247.

Denes-Raj, V., & Epstein, S. (1994). Conflict between intuitive and rational processing: When people behave against their better judgment. *Journal of Personality and Social Psychology, 66,* 819–829.

Epstein, S. (1983). The unconscious, the preconscious, and the self-concept. In J. Suls & A. Greenwald (Eds.), *Psychological perspectives on the self* (Vol. 2, pp. 219–247). Hillsdale, NJ: Erlbaum.

Epstein, S. (1985). The implications of cognitive–experiential self-theory for research in social psychology and personality. *Journal for the Theory of Social Behavior, 15,* 283–310.

Epstein, S., Lipson, A., Holstein, C., & Huh, E. (1992). Irrational reactions to negative outcomes: Evidence for two conceptual systems. *Journal of Personality and Social Psychology, 62,* 328–339.

Fazio, R. H. (1990). Multiple processes by which attitudes guide behavior: The MODE model as an integrative framework. In M. P. Zanna (Ed.), *Advances in experimental social psychology* (Vol. 23, pp. 75–110). San Diego, CA: Academic Press.

Fiedler, K., & Armbruster, T. (1994). Two halfs may be more than one whole: Category-split effects on frequency illusions. *Journal of Personality and Social Psychology, 66,* 633–645.

Fiske, S. T., & Neuberg, S. L. (1990). A continuum of impression formation, from category-based to individuating processes: Influences of information and motivation on attention and interpretation. In M. P. Zanna (Ed.), *Advances in experimental social psychology* (Vol. 23, pp. 1–74). San Diego, CA: Academic Press.

Gelman, S. A., & Markman, E. M. (1987). Young children's inductions from natural kinds: The role of categories and appearances. *Child Development, 58,* 1532–1541.

Gilovich, T. (1990). Differential construal and the false consensus effect. *Journal of Personality and Social Psychology, 59,* 623–634.

Givon, T. (1989). *Mind, code, and context.* Hillsdale, NJ: Erlbaum.

Hamilton, D. L., & Sherman, S. J. (1996). Perceiving persons and groups. *Psychological Review*, *103*, 336–355.

Hastie, R., & Park, B. (1986). The relationship between memory and judgment depends on whether the judgment task is memory-based or on-line. *Psychological Review*, *93*, 258–268.

Herr, P. M. (1986). Consequences of priming: Judgment and behavior. *Journal of Personality and Social Psychology*, *51*, 1106–1115.

Herr, P. M., Sherman, S. J., & Fazio, R. H. (1983). On the consequences of priming: Assimilation and contrast effects. *Journal of Experimental Social Psychology*, *19*, 323–340.

Hesslow, G. (1983). Explaining differences and weighting causes. *Theoria*, *49*, 87–111.

Higgins, E. T., & Rholes, W. S. (1976). Impression formation and role fulfillment: A "holistic reference" approach. *Journal of Experimental Social Psychology*, *12*, 422–435.

Hilton, D. J., & Slugoski, B. R. (1986). Knowledge-based causal attribution: The abnormal conditions focus model. *Psychological Review*, *93*, 75–88.

Jones, E. E., & Nisbett, R. (1971). *The actor and the observer: Divergent perceptions of the causes of behavior*. Morristown, NJ: Erlbaum.

Kahneman, D., & Miller, D. T. (1986). Norm theory: Comparing reality to its alternatives. *Psychological Review*, *93*, 136–153.

Kahneman, D., & Tversky, A. (1973). On the psychology of prediction. *Psychological Review*, *80*, 237–251.

Klayman, J., & Ha, Y.-W. (1987). Confirmation, disconfirmation, and information in hypothesis-testing. *Psychological Review*, *94*, 211–228.

Koriat, A., Lichtenstein, S., & Fischhoff, B. (1980). Reasons for confidence. *Journal of Experimental Psychology: Human Learning and Memory*, *6*, 107–118.

Krueger, J., & Rothbart, M. (1988). Use of categorical and individuating information in making inferences about personality. *Journal of Personality and Social Psychology*, *55*, 187–195.

Kunda, Z. (1990). The case for motivated reasoning. *Psychological Bulletin*, *108*, 480–498.

Landman, J. (1988). Regret and elation following action and inaction: Affective responses to positive versus negative outcomes. *Personality and Social Psychology Bulletin*, *13*, 524–536.

LaPiere, R. T. (1934). Attitudes vs. actions. *Social Forces*, *13*, 230–237.

Lichtenstein, S., Earle, T. C., & Slovic, P. (1975). Cue utilization in a numerical prediction task. *Journal of Experimental Psychology: Human Perception and Performance*, *104*, 77–85.

Lichtenstein, S., Fischhoff, B., & Phillips, L. D. (1982). Calibration of probabilities: The state of the art in 1980. In D. Kahneman, P. Slovic, & A. Tversky (Eds.), *Judgment under uncertainty: Heuristics and biases* (pp. 306–334). Cambridge, England: Cambridge University Press.

Martin, L. L. (1986). Set/reset: Use and disuse of concepts in impression formation. *Journal of Personality and Social Psychology*, *51*, 493–504.

Martin, L. L., Ward, D. W., & Achee, J. W. (1993). Mood as input: People have to interpret the motivational implications of their moods. *Journal of Personality and Social Psychology*, *64*, 317–326.

Matthews, V. L., & Piper, G. W. (1974). *The Saskatoon*

smoking study: Habits and beliefs of children in grades seven and eight about smoking. Unpublished manuscript, University of Saskatchewan, Saskatoon, Saskatchewan, Canada.

McCloskey, M. (1983). Intuitive physics. *Scientific American*, *248*, 122–130.

McGill, A. L. (1989). Context effects in judgments of causation. *Journal of Personality and Social Psychology*, *57*, 189–200.

McGill, A. L. (1993). Selection of a causal background: Role of expectation versus feature mutability. *Journal of Personality and Social Psychology*, *64*, 701–707.

Miller, D. T. (1977). Altruism and threat to a belief in a just world. *Journal of Experimental Social Psychology*, *13*, 113–125.

Miller, D. T., & Turnbull, W. (1990). The counterfactual fallacy: Confusing what might have been with what should have been. *Social Justice Research*, *4*, 1–19.

Navon, D. (1977). Forest before trees: The precedence of global features in visual perception. *Cognitive Psychology*, *9*, 353–383.

Niedenthal, P. M., Tangney, J. P., & Gavanski, I. (1994). "If only I weren't" vs. "If only I hadn't": Distinguishing shame and guilt in counterfactual thinking. *Journal of Personality and Social Psychology*, *67*, 585–595.

Nisbett, R. E., & Ross, L. (1980). *Human inference: Strategies and shortcomings of social judgment*. Englewood Cliffs, NJ: Prentice-Hall.

Nisbett, R. E., Zukier, H., & Lemley, R. E. (1981). The dilution effect: Nondiagnostic information weakens the implications of diagnostic information. *Cognitive Psychology*, *18*, 248–277.

Petty, R. E., & Cacioppo, J. T. (1981). *Attitudes and persuasion: Classic and contemporary approaches*. Dubuque, IA: William C. Brown.

Petty, R. E., & Cacioppo, J. T. (1986). *Communication and persuasion: Central and peripheral routes to attitude change*. New York: Springer-Verlag.

Petty, R. E., & Wegener, D. T. (1993). Flexible correction processes in social judgment: Correcting for context-induced contrast. *Journal of Experimental Social Psychology*, *29*, 137–165.

Rosch, E. (1978). Principles of categorization. In E. Rosch & B. B. Lloyd (Eds.), *Cognition and categorization* (pp. 87–116). Hillsdale, NJ: Erlbaum.

Schwarz, N., & Bless, H. (1992a). Scandals and the public's trust in politicians: Assimilation and contrast effects. *Personality and Social Psychology Bulletin*, *18*, 574–579.

Schwarz, N., & Bless, H. (1992b). Constructing reality and its alternatives: An inclusion/exclusion model of assimilation and contrast effects in social judgment. In L. L. Martin & A. Tesser (Eds.), *The construction of social judgments* (pp. 217–245). Hillsdale, NJ: Erlbaum.

Sears, D. O. (1983). The person-positivity bias. *Journal of Personality and Social Psychology*, *44*, 233–240.

Sherman, S. J. (1980). On the self-erasing nature of errors of prediction. *Journal of Personality and Social Psychology*, *39*, 211–221.

Sloman, S. A. (1996). The empirical case for two systems of reasoning. *Psychological Review*, *119*, 3–22.

Sniezek, J. A., & Buckley, T. (1991). Confidence depends on level of aggregation. *Journal of Behavioral Decision Making*, *4*, 263–272.

Sniezek, J. A., Paese, P. W., & Switzer, F. S. (1990). The effect of choosing on confidence in choice. *Organizational Behavior and Human Decision Processes, 46,* 264–282.

Stapel, D. A., Koomen, W., & van der Pligt, J. (1996). The referents of trait inferences: The impact of trait concepts versus actor-trait links on subsequent judgments. *Journal of Personality and Social Psychology, 70,* 437–450.

Troutman, C. M., & Shanteau, J. (1977). Inferences based on nondiagnostic information. *Organizational Behavior and Human Performance, 19,* 43–55.

Trope, Y., & Liberman, A. (1996). Social hypothesis testing: Cognitive and motivational mechanisms. In E. T. Higgins & A. W. Kruglanski (Eds.), *Social psychology: Handbook of basic principles* (pp. 239–270). New York: Guilford Press.

Tulving, E. (1983). *Elements of episodic memory.* Oxford: Clarendon Press.

Tversky, A., & Kahneman, D. (1982). Judgments of and by representativeness. In D. Kahneman, P. Slovic, & A. Tversky (Eds.), *Judgment under uncertainty: Heuristics and biases* (pp. 84–100). New York: Cambridge University Press.

Tversky, A., & Koehler, D. J. (1994). Support theory: A nonextensional representation of subjective probability. *Psychological Review, 101,* 547–567.

Uleman, J. S. (1987). Consciousness and control: The case of spontaneous trait inferences. *Personality and Social Psychology Bulletin, 13,* 337–354.

Wedell, D. H., Parducci, A., & Geiselman, R. E. (1987). A formal analysis of ratings of physical attractiveness: Successive contrast and simultaneous assimilation. *Journal of Experimental Social Psychology, 23,* 230–249.

Zukier, H., & Jennings, D. L. (1983–1984). Nondiagnosticity and typicality effects in prediction. *Social Cognition, 2,* 187–198.

C

Stereotyping in Particular

11

The Continuum Model

TEN YEARS LATER

SUSAN T. FISKE
MONICA LIN
STEVEN L. NEUBERG

[People's windows on their impressions of others] have this mark of their own that at each of them stands a figure with a pair of eyes, or at least with a field-glass, which forms, again and again, for observation, a unique instrument, insuring to the person making use of it an impression distinct from every other. He and his neighbors are watching the same show, but one seeing more where the other sees less, one seeing black where the other sees white, one seeing big where the other sees small, one seeing coarse where the other sees fine. . . . [The windows] are, singly or together, as nothing without the posted presence of the watcher.

—HENRY JAMES, Preface, *The Portrait of a Lady* (1881/1983, pp. ix–x)

The continuum model was designed to describe the range of ways in which—the many "windows" from which—people form impressions of other people, while acknowledging that they all do share some fundamental processes; they all inhabit the same human "house." This chapter summarizes the continuum model and assesses its ongoing viability in light of the research exploring impression formation since the model's formal publication in 1990. The chapter works from the specific to the more general. It first reviews the model's history and its specific stages. Then the chapter examines the model's five core premises, highlighting some of the over 300 citations of it in the social-scientific literature since 1990. Finally, the chapter revisits some of the model's theoretical meta-assumptions,

clarifying where appropriate some misinterpretations of our positions.

THE CONTINUUM MODEL: HISTORY AND SPECIFIC STAGES

Historical Context

The central statement of the model (Fiske & Neuberg, 1990) dates back hardly 10 years, yet its origins date back farther. Fiske (1982) proposed the notion of "schema-triggered affect" to account for the immediate evaluation and affect associated with spontaneous social categorization. A 1984 grant proposal became the basis for a chapter (Fiske & Pavelchak, 1986) that delineated the subsequent empirical support for schema-triggered affect, contrasting category-based and piece-meal-based responses. Over the next several years, Fiske and Neuberg detailed the full model, making explicit the sequence of stages proposed, the core premises, and the support for both in the extant literature; the literature review was updated soon after (Riley & Fiske, 1991).

As its centerpiece, the model tackled a contradiction between the literature on impression formation and social cognition—a contradiction pitting elemental, algebraic approaches to impression formation against Gestalt, holistic, configural approaches (Asch, 1946). The elemental, piecemeal view of impression formation posited that people form evaluative impressions of others by computing a weighted average of the isolated evaluations of the targets' features (Anderson, 1981). For instance, a person known to be intelligent and altruistic should be evaluated favorably, because intelligence and altruism are each positively viewed characteristics (for most perceivers). Indeed, Anderson's information integration model—the standard bearer of the elemental approach—did quite well in predicting people's evaluations of others.

Researchers expressed two main concerns with this and similar models, however. First, many believed that the piecemeal processes articulated by such models are psychologically peculiar, and perhaps even impossible for people to perform. Second, the elemental models viewed the meaning of each characteristic as fixed, not influenced by the other characteristics possessed by the target. For instance, regardless of whether it is paired with "altruistic" or "cruel", the evaluation and meaning of "intelligent" is presumed to remain the same. This assumption conflicts with Gestalt, configural approaches, which posit that a characteristic's meaning can change in light of a target's other characteristics—that "intelligent" may mean something different and be valued differently, depending on whether it coexists with "altruistic" or "cruel" (for a review of this controversy, see Leyens & Fiske, 1994).

These critiques were taken quite seriously, and many espoused instead a modern, information-processing version of the Gestalt approach. As the social-cognitive literature developed, aspects of the Gestalt approach in-

formed researchers' understanding of social categorization processes—a view represented in schema, category, prototype, and stereotype models (for a review, see Fiske & Taylor, 1991, Ch. 6). Theorists proposed both a richer role for perceivers' prior knowledge in organizing their thinking about newly encountered people, and a more configural approach to understanding how elements of this prior knowledge might interact to create a more holistic meaning. This approach, too, garnered significant empirical support.

And so the debate between the two approaches raged, until it was declared unresolvable, given the theories and methods then available (Ostrom, 1977). Synthesizing the two approaches was the aim of the continuum model.

Sequence of Processes

Combining the social categorization and elemental approaches, the continuum model proposes that people can use a range of impression formation processes (see Figure 11.1), and that the utilized processes depend on two primary factors: the available information and the perceiver's motivation. We briefly outline this continuum of processes next.

Initial Categorization

Upon encountering an individual, perceivers rapidly categorize that individual on the basis of salient features. These features can take the form of physical characteristics, such as skin color or body shape; they can be a configuration of behavior that quickly and easily cues a social category, as when a smiling student strolls into one's office and is categorized as a friendly person; or they can be verbally transmitted category labels, as when a friend introduces a new acquaintance as an "electrical engineer." Many features can potentially elicit social categories, which then serve to organize and constrain the meaning and usefulness of subsequently identified features or attributes. Which features organize the others—taking on the role of category—depends on the cognitive and social context (Fiske & Neuberg, 1990, pp. 9–12).

The model proposes, however, that cer-

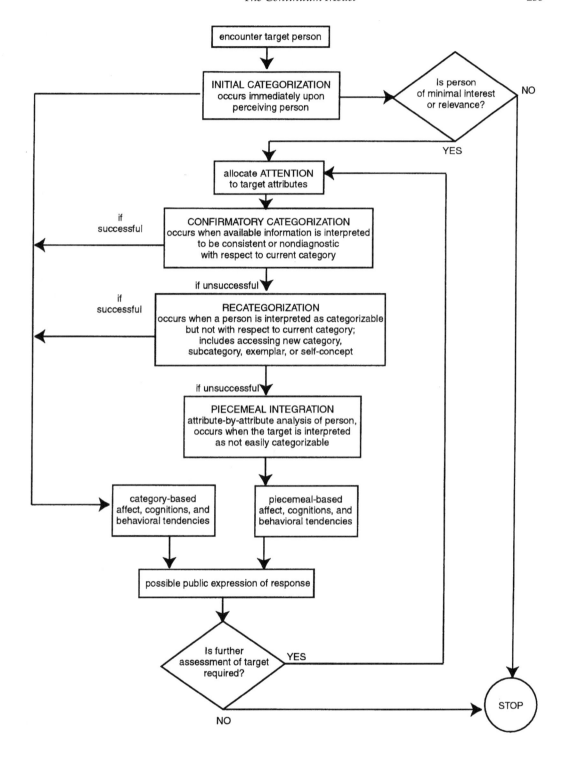

FIGURE 11.1. The continuum model of impression formation. It shows the range from category-based to individuating impression formation processes, as a function of attention and interpretation. Informational and motivational conditions determine the attentional and interpretive processes that result in the various impression formation processes. Copyright 1986 by Susan T. Fiske.

tain social categories—such as gender, ethnicity, and age—are "privileged," in that they can be easily applied to most people one encounters. Indeed, subsequent research has demonstrated that these categories are central and available to perceivers automatically, within milliseconds (see Fiske, 1998, for a review). These social categories have two advantages over others: They are physically manifested and thus have temporal primacy (most of all in visual encounters), and they have important cultural meanings that are often relevant for people's immediate interaction goals. In any case, once perceivers categorize the encountered individual, they automatically tend to feel, think, and behave toward that individual in the same way they tend to feel, think, and behave toward members of that social category more generally, as research has amply demonstrated (Fiske, 1998).

Personal Relevance

The continuum model proposes that personal relevance determines whether a perceiver stays with the initial category-based impression (in the case of low-relevance circumstances) or tries to move beyond it (in the case of more relevant circumstances). The later sections reviewing the model's core premises and meta-assumptions will explore the role of motivation. Our inclusion of personal relevance assumes a rich array of motivations relevant to belonging, understanding, controlling, self-enhancing, and trusting. The term "personal relevance" in the model merely implies motivational relevance.

Attention and Interpretation

The central mediators of this model, attention and interpretation, determine whether (and how far) perceivers go beyond the initial category and its immediate cognitive, affective, and behavioral associates. To individuate, perceivers must examine other perceived attributes of the target, and they cannot do this unless they devote additional attentional resources to the task. "Attention to attributes mediates the extent to which people use relative stereotypic or relatively more individuat-

ing processes" (Fiske & Neuberg, 1990, p. 6). And how perceivers interpret the information they heed then determines whether the initial categorization remains plausible, or whether new (re)categorizations are needed.

Attention does not guarantee accuracy (however defined) or individuation, but it does permit processes more individuating than the split-second initial categorization. Some colleagues (to remain anonymous) have sometimes read the model as claiming that attention necessarily creates accuracy, but instead "the attention stage is especially important because it provides the raw material that *heavily influences* which of the alternative processes is utilized. . . . This single mediator is posited to *transmit the effect of both informational and motivational* influences on subsequent impression-formation processes" (Fiske & Neuberg, 1990, p. 6, emphasis added). Informational fit and motivational pressure determine the impression formation processes used; attention and interpretation enable information and motivation to have this influence.

Confirmatory Categorization

Upon receiving additional information, perceivers attempt to preserve the initial categorization. Originally, Fiske and Neuberg (1990) reviewed evidence that confirmatory categorization was encouraged by certain information conditions—namely, a label plus category-consistent attributes; a label plus mixed attributes; or a strong label plus judgment-irrelevant, category-irrelevant attributes. In addition, Fiske and Neuberg speculated that certain motivators (such as self-esteem threat) might *increase* the likelihood that a perceiver would view target information as consistent with the initial categorization, whereas other motivators (such as task outcome dependency, fear of invalidity, and accountability to an audience with unknown attitudes) might *reduce* the likelihood that a perceiver would view target information as consistent with the initial categorization. Since the publication of the original chapter, new evidence suggests not only that successful confirmatory categorization requires perceivers to attend effortfully to stereotype consistencies, but that such efforts indeed can be triggered by threats to oneself or one's ingroup (Fiske & Leyens, 1996) and by the need to justify one's power position (Goodwin, Gubin, Fiske, & Yzerbyt, 1998).

Recategorization

Sometimes people's interpretation of new target information reveals the initial categorization to be faulty in some way. When this happens, and when perceivers have sufficient motivation (and attentional resources), the perceivers recategorize: "Recategorization represents an attempt to find a different category that can be interpreted as adequately organizing the bulk of current information" (Fiske & Neuberg, 1990, p. 7). Subcategories, exemplars, self-references, and new superordinate categories all represent attempts to install a better-fitting category in place of the initial category. Some commentators (Oakes & Reynolds, 1997) have not noted that all these are categories too, and thus subject to the same interplay between prior knowledge and perceived information fit, within a given social (cultural and interactional) context. Originally, Fiske and Neuberg described information conditions that encourage recategorization: a weak initial category confronted by judgment-irrelevant, category-irrelevant attributes, or an initial category confronted with clearly inconsistent attributes. In addition, they speculated that motivations would determine the specificity of categories used.

Piecemeal Integration

The most individuating stage of the continuum model is described as integrating, attribute by attribute, each relevant piece of information into an overall assessment. The initial category, under this process, does not evaporate, but becomes just another attribute that contributes to the overall impression. Some particular research programs have obtained piecemeal-type results, but they tend to require participants to judge multitudes of targets, using standardized information that varies according to a limited number of criteria (e.g., Anderson, 1981; Fiske, 1980). Compa-

rable everyday examples include screening large quantities of admissions or job applications on a very few specified dimensions, with the aim of assigning each applicant some summary rating.

In retrospect, purely elemental, attribute-by-attribute processing does not strike us as capturing every type of individuating response. The original version of the model also suggested that, in theory, one can make piecemeal sense of a single person who is otherwise uncategorizable. In hindsight, we are convinced that this latter sort of process is rare: Rather than simply adding up (or averaging) people's good and bad points, people demonstrably construct naive theories to account for contradictory and novel combinations of attributes (Asch & Zukier, 1984; Kunda, Miller, & Claire, 1990; Leyens & Yzerbyt, 1992).

Public Expression and Further Assessment

The model closes with a perceiver's implicit or explicit decision to express the cognitions, affect, and behavior associated with the impressions resulting from processes along the continuum. Of course, such expressions can be made at any point along the way, even if a "final" impression has yet to be formed. Indeed, the further-assessment feedback loop captures the tendency for people to continue the thoughtful categorization–recategorization process (using the most recently accepted category as the foundation) as new information about the target becomes available or as they decide actively to seek more information. From the perspective of the continuum model, impression formation is a dynamic process that responds both to the motives of perceivers and to the information impinging upon them.

Conclusion

The stages of initial categorization, confirmatory categorization, recategorization, and piecemeal processing are mediated by attention and interpretation, both of which are influenced by information and motivation. The subsequent research literature suggests that initial categorization and recategorization occur most easily, but this conclusion awaits an overview of the model's broader premises.

EVIDENCE FOR THE CORE PREMISES OF THE MODEL

Five key premises underlie the continuum model. Contemporaneous support for the initial formulation of the model was strong (see Fiske & Neuberg, 1990), and its premises have been further supported by subsequent research on impression formation. The following review explores this subsequent research, but is not meant to be exhaustive; instead, it concentrates on relevant recent research addressing the model or its five premises:

1. Perceivers give priority to categorization over individuation.
2. Ease of information fit between category and attributes influences progress along the continuum.
3. Attention to attribute information mediates the use of various impression formation processes.
4. Motivational factors influence progress along the impression formation continuum, according to the social interdependence structure and the criteria set by the primary motivating agent.
5. Attention to and interpretation of attribute information mediate the motivational influences on impression formation.

Premise 1: Perceivers Give Priority to Categorizing Processes

The model's first premise assumes that perceivers typically use category-based processes before they use attribute-oriented processes, and that if the category-oriented processes work well enough, perceivers do not engage additional, more attribute-oriented processes. In the context of the model, the premise implies that current knowledge about the target is fitted to the contents associated with the perceiver's category to the degree tolerated by the perceiver's interaction purposes and context. These purposes are determined by situational and individual differences in motivations, but the basic point is that category-based processes have priority and will be used without additional information search, to the extent that the category is pragmatic in context (especially in providing guidelines for interaction). The priority of categorizing processes continues to receive research support.

First, people frequently use social categories to understand others, especially visually prominent categories such as gender, race, and age (Biernat & Vescio, 1993; Gardner, MacIntyre, & Lalonde, 1995; Hewstone, Hantzi, & Johnston, 1991; McCann, Ostrom, Tyner, & Mitchell, 1985; Stangor, Lynch, Duan, & Glas, 1992; Verkuyten, Masson, & Elffers, 1995; Zárate & Sandoval, 1995; Zebrowitz, Montepare, & Lee, 1993; for a review, see Fiske 1998). Indeed, perceivers can apply such social categories to targets quite quickly, usually in just fractions of a second after encountering them (Banaji & Hardin, 1996; Blair & Banaji, 1996; Devine, 1989; Dovidio, Evans, & Tyler, 1986; Fazio, Jackson, Dunton, & Williams, 1995; Gaertner & McLaughlin, 1983; Klinger & Beall, 1992; Lepore & Brown, 1997; Perdue & Gurtman, 1990; Wittenbrink, Judd, & Park, 1997; Zárate & Sandoval, 1995; Zárate & Smith, 1990; for reviews, see Dovidio & Gaertner, 1993; Fiske, 1998).

Moreover, once a perceiver categorizes a target, the category works quickly and efficiently, making immediately accessible its associated affective, cognitive, and behavioral responses without requiring the perceiver to engage in much effortful thought (Macrae, Bodenhausen, & Milne, 1995; Macrae, Milne, & Bodenhausen, 1994; Macrae, Stangor, & Milne, 1994). People categorize others in part because doing so provides a wealth of information at little cognitive cost.

Beyond providing information useful for impression formation, activated social categories can potentially bias attribute-oriented processing by eliciting selective perception, interpretation, inference, and memory (Heilman, 1995). In one study, for instance, men primed to think of women in stereotypical terms were not only more likely to ask a female job applicant more sexist questions and to exhibit more sexualized behavior toward her; they were also *slower* to recognize *non*sexist words in a lexical-decision task (Rudman & Borgida, 1995). Indeed, the biasing effects of social categories occur so effortlessly that it becomes difficult to ignore or disregard these effects, even under relatively ideal circumstances (Nelson, Acker, & Manis, 1996). Furthermore, active attempts to inhibit category-based thoughts before they interfere with subsequent judgments or behaviors may create a "rebound effect," whereby the stereotypic thoughts reappear with an insistence even greater than if they had never been suppressed (Macrae, Bodenhausen, Milne, & Jetten, 1994).

Of course, this is not to say that social categories always inhibit conceptual processing of category-inconsistent individuating information. For instance, perceivers can preferentially recall stereotype-inconsistent information when they have plenty of available attentional resources (Macrae, Hewstone, & Griffiths, 1993), and this preferential recall may enable perceivers to modify their otherwise category-based impressions (Stangor & Duan, 1991). When attentional resources are restricted, however, the biasing effects of active social categories almost always increase (e.g., Gilbert & Hixon, 1991; Harris-Kern & Perkins, 1995; Macrae et al., 1993), even when perceivers are motivated to form accurate impressions (Biesanz, Neuberg, Judice, Smith, & Asher, 1998; Pendry & Macrae, 1994). And because people often focus their attention on category-consistent information, their stereotypic expectations are easily reinforced (Leyens & Yzerbyt, 1992; Moberg, 1995; Wojciszke, 1994).

In sum, the propensity for category-based cognitive processing to prevail speaks to the powerful effects of categorization over individuation. Nevertheless, the priority perceivers give to categorizing processes does not preclude their ability to use more attribute-oriented processes. Indeed, with the continuum model, we have hoped both to convey our belief that people rely on various kinds of impression formation and to describe the set of processes we think encourage perceivers to use each.

Premise 2: Ease of Information Fit between Category and Attributes Determines the Processes People Use

The continuum model posits that different informational conditions elicit various impression formation processes, depending on the ease with which perceivers can fit a target's attributes to the presently available category.

When perceivers interpret a target's attributes as fitting the category, they respond to the target in ways reflecting the contents of that category. In contrast, when perceivers interpret a target's attributes as incompatible with the existing category, they are likely to move farther toward the individuating end of the continuum—first, by attempting to recategorize the target in a way that better takes account of target features perceived as relevant; and then, but only if necessary, performing a more piecemeal, attribute-by-attribute analysis. Recent research specifies information configurations that typically invoke different interpretations of category–attribute fit, leading to the impression formation processes of category confirmation, recategorization, and piecemeal integration.

The initial categorization process differs from the others in that it is an automatic, perceptual process; perceivers spontaneously categorize targets. However, when perceivers judge targets to be of sufficient motivational relevance, and subsequently encounter additional information about them, perceivers move to the more thoughtful portion of the continuum, beginning with the process labeled "confirmatory categorization." Here, reflecting on information they have about the target, perceivers assess whether the initial categorization still represents the target well enough for current purposes, given the target's prototypicality and the perceiver's sense of variability in the category (Haslam, Oakes, McGarty, Turner, & Onorato, 1995; Lambert, 1995; Perry, 1994). If the additional target information fits well with the initially selected category, the target's perceived membership in that social category becomes more salient and compelling, leading perceivers to respond in ways heavily aligned with the initial category (Hamilton, Sherman, & Ruvolo, 1990; Jackson, Hansen, Hansen, & Sullivan, 1993; Oakes, Turner, & Haslam, 1991).

When perceivers successfully confirm an initial categorization, they avoid the increased cognitive effort needed to shift toward more individuating processes. Nonetheless, perceivers may feel that the target's characteristics do not fit well with the initial categorization. When this happens, they may attempt to identify a different category, one better able to capture the whole of the target's characteristics. Fiske and Neuberg (1990) labeled this process "recategorization," and viewed it as occupying an intermediate position along the continuum of impression formation processes: Although recategorization still involves categorizing the target, it relies more heavily on additional target characteristics to do so. Perceivers can recategorize a target in several ways (see Fiske & Neuberg, 1990). They can access more differentiated subcategories, or subtypes, of the initial category (e.g., Eckes, 1994; for a review, see Fiske, 1998). For instance, a surprisingly passive man may be viewed as one of those "strong, silent types." Subcategorizing is probably the preferred method of recategorization, as it enables the perceiver to retain information from the initial categorization, often with the apparently incompatible target information as justification (Kunda & Oleson, 1995). People may also recategorize using exemplars ("He reminds me of Colin Powell") or self-reference ("He reminds me of the way I used to be"), or may even select a new category altogether, discarding those target characteristics seen as less important and generating a new category that effectively captures the remaining characteristics (Stangor et al., 1992). Regardless of the particular recategorization technique used, the perceivers' affective, cognitive, and behavioral tendencies will be those reflecting the contents of the newly accepted (re)category.

What factors lead perceivers to view new target information as incompatible with their previous categorizations? Obviously, the target characteristics themselves play a critical role: The more extremely inconsistent they are with the category, the more likely it is that people will attempt to recategorize or further individuate the target (Seta & Seta, 1993). In addition, certain social categories are less well developed and entrenched than others, and perceivers may be more likely to doubt the ability of such categories to account adequately for even minimally incompatible target characteristics. Furthermore, when a particularly credible source provides information that a target does not seem to fit the initial category, perceivers are more likely to presume the information to be accurate and reliable, and thus more likely to recategorize or further individuate the target (Macrae, Shepherd, & Milne, 1992). And certain motivations probably influence people's thresholds for accepting new target information as incompatible with existing categorizations; a later section explores such motives.

Finally, when perceivers cannot confirm the initial categorization or recategorize the target—and we think such instances are rare—they are likely to integrate the target information attribute by attribute in a piecemeal fashion (e.g., Kashima & Kerekes, 1994; Levine, Halberstadt, & Goldstone, 1996), *if* they possess sufficient time, attentional resources, and motivation. This is the most individuating of the impression formation processes, for the perceiver considers target-based attributes with minimal reference to a category label.

In summary, interpretation of category–attribute fit determines use of the impression formation continuum: When perceivers view a target's characteristics as fitting easily with the initially selected category, they form impressions consistent with that category; when perceivers cannot fit a target's characteristics with the initially selected category, they engage more individuating processes, such as recategorization or (in unusual cases) piecemeal integration.

Premise 3: Attention to Attribute Information Mediates Use of the Continuum

The third premise proposes that attention mediates the various types of impression formation: Increased attention to target attributes is necessary for perceivers to engage the more thoughtful individuating processes of impression formation.

Why is attention to attributes so important to the model? First, target characteristics suggest categories that may represent the target well. Second, once a category is in place, additional target characteristics become the critical data for examining interpretive fit (Premise 2). And third, when perceivers decide to go beyond the initial categorizations, these attributes become the relevant information base: When perceivers recategorize the target, they need do so in a way that accommodates the attributes, and when perceivers use piecemeal integration processes, the attributes become the pieces of information to be integrated.

This premise was supported originally by work indicating that attention to attributes, but not attention to the category, is correlated with individuation (Fiske, Neuberg, Beattie, & Milberg, 1987), as well as by early work on time pressure (Jamieson & Zanna, 1989; see Fiske & Neuberg, 1990, for a review). Recent research expands these points. People stereotype at the nadir of their circadian rhythm (Bodenhausen, 1990), when they have less capacity to attend. Time pressure, as noted, encourages stereotyping (e.g., Heaton & Kruglanski, 1991; Kaplan, Wanshula, & Zanna, 1993; Kruglanski & Webster, 1991; Pratto & Bargh, 1991). Arousal created by exercise can be distracting enough to encourage stereotyping (Kim & Baron, 1988). Noise that diminishes attentional capacity has similar effects (Kruglanski & Webster, 1991). Anxiety, which in part amounts to capacity-reducing "mental noise," also interferes with individuation (Wilder & Shapiro, 1989a, 1989b).

Increased attention mediates the individuating influence of informational inconsistency. People use more individuating processes when they discover that targets' characteristics are inconsistent with the way they have been categorized (e.g., Fiske et al., 1987). For instance, perceivers pay more attention to a target who violates their expectations than to a target who confirms them (Hilton, Klein, & von Hippel, 1991); this increased attention potentially leads to more individuating evaluations of the target. If people fail to elaborate disconfirming information about an individual target, they may not remember it and use it (Sekaquaptewa & von Hippel, 1994). Stereotype dilution occurs only when perceivers find it impossible to construe the attribute information as stereotype-consistent (De Dreu, Yzerbyt, & Leyens, 1995). Thus, only when attribute information is highly inconsistent and highly attended are more individuating processes likely to supersede category-based ones.

In the end, use of *category* information remains rather high across various information conditions (Fiske & Neuberg, 1990; Fiske, 1998). The changes in attention to and use of *attribute* information, however, are what mediate changes in impression formation. By retaining and emphasizing the crucial roles of both category and attribute information, the model proposes that category information has a constant role, while attribute information has a variable role, mediated by attention allocation.

Premise 4: Motivational Influences on Impression Formation Operate According to the Interdependence Structure and the Motivating Agent's Criteria

Thus far, the chapter has discussed impression formation in terms of the informational influences of prevailing category-based processes, interpretations of information configurations that guide use of the continuum, and differential attention to attribute information that mediate the processes. The model's fourth premise posits that motivations also influence impression formation. This premise is represented in Figure 11.1's inclusion of "personal relevance" as determining whether perceivers go beyond their split-second initial categorizations. Specifically, the premise proposes that outcome dependency (the perceived interdependence structure within a given situation) is crucial. For example, when a person from an underrepresented group suddenly comes in as department head, the department members are likely to adopt a goal of accurately understanding the person who controls many of their outcomes. If the same person is an irrelevant peer or a subordinate, they may not bother to attempt accuracy. Outcome dependency motivates effortful impression formation, in an attempt to be accurate about the person controlling outcomes—the person whom the model describes as the motivating agent.

Outcome dependency operates according to the particular motivating agent's criteria for providing the perceiver's desired outcomes. To continue the prior example, it matters whether a bigoted or an equity-oriented person is department head. With a bigot for a boss, people will stay with more category-based decisions about subordinates and peers than they will with an equity-oriented boss. Perceivers are impelled toward the categorizing or the individuating end of the continuum, precisely because of their motivations that arise from outcome dependency.

More formally, perceiver motivations can be analyzed structurally by focusing on the interdependence structure within the situation.

In particular, consider the structural features of outcome dependency: the motivating agent (who controls the outcomes) and the criteria set for attaining some desired outcome. The motivating agent—the target, a third party, or the perceiver's self—determines the specific criteria for attaining a desired outcome (or avoiding a feared outcome). Together, the motivating agent and the criteria shape the perceiver's goals during impression formation (Riley & Fiske, 1991).

Supporting research underscores how outcome dependency motivates changes toward individuation and toward categorization. Our own research indicates a robust effect, such that outcome dependency increases individuating attention—that is, attention to expectancy-disconfirming information—in the service of forming individual dispositional attributions about the target (Erber & Fiske, 1984; Neuberg & Fiske, 1987). If the perceiver is not initially biased, outcome dependency creates an accuracy goal that leads to open-minded information seeking (Neuberg, 1989). In another study, an outcome dependency decreased bias only among non-partisan (initially unbiased) perceivers. Non-partisan observers of a negotiation were more likely to notice compatible interests, were more accurate with their judgments, and were more evenhanded with their judgments than partisan (initially biased) negotiators (Thompson, 1995). These results imply that nonpartisan perceivers presumably have less at stake and so are less motivated to process information in terms of partisan categories.

Another example of outcome dependency shows its implications for behavior. If a perceiver expects short-term involvement in an interaction with another, tendencies toward behavioral confirmation may encourage more category-based processing. In one instance where perceivers were motivated to form stable, predictable social impressions of their targets' personality, "to check out [their] first impression," perceivers came to believe that their targets held the stereotypic traits expected of them (Snyder & Haugen, 1994). Other interaction goals, however, encourage more individuating processes. For instance, when perceivers are motivated to form accurate impressions of their targets, to get their targets to like them, or to create an easily flowing conversation, they are more respon-

sive to target attributes and more individuating in their impressions (Neuberg, 1989; Neuberg, Judice, Virdin, & Carrillo, 1993; Snyder & Haugen, 1994). Their outcomes, in the short term, depend on the target, for whom accuracy is doubtless a virtue.

Outcome dependency is clearest under conditions of cooperation, when people's outcomes are mutually contingent. Structured cooperative contact can decrease stereotyping, according to the contact hypothesis. Cooperation (mutual outcome dependency) facilitates individuation of outgroup members and reduces bias toward the group as a whole. In a study involving cooperative learning between a perceiver and a confederate posing as a former mental patient, perceivers expected traits that fit the stereotype of a former mental patient. However, those perceivers in the cooperative-learning sessions with the confederate subsequently judged the target more positively and adopted more positive views of the target's social group as a result, presumably because they had focused on the person's individual attributes (Desforges et al., 1991).

Perceivers' outcomes can also be contingent on third parties—persons who are outside the interaction but hold a stake in it. Being held accountable to a third party with unknown or unbiased views can make perceivers attend carefully, with the goal of accuracy (Tetlock, 1992; Tetlock & Lerner, Chapter 28, this volume). Information and accountability can moderate stereotype-driven processes during social decision making, such that perceivers who are held accountable attend to stereotype-inconsistent attributes (Hattrup & Ford, 1995). Moreover, accountability can influence perceivers who initially categorize a target at a superordinate level (e.g., "woman"), to process further any available attribute information regarding the target and to form a more differentiated, subtyped impression (e.g., "businesswoman") (Pendry & Macrae, 1996).

Outcome dependency on a third party—that is, accountability—can undercut even the effects of mood on stereotyping processes. In the absence of such motivations, angry perceivers rendered more stereotypic judgments, compared to neutral and sad perceivers, who did not significantly differ (Bodenhausen, Sheppard, & Kramer, 1994). Again, in the absence of accountability, happy perceivers used stereotypic processing (Bodenhausen, Kramer, & Susser, 1994). Nevertheless, when informed that they would be accountable for their judgments, even mood-manipulated participants greatly reduced their stereotypic thinking. Despite the pervasiveness of happy people rendering stereotyped judgments, they can avoid the influences of stereotypes in forming judgments when accountability (third-party outcome dependency) offers a motivational incentive (see also Bodenhausen, Macrae, & Sherman, Chapter 13, and Bless & Schwarz, Chapter 21, this volume).

Given the research presented, outcome dependency in various forms plays a part in attentional and interpretive processes by altering how the perceiver forms impressions. The particular interdependence structure, which includes the motivating agent and the criteria set by the agent, moves the perceiver's impression formation goals along the continuum. In other words, motivations arising from the interdependence structure push perceivers toward individuation or keep them toward the continuum's category-based end.

Premise 5: Attention to and Interpretation of Attributes Mediate Motivational Influences on Impression Formation

The preceding section suggests that perceivers' motivations stem from the interdependence structure, but exactly how do these motivations operate? From an analysis of the motivational implications of interdependence, as well as from the overall continuum model, the fifth premise proposes that motivational influences are mediated by attentional and interpretive responses to attributes. As with the impact of different information configurations on the continuum (Premise 3), attention is the necessary mediating mechanism, and interpretation determines the amount of perceived category–attribute fit (Premise 2). Again, available research supports this theoretical framework.

Perceiver outcome dependency or outcome control can influence how information relevant to a target is heeded and interpreted. As noted already, social information may be variously attended and may be interpreted stereotypically, given differential outcome dependency. Motivated to enhance prediction

and control over their situations, the outcome-dependent powerless attend to the powerful others who control their outcomes. Thus, powerless perceivers tend to formulate complex, potentially nonstereotyped (but not necessarily accurate) impressions (Dépret & Fiske, in press; Goodwin et al., 1998; Stevens & Fiske, 1998). On the other hand, the powerful, who are by definition less outcome-dependent on their subordinates, grant less individuating attention to those with less power, making them more vulnerable to stereotype-based information processing (Goodwin et al., 1998; Operario & Fiske, 1998; Zemore & Fiske, 1998). The powerful need not attend to target others to control their own outcomes; often cannot attend to others because they are attentionally overloaded; and, if they are high in need for dominance, do not desire to attend to others (Fiske, 1993a).

For people whose cooperative outcomes depend upon others, as noted, individuating attention rather than stereotyping attention appears especially likely (e.g., Erber & Fiske, 1984; Neuberg & Fiske, 1987). Are individuating processes equally likely when the interdependence structure is characterized by a negative contingency between outcomes—that is, by competition? One study investigated this likelihood by having participants expect to compete or not to compete with a fictitious other portrayed as competent or incompetent (Ruscher & Fiske, 1990). They then commented about the individual's attributes, some of which were consistent with the expectations and others of which were inconsistent. As predicted, competitors increased their attention to inconsistencies, rendered more dispositional inferences about the inconsistencies, and developed more varied, idiosyncratic impressions. When individual competition enters the interdependence structure, perceivers' goals are geared toward understanding the competitor's attributes—presumably to gain better, more accurate knowledge of the competitor, in order to enhance their chances of success.

Within competitive contexts, expectancies of the target and the nature of the information available both work to influence information processing. When perceivers form expectancies of an opponent's competence, they tend to limit their attention to the opponent's discrete attributes to aid them in matching the expectancy with the attributes, perhaps in an attempt to "size up the competition" more accurately (Miki, Tsuchiya, & Nishino, 1993). But when the target expectancy is less well formulated, because the available attribute information is initially nondiagnostic, competitors may interpret the attribute information as congruent with their stereotype-based beliefs.

Whereas interpersonal (one-on-one) competition facilitates individuating impressions of opponents, intergroup (group-on-group) competition tends to promote stereotyping of opponents. In one study, when a person was joined by others who would compete with that person, the competitors as a group managed their limited attentional resources by assigning greater priority to individuating each other as teammates (Ruscher, Fiske, Miki, & Van Manen, 1991). Expectancy information was manipulated, and those who competed alone were then compared to those who competed in teams. Results showed that individuating processes, reflected in attention to and dispositional inferences about expectancy-incongruent attributes, were apparent in interpersonal but not intergroup competition, a result also supported by Dépret and Fiske (in press). This suggests that one-on-one competition makes the goal of obtaining accurate impressions of opponents particularly more salient.

Indeed, a watered-down version of outcome dependency—simply expecting to interact with someone—can encourage accuracy-driven attention to a target's individual attributes in the service of one's goal. For example, perceivers exert greater effort making inferences about individuals with whom they expect to interact (Johnston, Hewstone, Pendry, & Frankish, 1994). Thus prospective interaction has sometimes been considered as a means to reduce inaccurate impressions. Although the prospect of interaction with a target can prevent inferential error by motivating perceivers with already biased impressions of the target to revise such impressions, it can also promote error by prompting perceivers to consume cognitive resources in planning their own behavior instead of changing their biases. Certain features of prospective interaction, such as role demands, goal familiarity, and partner novelty, determine whether

perceivers become preoccupied with preparing their own behavior, which in turn determines whether the prospective interaction prevents or promotes inferential error (Osborne & Gilbert, 1992). Attention to the target (specifically, to the target's attributes) and the perceiver's motivational goals apparently play key roles in the correction of biased impressions.

In summary, motivational influences, like informational influences, are also mediated by attentional and interpretive responses to attributes. Interdependence structure is a central source of motivations prompting either category-based or individuating responses, depending on the particular motivating agents and their established criteria. Thus, the variations in perceived type of interdependence directly affect a perceiver's attention to and interpretations of the information configuration.

Conclusion

The five core premises of the continuum model have aged gracefully. In particular, the evidence for each has expanded since the original literature review.

REVISITING SOME META-ASSUMPTIONS

Behind the explicit stages and more abstract core premises of the continuum model, there lurk some background perspectives that we now bring into the foreground. The crucial role of motivation is one, and the role of individual differences is closely related, reminding us of Henry James's admonition at the beginning of this chapter—"the posted presence of the watcher." What is more, the model has long assumed that expectations interplay with information; it is neither a fully social constructionist model nor a totally data-driven one. Finally, as an information-processing model, it can be implemented as serial or parallel processes, and this was made explicit in the original statement (Fiske & Neuberg, 1990). This section, then, addresses two issues of motives (situational and individual) and two issues of information (its interplay and its implementation).

Situational Motives Matter

Perceivers tend toward category-based processes as default processes. But depending on motivation ("personal relevance" in Figure 11.1), perceivers may end up anywhere on the impression formation continuum; they pay attention and form interpretations in accord with their motivations. As just noted, Fiske and Neuberg (1990) described motivations as stemming from a motivating agent—self, target, or a third party—who controls outcomes that matter to the individual. The content of the outcomes matters less than who controls them and what the criteria are for obtaining them. The direction and nature of the perceiver's attention are determined by the motivating agent. For example, when the motivating agent is the target, who must cooperate with the perceiver for both to obtain a desired outcome, the perceiver attends to the target with a goal of accuracy (e.g., Neuberg & Fiske, 1987). Or the motivating agent may be a third party who desires a particular outcome, as when an employee is accountable to an audience (e.g., the boss) with known values (Tetlock, 1992; Tetlock & Lerner, Chapter 28, this volume); this situation encourages attention and interpretation in accord with the motivating agent's desired outcome. And if the motivating agent is the self, attention and interpretation operate in the service of one's own values (Fiske & Von Hendy, 1992).

The original formulation of the model did not specify the range of motivations likely to influence impressions. Instead, it used illustrations from then-current literature, organized in terms of the self, perceiver, and target. Since that time, Stevens and Fiske (1995) have organized social motives in terms of social adaptation. A truly social view of interpersonal motivation starts with the premise that people need other people to survive; thus people are adapted to live in social groups. People whose core motives facilitate group life are more likely to be successful, in this view. Thus people are psychologically adapted to the social group as the immediate survival environment (see Caporael, 1997; Caporael & Brewer, 1991).

Reviewing the range of motivations identified by two dozen personality and social psychologists during this century fits well with this social survival perspective (for references, see Stevens & Fiske, 1995). Under various names, the most frequently identified motives include belonging, understanding, controlling, self-enhancing, and trusting; social-cognition researchers have investigated only some of these. The boundaries among these motives are not absolute but overlapping, and the list is not necessarily exhaustive or uniquely appropriate. Still, it emphasizes the social quality of the core motives, each of which is applicable here.

Belonging

The main motivational emphasis both previously and in our ongoing research has been on interdependence, which may be considered a major aspect of the core motive of belonging. People's need to be part of social groups and dyadic relationships enhanced their ancient survival skills and continues to enhance their mental and physical health in modern times (e.g., Baumeister & Leary, 1995). The other person or people are the context for adaptation and survival (Caporael, 1997). In this context, it is not surprising, then, that people try to maintain their relationships and social belonging by trying to form accurate (or at least good enough) impressions of the others on whom they depend. In the model's previous terms, the target is then the primary motivating agent—the one whose criteria must be met to obtain outcomes that matter (in this case, constructive interactions). In most cases, interdependence is facilitated by trying to get an accurate impression of the other, and a program of research has established that interdependence facilitates various specific individuating processes: (1) increased attention to stereotype-discrepant information; (2) increased dispositional inferences to it; and (3) more varied, idiosyncratic impressions (Dépret & Fiske, in press; Erber & Fiske, 1984; Goodwin et al., 1998; Neuberg & Fiske, 1987; Pendry & Macrae, 1994; Ruscher & Fiske, 1990; Ruscher et al., 1991; Snodgrass, 1992; Stevens & Fiske, 1998; for a review, see Fiske & Dépret, 1996).

The need to get along has been newly identified as a motive relevant to impression formation (Smith, Neuberg, Judice, & Biesanz, 1997; Snyder, 1992; Snyder & Haugen, 1994). For perceivers, the need to get along interferes with their attempting to confirm their stereotypes. For targets, the motive to get along encourages them to accommodate, and thus to confirm the perceivers' stereotypes. Getting along encourages people to go along with their partners' presumed attitudes, even if these are stereotypic (Chen, Shechter, & Chaiken, 1996; Ruscher, Hammer, & Hammer, 1996).

Essentially, people who are forming impressions comply with salient norms. If the local norms appear to promote stereotypes, people's impression formation processes and expressed impressions tend to be more stereotypic. The converse is true when individuating, egalitarian norms are salient (Blanchard, Crandall, Brigham, & Vaughn, 1994; Blanchard, Lilly, & Vaughn, 1991; Fiske & Von Hendy, 1992; Leippe & Eisenstadt, 1994; Pryor, Geidd, & Williams, 1995).

Accountability to a third party also motivates more effortful impression formation processes (Pendry & Macrae, 1996; Tetlock, Skitka, & Boettger, 1989; for a review, see Tetlock, 1992). To the extent that the third-party audience's views are known, perceivers conform their decision-making processes to those views. The third party's imagined views also embody perceived norms, so accountability is another form of social contingency. Thus there is evidence that interdependence, getting along, norms, and accountability forms of belonging all influence how impressions are formed along the continuum from more category-based to more individuating impressions.

Understanding

In social contexts, interdependent players must operate under shared understanding of the environment, group norms, and each other. The need to understand the social world, and the physical world as interpreted by the social world, is a core motive from infancy onward. This "cognitive drive" relies on the self as a motivating agent, as White (1959) so aptly described "effectance motivation" many years ago (see Stevens & Fiske, 1995, for more references). But all cognition is social (Ostrom, 1984; Resnick, Levine, & Teasley, 1991) and responds to shared social reality, so targets and third parties are motivating agents here as well. Explicit instructions to be accurate (Chen et al., 1996; Neuberg, 1989; Neuberg & Fiske, 1987) and situationally manipulated fear of invalidity (Freund, Kruglanski, & Shpitzajzen, 1985; Kruglanski & Freund, 1983; Kruglanski & Mayseless, 1988) cause people to form more effortful, potentially individuating impressions. (A later section discusses individual differences in needs for accurate understanding.) This relatively "cognitive" motive allows people to function better in groups by moving toward shared understandings.

Controlling

The need for control also has important cognitive elements, and in the context of the continuum model, it subsumes primarily those goals that relate to maintaining control over the self and the target. People who are deprived of control have been demonstrated to search for information in their social environment (e.g., Pittman & D'Agostino, 1989; for reviews, see Pittman, 1998; Pittman & Heller, 1987), even apart from the work on interdependence, just reviewed. Time pressure may be viewed as another form of control deprivation, and time pressure limits perceivers' abilities to move down the continuum toward more individuating impressions (for reviews, see Fiske, 1993b; Kruglanski & Webster, 1996). Time pressure can increase discrimination (Freund et al., 1985; Jamieson & Zanna, 1989; Kruglanski & Freund, 1983), as can the pressure to implement a decision (Gollwitzer & Kinney, 1989).

People who have social control strive to maintain it. Power can be defined as control of others' outcomes (for a review, see Dépret & Fiske, 1993). As noted earlier, people can maintain power by relying on stereotypic information and ignoring counterstereotypic information; stereotypes perpetuate asymmetrical power relations, and inaccuracy is presumably less costly for the powerful than for the powerless (Fiske, 1993a; Fiske & Dépret, 1996; Goodwin et al., 1998), who can confirm the stereotypic outcomes they expect (Claire & Fiske, 1998; Copeland, 1994).

Self-Enhancing

Motives to feel good or at least to improve the self carry a less cognitive, more affective flavor than the previous two (more cognitive) motives. The crucial phenomena appear to be threats to self-esteem. People whose collective high self-esteem is threatened are most likely to discriminate (Crocker & Luhtanen, 1990). Social identity theory (Tajfel & Turner, 1986) describes self-esteem maintenance as critical to intergroup perception; favoring the ingroup, which often entails at least relatively disadvantaging the outgroup (see Brewer & Brown, 1998), is the basis for a positive identity. Under threat, the individuating effects of interdependence break down (Dépret & Fiske, in press; Stevens & Fiske, 1998). And being insecure or anxious enhances stereotyping (Fiske, Morling, & Stevens, 1996; Stephan & Stephan, 1984; Wilder & Shapiro, 1989a, 1989b). Thus self-esteem maintenance and self-enhancement can require outgroup derogation. And, relatedly, Altemeyer's (1981, 1988) modern scale of authoritarianism incorporates personal threat as predicting categorical responses.

Self-enhancement motives can also, in contrast, discourage category-based responses. Theories of subtle racism—aversive racism (Gaertner & Dovidio, 1986), racial ambivalence (Katz & Hass, 1988), and modern racism (McConahay & Hough, 1976)—all presuppose that self-esteem can depend on an unprejudiced self-concept. The theories of modern sexism (Swim, Aikin, Hall, & Hunter, 1995), neosexism (Tougas, Brown, Beaton, & Joly, 1995), and ambivalent sexism (Glick & Fiske, 1996) make similar assumptions about sexism; they all focus on self-enhancement as underlying stereotyping and prejudice.

People's motivation to maintain self-esteem or to improve themselves (hence the term "self-enhancing," which covers both) arguably makes them strive to be better members of their group. This can entail category-based responses that favor the ingroup and (relatively) derogate the outgroup. Especially under threat, these responses motivate category confirmation processes. However, if egalitarian values are important to the self, the self-improvement form of self-enhancement can undercut stereotyping.

Trusting

People adapt better to immediate social groups when they are at least initially trusting of ingroup members. The impression formation literature has long demonstrated a positivity bias, such that perceivers expect positive things from others, all else being equal (e.g., Matlin & Stang, 1978; Parducci, 1968; Sears, 1983). These kinds of motives remain to be investigated for their bearing on category-based versus individuated processes. But a basic motive to trust the ingroup would seem related to individuating ingroup members, even given the effort required.

Conclusion

A variety of situational motives direct impression formation toward more categorizing or more individuating processes. Although different frameworks can parse social motives, one framework identifies core motives in terms of individuals' functioning adaptively in social groups, and describes the implications of these motives for impression formation.

Individual Differences in Motivation Matter

People come to their social encounters with different chronic goals, many of which influence the way they form impressions of others. This section briefly considers several such goals: personal need for structure, depression, need for cognition, fear of invalidity, and content-specific goals.

Personal Need for Structure

Some people, more than others, like their lives to be organized, simply structured, and predictable. These people value their routines and become uncomfortable or distressed when their sense of order is disrupted. Their cognitive activities often show a similar penchant for simple structure and order. For instance, people scoring high on the Personal Need for Structure Scale (Thompson, Nacarrato, & Parker, 1989, 1992) view themselves, others, and nonsocial objects in relatively simple ways (Neuberg & Newsom, 1993); they are especially likely to spontaneously generate potentially categorizing trait inferences (Moskowitz, 1993); they are more likely to overgeneralize failure experiences into learned helplessness (Mikulincer, Yinin, & Kabili, 1991); and they are more likely to fulfill responsibilities in a prompt fashion, thus avoiding the discomfort associated with a lack of completion (Neuberg & Newsom, 1993; Roman, Moskowitz, Stein, & Eisenberg, 1995).

Of more direct relevance to impression formation, people with strong desires for simple structure are more likely to assimilate new information to previously existing structures (Thompson, Roman, Moskowitz, Chaiken, & Bargh, 1994), to create simple stereotypes of new groups (Schaller, Boyd, Yohannes, & O'Brien, 1995), and to use simplifying social categories to understand others (Naccarato, 1988; Neuberg & Newsom, 1993). People who desire simple structure in their lives prefer the more category-based end of the impression formation continuum; they are perhaps aware that a thoughtful, individuating consideration of new target information carries with it the potential to prove one's existing categorizations inadequate. In sum, people who are dispositionally high in the need for structure want to preserve their initial category-based impressions when possible.

Mild Depression and the Desire for Control

Mildly depressed individuals are especially likely to use individuating processes, perhaps in an attempt to gain control over their lives (Edwards & Weary, 1993). Consistent with this interpretation, people who score highly on the Desire for Control Scale are especially likely to explore more deeply their social situations (Burger, 1992). In one study, for instance, such individuals were less likely to succumb to the simplifying correspondence bias and more likely to search their social situation for causes of another's behavior (Burger & Hemans, 1988). Of course, people who are *severely* depressed tend to view the world as uncontrollable, and may thus see little reason to expend scarce cognitive resources in an effort to understand others in a more individuated way. Indeed, severely depressed people tend to rely more heavily on category-oriented processing (Marsh & Weary, 1994).

Need for Cognition and Personal Fear of Invalidity

Some people enjoy solving life's puzzles, view thinking as fun, and appreciate discovering the strengths and weaknesses of their arguments. These people are high in the "need for cognition" (Cacioppo & Petty, 1982); they are less likely to use simplifying cognitive heuristics and more willing to expend extra efforts to assess fully their social circumstances (Cacioppo, Petty, Feinstein, & Jarvis, 1996). Although data are lacking, such individuals seem more likely to stray deeply into the individuating end of the impression formation continuum.

We would expect the same from people high in the "fear of invalidity" (Freund et al., 1985; Thompson et al., 1989, 1992), for a different but related reason. These individuals worry about making poor judgments. As such, they often set for themselves high thresholds for accepting any decision; in the absence of great confidence, they are reluctant to commit to decisions. People high in the fear of invalidity should thus be slow to apply simple categorizations for targets they encounter. Instead, they are likely to continue gathering information about the target, in the hope of forming a particularly accurate impression.

"Content" Goals

The chronic goals just noted might well be characterized as "process" goals, as they capture individual differences in the *ways* people like to think about their social worlds. Such goals work by directing perceivers' attention generally toward or away from target attributes, and perceivers care little about the content of the information they focus on (except, perhaps, for its relevance to the information previously collected or to the impressions previously formed). Other goals, in contrast, direct perceivers' attention toward specific kinds of information. People who are dispositionally anxious to please may seek information about others that is diagnostic of social approval; people who are dispositionally insecure in their self-views may seek information about others' weaknesses, so that they can boost themselves in the process; people seeking to land a spouse will focus disproportionately on such characteristics as fidelity, agreeableness, intelligence, social status, physical attractiveness, and age. In short, people think about others so that they can reach their goals more efficiently, and different target characteristics serve different social goals. Within the framework of the continuum model, "content" goals will influence which categories perceivers use for initial categorization, which target attributes come into focus, and the willingness of a perceiver to settle on a particular impression.

Conclusion

Recent research focusing on chronic social and epistemic goals can be profitably applied to the continuum model. Having considered situational and chronic motives, we now turn to information—specifically, its interplay with expectations and its implementation in the formal model.

Expectations Interplay with Information

The continuum model has been labeled by some as a "strong" social-constructivist model—one that "assumes that social perception *creates* social reality as much or more than it reflects social reality" (Jussim, 1991, p. 54; emphasis in original). Such a representation misses the essence of the model. Indeed, its original purpose was to begin explaining the interplay between features of the social perceiver on the one hand, and the information received from the target on the other. A target's characteristics influence how the target is categorized and when (or if) these categories are abandoned in the search for a more individuating understanding. A perceiver's expectations and goals influence which target characteristics come into focus and how they are interpreted. And the social context influences both what a target reveals and what a perceiver apprehends. Although we do indeed believe that perceivers sometimes see primarily what they want to see, we believe just as strongly that "there is a there out there" that strongly constrains social perception and impression formation processes. Our position was never one of advocating for a social-constructivist versus a social-realist view of impression formation. Rather, our interest has always been in understanding the mutual, interactive influences of the perceiver and the perceived.

Serial and Parallel Processes Both Fit the Continuum Model

In a recent paper, Kunda and Thagard (1996) proposed a parallel-constraint-satisfaction theory of impression formation, in which social stereotypes and target traits and behaviors constrain one another's meanings and together influence the impressions people form. They contrasted their theory with the continuum model and found the latter wanting, due primarily to its alleged serial nature and to the priority it ostensibly gives to social stereotype information over individuating information. Their critique rests on several misunderstandings of the continuum model. Indeed, Fiske and Neuberg (1990) considered (albeit briefly) the possibility that its proposals could be instantiated equally well by parallel or serial mechanisms.

Space prevents addressing all relevant issues here, so this section will briefly focus on two. First, the 1990 model stated quite clearly (as we have done again, earlier in the present chapter) that many different features of a target can take on the organizing role of social category. Although certain features, such as gender, race, and age, may gain preeminence because of their visual accessibility (and thus their temporal precedence), this need not be the case. Thus, although the model does claim that perceivers categorize targets, and that once targets are categorized, other features of the targets will often not demonstrate a similar impact, it does not limit the features that may serve as categories to those evoking common social stereotypes (as Kunda and Thagard imply). For instance, a target can be categorized on the basis of a single behavior, and as a result, the behavior will gain an enhanced amount of influence over the ultimate impression formed. Kunda and Thagard's claim that common social stereotypes need not have a greater impact on the perceiver's impressions than other target features is compatible with the continuum model.

Second, Kunda and Thagard (1996) criticize the serial nature of the impression formation processes located on our continuum, noting that a parallel model can account for the existing laboratory data at least as well. Several points apply: Information about others usually arrives (or is captured via our limited-capacity attentional system) sequentially; rarely do people in the real world simultaneously apprehend all the many pieces of information that Kunda and Thagard include in their modeling simulations. The continuum model was designed to capture this kind of active, thoughtful impression formation, and so we are unapologetic about its roughly serial nature. Note further that when the parallel-constraint-satisfaction model is made to accept information serially (as in Kunda and Thagard's simulation of the primacy effect), it begins to look much like the continuum model in the predictions it makes.

We should also note that Kunda and Thagard's (1996) critique of the serial nature of the continuum model rests on several unusual features of their own model. Their simulations presume that all information is available to the perceiver simultaneously, that each piece of information receives the identical amount of attention, and that perceivers do not form impressions until all the information is in. Such assumptions may approximate the conditions in sparse experimental paradigms, but they do not capture most impression formation in the real world. Indeed, their model would generate perceiver responses quite compatible with the predictions of the continuum model (1) if it received target features in the order in which they typically appear (e.g., physical features such as race and gender, followed by social behaviors, followed by inferences about the traits these behaviors represent); (2) if these features received different amounts of processing as a function of their frequency and recency of activation, the perceiver's goals and attentional capacity, and so forth; and (3) if the simulation were to "read out" the cognitive and affective responses in a more continuous manner. In particular, the flow from initial categorization through recategorization would be easily discerned if one were to model these more realistic conditions (see Bodenhausen et al., Chapter 13, this volume).

Moreover, the continuum model is entirely compatible with an implementation in which categorization processes and more attribute-based processes are set in motion simultaneously, but the categorization processes are faster and can constitute a "stop rule" for the more attribute-based processes if categorization results seem adequate for present purposes. In this parallel implementation (anticipated by Fiske & Neuberg, 1990), the categories and other attributes begin to interplay after the initial categorization, with the categorical processes carrying less relative weight as the attribute-oriented processes carry more relative weight, but both proceed in parallel.

In other respects, we have been necessarily brief here and certainly not as thorough as we would like. For instance, space does not allow us to explore the commonalities between the process of constraint satisfaction and the process of information fit assessment, or to address how the experimental procedures and demands of many laboratory studies might artifactually increase the apparent fit of Kunda and Thagard's data to their model.

Finally, although they are not alone in this, note that Kunda and Thagard (1996) fail to appreciate the dynamic nature of the continuum model. As we conceive of it, the impression formation process not only continually cycles back to the confirmatory categorization stage (using in later iterations the most recently accepted categorization as its foundation) as each piece of new information is attended, but also always evokes perceiver impressions appropriate to its last accepted categorization. Such a continually flowing system seems quite amenable to a parallel-processing mechanism—albeit one nested in a roughly serial information-gathering system.

In sum, the alleged incompatibilities between the parallel-constraint-satisfaction model and the continuum model are less real than they may appear. Indeed, an integration of the two models could capitalize on each model's strengths. The Kunda and Thagard model provides a mechanism by which target features can constrain one another's meanings; a means of capturing the flow from initial categorization to recategorization in a more obviously dynamic way; and a thoughtful consideration of how response modalities (e.g., inferences about traits versus behavioral expectations) might respond differently, given the identical target information. The continuum model posits the factors that influence which categories become activated; articulates how motivation and attention bring target information roughly serially into the system, and differentially focus the perceiver on some information at the expense of other information; and so on. Such an integration would move us beyond debate (serial processing vs. parallel processing) to a resolution (serial processing *and* parallel processing).

COMPARISONS WITH OTHER DUAL-PROCESS MODELS

In this chapter, we have first described the historical context and reviewed the specific stages of the continuum model; have then described its five core premises and some of the new research support for them; and, finally, have examined some of its meta-assumptions about situational and individual differences in motives, along with its emphasis on both expectations and information, and its compatibility with both serial and parallel implementations.

In conclusion, we wish to note the compatibility and contrast of the model with some other dual-process models reviewed in this volume. The continuum model is superficially closest to Brewer's model of impression formation (Brewer & Harasty, Chapter 12, this volume), in that both propose alternative sequences or stages of processing, with more category-based processes dominant. The essential differences (Fiske, 1988) include (1) Brewer's emphasis on distinct types of cognitive representations versus our emphasis on one type that is modified on-line; (2) her emphasis on distinct inference rules following each stage, versus our standard reliance on informational fit and motivational involvement at each stage; (3) our focus on attentional and interpretive processes as the single, unifying mediator; (4) Brewer's use of a branching model, versus our continuum; and (5) our more explicit emphasis on motivations and goals. Nevertheless, the similarities remain, in that both models synthesize a variety of literatures in person perception and stereotyping.

The continuum model also bears some resemblance to the heuristic–systematic model (Chen & Chaiken, Chapter 4, this volume) and the elaboration likelihood model (Petty & Wegener, Chapter 3, this volume) of attitudes. The similarities include the specification of more automatic, superficial processes versus more in-depth, analytic processes, with the joint role of informational and motivational factors in both. One of the major differences, of course, is that the continuum model focuses on the cues provided by people, not the cues provided by persuasive communications. Moreover, whereas categorization plays a major role in the continuum model, it is mostly absent in the heuristic-systematic model and the elaboration likelihood model. Like the two attitude models, the continuum model provides a role for multiple types of motivation, but its most frequently studied motivations have been those most relevant to interactions between people. The continuum model also has some similarities to another model of attitudes—namely, Fazio's "motivation and opportunity as determinants" (MODE) model (Fazio & Towles-Schwen, Chapter 5, this volume). Both models posit affective associations to attitude objects (in our case, people), which are quickly triggered upon each encounter. Although schema-triggered affect is a central theoretical feature of the continuum model (Fiske, 1982), research on this model has never pursued the processing dynamics of such affect, whereas the MODE research has pursued these implications in detail. In short, some common themes underlie the various dual-process models, but they fit different circumstances.

ACKNOWLEDGMENTS

The writing of this chapter was supported by National Science Foundation Grant No. 9421480 to Susan T. Fiske; by National Institute of Mental Health Grant No. MH45719 to Steven L. Neuberg; and by National Institute of Mental Health Training Grants No. MH18827 to the Personality and Social Psychology program at the University of Massachusetts, and No. MH15742, administered by the American Psychological Association; both training grants supported Monica Lin.

REFERENCES

Altemeyer, B. (1981). *Right-wing authoritarianism.* Winnipeg: University of Manitoba Press.
Altemeyer, B. (1988). *Enemies of freedom.* San Francisco: Jossey-Bass.
Anderson, N. H. (1981). *Foundations of information integration theory.* New York: Academic Press.

Asch, S. E. (1946). Forming impressions of personality. *Journal of Abnormal and Social Psychology, 41*, 303–314.

Asch, S. E., & Zukier, H. (1984). Thinking about persons. *Journal of Personality and Social Psychology, 46*, 1230–1240.

Banaji, M. R., & Hardin, C. (1996). Automatic stereotyping. *Psychological Science, 7*, 136–141.

Baumeister, R. F., & Leary, M. R. (1995). The need to belong: Desire for interpersonal attachments as a fundamental human motivation. *Psychological Bulletin, 117*, 497–529.

Biernat, M., & Vescio, T. K. (1993). Categorization and stereotyping: Effects of group context on memory and social judgment. *Journal of Experimental Social Psychology, 29*, 166–202.

Biesanz, J. C., Neuberg, S. L., Smith, D. M., & Asher, T. (1998). *When accuracy-motivated perceivers fail: Attentional load, personal need for structure, and the reemerging self-fulfilling prophecy.* Unpublished manuscript, Arizona State University.

Blair, I. V., & Banaji, M. R. (1996). Automatic and controlled processes in stereotype priming. *Journal of Personality and Social Psychology, 70*, 1126–1141.

Blanchard, F. A., Crandall, C. S., Brigham, J. C., & Vaughn, L. A. (1994). Condemning and condoning racism: A social context approach to interracial settings. *Journal of Applied Social Psychology, 79*, 993–997.

Blanchard, F. A., Lilly, T., & Vaughn, L. A. (1991). Reducing the expression of racial prejudice. *Psychological Science, 2*, 101–105.

Bodenhausen, G. V. (1988). Stereotypic biases in social decision making and memory: Testing process models for stereotype use. *Journal of Personality and Social Psychology, 55*, 726–737.

Bodenhausen, G. V., Kramer, G. P., & Susser, K. (1994). Happiness and stereotypic thinking in social judgment. *Journal of Personality and Social Psychology, 66*, 621–632.

Bodenhausen, G. V., Sheppard, L. A., & Kramer, G. P. (1994). Negative affect and social judgments: The differential impact of anger and sadness. *European Journal of Social Psychology, 24*, 45–62.

Brewer, M. B., & Brown, R. J. (1998). Intergroup relations. In D. T. Gilbert, S. T. Fiske, & G. Lindzey (Eds.), *The handbook of social psychology* (Vol. 2, 4th ed., pp. 554–594). New York: McGraw-Hill.

Burger, J. M. (1992). *Desire for control: Personality, social, and clinical perspectives.* New York: Plenum.

Burger, J. M., & Hemans, L. T. (1988). Desire for control and the use of attribution processes. *Journal of Personality, 56*, 531–546.

Cacioppo, J. T., & Petty, R. E. (1982). The need for cognition. *Journal of Personality and Social Psychology, 42*, 116–131.

Cacioppo, J. T., Petty, R. E., Feinstein, J. A., & Jarvis, W. B. G. (1996). Dispositional differences in cognitive motivation: The life and times of individuals varying in need for cognition. *Psychological Bulletin, 119*, 197–253.

Caporael, L. R. (1997). The evolution of truly social cognition: The core configurations model. *Personality and Social Psychology Review, 1*, 276–298.

Caporael, L. R., & Brewer, M. B. (1991). Reviving evolutionary psychology: Biology meets society. *Journal of Social Issues, 47*, 187–195.

Chen, S., Schechter, D., & Chaiken, S. (1996). Getting the truth or getting along: Accuracy- vs. impression-motivated heuristic and systematic processing. *Journal of Personality and Social Psychology, 71*, 262–275.

Claire, T., & Fiske, S. T. (1998). A systemic view of behavioral confirmation: Counterpoint to the individualist view. In C. Sedikides, C. Insko, & J. Schopler (Eds.), *Intergroup cognition and behavior* (pp. 205–232). Mahwah, NJ: Erlbaum.

Copeland, J. T. (1994). Prophecies of power: Motivational implications of social power for behavioral confirmation. *Journal of Personality and Social Psychology, 67*, 264–277.

Crocker, J., & Luhtanen, R. (1990). Collective self-esteem and ingroup bias. *Journal of Personality and Social Psychology, 58*, 60–67.

De Dreu, C. K. W., Yzerbyt, V. Y., & Leyens, J.-P. (1995). Dilution of stereotype-based cooperation in mixed-motive interdependence. *Journal of Experimental Social Psychology, 31*, 575–593.

Dépret, E. F., & Fiske, S. T. (1993). Social cognition and power: Some cognitive consequences of social structure as a source of control deprivation. In G. Weary, F. Gleicher, & K. Marsh (Eds.), *Control motivation and social cognition* (pp. 176–202). New York: Springer-Verlag.

Dépret, E. F., & Fiske, S. T. (in press). Perceiving the powerful: Intriguing individuals versus threatening groups. *Journal of Experimental Social Psychology.*

Desforges, D. M., Lord, C. G., Ramsey, S. L., Mason, J. A., Van Leeuwen, M. D., West, S. L., & Lepper, M. R. (1991). Effects of structured cooperative contact on changing negative attitudes toward stigmatized social groups. *Journal of Personality and Social Psychology, 60*, 531–544.

Devine, P. G. (1989). Stereotypes and prejudice: Their automatic and controlled components. *Journal of Personality and Social Psychology, 56*, 5–18.

Dovidio, J. F., Evans, N., & Tyler, R. B. (1986). Racial stereotypes: The contents of their cognitive representations. *Journal of Experimental Social Psychology, 22*, 22–37.

Dovidio, J. F., & Gaertner, S. L. (1993). Stereotypes and evaluative intergroup bias. In D. M. Mackie & D. L. Hamilton (Eds.), *Affect, cognition, and stereotyping* (pp. 167–193). San Diego, CA: Academic Press.

Eckes, T. (1994). Explorations in gender cognition: Content and structure of female and male subtypes. *Social Cognition, 12*, 37–60.

Edwards, J. A., & Weary, G. (1993). Depression and the impression-formation continuum: Piecemeal processing despite the availability of category information. *Journal of Personality and Social Psychology, 64*, 636–645.

Erber, R., & Fiske, S. T. (1984). Outcome dependency and attention to inconsistent information. *Journal of Personality and Social Psychology, 47*, 709–726.

Fazio, R. H., Jackson, J. R., Dunton, B. C., & Williams, C. J. (1995). Variability in automatic activation as an unobtrusive measure of racial attitudes: A bona fide pipeline? *Journal of Personality and Social Psychology, 69*, 1013–1027.

Fiske, S. T. (1980). Attention and weight in person perception: The impact of negative and extreme behavior.

Journal of Personality and Social Psychology, 38, 889–906.

Fiske, S. T. (1982). Schema-triggered affect: Applications to social perception. In M. S. Clark & S. T. Fiske (Eds.), *Affect and cognition: The 17th annual Carnegie Symposium on Cognition* (pp. 55–78). Hillsdale, NJ: Erlbaum.

Fiske, S. T. (1988). Compare and contrast: Brewer's dual-process model and Fiske et al.'s continuum model. In T. K. Srull & R. S. Wyer (Eds.), *Advances in social cognition: Vol. 1. A dual model of impression formation* (pp. 65–76). Hillsdale, NJ: Erlbaum.

Fiske, S. T. (1993a). Controlling other people: The impact of power on stereotyping. *American Psychologist, 48,* 621–628.

Fiske, S. T. (1993b). Social cognition and social perception. *Annual Review of Psychology, 44,* 155–194.

Fiske, S. T. (1998). Stereotyping, prejudice, and discrimination. In D. T. Gilbert, S. T. Fiske, & G. Lindzey (Eds.), *The handbook of social psychology* (Vol. 2, 4th ed., pp. 367–411). New York: McGraw-Hill.

Fiske, S. T., & Dépret, E. (1996). Control, interdependence, and power: Understanding social cognition in its social context. In W. Stroebe & M. Hewstone (Eds.), *European review of social psychology* (Vol. 7, pp. 31–61). New York: Wiley.

Fiske, S. T., & Leyens, J.-P. (1996). Let social psychology be faddish, or at least heterogenous. In C. McGarty & S. A. Haslam (Eds.), *Message of social psychology: Perspectives on mind in society* (pp. 92–112). Oxford: Blackwell.

Fiske, S. T., Morling, B. A., & Stevens, L. E. (1996). Controlling self and others: A theory of anxiety, mental control, and social control. *Personality and Social Psychology Bulletin, 22,* 115–123.

Fiske, S. T., & Neuberg, S. L. (1990). A continuum of impression formation, from category-based to individuating processes: Influences of information and motivation on attention and interpretation. In M. P. Zanna (Ed.), *Advances in experimental social psychology* (Vol. 23, pp. 1–74). New York: Academic Press.

Fiske, S. T., Neuberg, S. L., Beattie, A. E., & Milberg, S. J. (1987). Category-based and attribute-based reactions to others: Some informational conditions of stereotyping and individuating processes. *Journal of Experimental Social Psychology, 23,* 399–427.

Fiske, S. T., & Pavelchak, M. A. (1986). Category-based versus piecemeal-based affective responses: Developments in schema-triggered affect. In R. M. Sorrentino & E. T. Higgins (Eds.), *Handbook of motivation and cognition: Foundations of social behavior* (Vol. 1, pp. 167–203). New York: Guilford Press.

Fiske, S. T., & Taylor, S. E. (1991). *Social cognition* (2nd ed.). New York: McGraw-Hill.

Fiske, S. T., & Von Hendy, H. M. (1992). Personality feedback and situational norms can control stereotyping processes. *Journal of Personality and Social Psychology, 62,* 577–596.

Freund, T., Kruglanski, A. W., & Shpitzajzen, A. (1985). The freezing and unfreezing of impression primacy: Effects of the need for structure and the fear of invalidity. *Personality and Social Psychology Bulletin, 11,* 479–487.

Gaertner, S. L., & Dovidio, J. F. (1986). The aversive form of racism. In J. F. Dovidio & S. L. Gaertner (Eds.), *Prejudice, discrimination, and racism* (pp. 61–89). San Diego, CA: Academic Press.

Gaertner, S. L., & McLaughlin, J. P. (1983). Racial stereotypes: Associations and ascriptions of positive and negative characteristics. *Social Psychology Quarterly, 46,* 23–30.

Gardner, R. C., MacIntyre, P. D., & Lalonde, R. N. (1995). The effects of multiple social categories on stereotyping. *Canadian Journal of Behavioural Science, 27,* 466–483.

Gilbert, D. T., & Hixon, J. G. (1991). The trouble of thinking: Activation and application of stereotypic beliefs. *Journal of Personality and Social Psychology, 60,* 509–517.

Glick, P., & Fiske, S. T. (1996). The Ambivalent Sexism Inventory: Differentiating hostile and benevolent sexism. *Journal of Personality and Social Psychology, 70,* 491–512.

Gollwitzer, P. M., & Kinney, R. F. (1989). Effects of deliberative and implemental mind-sets on illusion of control. *Journal of Personality and Social Psychology, 56,* 531–542.

Goodwin, S. A., Gubin, A., Fiske, S. T., & Yzerbyt, V. (1998). *Power can bias impression formation: How powerholders stereotype by default and by design.* Unpublished manuscript, Boston College.

Hamilton, D. L., Sherman, S. J., & Ruvolo, C. M. (1990). Stereotype-based expectancies: Effects on information processing and social behavior. *Journal of Social Issues, 46,* 35–60.

Harris-Kern, M. J., & Perkins, R. (1995). Effects of distraction on interpersonal expectancy effects: A social interaction test of the cognitive busyness hypothesis. *Social Cognition, 13,* 163–182.

Haslam, S. A., Oakes, P. J., McGarty, C., Turner, J. C., & Onorato, R. S. (1995). Contextual changes in the prototypicality of extreme and moderate outgroup members. *European Journal of Social Psychology, 25,* 509–530.

Hattrup, K., & Ford, J. K. (1995). The roles of information characteristics and accountability in moderating stereotype-driven processes during social decision making. *Organizational Behavior and Human Decision Processes, 63,* 73–86.

Heaton, A. W., & Kruglanski, A. W. (1991). Person perception by introverts and extraverts under time pressure: Effects of need for closure. *Personality and Social Psychology Bulletin, 17,* 161–165.

Heilman, M. C. (1995). Sex stereotypes and their effects in the workplace: What we know and what we don't know. *Journal of Social Behavior and Personality, 10,* 3–26.

Hewstone, M., Hantzi, A., & Johnston, L. (1991). Social categorization and person memory: The pervasiveness of race as an organizing principle. *European Journal of Social Psychology, 21,* 517–528.

Hilton, J. L., Klein, J. G., & von Hippel, W. (1991). Attention allocation and impression formation. *Personality and Social Psychology Bulletin, 17,* 548–559.

Jackson, L. A., Hansen, C. H., Hansen, R. D., & Sullivan, L. A. (1993). The effects of stereotype consistency and consensus information on predictions of performance. *Journal of Social Psychology, 133,* 293–306.

James, H. (1983). *The portrait of a lady.* New York: Bantam. (Original work published 1881)

Jamieson, D. W., & Zanna, M. P. (1989). Need for structure in attitude formation and expression. In A. R. Pratkanis, S. J. Breckler, & A. G. Greenwald (Eds.), *Attitude structure and function* (pp. 383–406). Hillsdale, NJ: Erlbaum.

Johnston, L. C., Hewstone, M., Pendry, L., & Frankish, C. (1994). Cognitive models of stereotype change: Motivational and cognitive influences. *European Journal of Social Psychology, 24*, 237–265.

Jussim, L. (1991). Social perception and social reality: A reflection–construction model. *Psychological Review, 98*, 54–73.

Kaplan, M. F., Wanshula, L. T., & Zanna, M. P. (1993). Time pressure and information integration in social judgment: The effect of need for structure. In O. Svenson & A. J. Maule (Eds.), *Time pressure and stress in human judgment and decision making* (pp. 255–267). New York: Plenum Press.

Kashima, Y., & Kerekes, A. R. Z. (1994). A distributed memory model of averaging phenomena in person impression formation. *Journal of Experimental Social Psychology, 30*, 407–455.

Katz, I., & Hass, R. G. (1988). Racial ambivalence and value conflict: Correlational and priming studies of dual cognitive structures. *Journal of Personality and Social Psychology, 55*, 893–905.

Kim, H., & Baron, R. S. (1988). Exercise and the illusory correlation: Does arousal heighten stereotypic processing? *Journal of Experimental Social Psychology, 24*, 366–380.

Klinger, M. R., & Beall, P. M. (1992). *Conscious and unconscious effects of stereotype activation.* Paper presented at the 64th Annual Meeting of the Midwestern Psychological Association, Chicago.

Kruglanski, A. W., & Freund, T. (1983). The freezing and unfreezing of lay-inferences: Effects of impressional primacy, ethnic stereotyping, and numerical anchoring. *Journal of Experimental Social Psychology, 19*, 448–468.

Kruglanski, A. W., & Mayseless, O. (1988). Contextual effects in hypothesis testing: The role of competing alternatives and epistemic motivations. *Social Cognition, 6*, 1–20.

Kruglanski, A. W., & Webster, D. M. (1991). Group members' reactions to opinion deviates and conformists at varying degrees of proximity to decision deadline and use of environmental noise. *Journal of Personality and Social Psychology, 61*, 212–225.

Kruglanski, A. W., & Webster, D. M. (1996). Motivated closing of the mind: "Seizing" and "freezing." *Psychological Review, 103*, 263–283.

Kunda, Z., Miller, D. T., Claire, T. (1990). Combining social concepts: The role of causal reasoning. *Cognitive Science, 14*, 551–577.

Kunda, Z., & Oleson, K. C. (1995). Maintaining stereotypes in the face of disconfirmation: Constructing grounds for subtyping deviants. *Journal of Personality and Social Psychology, 68*, 565–579.

Kunda, Z., & Thagard, P. (1996). Forming impressions from stereotypes, traits, and behaviors: A parallel-constraint-satisfaction theory. *Psychological Review, 103*, 284–308.

Lambert, A. J. (1995). Stereotypes and social judgment: The consequences of group variability. *Journal of Personality and Social Psychology, 68*, 388–403.

Leippe, M. R., & Eisenstadt, D. (1994). Generalization of dissonance reduction: Decreasing prejudice through induced compliance. *Journal of Personality and Social Psychology, 67*, 395–413.

Lepore, L., & Brown, R. (1997). Category and stereotype activation: Is prejudice inevitable? *Journal of Personality and Social Psychology, 72*, 275–287.

Levine, G. M., Halberstadt, J. B., & Goldstone, R. L. (1996). Reasoning and the weighting of attributes in attitude judgments. *Journal of Personality and Social Psychology, 70*, 230–240.

Leyens, J.-P., & Fiske, S. T. (1994). Impression formation: From recitals to *symphonie fantastique*. In P. G. Devine, D. L. Hamilton, & T. M. Ostrom (Eds.) *Social cognition: Impact on social psychology* (pp. 39–75). San Diego, CA: Academic Press.

Leyens, J., & Yzerbyt, V. Y. (1992). The ingroup overexclusion effect: Impact of valence and confirmation on stereotypical information search. *European Journal of Social Psychology, 22*, 549–569.

Macrae, C. N., Bodenhausen, G. V., & Milne, A. B. (1995). The dissection of selection in person perception: Inhibitory processes in social stereotyping. *Journal of Personality and Social Psychology, 69*, 397–407.

Macrae, C. N., Bodenhausen, G. V., Milne, A. B., & Jetten, J. (1994). Out of mind but back in sight: Stereotypes on the rebound. *Journal of Personality and Social Psychology, 67*, 808–817.

Macrae, C. N., Hewstone, M., & Griffiths, R. J. (1993). Processing load and memory for stereotype-based information. *European Journal of Social Psychology, 23*, 77–87.

Macrae, C. N., Milne, A. B., & Bodenhausen, G. V. (1994). Stereotypes as energy-saving devices: A peek inside the cognitive toolbox. *Journal of Personality and Social Psychology, 66*, 37–47.

Macrae, C. N., Shepherd, J. W., & Milne, A. B. (1992). The effects of source credibility on the dilution of stereotype-based judgments. *Personality and Social Psychology Bulletin, 18*, 765–775.

Macrae, C. N., Stangor, C., & Milne, A. B. (1994). Activating social stereotypes: A functional analysis. *Journal of Experimental Social Psychology, 30*, 370–389.

Marsh, K. L., & Weary, G. (1994). Severity of depression and responsiveness to attributional information. *Journal of Social and Clinical Psychology, 13*, 15–32.

Matlin, M., & Stang, D. (1978). *The Pollyanna principle.* Cambridge, MA: Schenkman.

McCann, C. D., Ostrom, T. M., Tyner, L. K., & Mitchell, M. L. (1985). Person perception in heterogeneous groups. *Journal of Personality and Social Psychology, 49*, 1449–1459.

McConahay, J. B., & Hough, J. C., Jr. (1976). Symbolic racism. *Journal of Social Issues, 32*, 23–45.

Miki, H., Tsuchiya, H., & Nishino, A. (1993). Influences of expectancy of opponents competence upon information processing of their discrete attributes. *Perceptual and Motor Skills, 77*, 987–993.

Moberg, S. (1995). Impact of teachers' dogmatism and pessimistic stereotype on the effect of EMR-class label on teachers judgments in Finland. *Education and Training in Mental Retardation and Developmental Disabilities, 30*, 141–150.

Mikulincer, M., Yinon, A., & Kabili, D. (1991). Epistemic needs and learned helplessness. *European Journal of Personality, 5*, 249–258.

Moskowitz, G. B. (1993). Individual differences in social categorization: The influence of personal need for structure on spontaneous trait inference. *Journal of Personality and Social Psychology, 65,* 132–142.

Naccarato, M. E. (1988). *The impact of need for structure on stereotyping and discrimination.* Unpublished master's thesis, University of Waterloo, Waterloo, Ontario, Canada.

Nelson, T. E., Acker, M., & Manis, M. (1996). Irrepressible stereotypes. *Journal of Experimental Social Psychology, 32,* 13–38.

Neuberg, S. L. (1989). The goal of forming accurate impressions during social interactions: Attenuating the impact of negative expectancies. *Journal of Personality and Social Psychology, 56,* 374–386.

Neuberg, S. L., & Fiske, S. T. (1987). Motivational influences on impression formation: Outcome dependency, accuracy-driven attention, and individuating processes. *Journal of Personality and Social Psychology, 53,* 431–444.

Neuberg, S. L., Judice, T. N., Virdin, L. M., & Carrillo, M. A. (1993). Perceiver self-presentational goals as moderators of expectancy influences: Ingratiation and the disconfirmation of negative expectancies. *Journal of Personality and Social Psychology, 64,* 409–420.

Neuberg, S. L., & Newsom, J. T. (1993). Personal need for structure: Individual differences in the desire for simpler structure. *Journal of Personality and Social Psychology, 65,* 113–131.

Oakes, P. J., & Reynolds, K. J. (1997). Asking the accuracy question: Is measurement the answer? In R. Spears, P. Oakes, N. Ellemers, & S. A. Haslam (Eds.), *The social psychology of stereotyping and group life* (pp. 51–71). Oxford: Blackwell.

Oakes, P. J., Turner, J. C., & Haslam, S. A. (1991). Perceiving people as group members: The role of fit in the salience of social categorizations. *British Journal of Social Psychology, 30,* 125–144.

Operario, D., & Fiske, S. T. (1998). *Effects of trait dominance on powerholders' judgments of subordinates.* Unpublished manuscript, University of Massachusetts at Amherst.

Osborne, R. E., & Gilbert, D. T. (1992). The preoccupational hazards of social life. *Journal of Personality and Social Psychology, 62,* 219–228.

Ostrom, T. M. (1977). Between-theory and within-theory conflict in explaining context effects in impression formation. *Journal of Experimental Social Psychology, 13,* 492–503.

Ostrom, T. M. (1984). The sovereignty of social cognition. In R. S. Wyer, Jr., & T. K. Srull (Eds.), *Handbook of social cognition* (Vol. 1, pp. 1–38). Hillsdale, NJ: Erlbaum.

Parducci, A. (1968). The relativism of absolute judgments. *Scientific American, 219,* 84–90.

Pendry, L. F., & Macrae, C. N. (1994). Stereotypes and mental life: The case of the motivated but thwarted tactician. *Journal of Experimental Social Psychology, 30,* 303–325.

Pendry, L. F., & Macrae, C. N. (1996). What the disinterested perceiver overlooks: Goal-directed social categorization. *Personality and Social Psychology Bulletin, 22,* 249–256.

Perdue, C. W., & Gurtman, M. B. (1990). Evidence for the automaticity of ageism. *Journal of Experimental Social Psychology, 26,* 199–216.

Perry, E. (1994). A prototype matching approach to understanding the role of applicant gender and age in the evaluation of job applicants. *Journal of Applied Social Psychology, 24,* 1433–1473.

Pittman, T. S. (1998). Motivation. In D. T. Gilbert, S. T. Fiske, & G. Lindzey (Eds.), *The handbook of social psychology* (Vol. 1, 4th ed., pp. 549–590). New York: McGraw-Hill.

Pittman, T. S., & D'Agostino, P. R. (1989). Motivation and cognition: Control deprivation and the nature of subsequent information processing. *Journal of Experimental Social Psychology, 25,* 465–480.

Pittman, T. S., & Heller, J. F. (1987). Social motivation. *Annual Review of Psychology, 38,* 461–489.

Pratto, F., & Bargh, J. A. (1991). Stereotyping based on apparently individuating information: Trait and global components of sex stereotypes under attention overload. *Journal of Experimental Social Psychology, 27,* 26–47.

Pryor, J. B., Giedd, J. L., & Williams, K. B. (1995). A social psychological model for predicting sexual harassment. *Journal of Social Issues, 51,* 69–84.

Resnick, L. B., Levine, J. M., & Teasley, S. D. (Eds.). (1991). *Perspectives on socially shared cognition.* Washington, DC: American Psychological Association.

Riley, T., & Fiske, S. T. (1991). Interdependence and the social context of impression formation. *Cahiers de Psychologie Cognitive, 11,* 173–192.

Rudman, L. A., & Borgida, E. (1995). The afterglow of construct accessibility: The behavioral consequences of priming men to view women as sexual objects. *Journal of Experimental Social Psychology, 31,* 493–517.

Ruscher, J. B., & Fiske, S. T. (1990). Interpersonal competition can cause individuating processes. *Journal of Personality and Social Psychology, 58,* 832–843.

Ruscher, J. B., Fiske, S. T., Miki, H., & Van Manen, S. (1991). Individuating processes in competition: Interpersonal versus intergroup. *Personality and Social Psychology Bulletin, 17,* 595–605.

Ruscher, J. B., Hammer, E. Y., & Hammer, E. D. (1996). Forming shared impressions through conversation: An adaptation of the continuum model. *Personality and Social Psychology Bulletin, 22,* 705–720.

Schaller, M., Boyd, C., Yohannes, J., & O'Brien, M. (1995). The prejudiced personality revisited: Personal need for structure and formation of erroneous group stereotypes. *Journal of Personality and Social Psychology, 68,* 544–555.

Sears, D. O. (1983). The person-positivity bias. *Journal of Personality and Social Psychology, 44,* 233–240.

Sekaquaptewa, D., & von Hippel, W. (1994, May). *The role of prejudice in encoding and memory of stereotype-relevant behaviors.* Paper presented at the 66th Annual Meeting of the Midwestern Psychological Association, Chicago.

Seta, J. J., & Seta, C. E. (1993). Stereotypes and the generation of compensatory and noncompensatory expectancies of group members. *Personality and Social Psychology Bulletin, 19,* 722–731.

Smith, D. M., Neuberg, S. L., Judice, T. N., & Biesanz, J. C. (1997). Target complicity in the confirmation and disconfirmation of erroneous perceiver expectations: Immediate and longer term implications. *Journal of Personality and Social Psychology, 72,* 1396–1412.

Snodgrass, S. E. (1992). Further effects of role versus gender on interpersonal sensitivity. *Journal of Personality and Social Psychology, 62,* 154–158.

Snyder, M. (1992). Motivational foundations of behavioral confirmation. In M. P. Zanna (Ed.), *Advances in experimental social psychology* (Vol. 25, pp. 67–114). San Diego, CA: Academic Press.

Snyder, M., & Haugen, J. A. (1994). Why does behavioral confirmation occur?: A functional perspective on the role of the perceiver. *Journal of Experimental Social Psychology, 30,* 218–246.

Stangor, C., & Duan, C. (1991). Effects of multiple task demands upon memory for information about social groups. *Journal of Experimental Social Psychology, 27,* 357–378.

Stangor, C., Lynch, L., Duan, C., & Glas, B. (1992). Categorization of individuals on the basis of multiple social features. *Journal of Personality and Social Psychology, 62,* 207–218.

Stephan, W. G., & Stephan, C. W. (1984). The role of ignorance in intergroup relations. In N. Miller & M. B. Brewer (Eds.), *Groups in contact: The psychology of desegregation* (pp. 229–250). San Diego, CA: Academic Press.

Stevens, L. E., & Fiske, S. T. (1995). Motivation and cognition in social life: A social survival perspective, *Social Cognition, 13,* 189–214.

Stevens, L. E., & Fiske, S. T. (1996). *Forming motivated impressions of a powerholder: Accuracy under task dependency and misperception under evaluation dependency.* Unpublished manuscript, University of Massachusetts at Amherst.

Swim, J. K., Aikin, K. J., Hall, W. S., & Hunter, B. A. (1995). Sexism and racism: Old-fashioned and modern prejudices. *Journal of Personality and Social Psychology, 68,* 199–214.

Tajfel, H., & Turner, J. C. (1986). The social identity theory of intergroup behavior. In S. Worchel & W. G. Austin (Eds.), *Psychology of intergroup relations* (pp. 7–24). Chicago: Nelson-Hall.

Tetlock, P. E. (1992). The impact of accountability on judgment and choice: Toward a social contingency model. In M. P. Zanna (Ed.), *Advances in experimental social psychology* (Vol. 23, pp. 331–376). San Diego, CA: Academic Press.

Tetlock, P. E., Skitka, L., & Boettger, R. (1989). Social and cognitive strategies for coping with accountability: Conformity, complexity, and bolstering. *Journal of Personality and Social Psychology, 57,* 632–640.

Thompson, L. (1995). "They saw a negotiation": Partisanship and involvement. *Journal of Personality and Social Psychology, 68,* 839–853.

Thompson, E. P., Roman, R. J., Moskowitz, G. B., Chaiken, S., & Bargh, J. A. (1994). Accuracy motivation attenuates covert priming effects: The systematic processing of social information. *Journal of Personality and Social Psychology, 66,* 474–489.

Thompson, M. M., Naccarato, M. E., & Parker, K. E. (1989, June). *Assessing cognitive need: The development of the Personal Need for Structure and Personal Fear of Invalidity Scales.* Paper presented at the annual meeting of the Canadian Psychological Society, Halifax, Nova Scotia, Canada.

Tougas, F., Brown, R., Beaton, A. M., & Joly, S. (1995). Neo-sexism: Plus ça change, plus c'est pareil. *Personality and Social Psychology Bulletin, 21,* 842–849.

Verkuyten, M., Masson, K., & Elffers, H. (1995). Racial categorization and preference among older children in The Netherlands. *European Journal of Social Psychology, 25,* 637–656.

White, R. W. (1959). Motivation reconsidered: The concepts of competence. *Psychological Review, 66,* 297–333.

Wilder, D. A., & Shapiro, P. (1989a). Effects of anxiety on impression formation in a group context: An anxiety-assimilation hypothesis. *Journal of Experimental Social Psychology, 25,* 481–499.

Wilder, D. A., & Shapiro, P. (1989b). The role of competition-induced anxiety in limiting the beneficial impact of positive behavior by an out-group member. *Journal of Personality and Social Psychology, 56,* 60–69.

Wittenbrink, W., Judd, C. M., & Park, B. (1997). Evidence for racial prejudice at the implicit level and its relationship with questionaire measures. *Journal of Personality and Social Psychology, 72,* 262–274.

Wojciszke, B. (1994). Inferring interpersonal attitudes: Hypotheses and the information-gathering process. *European Journal of Social Psychology, 24,* 383–401.

Zárate, M. A., & Sandoval, P. (1995). The effects of contextual cues on making occupational and gender categorizations. *British Journal of Social Psychology, 34,* 353–362.

Zárate, M. A., & Smith, E. R. (1990). Person categorization and stereotyping. *Social Cognition, 8,* 161–185.

Zebrowitz, L. A., Montepare, J. M., & Lee, H. (1993). They don't all look alike: Individual impressions of other racial groups. *Journal of Personality and Social Psychology, 65,* 85–101.

Zemore, S. E., & Fiske, S. T. (1998). *Who's controlling me? The role of power in the self-regulation of prejudice.* Unpublished manuscript, University of Massachusetts at Amherst.

12

Dual Processes in the Cognitive Representation of Persons and Social Categories

MARILYNN B. BREWER
AMY S. HARASTY FEINSTEIN

Consider the following sentence ".James is a nurse." At first blush, this is a relatively simple propositional statement (the kind that was easy to parse in fifth-grade English grammar lessons). However, the meaning of this proposition is actually quite ambiguous with respect to the referent for the word "nurse." On the one hand," nurse" may refer to a *feature* of James—one of the things that is true of this particular person, along with his tall stature, sense of humor, and passion for classical music. On the other hand," nurse" may be intended to refer to a general occupational *category*, of which James is a specific exemplar or category member.[1]

The latter, category-based interpretation of the descriptive statement will arise in an information-processing context (e.g., a discussion about nurses, a hospital setting, or an occupational classification task) in which the category "nurse" is activated prior to information about James. In such a processing context, general knowledge (category stereotypes) about nurses will be used to select, interpret, and encode subsequent information about the particular individual. (General knowledge may include the belief that nurses

are usually women, in which case a special subtype of "male nurses" may be activated to guide further information processing in this instance.) Any new information acquired about James in this process will be stored with the category knowledge base, to be activated later whenever the concept "nurse" (or "male nurse") is accessed.

The alternative, person-based interpretation of the descriptive statement is be expected in an information-processing context in which James himself, as a unique individual, is the subject of discussion or the target of information gathering. In this case, the feature of being a nurse, and any subsequent information about James, will be processed in terms of prior knowledge about James (or about persons in general), integrated with other information about this specific person, and activated later whenever the concept "James" is accessed. Information about nurses as a category may not necessarily be activated at all in connection with James.

The dual-process model of impression formation (Brewer, 1988a) is intended to distinguish between these two modes of processing person information, the situations in which the two modes can be expected to be engaged, and the subsequent cognitive representations associated with the separate modes.[2]

The two modes of impression formation described in Brewer (1988a) reflect the difference between information processing that is top-down (from schema to data) and processing that is bottom-up (from data to representation). In an initial elaboration of the dual-process model, a construction metaphor served to capture the distinction between the two modes of impression formation as analogous to two different ways in which a physical structure (such as a piece of sculpture) can be created:

> In one mode, the constructor starts with a mold or frame and inserts new component elements into the existing framework, filling in some parts here, and adding some new elements there, but the final product is constrained by the structural features of the original mold. In the second mode, the constructor starts with the individual component elements, piecing them together in novel ways, constrained only by the possible structural relationships between new elements and those that have already been incorporated into the construction. . . . These two modes of construction are not entirely dissimilar. Both are limited by some common structural constraints, and even the piecemeal construction project is guided by some prior model of the structure to be produced. But . . . the products of the two construction modes are likely to differ significantly in content and structural properties. (Brewer, 1988b, pp. 178–179)

The term "category-based impression formation" describes the top-down process, where impression formation begins with categorization of the target individual and activation of a category schema; this schema then guides subsequent attention, interpretation, and encoding of incoming information about the individual. In effect, the category representation acts as a template against which new information is compared or contrasted. The term "personalized impression formation" (or "person-based impression formation") describes the contrasting mode, in which a representation of the target individual is "built up" from incoming information and subsequent inferences and generalizations.

The original schematic representation of the dual-process model is reproduced in Figure 12.1. The model assumes that the selection of processing mode occurs relatively early in the information-processing sequence, at the second choice point depicted in Figure 12.1. From this point on, the two modes of processing are separate and distinct processing "paths" that result in different types of cognitive representations of the information that has been encoded. It is possible for the two processes to occur in parallel, but the model assumes that such parallel processing will result in separate representations of the information, not in a single, integrated representation.

Once the mode is selected, processing of incoming information is determined jointly by the knowledge structures that have been accessed, the nature of the stimulus information, and the level of effort engaged by the perceiver. Category-based processing, depicted in the lower left-hand portion of Figure 12.1, begins with the activation of the relevant category stereotype or knowledge base and proceeds through a process of pattern matching (comparing attributes of the stimulus person to category attributes) until a satisfactory "fit" between the stimulus information and prior knowledge has been achieved. The resulting representation of the stimulus person will be more or less individuated (as a distinct category member), depending on how much person-specific attribute information has been attended to and encoded.

In the person-based processing mode, depicted in the lower right-hand portion side of Figure 12.1, prior knowledge is used to draw inferences directly from the attributes themselves about what kind of a person this is. The resulting personalized representation may be more or less complex, depending on how much information has been attended to and integrated into the impression that is formed.

The distinction between person-based and category-based information processing corresponds to the distinction between interpersonal and intergroup orientations toward social interactions, postulated in the literature on social identity theory (Brewer & Miller, 1984; Brown & Turner, 1981; Tajfel & Turner, 1986). The fact that individuals can be encoded either as representatives of a social type or apart from any category identity

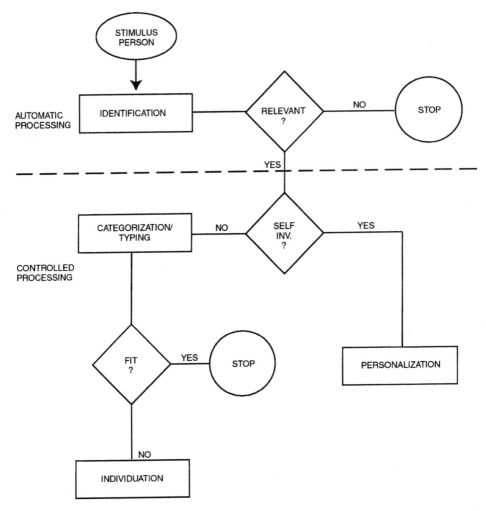

FIGURE 12.1. A schematic representation of the dual-process model. From Brewer (1988a, p. 5). Copyright 1988 by Lawrence Erlbaum Associates. Reprinted by permission.

creates an interesting dilemma for social programs designed to reduce intergroup prejudice and stereotyping through contact and familiarity. The rationale underlying the contact hypothesis is that extended interpersonal experiences with individual outgroup members will be generalized to the group as a whole. But as Rothbart and John (1985) and Hewstone and Brown (1986) have pointed out, generalization will occur only if those experiences are encoded and stored with information about the social category. According to the dual-process model, if interpersonal experiences are encoded in a person-based cognitive representation, they will be dissociated from category-based representations and hence are not likely to be generalized in any form to more inclusive social categories.

A particularly dramatic and poignant example of this phenomenon is represented by events in Bosnia-Herzegovina, where 20 years of close interpersonal contact (including intermarriage) between Serbs and Muslims did not prove sufficient to preclude the outbreak of virulent category-based hostilities and slaughter. Clearly, information encoded in the context of personal relationships did not get linked to the representation of those same persons as members of an outgroup social category.

PROCESSING MODES VERSUS LEVELS OF PROCESSING

Since its initial presentation in 1988, the dual-process model of impression formation has been frequently misrepresented in the social-cognitive literature. The most common misconstrual is to ignore the diverging pathways of the model and to equate the distinction between category-based and person-based representations with the categorization–individuation distinction (in effect, making the model equivalent to the continuum model of Fiske & Neuberg, 1990; see Fiske, Lin, & Neuberg, Chapter 11, this volume). This misrepresentation focuses only on the lower left-hand side of Figure 12.1 and assumes that the dual-process model privileges category-based processing over attribute-based ones in all impression formation (see, e.g., Kunda & Thagard, 1996). In actuality, the model does not give priority to either mode. The distinction between the two modes revolves around *what information is attended to and what prior knowledge is activated* at the time information is presented, and subsequent effects on *how that information is stored and organized in memory.*

A related misconception of the dual-process model is to equate category-based and person-based processing with heuristic processing and systematic, elaborative processing, respectively. The distinctions made by Brewer (1988a) between category-based and person-based representations were not intended to correspond to the products of relatively shallow, effortless versus elaborative, effortful information-processing modes. On the contrary, *both* modes of person perception can be *either* heuristic or elaborated (see Chen & Chaiken, Chapter 4, this volume).

As represented in the lower left-hand path of Figure 12.1, top-down, category-based processing can be more or less responsive to individuating information (attributes of the specific stimulus person). With superficial, effortless processing, the category representation or stereotype will be generalized in its entirety to the target individual, with little modification from person-specific information. With more effortful processing, data about the individual will be matched against features of the category prototype, mismatches will be identified and encoded, and a

more *individuated* impression will be developed.[3] Nonetheless, this individuation process is category-based, in that a prior category schema guides selection of information and ultimately constrains the features that are incorporated in the individual representation.

In the category-based processing mode, category information *biases* subsequent systematic processing of attribute information, so that the individuated impression is a product of both heuristic and systematic processes (Chaiken & Maheswaran, 1994). Category-relevant information (whether congruent or incongruent with the category stereotype) is more likely to be noticed, remembered, and incorporated in the individuated impression than is information that is unrelated to the initial categorization. And the individuated representation that is formed is "attached" to the general category knowledge base in memory (either as a representation of a category subtype or as an exceptional exemplar).

In person-based processing, on the other hand, category knowledge is not invoked, and category stereotypes are irrelevant to the processing of person attributes (except perhaps as the products of inferences drawn from the attribute information). This processing mode can also be relatively superficial or effortless. The well-documented "halo effects" from the person perception literature (e.g., Cooper, 1981) reflect how initial salient information about an individual (particularly information that has strong evaluative implications) can create expectancies that "short-circuit" processing of further information and dominate the impression formed. On the other hand, more motivated, thoughtful person-based processing can result in elaborated representations in which inconsistent pieces of information have been interpreted and incorporated in a coherent, differentiated representation (e.g., Asch & Zukier, 1984; Wyer & Srull, 1986).

The differences between simplistic and elaborated person representations correspond to attitudes formed through peripheral versus central processing routes in the elaboration likelihood model (see Petty & Wegener, Chapter 3, this volume). Crossing the distictinion in processing modes represented in Brewer's (1988a) dual-processing model with the distinction in processing styles represented by the elaboration likelihood model results in a 2

TABLE 12.1. A Taxonomy of Processing Modes and Levels

	Processing mode	
Processing level	Category-based	Person-based
Peripheral	Stereotyping	Simple
Central	Individuation	Complex

× 2 taxonomy of impression formation types, as depicted in Table 12.1. The distinction between stereotyping and subtyping or individuation corresponds to the different levels of processing represented in the lower left-hand pathway of Figure 12.1. The distinction between simple and differentiated person-based impressions represents a further elaboration of the lower right-hand pathway in terms of depth of processing.

The goal of the present chapter is to consider the implications of this two-way classification of processing modes for encoding, organization, and retrieval of information about persons. The primary emphasis is on effects associated with the distinction between category-based and person-based processing modes. Differences associated with the peripheral versus central routes of processing are discussed only as they are relevant within each processing mode.

COGNITIVE REPRESENTATIONS AND RETRIEVAL

One implication of the Brewer (1988a) dual-processing model is that different types of processing and encoding of social information result in different associative structures and different associative paths by which information is retrieved. Category-based processing should result in altered associative connections between new information and previous category knowledge, at the expense of any associations between other, category-irrelevant information about the individual person. Person-based processing, on the other hand, should strengthen intraindividual associative networks, with little or no effect on category-related knowledge. Research to test these propositions about the structure of cognitive representations uses information retrieval tasks as an indirect method of assessing how information has been organized in memory.

One line of relevant research uses recognition and recall of information about specific persons to determine whether information has been stored with a representation of that person or with a representation of the social category to which the person belongs. Another line of research has used an exemplar retrieval task to test the difference between traits and categories as components of person memory. Findings from each of these lines of research are reviewed below.

Encoding: Formation of Category-Based versus Person-Based Representations

Complex social situations, in which information about multiple individuals is presented simultaneously, provide one context in which the motivations for different processing modes can be examined. In such situations, it is not clear whether incoming information will be encoded and organized around individual persons or in terms of some other organizing framework, such as specific events, topics, or social categories (Ostrom, Pryor, & Simpson, 1981; Sedikides & Ostrom, 1988). Of particular interest are settings in which large groups of persons can be clustered into subcategories, in which case category-based processing competes directly with person-based processing as the basis for forming cognitive representations of the social situation.

When a multiperson group can be segregated into two or more salient subcategories, processing mode may be determined in part by the strength of prior knowledge about the specific persons and categories. If the category distinctions represent known social groups (e.g., gender, ethnicity, occupations, etc.) and the individual persons are unknown strangers, then it is not surprising to find that category-based processing dominates over personalized representations (e.g., Doise & Sinclair, 1973; Taylor, Fiske, Etcoff, & Ruderman, 1978). On the other hand, when category differences are based on socially meaningless cues (such as color of clothing), category-based representations may be less likely (Stangor, Lynch, Duan, & Glass, 1992).

When impressions are first being developed, it is an open question whether the formation of category-based impressions or of person-based impressions will be more effortful. Category-based processing requires combining larger amounts of information to extract fewer representations, relative to person-based processing, which "chunks" information into more subunits. Since both processes require effort, the functional significance of the category or the individual persons should be particularly important in determining which processing mode is engaged.

In a series of experiments utilizing the recognition confusion paradigm, Brewer, Weber, and Carini (1995) explored the conditions under which an arbitrary categorical distinction would induce category-based as opposed to person-based organization of social information. After viewing a 16-minute videotaped group discussion among six individuals (three dressed in red sweatshirts, three dressed in blue), subjects were tested for memory of who said what during the taped discussion. Following presentation of the video (and an intervening task), participants were presented with a set of facial photos of the six individuals from the tape (with sweatshirt color visible). They were then shown 24 one-sentence excerpts taken from the statements made in the videotape discussion (4 per speaker), and were asked to identity which individual had made each statement. The rate of intracategory recognition confusions in the memory test was used as a measure of category-based information processing (Taylor et al., 1978). Higher confusion rates signified category-based representations of the information.

One factor that influenced processing mode in this paradigm was the social significance of the category distinction represented by sweatshirt color. Category-based memory confusions were highest when the colors signified an ingroup–outgroup distinction under conditions of intergroup competition (Brewer et al., 1995, Experiment 2). Although the content of the discussion on the tape was irrelevant to the nature of the intergroup relationship, the presence of a competitive relationship between ingroup and outgroup apparently heightened the interest in category distinctions and created category expectancies that guided extraction of information at the category level.

Another factor that influenced processing mode was category distinctiveness. In general, information about members of a distinctive (minority) group was more likely to be processed in a category-based mode than information about members of a less distinctive (majority) group (Brewer et al., 1995, Experiment 3). Even though the videotape presented a group composed of three members of each category, knowing that one category was more unusual or distinctive led to greater intracategory recognition errors for members of that category than for participants who were identified as members of the majority category. One inference that can be made from these results is that distinctive social categories are considered more useful or functional as units for organizing and storing social information than are large, nondistinctive social categories.[4]

There is a problem with using the recognition confusion paradigm as a method for assessing whether category-based or person-based processing modes have been engaged at encoding. When rates of within-category recognition confusions are high, the evidence of category-based processing is unequivocal. However, when intracategory errors are low (accurate person recognition), it is not possible to distinguish whether accuracy is based on *individuated* (and category-based) or *personalized* (person-based) memories. The relative frequency of between- and within-category confusions provides one clue to which processing mode has been involved. If processing has been strictly person-based, within- and between-category errors should both occur at chance levels. If processing has been category-based, within-category errors should exceed chance to a greater extent than between-category errors.

In the Brewer et al. (1995) experiments reported above, between-category errors were infrequent and lower than within-category errors in all conditions. This suggests that information processing in this paradigm was generally category-based, and that differences in accuracy for individuated information reflected differences in depth of processing.

Analyses of the clustering of memory in a free-recall task (Brewer et al., 1995, Experiment 3) supported this conclusion. Minority ingroup members (who showed the greatest accuracy for information about individual members of their own category) demonstrated a high level of clustering of recalled information by category *and* by person. This pattern of recall suggested that minority group members first extracted category-based distinctions and then engaged further individuated impression formation processes for targets who were fellow minority ingroup members, but not for the majority outgroup. In this case, ingroup processing appeared to reflect effortful category-based individuation rather than an initially person-based processing mode.

Types versus Traits as Associative Networks

Brewer's (1988a) dual-process model also draws a distinction between traits and categories as different knowledge structures implicated in person perception. Categories are assumed to be configural representations consisting of visual, behavioral, and psychological characteristics shared by members of the category. Furthermore, category knowledge is hierarchically organized into subtypes and individual exemplars. The representation of individual category members derived from category-based processing is a product of placing those individuals within the category hierarchy.

Traits, on the other hand, reflect dimensions of evaluation along which the attributes of a particular object, concept, or person can be assessed. The object's placement on a particular trait dimension is represented as a feature of that object; as features, traits are subordinate to the object or category. Such trait evaluations are typical of the person-based processing mode of impression formation.

Support for the distinction between traits and categories (or types) comes from data collected by Brewer and Lui (1989), who used a nonverbal picture-sorting task to assess different representational forms. Participants in this study were given 140 facial photographs to categorize by way of a free-sort procedure. The persons depicted in the

photos differed systematically in age and sex, as well as in many other visual features. For some subjects, the sorting instructions suggested that the faces should be grouped according to similarity of "psychological traits or states"; for others, the instructions indicated that the grouping should be based on similarity of "character or personality type"; and still others were instructed to group faces according to similarity of "specific physical features."

The resulting clusterings of the 140 photographs (derived from aggregated co-occurrence matrices) differed as a function of the wording of the sorting instructions. Of particular importance for the present purposes, the values in the co-occurrence matrices produced by subjects in the physical-feature and character-type instructional conditions were highly correlated with each other ($r = .75$) and corresponded much less with the sortings produced by subjects in the trait condition ($r = .44$ in both cases). Furthermore, the sortings produced in both the physical-feature and character-type instructional conditions were hierarchically organized by age and sex; similarity in age and sex was the strongest predictor of the probability that two photos would be sorted into the same "character-type" group, suggesting that these person categories are subtypes of social categorizations based on age and gender. Sortings based on personality traits, on the other hand, were less likely to be organized in accord with age or sex of the stimulus picture.

Another finding that emerged from the Brewer and Lui (1989) study was that participants found it much more difficult to do sortings under the trait-sorting instructional condition than under the type-sorting condition. The task of sorting or clustering by types assumes a hierarchical structure in which individual persons can be nested within higher-order category clusters. This hierarchical structure appears to be appropriate for category-based processing; subtypes are nested within superordinate categories, and individual exemplars within subtypes. Trait concepts, on the other hand, do not appear to be superordinate categories in which individual exemplars are nested.[5]

These assumptions about the network structure of traits and types have implications for how traits and categories may function as cues for retrieval of known instances. The hierarchical structure of category information should provide a natural strategy for retrieval of person exemplars; category labels activate subtype representations, which in turn activate individual category members as exemplars. Once exemplars in the activated subtype are exhausted, the next accessible subtype in the structure is accessed, and so forth. Trait labels, on the other hand, should not engage a similar retrieval process. In this case, retrieval should involve searching through accessible person exemplars to determine whether the target trait is present. When a person exhibiting the trait is retrieved, other related individuals may be accessed as well (e.g., retrieving "my mother" may lead to accessing other family members). However, once these related associations are exhausted, the search for new exemplars should take longer. Furthermore, the accessibility of individual exemplars of trait concepts should be more influenced by personal familiarity than the retrieval of category exemplars should be, because person-based representations are more likely for familiar, close relationships than for individuals who are not known on a personal basis. People use trait terms more to describe themselves and intimate acquaintances (Hampson, 1983), whereas stereotypes are used to describe public figures who are familiar but not intimate (Klatzky & Andersen, 1988).

We (Harasty & Brewer, 1995) reported a preliminary study designed to test these predictions about the use of traits and types as retrieval strategies. The study involved a modified version of the unconstrained-recall task developed by Bousfield and Sedgewick (1944) (see also Gruenewald & Lockhead, 1980), as adapted by Bond and Brockett (1987) for the study of memory for acquaintances. The general paradigm is to time people while they freely recall instances of some general category from personal memory, and then later to have them sort the items into meaningful subgroups. The researchers then examine the response times between items that are part of the same subgrouping (within-group item transitions) compared to response times between items that fall into different subgroups (between-group transitions), as a measure of the use of subtyping to facilitate retrieval (and, indirectly, to infer the organizational structure of concepts in memory).

We (Harasty & Brewer, 1995) used this paradigm to examine whether the task of naming all the people one could think of who possess a specified trait versus the task of naming all the people one could think of who are members of a specified social category would produce different temporal patterns of exemplar retrieval. With respect to interitem response times, we hypothesized first of all that category-based retrieval should facilitate the speed and amount of retrieval overall, in comparison to trait-based retrieval. Second, we hypothesized an effect of the interaction between retrieval strategy and interitem transition type. Specifically, within-group interitem response times were predicted to be approximately the same for both retrieval strategies, but the transition between different subgroups was predicted to take longer for trait-based retrieval than for category-based retrieval.

Participants in the experiment were given 4 minutes to generate names of all the individuals they could think of in response to a given retrieval cue. Participants in the category retrieval condition were asked to name all the people they could think of who fit into the category "women." Participants in the trait retrieval condition were asked to name all the people they could think of who possessed the personality trait of "kindness."[6]

As participants recited the first names of these individuals into a tape recorder, an experimenter wrote each name onto a notecard. After completing a 5-minute filler task, participants were given the notecards in shuffled order and were asked to sort these names into subgroupings of individuals who "belonged together" (an unstructured sorting task). Finally, each participant rated each named individual on a 10-point personal closeness scale to indicate how well the participant and that individual knew each other. Together these procedures generated measures of the number of names retrieved, the number of subgroups represented among the retrieved exemplars, closeness ratings of the people named, and interitem response times (assessed from the tape recording).

As predicted, category-based retrieval led to significantly more names generated (mean = 40.12 vs. 21.70), more subgroups formed, and shorter average interitem response times. On the other hand, the average closeness rating of items generated in response to the trait cue was significantly higher (mean = 6.79) than that of items generated for the category cue (mean = 5.17).

Most important, there was a significant interaction between retrieval cue condition and type of interitem transition (within-group vs. between-group) in response times. The shape of this interaction is depicted in Figure 12.2. Within-subgroup interitem transition times were relatively short and equivalent for both the category and trait retrieval conditions. However, there was a significantly longer gap in making transitions to new subgroup exemplars in the trait retrieval condition than in the category retrieval condition.

Since this study involved only one example each of category and trait cues, respectively, there are many possible interpretations of the pattern of retrieval findings that were obtained, and the procedure provided only indirect evidence of the organizational structure of the cognitive representations involved. To bolster that inference, we compared the temporal patterns obtained from the category and trait cues to those obtained from a retrieval task in which search strategies are better known.

The same participants in our initial experiment (Harasty & Brewer, 1995) were given a separate exemplar task in which they were asked to name all the animals they could think of. In one condition, the naming task was unconstrained. Since animals constitute a system of "natural categories" with a known hierarchical structure, we assumed this condition would parallel the category cue condition for naming known persons. In a second condition, participants were asked to name all the animals they could think of in alphabetical order (beginning with all those whose names started with the letter "a," then all those starting with "b," etc.). This instruction was presumed to necessitate a search procedure in which names beginning with the appropriate letter would be accessed and then tested for having the property of referring to animals. As such, it was expected to parallel the search process involved in retrieving names associated with a trait cue.

Again, participants were tape-recorded as they generated animal names, and at the same time the names were written on notecards by an experimenter. Following the exemplar generation task, names generated by each subject in the alphabetical condition

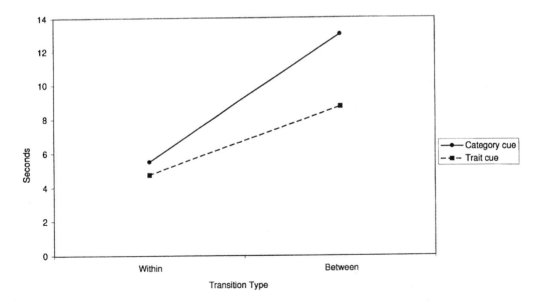

FIGURE 12.2. Interitem response times as a function of retrieval cue and transition type: Person names. From Harasty and Brewer (1995).

were subcategorized by letter of the alphabet. The names generated by each participant in the free-response condition were clustered into meaningful groupings by two coders who sorted the cards on which the subject's responses had been written, without knowledge of the response latencies involved in their production.

Not surprisingly, the number of items generated was significantly greater, and the speed of production was significantly faster, in the free-response retrieval condition than in the alphabetical-order condition. More importantly, there was a significant interaction between retrieval condition and transition type in interitem response times. The form of this interaction is depicted in Figure 12.3. The parallels between the data represented in Figures 12.2 and 12.3 are striking. These parallels support, at least indirectly, the mapping of temporal patterns of retrieval to inferred differences in cognitive structures that are consistent with the assumptions of the dual-process model.

INFORMATION PROCESSING

In addition to implications for the structure of cognitive representations and retrieval of information from stored knowledge, the dual-process model makes explicit assumptions about the processing of new information at acquisition. As mentioned earlier, these assumptions have to do with what information is attended to and what prior knowledge is activated at the time the information is encoded, depending on which processing mode is engaged. To refer again to Figure 12.1, there are two particularly important choice points that mark the difference between the two processing modes. The first is the distinction between initial classification (identification) of the target stimulus (which occurs before the point of divergence between the two modes) and whether social category knowledge is activated at early stages of processing (which occurs only in the category-based mode). The second is the difference between the two processing modes

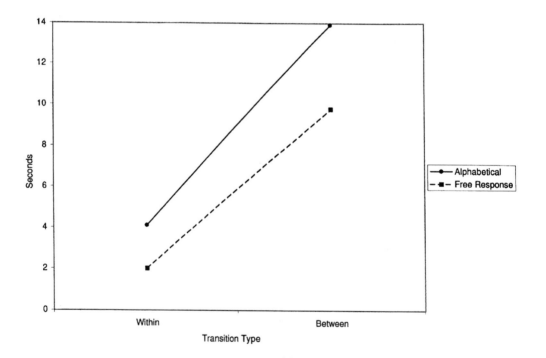

FIGURE12.3. Interitem response times as a function of retrieval instructions and transition type: Animal names. From Harasty and Brewer (1995).

in the role of individuating information about the target.

Classification versus Stereotyping

In the dual-process model, it is assumed that the choice point for category-based versus personalized processing modes occurs early in the information-processing sequence, immediately after the automatic stages of identification and initial classification of the target stimulus. According to the model, at this prior stage the target has been classified in terms of certain features (including age, sex, and race) that have become automatic. Feature identification occurs without effort or motivation to form an impression of the stimulus person. The perceiver's motives or processing goals determine whether there is any need for further processing; at this point, either it is terminated or more controlled, conscious processing begins. Both category-based and personalized processing modes are assumed to be controlled processes, although the perceiver may be relatively unaware of the influences that are guiding the impression being formed.

One implication of the difference between preconscious identification and later category-based processing is to draw a distinction between classification (identification) and stereotyping as aspects of person perception. There is some confusion in the social-cognitive literature in the use of these terms—as if the act of placing an individual in a social category were equivalent to the use of category stereotypes. Yet the recognition that an individual has a category-defining feature (such as femaleness or black skin) does not necessarily imply that impressions of that individual are derived from category stereotypes, or that category information has been activated or utilized in forming an impression. Within the dual-process model, recognizing that an individual is black does not necessarily activate the network of attributes associated with the social category of blacks, either because competing categories are more salient (weak activation of the black stereotype) or because the processing mode is personalized so that "black" is encoded as a feature, with no activation of the black category stereotype at all.

In the dual-process model, identification (classification) is simply feature recognition, which has no particular stereotyping content. Person categories (types), on the other hand, are feature configurations that are rich in stereotypic implications. If forced to make inferences based on taxonomic classifications alone (e.g., knowing only that a target person is male or female), the perceiver will draw on very generalized, abstract knowledge or on a particularly salient subtype within that taxonomic category as default options; however, if provided with more concrete information, the perceiver will readily abandon the standard stereotype in favor of more differentiated person types. A number of experimental studies support the contention that global, abstract attributes (such as "masculine" and "feminine") function very differently in person memory than do more concrete social stereotypes (e.g., Andersen & Klatzky, 1987; Pratto & Bargh, 1991; Pryor, McDaniel, & Kott-Russo, 1986).

As depicted in Table 12.1, category-based stereotyping may be a less effortful form of impression formation than individuated impression formation, but in the dual-process model it is still a higher-level representation engaging more associated systems and requiring more cognitive involvement than mere perceptual recognition or verbal labeling. Indeed, research on the "solo effect" suggests that category salience does not invariably lead to application of stereotypes (Taylor & Falcone, 1982; Oakes & Turner, 1986). Identification or classification as a preconscious, automatic process may well *prime* access and utilization of associated category stereotypes, but both stimulus characteristics and perceiver goals can intervene at the level of conscious processing to sever the connection between classification and stereotyping (Bargh, 1989; Brewer, 1996; Devine, 1989).

Research reported by Devine (1989, Experiment 2) has been cited as evidence that stereotypes are automatically activated when the category "black" is primed subliminally. But the primes used in the Devine experiment included a lot of stereotype content (e.g., "lazy," "welfare," "ghetto") in addition to the category cue. As Lepore and Brown (1997) point out, it is important to distinguish between automatic stereotype activation due to direct priming of content and that due to category activation alone (see also Ford, Stangor, & Duan, 1994, and Pratto & Bargh, 1991, for evidence that priming categories and priming stereotypes have different effects on impression formation). A number of studies conducted since the publication of Devine (1989) indicate that stereotype activation in response to category priming varies as a function of individual differences in attitudes (Fazio, Jackson, Dunton, & Williams, 1995; LePore & Brown, 1997; Locke, MacLeod, & Walker, 1994) and situational demands (Gilbert & Hixon, 1991). These findings support the contention that category identification and stereotype activation are separable processes.

The dual-process model assumes that category stereotypes will not be accessed when a strong interpersonal orientation characterizes the relationship between perceiver and target. In the latter case, relational qualities, such as cooperation, similarity, or power, will provide the schematic framework for information processing and impression formation (Baldwin, 1992; Fiske & Haslam, 1996). However, prejudices associated with social categorization can influence impressions formed in both category-based and person-based processing modes, albeit by different routes. As indicated above, categorization can prime particular stereotypes that then determine the course of category-based impression formation. However, category cues are also person attributes that enter into person-based impression formation processes. If these cues or features are directly associated with negative affect, negative evaluation will influence person-based processing through halo effects.

Research indicating that racial cues produce automatic evaluation (Dovidio & Gaertner, 1993; Fazio et al., 1995) suggests that this affective response occurs at the initial stage of identification, prior to selection of processing mode. This automatic activation of attitudes can play a role in subsequent processing in either route, via activation of negative category stereotypes or more directly in the processing of person-specific attributes. Prejudice biases information processing in either case, but corrections for bias should differ, depending on whether bias is operating through the content of negative stereotypes or through affective channels.

Distinguishing Category-Based Individuation from Person-Based Impressions

When effortful processing is engaged, both category-based and person-based modes result in individualized impressions of the target person. As indicated by the two paths in the lower portion of Figure 12.1, however, the dual-process model distinguishes between individuated impressions that are the product of category-based processing and personalized impressions that result from bottom-up person-based processing. One way to differentiate between these two types of impression formation is to trace the impact of category-relevant information on the impression that is formed.

In general, it has been found that expectancy-inconsistent information about an individual person induces more processing and is more memorable than expectancy-consistent information. However, this generalization has to be qualified by whether an expectancy is person-based (Hastie & Kumar, 1979) or category-based (Jones & McGillis, 1976). When expectancies are derived from category stereotypes, the effect of consistent and inconsistent information about individual category members depends on how deeply or elaborately the information is being processed. When processing is relatively effortless or peripheral, category-inconsistent information is ignored or assimilated, and the impression is dominated by stereotype-consistent attributes. However, when processing is more effortful and individuated, category-inconsistent attributes are noticed and incorporated in the impression of the target person (Neuberg & Fiske, 1987; Fiske & Neuberg, 1990; Pendry & Macrae, 1994). Nonetheless, at either end of the processing continuum, category-related information has more impact than category-irrelevant information. (This is consistent with the dual-process model's depiction of category-based processing as a feature-matching process in which category stereotypes serve as a sort of template.) It is only in the context of category-based processing that stereotype-inconsistent behaviors or attributes should be "surprising" and elicit additional processing attention.

When impressions are formed under a person-based processing mode, by contrast, stereotype-relevant attributes should not have any privileged status in the final impression. Instead, idiosyncratic person-based expectancies or relevance to relational goals should determine attention allocation, independent of category relevance of the information. Thus, one method for operationalizing the distinction between a person-based and a category-based individuated representation should be the prominence of category-irrelevant traits in the person description. Furthermore, recall of category-based impressions should be facilitated by cueing the category label, whereas such cues should have little effect on recall of personalized impressions.

Another difference between category-based individuation and person-based representations should be manifested in the relationship between traits and behaviors stored with the person representation. Petzold and Edeler (1995) identified three different models for how behavioral information and trait inferences about a particular person are organized in memory. Hierarchical-network models assume that behavioral acts are encoded in terms of the trait concepts they exemplify. Thus, traits are subordinate to person representations, and behaviors are clustered within traits. A second model assumes that individual behaviors are linked with individual traits in memory, but without any hierarchical organization. The third model assumes that individual behaviors and inferred traits are stored separately in memory, as two different associative paths within the person representation.

With top-down category-based processing, category-relevant traits should be used to encode and interpret specific behaviors of category members. Thus, memory for behaviors should be clustered with relevant traits, and trait cues should facilitate retrieval of associated behaviors, as expected in a hierarchical model (e.g., Wyer & Srull, 1981). With bottom-up person-based processing, however, traits are inferred from behaviors and may be stored separately and retrieved independently from memory (Anderson & Hubert, 1963; Allen & Ebbesen, 1981; Ostrom, Lingle, Pryor, & Geva, 1980). Petzold and Edeler (1995) used a recognition reaction time task, following presentation of person descriptions, to test decision time for inferring traits from behaviors and vice versa. They found strong evidence for separate representations of traits and behavioral information. However, the decision times for traits as cues showed systematic individual differences, which suggested that the organization of person memory may have differed among subjects in terms of the structural relationship between traits and behaviors. Such individual differences may reflect the product of person-based versus category-based processes.

CONCLUSION

Research since 1988, employing a variety of social-cognitive paradigms, provides support for the idea that person memory differs as a function of different processing modes. However, a number of aspects of the dual-process model have yet to be tested systematically.

The least well-articulated aspect of the model is the nature of the choice point that determines what processing mode is engaged in a particular social context. The consequences of adopting an "interpersonal" versus an "intergroup" orientation toward social interactions have received considerable research attention in the literature on social identity and intergroup relations (cf. Brewer & Brown, 1998), but relatively little research has been directed toward understanding the antecedents or determinants of which orientation is engaged at any specific time.

In the original formulation of the model (Brewer, 1988a), the critical factor was assumed to be some level of "self-involvement" with the target person.[7] Person-based processing is assumed to occur when the *relationship* between self and other is at stake, rather than knowledge of the properties of the other person as a social object. Here, again, the difference between processing *mode* and processing *level* becomes significant. Increasing the importance or relevance of a social judgment influences the level of processing (peripheral, low-effort vs. central, high-effort) that is likely to be engaged. But importance alone does not determine whether effortful processing is category-based or person-based. The latter depends on whether the judgment to be made is about attributes inherent in the target person or about relational qualities (Fiske & Haslam, 1996). Interdependence of outcomes, for example, has been shown to increase attention to individuating information (Neuberg & Fiske, 1987), but this can occur through either processing route. When interdependence increases the importance of assessment of the other's competence or abilities, for instance, category-based processing may be most efficient. When interdependence calls for judgments of interpersonal compatibility or complementarity, on the other hand, person-based processing is more likely to be engaged.

A second, closely related issue is the relationship between processing mode and *accuracy* of impressions. As discussed previously, biases and preconceptions can enter into forming impressions under either processing mode. Again, level of processing may be more significant than processing mode as a determinant of the match between the cognitive representation of an individual and the actual qualities of that individual.[8] There is one aspect of category-based processing, however, that does have some interesting implications for accuracy. Because category knowledge is brought to bear in making inferences about an individual target, impressions and judgments may be derived from a prior knowledge base that is richer in detail and associations than the information available about the person himself or herself. Once an individual has been matched to a category type, the generic representation of that category is merged with information about the specific person, with little (if any) discrimination between the two sources. As a consequence, the perceiver has a richer impression than that warranted by what has actually been extracted from incoming information about the target person. Overconfidence in one's judgments of others may well be a pervasive consequence of category-based processing and an important direction for future research on dual-processing models.

NOTES

1. Note that this same category–feature ambiguity will be true of other descriptive statements about James, including statements such as "James is black" or "James is male."

2. Brewer's dual-process model is unique in its explicit focus on the distinct cognitive representations derived from the alternative processing modes. The original formulation of the model re-

lied on traditional conceptions of cognitive representations as relatively fixed cognitive structures. But the theory is equally compatible with more recent connectionist models, in which representations are temporary patterns of activation of discrete processing units rather than intact cognitive structures (e.g., Smith, 1996). In fact, many of the assumptions of the dual-process theory fit better within a connectionist or distributed-memory framework, as suggested by Anderson (1988).

3. Again, the original formulation of the model presented the path from categorization to individuation as a sequential process, but there is no reason why category knowledge and individual attributes cannot be processed in parallel, as suggested by Kunda and Thagard's (1996) model.

4. Interestingly, this asymmetry of processing was reversed for observers who were themselves members of the minority category. Subjects who had been told previously that they were members of the distinct category showed more accurate memory for individuals in their ingroup and made more category-based errors in recognition of members of the majority outgroup.

5. If anything, traits appear to be categories for clusters of behaviors, not persons (Fleeson, Zirkel, & Smith, 1995).

6. The labels "women" and "kindness" were selected to be of roughly comparable levels of abstraction or superordinate category inclusiveness (cf. Hampson, John, & Goldberg, 1986).

7. This was later changed to "self-referencing" (Brewer, 1988b, p. 181).

8. There is, however, no simple relationship between elaborated processing and accuracy of judgments. Highly motivated cognition can result in judgment biases, and heuristic judgments can sometimes be quite accurate.

REFERENCES

Allen, R. B., & Ebbesen, E. B. (1981). Cognitive processes in person perception: Retrieval of personality trait and behavioral information. *Journal of Experimental Social Psychology, 17,* 119–141.

Andersen, S. M., & Klatzky, R. L. (1987). Traits and social stereotypes: Levels of categorization in person perception. *Journal of Personality and Social Psychology, 53,* 235–246.

Anderson, N. H. (1988). A functional approach to person cognition. In T. Srull & R. Wyer (Eds.), *Advances in social cognition* (Vol. 1, pp. 37–51). Hillsdale, NJ: Erlbaum.

Anderson, N. H., & Hubert, S. (1963). Effects of concomitant verbal recall on order effects in personality impression formation. *Journal of Verbal Learning and Verbal Behavior, 2,* 379–391.

Asch, S. E., & Zukier, H. (1984). Thinking about persons. *Journal of Personality and Social Psychology, 46,* 258–290.

Bargh, J. A. (1989). Conditional automaticity: Varieties of automatic influence in social perception and cognition. In J. Uleman & J. Bargh (Eds.), *Unintended thought* (pp. 3–51). New York: Guilford Press.

Baldwin, M. W. (1992). Relational schemas and the processing of social information. *Psychological Bulletin, 112,* 461–484.

Bond, C. F., & Brockett, D. R. (1987). A social context-personality index theory of memory for acquaintances. *Journal of Personality and Social Psychology, 52,* 1110–1121.

Bousfield, W. A., & Sedgewick, C. H. W. (1944). An analysis of sequences of restricted associative responses. *Journal of General Psychology, 30,* 149–165.

Brewer, M. B. (1988a). A dual process model of impression formation. In T. Srull & R. Wyer (Eds.), *Advances in social cognition* (Vol. 1, pp. 1–36). Hillsdale, NJ: Erlbaum.

Brewer, M. B. (1988b). Reply to commentaries. In T. Srull & R. Wyer (Eds.), *Advances in social cognition* (Vol. 1, pp. 177–183). Hillsdale, NJ: Erlbaum.

Brewer, M. B. (1996). When stereotypes lead to stereotyping: The use of stereotypes in person perception. In C. N. Macrae, C. Stangor, & M. Hewstone (Eds.), *Stereotypes and Stereotyping* (pp. 254–275). New York: Guilford Press.

Brewer, M. B., & Brown, R. J. (1998). Intergroup relations. In D. Gilbert, S. Fiske, & G. Lindzey (Eds.), *The handbook of social psychology* (Vol. 2, 4th ed., pp. 554–594). Boston: McGraw-Hill.

Brewer, M. B., & Lui, L. (1989). The primacy of age and sex in the structure of person categories. *Social Cognition, 7,* 262–274.

Brewer, M. B., & Miller, N. (1984). Beyond the contact hypothesis: Theoretical perspectives on desegregation. In N. Miller & M. Brewer (Eds.), *Groups in contact: The psychology of desegregation* (pp. 281–302). New York: Academic Press.

Brewer, M. B., Weber, J. G., & Carini, B. (1995). Person memory in intergroup contexts: Categorization versus individuation. *Journal of Personality and Social Psychology, 69,* 29–40.

Brown, R. J., & Turner, J. C. (1981). Interpersonal and intergroup behaviour. In J. Turner & H. Giles (Eds.), *Intergroup behaviour* (pp. 33–65). Oxford: Blackwell.

Chaiken, S., & Maheswaran, D. (1994). Heuristic processing can bias systematic processing: Effects of source credibility, argument ambiguity, and task importance on attitude judgment. *Journal of Personality and Social Psychology, 66,* 460–474.

Cooper, W. H. (1981). The ubiquitous halo. *Psychological Bulletin, 90,* 218–244.

Devine, P. G. (1989). Stereotypes and prejudice: Their automatic and controlled components. *Journal of Personality and Social Psychology, 56,* 5–18.

Doise, W., & Sinclair, A. (1973). The categorization process in intergroup relations. *European Journal of Social Psychology, 3,* 145–157.

Dovidio, J. P., & Gaertner, S. L. (1993). Stereotypes and evaluative intergroup bias. In D. Mackie & D. Hamilton (Eds.), *Affect, cognition, and stereotyping* (pp. 167–193). San Diego, CA: Academic Press.

Fazio, R. H., Jackson, J. R., Dunton, B. C., & Williams, C. J. (1995). Variability in automatic activation as an unobtrusive measure of racial attitudes: A bona fide

pipeline? *Journal of Personality and Social Psychology, 69,* 1013–1027.

Fiske, A., & Haslam, N. (1996). Social cognition is thinking about relationships. *Current Directions in Psychological Science, 5,* 143–148.

Fiske, S. T., & Neuberg, S. L. (1990). A continuum of impression formation, from category-based to individuating processes: Influences of information and motivation on attention and interpretation. In M. Zanna (Ed.), *Advances in experimental social psychology* (Vol. 23, pp. 1–74). San Diego, CA: Academic Press.

Fleeson, W., Zirkel, S., & Smith, E. E. (1995). Mental representations of trait categories and their influences on person perception. *Social Cognition, 13,* 365–397.

Ford, T. E., Stangor, C., & Duan, C. (1994). Influence of social category accessibility and category-associated trait accessibility on judgments of individuals. *Social Cognition, 12,* 149–168.

Gilbert, D. T., & Hixon, J. G. (1991). The trouble of thinking: Activation and application of stereotypic beliefs. *Journal of Personality and Social Psychology, 60,* 509–517.

Gruenewald, P. J., & Lockhead, G. R. (1980). The free recall of category examples. *Journal of Experimental Psychology: Human Learning and Memory, 6,* 225–240.

Hampson, S. E. (1983). Trait ascription and depth of acquaintance: The preference for traits in personality descriptions and its relation to target familiarity. *Journal of Personality and Social Psychology, 17,* 398–411.

Hampson, S. E., John, O. P., & Goldberg, L. R. (1986). Category breadth and hierarchical structure in personality: Studies of asymmetries in judgments of trait implications. *Journal of Personality and Social Psychology, 51,* 37–54.

Harasty, A. S., & Brewer, M. B. (1995, May). *Personality traits and social categories as retrieval cues.* Paper presented at the annual meeting of the Midwestern Psychological Association, Chicago.

Hastie, R., & Kumar, P. (1979). Person memory: Personality traits as organizing principles in memory for behaviors. *Journal of Personality and Social Psychology, 37,* 25–38.

Hewstone, M., & Brown, R. (1986). Contact is not enough: An intergroup perspective on the 'contact hypothesis.' In M. Hewstone & R. Brown (Eds.), *Contact and conflict in intergroup encounters* (pp. 1–44). Oxford: Blackwell.

Jones, E. E., & McGillis, D. (1976). Correspondent inferences and the attribution cube: A comparative appraisal. In J. Harvey, W. Ickes, & R. Kidd (Eds.), *New directions in attribution research* (Vol. 1, pp. 389–420). Hillsdale, NJ: Erlbaum.

Klatzky, R. L., & Andersen, S. M. (1988). Category-specificity effects in social typing and personalization. In T. Srull & R. Wyer (Eds.), *Advances in social cognition* (Vol. 1, pp. 91–101). Hillsdale, NJ: Erlbaum.

Kunda, Z., & Thagard, P. (1996). Forming impressions from stereotypes, traits, and behaviors: A parallel-constraint-satisfaction theory. *Psychological Review, 103,* 284–308.

LePore, L., & Brown, R. (1997). Category and stereotype activation: Is prejudice inevitable? *Journal of Personality and Social Psychology, 72,* 275–287.

Locke, V., MacLeod, C., & Walker, I. (1994). Automatic and controlled activation of stereotypes: Individual differences associated with prejudice. *British Journal of Social Psychology, 33,* 29–46.

Neuberg, S. L., & Fiske, S. T. (1987). Motivational influences on impression formation: Outcome dependency, accuracy-driven attention, and individuating processes. *Journal of Personality and Social Psychology, 53,* 431–444.

Oakes, P., & Turner, J. C. (1986). Distinctiveness and the salience of social category membership: Is there an automatic perceptual bias towards novelty? *European Journal of Social Psychology, 16,* 325–344.

Ostrom, T. M., Lingle, J., Pryor, J., & Geva, N. (1980). Cognitive organization of person impressions. In R. Hastie, T. Ostrom, E. Ebbesen, R. Wyer, D. Hamilton, & D. Carlston (Eds.), *Person memory: The cognitive basis of social perception* (pp. 3–38). Hillsdale, NJ: Erlbaum.

Ostrom, T. M., Pryor, J., & Simpson, D. (1981). The organization of social information. In E. T. Higgins, C. P. Herman, & M. Zanna (Eds.), *Social cognition: The Ontario Symposium* (Vol. 1, pp. 3–38). Hillsdale, NJ: Erlbaum.

Pendry, L. F., & Macrae, C. N. (1994). Stereotypes and mental life: The case of the motivated but thwarted tactician. *Journal of Experimental Social Psychology, 30,* 303–325.

Petzold, P., & Edeler, B. (1995). Organization of person memory and retrieval processes in recognition. *European Journal of Social Psychology, 25,* 249–267.

Pratto, F., & Bargh, J. A. (1991). Stereotyping based on apparently individuating information: Trait and global components of sex stereotypes under attention overload. *Journal of Experimental Social Psychology, 27,* 26–47.

Pryor, J., McDaniel, M., & Kott-Russo, T. (1986). The influence of the level of schema abstractness upon the processing of social information. *Journal of Experimental Social Psychology, 22,* 312–327.

Rothbart, M., & John, O. (1985). Social categorization and behavioral episodes: A cognitive analysis of the effects of intergroup contact. *Journal of Social Issues, 41*(3), 81–104.

Sedikides, C., & Ostrom, T. M. (1988). Are person categories used when organizing information about unfamiliar persons? *Social Cognition, 6,* 252–267.

Smith, E. R. (1996). What do connectionism and social psychology offer each other? *Journal of Personality and Social Psychology, 70,* 893–912.

Stangor, C., Lynch, L., Duan, C., & Glass, B. (1992). Categorization of individuals on the basis of multiple social features. *Journal of Personality and Social Psychology, 62,* 207–218.

Tajfel, H., & Turner, J. C. (1986). The social identity theory of intergroup behavior. In S. Worchel & W. Austin (Eds.), *Psychology of intergroup relations* (pp. 7–24). Chicago: Nelson-Hall.

Taylor, S. E., & Falcone, H. (1982). Cognitive bases of stereotyping: The relationship between categorization and prejudice. *Personality and Social Psychology Bulletin, 8,* 426–432.

Taylor, S. E., Fiske, S. T., Etcoff, N. L., & Ruderman, A. (1978). Categorical and contextual bases of person memory and stereotyping. *Journal of Personality and Social Psychology, 36,* 778–793.

Wyer, R. S., Jr., & Srull, T. K. (1981). Category accessibility: Some theoretical and empirical issues concerning the processing of social information. In E. T. Higgins, C. P. Herman, & M. Zanna (Eds.), *Social cognition: The Ontario Symposium* (Vol. 1, pp. 161–197). Hillsdale, NJ: Erlbaum.

Wyer, R. S., Jr., & Srull, T. K. (1986). Human cognition in social context. *Psychological Review, 93,* 322–359.

13

On the Dialectics of Discrimination

DUAL PROCESSES IN SOCIAL STEREOTYPING

GALEN V. BODENHAUSEN
C. NEIL MACRAE
JEFFREY W. SHERMAN

Over 35 years have passed since the historic moment when Martin Luther King, Jr., delivered his galvanizing speech entitled "I Have a Dream." In that speech, he expressed the hope that his children might "one day live in a nation where they will not be judged by the color of their skin, but by the content of their character." Explicit in this poignant comment is the assertion that there are two fundamentally different ways of judging others: either by relying on group-based assumptions, or by conducting an assessment of the personal qualities of each individual. This view has been at the heart of most social-psychological theories of stereotyping in social perception as well. For example, in the influential models of Brewer (1988) and Fiske and Neuberg (1990), a fundamental distinction is drawn between stereotyping and individuating or personalizing one's social impressions (see also Allport, 1954). In this chapter, we review the evidence for two qualitatively different pathways to social impressions, evaluate challenges to the validity of such distinctions, and consider how the dual-process models of stereotyping in social perception relate to other dual-process conceptualizations. We also consider in some detail other aspects of stereotyping that involve the interplay of two qualitatively different processes. The overall utility of a dual-process approach to stereotyping is then evaluated in light of these considerations.

STEREOTYPING VERSUS INDIVIDUATION: DISTINCT PATHS TO SOCIAL IMPRESSIONS

Occasionally we may have the disorienting experience of not being able to "make sense" of the sensory input impinging upon us, but most often we can construct a meaningful representation of whatever external stimuli happen to be at the focus of our attention. Following the lead of philosophers such as Immanuel Kant, perception researchers have long asserted that the seemingly effortless attainment of a coherent and meaningful interpretation of the external world is accomplished via the interaction of bottom-up and top-down processes (e.g., Bruner, 1951; Neisser, 1976; Palmer, 1975; Yates, 1985). Bottom-up processes rely upon the raw input acquired by the sensory systems to furnish information about low-level stimulus features (e.g., shape, color, loudness, saltiness, etc.), whereas top-down processes rely upon the memorial representations of the perceiver (e.g., general knowledge, previous experiences, attitudes, goals, etc.) to impose coherence and meaning on these stimulus features. In this sense, perceptions routinely go "beyond the information given" in the current stimulus array (Bruner, 1957). The notion of being judged by the color of one's skin similarly implies taking a simple, bottom-up feature (e.g., a person's African, Asian, or European skin tone) and imbuing it with surplus social meaning (e.g., assumptions about the person's behavioral proclivities, moral qualities, etc.) that may be unsubstantiated in the actual evidence available about the individual. This process is the sort of phenomenon that we are likely to have in mind when we speak of stereotyping.

The top-down versus bottom-up distinction has considerable intuitive appeal as an analogue for stereotyping versus individuation. However, some potentially thorny problems arise when the issue is viewed in this way (cf. McCauley, 1988). For instance, even if one were to ignore a person's race completely and judge him or her solely on the basis of the personality dispositions that are revealed in a careful observation of the person's behavior, one would of necessity still rely heavily on top-down processes of social perception. Indeed, top-down processes inform virtually all meaningful thoughts and impressions that arise (e.g., Murphy & Medin, 1985; Yates, 1985).

Another way of framing the issue is to distinguish between two different types of information to be used in impression formation—namely, categories versus attributes (e.g., Brewer, 1988; Fiske & Neuberg, 1990; for a review, see Fiske, Lin, & Neuberg, Chapter 11, this volume). From this perspective, stereotyping is equated with reliance upon categories (such as race or gender), while individuation is marked by reliance on personal attributes (such as personality traits or behaviors). One's overall impression of a social target can thus be based upon the target's social group membership (and the attributes stereotypically associated with the group in question) or on his or her personal attributes (which normally will include numerous nonstereotypic and/or counterstereotypic characteristics. Thus, the descriptive content and the evaluative content of one's overall impression may be quite different, depending upon whether categorical or attribute-based information is emphasized in the mental representation one forms of the target.

Stereotypes as Heuristics for Judgment

Attempts to understand when and how stereotypic judgments arise have led to the application of a related conceptual distinction between heuristic and systematic processing. Heuristic strategies for judgment, decision making, and problem solving are often contrasted with systematic or algorithmic ones (e.g., Kahneman, Slovic, & Tversky, 1982; Newell & Simon, 1972). The general spirit of this approach can be summarized as follows. Although there may be procedures available for reaching a decision or making a judgment that are likely to maximize decision quality, they are often cumbersome. Much simpler alternative strategies may be available that, although less likely to ensure a high-quality decision, nevertheless do a good enough job much of the time. These alternative strategies (i.e., heuristics) consist of simple inferential rules that reduce the number of considerations that must be taken into account in making a choice or a judgment. This framework has been successfully exploited in social-psychological domains (such as attitude change) by Chaiken and her associates (e.g., Chaiken, 1980, 1987; Chaiken, Liberman, & Eagly, 1989; Chaiken, Giner-Sorolla, & Chen, 1996; see Chen & Chaiken, this Chapter 4, volume). For example, when a person listens to a persuasive appeal and has some motivation to assess the validity of the speaker's position, the person may carefully attend to each argument and weigh and integrate it into an overall assessment. This systematic approach is contrasted with the use of simple heuristics (e.g., speaker credibility cues, audience reaction, etc.), which may provide a "quick and dirty" index of validity.

The same kinds of options are available in the context of many social judgments (Chaiken et al., 1989). One class of heuristics that is often available for social judgment consists of stereotypic beliefs about the target to be judged (Bodenhausen, 1988, 1990;

Bodenhausen & Wyer, 1985; Bodenhausen & Lichtenstein, 1987). If one must judge whether a young Latino is guilty of assault, for instance, one could pay careful, impartial attention to all available bits of evidence and, weighing their probative implications, render a judgment based on very systematic processing. Alternatively, one could use one's salient stereotypic beliefs about young Latinos to provide a quick, heuristic judgment ("They're aggressive, violence-prone people"), which may guide or dominate the processing of other available evidence (Bodenhausen, 1988; cf. Chaiken & Maheswaran, 1994). Once one has a framework for thinking about the available information, the requirements for making a judgment are substantially simplified (e.g., Macrae, Milne, & Bodenhausen, 1994).

Considering stereotypes to be heuristics for social judgment is not equivalent to viewing them as frameworks for general impression formation, because it remains possible that stereotypes can be used to guide judgments even when one has formed a relatively individuated impression of a social target. For example, consider the impression one might form of a gregarious, athletic, pizza-loving, female lawyer. An individuated impression of her will contain numerous facets, many of which may have some bearing on a decision that must be made about her (e.g., "Should I vote for her to become governor?"). If conditions permit, one may conduct a systematic assessment of her suitability for public office, based upon a relatively well-articulated mental impression of her. However, if one is pressed to make a judgment (perhaps after being ambushed by an opinion pollster), one may need to produce a quick response, and in this case one will be likely to rely on whatever heuristics are available to construct a reasonable response. If one's impression of the candidate is stereotype-dominated, then a stereotypic heuristic (e.g., "Lawyers can't be trusted") may be about the only readily available heuristic. If, instead, one has a richly individuated impression, then several distinct stereotypes may be available as heuristics. When many heuristic inference rules are potentially applicable, the most accessible one will probably be invoked (Chaiken et al., 1989). If a particular stereotypic belief is contextually salient (e.g., "Women can be trusted"), then it may form the dominant ba-

sis for the judgment. The important point is that an individuated mental representation of a person is not necessarily a guarantee that systematic judgments will be made about him or her.

Conditions of Stereotype Dominance

Whether general impressions or specific judgments are being considered, important insights are gained by placing the categorization–individuation distinction in the framework of heuristic versus systematic processes. In particular, this framing facilitates the generation of clear predictions about the conditions under which perceivers are likely to rely on stereotypes versus individuating information in social perception. In fact, a small set of factors has been repeatedly linked to the likelihood of a stereotype dominating one's response to another person. These factors, to be discussed in turn, are (1) information fit, (2) perceiver motivation, and (3) perceiver attentional capacity. As we will see, these moderating variables are largely convergent with the ones proposed in a wide variety of dual-process models.

Fit

A principal tenet of both Brewer's (1988) dual-process model and the continuum model (Fiske & Neuberg, 1990) is the notion that a stereotype will only be applied to a target when the other available information about him or her is congenial with the implications of the stereotype (see also Oakes, Haslam, & Turner, 1994). If one meets a librarian who rides a Harley-Davidson, smokes cigars, and has a pierced nose, one may be unlikely to assume that this person is just another typical librarian. These theoretical models predict that when fit is observed to be poor, individuation processes will ensue (Fiske, Neuberg, Beattie, & Milberg, 1987). Similar constraints are likely to hold in the context of other dual-process models. For example, in the persuasion model developed by Chaiken (1987), reliance on a simple heuristic such as "Experts can be trusted" might occur in many circumstances, but probably not when the expert is babbling incoherently or making patently absurd claims (e.g., "Toxic waste should be dumped freely into the environment because it causes cancer and costs taxpayers billions of dollars"). In this case, the fit between the heuristic cue and the message cues is simply too discrepant.

The question of crucial importance is what kinds and amounts of stereotype-inconsistent information are necessary before perceivers note the poor fit and abandon their preconceptions. Also important is the question of whether stereotype-irrelevant information undermines perceptions of fit. It seems to be the case that perceivers are quite capable of overlooking aspects of the available information that are not stereotype-consistent, as well as of assimilating a wide range of essentially ambiguous information to their stereotypic expectations (e.g., Darley & Gross, 1983; Kunda & Sherman-Williams, 1993; for reviews, see Fiske, 1998; Hamilton & Sherman, 1994). However, when expectancies are clear-cut and the available information strongly and unambiguously contradicts them, such information will probably not be overlooked; indeed, it may be particularly likely to attract attention and be quite memorable (e.g., Hastie & Kumar, 1979; Sherman, Lee, Bessenoff, & Frost, 1998), as in the case of the biker/librarian.

Motivation

Stereotyping is usually characterized as a less effortful strategy for the pursuit of social perception goals. Individuation, which requires building a new impressional framework based on the novel feature conjunctions that are ascribed to the target person, is more effortful. The metaphor of the "cognitive miser" (Fiske & Taylor, 1984) emphasizes the idea that under many circumstances, social perceivers prefer not to engage in extensive mental effort. As such, the effortful process of individuation will be relatively unappealing, and perceivers will be content to rely on stereotypic preconceptions. This notion fits with Simon's (1957) famous characterization of humans as "satisficers" rather than optimizers. People want to do a good enough job to get by, but usually no more than that.

Of course, there are some circumstances in which the stakes are higher, and the potential costs of errors in social perception loom large. Under such conditions, the extra motivation for accuracy may lead social perceivers to be more likely to avoid forming stereotypic impressions or relying on stereotypes as judgmental heuristics. Similar claims are offered in a host of dual-process models. Persons processing persuasive messages are more likely to rely on message cues than on peripheral cues when they are highly motivated (e.g., Petty & Cacioppo, 1979; see Petty & Wegener, Chapter 3, this volume). People are more likely to think carefully about the costs and benefits of various courses of action in a given situational context, rather than simply relying on a spontaneous assessment of the situation, when motivation levels are high (Fazio, 1990; see Fazio & Towles-Schwen, Chapter 5, this volume). And people are more likely to make adjustments to dispositional inferences, in recognition of the operation of situational constraints, when they are accuracy-motivated (see Gilbert & Malone, 1995). Thus, it would seem to be a general principle of social information processing that perceivers are likely to rely on relatively simple strategies for judgment, inference, and behavioral choice, unless the situation creates extra motivational energy for the effort required by more systematic forms of thinking (Chaiken et al., 1989).

In the realm of stereotyping, various motivational factors have been shown to be important in moderating the extent of perceivers' reliance on stereotypes in construing the social world. Fiske and her colleagues have led the charge in investigating the role of various forms of social interdependence in motivating accurate, individuated social impressions (e.g., Erber & Fiske, 1984; Fiske, 1993; Fiske & Dépret, 1996; Ruscher & Fiske, 1990; for a review, see Fiske et al., Chapter 11, this volume). When people's outcomes are on the line, they are willing to take the trouble to form an individuated impression of others who might affect those outcomes. Accountability pressures (e.g., Tetlock, 1992; Tetlock & Lerner, Chapter 28, this volume) also promote more detailed, less globally stereotypic social judgments (Bodenhausen, Kramer, & Süsser, 1994; Nelson, Acker, & Manis, 1996; Pendry & Macrae, 1996). When people feel they must be able to defend their choices and judgments, they are more likely to attend effortfully to a broader range of information, rather than rely on simple preconceptions. And the specific motivation to avoid stereotyping and prejudice can also promote less stereotypic responses, at least under some circumstances (see Bodenhausen & Macrae, 1998; Devine & Monteith, Chapter 17, this volume).

Conversely, certain situational and dispositional variables are associated with lowered motivation for systematic thinking. Kruglanski and Webster (1996) have shown that certain epistemic orientations are reliably linked to a preference for quick conclusions. In particular, the need for cognitive closure is an orientation (varying across both persons and situations) that is associated with a sense of urgency in the attainment of closure regarding a decision or judgment. When this need is high, stereotyping will be likely to prevail over individuation (e.g., Kruglanski & Freund, 1983). Variables such as time pressure, noise, and fatigue are examples of some antecedents of the need for cognitive closure.

Mood states have also been linked to perceivers' motivation for effortful thinking (e.g., Schwarz, 1990; see Bless & Schwarz, Chapter 21, this volume). Happiness is associated with feelings of contentment, which may undermine motivation for effortful thinking; instead, happy people may be content to rely on stereotypic preconceptions (Bodenhausen, Kramer, & Süsser, 1994). Sadness, on the other hand, may be associated with motivation to understand one's problematic environment better (e.g., Weary, 1990; Weary & Edwards, 1994), leading to greater attention to individuating information (Bless, Schwarz, & Wieland, 1996; Bodenhausen, Sheppard, & Kramer, 1994; Edwards & Weary, 1993) or to a greater likelihood of correcting initial stereotypic biases (Lambert, Khan, Lickel, & Fricke, 1997). Although some researchers have contended that these kinds of mood effects are not primarily motivational in origin (e.g., Mackie & Worth, 1989), the overall pattern of evidence suggests that motivation is playing at least some role in producing these effects (for reviews, see Bless, Schwarz, & Kemmelmeier, 1996; Bodenhausen, 1993). It thus appears that a variety of motivational factors can moderate the tendency to engage in stereotyping versus individuation.

Capacity

The third major moderator of stereotyping versus individuation is attentional capacity. Miller (1956) decreed that we humans can only manage to deal effectively with about 7 ± 2 chunks of information at a time. The "bottleneck" of attention (Simon, 1994) thus limits our very ability to engage in complex, individuated thinking. Crucially, whenever circumstances reduce our available capacity, they also reduce the possibility of our conducting a thorough, systematic assessment of social targets. Cognitive capacity is widely proposed as a moderator of systematic thinking in persuasion models (Chaiken et al., 1989; Petty & Cacioppo, 1986), attitude–behavior models (Fazio, 1990), and attribution models (Gilbert, Pelham, & Krull, 1988; Trope & Alfieri, 1997; for a review, see Trope & Gaunt, Chapter 8, this volume).

Numerous variables appear to promote stereotyping by reducing perceivers' capacity for engaging in more systematic assessments of others. Mental busyness and distraction are associated with greater use of activated stereotypes (Gilbert & Hixon, 1991; Macrae, Hewstone, & Griffiths, 1993). Similarly, when a judgment situation is especially demanding or difficult, or when judgment-relevant information is superabundant, people may fall back on simple strategies such as stereotype-based heuristics as a way of coping with this complexity (Bodenhausen & Lichtenstein, 1987; Pratto & Bargh, 1991). Attentional capacity also shows diurnal fluctuations, with some individuals having relatively greater capacity for cognitive tasks earlier in the day and others later (Broadbent, Broadbent, & Jones, 1989; May, Hasher, & Stoltzfus, 1993; Revelle, 1993). When circadian arousal levels are at their daily nadir and attentional resources are correspondingly scarce, people are more likely to rely on stereotypes in making judgments, if the stereotypes are descriptively relevant to the dimension of judgment (Bodenhausen, 1990). It is also the case that excessive amounts of arousal can disrupt focused attention, and high arousal levels have also been linked to heightened stereotyping (see Baron, Inman, Kao, & Logan, 1992; Kim & Baron, 1988; Stephan & Stephan, 1985; Wilder & Simon, 1996).

Overall, the research we have summarized supports the view that stereotyping is often the default process of social perception, and that it is only superseded by individuating strategies when there is sufficient motivation and attentional capacity. As such, both motivation and capacity can be regarded as necessary conditions for individuation. In other words, the extent of systematic thinking = f(motivation × capacity). If either component is too low, stereotyping will be likely to prevail. For instance, even individuals who are highly motivated to form accurate, individuated impressions are unable to do so if their attentional capacity is constrained (Osborne & Gilbert, 1992; Pendry & Macrae, 1994). Similarly, one may have ample capacity, but lacking any motivation to think deeply about the social world, one will probably be content to rely on stereotypes. Stereotypic thinking is thus conceived of as the dominant tendency that is only overridden when circumstances are right (Fiske & Neuberg, 1990).

This view does not imply, however, that limitations of motivation or capacity are the principal or root cause of stereotyping (cf. Oakes & Turner, 1990). It simply specifies the conditions under which people are most likely to go beyond a merely stereotypic reaction. To be sure, there are numerous reasons why stereotyping occurs in the first place, and we have summarized a number of them elsewhere (Bodenhausen & Macrae, 1996). Undoubtedly, stereotypes are valuable in large part because they enrich people's representations of others via top-down inference processes (Bodenhausen, 1992; Medin, 1988). It is important to realize that this fact in no way contradicts the cognitive miser viewpoint, although it is sometimes presented as inconsistent with it. In fact, it is at the very heart of this metaphor. By relying on stereotypes to form impressions or judgments of others, people rely on precomputed, preorganized frameworks that provide a potentially rich set of knowledge at the cost of relatively little effort. Moreover, the cognitive capacity saved by relying upon stereotypes is available for facilitating other goals people may happen to be pursuing (Macrae, Milne, & Bodenhausen, 1994; Sherman et al., 1998). Stereotypes are efficient tools for social perception, and the dual-process approach has been a success in providing a theoretically coherent specification of some of the major determinants of their use.

CHALLENGES TO DUAL-PROCESS MODELS

Although dual-processing approaches to stereotyping have produced an impressive array of empirical findings, they are not without their critics. Both the theoretical underpinnings and the empirical support for dual-process models have been challenged. We now consider some of these challenges in detail.

Are Categories and Attributes Distinct Concepts?

Although the distinction between categories and personal attributes is intuitively compelling, it is problematic in practice. To say that "race" is a category, but "extravert" is not, is simply not justifiable (for evidence of the categorical nature of personality descriptors, see Hampson, John, & Goldberg, 1986; John, Hampson, & Goldberg, 1991). Any concept that we might think of as a personality attribute (e.g., "extraverted," "assertive," "optimistic") can also be used as the basis for defining a social category (e.g., "extraverts," "assertive people," "optimists," etc.). As such, the distinction between stereotypic and individuating information becomes difficult to maintain.

Nevertheless, there are important differences between social categories and trait-based categories. First, there is a wide disparity in the degree of consensuality with which people have accepted the two kinds of information as valid means of distinguishing between groups of people. It has been argued that the essential criteria for group membership are that individuals define themselves and are defined by others as members of some category (e.g., Tajfel & Turner, 1986). It is clear that people frequently define themselves as members of social categories (e.g., African Americans) that are distinct from other social categories (e.g., European Americans). It is also clear that people are less likely to define themselves as members of trait categories (assertive people) that are distinct from other trait categories (unassertive people). Rather, we typically rely on trait knowledge to distinguish ourselves from other *individuals* who do not share our particular trait. Thus, whereas social categories are used to distinguish groups of people from one another, traits are used to distinguish individuals from one another.

The research of Andersen and Klatzky (1987; Klatzky & Andersen, 1988) suggests another important difference between social categories and trait categories. Whereas trait categories are typically descriptively unidimensional, stereotype categories are usually much richer and multifaceted. Therefore, trait categories distinguish between people along a single dimension, whereas stereotypes typically distinguish groups from one another on multiple dimensions. Relatedly, members of the same social categories are similar to one another along more dimensions than are members of the same trait categories. This difference has a number of important implications for social perception. For example, we might expect there to be greater inductive potential within social categories than trait categories. A person who knows something about one member of a stereotyped social group can infer that other members of the group may be the same way. The person may be less willing to make such assumptions about members of trait-based categories, particularly along dimensions that are unrelated to the central trait in question (Quattrone & Jones, 1980). These differences in inductive potential are clearly related to issues of perceived group variability, and thus will influence perceivers' willingness to infer attributes of an individual based on his or her group membership and attributes of a group based on any particular member (Park & Hastie, 1987). As a result, perceivers will be more likely to view stereotyped social categories than trait categories as "natural kinds" with underlying essences that are meaningful and unalterable (Rothbart & Taylor, 1992).

The disparity in between-group differences and within-group similarities between social and trait categories should also influence the usefulness and efficiency of the different types of categories during social perception. Categories that produce a stronger ratio of within-category similarity to between-category differences ought to be relied on more heavily (e.g., Turner, Hogg, Oakes,

Reicher, & Wetherell, 1987). In fact, Andersen, Klatzky, and Murray (1990) demonstrated a number of processing advantages associated with the application of social categories versus trait categories. This sort of evidence may go a long way in supporting the assumption of the dual-process models that so-called "individuating information" is indeed qualitatively distinguishable from stereotypic information.

Are Categorization and Individuation Distinct Processes?

Dual-process models argue not only that categories and attributes are distinct concepts, but that the applications of category-based and individuating information involve fundamentally distinct cognitive processes. However, both Smith and Zárate (1992) and Kunda and Thagard (1996) have questioned this assumption. Smith and Zárate's (1992) challenge comes in the form of an exemplar-based model of social judgment. According to this model, impressions of a target are based on the exemplars that are activated by the target. Exemplar activation is driven by the aspects of the target to which perceivers' attention is drawn. If attention is primarily focused on the "femaleness" of a target, other female exemplars will be activated, and these will direct the impressions formed of the target. In contrast, if the assertiveness of the target's behavior is the focus of attention, assertive behavioral exemplars will be retrieved and will guide impression formation. Thus, we might say that in the former case perceivers are relying on categorical information about the target's sex to judge her, whereas in the latter case they are relying on individuating information about her assertiveness. However, in both cases impressions are based on retrieved individual exemplars. In this view, there is no qualitative difference between the processes involved in forming category-based and individuated impressions.

Kunda and Thagard (1996) outline a similar model, which based on the activation of interconnecting nodes in a spreading-activation network. The medium of the mental representation is different than in Smith and Zárate's model, but many of the most important assumptions are the same. In particular, the extent to which impressions are based on categorical or individuating information depends primarily on the amount of attention that is directed at each type of information. If both types of information receive attention, then the impression is determined by the way the networks pertaining to the categorical and individuating information interact and eventually settle on a stable pattern of activation. As in Smith and Zárate's model, the underlying cognitive processes involved in categorization and individuation are the same.

Despite the interesting claims of these models, we believe that there are legitimate bases for distinguishing between categorization and individuation processes. For one thing, when deciding (for example) that a man is unfriendly because he is a skinhead, the perceiver need do nothing more than rely on a simple, preexisting association in memory between the category and trait. In contrast, when deciding that a man is unfriendly because he pushed his way through a crowd, the perceiver engages in an active inference process that involves the creation of new knowledge. That is, the perceiver must (1) characterize the pushing behavior on some trait-relevant dimension, and (2) decide whether the identified characteristic reflects an enduring personality trait of the actor. This is true even if impressions are based on retrieved exemplars or parallel-constraint-satisfaction processes. For example, in an exemplar-based model, the trait meaning still must be extracted from the behavioral exemplars activated by the pushing incident in a way that is not necessary when "skinhead" exemplars are activated by the skinhead. In the latter case, there is still a simple association between the retrieved skinheads and unfriendliness. Thus there is a fundamental distinction between the kinds of associative processes inherent in stereotyping and the kinds of inference processes that occur during behavioral encoding (Sherman, 1996).

We do not wish to suggest that inference processes play no role in stereotype application. In the example above, the perceiver will still need to infer (at some level) that the man encountered is a skinhead before a stereotype can be applied. However, inferring the presence or absence of a categorical feature (particularly a perceptually available feature) is not equivalent to inferring the descriptive meaning and trait implications of a behavioral act. Although inferring traits from behaviors may be a relatively spontaneous process (e.g., Carlston & Skowronski, 1994), it nevertheless may typically require more cognitive effort than categorizing and stereotyping. This is most clearly demonstrated by the fact that stereotypes become relatively more influential than individuating information in conditions of low motivation or cognitive capacity (as described above). One would not expect to find these effects if there were no differences in the difficulty of the processes involved in categorization and individuation.

Redefining Stereotyping and Individuation

Even if there were indeed no meaningful distinction to be drawn between categories and attributes, there are other bases for distinguishing between stereotyping and individuation. Rather than conceiving of the distinction between stereotyping and individuation in terms of qualitative differences in the types of informational input (i.e., categories vs. attributes), we may find it more defensible to think about differences in the *products* of impression formation that characterize stereotyping versus individuation. Specifically, we might say that stereotyping occurs when impressions are dominated by any particular preexisting mental category (which will most often, but perhaps not always, be one of the richer, more vivid sorts of categories identified as "stereotypes" by Andersen & Klatzky, 1987). In contrast, individuation occurs when impressions are not dominated by any particular category, but are based instead upon numerous distinct categories (Langer, Bashner, & Chanowitz, 1985). These various categories could include relatively unidimensional trait concepts (e.g., "gregarious," "athletic") as well as richer, more vivid social types (e.g., "female," "lawyer"). If one's impression of the gregarious, athletic, pizza-loving, female lawyer takes all of these facets into account, then individuation has occurred. However, if one responds to the hypothetical target primarily in terms of her gender or her occupation (or, for that matter, her athleticism) and constructs a mental image of her that relies primarily on default assumptions associated with this dominant category, then stereotyping can be said to have occurred.

From this standpoint, an individuated or personalized impression results from taking into account the unique conjunction of attributes (or categories) ascribed to the person, whereas a stereotypic impression results from using a single category as a framework for construing the person. In the latter case, the person is likely to be perceived as largely interchangeable with other members of the dominant category. The major differences, then, between stereotyping and individuation lie (1) in the number of organizing themes that are present; and (2) in whether the organizing framework is primarily a precomputed representation that is simply retrieved from memory (and to which other information is assimilated), or one that must be newly constructed in order to accommodate the novel constellation of qualities that constitute the content of the person's individual character.

Sometimes the dominant categorization guiding impression formation may be a subtype (e.g., "women lawyers"; see Macrae, Bodenhausen, & Milne, 1995). Although this sort of impression is more sensitive than simply judging the target in terms of her gender, for example, it is nevertheless an instance of stereotyping, because the target is still being construed by reference to membership in a particular category that includes multiple, substantially interchangeable exemplars (otherwise, there would be no subtype). An individuated impression should refer to other qualities that are not necessarily assumed to be shared by members of the subtype. From this perspective, the dominance of a single impressional framework when many alternative categories are applicable is the characteristic feature of stereotyping. And dominance occurs not only when other information is simply neglected, but also when the other information is assimilated to the implications of the dominant category (e.g., Duncan, 1976; Kunda & Sherman-Williams, 1993; Sagar & Schofield, 1980) or is actively inhibited (e.g., Dijksterhuis & van Knippenberg, 1996; Macrae et al., 1995; see Bodenhausen & Macrae, 1998). We assume that certain types of categories are more likely to achieve impressional dominance than others. Specifically, richer, more vivid social categories such as the ones studied by Andersen and Klatzky (1987) are much more likely to serve as the primary frameworks for our impres-

sions of others than are trait categories. In that sense, the continuum model's distinction between categorization and individuation is maintained in spirit, but the potential conceptual problems of distinguishing between an attribute and a category are circumvented.

Do Categories Dominate Individuating Information?

The formulation above maintains one critical distinction between categorization and individuation, even if we were to accept that there are otherwise no definitional or processing-based differences between attributes/individuation and categories/categorization. This distinction is that multidimensional social categories are more likely to dominate an impression than are unidimensional trait categories. However, even this assumption has recently been challenged by Kunda and Thagard (1996), who state that "we do not give stereotypes a special processing role but rather treat them as no different from other information about people such as their traits and behavior" (p. 286) and that "whenever stereotypes and individuating information are both observed, they will jointly influence impressions" (p. 300). Thus, rejecting the dominance of stereotype-based over individuating information, they propose instead a model in which all known information about a target is used to construct a mental impression. Whether it is membership in a social group, abstract trait information, or specific behaviors, each type of social information is assumed to be of equal *a priori* importance in the overall impression. The various pieces of information mutually constrain each other's meaning through a parallel-constraint-satisfaction process (e.g., Holyoak & Thagard, 1989). Specifically, through an iterative process, all concepts that are noticed in the stimulus input become activated, and activation (as well as inhibition) spreads both among the observed characteristics and to other concepts that are semantically linked to the observed characteristics. Eventually the activation pattern settles into a reasonably stable pattern, and this pattern of concepts, activated to various degrees, constitutes the mental impression of the target.

There can be no doubt that parallel-constraint-satisfaction models have provided appealing accounts for a variety of phenomena, such as letter perception (McClelland & Rumelhart, 1981) and discourse comprehension (Kintsch, 1988). Whether they provide a better account for social impression formation and judgment than the dual-process approaches that we have summarized above is a question that warrants further consideration. Kunda and Thagard (1996) claim that their approach can account for all phenomena that the serial, dual-process models can account for, plus many others that the serial approaches cannot. Below we consider the strength of their case.

The most fundamental difference between the parallel-constraint-satisfaction model proposed by Kunda and Thagard and its rivals concerns the question of whether stereotypes really are likely to dominate social impressions. Kunda and Thagard say, unequivocally, "no." Several empirical findings are relevant to this issue, as well as some general theoretical and ecological observations. First we consider the often reported finding that stereotypes become impotent in the presence of specific individuating information (e.g., Locksley, Borgida, Brekke, & Hepburn, 1980; Nisbett, Zukier, & Lemley, 1981; see Kunda & Thagard, 1996, for a thorough review). These studies suggest that when individuating information is available, stereotypes have little if any influence on social judgments. This is especially true when the individuating information is highly diagnostic with respect to the judgment, but may also sometimes be true even when the information is nondiagnostic (see Hilton & Fein, 1989). Reporting the results of a meta-analysis, Kunda and Thagard note that in studies that orthogonally varied both stereotype and individuating information, the effect of the individuating information is substantially larger. From this perspective, the concern that people may often be judged not by their individual qualities, but rather by the color of their skin or other social stereotypes, seems misplaced. Kunda and Thagard conclude, "It is difficult to see how one can maintain the view that stereotypes dominate impressions in the face of such findings" (p. 303).

Methodological Issues

Several factors deserve further consideration before we accept the conclusion that stereo-types become relatively impotent in the face of individuating information. First, some of the studies that show these effects investigated very weak stereotypes, such as "Engineering students have a higher tolerance for electric shock" (Nisbett et al., 1981). It is not hard to see that such stereotypes might be easily dominated by other information. Be that as it may, many other studies did in fact use stronger, better-established stereotypes (e.g., gender, sexual orientation, race, etc.). However, these stereotypes were often activated in relatively pallid ways. Beckett and Park (1995) noted that many studies documenting the absence of stereotyping effects in the presence of individuating information made use of vivid, salient manipulations of individuating information, but that the category information was not made salient. In an extension of earlier work by Locksley, Hepburn, and Ortiz (1982), Beckett and Park found that gender stereotypes exerted little effect on assertiveness judgments when gender was conveyed in the same pallid way it was manipulated by Locksley et al. However, when target gender was manipulated via photographs, gender clearly influenced assertiveness judgments. With salient visual cues to category membership (as is commonly the case in real-life interactions), stereotypic expectancies did influence social judgments substantially.

More generally, the experimental context in most of the studies reviewed by Kunda and Thagard produces a strong demand that research participants attend to and use the presented individuating information. Gricean norms of communication clearly imply that in conversation, one should only provide information if it is relevant (Grice, 1975). By extension, it is reasonable for experimental participants to assume that if the researcher has provided them with individuating information, they must be expected to use it (Schwarz, 1994; see also Leyens, Yzerbyt, & Schadron, 1994). Thus, it would not be too surprising that concrete information that is explicitly brought to participants' awareness with an implicit guarantee of relevance would have a notable impact on judgments. Finally, as Brown (1986) has argued, the lack of effects seen with many kinds of stereotypes can also plausibly be attributed to social desirability biases. Well-educated undergraduates may often be quite reluctant to furnish stereotypic reactions and may well be on their guard to censor such responses when their behavior is being monitored by a researcher.

Interpreting the Data

There is further reason to question whether the data summarized by Kunda and Thagard (1996) do support the conclusion that individuating information has dominated the use of stereotypes in this research literature. As a case in point, consider the influential research of Locksley et al. (1980). The Locksley et al. studies showed that a man was rated as more assertive than a woman was only when no diagnostic information was presented about the targets. When diagnostic behaviors were presented, the man and woman were viewed as equally assertive. Although this pattern is often taken as clear evidence for the relative impotence of stereotypes, such an interpretation is not universally accepted. The problem is that the null effect could very well represent a contrast effect, whereby the assertive act by the woman was seen as more assertive than the same act when performed by a man (in fact, this was true in the Locksley et al. study). In some cases, such contrasting processes may produce counterstereotypical judgments when combined with the trait implications of the stereotype (e.g., Biernat & Manis, 1994; Linville & Jones, 1980). However, in other cases, the contrast effect may simply cancel out the effects of the stereotype and produce null effects on target judgments (as in the case of Locksley et al., 1980). Thus, the application of stereotypes may indeed have occurred in many of the very studies that are commonly presented as demonstrating an absence of stereotyping effects.

The relevance of contrast effects to Kunda and Thagard's model could be questioned, given that in many cases, such effects may reflect the use of effortful causal reasoning on the part of perceivers. For example, perceivers may reason that in order to overcome socially accepted norms of passive behavior for women, a woman must be *especially* assertive. Kunda and Thagard regard relatively controlled thought processes of this sort as lying outside the explanatory reach of the parallel-constraint-satisfaction model. Although it is debatable whether most contrast effects do in fact involve conscious reasoning strategies, such a stance does have significant implications

for the generalizability of Kunda and Thagard's model. Specifically, it is not a trivial fact that contrast processes are more likely to occur in response to stereotype-inconsistent than to stereotype-consistent behaviors (see Kobrynowicz & Biernat, 1998). Perceivers are generally more likely to seek causal explanations for unexpected than for expected behaviors (e.g., Crocker, Hannah, & Weber, 1983; Hastie & Kumar, 1979), and they are more likely to make situational attributions for stereotype-inconsistent than for stereotype-consistent behaviors (e.g., Maass, Milesi, Zabbini, & Stahlberg, 1995). Stereotype-consistent behaviors tend to be attributed (if attributions are made at all) to the internal properties of the actor (Bodenhausen & Wyer, 1985; Yzerbyt, Rogier, & Fiske, 1998). These attributional biases diminish the trait implications of inconsistent behaviors and help to maintain the stereotype. Therefore, if the parallel-constraint-satisfaction model is limited to explaining relatively automatic, mindless processes of impression formation (as Kunda and Thagard themselves assert), then it will primarily be useful for predicting how stereotypes and stereotype-confirming information will be weighted. It may be of less use for understanding how inconsistent information is integrated into an overall impression, since this integration typically involves effortful rather than automatic processes.

Further Support for Stereotype Dominance

To focus on the relative weight given to stereotypes and individuating information as the sole indicator of stereotype dominance does not tell the whole story. Other relevant sources of data clearly demonstrate the dominance of stereotypes in impression formation. For example, Sherman (1996) showed that the availability of a stereotype reduced the extent to which perceivers retrieved previously encountered individuating information as they were making target judgments. Trope and Thompson (1997) further showed that perceivers with an available stereotype were less likely to seek out individuating information about a target. These studies demonstrate that stereotypes provide people with a sense of informational validity that decreases their interest in available individuating information.

To the extent that judgments are based

on what people can remember about a target, stereotypes may be particularly likely to predominate. For a variety of reasons, stereotype-consistent individuating information is more easily retrieved from memory than is stereotype-inconsistent and irrelevant information (e.g., Dijksterhuis & van Knippenberg, 1996; Rothbart, Sriram, & Davis-Stitt, 1996; Sherman et al., 1998; van Knippenberg & Dijksterhuis, 1996). In this case, stereotypes dominate judgments by influencing the subset of individuating information that is most available in memory.

Finally, as noted above, an extensive research literature has developed from within the framework of a dual-process conceptualization of stereotyping versus individuation. The hallmark of this literature is the demonstration that stereotypes are particularly likely to dominate impressions and judgments under conditions of low capacity and/or motivation. The parallel-constraint-satisfaction model is hard pressed to account for this pattern of findings. Consequently, Kunda and Thagard (1996) attempt to dismiss the evidence as equivocal. Conceding that the available studies indeed do show that "reduction in cognitive resources increases reliance on stereotypes" (p. 302), they argue that it may well be the case that these resource constraints increase reliance upon individuating information also. It is certainly a counterintuitive notion to claim that information-processing constraints will increase the use of all types of impression-relevant information. But even if this assertion were correct, it still cannot explain why judgments should shift more in the direction of the stereotype under conditions of resource constraint. Thus, it seems that the parallel-constraint-satisfaction model cannot account for one of the principal empirical patterns through which the dual-process models are substantiated. Stereotypes *do* dominate social impressions and judgments, and they do so under the conditions specified by the dual-process models.

As for phenomena that the parallel-constraint-satisfaction model can explain but the dual-process, serial models cannot, Kunda and Thagard emphasize evidence showing that the effects of stereotypes depend on the nature of the judgment task (Kunda, Sinclair, & Griffin, 1997). Specifically, they note that "individuating information undermines the effects of stereotypes on ratings of the target's traits but does not undermine the effects of stereotypes on predictions about the same target's future trait-related behavior" (pp. 300–301). In actuality, exactly this pattern has been offered as support for the dual-process approach (Bodenhausen & Lichtenstein, 1987; Bodenhausen & Wyer, 1985). Because of the relative simplicity of trait ratings, given clear evidence bearing on them, Bodenhausen and Lichtenstein argued that it takes relatively little motivation or capacity to make evidence-based trait judgments. As previously noted, trait inferences have been shown to occur relatively spontaneously in a wide range of experiments (e.g., Carlston & Skowronski, 1994; Lupfer, Clark, & Hutcherson, 1990; Newman, 1991; Uleman, Hon, Roman, & Moskowitz, 1996). More complicated or effortful forms of inference, such as predictions of future behavior or judgments of guilt, may be much more likely to recruit stereotypes as judgmental heuristics, in the absence of sufficient motivation and/or processing capacity. It remains debatable whether there are significant empirical phenomena that are better explained by Kunda and Thagard's model than by dual-process models.

Ecological Issues: On the Seriality of Impression Formation

A broader problem with the parallel-constraint-satisfaction model is that in proposing simultaneous, mutual constraint of stereotypes and individuating information, the model seemingly overlooks the largely serial fashion in which social information is acquired in everyday life. As Brewer (1988) has emphasized, stereotypic categories such as ethnicity, age, gender, or occupation are often readily apparent upon one's first encountering a person. The stereotypes associated with these features can be activated very quickly and automatically (e.g., Banaji & Greenwald, 1995; Bargh, 1997 and Chapter 18, this volume; Devine, 1989; Macrae, Bodenhausen, Milne, Thorn, & Castelli, 1997), setting up expectations that can bias and constrain interpretations of subsequently encountered information (e.g., Dunning & Sherman, 1997; Kunda & Sherman-Williams, 1993; Sagar & Schofield, 1980) and leading to the preferential search for stereotype-confirming information (e.g., Johnston & Macrae, 1994; Snyder & Cantor, 1979; Trope & Thompson, 1997). In contrast, we have already argued that forming individuated impressions of others based on their behaviors requires a more demanding inference process. Moreover, first encounters are often relatively superficial, providing minimal individuating information in any case. Thus, the possibility of *mutual* constraint is undermined by the typical sequence of *serial* information acquisition. Often it is only with more time that perceivers can observe a range of individuating behaviors and draw trait inferences, and by then their impressions may have already been colored by stereotypic beliefs.

The parallel-constraint-satisfaction model does assume that the first information that one encounters is likely to have greater influence than subsequent information. In fact, it explains Asch's (1946) classic demonstration of primacy effects in impression formation in this fashion. However, participants in Asch's studies actually did receive trait descriptors in virtually immediate succession, so if there were ever a situation where mutual parallel constraint of impressions should occur, it should be in this sort of context. Yet Kunda and Thagard suggest that the activation network settles after each trait is encountered, thereby giving greater weight to initial information by biasing the "start values" for activation levels on subsequent iterations. This assumption, of course, introduces a substantial serial component to their model. It is a sort of escape hatch for explaining stereotype dominance when it occurs, but stereotype dominance is nevertheless regarded as exceptional rather than typical. We disagree, given the temporal priority that stereotypes have under a wide array of natural information acquisition conditions and the importance they have in providing a rich, precomputed model of the individuals we encounter. As Medin (1988, p. 124) has noted, "some properties may not be simply more salient than others, but also more *central*" (emphasis in original; see also Asch, 1946; Asch & Zukier, 1984). These central properties are much more likely to constrain the interpretation of the other information than vice versa. As Andersen and Klatzky (1987) have demonstrated, social

stereotypes are much more likely, in the typical case, to provide a rich central theme for thinking of others than are personality trait concepts (and, we would add, individual behaviors). All person information is not equal. To deny this reality may add simplicity to the parallel-constraint-satisfaction model, but it results in conclusions that are markedly at odds with the experiences of members of stigmatized groups, who routinely report being judged "by the color of their skin" or other stigma markers, rather than by their individual character.

Kunda and Thagard's model is of course not without virtues. It may be a rather accurate model of the processes that occur when people read concise, verbally presented person descriptions provided by researchers under a variety of circumstances. But what it is modeling may be more akin to text comprehension (Kintsch, 1988) than to social impression formation and judgment, which come packaged with abundant motivations to use and preserve stereotypic preconceptions of social groups. We believe that the dual-process, serial models do a better job of accounting for this reality than the parallel-constraint-satisfaction model that they have proposed.

FURTHER DUALITIES OF SOCIAL STEREOTYPING

In addition to distinguishing between stereotyping and individuation, it is useful to make further distinctions when considering the nature of stereotyping and its avoidance. Specifically, within the domain of stereotyping, it may be important to distinguish between *implicit* and *explicit* forms of stereotype activation and use (cf. Greenwald & Banaji, 1995). Similarly, stereotype avoidance may be subdivided into two subtypes: (1) the motivated thoroughness of individuation that we have focused on above, and (2) stereotype inhibition and correction (Bodenhausen & Macrae, 1998). In this section, we consider this latter distinction in some detail.

The Goal of Control: Alternative Pathways to Stereotype Avoidance

As we have already noted, dual-process models of person perception (Brewer, 1988; Fiske

& Neuberg, 1990) have provided some valuable insights into the motivational and cognitive determinants of stereotyping. The route to stereotype avoidance in these models is quite straightforward: Individuated (i.e., nonstereotypic) evaluations and impressions can be promoted through the allocation of attention to a person's idiosyncratic constellation of attributes and behaviors. However, various other approaches can be employed in the service of this goal. One favored tactic, for example, involves trying to expunge stereotypic thoughts and recollections from mind, thereby denying them the possibility of free behavioral expression. This mental exorcism is realized through the operation of cognitive inhibition—a process that has recently attracted considerable attention from researchers (e.g., Devine, 1989; Bodenhausen & Macrae, 1998; Wegner, 1994). Of relevance in the present context is the observation that dual-process models of cognitive functioning provide valuable insight into how inhibitory mechanisms can moderate the expression versus repression of social stereotypes.

It is only perhaps within the last 10 years or so that researchers have explicitly explored how inhibitory mechanisms can inform our understanding of aspects of the stereotyping process (see Bodenhausen & Macrae, 1996, 1998; Bodenhausen, Macrae, & Milne, 1998; Devine, 1989; Dijksterhuis & van Knippenberg, 1996; Macrae, Bodenhausen, Milne, & Ford, 1997; Macrae, Bodenhausen, Milne, & Jetten, 1994; Macrae, Bodenhausen, Milne, & Wheeler, 1996; Monteith, 1993). The impetus for much of this work was undoubtedly Devine's (1989) seminal article on the cognitive dynamics of prejudice. Devine's theoretical argument is an important one, implicating as it does the dual operation of automatic and controlled processes in stereotyping (see Devine & Monteith, Chapter 17, this volume). Following the (automatic) activation of stereotypic material in memory, egalitarian perceivers are believed to sanitize their outputs (e.g., behaviors, utterances) by inhibiting the unwanted contents of consciousness. That is, to prevent stereotypic thoughts from turning into prejudiced actions, low-prejudice perceivers are believed to remove unwanted items from mind through the operation of inhibitory processes (i.e., mind control). Once these items are banished from consciousness,

it is assumed that they can no longer exert an untoward influence on behavioral outputs (but see Macrae, Bodenhausen, et al., 1994; Macrae et al., 1996). For Devine (1989), then, prejudice can best be understood by analyzing the dual components of the stereotyping process: namely, the *automatic* activation and *controlled* inhibition of stereotypic thoughts (see also Monteith, 1993).

Inhibiting stereotypic thoughts, feelings, and reactions is quite a distinct goal from individuating a social target. To explain exactly how perceivers can attain the goal of mind control, it is relatively commonplace for researchers to propose dual-process models of cognitive functioning. One of the most prominent and influential examples of this type, for instance, is Wegner's (1994) "ironic-process" theory of mental control. According to this model, mind control is realized through the simultaneous operation of two cognitive processes: an *automatic* (ironic) monitoring process; and a *controlled* operating process. Following the onset of a conscious intention not to think about a particular topic (e.g., the belief that blondes are dumb), an automatic monitoring process is believed to scan consciousness, searching for any failures or lapses in mental control. When such a failure is detected, a controlled operating process (i.e., cognitive inhibition) is then instigated, the task of which is to remove the errant thought from mind. Mental tranquility is restored when the unwanted item (e.g., "Blondes are dumb") is replaced by a more palatable alternative (e.g., "That apple pie smells nice").

Closer inspection of Wegner's (1994) model reveals how the availability of attentional resources modulates the efficiency of the dual processes that drive mind control. Whereas the ironic monitoring process runs in a largely effortless manner, the controlled operating process, in contrast, makes more notable demands on perceivers' attentional resources. In other words, whereas detecting failures in mental control is a relatively easy affair, doing something about them is a considerably more troublesome task. When attentional resources are in plentiful supply, there is little to worry about. Unwanted items are replaced in consciousness by suitable distractors, and everything in the (mental) garden is rosy. However, when attentional resources are depleted, the process of mental control is seriously impaired. Indeed, under these conditions, thought control can backfire, prompting the rather paradoxical effect that perceivers become preoccupied with the very items they are trying to dismiss. Rebound effects of this sort have been documented for an impressive variety of mental contents, ranging from lost loves to obsessive ruminations to thoughts of white bears (see Wegner, 1994). Importantly, comparable effects have also emerged in person perception, with stereotypic thoughts reappearing in mind following the cessation of a period of intentional mind control (Macrae, Bodenhausen, et al., 1994; Macrae et al., 1996).

The utility of dual-process models of cognitive functioning resides in their ability to identify factors that moderate the expression of social stereotypes, including factors regulating stereotype suppression. Whether perceivers subvert stereotyping by focusing on a target's unique constellation of attributes (i.e., individuation), or by suppressing stereotypic thoughts and recollections in consciousness, attentional resources are required in each case to fuel the relevant cognitive routines. Avoiding the expression of stereotypes, it would seem, is an attentional-demanding affair.

If stereotyping can be circumvented via either individuation or suppression, when do perceivers implement these competing processing strategies? One potentially important factor is the strength of an activated stereotype. When an activated stereotype is strong (e.g., "skinhead"), and the associated categorical information (e.g., "dangerous") is deemed to be highly diagnostic, it may be futile to try to prevent stereotyping by focusing attention on a target's personalized attributes (e.g., "This skinhead has a pet canary"). Under these circumstances, the insistent stereotype-based material in memory may prevail and continue to color one's target-based judgments. To avoid stereotyping, a better strategy may be to attempt to remove the unwanted stereotypic material from mind through the process of intentional suppression, or to adjust one's judgments and reactions directly, in order to correct for stereotypic biases (e.g., Wilson & Brekke, 1994). For weak stereotypes (e.g., "golfers"), however, the opposite may be true. As the available stereotypic asso-

ciates (e.g., "wears tartan pants") are unlikely to have an overwhelming influence on judgmental outcomes, one's attentional resources may be spent more profitably in inspecting the target's unique attributes and qualities (e.g., "This golfer plays the banjo"). How attention is cognitively deployed, then, may be influenced by the strength of an activated stereotype and the judgmental potency of the available associates. For strong stereotypes, suppression may be the antidote to categorical thinking; for weak stereotypes, discrimination may be prevented by instead focusing attention on a target's personalized behaviors. Although speculative, these predictions can readily be derived from extant dual-process models of person perception, thereby revealing the empirical value of these approaches. Having provided a theoretical framework for informing our understanding of when people stereotype others, we believe that these models can also furnish insight into the equally important question of how stereotyping can be avoided. One task for future research on person perception will be to explore the largely uncharted waters that surround this topic.

CONCLUSIONS

The dual-process approach to stereotyping in impression formation and social judgment has yielded systematic insights into the fundamental nature of these phenomena, especially regarding the moderating variables that determine whether or not stereotypes exert a noteworthy influence on our reactions to others. The idea at the heart of the dual-process approaches–namely, that stereotyping represents a form of social information processing that is conceptually distinct from and inherently less demanding than individuation—has been the target of interesting recent theoretical challenges. On balance, however, we regard these challenges as less than convincing. We have attempted to document the success of the dual-process approaches in generating a rich set of predictions (and supporting evidence) concerning the determinants of stereotyping by reference to a parsimonious set of underlying assumptions. This body of evidence strongly suggests that the dual-process models have important insights to offer us in our attempts to understand the nature of stereotyping and stereotype-based discrimination.

The value of this analysis is also enhanced by recognizing that its underlying principles cohere with theoretical models designed to address a disparate variety of phenomena in other domains of social psychology. Indeed, the present volume is a testament to the fruitfulness of dual-process models and to the core insights that they share in attempting to understand the cognitive underpinnings of social behavior.

REFERENCES

Allport, G. W. (1954). *The nature of prejudice*. Reading, MA: Addison-Wesley.

Andersen, S. M., & Klatzky, R. L. (1987). Traits and social stereotypes: Levels of categorization in person perception. *Journal of Personality and Social Psychology, 53*, 235–246.

Andersen, S. M., Klatzky, R. L., & Murray, J. (1990). Traits and social stereotypes: Efficiency differences in social information processing. *Journal of Personality and Social Psychology, 59*, 192–201.

Asch, S. E. (1946). Forming impressions of personality. *Journal of Abnormal and Social Psychology, 41*, 303–314.

Asch, S. E., & Zukier, H. (1984). Thinking about persons. *Journal of Personality and Social Psychology, 46*, 1230–1240.

Banaji, M. R., & Greenwald, A. G. (1995). Implicit gender stereotyping in judgments of fame. *Journal of Personality and Social Psychology, 68*, 181–198.

Bargh, J. A. (1997). The automaticity of everyday life. In R. S. Wyer, Jr. (Ed.), *Advances in social cognition: Vol. 10. The automaticity of everyday life* (pp. 1–61). Mahwah, NJ: Erlbaum.

Baron, R. S., Inman, M. L., Kao, C. F., & Logan, H. (1992). Negative emotion and superficial social processing. *Motivation and Emotion, 16*, 323–346.

Beckett, N. E., & Park, B. (1995). Use of category versus individuating information: Making base rates salient. *Personality and Social Psychology Bulletin, 21*, 21–31.

Biernat, M., & Manis, M. (1994). Shifting standards and stereotype-based judgments. *Journal of Personality and Social Psychology, 66*, 5–20.

Bless, H., Schwarz, N., & Kemmelmeier, M. (1996). Mood and stereotyping: Affective states and the use of general knowledge structures. In W. Stroebe & M. Hewstone (Eds.), *European review of social psychology* (Vol. 7, pp. 63–93). Chichester, England: Wiley.

Bless, H., Schwarz, N., & Wieland, R. (1996). Mood and the impact of category membership and individuating information. *European Journal of Social Psychology, 26*, 935–960.

Bodenhausen, G. V. (1988). Stereotypic biases in social decision making and memory: Testing process models of stereotype use. *Journal of Personality and Social Psychology, 55*, 726–737.

Bodenhausen, G. V. (1990). Stereotypes as judgmental heuristics: Evidence of circadian variations in discrimination. *Psychological Science, 1*, 319–322.

Bodenhausen, G. V. (1992). Information-processing functions of generic knowledge structures and their role in context effects in social judgment. In N. Schwarz & S. Sudman (Eds.), *Context effects in social and psychological research* (pp. 267–277). New York: Springer-Verlag.

Bodenhausen, G. V. (1993). Emotion, arousal, and stereotypic judgments: A heuristic model of affect and stereotyping. In D. M. Mackie & D. L. Hamilton (Eds.), *Affect, cognition, and stereotyping: Interactive processes in group perception* (pp. 13–37). San Diego, CA: Academic Press.

Bodenhausen, G. V., Kramer, G. P., & Süsser, K. (1994). Happiness and stereotypic thinking in social judgment. *Journal of Personality and Social Psychology, 66*, 621–632.

Bodenhausen, G. V., & Lichtenstein, M. (1987). Social stereotypes and information-processing strategies: The impact of task complexity. *Journal of Personality and Social Psychology, 52*, 871–880.

Bodenhausen, G. V., & Macrae, C. N. (1996). The self-regulation of intergroup perception: Mechanisms and consequences of stereotype suppression. In C. N. Macrae, C. Stangor, & M. Hewstone (Eds.), *Stereotypes and stereotyping* (pp. 227–253). New York: Guilford Press.

Bodenhausen, G. V., & Macrae, C. N. (1998). Stereotype activation and inhibition. In R. S. Wyer, Jr. (Ed.), *Advances in social cognition: Vol. 11. Stereotype activation and inhibition* (pp. 1–52). Mahwah, NJ: Erlbaum.

Bodenhausen, G. V., Macrae, C. N., & Milne, A. B. (1998). Disregarding social stereotypes: Implications for judgment, memory, and behavior. In J. M. Golding & C. M. MacLeod (Eds.), *Directed forgetting: Interdisciplinary perspectives* (pp. 349–368). Mahwah, NJ: Erlbaum.

Bodenhausen, G. V., Sheppard, L., & Kramer, G. P. (1994). Negative affect and social judgment: The differential impact of anger and sadness. *European Journal of Social Psychology, 24*, 45–62.

Bodenhausen, G. V., & Wyer, R. S., Jr. (1985). Effects of stereotypes on decision making and information-processing strategies. *Journal of Personality and Social Psychology, 48*, 267–282.

Brewer, M. B. (1988). A dual-process model of impression formation. In T. K. Srull & R. S. Wyer, Jr. (Eds.), *Advances in social cognition: Vol. 1. A dual-process model of impression formation* (pp. 1–36). Hillsdale, NJ: Erlbaum.

Broadbent, D. E., Broadbent, M. H. P., & Jones, J. L. (1989). Time of day as an instrument for the analysis of attention. *European Journal of Cognitive Psychology, 1*, 69–94.

Brown, R. (1986). *Social psychology* (2nd ed.). New York: Free Press.

Bruner, J. (1951). Personality dynamics and the process of perceiving. In R. R. Blake & G. V. Ramsey (Eds.), *Perception: An approach to personality* (pp. 121–147). New York: Ronald Press.

Bruner, J. (1957). On perceptual readiness. *Psychological Review, 64*, 123–152.

Carlston, D. E., & Skowronski, J. J. (1994). Savings in relearning of trait information as evidence for spontaneous inference generation. *Journal of Personality and Social Psychology, 66,* 840–856.

Chaiken, S. (1980). Heuristic versus systematic information processing and the use of source versus message cues in persuasion. *Journal of Personality and Social Psychology, 39,* 752–766.

Chaiken, S. (1987). The heuristic model of persuasion. In M. P. Zanna, J. M. Olson, & C. P. Herman (Eds.), *Social influence: The Ontario Symposium* (Vol. 5, pp. 3–39). Hillsdale, NJ: Erlbaum.

Chaiken, S., Giner-Sorolla, R., & Chen, S. (1996). Beyond accuracy: Defense and impression motives in heuristic and systematic information processing. In P. M. Gollwitzer & J. A. Bargh (Eds.), *The psychology of action: Linking cognition and motivation to behavior* (pp. 553–578). New York: Guilford Press.

Chaiken, S., Liberman, A., & Eagly, A. (1989). Heuristic and systematic information processing within and beyond the persuasion context. In J. S. Uleman & J. A. Bargh (Eds.), *Unintended thought* (pp. 212–252). New York: Guilford Press.

Chaiken, S., & Maheswaran, D. (1994). Heuristic processing can bias systematic processing: Effects of source credibility, argument ambiguity, and task performance on attitude judgment. *Journal of Personality and Social Psychology, 66,* 460–473.

Crocker, J., Hannah, D. B., & Weber, R. (1983). Person memory and causal attributions. *Journal of Personality and Social Psychology, 44,* 55–66.

Darley, J. M., & Gross, P. (1983). A hypothesis-confirming bias in labeling effects. *Journal of Personality and Social Psychology, 44,* 20–33.

Devine, P. G. (1989). Stereotypes and prejudice: Their automatic and controlled components. *Journal of Personality and Social Psychology, 56,* 5–18.

Dijksterhuis, A., & van Knippenberg, A. (1996). The knife that cuts both ways: Facilitated and inhibited access to traits as a result of stereotype activation. *Journal of Experimental Social Psychology, 32,* 271–288.

Duncan, B. L. (1976). Differential social perception and attribution of intergroup violence: Testing the lower limits of stereotyping of blacks. *Journal of Personality and Social Psychology, 34,* 590–598.

Dunning, D., & Sherman, D. A. (1997). Stereotypes and tacit inference. *Journal of Personality and Social Psychology, 73,* 459–471.

Edwards, J. A., & Weary, G. (1993). Depression and the impression-formation continuum: Piecemeal processing despite the availability of category information. *Journal of Personality and Social Psychology, 64,* 636–645.

Erber, R., & Fiske, S. T. (1984). Outcome dependency and attention to inconsistent information. *Journal of Personality and Social Psychology, 47,* 709–726.

Fazio, R. H. (1990). Multiple processes by which attitudes guide behavior: The MODE model as an integrative framework. In M. P. Zanna (Ed.), *Advances in experimental social psychology* (Vol. 23, pp. 75–109). San Diego, CA: Academic Press.

Fiske, S. T. (1993). Controlling other people: The impact of power on stereotyping. *American Psychologist, 48,* 621–628.

Fiske, S. T. (1998). Stereotyping, prejudice, and discrimination. In D. T. Gilbert, S. T. Fiske, & G. Lindzey (Eds.), *Handbook of social psychology* (4th ed.). New York: McGraw-Hill.

Fiske, S. T., & Dépret, E. (1996). Control, interdependence, and power: Understanding social cognition in its social context. In W. Stroebe & M. Hewstone (Eds.), *European review of social psychology* (Vol. 7, pp. 31–61). Chichester, England: Wiley.

Fiske, S. T., & Neuberg, S. L. (1990). A continuum of impression formation, from category-based to individuating processes: Influences of information and motivation on attention and interpretation. In M. P. Zanna (Ed.), *Advances in experimental social psychology* (Vol. 23, pp. 1–74). San Diego, CA: Academic Press.

Fiske, S. T., Neuberg, S. L., Beattie, A., & Milberg, S. (1987). Category-based and atttribute-based reactions to others: Some informational conditions of stereotyping and individuating processes. *Journal of Experimental Social Psychology, 23,* 399–427.

Fiske, S. T., & Taylor, S. E. (1984). *Social cognition* (1st ed.). New York: McGraw-Hill.

Gilbert, D. T., & Hixon, J. G. (1991). The trouble of thinking: Activation and application of stereotypic beliefs. *Journal of Personality and Social Psychology, 60,* 509–517.

Gilbert, D. T., & Malone, P. S. (1995). The correspondence bias. *Psychological Bulletin, 117,* 21–30.

Gilbert, D. T., Pelham, B. W., & Krull, D. S. (1988). On cognitive busyness: When person perceivers meet persons perceived. *Journal of Personality and Social Psychology, 54,* 733–740.

Greenwald, A. G., & Banaji, M. R. (1995). Implicit social cognition: Attitudes, self-esteem, and stereotypes. *Psychological Review, 102,* 4–27.

Grice, H. P. (1975). Logic in conversation. In P. Cole & J. L. Morgan (Eds.), *Syntax and semantics* (Vol. 3, pp. 41–58). New York: Academic Press.

Hamilton, D. L., & Sherman, J. W. (1994). Stereotypes. In R. S. Wyer, Jr., & T. K. Srull (Eds.), *Handbook of social cognition* (2nd ed., Vol. 2, pp. 1–68). Hillsdale, NJ: Erlbaum.

Hampson, S. E., John, O. P., & Goldberg, L. R. (1986). Category breadth and hierarchical structure in personality: Studies of asymmetries in judgments of trait implications. *Journal of Personality and Social Psychology, 51,* 37–54.

Hastie, R., & Kumar, P. (1979). Person memory: Personality traits as organizing principles in memory for behaviors. *Journal of Personality and Social Psychology, 37,* 25–38.

Hilton, J. L., & Fein, S. (1989). The role of typical diagnosticity in stereotype-based judgments. *Journal of Personality and Social Psychology, 57,* 201–211.

Holyoak, K. J., & Thagard, P. (1989). Analogical mapping by constraint satisfaction. *Cognitive Science, 13,* 295–355.

John, O. P., Hampson, S. E., & Goldberg, L. R. (1991). The basic level in personality-trait hierarchies: Studies of trait use and accessibility in different contexts. *Journal of Personality and Social Psychology, 60,* 348–361.

Johnston, L. C., & Macrae, C. N. (1994). Changing social stereotypes: The case of the information seeker. *European Journal of Social Psychology, 24,* 581–592.

Kahneman, D., Slovic, P., & Tversky, A. (Eds.). (1982). *Judgment under uncertainty: Heuristics and biases.* Cambridge, England: Cambridge University Press.

Kim, H.-S., & Baron, R. S. (1988). Exercise and illusory correlation: Does arousal heighten stereotypic processing? *Journal of Experimental Social Psychology, 24,* 366–380.

Kintsch, W. (1988). The role of knowledge in discourse comprehension: A construction–integration model. *Psychological Review, 95,* 163–182.

Klatzky, R. L., & Andersen, S. M. (1988). Category-specificity effects in social typing and personalization. In T. K. Srull & R. S. Wyer, Jr. (Eds.), *Advances in social cognition: Vol. 1. A dual-process model of impression formation* (pp. 91–101). Hillsdale, NJ: Erlbaum.

Kobrynowicz, D., & Biernat, M. (1998). Considering correctness, contrast, and categorization in stereotyping phenomena. In R. S. Wyer, Jr. (Ed.), *Advances in social cognition: Vol. 11. Stereotype activation and inhibition* (pp. 109–126). Mahwah, NJ: Erlbaum.

Kruglanski, A. W., & Freund, T. (1983). The freezing and unfreezing of lay-inferences: Effects on impressional primacy, ethnic stereotyping, and numerical anchoring. *Journal of Experimental Social Psychology, 19,* 448–468.

Kruglanski, A. W., & Webster, D. M. (1996). Motivated closing of the mind: "Seizing" and "freezing." *Psychological Review, 103,* 263–283.

Kunda, Z., & Sherman-Williams, B. (1993). Stereotypes and the construal of individuating information. *Personality and Social Psychology Bulletin, 19,* 90–99.

Kunda, Z., Sinclair, L., & Griffin, D. (1997). Equal ratings but separate meanings: Stereotypes and the construal of traits. *Journal of Personality and Social Psychology, 72,* 720–734,

Kunda, Z., & Thagard, P. (1996). Forming impressions from stereotypes, traits, and behaviors: A parallel-constraint-satisfaction theory. *Psychological Review, 103,* 284–308.

Lambert, A. J., Khan, S., Lickel, B., & Fricke, K. (1997). Mood and the correction of positive versus negative stereotypes. *Journal of Personality and Social Psychology, 72,* 1002–1016.

Langer, E., Bashner, R., & Chanowitz, B. (1985). Decreasing prejudice by increasing discrimination. *Journal of Personality and Social Psychology, 49,* 113–120.

Leyens, J.-P., Yzerbyt, V., & Schadron, G. (1994). *Stereotypes and social cognition.* London: Sage.

Linville, P., & Jones, E. E. (1980). Polarized appraisals of out-group members. *Journal of Personality and Social Psychology, 38,* 689–703.

Locksley, A., Borgida, E., Brekke, N., & Hepburn, C. (1980). Sex stereotypes and social judgment. *Journal of Personality and Social Psychology, 39,* 821–831.

Locksley, A., Hepburn, C., & Ortiz, V. (1982). Social stereotypes and judgments of individuals: An instance of the base-rate fallacy. *Journal of Experimental Social Psychology, 18,* 23–42.

Lupfer, M. B., Clark, L. F., & Hutcherson, H. W. (1990). Impact of context on spontaneous trait and situational attributions. *Journal of Personality and Social Psychology, 58,* 239–249.

Maass, A., Milesi, A., Zabbini, S., & Stahlberg, D. (1995). Linguistic intergroup bias: Differential expectancies or in-group protection? *Journal of Personality and Social Psychology, 68,* 116–126.

Mackie, D. M., & Worth, L. T. (1989). Processing deficits and the mediation of positive affect in persuasion. *Journal of Personality and Social Psychology, 57,* 27–40.

Macrae, C. N., Bodenhausen, G. V., & Milne, A. B. (1995). The dissection of selection in person perception: Inhibitory processes in social stereotyping. *Journal of Personality and Social Psychology, 69,* 397–407.

Macrae, C. N., Bodenhausen, G. V., Milne, A. B., & Ford, R. (1997). On the regulation of recollection: The intentional forgetting of stereotypical memories. *Journal of Personality and Social Psychology, 72,* 709–719.

Macrae, C. N., Bodenhausen, G. V., Milne, A. B., & Jetten, J. (1994). Out of mind but back in sight: Stereotypes on the rebound. *Journal of Personality and Social Psychology, 67,* 808–817.

Macrae, C. N., Bodenhausen, G. V., Milne, A. B., & Wheeler, V. (1996). On resisting the temptation for simplification: Counterintentional consequences of stereotype suppression on social memory. *Social Cognition, 14,* 1–20.

Macrae, C. N., Bodenhausen, G. V., Milne, A. B., Thorn, T. M. J., & Castelli, L. (1997). On the activation of social stereotypes: The moderating role of processing objectives. *Journal of Experimental Social Psychology, 33,* 471–489.

Macrae, C. N., Hewstone, M., & Griffiths, R. J. (1993). Processing load and memory for stereotype-based information. *European Journal of Social Psychology, 23,* 77–87.

Macrae, C. N., Milne, A. B., & Bodenhausen, G. V. (1994). Stereotypes as energy-saving devices: A peek inside the cognitive toolbox. *Journal of Personality and Social Psychology, 66,* 37–47.

May, C. P., Hasher, L., & Stoltzfus, E. R. (1993). Optimal time of day and the magnitude of age differences in memory. *Psychological Science, 4,* 326–330.

McCauley, C. (1988). The content of awareness and top-down versus bottom-up processes. In T. K. Srull & R. S. Wyer, Jr. (Eds.), *Advances in social cognition: Vol. 1. A dual process model of impression formation* (pp. 111–118). Hillsdale, NJ: Erlbaum.

McClelland, J. L., & Rumelhart, D. E. (1981). An interactive activation model of context effects in letter perception: Part I. An account of basic findings. *Psychological Review, 88,* 375–407.

Medin, D. L. (1988). Social categorization: Structures, processes, and purposes. In T. K. Srull & R. S. Wyer, Jr. (Eds.), *Advances in social cognition: Vol. 1. A dual-process model of impression formation* (pp. 119–126). Hillsdale, NJ: Erlbaum.

Miller, G. A. (1956). The magical number seven, plus or minus two: Some limits on our capacity for processing information. *Psychological Review, 63,* 81–97.

Monteith, M. J. (1993). Self-regulation of prejudiced responses: Implications for progress in prejudice-reduction efforts. *Journal of Personality and Social Psychology, 65,* 469–485.

Murphy, G. L., & Medin, D. L. (1985). The role of theories in conceptual coherence. *Psychological Review, 92,* 289–316.

Neisser, U. (1976). *Cognition and reality: Principles and implications of cognitive psychology.* San Francisco: W. H. Freeman.

Nelson, T. E., Acker, M., & Manis, M. (1996). Irrepressible stereotypes. *Journal of Experimental Social Psychology, 32,* 13–38.

Newell, A., & Simon, H. A. (1972). *Human problem solving*. Englewood Cliffs, NJ: Prentice-Hall.

Newman, L. S. (1991). Why are traits inferred spontaneously?: A developmental approach. *Social Cognition, 9*, 221–253.

Nisbett, R. E., Zukier, H., & Lemley, R. E. (1981). The dilution effect: Nondiagnostic information weakens the implications of diagnostic information. *Cognitive Psychology, 13*, 248–277.

Oakes, P., Haslam, S. A., & Turner, J. C. (1994). *Stereotyping and social reality*. Oxford: Blackwell.

Oakes, P., & Turner, J. C. (1990). Is limited information processing capacity the cause of social stereotyping? In W. Stroebe & M. Hewstone (Eds.), *European review of social psychology* (Vol. 1, pp. 111–135). Chichester, England: Wiley.

Osborne, R. E., & Gilbert, D. T. (1992). The preoccupational hazards of social life. *Journal of Personality and Social Psychology, 62*, 219–228.

Palmer, S. E. (1975). Visual perception and world knowledge. In D. A. Norman, D. E. Rumelhart, & the LNR Research Group (Eds.), *Explorations in cognition*. San Francisco: Freeman.

Park, B., & Hastie, R. (1987). Perception of variability in category development: Instance- versus abstraction-based stereotypes. *Journal of Personality and Social Psychology, 53*, 621–635.

Pendry, L. F., & Macrae, C. N. (1994). Stereotypes and mental life: The case of the motivated but thwarted tactician. *Journal of Experimental Social Psychology, 30*, 303–325.

Pendry, L. F., & Macrae, C. N. (1996). What the disinterested perceiver overlooks: Goal-directed social categorization. *Personality and Social Psychology Bulletin, 22*, 249–256.

Petty, R. E., & Cacioppo, J. T. (1979). Issue involvement can increase or decrease persuasion by enhancing message-relevant cognitive responses. *Journal of Personality and Social Psychology, 37*, 1915–1926.

Petty, R. E., & Cacioppo, J. T. (1986). The elaboration likelihood model of persuasion. In L. Berkowitz (Ed.), *Advances in experimental social psychology* (Vol. 19, pp. 123–205). Orlando, FL: Academic Press.

Pratto, F., & Bargh, J. A. (1991). Stereotyping based on apparently individuating information: Trait and global components of sex stereotypes under attention overload. *Journal of Experimental Social Psychology, 27*, 26–47.

Quattrone, G. A., & Jones, E. E. (1980). The perception of variability within in-groups and out-groups: Implications for the law of small numbers. *Journal of Personality and Social Psychology, 38*, 141–152.

Revelle, W. (1993). Individual differences in personality and motivation: "Non-cognitive" determinants of cognitive performance. In A. Baddeley & L. Weiskrantz (Eds.), *Attention: Selection, awareness, and control* (pp. 346–373). Oxford: Oxford University Press.

Rothbart, M., Sriram, N., & Davis-Stitt, C. (1996). The retrieval of typical and atypical category members. *Journal of Experimental Social Psychology, 32*, 309–336.

Rothbart, M., & Taylor, M. (1992). Category labels and social reality: Do we view social categories as natural kinds? In G. R. Semin & K. Fiedler (Eds.), *Language, interaction, and social cognition* (pp. 11–36). London: Sage.

Ruscher, J. B., & Fiske, S. T. (1990). Interpersonal competition can cause individuating impression formation. *Journal of Personality and Social Psychology, 58*, 832–842.

Sagar, H. A., & Schofield, J. W. (1980). Racial and behavioral cues in black and white children's perceptions of ambiguously aggressive acts. *Journal of Personality and Social Psychology, 39*, 590–598.

Schwarz, N. (1990). Feelings as information: Informational and motivational functions of affective states. In E. T. Higgins & R. M. Sorrentino (Eds.), *Handbook of motivation and cognition: Foundations of social behavior* (Vol. 2, pp. 527–561). New York: Guilford Press.

Schwarz, N. (1994). Judgment in a social context: Biases, shortcomings, and the logic of conversation. In M. P. Zanna (Ed.), *Advances in experimental social psychology* (Vol. 26, pp. 123–162). San Diego, CA: Academic Press.

Sherman, J. W. (1996). Development and mental representation of stereotypes. *Journal of Personality and Social Psychology, 70*, 1126–1141.

Sherman, J. W., Lee, A. Y., Bessenoff, G. R., & Frost, L. A. (1998). Stereotype efficiency reconsidered: Encoding flexibility under cognitive load. *Journal of Personality and Social Psychology, 75*, 589–606.

Simon, H. A. (1957). *Models of man*. New York: Garland Press.

Simon, H. A. (1994). The bottleneck of attention: Connecting thought with motivation. In W. D. Spaulding (Ed.), *Nebraska Symposium on motivation: Vol. 41. Integrative views of motivation, cognition, and emotion* (pp. 1–21). Lincoln: University of Nebraska Press.

Smith, E. R., & Zárate, M. A. (1992). Exemplar-based model of social judgment. *Psychological Review, 99*, 3–21.

Snyder, M., & Cantor, N. (1979). Testing hypotheses about other people: The use of historical knowledge. *Journal of Experimental Social Psychology, 15*, 330–342.

Stephan, W. G., & Stephan, C. W. (1985). Intergroup anxiety. *Journal of Social Issues, 41*(3), 157–175.

Tajfel, H., & Turner, J. C. (1986). The social identity theory of intergroup behavior. In S. Worchel & W. G. Austin (Eds.), *Psychology of intergroup relations* (pp. 7–24). Chicago: Nelson-Hall.

Tetlock, P. E. (1992). The impact of accountability on judgment and choice: Toward a social contingency model. In M. P. Zanna (Ed.), *Advances in experimental social psychology* (Vol. 25, pp. 331–376). San Diego, CA: Academic Press.

Trope, Y., & Alfieri, T. (1997). Effortfulness and flexibility of dispositional inference processes. *Journal of Personality and Social Psychology, 73*, 662–674.

Trope, Y., & Thompson, E. P. (1997). Looking for truth in all the wrong places: Asymmetric search of individuating information about stereotyped group members. *Journal of Personality and Social Psychology, 73*, 229–241.

Turner, J. C., Hogg, M., Oakes, P. J., Reicher, S., & Wetherell, M. S. (1987). *Rediscovering the social group: A self-categorization theory*. Oxford: Blackwell.

Uleman, J. S., Hon, A., Roman, R. J., & Moskowitz, G. B. (1996). On-line evidence for spontaneous trait inferences at encoding. *Personality and Social Psychology Bulletin, 22,* 377–394.

van Knippenberg, A., & Dijksterhuis, A. (1996). A posteriori stereotype activation: The preservation of stereotypes through memory distortion. *Social Cognition, 14,* 21–153.

Weary, G. (1990). Depression and sensitivity to social information. In B. S. Moore & A. M. Isen (Eds.), *Affect and social behavior* (pp. 207–230). Cambridge, England: Cambridge University Press.

Weary, G., & Edwards, J. (1994). Social cognition and clinical psychology: Anxiety, depression, and the processing of social information. In R. S. Wyer, Jr., & T. K. Srull (Eds.), *Handbook of social cognition* (2nd ed., Vol. 2, pp. 289–338). Hillsdale, NJ: Erlbaum.

Wegner, D. M. (1994). Ironic processes of mental control. *Psychological Review, 101,* 34–52.

Wilder, D. A., & Simon, A. F. (1996). Incidental and integral affect as triggers of stereotyping. In R. M. Sorrentino & E. T. Higgins (Eds.), *Handbook of motivation and cognition: Vol. 3. The interpersonal context* (pp. 397–419). New York: Guilford Press.

Wilson, T. D., & Brekke, N. (1994). Mental contamination and mental correction: Unwanted influences on judgments and evaluations. *Psychological Bulletin, 116,* 117–142.

Yates, J. (1985). The content of awareness is a model of the world. *Psychological Review, 92,* 249–284.

Yzerbyt, V. Y., Rogier, A., & Fiske, S. T. (in press). Social attribution and subjective essentialism: On translating situational constraints into stereotypes. *Personality and Social Psychology Bulletin.*

D

One or Two Processing Modes in Social Cognition?

14

Separate or Equal?

BIMODAL NOTIONS OF PERSUASION AND A SINGLE-PROCESS "UNIMODEL"

ARIE W. KRUGLANSKI
ERIK P. THOMPSON
SCOTT SPIEGEL

Of the plethora of topics studied by social psychologists, persuasion must surely be among the "nearest and dearest" to the heart of our discipline. This has been particularly true because of the traditionally cognitive flavor of many social-psychological explanations. Social psychology's essential concern is with how people affect one another; persuasion reflects that concern in reference to people's minds. It thus addresses a cognitive aspect of social influence—always of quintessential interest to social psychologists, and more so now than ever. Indeed, over the last two decades the topics of persuasion and attitude change have received a considerable amount of research attention, which has yielded exciting conceptual developments and a rich crop of intriguing findings.

Over time, research in the area has increasingly zeroed in on the underlying processes of persuasion phenomena. Early treatments of the topic (e.g. Hovland, Janis, & Kelley, 1953; see review by McGuire, 1969) merely hinted at issues of process; they focused instead on the *listing* of variables relevant to persuasion, organized within a broader system of appropriate categories. A particularly influential classification system grew out of Laswell's (1948, p. 37) comprehensive question: "Who says what in which channel to whom with what effect?" Contemporary persuasion research remains indebted to Laswell's classification (as witnessed by the currently popular distinction between the contents of message arguments (the "what" in Laswell's scheme) and source factors (the "who" in Laswell's scheme). Yet the emphasis in persuasion research has undoubtedly shifted from the mere listing and interrelating of variables to exploring the basic cognitive and motivational processes underlying persuasion.

Significant milestones on this road have been McGuire's (1968, 1969, 1972) reception-yielding model, as well as the cognitive-response model of persuasion (Greenwald, 1968; Petty, Ostrom, & Brock, 1981; see Eagly & Chaiken, 1993, for discussion). Yet the gist of current persuasion work derives from two major theoretical frameworks: Petty and Cacioppo's elaboration likelihood model (ELM; Petty & Cacioppo, 1986; see Petty &

Wegener, Chapter 3, this volume), and Chaiken and Eagly's heuristic–systematic model (HSM; Chaiken, Liberman, & Eagly, 1989; see Chen & Chaiken, Chapter 4, this volume). Though they differ significantly in some respects (for recent comparisons, see Petty, 1994; Eagly & Chaiken, 1993), the ELM and the HSM share a fundamental commonality: They both posit that persuasion may be accomplished via two qualitatively dissimilar ways of processing. In the ELM, these are the "central" and "peripheral" routes; in the HSM, they are the "systematic" and "heuristic" modes. While some differences exist (particularly in the specifics of heuristic-mode vs. peripheral-route processing; see Chaiken, 1987), both models have emphasized that conditions promoting the cognitive elaboration of argument information will promote opinion change via the *central* route or *systematic* mode, whereas conditions that restrict the effortful elaboration of such information will promote attitude change through information external to the semantic contents of the message arguments; this represents opinion change via the *peripheral* route or *heuristic* mode.

It is difficult to overstate these dual-process models' contribution to understanding persuasion. Not only have they clarified why classical persuasion variables (e.g., source expertise) may yield different outcomes in disparate circumstances (Petty, 1994), but they have also furnished invaluable insights into the complex ways in which these variables interact with others (e.g., recipients' involvement in the issue), and they have established a fruitful link between persuasion research and recent advances in social cognition (e.g., see Chaiken et al., 1989). Nonetheless, the present approach differs substantially from the dual-mode paradigm. Specifically, it proposes an integration of its two component processes into one, thereby introducing a "unimodel" of persuasion. This is accomplished by (1) adopting a more abstract level of analysis wherein the two persuasive modes (of either the ELM or the HSM) are treated as special cases of the same underlying process; and (2) "deconstructing" the Laswellian partition between the processing of message contents and of source factors, highlighting their similarities instead.

In what follows, we briefly note the common elements of the ELM and the HSM. We then present our own "unimodel" of persuasion, based on the lay epistemic theory (LET; Kruglanski, 1989), and indicate how it differs from the dual-mode approaches. In light of this discussion, we reexamine notions and empirical findings that have previously been interpreted in support of the dual-mode paradigm. It turns out that discussions by the dual-mode theorists already implicitly suggest that the two modes of persuasion are actually quite similar in many ways. Moreover, when viewed from the unimodel perspective, prior studies cited in support of qualitatively different processes of persuasion may have failed to control for important parameters of persuasion. We identify those parameters and outline a research program that will compare predictions of the dual-mode approaches with those derived from our "unimodel."

THE ELM AND HSM FRAMEWORKS

The ELM assumes that "there are two routes to persuasion that operate in different circumstances, and there are different consequences of each route to persuasion. . . . [Hence, the ELM] focuses on different persuasion processes that can operate in different situations" (Petty, 1994, p. 3). In fact, the model proposes a continuum of elaboration likelihood bounded at one end by the total absence of thought about issue-relevant information available in a persuasion situation, and at the other end by complete elaboration of *all* the relevant information (Petty, 1994, p. 1). Extensive elaboration of issue-relevant information is characteristic of persuasion via the central route; persuasion through cues irrelevant to the message contents occurs via the peripheral route.

Chaiken et al. (1989) define systematic processing as a "comprehensive, analytic orientation in which perceivers assess all informational input for its relevance and importance to their judgment task, and integrate all useful information in forming their judgments" (p. 212). By contrast, heuristic processing is viewed as a more limited processing mode that demands much less cognitive effort and capacity than systematic processing:

"When processing heuristically, people focus on that subset of available information that enables them to use simple inferential rules, schemata, or cognitive heuristics to formulate their judgments and decisions" (p. 213). Heuristic processing is furthermore regarded as "more exclusively theory-driven than systematic processing," and the mode-of-processing distinction is assumed to be "not merely quantitative" (p. 213), but rather qualitative. Specifically, heuristic processing is "more exclusively theory-driven because recipients utilize minimal informational input in conjunction with simple (declarative or procedural) knowledge structures to determine message validity quickly and efficiently" (p. 216).

Undoubtedly, the ELM and HSM formulations differ in some important respects. These are explicitly treated in Eagly and Chaiken (1993, Ch. 7) and Petty (1994, p. 4) and will not be revisited here. Instead, we highlight those aspects that the two dual-mode frameworks share. First, both posit the existence of two *qualitatively* different modes of persuasion, of which one is more thorough and extensive than the other. Second, both assume that engagement in the more extensive processing mode (i.e., the central route or the systematic mode) depends on sufficient motivation and ability to process information. Third, they both assume that the more extensive mode of persuasion is typically more of a "bottom-up" process, whereas the less extensive mode is more of a "top-down" process. Fourth, both models agree that persuasion accomplished via the more extensive mode (central or systematic) is more persistent, more closely linked to subsequent behavior, and more resistant to persuasion than that accomplished via the less extensive mode (peripheral or heuristic). Fifth, both models presume that the two modes of persuasion can co-occur, although the exact manner of their co-occurrence is depicted somewhat differently in the ELM and the HSM formulations. Though it permits co-occurrence, the ELM adheres nonetheless to the notion of a continuum whereby a tradeoff (hence, a negative correlation) governs the use of the two modes. In addition, the ELM allows that peripheral cues may affect the central processing of information (e.g., when a cue influences the degree of elaboration accorded the mes-

sage arguments). The HSM shares in this (biasing) assumption, but also allows orthogonality in use of the two modes, so that they can either augment each other or clash in their influence on the communication recipient.

Both the ELM and the HSM assume that the desire to hold accurate attitudes and opinions is a common motivation in persuasion contexts. Similarly, both models assume that in addition to accuracy strivings, extensive processing (i.e., central or systematic) can also be affected by alternative motivations. The HSM posits that the same motivations that affect systematic processing also have an impact on heuristic processing, whereas the ELM does not address the motivational underpinnings of peripheral processing. But let us now turn to our main issue: a single-mode model of persuasion, proposed as an alternative to the dual-mode frameworks.

AN ALTERNATIVE TO THE DUAL-MODE CONCEPTIONS: THE PERSUASIVE UNIMODEL

As noted above, our single-route model of persuasion is based on LET (Kruglanski, 1980, 1989), a theory of processes governing the formation of subjective knowledge. Such knowledge may come in various shapes or forms (e.g., as judgments, opinions, attitudes, or impressions that individuals may acquire and/or alter under the appropriate circumstances). Thus, in agreement with Chaiken et al. (1989), we view persuasion as integrally related to the general epistemic process of judgment formation. What might such a process consist of? We assume that it is a process of hypothesis testing and inference, in the course of which persons acquire beliefs on the basis of relevant information. This hypothesis-testing process may be affected by various factors related to the following basic parameters of persuasion: (1) the structure of evidence whereby conclusions are reached; (2) cognitive-ability factors, which affect the extent (or "depth") as well as the direction of the inferential activity; and (4) motivational factors, which also potentially affect its extent and direction. In other words, our single-route model of persuasion does stipulate a variety of influences on the persuasion process. It differs from the dual-mode notions, however, in claiming that these same influences hold regardless of whether persuasion is accomplished via peripheral cues/heuristics or via the contents of message arguments.

The Structure of Evidence: A Matter of Relevance

According to LET, "evidence" refers to information relevant to a conclusion. "Relevance," in turn, implies prior conditional ("if–then") linkage between general categories, such that affirmation of one in a specific case (the evidence) changes a person's belief in the other (the conclusion). Such prior linkage is subjective: It is assumed to be mentally represented in a given knower's mind and constitutes a personal belief to which he or she subscribes. For example, an individual may be convinced that "A candidate who lacks any political experience will make a poor president." Alternatively, he/she may subscribe to a conditional probability: "Given that a candidate lacks experience, the chances of his or her being a good president are low [say, 10%]." In both cases, granting our knower's beliefs, the lack of a political experience becomes *relevant evidence* for the candidate's expected presidential performance.

More formally speaking, the conditional belief linking (hence rendering relevant) the evidence to the conclusion is the "major premise" of a syllogism. Affirmation of the evidence in a particular instance—for example, compelling information that a specific Candidate X (say, Steve Forbes) indeed lacked any political experience—is referred to as the "minor premise." Jointly, the two premises yield the (logical or probabilistic) conclusion concerning Candidate X's future presidential failures.

Such interpretation of the evidence concept is compatible with major analyses of this topic within the philosophy of inference (e.g., Achinstein, 1983; Carnap, 1962, Sec. 86; Hempel, 1965; Glymour, 1980). More to the point, it is highly congruent with treatment of this topic within major social-psychological models of persuasion. Most explicit recognition of those evidential properties is accorded by the probabilistic models of belief inference

proposed by McGuire (1960) and Wyer (1970, 1974), and in the Bayesian analysis offered by Fishbein and Ajzen (1975, pp. 181–188). However, those notions are implicit in other models as well, such as dissonance or balance theories (for discussion, see Kruglanski & Klar, 1987; Kruglanski, 1989, Ch. 5).

Of particular importance to the present discussion, the foregoing notion of evidence provides the integrative "glue" for combining the dual modes of persuasion into one. Specifically, we propose that the distinction between heuristics/cues on the one hand and message arguments on the other reflects a difference in *evidential contents* relevant to a conclusion, rather than a qualitative difference in the persuasive process as such. In other words, heuristics/cues and message arguments are presently viewed as special cases of the category of "persuasive evidence." Such evidence, in turn, rests on an "if–then" linkage that a recipient assumes to exist between a given informational category and a conclusion.

Consider a communication by Dr. Smith, a noted environmental specialist, in which she asserts: "The use of freon in household appliances destroys the ozone layer, and therefore ought to be prohibited." The argument may appear persuasive to a recipient whose background knowledge includes the assumptions that "Anything that poses a health hazard should be prohibited" and "The thinning of the ozone layer poses a health hazard." Those assumptions yield the major premise of a syllogism, whereby "*If* something contributes to the thinning of the ozone layer, [*then*] it should be prohibited." Dr. Smith's specific argument supplies the minor premise—namely, "The use of freon in everyday appliances does destroy the ozone layer." In other words her pronouncement constitutes the "evidence" that, granting the major premise, implies the conclusion: "The use of freon ought to be prohibited." Such processing of a message argument from evidence to conclusion has been typically considered characteristic of persuasion via the central route or the systematic mode.

Consider now a recipient who does not necessarily assume either that "Thinning of the ozone layer poses a health hazard" or that "Anything posing a health hazard should be prohibited," yet strongly subscribes to the assumption that "*If* an opinion is offered by an expert, [*then*] it is valid." Again, this assumption may serve as the major premise of a syllogism, and the realization "Dr. Smith is an expert" may serve as the minor premise, furnishing evidence that (granting the major premise) leads to this conclusion: "Dr. Smith's opinion [that the use of freon ought to be prohibited] is valid." Such reliance on source attributes (e.g., expertise) has been typically considered characteristic of persuasion accomplished via the peripheral route or the heuristic mode. Yet from the present perspective, the two persuasion types (central/systematic and peripheral/heuristic) are fundamentally similar, in that both are mediated via "if–then" or syllogistic reasoning from evidence to conclusion.

Even though LET identifies "if–then" or rule-based reasoning from evidence to conclusion as essential to all instances to persuasion, this does not mean that all such instances are equal in all other respects. A major way in which they may differ is in the *extent* of information processing en route to constructing the evidence. At times, the premises of a pertinent syllogism that serve as evidence are highly accessible or salient for the individual, whereas at other times they may have to be effortfully gleaned from a thicket of informational detail in which they are embedded. At times, an individual may stop at generating a single set of (major and minor) premises; at other times, he or she may generate numerous such sets (ie., may consider multiple lines of evidence related to a given conclusion). Thus, LET posits that different instances of persuasion may differ *quantitatively* in the extent of information processing, but that they are *qualitatively similar* in terms of the way information functions as persuasive evidence. In turn, extent of processing is intimately tied to motivational and cognitive-ability considerations, which are discussed later.

DO OTHER DIFFERENCES EXIST BETWEEN THE TWO PROCESSING MODES (OR "ROUTES")?

Relevance to Conclusions

Although the structure of evidence seems to be the same for heuristics/cues and for message arguments, might it be the case that heuristics/cues systematically differ from message arguments in their *degree of relevance* to the persuasive conclusion? If they could be shown to do so, one could argue that persuasion accomplished via cues/heuristics is in some sense different from that accomplished via message arguments—and, after all, *some* systematic difference between the two is a necessary precondition for arguing that they differ in the quality of the mediating process. A moment's reflection suggests, however, that heuristics/cues as a class should not systematically differ from message arguments (as a class) in their relevance to persuasive conclusions. Specifically, both different heuristics/cues and different message arguments may vary in their relevance to a conclusion; hence no general difference between the category of heuristics/cues and that of message arguments should be expected.

Thus, Chaiken's (1987; see also Chaiken et al., 1989; Eagly & Chaiken, 1993) work on the reliability of heuristics indicates that heuristics may differ from each one another in perceived relevance. A more "reliable" heuristic in Chaiken's work is one that is more strongly linked (or, in present terms, is more relevant) to the persuasive conclusion. For instance, in a study by Chaiken (1987) "high-reliability" participants read sentences compatible with the liking–agreement heuristic (e.g., "When people want good advice, they go to their friends"), whereas "low-reliability" participants read sentences that undermined the liking–agreement heuristic (e.g., "Best friends do not necessarily make the best advisors"). It seems reasonable to think of such reliability manipulations as affecting the perceived linkage between friendship and the goodness of advice—that is, as affecting the relevance of the former to the latter. In other words, the reliability manipulation may have affected the participants' estimate of conditional probability that one category in the major premise (advice's being offered by a friend) would lead to another (the advice's being good).

Just as may be the case with different cues/heuristics, different message arguments may also differ widely in perceived relevance. For instance, the "strong arguments" in Petty and Cacioppo's work seem more relevant than the "weak arguments" to the conclusion that an issue merits a positive attitude. In short, the degree of evidential relevance seems uncorrelated, in principle, with the distinction between heuristics/cues and message argument: It should be possible to have highly relevant or not-so-relevant message arguments, and the same should be true of heuristics/cues.

Cognitive Ability

The ELM and the HSM alike stress that persuasion depends importantly on the recipient's cognitive ability. We deem it important to differentiate further between a "software" aspect of ability, called "capability," and a "hardware" aspect, called "capacity." These are considered in turn.

Capability

"Capability" refers to the knower's possession of active cognitive structures wherein the reasoning process from evidence to conclusion may be carried out. In this sense, the term refers to the epistemic "software" stored in the individual's memory and selected or rendered operative in specific circumstances. Specifically, beliefs representing the major and the minor premises need to be mentally represented, or "available" in the individual's mental repertory, as well as activated to some above-threshold degree of "accessibility" (Higgins, 1996). For instance, a physician concluding from a magnetic resonance imaging (MRI) scan that a patient has a slipped disk must have available and accessible (1) the mental representation linking a specific MRI pattern with disk slippage, and (2) the representation asserting that the specific imaging pattern has indeed turned up.

Availability and accessibility of mental representations may both affect the extent of information processing and bias its direction. Extent may be affected, for example, if a knower possessed multiple beliefs (vs. only a few) of the major-premise type linking different types of evidence to conclusions on a given topic. This may require the processing of different types of evidence, enhancing the amount (and duration) of processing. Occa-sionally, such evidence may give rise to conflicting inferences, requiring even further processing.

The "biasing effect" of mental representations (prior knowledge) refers to the fact that the presence of specific premises may direct the knower's attention selectively to categories those premises specify. A premise specifying that "Only unlit streets in New York are dangerous" (i.e., "Only *if* unlit, [*then*] a street is dangerous") may bias the individual's attention toward the degree of lighting, whereas a premise specifying that "only the stretch between 70th and 90th Streets on the West Side is dangerous" may direct one's attention to the street number, the direction, and so on.

Is it possible, then, that cues/heuristics *as a category* are more (or less) mentally available or accessible than message arguments *as a category*? Again, if it could be shown that they are, *some* systematic difference between the two could be claimed—a precondition for positing a *qualitative* difference. The answer, however, seems to be no. Comments by dual-process theorists already imply that both cues/heuristics and (premises relevant to) message arguments may differ in their availability or accessibility. The HSM in particular stresses the role played by the availability and accessibility of heuristics in persuasion. For instance, Chaiken et al. (1989, p. 217) note that "Heuristic processing depends . . . on whether cognitively available heuristics are activated or accessed from memory." By implication, some heuristics may be more strongly activated, and hence may be more accessible than others. Chaiken et al. (1989) also recognize that similar availability and accessibility considerations apply to systematic processing. Hence, "systematic processing [depends] upon . . . cognitive factors (e.g., the *accessibility* of knowledge structures that influence perceivers' interpretation and evaluation of information)" (p. 217; emphasis added). Both Chaiken et al. (1989) and Petty and Cacioppo (1986) recognize the relevance of availability considerations to systematic or central processing in their discussion of the effects of prior knowledge effects (Wood, 1982; Wood & Kallgren, 1988; Wood, Kallgren, & Preisler, 1985). Specifically, when activated from memory, available message-related knowledge may affect processing by generating pertinent evidence for the recipient's consideration (Wood, Biek, Nations, & Chaiken, 1994; Biek, Wood & Chaiken, 1995). Obviously, so should the activation of relevant knowledge related to a cue or a heuristic.

It thus seems fair to conclude that the availability and accessibility of relevant knowledge play an important part in persuasion, regardless of whether it is accomplished via the processing of message contents (i.e., via the central route or the systematic mode) or whether it is accomplished via peripheral cues or heuristics. Moreover, no systematic correlation seems to exist between the availability or accessibility of evidence and it's being based on cues/heuristics versus message arguments.

Capacity and the Length/Complexity of Cues/Heuristics and Message Arguments

The "hardware" aspect of cognitive ability refers to the "state of the machine" (e.g., given the individual's degree of alertness, energy level, or cognitive load). It connotes, in other words, attentional-capacity limitations on the amount of processing the knower is capable of carrying out at any given moment (Kahneman, 1973). Thus, under conditions that may tax cognitive capacity, the knower should be less able to process extensive bodies of complex information than under conditions where his or her capacity is relatively unencumbered. But are message arguments, in fact, necessarily lengthier or more complex than are cues/heuristics? Whereas this may have been typical of past persuasion research, a further examination indicates that it need not be so. In this connection, Petty and Cacioppo (1986) aptly note that "In addition to the relatively simple acceptance/rejection rules . . . attitude change may be affected by more complex reasoning processes, such as those based on balance theory . . . or certain attributional principles." Furthermore, information relevant to a heuristic or a cue (e.g., the communicator's expertise) may not be given simply or directly, but rather may be imbedded within lengthy and complex communications from which the heuristic "gist" may need to be laboriously distilled. Finally, whereas some message arguments may be lengthy or complex, others (e.g., "Crest fights plaque," "Mercedes affords quiet ride") may be terse and simple-minded. Again, then, no necessary correlation seems to exist between an important persuasion parameter—the length or complexity of evidence, in this case—and its content being classifiable as a cue/heuristic or a message argument.

To summarize our arguments concerning cognitive ability to this point, whereas the ELM and the HSM discuss ability factors in general, we deem it important to distinguish between ability factors having to do with the availability and/or accessibility of premises that lend persuasive force to various types of information (the "software" aspect) and ability factors having to do with the knower's attentional capacity at a given time (the "hardware" aspect). These two types of ability are determined by very different factors, and hence it is important to keep them apart. Moreover, in the dual-mode literature the implication that peripheral or heuristic processing occurs under "low-ability" conditions seems to refer to the "hardware" aspect only; the notion appears to be that when capacity is limited, only heuristic/peripheral but not central/systematic processing is possible. There is no implication of systematic differences between the two modes in the availability/accessibility of background knowledge—that is, in the "software" aspect of ability. Yet, as we have shown, neither the "hardware" nor the "software" aspect of cognitive ability seems to differentiate systematically between peripheral/heuristic processing on the one hand and systematic/central processing on the other. Hence ability considerations seem largely irrelevant to the processing mode (via heuristics or message argument contents).

Capacity and the Order of Presentation

Persuasion researchers have long known that the order of presentation—that is, the specific location of arguments in the informational sequence proffered to recipients—matters a great deal to the persuasiveness of those arguments (Hovland, 1957). Because it is assumed that the earlier information may partially deplete cognitive capacity (e.g., by instilling mental fatigue), it is thought that in cases where such capacity is limited to begin with, the late-appearing information may be given "short shrift" and be processed only superficially. Is it possible, then, that heuristics/cues and message arguments systematically differ in their order of presentation? Specifically, might it be the case that the cue information (e.g., information about the source) generally "hits" the recipients first, before the message information does? Whereas some heuristics/cues (e.g., the communicator's race, age, and gender) may be very salient and readily encoded by the recipient (Brewer, 1988; but see Smith, 1988), it is unlikely that all of them are. Even the ones just noted are salient only in face-to-face encounters with the communicator, but not necessarily in more detached communicative situations. In reading a magazine article, for example, one is often exposed to the message first, and only at the end to information about the source and its qualifications. Similarly, it is easy to conceive of situations wherein the arguments come first, and only subsequently one finds out that they represent a majority position or a minority position (affording an application of the "consensus heuristic"). Thus, the order of presentation does not seem to be systematically related to whether the evidence consists of cues/heuristics or message arguments. More generally, it seems fair to conclude that cognitive-capacity considerations are unrelated to whether persuasion is accomplished via cues/heuristics or message arguments.

Motivation

Types of Motivations

In fundamental agreement with the ELM and HSM, LET assumes that persuasion can be substantially affected by motivation (see Kruglanski, 1989, 1990; Kruglanski & Webster, 1996). It further assumes that a variety of different motivations may influence persuasion, even as they may influence alternate judgment formation processes. These motivations have an impact on persuasion (or judgment formation) *because* their objects pertain to (intrinsic or extrinsic) aspects of the epistemic activity. For instance, the need for cognition (Cacioppo & Petty, 1982; Thompson, Chaiken, & Hazlewood, 1993) pertains to the

appeal of thinking and information processing, both of which are intrinsic to the epistemic endeavor as such. Other motivations may pertain to the end products of the epistemic activity, and hence are extrinsic to it. The need for nonspecific cognitive closure (Kruglanski, 1996a; Kruglanski & Webster, 1996) pertains to one extrinsic goal of the epistemic activity—the possession of *any* definite or assured knowledge on a topic. The need for valid or accurate knowledge represents another concern about the type of knowledge ultimately formed. Though often the need for valid knowledge may lower the need for closure, this need not invariably be so (for discussion, see Kruglanski, 1996a; Kruglanski & Webster, 1996). Other extrinsic goals of the epistemic activity are implicated in the needs for various specific types of cognitive closures (Kruglanski, 1989, 1990). Such specific closures represent contents that appeal to the knower for some reason, constituting particular preferential conclusions. These may encompass a broad range of possible motivations, including self-esteem concerns, impression management concerns, concerns with one's economic and physical well-being, concerns with one's good fortunes in "love and war," and so on.

In short, according to LET, persuasion may be affected by a broad range of motivations. These include the three motivations specified in the HSM (i.e., accuracy, defense, and impression-management), but also include such motivations as need for nonspecific closure, need for cognition, and needs for sundry specific closures, at least some of which (e.g., safety or health concerns or aggressiveness toward others) would seem different from defensiveness and impression management motives as these are generally understood.

Motivational Effects

The LET assumes that, generally speaking, all epistemic motivations affect the same broad parameters of the judgment formation process. These include initiation of a judgment formation activity by a noticed discrepancy between an actual and a desired epistemic state (whose specific nature depends on the momentarily operative motivation) and its termination when the discrepancy has been removed (see also Chaiken et al., 1989). Beyond initiating and terminating the epistemic activity during a persuasive encounter, motivation may importantly affect its particular *course*, including its extent and direction. These may depend on both the quality and the magnitude of the underlying motivation for the activity. For example, the higher the need for nonspecific closure (i.e., the greater its magnitude), the *less* extensive the information processing. By contrast, the higher the motivation for accuracy or for the avoidance of closure, the more extensive the information processing (for more extensive discussion, see Kruglanski, 1996b).

Motivation may also affect the direction of cognitive activity accompanying persuasion or judgment. Because a goal constitutes a cognitive structure (Bargh & Gollwitzer, 1994; Kruglanski, 1996b; Srull & Wyer, 1986), its activation may spread to associated cognitions, increasing their accessibility (Higgins, 1996). This in turn may affect the construal of subsequent events (Higgins, Rholes & Jones, 1977). Motivation may also affect selective attention to relevant stimuli (Higgins, 1996). The attention-grabbing properties of goal-relevant objects have been demonstrated in several studies (Berscheid, Graziano, Monson, & Dermer, 1976; Erber & Fiske, 1984; Ruscher & Fiske, 1990; Taylor & Fiske, 1978).

Most importantly for the present argument, we assume that the foregoing motivational effects will apply equally, regardless of whether the persuasion process is propelled by evidence contained in the message itself or by evidence external to the message (i.e., cues or heuristics). If, as is presently assumed, information related to heuristics/cues is not necessarily briefer or less complex than message arguments, processing the latter (vs. the former) should not necessarily require greater effort or higher motivation. Furthermore, both heuristically mediated conclusions, and those following from message arguments may be desirable or undesirable to the listener (e.g., Giner- Sorolla & Chaiken, 1997). Hence, information processing in both cases may be similarly biased by directional motivations or needs for specific closure (Kruglanski, 1989, 1990).

The relevant discussions in the dual-mode literature seem to concur in this conclu-

sion. Consider recent versions of the HSM (see Chaiken et al., 1989; Eagly & Chaiken, 1993), which accord particular prominence to motivational factors and distinguish in particular among three major goals pertinent to persuasion. These are accuracy (often aroused by considerations of personal relevance), defense, and impression management. Do these motivations interact with the evidential category's being heuristics/cues or message arguments (i.e., with processing mode, in HSM terms)? Chaiken et al. (1989) explicitly deny it at several points. According to Chaiken et al., the accuracy motivation, for example, may underlie both systematic and heuristic processing (1989, p. 214), as personal relevance influences not only systematic processing but also heuristic processing (1989, p. 226; see also Darke et al., in press). Similarly, defense and impression management as motivations can underlie systematic and heuristic processing alike (Chaiken et al., 1989, p. 235; see also Chen, Shechter, & Chaiken, 1996; Chaiken, Wood, & Eagly, 1996; Giner-Sorolla & Chaiken, 1997). In short, "the multiple-mode HSM views processing mode and processing goals as orthogonal; heuristic and systematic processing occur in the service of the individual's processing goal whatever that goal may be" (Chaiken et al., 1989, p. 235).

As already noted, our LET-based account points to the very same conclusion, and suggests moreover that the *way* the two modes are affected by motivation is essentially the same. Again, the HSM position seems in accord with this analysis. For instance, the accuracy motivation (often aroused by personal relevance of the issue) is generally thought to intensify systematic (or central) processing; yet, according to the HSM, it should do the same for heuristic processing. As Chaiken et al. (1989) put it, "motivational variables such as personal relevance do not influence only the magnitude of systematic processing. These variables should also enhance the likelihood of heuristic processing because they . . . increase the vigilance with which people search (the setting or their memories) for relevant heuristic cues" (p. 226).

Alternative, epistemically relevant motivations—for example, the defense and impression management motivations identified by Chaiken et al. (1989), the need for closure

(Kruglanski, 1996a; Kruglanski & Webster, 1996; Webster & Kruglanski, 1998), and the need for cognition (Cacioppo & Petty, 1982)—should also have similar effects on cue/heuristic-based or message-based processing. For instance, a defensive motivation should bias the processing of message arguments in an ego-defensive direction, and it should similarly bias the processing of heuristically relevant information (e.g., by leading a recipient to seek out or attend to negative information about a source whose position is ego-damaging to the recipient; see Giner-Sorolla & Chaiken, 1997). The need for closure should curtail the processing of message arguments, but also that of heuristics/cues; and the need for cognition should enhance the processing of both types of information. And so forth.

In sum, peripheral cues or heuristics as a category do not seem to be affected by motivation any differently than message arguments are. Consistent with our unimodel, the evidential category (heuristics/cues or message arguments) does not seem to interact with the motivational dimension of persuasion.

THE UNIMODEL AND THE DUAL-MODE APPROACHES: TAKING STOCK OF COMMONALITIES AND DISTINCTIONS

Let us take stock now and summarize the commonalities between our unimodel and the dual-mode frameworks, as well as those aspects where the unimodel is unique. To start with a commonality, just like the dual-mode approaches, the unimodel is based on the assumption that persuasion often requires cognitive ability and motivation. Furthermore, we too assume that the extent or depth to which persuasive information is processed may vary across persons and circumstances, and we agree that such depth of processing may depend a great deal upon motivational and cognitive-ability factors. Similarly, we agree that the extent of processing may importantly affect such aspects of persuasion as persistence, resistance to counterarguments, and relation to behavior. So much for commonalities.

As to differences, we have further differentiated between the "software" and the "hardware" aspects of cognitive ability, and the range of motivations we have considered as potentially relevant to persuasion is broader than the range of motivations typically discussed in the dual-mode literature. However, the main distinguishing feature of the unimodel is that it considers heuristics/cues and message arguments as *functionally equivalent* in the persuasion process. Specifically, it considers both as constituting evidential content relevant to a conclusion, rather than as demarcating a qualitative discontinuity in the persuasive process as such. According to this argument, then, a uniform process mediates persuasion regardless of whether the evidence resides in the message arguments as such or in aspects of the persuasive context external to the message. Our process uniformity argument assumes that heuristics/cues do not systematically differ from message arguments on such persuasively relevant informational parameters as evidential relevance, length/complexity, or order of presentation. Furthermore, heuristics/cues should not in principle interact with such extrainformational parameters of persuasion as cognitive ability or motivation. Thus, although we agree that the extent or depth of processing persuasive information is important, we emphasize that the extent of processing need not be correlated with whether the information is heuristic/cue-related or message-argument-related.

As indicated throughout, many of the arguments for our unimodel have been garnered from explicit analysis of these issues by the dual-mode theorists. It seems, then, that we may be in fundamental agreement on the central issues, even though the conclusions we reach seem rather different. What may account for this a divergence? A strong possibility is that this has a great deal to do with the extensive body of empirical evidence seemingly supporting the dual-mode conception. We now turn to examine this evidence more closely.

THE EMPIRICAL EVIDENCE

Ample empirical findings (for reviews, see Petty & Cacioppo, 1986; Petty, 1994; Eagly & Chaiken, 1993) suggest that the type of evidential content (i.e., heuristic cues vs. mes-

sage arguments) does in fact interact ubiqui-
tously with major persuasion determinants in
regard to such significant persuasive outcome
variables as attitude change, its persistence
over time, resistance to counterarguments,
and the attitude—behavior relation. Insofar
as these interactions suggest that heuristics/
cues "behave" differently from message arguments, a dual-mode conception seems to be
warranted. Let us reconsider these interactions, however, from the unimodel perspective. To do so, it may be useful to distinguish
between two categories of interactions: (1)
"inferred" interactions—that is, cases where a
third factor's effect was empirically obtained
in research incorporating one evidence type
only (say, message arguments), and the implicit (albeit so far untested) assumption was
that such an effect would fail to appear with
the second evidence type (say, with cues or
heuristics); and (2) "manifest" interactions,
wherein the two evidence types were actually
observed to exert patently different effects at
different levels of a third factor (e.g., personal
relevance or involvement). We now consider
these findings and reinterpret them in terms
of our unimodel.

Inferred Interactions

The category of inferred interaction is exemplified by research on distraction (for a review, see Petty & Cacioppo, 1986, pp. 139–
141). Thus, in the classical work by Petty,
Wells, and Brock (1976), distraction was
found to enhance persuasion by low-quality
arguments and to decrease persuasion by
high-quality arguments. Petty and Cacioppo
(1986) concluded that "distraction is one
variable that affects a person's ability to process a message in a relatively objective manner" (p. 141). Though in agreement with this
conclusion, the present perspective raises the
question whether distraction may not similarly interfere with the processing of heuristic-
or cue-related information.

In a study by Schumann, Petty, and
Cacioppo (1985), repetition of message arguments extolling the positive properties of a
new pen increased the correlation between a
positive attitude toward the writing instrument and the intention to purchase it. Yet it is
unclear whether repetition of cue- or heuris-
tic-based evidence (and hence the opportunity

to process it more thoroughly) may not have
affected the attitude–behavior correlation
similarly. Again, then, the interaction between evidence content and repetition was
only inferred here rather than directly observed.

Cacioppo, Petty, Kao, and Rodriguez
(1986) found that "attitudes toward the candidates in the 1984 presidential election predicted voting intentions and reported behavior better for people who were high rather
than low in their 'need for cognition'" (Petty
& Cacioppo, 1986, p. 180). The authors concluded that when dispositional factors enhance people's motivation or ability to elaborate issue-relevant information, attitude–
behavior correlations are higher. Yet the need
for cognition might also enhance people's motivation and/or ability to process heuristic- or
cue-related information; hence it might increase attitude–behavior correlations for persuasion based on the latter type of evidence as
well.

In research by Petty, Cacioppo, and
Heesacker (1985), source credibility and message quality were deliberately confounded.
Participants received either a high-quality
message (in support of senior comprehensive
exams) delivered by a prestigious source or a
low-quality message from a low-prestige
source. Half the participants were exposed to
a high-relevance manipulation (the advocacy
was said to involve a change in policy at the
participants' own university), and the other
half to a low-relevance manipulation (the
change was said to be occurring at a remote
university). It was found that in the high-
relevance condition, the more positive attitude formed in the strong-message/source
(versus weak-message/source) condition per-
sisted over a period of 10–14 days following
exposure to the advocacy, whereas it did not
persist in the low-relevance condition. Petty
and Cacioppo (1986) concluded accordingly
that "subjects who formed their initial attitudes based on a careful consideration of issue relevant arguments (high relevance)
showed greater persistence of attitude change
than those subjects whose initial attitudes
were based primarily on the source cue (low
relevance)" (p. 178). Yet because of the con-
founding in this study of source prestige and
message quality, we may not know for certain
that an interaction occurred between the form

of evidence (heuristic/cue vs. message argument) and personal relevance in regard to the persistence of attitude. In this sense the interaction was *inferred* rather than explicitly manifested, and it was assumed that in the high-relevance condition recipients processed primarily message arguments rather than heuristics/cues (cf. Petty, Cacioppo, & Goldman, 1981). If, however, high-relevance participants were generally attentive to information, they may have carefully processed heuristic/cue-related information as well (e.g., information about source expertise or prestige). Moreover, it is possible in general that the care and thoroughness of processing, rather than the type of information processed (i.e., heuristics/cues vs. message arguments), are what critically determine the persistence of attitude change. Regardless of the type of information processed, thorough processing may establish multiple connections between the information and/or the conclusions it yields and numerous retrieval cues, hence increasing the likelihood that the attitude will be accessed on subsequent occasions.

Finally, Petty and Cacioppo (1986) cite previous work (e.g., by McGuire, 1964, as well as Burgoon, Cohen, Miller, & Montgomery, 1978) as demonstrating that "attitudes can be made more resistant by motivating or enabling people to engage in additional thought about the reasons or arguments supporting their attitudes" (p. 182). We agree, but also add that this should be true regardless of the type of evidence (cue/heuristic vs. message argument) on which the attitudes are based. As Petty and Cacioppo (1986) acknowledge, thus far these issues have not been adequately addressed in empirical research (see also Eagly & Chaiken, 1993).

Manifest Interactions

If the inferred-interaction studies afford a degree of ambiguity as to whether heuristic/cue-based versus message- argument-based persuasion is affected differently by various factors, the manifest-interaction studies answer the question directly in the affirmative. Typical of this research is the classic study by Petty, Cacioppo, and Goldman (1981), where personal relevance of the issue, argument quality, and source expertise were manipulated orthogonally to one another. The data indicated clearly that personal relevance had opposite effects in regard to source expertise versus argument quality: Whereas argument quality was a more important determinant of persuasion for high- than for low-relevance participants, source expertise was the more important determinant for low- than for high-relevance participants. Taken at face value, these results and many similar findings reported in the literature (see Petty & Cacioppo, 1986; Eagly & Chaiken, 1993) appear to constitute powerful support for the dual-process model. They imply that the type of evidence does in fact matter, and that cues/heuristics versus message arguments are affected in opposite ways by persuasively relevant factors. But let us take a closer look.

Consider the research by Petty, Cacioppo, and Goldman (1981) again. In that experiment, cue/ heuristic information (regarding source expertise) (1) was presented to participants prior to the message arguments, and (2) was considerably briefer and probably less complex (e.g., in terms of sheer number of words) than the message argument information. As a consequence, it seems plausible that the cue/heuristic information in this case was much easier to process than the message argument information. If we take seriously the possibility that the amount of information (i.e., length or complexity of the communication) and its ordinal position, constitute important persuasion determinants, this may account for the results obtained in terms that are unrelated to the type of evidence. It is entirely possible, in other words, that the reason the message arguments exerted greater impact under conditions of high versus low involvement is that they were more extensive and appeared later in the sequence, which would have made them more difficult to process. Both of these factors could have made them particularly likely to benefit from the enhanced epistemic motivation in the high-involvement condition. Similarly, because the extensive and/or later-appearing message arguments were not processed carefully in the low-involvement condition, the brief, easy-to-process, and early-appearing heuristics/cues may have enjoyed a persuasive advantage in this situation. The reason the heuristics/cues failed to exert an effect in the high-involvement condition may have been related to their loss of salience or recency—effects discussed by Petty (1994). According to the present interpretation, however, this loss of impact may have had little to do with the cues' being external or unrelated to the message, and could easily have applied to brief message arguments presented early in the sequence. In other words, *any* brief information presented early may lose its persuasive impact when it is followed by further, more extensive information, which is subjected to extensive processing under high-motivation conditions.

The foregoing features of the Petty, Cacioppo, and Goldman (1981) research seem typical of much of the research conducted on the ELM and the HSM. A cursory examination of such work reveals similar covariation patterns between important informational parameters and type of evidential content. Thus, Petty's (1994) "state-of-the-art" review describes six major ELM studies (Heesacker, Petty, & Cacioppo, 1983; Petty & Cacioppo, 1984; Petty, Cacioppo, & Goldman, 1981; Petty, Cacioppo, & Schumann, 1983; Petty, Harkins, & Williams, 1980; and Wells & Petty, 1980). Similarly, Chapter 7 in Eagly and Chaiken's (1993) volume discusses seven influential HSM studies (Axsom, Yates, & Chaiken, 1987; Chaiken, 1979, 1980; Chaiken & Eagly, 1983; Chaiken & Maheswaran, 1994; Maheswaran & Chaiken, 1991; and Ratneshwar & Chaiken, 1991). In *all* of this research, the message arguments seem to have been considerably more extensive, elaborate, and/or easy to process than the heuristics/cues. Furthermore, in 10 of the 13 studies the heuristics/cues were presented *before* the message arguments, and in the remaining 3, they were presented simultaneously with the message arguments (e.g., in the Wells & Petty [1980] research the cues consisted of the communicator's head movements as he was delivering the message arguments). If our analysis is correct, controlling for informational extent and ordinal position should eliminate the apparent differences in the ways cues/heuristics versus message arguments have interacted with various factors known to affect persuasion (e.g., involvement) in past research. In the following section we outline a research program aimed at exercising such control, and hence at providing evidence relevant to the unimodel.

TESTING THE UNIMODEL: A RESEARCH PROGRAM

As the foregoing discussion implies, the unimodel yields manifold empirical implications based on its central assumption of a unitary process governing persuasion based on heuristics/cues and on message arguments alike. In what follows, we outline a programmatic series of studies designed to test those implications. This research program (currently being carried out in our laboratory) revolves around two informational variables: (1) length/complexity of the heuristic/cue related or message-argument-related information presented to recipients; and (2) the order of presentation of these two information types. As already noted, we assume that in past research these variables tended to covary with the distinction between heuristics/cues and message arguments. Accordingly, we intend to dissolve this covariation by manipulating each variable within each information type. We will examine the interaction between these informational variables and epistemically relevant factors having to do with recipients' motivation or ability to process the information presented. In keeping with tradition, the major motivational variable to be manipulated will be the recipients' issue involvement. Similarly, the two major ability-related factors to be studied will be distraction and repetition of the information. Our research will focus upon several fundamental aspects of persuasion—namely, the degree of attitude change, its persistence over time, its resistance to counter arguments, and its relation to behavior.

Varying the Length/Complexity of Heuristic/Cue Information

One line of research will explore the possibility that the amount of heuristic/cue information constitutes an important determinant of persuasion. We hypothesize that the length or extent of such information will interact with contextual factors that are known to promote cognitive elaboration, and that in past research have differentially moderated the persuasive impact of different information types (i.e., heuristics/cues vs. message arguments) when information type has been confounded with information length (i.e., when heuristics/

cues have been brief and message arguments have been long). Specifically, we predict that when the heuristic/cue information is as extensive as the message information has typically been, contextual variables such as issue involvement, distraction, and repetition will moderate the impact of the persuasive implications of that information (e.g., implications of the source's being expert or inexpert) in the same way as they have moderated the impact of the implications of message arguments (i.e., implications of the arguments' being strong or weak). We predict that when issue involvement is high (vs. low), or when recipients are not distracted (vs. distracted), or when information is repeated (vs. not repeated), the persuasive impact of lengthy heuristic/cue information, compared to that of short heuristic/cue information, will be relatively high. Such evidence would be more consistent with the unimodel's assumption of process uniformity across information types than with previous assumptions of qualitatively different processing operations for message arguments versus heuristcs/cues.

*Experiment 1: The Interactive Effects
on Persuasion of Issue Involvement and Amount
of Heuristic/Cue Information*

An experimental study will manipulate the following independent variables: (1) amount of heuristic/cue information about the source (small or large); (2) type of heuristic/cue information (the source is expert or inexpert); (3) the recipients' issue involvement (high or low). Issue involvement will be manipulated in the usual manner—that is, by leading the participants to believe that the proposed advocacy (e.g., comprehensive examinations for college seniors) will or will not affect them personally. In the "small" version of the heuristic/cue information, the expertise of the source will be conveyed in a single sentence. In the "large" version, the information will be communicated in a one-page resume; listing the educator's various academic credentials and activities. In all experimental conditions, the heuristic/cue information will be followed by a message supposedly delivered by the source and arguing a given position. The main prediction is that when the amount of heuristic/cue information is large, attitudinal

differentiation between the expert and the inexpert source will be larger under conditions of high versus low issue involvement. By contrast, when the amount of heuristic/cue information is small, attitudinal differentiation between the expert and inexpert sources will be greater under conditions of low versus high involvement. Note that, strictly speaking, these predictions contrast with those of the traditional dual-model perspectives, which imply generally stronger effects of peripheral cues/heuristics (regarding source expertise) under low (vs. high) involvement.

*Experiment 2: The Interactive Effects
on Persuasion of the Amount of Heuristic/Cue
Information and Distraction*

Another experiment will test the hypothesis that under the appropriate conditions, cognitive distraction (a variable previously shown to interfere with the processing of message arguments; see Petty et al., 1976) will interfere similarly with the processing of heuristic/cue information and consequently will reduce its efficacy in producing attitude change. The design of the study will be a 2 × 2 × 2 factorial with these independent variables: (1) amount of heuristic/cue information about the source (small or large), (2) type of heuristic/cue information (the source is expert or inexpert), and (3) distraction (present or absent).

The amount of heuristic/cue information will be manipulated as in Experiment 1. Unlike this experiment, however, all participants will receive the high-involvement instructions, in order to establish a relatively high baseline level of effortful processing that may be then reduced via cognitive distraction. Participants assigned to the distraction condition will be shown a nine-digit number prior to reading the educator's resume; and will be instructed to silently rehearse that number until asked to write it down later during the session. No such manipulation will take place for participants in the no-distraction condition. It is predicted that when the amount of heuristic/cue information is large, attitudinal differentiation between the expert and inexpert sources will be greater in the no-distraction condition than in the distraction condition. Distraction should have less of an effect on attitudinal differentiation when the amount of information is small, because the processing of this information should be relatively easy, and hence less susceptible to interference by a distracting activity. Note that the traditional dual-process models of persuasion have emphasized the importance of available cognitive capacity (reduced by the competing attentional demands of the distracting activity) for systematic or central processing, but not for the processing of peripheral cues or heuristics. Confirmation of our prediction for a detrimental effect of distraction on the persuasive impact of a large (but not a small) amount of source information would yield further evidence for our alternative model of process uniformity.

Experiment 3: The Interactive Effects
on Persuasion of the Amount of Heuristic/Cue
Information and Repetition

The repetition of message arguments has been found to increase persuasion under the appropriate conditions (Cacioppo & Petty, 1980, 1985, 1989). If our analysis is correct, it should have a similar effect for the presentation of cue- or heuristic-related information. An experiment testing these notions will employ a $2 \times 2 \times 2$ factorial design with these independent variables: (1) number of presentations of heuristic/cue information (once vs. three times), (2) amount of heuristic/cue information (long vs. short), and (3) type of heuristic/cue information (the source is expert or inexpert). To create conditions favoring repetition effects, all participants will receive the persuasion- relevant information under conditions of relatively low issue involvement. In all cases, the heuristic/cue information about the source will be followed by the same relatively lengthy message argument. In this experiment, both the heuristic/cue information and the message arguments will be presented auditorily on Walkman-type personal cassette players. Half the participants will hear the heuristic/cue information once, and the others will hear it three times. To justify the repetition of the heuristic/cue information for some participants, we may tell all participants that they are helping the local college radio station check the quality of different sound mixes for a public information program being prepared on the topic of man-

datory comprehensive exams. The main prediction is that when the heuristic/cue information about the source is relatively long, the attitudinal differentiation between the expert and inexpert sources will be enhanced by repetition. For the brief heuristic/cue information, we may get either a weaker repetition effect (because the information is easy enough to process the first time around) or a reversal of the effect (because of tedium, reactance, or negative affect) (Petty & Cacioppo, 1986). Dual-process researchers have found that moderate repetition of (extensive) argument information increases the extent of its impact, and is mediated by the number of favorable (relative to unfavorable) relevant thoughts recipients generate (Cacioppo & Petty, 1989). We predict that such mediation will be enhanced by repetition when heuristic/cue information is extensive, but not (or less so) when such information is brief. This should provide additional support for our unimodel's emphasis on informational properties that enhance or undermine ease of processing, rather than on the Laswellian distinction between information source and message factors per se.

If the predictions outlined in Experiments 1 through 3 are supported, we will have obtained evidence that when the amount of cue/heuristic information is controlled for, it interacts with variables such as issue involvement, distraction, and repetition in the same way that message argument information has in prior research. Specifically, (1) in large amounts such information may exert greater persuasive impact under conditions of high (vs. low) issue involvement on the part of the communication recipients; (2) under high-involvement conditions, the impact of such information may be more vulnerable to the effects of cognitive distraction; and (3) in the absence of a strong processing motivation, the persuasive impact of such information may be enhanced by repetition. Though in the experiments outlined thus far the focus will be on the dependent variable of attitude change per se, follow-up experiments may be carried out to examine the persistence of change, resistance to counterpersuasion, and attitude–behavior relations. We predict that all the foregoing variables will be positively affected by the extent to which the heuristics/cues presented are processed. Specifically, resistance, persistence, and attitude–behavior relations should be more pronounced where a large amount of cue/heuristic information is processed under conditions of high issue involvement, when such information is presented repeatedly under conditions of low involvement, and when its processing is not interfered with by distraction. Finally, Experiments 1–3 should be replicated conceptually by manipulating the amount of message argument information (rather than of cue/heuristic information). We predict that the amount of message argument information will interact with contextual factors of involvement, distraction, and message repetition in an identical manner to that hypothesized for the amount of cue/heuristic information.

Persuasive Effects of the Ordinal Position of Cue/Heuristic versus Message Arguments

As noted earlier, in prior persuasion research cue/heuristic information has typically been presented before message argument information. The present study set is designed to investigate whether the order of presentation may account in part for findings of greater persuasive impact of message arguments (vs. heuristics/cues) under conditions conducive to effortful cognitive elaboration, and a relatively greater persuasive impact of heuristics/ cues information under conditions that promote superficial processing. We suspect that it may. Specifically, we propose that when either message argument or cue/heuristic information is positioned later (vs. earlier) in the sequence, it will be affected more by the contextual factors of issue involvement, distraction, or repetition, because earlier-presented information of either type may be processed relatively extensively and carefully.

Experiment 4: Interaction between Order of Presentation and Issue Involvement

Accordingly, our fourth experiment will examine the notion that moderately extensive cue/heuristic information, or equally extensive message information, will be affected more by issue involvement when it occurs later in a presentation than when it comes first. As already suggested, our underlying rationale is that even fairly uninvolved recipients will attend sufficiently to information presented early on. However, highly involved recipients are more likely also to attend to information appearing later, as their heightened concern with forming veridical attitudes may prompt them to consider all available and potentially relevant information. As a consequence, they are more likely than uninvolved recipients to respond to the persuasive implications of that information. Specifically, we predict that regardless of the type of information, variations in the persuasive implications of later-appearing information will have greater attitudinal impact under conditions of high (vs. low) involvement; thus, the extent to which high expertise (vs. low expertise) or strong arguments (vs. weak arguments) conveyed by later-appearing information result in greater acceptance of the advocated position will be more pronounced when issue involvement is high than when it is low. Our predictions here contrast with those one would extrapolate from the current dual-process models, which tend to emphasize how high levels of issue involvement foster persuasion through heightened cognitive processing of message arguments, but not through such processing of heuristics/cues.

Experiment 5: Interaction between Order of Presentation and Distraction

An experiment will examine the impact of distraction on heuristics/cues and message arguments as a function of their ordinal position. The main prediction is that the persuasive impact of both heuristic/cue information (the source is expert or inexpert) and argument quality (high or low) will be moderated by an interaction between order of presentation and distraction. Specifically, distraction should reduce the persuasive impact of variations in later-appearing information more than it will reduce the impact of variations in early-appearing information. When the message arguments follow the heuristic/cue information, strong arguments will produce greater agreement than weak arguments in the no-distraction condition than in the distraction condition. Conversely, when heuristic/cue information follows the message arguments, material implying high source expertise will produce greater agreement than material implying low source expertise in the no-distraction condition than in the distraction condition.

Experiment 6: Interaction between Order of Presentation and Repetition

A study may examine the impact, under conditions of low issue involvement, of repetition of heuristics/cues and of message arguments as a function of their ordinal position. The main prediction is that both heuristic/cue information (the source is expert or inexpert) and argument quality (high or low) will interact (in their effects on persuasion) with order of presentation and repetition. Specifically, both the heuristics/cues and the message arguments will benefit more from repetition (as evidenced by greater attitudinal differentiation between expert and inexpert sources and between high- and low-quality arguments) when the relevant information is positioned later versus earlier in the sequence.

Even though the variable of order of presentation has not figured prominently in current dual-process models of attitude change, it has in the past been of some considerable theoretical interest (Cohen, 1957; Hovland, 1957). In our own analysis of the contemporary persuasion literature we propose that presentation order has been correlated gratuitously with information type (message arguments vs. heuristics/cues) in the typical experimental procedure. If the predictions investigated in Experiments 4 through 6 are supported, we will have obtained evidence that the order in which information is presented interacts with context variables to affect persuasion similarly, regardless of whether the information consists of heuristics/cues or message arguments. Thus, regardless of information type, the persuasive impact of later-appearing information (resembling the positioning of message-arguments in most prior persuasion research) will benefit more from high issue involvement, will be more susceptible to disruption by distraction under high-involvement, and will benefit more from repetition under low-involvement conditions. In appropriate follow-up experiments examining the persistence of change, resistance to

counterpersuasion, and attitude-behavior relations, we predict that the foregoing variables will be positively affected by the extent to which information of both of types will be processed. Specifically, resistance, persistence, and attitude–behavior relations should all be more pronounced when the later-appearing information (more so than the early information) is processed under conditions of high issue involvement, when its processing under high-involvement conditions is not interfered with by distraction, and when such information is presented repeatedly under low-involvement conditions.

Effects of Issue Involvement within and between Information Types

Whereas the research described thus far will examine the variables of informational amount and ordinal position separately, the next set of studies will conjoin them in a manner resembling prior persuasion research. Each of the following three studies will present first a meager amount of persuasively relevant information, followed by a relatively extensive quantity of additional persuasive information. However, here the similarity to prior work will end. Thus, one of our studies will "turn the tables" on the typical persuasion paradigm, wherein brief cue/heuristic information is followed by extensive message argument information, and will instead place brief message argument information before extensive cue/heuristic information. The next two studies will abandon the *between-information-type* format, in which both heuristics/cues and message arguments are presented to recipients. If the unimodel is correct in positing that the critical variables affecting persuasion are amount of information and order of presentation, they should function similarly in a *within-information-type* format, wherein both the early-appearing brief information and the late-appearing extensive information belong in the same Laswellian category. To test those ideas, in one experiment both informational sets will consist of message arguments, whereas in another experiment they will both consist of cues/heuristics. In all three studies, the contextual factor of issue involvement will be manipulated orthogonally to the pertinent informational variations. Our main prediction is that regardless of type (i.e., whether it concerns message arguments or heuristic cues), the lengthier, later-appearing information will result in greater attitudinal differentiation under high-involvement conditions, and the briefer, early-appearing information will result in greater such differentiation under low-involvement conditions.

CONCLUSIONS

In this chapter we have outlined an integrative "unimodel" of persuasion, which is offered as a generalized alternative to prevalent dual-mode approaches. Even though it may differ from those approaches in its ultimate conclusions, our analysis has fundamental commonalities with the dual-process models, and in fact it builds upon (and in many cases grows out of) insights and arguments offered by the dual-process theorists. As we see it, the unimodel offers three fundamental advantages to persuasion researchers: (1) parsimony; (2) generative potential; and (3) a novel, highly flexible view of persuasion, of potentially considerable practical significance. The parsimony advantage resides in the synthesis that the unimodel affords not only in regard to the dual-mode notions as such, but also in regard to Laswell's fundamental distinction among the "who", the "what" and the "whom" of persuasion. According to the present analysis, the entire persuasion process occurs in the recipient's head; hence his or her characteristics (Laswell's "whom" category) may not be considered apart from his or her particular beliefs about the source (i.e., the "who" category) and about the message (i.e., the "what" category). If, furthermore, the latter two categories refer to functionally equivalent information types whereby persuasion may be accomplished (as has been argued throughout this chapter), the commonality between them may overshadow their differences as far as the underlying process of persuasion is concerned.

Critics may object at this juncture that the distinction between the processing modes isn't really about different information types (i.e., related to Laswell's "who" and "what" categories) but rather about more versus less elaborate (or more or less simple) processing, captured by the continuum notion in the

ELM and strongly implied in the HSM as well (see Petty & Wegener, Chapter 3, this volume). In fairness, however, this isn't quite the way the two processing modes have been characterized in the literature thus far. First, in most published research, peripheral cues or heuristics have been juxtaposed with the contents of message arguments, suggesting that the distinction does in fact relate to different information types rather than merely to the extent of elaboration. In fact, the notion of "peripheral cues" or "heuristics" as such (rather than heuristic *processing*) is invoked quite often in the dual-mode literature. Moreover, a major dual-mode theorist has recently affirmed that "heuristic processing is about information ... of general relevance to a judgment ... while systematic processing concerns information that is more specifically related to particular judgment called for" (S. Chaiken, personal communication, Oct. 21, 1997), again implying that the distinction between processing modes does in fact have to do with different information types (i.e., general vs. specific). Also, in studies conducted within the HSM framework (e.g., Maheswaran & Chaiken, 1991, pp. 17–18), systematic processing is operationally defined in terms of attribute-related thoughts, where attribute characteristics are depicted in the message; by contrast, heuristic processing is said to consist of consensus-related thoughts. These definitions suggest that it is the *thought content* that identifies the two types of processing.

Besides, the extent-of-elaboration distinction (which LET thoroughly accepts) seems incompatible with the notion that the two modes differ *qualitatively*. By its essence, the extent-of-elaboration distinction seems *quantitative*. After all, the extent-of-elaboration continuum can be subdivided into any number of segments, rendering somewhat arbitrary a conception of *two* qualitatively distinct modes of processing. Also, if extent of processing (or degree of simplicity) was all there was to the dual-mode distinction, it would not seem justifiable to maintain (as do both the ELM and the HSM theorists) that the two processing modes can co-occur. Logically, if the processing is extensive it can not be simultaneously restricted, and vice versa. In view of all these considerations, it seems fair to conclude, that as generally understood, the dual-mode theories do in fact link each processing mode with a different type of information. By contrast, within our unimodel those two information types are treated as different types of evidence contents, which are functionally equivalent in their persuasive role.

The current proposal also demonstrates the rich generative potential of the unimodel. The specific studies outlined above actually constitute basic research paradigms that can readily be extended to diverse follow-up investigations within the present conceptual framework. It is noteworthy that such studies are quite novel in their approach and often turn existing procedures of persuasion research "on their heads." It is also noteworthy that the unimodel affords numerous additional lines of empirical inquiry, a detailed description of which is beyond the scope of this chapter. These further avenues of research may incorporate variables affecting the extent of information processing (regardless of information type) not previously considered, such as the need for cognition (Cacioppo & Petty, 1982; Thompson et al., 1993) or the need for closure (Webster & Kruglanski, 1994). They could demonstrate the role of premise availability/accessibility in persuasion for the different evidence types (i.e., heuristics/cues and message arguments), and they could probe the general conditions under which either type of evidence affects the processing of the other.

Finally, the unimodel perspective on the persuasion process offers exciting new possibilities to potential communicators. It suggests that brief and superficial persuasion may be accomplished via simplistic message arguments as well as via message-unrelated cues or heuristics. More importantly, perhaps, it implies that when recipients are relatively motivated and able to process information in general, but are too unfamiliar with the topic at hand to appreciate the logic or complexities of issue-related arguments, persuasion agents may still be able to produce robust attitude change that is persistent over time, resistant to counterpersuasive appeals, and linked to behavior, by presenting, for example, extensive evidence for the expertise of the source that recipients may incorporate into their attitudes. In this sense, the unimodel relaxes the constraints inherent in the dual-mode approaches and offers a more flexible view of persuasion, wherein the same fundamental outcomes of persuasion may be attained via different means, contingent on the particular epistemic characteristics of the persuasion recipients.

ACKNOWLEDGMENTS

Work in this chapter was supported by National Science Foundation Grant No. SBR 9417422, National Institute of Mental Health (NIMH) Grant No. 1R01 MH 52578, and NIMH Research Scientist Award No. KO5 MH 01213 to Arie W. Kruglanski.

REFERENCES

Achinstein, P. (1983). Concepts of evidence. In P. Achinstein (Ed.), *The concept of evidence* (pp. 81–107). New York: Oxford University Press.

Axsom, D., Yates, S., & Chaiken, S. (1987). Audience response as a heuristic cue in persuasion. *Journal of Personality and Social Psychology, 53*, 30–40.

Bargh, J. A., & Gollwitzer, P. M. (1994). Environmental control of goal-directed action: Automatic and strategic contingencies between situations and behavior. In W. D. Spaulding (Ed.), *Nebraska Symposium on Motivation: Vol. 41. Integrative views of motivation, cognition, and emotion* (pp. 71–124). Lincoln: University of Nebraska Press.

Berscheid, E., Graziano, W., Monson, T., & Dermer, M. (1976). Outcome dependency: Attention, attribution, and attraction. *Journal of Personality and Social Psychology, 34*, 978–989.

Biek, M., Wood, W., & Chaiken, S. (1996). Working knowledge, cognitive processing, and attitudes: On the determinants of bias. *Personality and Social Psychology Bulletin, 22*, 547–556.

Brewer, M. B. (1988). A dual process model of impression formation. In T. K. Srull & R. S. Wyer (Eds.), *Advances in social cognition* (Vol. 1, pp. 1–36). Hillsdale, NJ: Erlbaum.

Burgoon, M., Cohen, M., Miller, M., & Montgomery, C. (1978). An empirical test of a model of resistance to persuasion. *Human Communication Research, 5*, 27–39.

Cacioppo, J. T., & Petty, R. E. (1980). Persuasiveness of communications is affected by exposure frequency and message quality: A theoretical and empirical analysis of persisting attitude change. In J. H. Leigh & C. R. Martin (Eds.), *Current issues and research in advertising* (pp. 97–122). Ann Arbor: University of Michigan Press.

Cacioppo, J. T., & Petty, R. E. (1982). The need for cognition. *Journal of Personality and Social Psychology, 42*, 116–131.

Cacioppo, J. T., & Petty, R. E. (1985). Central and peripheral routes to persuasion: The role of message repetition. In L. F. Alwitt & A. A. Mitchell (Eds.), *Psychological processes and advertising effects: Theory, research, and application* (pp. 91–111). Hillsdale, NJ: Erlbaum.

Cacioppo, J. T., & Petty, R. E. (1989). Effects of message repetition on argument processing, recall, persuasion. *Basic and Applied Social Psychology, 10*, 3–12.

Cacioppo, J. T., Petty, R. E., Kao, C. F., & Rodriguez, R. (1986). Central and peripheral routes to persuasion: An individual difference perspective. *Journal of Personality and Social Psychology, 51*, 1032–1043.

Carnap, R. (1962). *Logical foundations of probability.* Chicago: University of Chicago Press.

Chaiken, S. (1979). Communicator physical attractiveness and persuasion. *Journal of Personality and Social Psychology, 37*, 1387–1397.

Chaiken, S. (1980). Heuristic versus systematic information processing and the use of source versus message cues in persuasion. *Journal of Personality and Social Psychology, 39*, 752–766.

Chaiken, S. (1987). The heuristic model of persuasion. In M. P. Zanna, J. M. Olson, & C. P. Herman (Eds.), *Social influence: The Ontario Symposium* (Vol. 5, pp. 3–39). Hillsdale, NJ: Erlbaum.

Chaiken, S., & Eagly, A. H. (1983). Communication modality as a determinant of persuasion: The role of communicator salience. *Journal of Personality and Social Psychology, 45*, 241–256.

Chaiken, S., Liberman, A., & Eagly, A. H. (1989). Heuristic and systematic information processing within and beyond the persuasion context. In J. S. Uleman & J. A. Bargh (Eds.), *Unintended thought* (pp. 212–252). New York: Guilford Press.

Chaiken, S., & Maheswaran, D. (1994). Heuristic processing can bias systematic processing: Effects of source credibility, argument ambiguity, and task importance on attitude judgment. *Journal of Personality and Social Psychology, 66*, 460–473.

Chaiken, S., Wood, W., & Eagly, A. H. (1996). Principles of persuasion. In E. T. Higgins & A. W. Kruglanski (Eds.), *Social psychology: Handbook of basic principles* (pp. 702–742). New York: Guilford Press.

Chen, S., Shechter, D., & Chaiken, S. (1996). Getting at the truth or getting along: Accuracy versus impression-motivated heuristic and systematic processing. *Journal of Personality and Social Psychology, 71*, 262–275.

Cohen, A. R. (1957). Need for cognition and order of communication as determinants of opinion change. In C. I. Hovland (Ed.), *The order of presentation in persuasion* (pp. 79–192). New Haven, CT: Yale University Press.

Darke, P. R., Chaiken, S., Bohner, G., Einwiller, S., Erb, H., & Hazlewood, D. (in press). Accuracy motivation, consensus information, and the law of large numbers: Effects on attitude judgment in the absence of argumentation. *Personality and Social Psychology Bulletin.*

Eagly, A. H., & Chaiken, S. (1993). *The psychology of attitudes.* Fort Worth, TX: Harcourt Brace Jovanovich.

Erber, R., & Fiske, S. T. (1984). Outcome dependency and attention to inconsistent information. *Journal of Personality and Social Psychology, 47*, 709–726.

Fishbein, M., & Ajzen, I. (1975). *Belief, attitude, intention, and behavior: An introduction to theory and research.* Reading, MA: Addison-Wesley.

Giner-Sorolla, R., & Chaiken, S. (1997). Selective use of heuristic and systematic processing under defense motivation. *Personality and Social Psychology Bulletin, 23*, 84–97.

Glymour, C. N. (1980). *Theory and evidence.* Princeton, NJ: Princeton University Press.

Greenwald, A. G. (1968). Cognitive learning, cognitive response to persuasion, and attitude change. In A. G. Greenwald, T. C. Brock, & T. M. Ostrom (Eds.), *Psychological foundations of attitudes* (pp. 147–170). New York: Academic Press.

Heesacker, M., Petty, R. E., & Cacioppo, J. T. (1983). Field dependence and attitude change: Source credibility can alter persuasion by affecting message-relevant thinking. *Journal of Personality, 51*, 653–666.

Hempel, C. G. (1965). *Aspects of scientific explanation.* New York: Free Press.

Higgins, E. T. (1996). Knowledge activation, application, and salience. In E. T. Higgins & A. W. Kruglanski (Eds.), *Social psychology: Handbook of basic principles* (pp. 133–168). New York: Guilford Press.

Higgins, E. T., Rholes, W. S., & Jones, C. R. (1977). Category accessibility and impression formation. *Journal of Experimental Social Psychology, 13*, 141–154.

Hovland, C. I. (Ed.). (1957). *The order of presentation in persuasion.* New Haven, CT: Yale University Press.

Hovland, C. I., Janis, I. L., & Kelley, H. H. (1953). *Communication and persuasion: Psychological studies of opinion change.* New Haven, CT: Yale University Press.

Kahneman, D. (1973). *Attention and effort.* Englewood Cliffs, NJ: Prentice-Hall.

Kruglanski, A. W. (1980). Lay epistemo-logic—process and contents: Another look at attribution theory. *Psychological Review, 87*, 70–87.

Kruglanski, A. W. (1989). *Lay epistemics and human knowledge: Cognitive and motivational bases.* New York: Plenum.

Kruglanski, A. W. (1990). Motivations for judging and knowing: Implications for causal attribution. In E. T. Higgins & R. M. Sorrentino (Eds.), *Handbook of motivation and cognition: Foundations of social behavior* (Vol. 2, pp. 333–368). New York: Guilford Press.

Kruglanski, A. W. (1996a). Motivated social cognition: Principles of the interface. In E. T. Higgins & A. W. Kruglanski (Eds.), *Social psychology: Handbook of basic principles* (pp. 493–520). New York: Guilford Press.

Kruglanski, A. W. (1996b). Goals as knowledge structures. In P. M. Gollwitzer & J. A. Bargh (Eds.), *The psychology of action: Linking cognition and motivation to behavior* (pp. 599–618). New York: Guilford Press.

Kruglanski, A. W., & Klar, Y. (1987). A view from a bridge: Synthesizing the consistency and attribution paradigms from a lay epistemic perspective. *European Journal of Social Psychology, 17*, 211–241.

Kruglanski, A. W., & Webster, D. M. (1996). Motivated closing of the mind: "Seizing" and "freezing." *Psychological Review, 103*, 263–283.

Laswell, H. D. (1948). The structure and function of communication in society. In L. Bryson (Ed.), *Religion and civilization series: Vol 3. The communication of ideas* (pp. 37–51). New York: Harper & Row.

Maheswaran, D., & Chaiken, S. (1991). Promoting systematic processing in low motivation settings: The effect of incongruent information on processing and judgment. *Journal of Personality and Social Psychology, 61*, 13–25.

McGuire, W. J. (1960). A syllogistic analysis of cognitive

relationships. In C. I. Hovland & M. J. Rosenberg (Eds.), *Attitude organization and change: An analysis of consistency among attitude components* (pp. 65–111). New Haven, CT: Yale University Press.

McGuire, W. J. (1964). Inducing resistance to persuasion: Some contemporary approaches. In L. Berkowitz (Ed.), *Advances in experimental social psychology* (Vol. 1, pp. 191–229). New York: Academic Press.

McGuire, W. J. (1968). Personality and attitude change: An information-processing theory. In A. G. Greenwald, T. C. Brock, & T. M. Ostrom (Eds.), *Psychological foundations of attitudes* (pp. 171–196). New York: Academic Press.

McGuire, W. J. (1969). The nature of attitudes and attitude change. In G. Lindzey & E. Aronson (Eds.), *Handbook of social psychology* (2nd ed., Vol. 3, pp. 136–314). Reading, MA: Addison-Wesley.

McGuire, W. J. (1972). Attitude change: The information processing paradigm. In C. G. McClintock (Ed.), *Experimental social psychology* (pp. 108–141). New York: Holt, Rinehart, & Winston.

Petty, R. E. (1994). Two routes to persuasion: State of the art. In G. d'Ydewalle, P. Eelen, & P. Berteleson (Eds.), *International perspectives on psychological science* (Vol. 2, pp. 229–247). Hillsdale, NJ: Erlbaum.

Petty, R. E., & Cacioppo, J. T. (1984). The effects of involvement on responses to argument quantity and quality: Central and peripheral routes to persuasion. *Journal of Personality and Social Psychology, 46,* 69–81.

Petty, R. E., & Cacioppo, J. T. (1986). The elaboration likelihood model of persuasion. In L. Berkowitz (Ed.), *Advances in experimental social psychology* (Vol. 19, pp. 123–205). San Diego, CA: Academic Press.

Petty, R. E., Cacioppo, J. T., & Goldman, R. (1981). Personal involvement as a predictor of argument-based persuasion. *Journal of Personality and Social Psychology, 41,* 847–855.

Petty, R. E., Cacioppo, J. T., & Heesacker, M. (1985). *Persistence of persuasion: A test of the elaboration likelihood model.* Unpublished manuscript, University of Missouri–Columbia.

Petty, R. E., Cacioppo, J. T., & Schumann, D. (1983). Central and peripheral routes to advertising effectiveness: The moderating role of involvement. *Journal of Consumer Research, 10,* 135–146.

Petty, R. E., Harkins, S. G., & Williams, K. D. (1980). The effects of group diffusion of cognitive effort on attitudes: An information processing view. *Journal of Personality and Social Psychology, 38,* 81–92.

Petty, R. E., Ostrom, T. M., & Brock, T. C. (Eds.). (1981). *Cognitive responses in persuasion.* Hillsdale, NJ: Erlbaum.

Petty, R. E., Wells, G. L., & Brock, T. C. (1976). Distraction can enhance or reduce yielding to propaganda: Thought disruption versus effort justification. *Journal of Personality and Social Psychology, 34,* 874–884.

Ratneshwar, S., & Chaiken, S. (1991). Comprehension's role in persuasion: The case of its moderating effect on the persuasive impact of source expertise. *Journal of Consumer Research, 18,* 52–62.

Ruscher, J. B., & Fiske, S. T. (1990). Interpersonal competition can cause individuating processes. *Journal of Personality and Social Psychology, 58,* 832–843.

Schumann, D., Petty, R. E., & Cacioppo, J. T. (1985). *Effects of involvement, repetition, and variation on responses to advertisements.* Unpublished manuscript, University of Missouri–Columbia.

Smith, E. R. (1988). Impression formation in a general framework of social and nonsocial cognition. In T. K. Srull & R. S. Wyer, Jr. (Eds.), *Advances in social cognition* (Vol. 1, pp. 165–176). Hillsdale, NJ: Erlbaum.

Srull, T. K., & Wyer, R. S., Jr. (1986). The role of chronic and temporary goals in social information processing. In R. M. Sorrentino & E. T. Higgins (Eds.), *Handbook of motivation and cognition: Foundations of social behavior* (Vol. 1, pp. 503–549). New York: Guilford Press.

Taylor, S. E., & Fiske, S. T. (1978). Salience, attention, and attribution: Top of the head phenomena. In L. Berkowitz (Ed.), *Advances in experimental social psychology* (Vol. 11, pp. 249–288). New York: Academic Press.

Thompson, E. P., Chaiken, S., & Hazlewood, J. D. (1993). Need for cognition and desire for control as moderators of extrinsic reward effects: A person x situation approach to the study of intrinsic motivation. *Journal of Personality and Social Psychology, 64,* 987–999.

Webster, D. M., & Kruglanski, A. W. (1994). Individual differences in need for cognitive closure. *Journal of Personality and Social Psychology, 67,* 1049–1062.

Webster, D. M., & Kruglanski, A. W. (1998). Cognitive and social consequences of the need for cognitive closure. *European Review of Social Psychology.*

Wells, G. L., & Petty, R. E. (1980). The effects of overt head movements on persuasion: Compatibility and incompatibility of responses. *Basic and Applied Social Psychology, 1,* 219–230.

Wood, W. (1982). Retrieval of attitude-relevant information from memory: Effects on susceptibility to persuasion and on intrinsic motivation. *Journal of Personality and Social Psychology, 42,* 798–810.

Wood, W., Biek, M., Nations, C., & Chaiken, S. (1994). [Resistance to change and working knowledge: Knowledgeable people are objective, critical information processors]. Unpublished raw data, Texas A&M University.

Wood, W., & Kallgren, C. A. (1988). Communicator attributes and persuasion: Recipients' access to attitude-relevant information in memory. *Personality and Social Psychology Bulletin, 14,* 172–182.

Wood, W., Kallgren, C. A., & Preisler, R. M. (1985). Access to attitude-relevant information in memory as a determinant of persuasion: The role of message attributes. *Journal of Experimental Social Psychology, 21,* 73–85.

Wyer, R. S., Jr. (1970). Quantitative prediction of belief and opinion change: A further test of a subjective probability model. *Personality and Social Psychology, 16,* 559–570.

Wyer, R. S., Jr. (1974). *Cognitive organization and change: An information processing approach.* Hillsdale, NJ: Erlbaum.

15

Parallel Processing of Stereotypes and Behaviors

ZIVA KUNDA

When you come across a person with dark skin, what you "see," with little thought or inference, is an African American. Even very brief or subliminal exposure to photographs of African Americans can suffice to provoke you into automatically activating the stereotype of African Americans, along with your affective reactions to this group (e.g., Bargh, Chen, & Burrows, 1996; Chen & Bargh, 1997; Fazio, Jackson, Dunton, & Williams, 1995).

In the same manner, when you come across a person in the act of shoving another, what you will "see," with little thought or inference, is an aggressive person engaged in an aggressive act. You may make such trait inferences spontaneously even if you have no intention of making them, and even if your cognitive resources are taxed by other demanding tasks (for reviews, see Gilbert, 1989; Uleman, Chapter 7, this volume; Uleman, Newman, & Moskowitz, 1996).

What, then, do you "see" when you come across a person with dark skin in the act of shoving another? In a recent article, Paul Thagard and I proposed that in such circumstances, the stereotype implied by the person's skin color and the trait implied by the person's behavior will be activated automatically and simultaneously, will constrain each other's meaning, and will jointly determine

your impressions of the person (Kunda & Thagard, 1996). In the context of the aggressive act, this person may be seen as a particularly menacing kind of African American, perhaps an African American thug. And, in the context of the African American stereotype, the shove may be seen as particularly hostile and violent. The juxtaposition of this stereotype with this behavior may therefore result in an impression of greater aggressiveness than would have emerged if either piece of information had been presented alone. Any other information noticed about the person—gender, attire, attractiveness, accent—will also contribute to and figure in your impressions of this person.

Thagard and I proposed that impression formation can be viewed as emerging from a process of parallel constraint satisfaction, in which all information observed about a person simultaneously contributes to a perceiver's impressions (Kunda & Thagard, 1996). Much like Gestalt psychologists, most notably Asch (Asch, 1946, 1952/1987; Asch & Zukier, 1984), we assumed that the perceiver blends the many attributes of an observed person into a coherent impression that takes into account each attribute as well as the associations among attributes. In the process, the meaning of each attribute may be influenced by the meanings of related attributes that are activated at the same time. The impact of each piece of observed information on one's overall impression of the person depends only on the pattern of associations between that observation and other attributes. Observations that are strongly associated with aggressiveness, whatever their source, will contribute more to one's impressions of the person as aggressive than will observations that are only weakly associated with aggressiveness. Thagard and I showed that this parallel-constraint-satisfaction model can account for most findings reported in the literature on how people form impressions from stereotypes and individuating information.

An important aspect of the parallel-constraint-satisfaction model is that it treats all sources of information as equal in status (Kunda & Thagard, 1996). It does not matter whether "aggressive" is activated by a stereotype or by a behavior; the only thing that matters is how strongly it is activated. In this, the model differs importantly from two other influential models: Brewer's (1988) dual-process model and Fiske and Neuberg's (1990) continuum model of impression formation (see also Brewer & Harasty, Chapter 12, and Fiske, Lin, & Neuberg, Chapter 11, this volume). Both these models assume that one class of information, stereotypes, will often dominate impressions, carrying greater weight than any individuating information such as behavior or attire. Stereotypes will have this privileged, dominant role unless one is strongly motivated to gain deep understanding of a person, or unless the fit between the stereotype and the individuating information is poor (Brewer, 1988; Fiske & Neuberg, 1990). Despite these basic differences, there are broad areas of agreement between these models and the parallel-constraint-satisfaction model. I first outline these areas of agreement, and then return to a discussion of the remaining differences and the evidence bearing on them.

THE MOTIVATED PERCEIVER

All models agree that when a perceiver really cares about a person and is motivated to gain deep understanding of him or her, all information known to characterize this person will figure in the perceiver's impressions. The dual-process model assumes that when one is personally involved with a person, perhaps because one's relationship with this person is at stake, one will engage in person-based processing whereby, much as in the parallel-constraint-satisfaction model, stereotypes function as one of many equal-status attributes of the individual that all contribute to impressions (Brewer, 1988; Brewer & Harasty, Chapter 12, this volume). Similarly, the continuum model assumes that when one is motivated to arrive at an accurate impression of a person, perhaps because one depends on this person for important outcomes, one will engage in piecemeal integration whereby membership in a stereotyped group becomes just one of the many attributes that contribute to overall impressions (Fiske & Neuberg, 1990; Fiske et al., Chapter 11, this volume). Computer simulations of relevant empirical data have demonstrated that the parallel-constraint-satisfaction model provides a good account of how these diverse sources of information may be integrated (Kunda & Thagard, 1996). There now seems to be broad agreement that when stereotypes and individuating information are integrated, this may occur through parallel satisfaction of the constraints imposed by each kind of information (Brewer & Harasty, Chapter 12, and Fiske et al., Chapter 11, this volume).

There remain some differences in assumptions about the immediacy with which perceivers engage in such integration when they do engage in it, and about the automaticity of such integration processes. The parallel-constraint-satisfaction model and the dual-process model assume that perceivers will be thrown into integration mode almost immediately. The continuum model assumes, instead, that perceivers will arrive at the individuation stage where integration takes place only after cycling through a series of more category-based processes, such that one's impression is initially dominated by a single category and gradually accommodates more individuating information (Fiske & Neuberg, 1990; Fiske et al., Chapter 11, this volume). However, I am aware of no evidence indicating that perceivers go through this proposed sequence of processes.

The continuum model also differs from the remaining two models in that it assumes that piecemeal integration of individuating information requires more thoughtful, effortful processing than does category-based inference (Fiske & Neuberg, 1990; Fiske et al., Chapter 11, this volume). Thus, it assumes that perceivers will be able to perform such integration only when they have sufficient time and resources to engage in controlled processes. Bodenhausen, Macrae, and Sherman (Chapter 13, this volume) share this assumption (I shall return later to a critical discussion of the evidence on which this assumption is based). In contrast, Brewer and Harasty (Chapter 12, this volume) assume that inferences from stereotypes and from individuating information can both occur either automatically or through effortful processing; the depth with which each piece of evidence is processed depends not on its source but on the perceiver's state of mind. The parallel-constraint-satisfaction model shares this assumption. It assumes that behaviors and stereotypes can be integrated automatically and can influence each other's meaning and overall impressions through automatic priming and inhibition of associated constructs (Kunda & Thagard, 1996). This assumption is based on findings showing that an individual's race or gender can prompt automatic stereotype activation (e.g., Bargh et al., 1996; Chen & Bargh, 1997; Fazio et al., 1995) and that an individual's behavior can prompt automatic trait activation (e.g., Gilbert, Pelham, & Krull, 1988; Trope, 1986).

Although Thagard and I (Kunda & Thagard, 1996) focused on modeling such relatively automatic processes, we also noted that perceivers may resort to more controlled causal reasoning when puzzled by the information at hand, challenged by the demands of their task, or driven by their needs. Controlled causal reasoning can also involve parallel processing, whereby the causal implications of each piece of evidence are considered simultaneously and are integrated into a coherent explanation (Read & Miller, 1993; Thagard, 1989). Both automatic and effortful impression formation are assumed to be based on stereotypic as well as behavioral information. These assumptions have much in common with the model of attribution developed by Trope and his colleagues, which assumes that situational, stereotypic, and behavioral information are all integrated simultaneously and automatically to deter-

mine how the behavior is identified, but may also figure in more controlled processing to determine how the behavior is explained (for a review, see Trope & Gaunt, Chapter 8, this volume).

Despite these differences among the models of impression formation, all models agree that when we form impressions of people we are interested in—people we care about, people we depend upon, people with whom we have meaningful relationships—our impressions will be based on information gleaned from the social categories to which the people belong as well as from their behavior, appearance, and any other individuating information we have about them. Thus, when forming impressions of a new boss or coworker, a potential romantic partner or roommate, or someone interested in babysitting our children or painting our house, we will make use of all information available to us about this person. There seems to be an emerging consensus that the parallel-constraint-satisfaction model provides a good account of impression formation in these important interpersonal situations.

THE DISINTERESTED PERCEIVER

The differences between the parallel-constraint-satisfaction model on the one hand, and the dual-process and continuum models on the other hand, center on how we form impressions of strangers in whom we have little interest—for instance, the unfamiliar African American, woman, or police officer observed smiling in the hallway, shouting at a coworker, pushing ahead at the bank, or disciplining a child. The parallel-constraint-satisfaction model assumes that in such cases, too, all observed information will simultaneously influence one's impressions. In contrast, the dual-process and continuum models assume that in the case of strangers in whom we have little interest, stereotypes have a privileged status and will dominate impressions: Our initial impression will be based on a single, dominating stereotype, and any other information will be interpreted through the lenses of this stereotype (Bodenhausen et al., Chapter 13, this volume; Brewer, 1988; Fiske & Neuberg, 1990).

As Brewer and Harasty (Chapter 12, this

volume) note, this stereotype-dominated, top-down process has much in common with the process of integration outlined above. In both, individuating information will be shaped and disambiguated in line with the connotations of the stereotype. The difference lies in the assumption that in this case the disambiguation is driven by a single dominating construct along a one-way street. Behavioral information is not granted comparable power to influence and shape the meaning of stereotypic information, and although each person belongs to multiple stereotyped groups, only one of the applicable stereotypes can dominate impressions at any particular time. I see little reason to expect such one-way domination by a single stereotype when the person's membership in multiple stereotyped groups and the person's behavior and appearance are all noticed simultaneously.

However, if one piece of information is noticed first, it can exert a greater impact on impressions than it might have otherwise. If one notices or is told about a person's gender or ethnicity before one has had the opportunity to observe this person in action, beliefs activated by gender or ethnic stereotypes may have an especially powerful impact on the interpretation of subsequently encountered behaviors. I would also suggest that, for the same reasons, if one observers or is told about a person's behavior before finding out his or her ethnicity or profession, the behavioral information may similarly dominate impressions. Thagard and I demonstrated that the parallel-constraint-satisfaction model can simulate such order effects (Kunda & Thagard, 1996).[1] Therefore, knowing which information is observed first can take us a long way toward knowing which information is likely to dominate impressions.

Which information do we typically notice first? Both Fiske et al. (Chapter 11, this volume) and Bodenhausen et al. (Chapter 13, this volume) take it as a foregone conclusion that information related to group membership is typically observed first. One first notice gender and race; behaviors and other indicators of the contents of one's character are noticed only later, if at all. Moreover, people are rarely capable of noticing multiple pieces of information simultaneously. However, neither group of authors provides any evidence for these assumptions. Nor am I aware of any

research examining how many pieces of information a perceiver notices when encountering a person, and whether any kind of information—stereotypes or behaviors—comes into awareness before other kinds. Lacking relevant data, I can only point out that individuals are often observed in action—you see a woman shouting, an African American smiling, an elderly person watching birds. In addition to noting behaviors and facial expressions, even a brief glance can take in information about how well dressed the person is, how attractive, how well groomed, how muscular, and so on. Upon encounter, do we "see" a woman, or do we "see" a happy, attractive, well-dressed, professional woman? And will our initial, instantaneous impression of such a person be the same as our initial, instantaneous impression of a fidgety, unkempt, overweight woman? Will our spontaneous gut reaction to an African American man observed playing with a child in the park be the same as our spontaneous gut reaction to an African American man observed shouting crude insults at a cashier in a variety store? Do we wish to argue that racial identity will be observed and processed prior to and independently of such behaviors? Until we have relevant data, I would like to propose that it is at least plausible that we often observe such diverse sources of information simultaneously and integrate them automatically.

Evidence for the Privileged Status of Stereotypes

Advocates of the assumption that stereotypes dominate the impressions formed by disinterested perceivers base this assumption on two major kinds of evidence: the fact that stereotype activation and use are pervasive (Fiske & Neuberg, 1990; Fiske et al., Chapter 11, this volume) and the fact that inference from stereotypes is less effortful than inference from behavior (Bodenhausen et al., Chapter 13, and Fiske et al., Chapter 11, this volume). Below I explain why the first of these claims is irrelevant and the second unproved.

As noted by Fiske and her colleagues, there is a considerable amount of evidence showing that stereotypes can be activated spontaneously and immediately upon exposure to a stereotyped individual, and can be applied to one's impressions of others with little effort or intention. Stereotype use is undoubtedly pervasive. However, this does not imply that stereotypes will dominate impressions. Indeed, the parallel-constraint-satisfaction model, which explicitly assumes automatic activation and use of stereotypes, can account for all such findings without granting a privileged status to stereotypes. Moreover, there is also considerable evidence for spontaneous and automatic activation of traits upon observation of relevant behaviors, and for pervasive use of individuating information when forming impressions (for reviews, see Gilbert, 1988; Kunda & Thagard, 1996; Uleman et al., 1996). The use of stereotypes is pervasive, but so is the use of behavioral information. Neither of these lines of work alone can point to the dominance of one of these kinds of information over the other.

The second major argument for the privileged status of stereotypes is based on the claim that inference from stereotypes is less effortful than inference from behaviors. The disinterested observer, the argument goes, invests little effort and resources in impression formation, and, therefore falls back on quick and easy stereotypic thinking rather than engaging in more effortful assessment of individuating information (Fiske et al., Chapter 11, and Bodenhausen et al., Chapter 13, this volume). This view has gained broad acceptance despite the fact that the evidence for it is at best inconclusive (Kunda & Thagard, 1996). Here's why. The conclusion that stereotype use is more effortful than the use of individuating information rests on findings showing that stereotype use increases when cognitive capacity is reduced: People's impressions of stereotyped individuals become more stereotypic when they are cognitively busy, tired, or under time pressure (e.g., Bodenhausen, 1990; Kruglanski & Freund, 1983; Pendry & Macrae, 1994).

However, such findings speak to only half of the argument. To support the claim that stereotype use requires less effort than the use of individuating information, it is necessary to show not only that reliance on stereotypes *increases* when cognitive resources are limited, but also that reliance on individuating information *decreases* under the same circumstances; if the use of individuating information is indeed effortful, it should be disrupted when resources are taxed. To demonstrate such disruption of individuating information under high cognitive load, it is necessary to provide participants with different kinds of individuating information (e.g., strong and weak evidence of guilt) and to show that people become less sensitive to this information when their mental capacity is strained. Unfortunately, none of the studies examining the impact of mental capacity on stereotype use has done so; all have relied on a single description of a target person, which was presented to different participants as associated with members of differently stereotyped groups. To conclude from such data that cognitive load disrupts the use of individuating information while increasing stereotype use amounts to claiming a 2×2 interaction from a design that has varied only one of the independent variables. Logically, it remains plausible that the full design will reveal two main effects rather than an interaction: Cognitive load may increase the use of individuating information just as much as it increases stereotype use.

Bodenhausen et al. (Chapter 13, this volume) dismiss this possibility as counterintuitive. Obviously, my own intuitions differ. I find it quite plausible that when preoccupied, people will rely more heavily on each straightforward piece of relevant information rather than attempting a more complex and thoughtful reconciliation of the diverse pieces of evidence, a process that may blunt the impact of each. But this debate cannot be resolved by waving hands and intuitions; it needs to be resolved by data, and the appropriate data have not yet been collected. Until they are, the evidence that stereotype use is less effortful than the use of individuating information is at best inconclusive.

More recent evidence marshaled by Bodenhausen et al. (Chapter 13, this volume) in support of the dominant status of stereotypes in impression formation is equally one-sided. These authors cite studies showing that when stereotypes are available, people are less likely to retrieve or seek out individuating information about members of the stereotyped group (Sherman, 1996; Trope & Thompson, 1997). These findings are interesting and important, but they do not speak to the dominant role of stereotypes. This is because they do not address the question of how information retrieval and search will be influenced when behavioral information is made available. Thus, Trope and Thompson (1997) found that people attempting to determine a target person's attitudes addressed fewer questions to this person if they knew that he or she belonged to a group whose stereotype implied the attitude in question. Imagine a comparable study in which, instead of being informed about the target's group membership, perceivers were informed that the target had performed a behavior that implied the attitude. Can we suppose that this, too, would reduce the amount of questions asked of the target? Would it reduce perceivers' interest in finding out which stereotyped groups the target belonged to? And if so, would we still wish to argue that stereotypes have a more privileged status than behavioral information?

In short, to argue about the relative power of stereotypes and individuating information to shape impressions, it is not enough to demonstrate that the power of stereotypes is considerable. The power of individuating information may be every bit as considerable. Based on currently available data, there is little reason to assume otherwise. Moreover, what data there are suggest that behavioral evidence may, if anything, exert a more powerful impact on impressions than do stereotypes. A meta-analysis of studies in which behavioral information and group membership were varied orthogonally revealed that the impact of behavioral information on impressions was substantially larger than the impact of stereotypes (Kunda & Thagard, 1996). One may question, however, whether the impact of stereotypes was muted because they were overpowered by behavioral evidence or because people were simply reluctant to use stereotypes so as to avoid appearing discriminatory (Bodenhausen et al., Chapter 13, this volume). Therefore, although these data show that stereotypes do not figure heavily in people's public evaluations of stereotyped individuals in the presence of individuating information about these individuals, it remains unclear whether this is because the impact of stereotypes is overpowered by the impact of behavior or because the impact of stereotypes is suppressed by efforts to provide socially desirable responses.

Note, though, that the same interpretive problems complicate the understanding of the central findings voiced in support of stereotype dominance—namely, that stereotypes figure more heavily in judgment when people's mental capacity is strained. For example, Bodenhausen (1990) argued that people rely more heavily on their stereotypes when tired than when alert because they fall back on the quick and easy stereotypic heuristics when they are tired. Alternatively, it may be that people censor and curtail their use of stereotypes as suggested by Bodenhausen et al. (Chapter 13, this volume) when they are capable of doing so—namely, when they are alert and have ample cognitive resources. When resources are drained by fatigue, such effortful stereotype inhibition breaks down, and stereotypes figure more heavily in judgment. Thus, cognitive load may result in more stereotypic judgments not because it disrupts the effortful use of individuating information, as is commonly assumed, but rather because it disrupts the effortful inhibition of stereotypes (cf. Devine, 1989). More subtle measures of stereotype activation and use are needed to shed light on these issues. Happily, the field appears to be moving toward focusing on such subtle measures.

In sum, the field may have been too quick to accept the conclusion that stereotypes dominate the impressions of disinterested observers; although it is conceivable that appropriately designed studies will ultimately support this position, no such studies exist yet. And it remains just as plausible that behavioral evidence exerts at least as much impact on impressions as do stereotypes. It is likely that stereotypes dominate impressions on some occasions if the stereotyped category is noticed before other information is observed or if it is especially strongly associated with a given trait. But it seems just as likely that behavior will dominate impressions on other occasions if it is noticed first or is especially strongly associated with a given trait. Most likely, the extent to which an observation about a person—be it membership in a stereotyped category, behavior, attire, or anything else—figures in one's impressions of that person depends not on the source of that information, but on the strength of its associations with other information and on whether it was observed before, after, or at the same time as other pertinent observations.

FUTURE DIRECTIONS

It is important to keep in perspective the remaining disagreements about how disinterested perceivers form impressions of personally irrelevant strangers. One should bear in mind that there appears to be little disagreement on how people form impressions of individuals who are relevant and important to them. Given the general agreement about how people form impressions of others who matter to them, we may be able to gain better insight into the motivated perceiver by pooling the strengths of the different models (cf. Fiske et al., Chapter 11, this volume). The parallel-constraint-satisfaction model assumes that all information that is observed at the same time will be considered and integrated simultaneously, and it provides a precise account of the mechanisms for integrating observed information. But it does not address the question of what determines which information will be noticed; although it seems likely that one can pick up many kinds of information at a glance, it also seems likely that one will typically not notice everything there is to notice about each person, and that different people may notice and respond to different aspects of the same individual. Fiske, Neuberg, and their colleagues (Fiske & Neuberg, 1990; Fiske et al. Chapter 11, this volume) make the important point that goals may often influence which information is noticed and may determine how much attention is allocated to each piece of information. Their research has focused predominantly on accuracy goals, and has suggested that one becomes motivated to view another person as accurately as possible when one is under this person's power or when one depends upon this person for important outcomes.

It is also important to explore whether other goals can influence which of an individual's many attributes may be activated and used on a given occasion. Devine's (1989) seminal article highlighted the potential role of one important goal—the motivation to avoid prejudice. There is some evidence that people so motivated do tend to engage in less stereotypic thinking (Monteith, 1993; Sherman & Gorkin, 1980), but little evidence that the motivation to avoid prejudice also reduces the activation of stereotypes and their application to stereotyped

individuals (for a review, see Bargh, Chapter 18, this volume).

Other goals, however, have been shown to provoke stereotype inhibition. One recent series of studies found that individuals motivated to think highly of a Black person (because this person had praised their performance) inhibited the stereotype of Black people which, if activated, might have cast doubts on this person's competence; they showed lower stereotype activation than did individuals who had received the same praise from a White person. Similarly, individuals motivated to discredit a Black doctor (because he had criticized them) inhibited the stereotype of doctors, which, if activated, might have boosted this person's credibility. Moreover, motivation was shown to influence which of the stereotypes applicable to a given individual was activated: People praised by a black doctor inhibited the stereotype of Blacks while activating the stereotype of doctors, whereas people criticized by the same Black doctor inhibited the stereotype of doctors while activating the stereotype of Blacks (Sinclair, 1998; Kunda & Sinclair, in press). A Black doctor may be viewed as a doctor after delivering praise, but as a Black person after delivering criticism. The finding that such directional goals may lead to the inhibition of the very level of stereotype activation holds the promise that the motivation to control prejudice may do the same.

Another area worth pursuing is the dynamic process of impression formation as it develops over time (Fiske et al., Chapter 11, this volume). Much of the research to date has focused on very brief, often subliminal, exposure to very sketchy information—a word or a photograph. Such research may capture what happens in the first moments of an encounter with a stereotyped individual. But what happens as the interaction continues? Recent studies suggest that stereotype activation may recede over time (Adams & Kunda, 1995). Participants watching a videotaped interview with a Black person showed increased activation of the stereotype of Black people when activation was assessed within 30 seconds of the start of the interview, but not when activation was assessed 12 minutes into the interview. Unfortunately, this does not mean that the stereotype of Black people will be put completely to rest as one gets to know a Black individual, because even after it has dissipated, this stereotype can still be re-activated in response to the stereotyped individual's behavior. Another study found that the no longer activated stereotype of Black people was reactivated in perceivers' minds when they discovered that the Black person they had been observing disagreed with them on an important issue (Davies, Kunda, & Spencer, 1998). It is of great interest to determine what other factors can provoke the resurrection of stereotypes that have already dissipated.

Regardless of one's theoretical perspective, exploring the dynamic nature of impression formation as it is shaped by perceivers' motives and as it evolves over time promises to be an exciting enterprise.

ACKNOWLEDGMENTS

Preparation of this chapter was supported by a grant from the Social Sciences and Humanities Research Council of Canada. I thank Shelly Chaiken, Steven Spencer, and Yaacov Trope for their comments on an earlier version of this chapter.

NOTE

1. To make this point, we (Kunda & Thagard, 1996) simulated the classic (Asch, 1946) experiment demonstrating that the order in which trait descriptors are presented can influence one's impressions of the described individual. Bodenhausen et al. (Chapter 13, this volume) contend that this is precisely the kind of situation where our model compels us to expect parallel rather than serial processing, because the traits are presented in "virtually immediate succession." I disagree. There is ample evidence that the automatic priming effects that are assumed to drive such disambiguation processes can take place within fractions of seconds (see, e.g., Blair & Banaji, 1996). An observation that precedes other observations by as little as a second or two can therefore carry disproportionate weight.

REFERENCES

Adams, B. D., & Kunda, Z. (1995). *Stereotypes recede over time.* Paper presented at the annual conference of the American Psychological Association, Toronto.

Asch, S. E. (1946). Forming impressions of personality. *Journal of Abnormal and Social Psychology, 41,* 303–314.

Asch, S. E. (1987). *Social psychology.* Oxford: Oxford University Press. (Original work published 1952)

Asch, S. E., & Zukier, H. (1984). Thinking about persons. *Journal of Personality and Social Psychology, 46,* 1230–1240.

Bargh, J. A., Chen, M., & Burrows, L. (1996). Automaticity of social behavior: Direct effects of trait construct and stereotype activation on action. *Journal of Personality and Social Psychology, 71,* 230–244.

Blair, I. V., & Banaji, M. R. (1996). Automatic and controlled processes in stereotype priming. *Journal of Personality and Social Psychology, 70,* 1142–1163.

Bodenhausen, G. V. (1990). Stereotypes as judgmental heuristics: Evidence of circadian variations in discrimination. *Psychological Science, 1,* 319–322.

Brewer, M. B. (1988). A dual process model of impression formation. In T. K. Srull & R. S. Wyer, Jr. (Eds.), *Advances in social cognition* (Vol. 1, pp. 1–36). Hillsdale, NJ: Erlbaum.

Chen, M., & Bargh, J. (1997). Nonconscious behavioral confirmation processes: The self-fulfilling consequences of automatic stereotype activation. *Journal of Experimental Social Psychology, 33,* 541–560.

Davies, P., Kunda, Z., & Spencer, S. (1998). *When individual differences turn into cultural divides: How conflicts affect stereotyping.* Paper presented at the annual conference of the American Psychological Society, Washington, DC.

Devine, P. G. (1989). Stereotypes and prejudice: Their automatic and controlled components. *Journal of Personality and Social Psychology, 56,* 5–18.

Fazio, R. H., Jackson, J. R., Dunton, B. C., & Williams, C. J. (1995). Variability in automatic activation as an unobtrusive measure of racial attitudes: A bona fide pipeline? *Journal of Personality and Social Psychology, 69,* 1013–1027.

Fiske, S. T., & Neuberg, S. L. (1990). A continuum of impression formation, from category-based to individuating processes: Influences of information and motivation on attention and interpretation. In M. P. Zanna (Ed.), *Advances in experimental social psychology* (Vol. 23, pp. 1–74). San Diego, CA: Academic Press.

Gilbert, D. T. (1989). Thinking lightly about others: Automatic components of the social inference process. In J. A. Bargh & J. S. Uleman (Eds.), *Unintended thought* (pp. 189–211). New York: Guilford Press.

Gilbert, D. T., Pelham, B. W., & Krull, D. S. (1988). On cognitive busyness: When person perceivers meet persons perceived. *Journal of Personality and Social Psychology, 54,* 733–740.

Kruglanski, A. W., & Freund, T. (1983). The freezing and unfreezing of lay-inferences: Effects on impressional primacy, ethnic stereotyping, and numerical anchoring. *Journal of Experimental Social Psychology, 19,* 448–468.

Kunda, Z., & Sinclair, L. (in press). Motivated reasoning with stereotypes: Activation, application, and inhibition. *Psychological Inquiry.*

Kunda, Z., & Thagard, P. (1996). Forming impressions from stereotypes, traits, and behaviors: A parallel-constraint-satisfaction theory. *Psychological Review, 103,* 284–308.

Monteith, M. J. (1993). Self-regulation of prejudiced responses: Implications for progress in prejudice-reduction efforts. *Journal of Personality and Social Psychology, 65,* 469–485.

Pendry, L. F., & Macrae, N. (1994). Stereotypes and mental life: The case of the motivated but thwarted tactician. *Journal of Experimental Social Psychology, 30,* 303–325.

Read, S. J., & Miller, L. C. (1993). Rapist or "regular guy": Explanatory coherence in the construction of mental models of others. *Personality and Social Psychology Bulletin, 19,* 526–541.

Sherman, J. W. (1996). Development and mental representation of stereotypes. *Journal of Personality and Social Psychology, 70,* 1126–1141.

Sherman, S. J., & Gorkin, L. (1980). Attitude bolstering when behavior is inconsistent with central attitudes. *Journal of Experimental Social Psychology, 16,* 388–403.

Sinclair, L. M. (1998). *Justifying desired impressions of evaluators: Motivated activation, application, and inhibition of stereotypes.* Unpublished doctoral dissertation, University of Waterloo, Ontario, Canada.

Thagard, P. (1989). Explanatory coherence. *Behavioral and Brain Sciences, 12,* 435–467.

Trope, Y. (1986). Identification and inferential processes in dispositional attribution. *Psychological Review, 93,* 239–257.

Trope, Y., & Thompson, E. P. (1997). Looking for truth in all the wrong places?: Asymmetric search of individuating information about stereotyped group members. *Journal of Personality and Social Psychology, 73,* 229–241.

Uleman, J. S., Newman, L. S., & Moskowitz, G. B. (1996). People as flexible interpreters: Evidence and issues from spontaneous trait inference. In M. P. Zanna (Ed.), *Advances in experimental social psychology* (Vol. 28, pp. 211–279). San Diego, CA: Academic Press.

16

Associative and Rule-Based Processing

A CONNECTIONIST INTERPRETATION
OF DUAL-PROCESS MODELS

ELIOT R. SMITH
JAMIE DeCOSTER

As the other chapters in this volume demonstrate, dual-process models offer powerful accounts for empirical phenomena in several areas of social psychology, including such core topics as processing persuasive messages and forming impressions of other people. Our goals in this chapter are, first, to point out some of the most important common features shared by these existing models; and, second, to describe in general terms how these models may be integrated within a new connectionist framework. We believe that this novel conceptualization can account for the broad patterns of empirical findings in different content domains, bringing them under a common umbrella and potentially highlighting previously unrecognized parallels. We also believe that our model not only yields important new insights in many of these domains, but opens up new topics for investigation. Although connectionist models have been widely applied in cognitive, developmental, and other areas of psychology, they are only beginning to be investigated within social psychology. Examination of the implications of connectionism for dual-process theories, which are some of the best-developed theories in all of

social psychology, should provide an example of the power and potential fruitfulness of connectionist models for our field.

COMMON FEATURES
OF DUAL-PROCESS MODELS

Dual-process models have been advanced in numerous specific areas of social psychology and cognitive psychology (see Epstein and Pacini, Chapter 23, this volume, or Abelson, 1994, for lists). Many of these models (though not all models using the term "dual-process," some of which rest on different distinctions) share central features and, we will argue, amount to only minor variations on a common set of themes. Using Chaiken's (1980) model as an example, we contend that these models all share three basic assumptions:

1. One type of processing involves the use of simple, well-learned, and readily accessible decision rules, such as "Experts are always right," "The majority is correct," or "Statistics don't lie." This type of low-effort processing (termed "heuristic" by Chaiken) is

the default processing mode; people will process in this way unless special circumstances intervene.

2. People can also perform a second type of processing, termed "systematic" by Chaiken. This involves the active, effortful scrutiny of all relevant information, and therefore demands considerable cognitive capacity. For example, people may evaluate arguments by considering their logical coherence or by comparing them to existing knowledge. Systematic processing (compared to heuristic) leads to attitude change that is more enduring and more resistant to further persuasion attempts. When it occurs, systematic processing takes place simultaneously with, and in addition to (rather than replacing), heuristic processing.

3. When will systematic processing take place? As described by Chen and Chaiken (Chapter 4, this volume), a person may have any of several goals activated in a given situation: to form valid attitudes that will accurately guide thought and action; to defend currently held attitudes that are congruent with the person's interests or important self-definitions; or to hold attitudes and beliefs that will serve current social goals (such as creating a positive impression on others). People process systematically to the extent that they (a) feel an unusually great need to be accurate, to defend an attitude, or to create a positive impression; and (b) have enough time and cognitive capacity to permit more effortful processing.

Chaiken's model and virtually all of the dual-process models described in this book share similar assumptions about the nature of low-effort processing, the nature of more effortful processing, and the conditions (particularly cognitive capacity and motivation) that determine which type of processing is used. (For more detailed discussion of the parallels among a subset of these models, see Smith, 1994.) The models do differ in some details—particularly in whether the two types of processing operate simultaneously (as Chaiken assumes), in sequence, or as alternatives, and in whether motivational or capacity determinants of more effortful processing are emphasized. Still, the similarities are more important than these detailed differences among the models.

One additional dual-process model also shares the same general assumptions. We briefly describe it here, because it is not otherwise represented in this volume, but is important for its coverage of a distinct set of topics and for its background in cognitive rather than social psychology. In addition, we adopt this model's terminology because the terms seem most descriptive of the two basic processing modes.

Sloman (1996) has outlined a two-process model of reasoning and problem solving, though without citing any of the social-psychological work represented in this volume except for Epstein's. His two processes are labeled "associative" and "rule-based." Associative processing is quick, intuitive, and relatively effortless. It involves the retrieval of information that has become associated with currently available cues. Associations are structured by similarity and patterns of temporal co-occurrence, rather than by logic. Thus, in the associative mode people use concepts that are related through well-learned associations to cues found in a problem or stimulus. In the area of categorization, this process gives rise to similarity-based categorization, whether based on previously learned category exemplars or on abstract prototypes.

In contrast, rule-based processing involves the use of symbolically represented rules to manipulate problems and derive solutions. The laws of logic and causal inference, rather than simple associations, are brought to bear. These rules are abstract, incorporating variables that can be bound to specific contents. Importantly, this mode is assumed to make use of explicit symbolic representations of rules in the course of processing; it *uses* or *follows* rules (Sloman, 1996), explicitly representing them and using them to guide processing. This contrasts with simply *conforming* to rules or exhibiting behavior that can be described by rules, in the sense that a thrown ball conforms to the law of gravity. Rule-based processing underlies theory-based categorization, including the occasions when a theory overrides similarity-based categorization.

Sloman holds that in general the two modes work together, not as alternatives. Sometimes the two modes provide different answers; in other cases they work more cooperatively. For example, in proving a mathematical theorem, one "sees" intuitively what step is needed next and then uses symbolic rules to check that the proposed step actually works.

Table 16.1 summarizes the common points of several dual-process models to illustrate what we see as their essential similarity. These models all fit an outline like the following.

Associative Mode

The fundamental process involved in the associative mode of processing is the automatic access from memory, based on a cue that is salient in the current stimulus or context, of knowledge or affective reactions that have become associated with that cue. The learning of such an association is assumed to take repeated experiences over a long time—a point on which Devine (1989), Fazio (1986), and Sloman (1996) are particularly clear. Activation of the knowledge is automatic and preconscious, so that it becomes subjectively part of the stimulus information (rather than being seen as part of the perceiver's own evaluation or interpretation of it). This emphasis is perhaps clearest in Fazio's (1986) and Epstein's (1991) models. The associated knowledge, once activated, has the potential to affect judgments and behavior.

Using this mode, people automatically access such things as their well-learned attitudes toward specific attitude objects (Fazio, 1986); stereotypes that are culturally associated with particular social groups (Devine, 1989; Brewer, 1988; Fiske & Neuberg, 1990);

TABLE 16.1. Summary of Key Points of Existing Dual-Process Models

Model and domain of application	Terminology and properties of low-effort processing mode	Terminology and properties of high-effort processing mode	Assumptions about relations between processing modes
Chaiken (1980); Petty & Cacioppo (1981): Persuasion	Heuristic: Use learned associations of salient cues (e.g., source attractiveness or message length) with positive–negative evaluations.	Systematic: Effortfully search for relevant information and logically evaluate arguments.	Systematic processing occurs when need for subjective confidence is especially high and processing resources are available. Both modes occur simultaneously.
Fazio (1986): Attitude access	Associative: Use evaluation associated with attitude object through repeated pairings.	Construct attitude: Search for and summarize attitudinally relevant information.	Associative processing occurs when strongly associated attitude exists. Modes are alternatives.
Brewer (1988); Fiske & Neuberg (1990): Person perception	Categorization: Use information and evaluations associated with person's salient category membership (gender, race, etc.).	Individuation: Process and summarize multiple individual characteristics.	Individuation requires specific motivation (e.g., due to interdependence) or perceived lack of fit to category. Modes are alternatives.
Gilbert (1989): Person perception, attributional inference	Correspondent inference: Use trait associated (through semantic similarity) with person's observed behaviors.	Attributional thinking: Process range of attributionally relevant information, such as situational causes of behavior.	Attributional thinking requires cognitive capacity. Modes are sequential stages; attribution follows correspondent inference.
Trope & Gaunt (Chapter 8, this volume): Attributional inference	Assimilative identification: Use context automatically to help identify behaviors.	Diagnostic evaluation: Consider context as potential alternative explanation for behavior.	Context always affects judgment, but diagnostic evaluation requires motivation and capacity.

concepts that suggest particular solutions to reasoning or categorization problems (Sloman, 1996); traits that are related to observed behaviors performed by oneself or others (Bem, 1967; Gilbert, 1989); associations with the situational context to aid in the identification of behaviors (Trope & Gaunt, Chapter 8, this volume); or favorable or unfavorable evaluations of persuasive messages based on easily noticed cues, such as message length or source attractiveness (Chaiken, 1980; Petty & Cacioppo, 1981). Once accessed, these knowledge structures, often with an affective or emotional tinge, can affect people's thoughts, feelings, or overt behaviors.

Rule-Based Mode

In general, these dual-process models assume that rule-based processing is consciously controlled and effortful, involving search, retrieval, and use of task-relevant information (see Petty & Cacioppo, 1981; Sloman, 1996; or Fiske & Neuberg, 1990). The "rules" that govern processing in this mode range from formal or normative rules (like those of logic) to informal maxims (e.g., "Consider people as unique individuals, rather than just stereotyping them"). Rule-based processing is assumed to be strategic, and its exact nature will vary depending on the specifics of the task, the individual's goals, and situational constraints. When it occurs, this type of processing generally gives rise to a higher level of perceived validity and to longer-lasting effects (Chaiken, Liberman, & Eagly, 1989).

Using this mode, people may consider the details of persuasive arguments and evaluate their validity on the basis of logic and general knowledge (Chaiken, 1980; Petty & Cacioppo, 1981); use logical or mathematical reasoning to solve problems (Sloman, 1996); engage in attributional thinking to determine the causes of their own or others' behaviors (Gilbert, 1989; Trope & Gaunt, Chapter 8, this volume); summarize a number of known facts about a person or object into an individuated impression or attitude (Brewer, 1988; Fiske & Neuberg, 1990; Fazio, 1986); or effortfully override automatically generated judgments with alternative responses deemed more appropriate (Martin, Seta, & Crelia, 1990; Devine, 1989).

Relations between Modes

The dual-process models outlined above generally agree on the characterizations of the two processing modes themselves. However, differences among the models are more evident in their accounts of the relations between the processing modes. First, the models differ somewhat in their emphasis on the role of motivation versus cognitive capacity in determining how people process. Several models put greater stress on motivation, though they make varying assumptions about the specific nature of the relevant motives (Brewer, 1990; Fiske & Neuberg, 1988; Fazio, 1986). Other models emphasize factors affecting cognitive capacity, whether in the form of time pressure, distraction from external stimuli or simultaneous tasks, or resources such as task-relevant background knowledge (Gilbert, 1989; Sloman, 1996; Trope & Gaunt, Chapter 8, this volume). Still other models give relatively equal weight to motivation and ability (Chaiken, 1980; Petty & Cacioppo, 1981; Martin et al., 1990; Devine, 1989). Despite differences in emphasis, all these dual-process theorists would presumably agree that both capacity and motivation are in fact required.

The theories also differ somewhat in their account of the temporal and logical relationships between the two processing modes. Some models hold that the two are alternatives—that people process either one way or the other, but not both (Petty & Cacioppo, 1981; Fazio, 1986; Brewer, 1988). Other models assume sequential processing, with automatic associative processing occurring first and rule-based processing optionally following (Fiske & Neuberg, 1990; Gilbert, 1989; Martin et al., 1990; Wegener & Petty, 1995; Devine, 1989). Still other theories hold that both processing modes occur simultaneously (Chaiken, 1980; Sloman, 1996; Epstein, 1991). In this case their effects may be additive (if they lead to the same conclusions), or associative processing may bias ongoing rule-based processing, or the two modes may work in opposition (see Chen & Chaiken, Chapter 4, this volume).

NEW DUAL-PROCESSING MODEL

With this overview of the models' similarities as background, we now present a new connectionist-inspired dual-processing model that is intended to integrate these specific theories. In this section, we first present the structural basis of the two processing modes— two memory systems with systematically different properties. Then we describe how the associative and rule-based processing modes use each of these systems.

Dual Memory Systems

In recent years, theorists have advanced generally similar proposals focused on the idea that humans have two separate memory systems with distinct properties (Alvarez & Squire, 1994; Milner, 1989; Murre, 1995; see Schacter & Tulving, 1994, for additional discussion). A major article by McClelland, Mc-Naughton, and O'Reilly (1995) presents one such proposal on which we will focus. As a rationale for their theory, the authors argue that human memory must meet two conflicting demands that are functionally incompatible. One demand is to record information slowly and incrementally, so that the total configuration in memory reflects a large sample of experiences. This is important so that general expectancies and long-term organized knowledge can be based on the average, typical properties of the environment. This slow-learning memory system matches the typical properties assumed for schemas in social and cognitive theories (see Fiske & Taylor, 1991; Rumelhart, Smolensky, McClelland, & Hington, 1986). A second demand is for rapid learning of new information, so that a novel experience can be remembered after a single occurrence. After all, people can at least sometimes learn things after hearing them once.

As a solution to this problem, McClelland et al. (1995) propose that these demands are handled by independent "slow-learning" and "fast-binding" memory systems.[1] This idea may seem unparsimonious, but many types of psychological and neuro-psychological evidence, described in detail in McClelland et al. (1995), point to the existence of two memory systems with the postulated properties. For example, this model makes sense of the patterns of memory impairment exhibited by patients with damage in specific brain areas (Squire, 1992).

McClelland et al. (1995) hold that the slow-learning system learns only gradually and incrementally with experience, and is more automatic and less sensitive to the allocation of conscious attention. In contrast, the fast-binding system learns rapidly in order to acquire new memories quickly. The latter system is responsible for one-shot learning, particularly about novel and unexpected events and stimuli, in a way that depends on selective attention and thus on conscious awareness.

The two systems interact in several ways. One key process is "consolidation," by which a newly formed memory is transferred by repeated presentations from the fast-binding to the slow-learning system. Consolidation is known, on independent grounds, to take considerable time in humans (weeks to years), and the authors suggest that it is necessarily slow so that new knowledge can be integrated into the stably structured representations maintained in the slow-learning system without disrupting previous knowledge.

Thus, one memory system is responsible for learning stable, general representations of the typical properties of the environment (i.e., schematas) and using them preconsciously to interpret new information by categorizing, filling in unobserved details, and the like. The other system is responsible for constructing new representations (i.e., episodic memories) that bind together information about different aspects of an object or experience in its context (Wiles & Humphreys, 1993). This second system seems to mediate conscious, explicit recollection. In addition to differences in speed and conscious accessibility, McClelland et al. (1995) hold that the two systems differ in the type of information to which they attend. The slow-learning system is chiefly concerned with regularities, so it primarily records what is typical and expected. In contrast, the fast-binding system records the details of events that are novel and interesting; it attends more to the unexpected and unpredicted.

Dual Modes of Processing

Our model of two processing modes has similarities to an earlier formulation by Smolensky (1988). It also draws heavily on the evidence regarding dual modes of processing in many areas of social and cognitive psychology (reviewed earlier), as well as the recent evidence and theorizing (just discussed) regarding the properties of two memory systems. In brief, we believe that the associative processing mode is based directly on the properties of the slow-learning system and operates essentially as a pattern completion mechanism. After knowledge has been accumulated from a large number of experiences, this memory system can quickly and automatically fill in information about characteristics that have previously been observed or affective reactions that have previously been experienced in situations that resemble the current one.

The rule-based processing mode uses symbolically represented and culturally transmitted knowledge as its "program" (Smolensky, 1988). It rests on human linguistic abilities, which in turn draw on both underlying memory systems. The slow-learning system is needed to store long-term, stable knowledge (e.g., knowledge of the meanings of words), while the fast-binding system is crucial for its ability to construct and store new structures rapidly (e.g., building a representation of the meaning of a sentence as it is comprehended).

*Properties of the Associative
Processing Mode*

Associative processing takes the form of pattern completion or similarity-based retrieval in a connectionist schematic memory. This mode provides information both quickly and automatically. Associative processing operates preconsciously (Bargh, 1994); we are generally only aware of the results of this processing, not of its performance. The associative mode generates what are experienced as intuitive and affective responses to objects or events. We may look at a mug and know that it is used to hold coffee, or we may look at a friend and feel warmth and affection.

Associative processing is reproductive rather than productive; it uses currently available cues to retrieve representations stored on past occasions when similar cues were present. Through associative processing, information that has been repeatedly linked to an object in the past is automatically brought to mind whenever we perceive or think about the object again. This information can fill in

unobserved details or can even change the way we perceive existing features of an object. The term "association" may suggest a learned connection between two items or concepts, as when people study word pairs such as "table–blue" in a paired-associates learning task and then try to recall one word, given the other as a cue. However, associative processing is better regarded as performing a *pattern completion* function. An associative memory system can learn an entire set of characteristics that frequently co-occur, such as the visual appearance of a hammer, its name, the actions one performs with it, one's emotional reactions to it, and so on. This entire configuration can then be retrieved or reconstructed when a subset of the characteristics (say, just the name) is again encountered; the complete pattern is brought forth from a sufficiently distinctive part.

Associative processing uses general, overall similarity between the cues and stored memory representations as the basis for retrieval. Past knowledge can be used because of superficial or irrelevant similarities to the current cues, rather than only for structurally important or logical reasons (see Gilovich, 1981, and Lewicki, 1985, for social-psychological demonstrations of this property).

As described here, associative processing is a natural result of the operations of a connectionist memory system. Recurrent-network models are especially well suited to the task. Using appropriate connectionist learning rules, recurrent networks can construct representations of the "typical" properties of a set of input patterns. When a novel input pattern is then presented, the network's state will evolve over time into the previously learned pattern that the input most closely resembles (McClelland & Rumelhart, 1986). Technically, the learned configuration acts as an attractor state of the network's activity (McClelland & Rumelhart, 1986; Smith, 1996). An associative processor thus uses the new stimuli as cues and can access its memory to fill in unobserved details or even to correct expectation-inconsistent information. Elsewhere (Smith & DeCoster, 1998), we demonstrate that a recurrent connectionist network can function in this way—for example, by learning a "group stereotype" (the typical properties of a set of stimuli) from exposure to input patterns representing a number of specific group members. When given a new member of the same group, the network infers that this individual possesses the group's typical characteristics.

Properties of the Rule-Based Processing Mode

The defining feature of rule-based processing is that it uses symbolically represented knowledge as rules to guide processing. Unlike a data base of associative knowledge that must be built up over a long period of time, symbolic knowledge can be rapidly learned from a single experience. Symbolic knowledge can then be used as rules to guide inferences and judgments—in other words, as the "program" for rule-based processing. This interpretive process is necessarily sequential and relatively slow (in contrast to the fast parallel-constraint-satisfaction process that can be used with associative knowledge representations). The reason is that only one rule can be explicitly used to guide processing at a time.

Symbolic rules may be socially learned, by comprehending language input from other individuals, the mass media, or other cultural sources. We humans do not have the ability to directly transmit what we think or experience to each other, so we must choose commonly accepted symbols (words) to express ourselves. Each time that we talk to another person, we have to fit what we want to say into words. Most knowledge shared between individuals therefore exists in symbolic form. Symbolic rules may also be constructed through explicit, conscious thought by an individual, rather than being socially learned. In either case, we can learn symbolic information after just a single exposure. The process of learning, however, requires conscious attention and can be strategically directed and controlled—in contrast to learning in the associative memory system, which is more automatic and less dependent on attention.

Because the rule-based processing mode rests on culturally shared rules, its results have greater perceived validity (Smolensky, 1988). We are more likely to trust a statement made by someone when it is based on logical reasoning than when it is based on intuition. It is the wide sharing of the rules of logical inference that generates this feeling of validity (Levine, Resnick, & Higgins, 1993). Ultimately, validity stems from consensus. When many of us agree on a rule or on a conclusion generated by applying shared rules, we tend to attribute the agreement to objective reality rather than to possible errors or misinterpretations made by the individuals concerned.

We have stated earlier that associative processing rests directly on the properties of the slow-learning system and can be easily modeled with standard and well-understood types of connectionist networks. In contrast, connectionist models of symbolic processing, which underlie the rule-based system, have been the subject of great controversy to date. Some early models were naive and inadequate in various ways, and elicited vigorous criticism. Critics even claimed that the failings of these models demonstrated that in principle connectionist networks cannot account for human linguistic abilities (e.g., Pinker & Prince, 1988). However, modern work is gradually remedying many of the earlier theories' defects. A full connectionist account of symbolic processing is clearly not yet at hand, but strides are being made in this direction (see Seidenberg, 1997, for a review).

Fundamental Differences between the Two Processing Modes

This model embodies the assumption that the two processing modes tap separate data bases representing knowledge in distinct formats. The associative mode draws solely on links between features built up over time in the slow-learning memory system. Rule-based processing, while it also makes use of the slow-learning memory system for the storage of long-term knowledge of word meanings and the like, also uses the fast-binding memory for holding symbolically encoded propositions and other linguistic materials. Many dual-process models within social psychology, while recognizing that the two processing modes differ in efficiency, automaticity, and conscious awareness, nevertheless have held that both forms of processing are of essentially the same kind. For example, both have been thought of as "schematic processing" in more and less efficient versions (see Fiske & Taylor, 1991). From our perspective, the two modes differ much more fundamentally. The two processing modes are not accurately characterized as involving just "more or less extensive processing"; rather, they embody qualitatively different types of processing (but see Kruglanski, Thompson, & Spiegel, Chapter 14, this volume, for a different view).

Each processing mode has its own strengths. Associative processing provides useful information, including evaluations and affective reactions, very quickly and without much attention from the perceiver. Because this type of processing relies on similar past experiences, knowledge can easily be used to make judgments about new objects. The system can also learn to operate in any environment; given enough experience, an associative processor can extract useful information about an environment simply through exposure to its regularities. Rule-based processing is useful because it can retain information after a single exposure. It also allows knowledge to be transmitted from one individual to another, and ultimately provides a format for the long-term external storage of data in the form of cultural traditions and written documents. The social sharing of knowledge allows for the creation of standardized systems of information, allowing people to answer questions in ways that can generally be seen as true within delimited cultural groups.

Alternative, Sequential, or Simultaneous Processing?

Like Chaiken (1980), Epstein (1991), and Sloman (1996), we assume that the two processing modes generally operate simultaneously rather than as alternatives or in sequence. However, because rule-based processing is assumed to be slower than associative processing, it may be argued that both processing modes operate initially but then the fast associative processing finishes, leaving only rule-based processing. Such a partial-overlap model would be difficult to distinguish empirically from a pure sequential model in which first associative processing and then rule-based processing take place, without any overlap. In terms of our model, both partial overlap and sequential processing seem unlikely. True, rule-based processing is relatively slow, but as rule applications generate new concepts and representations, those will elicit associative retrieval

from the slow-learning memory system. In other words, the relative automaticity of associative processing means that it will continue to operate, rather than ceasing before rule-based processing begins (in the sequential model) or is completed (in the partial-overlap model). In support of this interpretation, Chen and Chaiken (Chapter 4, this volume) have found evidence of the ongoing impact of associative processing during persuasion.

Roles of Motivation and Capacity in Determining Processing

In many cases, associative and rule-based processing will arrive at the same answer. This can occur, for instance, when people originally use a symbolic rule but over time learn to produce the same response associatively (e.g., Logan, 1988). However, there will also be times when the two modes produce different responses. In fact, Sloman (1996) treats this type of "simultaneous contradictory belief" as a key criterion for demonstrating two independent processing systems. For example, in certain types of logic puzzles, two different answers seem appealing (though for different reasons). Conflicting answers arising from the two systems have also been extensively investigated in the domain of persuasion, where a message may be constructed that contains strong or weak arguments, together with cues that lead people to agree or disagree with it through well-learned associations (Chaiken, 1980). A message containing weak arguments, for example, may be presented by an attractive or an expert source. When the two modes tend to give different responses, what factors affect the way people weight them and arrive at an overall response? The dual-process models reviewed earlier point to motivation and capacity as key factors.

As we have outlined earlier in this chapter, using the rule-based system is subjectively effortful, requiring attentional resources. Thus, if people are not motivated to use rules, the response will generally be controlled by the relatively effortless associative system. Several distinct motives may spur rule-based processing. Perhaps the most obvious of these is a desire for accuracy. The socially shared and subjectively valid nature of rule-based processing means that people believe it provides more accurate answers than low-effort associative processing (Chaiken et al., 1989). However, other motives can also encourage rule-based processing. Chen and Chaiken (Chapter 4, this volume) discuss the processing effects of motivation to defend important existing beliefs or attitudes, or to meet important social goals such as creating a positive impression on others. Note that rule-based processing driven by these motives may not be evenhanded and unbiased; in fact, it may decrease (rather than increase) the accuracy of overall conclusions, compared to the results of associative processing.

Cognitive capacity as well as motivation is required for rule-based processing. "Capacity" refers to available processing time as well as attentional resources. Rule-based processing generally takes longer than the associative system to operate (Logan, 1988), and because it requires attention, it is more subject to disruption by distraction or interference. Thus, responses that are made quickly or when the perceiver is busy or distracted are likely to be controlled by the associative system. However, given adequate time and freedom from distraction, rule- based responses (because of their greater subjective validity) may override associative responses (Chaiken et al., 1989).

Implications for Specific Topic Areas

The unified conceptualization presented here has implications for several prominent dual-process theories within social psychology. These are briefly described here, followed by a few additional implications for significant research issues within social psychology.

Chaiken's Dual-Process Model of Persuasion

Chaiken's (1980) model is closely aligned with our perspective in most ways. For example, it assumes that the two modes operate simultaneously, and it takes a broad view of the potential motives that can encourage systematic processing. One terminological difference is Chaiken's use of the term "simple decision rules" or "heuristics" to describe the representations that guide processing in the heuristic or associative mode. The term "rule" should probably be avoided in this context, for a key assumption of the current model is that associations and rules are quite different. If the representations used in heuristic processing were described as "well-learned associations" rather than as "rules," the distinction would be clearer.

Petty and Cacioppo's Dual-Process Model of Persuasion

Petty and Cacioppo's (1981) model overlaps greatly with Chaiken's, as numerous reviews have observed. One key difference is that the central and peripheral processing modes are characterized as endpoints of a processing continuum, and thus effectively as alternatives. Instead, from the perspective of our theory, the two processing modes can operate simultaneously (as in Chaiken's model). Another difference is the model's general emphasis on accuracy motivation as the driving force behind effortful processing.

Fazio's Model of Attitude Access

The two postulated modes of attitude access in Fazio's (1986) model (i.e., using a well-learned association vs. effortfully retrieving relevant information and constructing an attitude) probably operate simultaneously instead of as alternatives. Thus, a previously formed attitude may be associatively retrieved and bias a simultaneously occurring search for further information. Also, this model has emphasized the capacity requirements of the effortful attitude construction process, but we should note that motivation is also required.

Models of Categorization and Individuation in Person Perception

The models of Brewer (1988) and Fiske and Neuberg (1990) maintain that the two types of processing occur sequentially, with relatively effortless categorization preceding more effortful individuation. From the perspective of our model, the two forms of processing occur simultaneously.

Gilbert's Dual-Process Model of Person Perception

Gilbert's (1989) model holds that attributional reasoning may follow, and possibly correct, an initial correspondent inference. Gilbert's research emphasizes that the correction process requires more resources than does correspondent inference, though he has acknowledged that motivation is also required. From our perspective, however, the two processes occur simultaneously rather than in sequence.

Trope's Model of Attributional Inference

Trope and Gaunt's (Chapter 8, this volume) presentation is generally consistent with our model, although, like Gilbert (1989), they have focused more on the role of capacity than on that of motivation.

Martin's Dual-Process Model of Social Judgment and Correction

Martin's model (Martin et al., 1990) recognizes the requirements of both motivation and capacity to correct for automatically occurring judgmental effects. However, like Gilbert's two-stage model of person perception, it holds that the processes occur sequentially, whereas from our perspective simultaneous operation seems more likely.

Devine's Model of Stereotyping and Suppression

Exactly the same points may be made regarding Devine's (1989) model. Both motivation (stemming from guilty feelings about using stereotypes) and capacity are stressed, but automatic access to stereotypes and conscious suppression processes should probably be considered to occur simultaneously rather than sequentially.

Our proposal may also solve a puzzle that is implicit in Devine's theory. Her model (among others) assumes that people possess "implicit" beliefs (e.g., as group stereotypes) that contradict their "explicit" (i.e., verbalizable, consciously held) beliefs. How an assumed single memory system can represent both of these contradictory beliefs is not made clear. Under our model, stereotypes are represented by associations built up in a connectionist distributed memory, while explicit beliefs are symbolically represented; this solves the representational puzzle. The term "association" is probably clearer in cases like this than clumsy terms such as "implicit beliefs," because of the qualitative difference be-

tween associations and explicit symbolically represented beliefs.

Epstein's Cognitive–Experiential Self-Theory

Epstein's (1991) model generally fits well with the outlines of the model advanced here, except that he gives more attention to capacity than to the motivational determinants of rational processing. Epstein also emphasizes that the results of processing in the experiential mode (which we term "associative") are particularly subjectively compelling. We agree that in some cases, such as food preferences, experientially based reactions override rational responses. However, in general validity arises from social sharing, and therefore it is higher for the rational system (Levine et al., 1993). Moreover, reactions that are initially generated by the rule-based/rational system come over time to be embodied in associations. This process means that socially shared reactions will generally also have the phenomenologically "given" quality that the preconscious associative (or experiential) system affords. The idea "Spinach is good for you," originally derived from symbolic, socially shared knowledge, eventually becomes just as compelling and subjectively valid as the idea "Spinach tastes awful."

Sloman's Dual-Process Model of Reasoning

Sloman's (1996) model fits well with the one we advance here, except that (like Epstein) he emphasizes cognitive capacity, failing to discuss the necessity for motivation for rule-based processing.

Explanations for Various Dissociations

Besides its implications for existing dual-process models, our theory may also explain some frequently observed dissociations between measures that appear to be closely related. In general, the explanation involves the assumption that one measure taps the associative processing system (and therefore the contents of the slow-learning memory system), while the other measure is generated by rule-based processing.

For example, a well-known dissociation is commonly seen between judgment and explicit memory (usually recall) of the information upon which the judgment was based. A perceiver may encounter a mix of positive and negative information about a target person, and then may both report an overall evaluation of the person and attempt to recall the provided information. In many cases, the correlation between the judgment and the recalled information (weighted by its evaluative implications) is near zero (Hastie & Park, 1986). From the perspective of our model, the judgment reflects the net association of the target person with positivity or negativity—an association that is gradually built up "on-line" as the information is initially processed. Thus, this information is held in the slow- learning memory system. In contrast, explicit recall draws on the content of the fast-learning memory system. The typical dissociation is thus explained as a function of the considerable degree of independence between the two memory systems.

Another dissociation is often found between explicit memory and repetition priming. Having processed a particular stimulus in a particular way facilitates a repetition of that same processing for a long period of time (Tulving, Schacter, & Stark, 1982; Smith, Stewart, & Buttram, 1992). This facilitation is generally found to be independent of measures of explicit memory, such as the ability to recognize that the stimulus has been previously processed. We explain this dissociation by attributing repetition priming to small changes in connection weights in slow-learning memory, whereas explicit recall or recognition draws on the fast-learning memory system (see Schacter & Tulving, 1994; Wiles & Humphreys, 1993).

CONCLUSIONS

We would like to emphasize two main points based on our conceptualization of dual-process models within a connectionist framework.

First, this way of thinking makes it very clear that the two processing modes are qualitatively different, both in terms of the data bases on which they draw and in terms of their operating principles. The associative mode draws on representations that may be perceptual or affective in nature, that are not necessarily linguistically encoded, and that are structured and interrelated by the principles of association (i.e., similarity and contiguity). The representations are the substrate for an automatic, preconscious pattern completion mechanism. This "subconceptual" processing is context-sensitive and flexible, such that its operation cannot be fully captured by a conceptual-level description (Smolensky, 1988; Clark, 1993). In contrast, rule-based processing draws on symbolic representations, which are structured and interrelated by the laws of language and logic (Smolensky, 1988). Processing in this mode is sequential and generally accessible to consciousness.

The fundamental differences between the processing modes bear emphasis, because many current theories in social psychology assume that all mental representations are composed of conceptual-level or semantically meaningful units (schemas, or nodes joined by associative links). Therefore, both processing modes are assumed to draw on a common data base or memory store of representations. Two types of processing may be assumed to differ in speed, efficiency, and availability to conscious awareness, but nevertheless to follow basically the same principles. For example, effortless "heuristic" processing and conscious "systematic" processing may both be considered to involve the "application of schemas" to input information, with the schemas drawn from the same memory repository; the two types of processing may be thought to differ only in speed and efficiency. Or the two modes may be considered to involve simply "more extensive" or "less extensive" processing, with the processing assumed to be of the same sort in either case. We reject these views, as do other theorists who have pointed out the fundamental differences between the two processing modes (see especially Epstein & Pacini, Chapter 23, this volume; Sloman, 1996).

The second major point that we wish to emphasize is the value of the connectionist approach in providing theoretical integration. Integration does not mean that differences among specific dual-process models are to be ignored. Clearly, each of the models discussed in this volume involves a number of specific details, and each has been fine-tuned to account for empirical findings in its own topic domain. Our connectionist approach abstracts from that level of detail, though the details are important for understanding how people process persuasive messages, form attitudes, suppress stereotypes, and so on. However, we believe that putting the diverse models into a common framework provides new insights and ultimately will benefit theorists in each area by providing multiple sources of strong constraints. If the basic nature of the two processing modes is constant across all these empirical domains, then a theorist working in a particular area can directly make use of findings from other areas, drawing on a common framework that is supported not only by research in all those areas but also by more basic work in memory (e.g., McClelland et al., 1995) and cognitive science (e.g., Smolensky, 1988). In this way, theoretical integration promises to strengthen researchers' ability to elucidate the special and unique processes that operate in each particular area, not to blur all such distinctions.

This integrative approach should also encourage the application of dual-process models to additional areas of social and cognitive psychology. Within social psychology, for example, it is possible to imagine dual-process models of conflict in close relationships, or bystanders' decisions to intervene and offer help in emergencies, or stereotype change through intergroup contact. As an illustration, it may be reasonable to assume that stereotypes can sometimes change in a relatively automatic way through the gradual buildup of new associations over time, driven by repeated contacts with group members and observations of their counter-stereotypic attributes. Alternatively, stereotypes may change when people consciously and effortfully reflect on their stereotypes and the new evidence provided by contact to change their explicit, verbalizable beliefs, perhaps bringing attributional principles to bear (e.g., deciding that a group's stereotypic tendencies to criminality may reflect that group's poor economic standing because of prevalent societal discrimination). If researchers can draw on theories and research methods from other areas in which dual-process models have been applied, rapid progress may be made in understanding difficult issues in diverse domains such as stereotype change. For example, researchers can apply thought-listing tasks and/or distraction manipulations (which have often been used in persuasion studies) to clarify which type of process contributes to stereotype change under what conditions.

Theoretical integration represents an increasingly important trend in psychology. In the past, theories in social psychology were typically formulated for specific topic areas (e.g., attribution, attitude change, etc.) and used topic-specific theoretical constructs. As a result, such theories tended to be incommensurable and could not easily be placed within more comprehensive conceptual frameworks (see Smith, 1998). The social cognition movement of the 1970s and 1980s brought a strong trend toward increased integration within social psychology, as theories in various topic areas drew on a common conceptual vocabulary (of schemas, exemplars, prototypes, automatic and controlled processing, and the like; Devine, Hamilton, & Ostrom, 1994). This vocabulary was largely shared with cognitive psychology as well, so the integration went beyond the boundaries of social psychology. In important ways, the emergence of connectionism takes the same process one step further. Connectionist models are being used in many areas of psychology, including most notably cognitive psychology (Humphreys, Bain, & Pike, 1989), developmental psychology (Elman et al., 1996), and psycholinguistics (Seidenberg, 1997). Beyond psychology, the trend includes social anthropology (Hutchins, 1995), cognitive neuroscience (McClelland et al., 1995), and philosophy (Clark, 1997). These trends suggest that connectionism is particularly conducive to broadly integrative theorizing. Thus, to the extent that social psychologists participate in the development and testing of theoretical models that are framed in connectionist language, they will be participating in an integrative and cumulative enterprise that ultimately promises to unify psychology with several of its neighbor disciplines.

ACKNOWLEDGMENTS

Preparation of this chapter was made possible by National Institute of Mental Health Grants No. R01 MH46840 and No. K02 MH01178. Thanks to Shelly Chaiken, Leonel and Teresa Garcia-Marques, Dan Gilbert, Sarah Queller, Güaun Semin, Steve Sloman, and Janet Swim for helpful comments that contributed to this presentation of our ideas.

NOTE

1. Note that these proposed memory systems are not equivalent to short-term and long-term memory; both are long-term in nature. Most current models hold that short-term memory is not a separate store, but is the activated portion of information held in long-term memory.

REFERENCES

Abelson, R. P. (1994). A personal perspective on social cognition. In P. G. Devine, D. L. Hamilton, & T. M. Ostrom (Eds.), *Social cognition: Impact on social psychology* (pp. 15–37). San Diego, CA: Academic Press.

Alvarez, P., & Squire, L. R. (1994). Memory consolidation and the medial temporal lobe: A simple network model. *Proceedings of the National Academy of Sciences USA, 91,* 7041–7045.

Bargh, J. A. (1994). The four horsemen of automaticity: Awareness, intention, efficiency, and control in social cognition. In R. S. Wyer, Jr. & T. K. Srull (Eds.), *Handbook of social cognition* (2nd ed., Vol. 1, pp. 1–40). Hillsdale, NJ: Erlbaum.

Bem, D. J. (1967). Self-perception: An alternative interpretation of cognitive dissonance phenomena. *Psychological Review, 24,* 183–200.

Brewer, M. B. (1988). A dual process model of impression formation. In T. K. Srull & R. S. Wyer, Jr. (Eds.), *Advances in social cognition* (Vol. 1, pp. 1–36). Hillsdale, NJ: Erlbaum.

Chaiken, S. (1980). Heuristic versus systematic information processing and the use of source versus message cues in persuasion. *Journal of Personality and Social Psychology, 39,* 752–766.

Chaiken, S., Liberman, A., & Eagly, A. H. (1989). Heuristic and systematic information processing within and beyond the persuasion context. In J. S. Uleman & J. A. Bargh (Eds.), *Unintended thought* (pp. 212–252). New York: Guilford Press.

Clark, A. (1993). *Associative engines: Connectionism, concepts, and representational change.* Cambridge, MA: MIT Press.

Clark, A. (1997). *Being there: Putting brain, body, and world together again.* Cambridge, MA: MIT Press.

Devine, P. G. (1989). Stereotypes and prejudice: Their automatic and controlled components. *Journal of Personality and Social Psychology, 56,* 5–18.

Devine, P. G., Hamilton, D. L., & Ostrom, T. M. (Eds.). (1994). *Social cognition: Impact on social psychology.* San Diego, CA: Academic Press.

Elman, J. L., Bates, E. A., Johnson, M. H., Karmiloff-Smith, A., Parisi, D., & Plunkett, K. (1996). *Rethinking innateness.* Cambridge, MA: MIT Press.

Epstein, S. (1991). Cognitive–experiential self-theory: An integrative theory of personality. In R. Curtis (Ed.), *The relational self: Theoretical convergences of psychoanalysis and social psychology* (pp. 111–137). New York: Guilford Press.

Fazio, R. H. (1986). How do attitudes guide behavior? In R. M. Sorrentino & E. T. Higgins (Eds.), *Handbook of motivation and cognition: Foundations of social behavior* (Vol. 1, pp. 204–243). New York: Guilford Press.

Fiske, S. T., & Neuberg, S. L. (1990). A continuum of impression formation, from category-based to individuating processes: Influences of information and motivation on attention and interpretation. In M. P. Zanna (Ed.), *Advances in experimental social psychology* (Vol. 23, pp. 1–74). San Diego, CA: Academic Press.

Fiske, S. T., & Taylor, S. E. (1991). *Social cognition* (2nd ed.). New York: McGraw-Hill.

Gilbert, D. T. (1989). Thinking lightly about others: Automatic components of the social inference process. In J. S. Uleman & J. A. Bargh (Eds.), *Unintended thought* (pp. 189–211). New York: Guilford Press.

Gilovich, T. (1981). Seeing the past in the present: The effect of associations to familiar events on judgments and decisions. *Journal of Personality and Social Psychology, 40,* 797–807.

Hastie, R., & Park, B. (1986). The relationship between memory and judgment depends on whether the judgment task is memory-based or on-line. *Psychological Review, 93,* 258–268.

Humphreys, M. S., Bain, J. D., & Pike, R. (1989). Different ways to cue a coherent memory system: A theory for episodic, semantic, and procedural tasks. *Psychological Review, 96,* 208–233.

Hutchins, E. (1995). *Cognition in the wild.* Cambridge, MA: MIT Press.

Levine, J. M., Resnick, L. B., & Higgins, E. T. (1993). Social foundations of cognition. *Annual Review of Psychology, 44,* 585–612.

Lewicki, P. (1985). Nonconscious biasing effects of single instances of subsequent judgments. *Journal of Personality and Social Psychology, 48,* 563–574.

Logan, G. D. (1988). Toward an instance theory of automatization. *Psychological Review, 95,* 492–527.

Martin, L. L., Seta, J. J., & Crelia, R. A. (1990). Assimilation and contrast as a function of people's willingness and ability to expend effort in forming an impression. *Journal of Personality and Social Psychology, 59,* 27–37.

McClelland, J. L., McNaughton, B. L., & O'Reilly, R. C. (1995). Why there are complementary learning systems in the hippocampus and neocortex: Insights from the successes and failures of connectionist models of learning and memory. *Psychological Review, 102,* 419–457.

McClelland, J. L., & Rumelhart, D. E. (1986). A distributed model of human learning and memory. In J. L. McClelland & D. E. Rumelhart (Eds.), *Parallel distributed processing: Explorations in the microstructure of cognition* (Vol. 2, pp. 170–215). Cambridge, MA: MIT Press.

Milner, P. (1989). A cell assembly theory of hippocampal amnesia. *Neuropsychologia, 27,* 23–30.

Murre, J. (1995). Transfer of learning in backpropagation and in related neural network models. In J. P. Levy, D. Bairaktaris, J. A. Bullinaria, & P. Cairns (Eds.), *Connectionist models of memory and language* (pp. 73–94). London: UCL Press.

Petty, R. E., & Cacioppo, J. T. (1981). *Attitudes and persuasion: Classic and contemporary approaches.* Dubuque, IA: William C. Brown.

Pinker, S., & Prince, A. (1988). On language and connectionism: Analysis of a parallel distributed processing model of language acquisition. In S. Pinker & J. Mehler (Eds.), *Connections and symbols* (pp. 73–193). Cambridge, MA: MIT Press.

Rumelhart, D. E., Smolensky, P., McClelland, J. L., & Hinton, G. E. (1986). Schemata and sequential thought processes in PDP models. In J. L. McClelland & D. E. Rumelhart (Eds.), *Parallel distributed processing: Explorations in the microstructure of cognition* (Vol. 2, pp. 7– 57). Cambridge, MA: MIT Press.

Schacter, D. L., & Tulving, E. (Eds.). (1994). *Memory systems 1994.* Cambridge, MA: MIT Press.

Seidenberg, M. S. (1997). Language acquisition and use: Learning and applying probabilistic constraints. *Science, 275,* 1599–1603.

Sloman, S. A. (1996). The empirical case for two systems of reasoning. *Psychological Bulletin, 119,* 3–22.

Smith, E. R. (1994). Procedural knowledge and processing strategies in social cognition. In R. S. Wyer, Jr. & T. K. Srull (Eds.), *Handbook of social cognition* (2nd ed., Vol. 1, pp. 99–151). Hillsdale, NJ: Erlbaum.

Smith, E. R. (1996). What do connectionism and social psychology offer each other? *Journal of Personality and Social Psychology, 70,* 893–912.

Smith, E. R. (1998). Mental representation and memory. In D. Gilbert, S. Fiske, & G. Lindzey (Eds.), *Handbook of social psychology* (4th ed., Vol. 1, pp. 391–445). New York: McGraw-Hill.

Smith, E. R., & DeCoster, J. (1998). Knowledge acquisition, accessibility, and use in person perception and stereotyping: Simulation with a recurrent connectionist network. *Journal of Personality and Social Psychology, 74,* 21–35.

Smith, E. R., Stewart, T. L., & Buttram, R. T. (1992). Inferring a trait from a behavior has long-term, highly specific effects. *Journal of Personality and Social Psychology, 62,* 753–759.

Smolensky, P. (1988). On the proper treatment of connectionism. *Behavioral and Brain Sciences, 11,* 1–74.

Squire, L. R. (1992). Memory and the hippocampus: A synthesis from findings with rats, monkeys, and humans. *Psychological Review, 99,* 195–231.

Tulving, E., Schacter, D. L., & Stark, H. (1982). Priming effects in word-fragment completion are independent of recognition memory. *Journal of Experimental Psychology: Learning, Memory, and Cognition, 8,* 336–342.

Wegener, D. T., & Petty, R. E. (1995). Flexible correction processes in social judgment: The role of naive theories of correction for perceived bias. *Journal of Personality and Social Psychology, 68,* 36–51.

Wiles, J., & Humphreys, M. S. (1993). Using artificial neural nets to model implicit and explicit memory test performance. In P. Graf & M. E. J. Masson (Eds.), *Implicit memory: New directions in cognition, development, and neuropsychology* (pp. 141–165). Hillsdale, NJ: Erlbaum.

III

Issues of Cognitive Control
in Processing and Judgment

17

Automaticity and Control in Stereotyping

PATRICIA G. DEVINE
MARGO J. MONTEITH

Interest in the nature of the more or less intentional or rational processes in thought and behavior has a long and rich tradition in psychology. It formed, for example, the cornerstone of Freud's classic theorizing about the nature of personality. But interest in the fundamental nature of human thought was also of central concern to classic philosophers, whose continuing impact on modern-day psychological theorists is considerable (see Gilbert, 1991). Empirical efforts to examine the less intentional (unconscious) components of thought and behavior were often frustrated by the absence of methodologies that could reveal such influences. In the 1970s, however, great strides were made in cognitive psychology in terms of both theory and methods that made it possible to explore independently the influence of intentional (conscious) and unintentional (unconscious) components of human thought and behavior (Posner & Snyder, 1975; Shiffrin & Schneider, 1977; Neely, 1977). These efforts gave birth to dual-processing theories that distinguished between automatic and controlled information processing.

"Automatic processes" were initially defined as processes that occur without intention, effort, or awareness, and without interfering with other concurrent cognitive processes (Posner & Snyder, 1975; Shiffrin & Schneider, 1977; Jacoby, Lindsay, & Toth, 1992; Johnson & Hasher, 1987; Logan & Cowan, 1984). In short, they were thought to be involuntary and inescapable. "Controlled processes," in contrast, were defined as possessing the opposite qualities. Thus, they were considered to be intentional, to be under the individual's control, to be effortful, and to entail conscious awareness. Although controlled processes were thought to be capacity-limited, they were considered to be more flexible than automatic processes. Their intentionality and flexibility were believed to make them useful for decision making and the initiation of new behaviors.

Dual-processing theories led to important advances in the understanding of information processing generally, and had a major impact on cognitive psychologists. However, their impact was much more widespread, also influencing theory and research that were emerging at the interface of social and cognitive psychology. The insights of dual-process theories were quickly applied to a wide array of social-psychological phenomena that had previously been difficult to explain fully. Specifically, various aspects of social thought or behavior appeared to have unintended or automatic influences that extant theories were not equipped to explain. For example, the conditions under which highly credible sources influenced the persuasion process became clearer under the illumination of dual-process reasoning (Chaiken, 1987; Petty & Cacioppo, 1986). Similarly, the tendency to make dispositional attributions quickly and to correct later for possible situational influences has also been accounted for in terms of automatic processes that can be controlled only when sufficient cognitive capacity is available for the correction process (Gilbert, 1989; Trope & Alfieri, 1997). Indeed, the present volume provides strong testimony to the widespread and productive impact of conceptualizing many social-psychological phenomena in terms of their automatic and controlled components.

In the present chapter, we consider the distinction between automatic and controlled processes as it has been applied to stereotyping. It has long been assumed in the stereotyping literature that stereotypes play a central and pervasive role in social perception (Allport, 1954; Lippman, 1922). Stereotypes, it is frequently argued, ease the burden of the social perceiver in responding to a potentially overwhelming and complex social environment (see Hamilton & Sherman, 1994, for a review). Allport (1954, p. 21) suggested that "the mind tends to categorize environmental events in the 'grossest' manner compatible with action." The rationale for this suggestion is that such categorizations take little effort and facilitate adjustment to the environment. More contemporarily, Macrae, Milne, and Bodenhausen (1994, p. 37) have suggested that stereotypes "serve to simplify perception, judgment, and action. As energy saving devices, they spare perceivers the ordeal of responding to an almost incomprehensively complex social world." As such, stereotypes came to be viewed as cognitive structures that were automatically applied to members of stigmatized groups.

As early as 1954, Allport suggested that "It seems a safe generalization to say that an ethnic label arouses a stereotype which in turn leads to rejective behavior" (p. 333). Following in the tradition of Allport's (1954) classic writings, many theorists have assumed that stereotype activation automatically and inevitably follows when one comes in contact with a member of the stereotyped group (Brewer, 1988; Devine, 1989; Dovidio, Evans, & Tyler, 1986; Fiske & Neuberg, 1990).

Emerging from this type of analysis was the discouraging possibility that stereotype activation ultimately results in biased and prejudiced responses that are not amenable to control. That is, stereotype application was also assumed to be rather automatic. This type of reasoning led some to argue that prejudice is an inevitable consequence of these normal, even adaptive, categorization processes (Fox, 1992; cf. Billig, 1985). And, indeed, the research literature is replete with evidence that stereotypes often result in biased judgments of and behaviors toward targets of stereotypes (see Hamilton & Sherman, 1994, for a review).

Others, however, were more reluctant to accept the fatalism implied by the inevitability-of-prejudice conclusions. The inevitability-of-prejudice perspective functionally eliminates the possibility that the potentially destructive and biasing effects of stereotypes on social perception and behavior can be controlled or otherwise avoided. A review of the stereotyping literature reveals an ongoing tension between stereotypes' apparently adaptive functions in simplifying social perception and their potentially destructive and biasing effects. That is, however easily stereotypes are activated, there are many circumstances under which, and some social perceivers for whom, stereotype application is considered unacceptable.

Allport (1954) also anticipated that such quick categorizations may not always be compatible with a perceiver's goals, and thus anticipated more contemporary concerns over whether and how control over automatically activated stereotypes can be accomplished. According to Allport, perceivers will sometimes "put the brakes on their prejudices" (1954, p. 332). Increasing concern over the potentially destructive and biasing effects of stereotypes has motivated interest in identifying strategies to reduce or eliminate the pernicious impact of stereotypes on social thought and behavior. Indeed, a central assumption made by several theorists is that stereotypic thinking can be overridden under favorable conditions (i.e., that perceivers have the motivation and ability to "apply the brakes") (Devine, 1989; Fiske, 1989; Higgins & King, 1981; Kruglanski & Freund, 1983; Jamieson & Zanna, 1989; but see Bargh, Chapter 18, this volume; Wilson & Brekke, 1994).

Fiske (1989, p. 277) noted, for example, that "The idea that categorization is a natural and adaptive, even dominant, way of understanding other people does not mean that it is the only option available." Concern over assumptions that prejudice may be an inevitable consequence of ordinary thought processes is a key component of the contemporary leading models of person perception processing (Brewer, 1988; Brewer & Harasty, Chapter 12, this volume; Fiske & Neuberg, 1990; Fiske, Lin, & Neuberg, Chapter 11, this volume). These models contend that social perceivers categorize or stereotype others initially, but *can* avoid stereotypic biases by replacing such categorical processing with more individuated processing. This more controlled, intentional type of processing is only likely to occur, however, when sufficient motivation and ability are present. Thus, in such models, stereotyping is the quickly and effortlessly applied default process, which precedes any conscious, goal-driven processes. Such efficient processing can only be corrected or nullified, according to these models, by more careful, elaborated processing. These types of conceptualizations paved the way for social psychologists to think of stereotype activation and the use of stereotypes in terms of their automatic and controlled components (e.g., Devine, 1989). Specifically, in the stereotyping context, these dual processes have been conceptualized as involving relatively nonthoughtful, effortless categorization processes on the one hand, and relatively thoughtful, effortful correction processes on the other.

The importance of exploring the role of automatic and controlled processes in stereotyping stems from both theoretical and practical considerations. Theoretically, it is of interest to understand the conditions under which stereotypes are and are not activated, and the ways in which control over stereotype activation and application can be achieved. Practically, understanding the possible controllability of stereotype activation and use has implications for a variety of social and interpersonal settings in which stereotypes can have serious and pernicious consequences, particularly for those who are the objects of stereotypes (Fiske, 1989; Jones, Farina, Hastorf, Markus, & Scott, 1984). Dual-process conceptions of stereotype activation

and use (or control over use) have witnessed an explosion of research activity in the recent years (e.g., Blair & Banaji, 1996; Devine, 1989; Devine & Elliot, 1995; Dovidio, Kawakami, Johnson, Johnson, & Howard, 1997; Fazio, Jackson, Dunton, & Williams, 1995; Gilbert & Hixon, 1991; Sinclair & Kunda, 1997). There is little doubt that the research investigating automatic and controlled processes related to stereotype activation and use has been productive. Indeed, in the last decade progress has been made quickly. In reviewing this progress, we believe that the time is ripe for reflecting on what has been learned, as well as for considering issues in need of additional theoretical and empirical attention.

Our main goal in this chapter is to review what has been learned about the automatic and controlled processes involved in stereotype activation and use. In addition, we hope to identify areas in which our knowledge is still rather preliminary, and thus to highlight some productive avenues for future research. As reflected in what follows, the dual-process approach to the study of stereotypes has been guided by several important and interrelated questions: Is stereotype activation unconditionally automatic? When will activated stereotypes be applied in the context of social judgment and behavior? When activated, can stereotype application be controlled or otherwise avoided? Can stereotype activation be inhibited or prevented? What are the mechanisms underlying the control of stereotyping? The chapter is organized around two companion themes: the automaticity of stereotype activation and use and the controllability of stereotype use and activation.

THE AUTOMATICITY OF STEREOTYPE ACTIVATION AND USE

Making the Case for Automatic Stereotype Activation: Illustrative Research

The earliest applications of the distinction between automatic and controlled processes to the study of stereotypes assumed, in line with the then prevailing cognitive theories, that stereotype activation is automatic. Devine (1989), for example, argued that stereotype activation does not require intention, attention, or capacity; thus, when the appropriate cues are present (e.g., race, gender), stereotype activation should inevitably follow. To test this assumption empirically, Devine (1989, Experiment 2) adapted a procedure for activating cognitive constructs developed by Bargh and Pietromonico (1982), in which primes related to a construct are presented in participants' parafoveal visual field. As a result, participants are not consciously aware of the content of the primes, thus establishing one key feature of automaticity. This procedure, however, should make the construct more accessible and thus more likely to be used to interpret subsequently presented behaviors that are relevant but ambiguous with respect to the primed construct.

In Devine's research, the primes were terms related to the stereotype of blacks (e.g., group membership labels, group physical and trait characteristics), and the participants varied in their self-reported level of prejudice. The level of stereotype priming was also manipulated in this study, and high levels of stereotype priming were expected to increase the accessibility of the black stereotype more than low levels of priming were. After the priming task, participants formed an impression of a target person who engaged in ambiguously hostile behaviors (Srull & Wyer, 1979). Evaluation of ambiguously hostile behaviors was examined because pretesting indicated that hostility is a core element of the stereotype of blacks, and this stereotype has guided research on intergroup perception (e.g., Duncan, 1976). Importantly, no words directly related to hostility were included in the priming phase of the study, so that any priming effects would be due to stereotype activation rather than to a direct priming of the hostility construct. Devine expected and found that the target was rated as more hostile by both low- and high-prejudice participants when priming was high than when it was low. Devine interpreted these data as suggesting that stereotype activation is automatic for both low- and high-prejudice individuals.

Studies using alternative procedures have also suggested that gender and age stereotypes can be activated automatically (e.g., Banaji & Hardin, 1996; Purdue & Gurtman, 1990). For example, Purdue and Gurtman (1990, Experiment 2), using a masked priming procedure to prevent participants from being aware of the age-related primes, provided evidence that age stereotypes are automatically activated. Specifically, the labels "old" and "young" were presented for brief intervals (55 milliseconds [ms] and followed by a pattern mask. Participants were then presented with negative and positive trait terms (e.g., "irritable," "stubborn," "logical," "clever") and were asked to make evaluative judgments of the words (i.e., "Is this generally a good or bad quality for a person to possess?"). Purdue and Gurtman found that evaluative judgments about negative traits were made more quickly when the traits were preceded by the label "old" than when they were preceded by the label "young." These findings were interpreted as a form of automatic ageism. The logic of the studies by Devine (1989) and by Purdue and Gurtman (1990) was that if participants were not aware of the priming of stereotypes, their reactions could not reflect controlled processes.

Instead of preventing conscious awareness of the primes, as was done in the studies just reviewed, Banaji and Hardin (1996) limited the possibility for controlled processing by using an extremely brief interval between the prime and targets (300-ms stimulus-onset asynchrony, or SOA). Conventional wisdom had previously held that SOAs under 500 ms were too brief to allow the operation of controlled processes (Neely, 1977, 1991). In their studies, participants were presented with a sequence of two words and were asked to make a judgment about the second word. In their first study, the first word (i.e., prime) in the sequence was related to gender (e.g., "doctor" or "father" vs. "nurse" or "mother"), and the second word (i.e., target) was a masculine or feminine pronoun (e.g., "he" or "him" vs. "she" or "her"). In the second study, the second word was a gender specific pronoun, a gender-neutral pronoun (e.g., "it," "me") or a nonpronoun (e.g., "do," "all," "is"). Participants were instructed to ignore the prime word and to judge whether the target pronoun was a male or female pronoun (Experiment 1) or a pronoun or not a pronoun (Experiment 2). Banaji and Hardin (1996) found that judgments about consistent prime–target pairings (e.g., "doctor–he") were made more quickly than inconsistent pairings (e.g., "doctor–she") in both studies. These effects were independent of participants' explicit beliefs about gender and of their awareness of the prime–target relation. Banaji and Hardin argued that finding automatic stereotyping with a gender-irrelevant task (i.e., judgments about whether the target was a pronoun or not in Experiment 2) is particularly powerful in demonstrating the automatic activation of gender stereotypes.

Is Stereotype Activation Truly Automatic?

The illustrative research just summarized, as well as other studies, underscores how the possibility that stereotypes could unconsciously, effortlessly, and unintentionally be activated and influence social thought and behavior has captured the imagination of many social psychologists (Banaji & Greenwald, 1994, 1995; Banaji, Hardin, & Rothman, 1993; Bargh, Chapter 18, this volume; Bargh, Chen, & Burrows, 1996; Blair & Banaji, 1996; Chen & Bargh, 1997; Devine, 1989; Dovidio et al., 1986, 1997; Fazio et al., 1995; Gilbert & Hixon, 1991; Lepore & Brown, 1997; Macrae, Milne, & Bodenhausen, 1994; Perdue & Gurtman, 1990; Pratto & Bargh, 1991; Wittenbrink, Judd, & Park, 1997). Although many researchers have suggested that their stereotype-related findings are indicative of truly automatic processes, Bargh (1989, 1994) has cogently argued that the dichotomy between automatic and controlled processing, especially as applied in social psychology, is misleading. The initial source of the theoretical confusion was the early assumption that automatic and controlled processes were mutually exclusive and exhaustive processes. In careful examinations of the literature on automaticity, Bargh (1989, 1994) has suggested not only that the dichotomy is misleading, but that automaticity is more complex than researchers typically assume. Theoretically, to be considered truly automatic, a cognitive process has to meet all four criteria of automaticity; that is, it has to be unintentional, involuntary (uncontrollable), and effortless, and to occur outside of conscious awareness.

Bargh's (1989, 1994) reviews have clearly revealed that, in practice, researchers have not been as stringent as this in their identification of processes as automatic. In the social-cognitive literature generally, and the stereotyping literature in particular, a process has

often been labeled "automatic" if it satisfies any of the four criteria. Thus, if a process is effortless and occurred without awareness (e.g., Devine, 1989; Purdue & Gurtman, 1990), or occurs without explicit intentions (e.g., Banaji & Hardin, 1996), it has been considered automatic. Because awareness, attention, intention, and control do not necessarily co-occur and may occur in various combinations, Bargh (1994) has recommended that researchers be more explicit and precise in their identification of processes as automatic.

Indeed, equating all these types of automaticity has produced some confusion concerning what is meant by "automaticity," and has led to erroneous conclusions about the likelihood that a process can be controlled. In the context of stereotyping, for example, demonstrations of the unintended and efficient activation of racial or gender stereotypes led many to conclude that stereotyping is uncontrollable (see Bargh, Chapter 18, this volume, for an argument supporting the uncontrollability of stereotyping). This type of reasoning has potentially perilous implications. For example, Fiske (1989) argued that assumptions that stereotyping is automatic (i.e., inevitable and uncontrollable) have serious implications for judgments of responsibility in legal settings such as discrimination cases. After all, people cannot be held responsible for what they cannot control.

In addressing these issues, Bargh (1989) provided an elaborated analysis of automaticity, which illustrates that all automatic processing is conditional because it is dependent on a specific set of circumstances. Specifically, Bargh identified three classes of automaticity. "Preconscious" automatic processes occur prior to conscious awareness and only require the presence of a triggering stimulus to initiate them. "Postconscious" automaticity requires some type of conscious processing of relevant stimuli, but the outcome of this processing is unintended (e.g., nonconscious consequences of conscious thought and the effects of recent construct priming). "Goal-dependent" automaticity requires intentional, goal-directed processing, the outcomes of which may or may not be intended (e.g., making trait inferences when one's goal is to memorize sentences containing behaviors; well-practiced procedures that one intentionally employs in social judgment or as part of a complex skilled action, such as driving or typing). In the stereotyping literature, the types of automaticity most often explored in experimental settings have been of the preconscious (e.g., Chen & Bargh, 1997; Devine, 1989; Purdue & Gurtman, 1990) and postconscious (e.g., Banaji & Greenwald, 1995; Banaji & Hardin, 1996; Banaji et al., 1993; Blair & Banaji, 1996; Macrae, Milne, & Bodenhausen, 1994) varieties.

The complex nature of automaticity and its conditional nature have been explored in studies designed to push the limits of the automaticity analysis of stereotype activation and application. These findings have begun to bear out Bargh's cautionary statements regarding the application of the label "automaticity." For example, several studies have obtained evidence suggesting that stereotype activation is not unconditionally automatic when individuals are exposed to members of stigmatized groups or the symbolic equivalent (e.g., Blair & Banaji, 1996; Fazio et al., 1995; Gilbert & Hixon, 1991; Lepore & Brown, 1997; Sinclair & Kunda, 1997; Wittenbrink et al., 1997). Such findings ultimately encourage not only careful analysis of automaticity, but careful thinking about the nature of control over stereotype activation and use.

Gilbert and Hixon (1991), for example, demonstrated that stereotype activation could be prevented when perceivers' cognitive resources were drained. This finding is important for the automaticity analysis of stereotype activation, because one of the defining features of automatic processing is that it is not limited by available capacity. In Gilbert and Hixon's study, participants completed a word fragment completion task under conditions in which half of the participants were made cognitively busy (i.e., told to remember an eight-digit number), but the others were not made busy. The word fragments were presented via videotape by an Asian assistant. Some of the words could be completed in a stereotypic manner (e.g., "s_y" could be "shy"; "r_ce" could be "rice," etc.), and hence this task was used as a measure of stereotype activation. Gilbert and Hixon reasoned that to the extent that the presence of the Asian assistant automatically activated stereotypes, the number of stereotypic completions should be equivalent for the busy and

not-busy participants. In contrast with the automaticity-of-stereotype-activation analysis, Gilbert and Hixon found that cognitively busy participants generated fewer stereotypic completions than participants who were not cognitively busy during the word fragment completion task (see also Spencer, Fein, Wolfe, Hodgson, & Dunn, in press).

More recent studies continue to highlight the complexity of automaticity and control. For example, Sinclair and Kunda (1997, Study 3) showed that the tendency for stereotype activation or inhibition to occur depended on the type of feedback participants received from the target. In this research, participants were either criticized or praised by a negatively stereotyped (black) evaluator, and stereotype activation (word fragment completion task as in Gilbert & Hixon, 1991) and application (evaluative judgments of the target) were measured. Participants who had been criticized by the black evaluator showed evidence of stereotype activation (i.e., above baseline) and applied the stereotype in their judgments of the evaluator, apparently to discredit him. Participants who had been praised by the black evaluator showed an apparent motivated inhibition of stereotype activation (i.e., stereotype activation was below baseline), presumably reflecting an effort to avoid discrediting the evaluator. The point at which the inhibition or reduced accessibility of the stereotype occurs, and the exact mechanisms producing this effect, are not yet well specified. However, generally supporting their motivational account, Sinclair and Kunda found that participants' evaluative judgments of the black evaluator were mediated by the extent to which the black stereotype had been activated.

The pattern of findings, however, was different when the participants were detached observers rather than direct recipients of the criticism or praise (e.g., Study 4, in which participants observed others being praised or criticized by a black evaluator). Specifically, detached observers showed evidence of stereotype activation in both the criticism and praise conditions, but their judgments of the negatively stereotyped evaluator were not related to the activated stereotype. Apparently these participants did not use their activated stereotypes in making their judgments of the evaluator. Sinclair and Kunda suggested that the selective application and inhibition of stereotypes resulted from self-protective motives of the recipients who actually received negative or positive feedback from black evaluators; the detached observers would not have had such self-protective motives engaged. These findings suggest that the activation and inhibition of stereotypes may be fairly flexible and may occur in the service of specific motives.

In other recent work, Blair and Banaji (1996) showed that intentional processes could operate at SOAs previously thought to preclude the possibility for controlled processing. More specifically, Blair and Banaji (1996) used a priming paradigm to demonstrate that the extent to which stereotypes are automatically activated can be modified by the conscious intention to replace stereotypic thoughts with counterstereotypic thoughts. In their studies, male and female names were presented on a computer screen following the presentation of a trait or nontrait word that was either stereotypically masculine or feminine (e.g., "dependent" or "nurse," followed by "Jane" or "James"). Blair and Banaji (Experiments 3 and 4) explicitly provided some participants with counterstereotypical expectancies. Participants were told that following a stereotypically male word, they should expect a female name, and following a female word, they should expect a male name. The names were presented at one of two different intervals following the trait primes. For some participants, the interval was very brief (350 ms in Experiment 3, and 250 ms in Experiment 4). For other participants, the interval was increased to 2,000 ms, which provided enough time for participants to reflect on their expectancies consciously.

The results showed that, as expected, participants were able to reverse the stereotype-priming effect with the longer interval. In other words, participants in this condition identified female names more quickly than male names following male words, and male names more quickly than female names following female words. Their findings also showed that in the 250- and 350-ms intervals conditions, the counterstereotype expectancy moderated the stereotype-priming effect. That is, although participants did not have enough time to apply their expectancy and reverse the stereotype-priming effect consciously, they also did not show the patterns of facilitation

that result from automatic stereotype activation.

In sum, it appears that when demands are placed on perceivers' cognitive resources (Gilbert & Hixon, 1991; Spencer et al., in press) stereotype activation can be prevented. When people are sufficiently motivated, recent evidence suggests that stereotype activation can be inhibited (Sinclair & Kunda, 1997). One reason why such findings are important is that if stereotypes are not activated or are effectively inhibited, they cannot be used in subsequent judgments or behaviors. In addition, intentions can override the effects of automatic stereotype activation even under conditions that were previously thought to preclude controlled processing (Blair & Banaji, 1996). These types of findings pose a serious challenge to the notion that stereotypes are unconditionally and inevitably activated in the presence of members of a stereotyped group. As such, they suggest that the automatic–controlled dichotomy may, as Bargh has argued, ultimately be misleading regarding both the nature of stereotype activation and the possibility of control over stereotyping processes.

In sum, theoretical arguments and accumulating findings suggest that automaticity of stereotype activation is considerably more complex than researchers once thought. This work has made it increasingly clear that there are limits to what was once presumed to be rather inevitable. Specifically, the mere presence of members of stereotyped groups (or their symbolic equivalents) does not *necessarily* result in stereotype activation. We expect that future research will further explore the limits of the automaticity of stereotype activation. Nevertheless, the cumulative evidence also suggests that—despite the fact that stereotype activation is not unconditionally automatic—it is often unintended and efficient. In short, it is very likely. Given its high likelihood, the social injustices that result from stereotype use can be avoided only if perceivers can effectively control their stereotyping. It is to issues of control that we now turn.

CONTROLLED PROCESSING AND THE CONTROL OF STEREOTYPING

Just as the previous thinking about automatic and controlled processes as they apply to stereotypes proved to be somewhat misleading in terms of understanding the automaticity of stereotyping, the initial thinking also seems to have overlooked some important issues related to stereotype control. Specifically, the either–or reasoning (i.e., a process is either automatic or controlled) appears to have led researchers astray in two ways that are relevant to issues of stereotype control. First, as we have pointed out previously, it spawned the erroneous conclusion that stereotyping is frequently uncontrollable (but see Bargh, Chapter 18, this volume). That is, because stereotype activation was found to have certain properties of automaticity (e.g., lacking intention and being efficient), it was also assumed to be uncontrollable (see Bargh, 1994). Furthermore, stereotype application following stereotype activation was assumed to be uncontrollable in situations that do not afford the motivation and ability to engage in controlled processing. These sorts of assumptions seem to have discouraged researchers from investigating certain issues in relation to stereotype control. For example, if one assumes that stereotype activation is uncontrollable, why would one pursue investigations of the potential controllability of stereotype activation?

A second shortcoming of the either–or reasoning is that it has not been conducive to stimulating research on the exact nature of control. Specifically, research to date that has investigated issues of stereotype control has focused on the question of whether control can be achieved over stereotypic responses (e.g., Devine, 1989; Gilbert & Hixon, 1991; Kruglanski & Freund, 1983). However, it has not been as concerned with identifying the precise mechanisms through which control is achieved. This seems to be an unfortunate albeit natural consequence of rigid adherence to the dual-process conception, in that the dichotomy has focused attention on the question of "Is it automatic or controlled?" Such a focus seems to have discouraged investigators from attempting to understand the microprocesses involved in implementing control efforts, the points at which particular control strategies are implemented, and the efficacy of these control strategies.

It seems appropriate at this juncture, therefore, to focus greater attention on issues related to the controllability of stereotyping. Our goal for the remainder of this chapter is

to provide a framework for thinking about control strategies that is organized on the basis of *when* control attempts are exerted (i.e., do these occur after stereotypes have been activated, during their activation, or before their activation?), *how* control may be achieved (i.e., what are the mechanisms and strategies used under various conditions?), and *who* is likely to attempt control.

There are three ways in which control is relevant to the question of whether stereotyping will occur. First, a person can override the influence of an activated stereotype with responses based on controlled processing.[1] In other words, although the stereotype is fully activated, a stereotype-consistent response is prevented by overriding it with a response that is based on more cautious, careful processing. Second, a person can stop or interrupt stereotype activation once it has started, so that a stereotypic response may be averted. In this case, controlled processes are brought to bear earlier, exerting an influence over the activation process itself so as to stop or interrupt it. Then a controlled process is used to generate a nonstereotypic response. Third, control can be exercised over prejudiced responses by preventing stereotype activation from occurring in the first place. We address each of these possible avenues for stereotype control below.

Overriding Responses Resulting from Stereotype Activation

As we have already noted, a good deal of evidence indicates that activated stereotypes need not be applied in the generation of social judgments and behaviors. Bargh (1994) has nicely summarized this point by stating that "the use of automatically supplied input in consciously produced judgmental output is not mandatory" (p. 30). Perceivers have a choice in how they respond toward others (Fiske, 1989). Certain conditions must be met, however, for that choice to be realized and for some form of controlled-processing strategy to be spurred into action.

First, one must be aware of the potential influence of the stereotype. This condition is rather obvious; one cannot counteract the outcome if one is unaware of the need for counteraction. Second, one must have the available cognitive resources to initiate the controlled processing necessary for overriding responses resulting from stereotype activation (Bodenhausen, 1990; Bodenhausen & Lichtenstein, 1987; Bodenhausen & Wyer, 1985; Devine, 1989; Fiske & Pavelchak, 1986; Gilbert & Hixon, 1991; Jamieson & Zanna, 1989; Kruglanski & Freund, 1983; Pratto & Bargh, 1991). Finally, one must be sufficiently motivated to initiate some strategy to override stereotypic responses.

This motivation to override stereotypic responses may be situationally induced in a variety of ways. For example, the situational salience of social norms suggesting that prejudice and stereotyping are inappropriate may encourage even those with prejudiced tendencies to monitor their responses and to override prejudiced responses with less prejudiced responses (Gaertner & Dovidio, 1986; Monteith, Deneen, & Tooman, 1996; Plant & Devine, 1998). Explicit instructions to avoid stereotypic responses may instigate control efforts as well (Macrae, Bodenhausen, Milne, & Jetten, 1994). Being dependent on members of stereotyped groups who control one's outcomes also gives rise to careful processing and reduced stereotyping (Erber & Fiske, 1984; Neuberg & Fiske, 1987). When the stakes are high, people do not want to risk reliance on potentially inaccurate social perceptions resulting from stereotype use. Finally, situations that induce the motivation to be accurate (Brewer, 1988; Brewer & Harasty, Chapter 12, this volume; Neuberg, 1989; Fiske & Neuberg, 1990; Fiske et al., Chapter 11, this volume), or that make one feel accountable (Tetlock & Kim, 1987) for one's judgments and behaviors, encourage a reliance on controlled processes during response generation.

Presumably, even persons who hold high-prejudice attitudes toward members of the stereotyped group, and who therefore have no personal qualms about the application of stereotypes, can be roused to engage in controlled processing in situations that create the motivation to do so (Plant & Devine, 1998). However, the motivation is likely to be more cross-situationally salient among individuals who are internally motivated to override the effects of automatic processes. Specifically, responding in prejudiced ways poses a conflict with the personal beliefs and egalitarian ideals held by low-prejudice individuals (Devine,

Monteith, Zuwerink, & Elliot, 1991; Monteith, Devine, & Zuwerink, 1993; Monteith, 1996a; Plant & Devine, 1998). Therefore, low-prejudice individuals' internal motivation to avoid stereotypic responses will prompt them to take the necessary steps to avoid such responses (Devine, 1989; Devine & Monteith, 1993; Monteith, 1993).

There may be many routes to the same ultimate outcome of reducing the impact of stereotypes on social thought and behavior. The problem of stereotype control following stereotype activation thus may very well be a problem of identifying the best alternative(s) for meeting this goal. In what follows, we review the various control strategies that researchers have suggested perceivers may use; we also speculate about the conditions under which these control strategies are likely to be instigated. Additional empirical work will be needed to establish with greater certainty when and why particular control strategies are instigated by whom. In addition, research will need to address the comparative efficacy of alternative strategies—both individually and jointly.

Gathering Additional Information

Perceivers can avoid stereotypic responses by taking the more effortful and time-consuming route of gathering individual pieces of information about the target, rather than relying on activated stereotypes. In other words, the perceiver can gather information about a target that goes beyond the category-based (and associated stereotypic) information that is immediately available from basic perceptual processing. The two leading models of person impression formation (Brewer, 1988; Brewer & Harasty, Chapter 12, this volume; Fiske & Neuberg, 1990; Fiske et al., Chapter 11, this volume) each suggest that information gathering can be more or less thorough. In general, the less information gathered, the more likely it is that the resulting impression will be category-based (i.e., stereotypic). If stereotypic responses are to be avoided, perceivers need to engage in a type of processing that yields a highly individualized impression. For example, in Fiske and Neuberg's model, the final stage of processing entails piecemeal integration, whereby information is gathered and integrated in an attribute-by-attribute manner. In Brewer's model, category-based impressions of individuals are avoided through a bottom-up type of processing called "personalization," in which the individual (rather than the category) serves as the basis for organizing all of the information that has been gathered. According to these models, such elaborated processing will only occur when perceivers are sufficiently motivated to engage in such processing (e.g., because of personal or situational motivations or task demands).

Recent evidence suggests that the internal motivation to avoid prejudiced responses prompts people to attend to individuating information. Specifically, Sherman, Stroessner, and Azam (1997) found that low-prejudice individuals' judgments of a gay target were closely related to individuating information presented about the target, whereas high-prejudice participants' judgments were not. Even high-prejudice individuals, who are not internally motivated to respond without prejudice (Plant & Devine, 1998), may be motivated to attend to individuating information under some circumstances, such as when they are dependent on the target for desired outcomes (see Fiske, 1993).

The relatively effortful and time-consuming practice of gathering information to avoid relying on initially activated stereotypes is a control strategy that is probably used in impression formation and target evaluation situations. More generally, this strategy may be used when perceivers are forming judgments or evaluations relevant to public policies that affect the stereotyped group (e.g., "What do I think about this affirmative-action policy?"). If there is insufficient information or time to gather and process the information, perceivers may rely instead on a different control strategy for generating a nonprejudiced response (e.g., generating a response that a perceiver believes is egalitarian).

Replacement with Egalitarian Responses

In certain situations, stereotypic responses that initially come to mind can be overridden and replaced with more egalitarian responses that apparently come to mind through more careful and cautious responding. For example, in Devine's (1989) research, low-prejudice individuals provided nonstereotypic, egalitarian descriptions of their beliefs about blacks when they had ample time to generate those descriptions. In contrast, when limits were placed on low-prejudice participants' cognitive capacity, they showed evidence of stereotype application. Likewise, Monteith (1993) found that low-prejudice participants provided unfavorable (nonstereotypic) evaluations of jokes about gays, but only when they had experienced an earlier experimental manipulation that was designed to instigate controlled processing in the generation of prejudice-related responses. In both sets of research, a stereotype control strategy was implemented among the low-prejudice participants only. However, one can imagine other situations (e.g., in the presence of social norms prohibiting prejudiced expressions) that likewise would encourage high-prejudice individuals to override stereotypic responses with more egalitarian ones (cf. Plant & Devine, 1998).

This particular control strategy can be used only when there is a clear, egalitarian alternative to responding in a prejudiced manner. To be sure, there are many such situations in everyday life, including ones that parallel the Devine (1989) and Monteith (1993) measures (e.g., when people describe their beliefs about blacks, and when they respond to jokes made at the expense of stereotyped groups) and other situations (e.g., when people choose a partner for completing a task). However, precisely what sort of response is "egalitarian" may not be entirely clear in other situations (Devine, Evett, & Vasquez-Suson, 1996). Also, in other situations that require one to gather and integrate a good deal of information (e.g., evaluating a job applicant), alternative control strategies may be necessary instead of or in addition to a reliance on egalitarian beliefs.

Correction

After stereotypes have been activated, perceivers may attempt to assess the likely impact of the stereotypes on their responses, and to adjust their responses in a direction opposite to the presumed influence of the stereotype (Wilson & Brekke, 1994; Wegener & Petty, 1997). This is a frequently discussed strategy for mitigating the unfair use of stereotypes and judgments. For correction processes to operate, perceivers must (1) believe that bias is operating, (2) be motivated to make corrections, and (3) have naive theories about the direction and magnitude of the biasing effect of stereotypes on responses. For example, Wegener and Petty (1997) have argued, according to their flexible-correction model, that perceivers can correct for the perceived influence of a variety of factors (e.g., transient moods, social norms, salient beliefs, motives) on a wide array of outcomes (e.g., attributions, impressions, persuasion, etc.). In the domain of stereotyping, Wegener and Petty have suggested that people may vary in both whether they believe that their judgments are biased by stereotypes and whether they are motivated to initiate processes to correct for such biases. In particular, these authors suggest that low-prejudice people who are motivated to correct for unfair bias are the ones most likely to manifest such correction processes. This strategy for overriding stereotypic responses is likely to occur in situations that call for considered evaluations and judgments of others (e.g., evaluating job applicants, grading students' papers, forming impressions of others). To the extent that people can adjust for such biases, correction holds promise for correcting unintended effects of activated stereotypes. Subsequent work addressing the nature of people's naive theories concerning the impact of stereotypes on judgments and behaviors, whether accurate or not, may help to elucidate the challenges of combating the influence of stereotypes—at least as understood by naive social perceivers.

Suppression

Another control strategy—one that has received a good deal of empirical and theoretical attention in recent work—is suppression (see Wegner, 1994). Specifically, in an attempt to control prejudiced responses, people may try to banish stereotypic thoughts from the mind (i.e., to suppress stereotypic thoughts) and to replace them with alternative, "distracter" thoughts. How does this control strategy differ from those discussed above? To the extent that individuating information or

egalitarian thoughts are used as the distracter thoughts, the strategies have some similarity. The important divergence is that the active effort to avoid and banish stereotypic thoughts from the mind is argued to have undesirable outcomes.

Specifically, recent findings have underscored the possibility that this control strategy may have unintended effects, such that stereotypic thoughts become more accessible than if suppression had never been attempted (Macrae, Bodenhausen, Milne, & Jetten, 1994; Macrae, Bodenhausen, & Milne, in press; Wegner, Erber, & Bowman, 1993, as cited in Wegner, 1994). In other words, stereotypic thoughts may "rebound," and subsequently exert undue influences on social thought and behavior. Such paradoxical outcomes have been explained using Wegner's model of mental control (Macrae, Bodenhausen, et al., 1994; Wegner, 1994; Wegner & Erber, 1992). According to this model, control is effectively achieved as long as the perceiver is able to persist in an effortful search for distracter thoughts to replace the unwanted (stereotypic) thoughts. However, while this search-and-replace process occurs, an ironic monitoring process supposedly searches consciousness for evidence of the stereotypic thoughts, which causes these thoughts to be repeatedly primed and thus increases their accessibility. Therefore, if the functioning of the operating process is undermined (e.g., due to cognitive load; Wegner, 1994), or if the conscious intention to avoid the unwanted thought is relaxed (Macrae, Bodenhausen, et al., 1994), stereotypic thoughts may rebound. The interesting findings obtained in this line of research suggest that the more people try to reduce their stereotypic thinking through suppression, the more they will fail to do so (e.g., Macrae, Bodenhausen, et al., 1994).

Because stereotype suppression as a control strategy emphasizes the potential drawbacks of attempts to avoid thinking about stereotypes while simultaneously thinking about something else, there is the possibility that this control strategy is applied in *all* situations in which perceivers are aware that stereotypes will potentially influence their responses. However, this suggestion is difficult to reconcile with the findings from a variety of experiments in which control efforts have been successful. It appears that there are important boundary conditions to stereotype rebound that initial research on the topic was not designed to detect. For example, recent evidence that low-prejudice individuals do not appear to be prone to stereotype rebound (Monteith, Spicer, & Tooman, 1997; Pressly & Devine, 1997), and that high-prejudice participants are not prone to it under certain circumstances (Monteith, Spicer, & Tooman, 1997) leads us to conclude that there are important moderating influences on the stereotype rebound effect (see Monteith, Sherman, & Devine, 1998). For instance, when stereotype suppression is well practiced (as may be the case for low-prejudice individuals) or is paired with certain other control strategies (e.g., simultaneous stereotype suppression and individuation of targets), control efforts may succeed.

Potential Obstacles to Successful Control

Individuals may experience success in their attempts to override the influence of stereotypes by employing the control strategies described above, either individually or collectively. However, the inherent nature of many of the situations in which control is necessary for avoiding bias creates a variety of potential obstacles to successful control.

First, the criteria for detecting the potential for bias may be ambiguous. That is, perceivers must first be aware that stereotypes may influence their responses before efforts to correct such responses can be instigated. The challenge for social perceivers, however, is that there are often no clear-cut criteria for knowing when judgments will potentially be biased. This challenge is discussed by Wilson and Brekke (1994) in connection with what they call "mental contamination." These theorists underscore the possibility that judgments, emotions, or behaviors will be biased in unwanted ways because people do not detect the potential for bias.

The failure to detect bias may occur in part because people have limited access to their mental processes (Wilson & Brekke, 1994; Nisbett & Wilson, 1977), so that the mental processes leading to bias can occur without ever being consciously detected. This failure in detection is illustrated well in the context of stereotyping in Banaji and her colleagues' research on implicit (or unconscious) stereotyping (Banaji & Greenwald, 1995; Banaji et al., 1993; Greenwald & Banaji, 1995). For example, Banaji et al. (1993) found that participants who were primed with the construct "dependence" subsequently rated a female target as more dependent than did participants in a neutral-priming condition. Similar, though less strong, priming effects were observed in connection with the construct "aggressive" and judgments of a male target's aggressiveness. As Banaji et al. concluded, such implicit stereotyping findings "suggest that stereotyped information may be an especially potent source of discrimination when it is not consciously attended to at the time of judgment" (p. 279). Further emphasizing people's potential inability to take control over their prejudiced responses, Banaji et al. asserted that "Implicit stereotyping effects undermine the current belief about the role of consciousness in guaranteeing equality in the treatment of individuals irrespective of sex, class, color, and national origin" (p. 280).

People also may fail to detect their potential for bias because, although they are aware that certain mental processes can result in stereotype use, they underestimate their own susceptibility to such bias or overestimate their own ability for mental control (Wilson & Brekke, 1994). This leads us to the second potential obstacle to successful control, which is that the rules for overriding biased responses may be ambiguous or not well specified. The problem here is that people need to know precisely how much and in what direction they are being influenced by activated stereotypes to override their responses, so that completely unbiased responses can be provided. However, people rarely come to situations equipped with a set of formulas for computing the direction and magnitude of potential bias. Thus, people may underadjust or even overadjust their responses (as has been found in reversals of classic priming effects; Lombardi, Higgins, & Bargh, 1987; Martin, 1986). Moreover, even if people have clear theories about how their responses may be biased by stereotypes, there is no guarantee that they are correct. Wegener and Petty (1997) have shown that adjustments can be systematically related to participants' naive theories about bias, but that these theories are sometimes incorrect.

A third difficulty is that the criteria for evaluating success at achieving control can be ambiguous, so people may have difficulty learning how to implement strategies of control successfully across situations. In some cases, success at achieving control may be fairly clear, such as when a person does not laugh at a stereotypic joke. However, other situations may be inherently more ambiguous, such as when a teacher is evaluating a student's performance (e.g., Darley & Gross, 1983) or a person is engaged in an interpersonal interaction with a member of a stereotyped group (Devine et al., 1996). In such situations, accurate feedback about the degree of success may not be readily available or easily determined. The world outside the laboratory does not readily supply a control condition against which a person can evaluate the success of his or her control efforts.

Because research designed to examine the processes of control is relatively new, a high priority for future work is to examine systematically the extent to which these potential obstacles undermine control efforts. Early work has focused on documenting failures of control, and, as such, the research has been designed so as to maximize the likelihood of failure by creating insurmountable obstacles to control. What is not clear at present is how often such failures occur in naturally occurring environments. Are natural social perceivers as prone to control failures as their counterparts in the social-psychological laboratory? It seems imperative that future research on control be designed so as to provide an answer to this question.

Interrupting Stereotype Activation and Generating Nonprejudiced Responses

Although overriding stereotypic responses using controlled processing represents one way to achieve stereotype control, there are clearly situations in which individuals will be unable to implement this type of control (see Bargh, Chapter 18, this volume, for an extreme position). When people are unaware of the potential influence of stereotypes, or unable to muster up the cognitive resources or motivation to override their stereotypic responses, they will be unable to control their prejudiced responses. Even among those people who are most internally motivated to control their prejudices (i.e., low-prejudice individuals), the typical day is very rushed and multifarious. Thus, the type of constant vigilance needed to detect possible stereotype use is unlikely, not to mention the improbability of having continually available the cognitive resources needed to override stereotypic responses. According to this reasoning, even the best-intentioned individuals are likely to be prone to generating prejudiced responses (e.g., Devine et al., 1991).

However, in this section we argue that processes of learning and self-regulation may enable individuals to gain control over their prejudiced responses, even when the situation seems to favor a prejudiced response. As an introduction to our argument, consider the following scenario: Paula (who is white) is tired, hungry, and rushed as she shops for groceries on the way home from work. She is also frustrated, as she cannot find an item that she needs. It is in this state that she makes a stereotypic inference that is frequently made in relation to black persons (see Feagin, 1991). Specifically, she assumes that a black woman in the store is an employee rather than a fellow shopper, and she asks the woman where the sought-for item is located. Paula realizes her mistake at the same time the woman informs her that she does not in fact work in the store. Paula resumes her search for the item, feeling guilty about her faulty and insulting stereotypic inference, and wondering how she could have made such a blunder. Thus far, this scenario illustrates the failure to override a stereotypic response with a nonprejudiced response. However, the fact that Paula has experienced guilt over her stereotypic response and spent even a few seconds considering her error is extremely important for the likelihood that she will make the same sort of stereotypic inference in the future. The next time Paula is in the grocery store (or, for that matter, a different store) and circumstances conspire (e.g., she is tired and hurried) to create the ideal situation for stereotype use, she should be less likely to do so. This is because Paula's previous experience should have resulted in a building of associations among a store environment, her stereotypic inference, and the guilt she experienced in relation to that inference. As a consequence of these associations, the next time a stereotypic response is possible, Paula essentially should "think twice."

This scenario illustrates how processes of learning and self-regulation may help individuals to detect situations in which they may engage in a prejudiced response, to interrupt ongoing processing (i.e., stereotype activation), and then to generate a nonprejudiced response based on more thoughtful processing. We now provide a more detailed theoretical account of the precise nature of these processes—an account based on the model of self-regulation of prejudiced responses (Monteith, 1993).

Prerequisites to Self-Regulating Prejudiced Responses

There are two important prerequisites to the self-regulation of prejudiced responses. First, individuals must recognize that they have relied on a stereotype in an initial situation for that experience to affect the subsequent likelihood of a similar use of a stereotype. That is, people must "catch" themselves engaging in responses that are discrepant from how they believe they should respond. People's awareness of their proneness to such prejudice-related discrepant responses has been examined in a variety of studies (Devine et al., 1991; Monteith, 1996a, 1996b; Monteith et al., 1993; Plant & Devine, in press; Pressly & Devine, 1992; Zuwerink, Devine, Monteith, & Cook, 1996). This research has revealed that approximately 80% of participants report that they are prone to responding in ways that are more prejudiced than their personal beliefs suggest are appropriate. In addition, other research (Amodt & Devine, 1994) has indicated that people who actually engaged in a prejudiced response subsequently did realize its inconsistency with their beliefs about how they should respond, without any encouragement to come to this realization on the part of the experimenter. Thus, it seems likely that individuals will realize their prejudiced responses with at least a fair amount of frequency, which will help in setting the stage for the subsequent self-regulation of those responses.

The second prerequisite to self-regulating prejudiced responses is that some form of punishment must be experienced when one engages in a stereotypic or prejudiced response. As will become clearer shortly, the ex-

perience of punishment is essential for the subsequent instigation of self-regulatory mechanisms. The discrepancy-related research described above has revealed that low-prejudice individuals experience strong feelings of negative self-directed affect (e.g., guilt) in relation to their stereotypic responses, which serve as a self-punishment. These feelings result because low-prejudice individuals experience a strong sense of moral obligation to avoid stereotypic responses. In contrast, high-prejudice individuals experience less of this obligation (Monteith & Walters, 1998), so that they experience modest levels of guilt at best in relation to their stereotypic responses. Importantly, these differences between low- and high-prejudice individuals carry with them the implication that low- but not high-prejudice individuals are likely to self-regulate their prejudiced responses.

The Process of Self-Regulation: Learning to Control Prejudiced Responses

Exactly how can individuals interrupt stereotype activation so that nonprejudiced responses can be provided? According to the model of self-regulation of prejudiced responses (Monteith, 1993), individuals' social histories are thought to provide them with opportunities to learn from their mistakes, to identify situations in which they are especially likely to commit the same mistakes, and therefore to avoid making those mistakes.

Specifically, based on the work of Devine (1989) and Devine et al. (1991), the model posits that group membership cues (e.g., members of stereotyped groups) can spontaneously activate stereotypes and result in a prejudiced response that is discrepant from how one believes one should respond (hereafter referred to as a "discrepant response"). As explained earlier, realizing that one's response violates internally derived standards for responding produces feelings of guilt. Theoretically, the experience of guilt serves as a punishment for engaging in the prejudiced response (see Gray, 1982; Fowles, 1980) and motivates discrepancy reduction efforts (see Aronson, 1968; Bandura, 1986; Bandura & Jourdan, 1991; Duval, Duval, & Mulisis, 1992; Duval & Wicklund, 1972; Festinger, 1957; Rokeach, 1973).

According to the self-regulation model, another consequence of awareness of a prejudice-related discrepant response is heightened self-focused attention, which then instigates attempts to regulate or control subsequent discrepancy-relevant responses (see Pyszczynski & Greenberg, 1986, 1987). Exactly how can this control be achieved? At this point, Monteith (1993) extrapolated from Gray's (1982; see also Patterson & Newman, 1993) neuropsychological model of motivation and learning, in order to understand how control might be gained over spontaneously generated prejudiced responses. As inferred from Gray's work, awareness of a discrepant response should activate the "behavioral-inhibition system" (BIS). The activation and operation of this system are of central importance for understanding how stereotype activation can be interrupted and controlled in the future.

Specifically, BIS activation results in a brief increase in arousal and an automatic, momentary pausing or interruption of ongoing behavior (i.e., "behavioral inhibition") (Gray, 1982; Fowles, 1980; Patterson & Newman, 1993). Then the behavioral sequence that resulted in the "faulty" (i.e., discrepant) response is allotted enhanced attention, so that the person can determine what went wrong. In addition, exploratory/investigative behavior should be initiated to search for indications of the discrepant response, so that the individual can identify environmental stimuli that were present when the discrepant response occurred. Importantly, these attentional and investigative consequences should work in concert, in order for an association to be created among cues present when the discrepant response occurred, the discrepant response itself, and the punishment (i.e., guilt) that results from engaging in the prejudiced response. In other words, through a process that Patterson and Newman (1993) call "retrospective reflection," cues for punishment can be established.

The operation of the BIS and the establishment of cues for punishment are critical to the subsequent self-regulation of prejudiced responses. Specifically, when automatic processes give rise to stereotype activation on subsequent occasions, and previously established cues for punishment are present, a "warning signal" of sorts should be sounded. This should cause the BIS to be activated, resulting in increased arousal and behavioral inhibition (i.e., a slowing of ongoing behavior).

Consequently, the response generation process should be slowed and executed more carefully (see Gray, 1982; Patterson & Newman, 1993). Thus, rather than relying on automatic processes when generating a response, the person should initiate controlled processes. This ultimately should allow the person to inhibit stereotype-based (prejudiced) responses, and to bring personal beliefs to mind as a basis for responding instead.

In sum, the critical elements of how control is achieved over stereotypes, according to the self-regulation model, is that external stimuli that have come to serve as cues for punishment that trigger inhibitory mechanisms. Through behavioral inhibition, the automatic processing that would otherwise give rise to a prejudiced response is disrupted, and the individual has the opportunity to generate a nonprejudiced response based on controlled processing (i.e., through individuation, generation of an egalitarian response, etc.). Control is exerted both in the interruption of stereotype activation and in the generation of a personally acceptable response.

Research to date is consistent with the notion that control can be achieved over prejudiced responses in the ways described by the self-regulation model. For example, low-prejudice subjects who believed they engaged in prejudiced responses experienced guilt, showed heightened self-focus and attention to discrepancy-relevant information (Monteith, 1993, Experiment 1), and showed evidence of more careful and deliberate subsequent responding (Monteith, 1993, Experiment 2). Moreover, after experiencing a prejudice-related discrepancy, low-prejudice individuals were less likely to generate a prejudiced response in a subsequent task than subjects who did not experience such a discrepancy. Presumably, subjects who believed they had previously responded in a prejudiced manner were able to regulate their responses in the subsequent task, so that automatic, prejudiced responses were inhibited and belief-based (low-prejudice) responses were generated instead.

Additional research is clearly needed to examine this potential form of control further. For example, when cues for punishment have been established in an initial situation, does their presence days later decrease the likelihood of a prejudiced response—as suggested by the model? How similar do the cues have to be across situations to be effective? How long does it take individuals to learn to regulate their responses? What factors facilitate versus or obstruct self-regulation efforts? How applicable is the self-regulation model to non-college-student samples? These and other questions require exploration. Nevertheless, there are at present theoretically and empirically based reasons for suspecting that individuals can learn to interrupt the stereotype activation process before stereotypic responses are generated.

Controlling Stereotype Activation

The third form of stereotype control that we discuss is the actual control (prevention) of stereotype activation. This form of control should obviously be more effective than any other form of control, because stereotypes cannot possibly influence responses if they have not been activated. How can people avoid the activation of stereotypes? One possibility is that the stereotype is not learned well enough to be automatically activated in the first place. To be sure, the ease with which stereotypes come to mind differs across individuals and especially across target groups. In some cases, stereotypes will not come to mind spontaneously. Of greater relevance to the goals of this chapter are instances in which stereotypes that were at one time activated in a rather automatic manner (e.g., without intention or awareness) have, through some controlled effort, become cognitive constructs that no longer are activated in this way.

The questions of whether and how controlled processing can be implemented so that stereotype activation is prevented in the end are questions that only recently have begun to be investigated. We believe that these issues may have been relatively neglected because of popular thinking about automatic and controlled processes as mutually exclusive and noninteractive (but see Chen & Chaiken, Chapter 4, this volume). Only very recent thinking explicitly considers the possibility that there may be an interplay between automatic and controlled processes. As Blair and Banaji have argued (1996), "Researchers must be sensitive to the complexity with which automatic and controlled processes interact to produce a response" (p. 1159). Similarly, Bargh (1994) has noted that "mental

processes at the level of complexity studied by social psychologists are not exclusively automatic or exclusively controlled, but are in fact combinations of the features of each" (p. 3).

Because the suggestion that stereotype activation may be preventable through controlled processes has only been advanced quite recently, it has received scant empirical attention. Recent findings do support the notion that some individuals are able to avoid the activation of stereotypes under conditions that meet at least several of the criteria of automaticity (Fazio et al., 1995; Lepore & Brown, 1997; Wittenbrink et al., 1997). Such findings are consistent with the possibility that those individuals who do not show evidence of stereotype activation are able to control it in some way, and they raise the intriguing and exciting possibility that stereotyping can be controlled through the prevention of stereotype activation. Below, we review two possible avenues to controlling stereotype activation.

Long-Term Consequences of Practiced Self-Regulation

One possibility is that with practice at the self-regulation of prejudiced responses, stereotype activation not only is interrupted, but is prevented entirely. Specifically, two consequences should follow from the sort of self-regulation described by Monteith (1993). First, behavioral inhibition (i.e., a slowing of ongoing responding) should theoretically become a natural and immediate reaction to stereotype activation. That is, repeated and frequent inhibition following stereotype activation in the presence of cues for punishment should serve to automate the process of inhibition following stereotype activation. Second, the generation of nonprejudiced responses should be executed with increasing ease and speed, due to the frequent activation and use of nonprejudiced constructs (e.g., egalitarian beliefs) as a basis for responding. Thus, the long-term implications of practiced self-regulation may be that stereotype activation is prevented and replaced with the activation of and reliance on nonprejudiced patterns of responding.

The recent findings of Blair and Banaji (1996), described in detail earlier, are consistent with the possibility that individuals can prevent stereotype activation when they are motivated to control their stereotypic responses. Specifically, individuals who were given a counterstereotypic expectancy (i.e., expecting to see a male name after a female-related prime) were able to eliminate the typical stereotype-priming effect (e.g., facilitation when male names were paired with male-related primes). This was true even at very short SOAs (e.g., 250 ms). Although these findings do not unequivocally establish that stereotype activation was prevented (i.e., perhaps stereotypes were activated, and then some other control strategy intervened to prevent the typical stereotype priming), they are consistent with the possibility. That is, the stereotype-priming effect may have been eliminated because participants' motivation to avoid stereotypic responses served to prevent stereotypes from being activated.

Future research is needed to examine the precise mechanisms underlying Blair and Banaji's findings. Also, it will be important to examine the extent to which similar findings are observed when the source of motivation to control stereotypic responses is internal (i.e., stemming from a personal desire to control prejudice) rather than external (i.e., stemming from experimenter-supplied instructions). Finally, research will need to explore the extent to which practice at controlling prejudiced responses across time and situations helps individuals to avoid stereotype activation. Such future investigations may have the ultimate outcome of establishing that stereotype activation can be prevented among individuals who are motivated to practice the self-regulation of prejudiced responses.

The Influence of Chronically Accessible Egalitarian Goals

Gollwitzer and Moskowitz (1996) have recently argued that establishing the chronic goal to be egalitarian, through frequent and recent activation of the goal, should lead to the preconscious automatic activation of that goal (see Bargh, 1990) and to inhibition of stereotype activation. In a related study, Moskowitz, Wasel, Gollwitzer, and Schaal (1996) did not find evidence of stereotype activation among participants who had chronic

egalitarian goals when they were presented with pictures of members of stereotyped groups. Among participants without chronic egalitarian goals, stereotypes were activated upon viewing the pictures. Additional work seems necessary to identify the precise mechanisms underlying how chronic egalitarian goals have the effect of preventing stereotype activation.

CONCLUDING COMMENTS

Our goal in this chapter has been to review the extant literature on the automaticity and control in stereotyping. This review has revealed that issues of both automaticity and control with regard to stereotyping are multifaceted and do not lend themselves to easy generalizations at present. For example, although stereotype activation may not be unconditionally automatic, it is very efficient and likely to occur. Thus, for those who are so inclined, there is something to be controlled. Our review of the literature suggests that control appears to be possible, at least for certain types of responses under some circumstances (e.g., Devine, 1989; Monteith, 1993; Gilbert & Hixon, 1991; Sherman et al., 1997; Sinclair & Kunda, 1997). Such findings provide reason for optimism that control over stereotyping is possible, and they suggest reasons to further develop analyses of stereotype control mechanisms. However, in a provocative chapter in this volume (Chapter 18), John Bargh reviews much of the same evidence but comes to a more pessimistic conclusion about the efficacy of control efforts. Specifically, Bargh suggests that the challenges associated with controlling automatic stereotype activation are so formidable that successful stereotype control is unlikely, even when people's intentions are to avoid using stereotypes. To date, however, the research literature has not yielded unequivocal answers concerning just how much control people do or can exert over prejudiced responses.

From the existing work, which has focused largely on documenting failures of control, one might conclude (as Bargh has) that gaining control over stereotypes is unlikely. Alternatively, one could opt (as we do) for taking a more considered and thorough look at the processes and mechanisms involved in stereotype control. Indeed, one of our observations is that analysis and investigation of the mechanisms and processes involved in stereotype control are currently only in the earliest stages of development. As such, strong conclusions about the likely (in)efficacy of stereotype control efforts may be premature. Again, the purpose of our review has been to provide an overview of the various stereotype control strategies explored to date; our hope is that this review will help to stimulate additional research into these mechanisms, and perhaps will serve as a springboard for the development of alternative, potentially more effective stereotype control strategies.

In this context, we believe that the most exciting developments in the analysis of the controllability of stereotype activation and application are likely to be forthcoming as we move beyond strict dual-process conceptions to more elaborated analyses that afford the opportunity to think more complexly about both automaticity and control in stereotyping. It will be especially important to develop more complete analyses of the ways in which automatic and controlled processes interact to affect thought, judgment, and behavior. Although some theorists have acknowledged the interactive nature of automatic and controlled processes more than others, we see this as a particularly rich area for continued development. In moving the study of control forward, we strongly encourage the development of formal analyses of the sources of motivation to control stereotyping and prejudice and the link between these sources of motivation (e.g., internal vs. external; cf. Plant & Devine, 1998) and the nature of people's control efforts. That is, people are likely to be motivated to control stereotyping for a variety of reasons (e.g., because they personally believe it is wrong or because others will evaluate them negatively). To date, however, there exists no well-developed theoretical analysis of the alternative sources of motivation to control stereotype use, or of the ways such motivations may affect the consequences of successful or failed stereotype control efforts. It seems a safe generalization that without motivation, whatever its source, other issues of control are moot. To the extent that the source of motivation underlying control efforts determines the specific control strategies pursued, which may determine their short-

term and long-term ultimate efficacy, failure to attend to these issues will produce incomplete analyses of stereotype control.

Finally, in addition to the various new research directions we have highlighted throughout the section on control, we also encourage researchers to examine the implications of automaticity and control of stereotyping in the context of the interpersonal aspects of intergroup perception and behavior. Although the most important implications of stereotype activation and control are played out in the interpersonal arena, where failures to control can be most destructive, relatively little effort has been devoted to exploring issues of automaticity and control of stereotyping in such settings. Interpersonal, intergroup settings are likely to create additional challenges in controlling stereotypes (Devine et al., 1996; Devine & Vasquez, 1998). In short, we need to move beyond studying issues of automaticity and control of stereotypes in isolated social perceivers. Social perceivers, after all, need to manage not only their cognitive processes, but also the social context in which stereotyping is typically played out. Complete analyses of stereotype control will be forthcoming only when we take seriously both the intrapersonal and interpersonal challenges involved in controlling stereotypes. We eagerly await such developments.

ACKNOWLEDGMENTS

Preparation of this chapter was supported in part by an H. I. Romnes Fellowship to Patricia G. Devine and by National Institute of Mental Health FIRST Award No. 1R29MH56536-01 to Margo J. Monteith.

NOTE

1. In this chapter, our concern is with control as an alternative to automatic processing that can attenuate or otherwise help one to limit the impact of social stereotypes on perception, judgment, and behavior. However, controlled processing does not invariably produce attenuation of stereotype effects. Some people may be particularly motivated to think in stereotypic ways and may use controlled processing to promote stereotype use. In addition, Chen and Chaiken (Chapter 4, this volume) suggest how controlled or systematic processes may be biased by previous heuristic processing in

ways that can produce increased stereotyping. The argument following from the heuristic–systematic model's bias hypothesis is as follows: Ambiguous information about a target can be interpreted in stereotypic ways through systematic processing if perceivers have previously responded to the target heuristically and in line with the stereotype. Group membership, for example, can serve as a heuristic cue (e.g., in a business context, a woman must be a secretary) that may influence subsequence systematic processing, particularly when a perceiver is not fully aware of the previous heuristic processing of the target. Thus, even though processing of the target may be systematic (or controlled), stereotypic judgments may follow.

REFERENCES

Allport, G. W. (1954). *The nature of prejudice.* Reading, MA: Addison-Wesley.

Amodt, I. J., & Devine, P. G. (1994, May). *When personal standards collide with social pressure. Competing motivations and affective consequences.* Paper presented at the annual 1994 meeting of the Midwestern Psychological Association, Chicago.

Aronson, E. (1968). The theory of cognitive dissonance: A current perspective. In L. Berkowitz (Ed.), *Advances in experimental social psychology* (Vol. 4, pp. 1–34). New York: Academic Press.

Ausubel, D. P. (1955). Relationships between shame and guilt in the socializing process. *Psychological Review,* 62, 378–390.

Banaji, M. R., & Greenwald, A. G. (1994). Implicit stereotyping and unconscious prejudice. In M. P. Zanna & J. M. Olson (Eds.), *The psychology of prejudice: The Ontario Symposium* (Vol. 7, pp. 55–76). Hillsdale, NJ: Erlbaum.

Banaji, M. R., & Greenwald, A. G. (1995). Implicit gender stereotyping in judgments of fame. *Journal of Personality and Social Psychology,* 68, 181–198.

Banaji, M. R., & Hardin, C. D. (1996). Automatic stereotyping. *Psychological Science,* 7, 136–141.

Banaji, M. R., Hardin, C. D., & Rothman, A. J. (1993). Implicit stereotyping in person judgment. *Journal of Personality and Social Psychology,* 65, 272–281.

Bandura, A. (1986). *Social foundations of thought and action.* Englewood Cliffs, NJ: Prentice Hall.

Bandura, A., & Jourdan, F. (1991). Self-regulatory mechanisms governing the impact of social comparison on complex decision making. *Journal of Personality and Social Psychology,* 60, 941–951.

Bargh, J. A. (1989). Conditional automaticity: Varieties of automatic influence in social perception and cognition. In J. S. Uleman & J. A. Bargh (Eds.), *Unintended thought* (pp. 3–51). New York: Guilford Press.

Bargh, J. A. (1990). Automotives: Preconscious determinants of thought and behavior. In E. T. Higgins & R. M. Sorrentino (Eds.), *Handbook of motivation and cognition* (Vol. 2, pp. 93–130). New York: Guilford Press.

Bargh, J. A. (1994). The four horsemen of automaticity: Awareness, intention, efficiency, and control in social cognition. In R. S. Wyer, Jr., & T. K. Srull (Eds.), *Handbook in social cognition* (2nd ed., Vol. 1, pp. 1–40). Hillsdale, NJ: Erlbaum.

Bargh, J. A., Chen, M., & Burrows, L. (1996). Automaticity of social behavior: Direct effects of trait construct and stereotype activation on action. *Journal of Personality and Social Psychology,* 71, 230–244.

Bargh, J. A., & Pietromonaco, P. (1982). Automatic information processing and social perception: The influence of trait information presented outside of conscious awareness. *Journal of Personality and Social Psychology,* 43, 437–449.

Bargh, J. A., & Pratto, F. (1986). Individual construct accessibility and perceptual selection. *Journal of Experimental Social Psychology,* 22, 293–311.

Billig, M. (1985). Prejudice, categorization, and particularization: From a perceptual to a rhetorical approach. *European Journal of Social Psychology,* 15, 79–103.

Blair, I. V., & Banaji, M. R. (1996). Automatic and controlling processes in stereotype priming. *Journal of Personality and Social Psychology,* 70, 1142–1163.

Bodenhausen, G. V. (1990). Stereotypes as judgmental heuristics: Evidence of circadian rhythms in discrimination. *Psychological Science,* 1, 319–322.

Bodenhausen, G. V., & Lichtenstein, M. (1987). Social stereotypes and information processing strategies: The importance of task complexity. *Journal of Personality and Social Psychology,* 52, 871–880.

Bodenhausen, G. V., & Macrae, C. N. (1998). Stereotype activation and inhibition. In R. S. Wyer, Jr. (Ed.), *Advances in social cognition* (Vol. 11, pp. 1–62). Mahwah, NJ: Erlbaum.

Bodenhausen, G. V., & Wyer, R. S., Jr. (1985). Effects of stereotypes on decision making and information processing strategies. *Journal of Personality and Social Psychology,* 48, 267–282.

Brewer, M. B. (1988). A dual process model of impression formation. In R. S. Wyer, Jr., & T. K. Srull (Eds.), *Advances in social cognition* (Vol. 1, pp. 1–36). Hillsdale, NJ: Erlbaum.

Carver, C. S., & Scheier, M. F. (1990). Origins and functions of positive and negative affect: A control process view. *Psychological Review,* 97, 19–35.

Chaiken, S. (1987). The heuristic–systematic model of persuasion. In M. P. Zanna, J. M. Olson, & C. P. Herman (Eds.), *Social influence: The Ontario Symposium* (Vol. 5, pp. 3–39). Hillsdale, NJ: Erlbaum.

Chen, M., & Bargh, J. A. (1997). Nonconscious behavioral confirmation processes: The self-fulfilling consequences of automatic stereotype activation. *Journal of Experimental Social Psychology,* 33, 541–560.

Darley, J. M., & Gross, P. H. (1983). A hypothesis confirming bias in labeling effects. *Journal of Personality and Social Psychology,* 44, 20–33.

Devine, P. G. (1989). Stereotypes and prejudice: Their automatic and controlled components. *Journal of Personality and Social Psychology,* 56, 5–18.

Devine, P. G., & Elliot, A. J. (1995). Are racial stereotypes *really* fading?: The Princeton trilogy revisited. *Personality and Social Psychology Bulletin,* 21, 1139–1150.

Devine, P. G., Evett, S. R., & Vasquez-Suson, K. A. (1996). Exploring the interpersonal dynamics of intergroup contact. In R.M. Sorrentino & E. T. Higgins (Eds.), *Handbook of motivation and cognition: Vol. 3. The interpersonal context* (pp. 423–464). New York: Guilford Press.

Devine, P. G., & Monteith, M. J. (1993). The role of discrepancy-associated affect in prejudice reduction. In D. M. Mackie & D. L. Hamilton (Eds.), *Affect, cognition, and stereotyping: Interactive processes in intergroup perception* (pp. 317–344). San Diego, CA: Academic Press.

Devine, P. G., Monteith, M. J., Zuwerink, J. R., & Elliot, A. J. (1991). Prejudice with and without compunction. *Journal of Personality and Social Psychology, 60,* 817–830.

Devine, P. G., & Vasquez, K. A. (1998). The rocky road to positive intergroup relations. In J. Ebberhardt & S. T. Fiske (Eds.), *Racism: The problem and the response* (pp. 234–262). Thousand Oaks, CA: Sage.

Dovidio, J. F., Evans, N., & Tyler, R. B. (1986). Racial stereotypes: The contents of their cognitive representations. *Journal of Experimental Social Psychology, 22,* 22–37.

Dovidio, J. F., Kawakami, K., Johnson, C., Johnson, B., & Howard, A. (1997). On the nature of prejudice: Automatic and controlled processes. *Journal of Experimental Social Psychology, 33,* 510–540.

Duncan, B. L. (1976). Different social perception and attribution of intergroup violence: Testing the lower limits of stereotyping of blacks. *Journal of Personality and Social Psychology, 34,* 590–598.

Duval, S., & Wicklund, R. A. (1972). *A theory of objective self-awareness.* New York: Academic Press.

Duval, T. S., Duval, B. H., & Mulisis, J. (1992). Effects of self-focus, discrepancy between self and standard, and outcome expectancy favorability on the tendency to match self to standard or to withdraw. *Journal of Personality and Social Psychology, 62,* 340–348.

Erber, R., & Fiske, S. T. (1984). Outcome dependency and attention to inconsistent information. *Journal of Personality and Social Psychology, 47,* 709–726.

Fazio, R. H., Jackson, J. R., Dunton, B. C., & Williams, C. J. (1995). Variability in automatic activation as an unobtrusive measure of racial attitudes: A bona fide pipeline? *Journal of Personality and Social Psychology, 69,* 1013–1027.

Feagin, J. (1991). The continuing significance of race: Antiblack discrimination in public places. *American Sociological Review, 56,* 101–116.

Fein, S., & Spencer, S. J. (1997). Prejudice as self-image maintenance: Affirming the self through derogating others. *Journal of Personality and Social Psychology, 73,* 31–44.

Festinger, L. (1957). *A cognitive theory of dissonance.* Stanford, CA: Stanford University Press.

Fiske, S. T. (1989). Examining the role of intent: Toward understanding its role in stereotyping and prejudice. In J. S. Uleman & J. A. Bargh (Eds.), *Unintended thought* (pp. 253–283). New York: Guilford Press.

Fiske, S. T. (1998). Controlling other people: The impact of power on stereotyping. *American Psychologist, 48,* 621–628.

Fiske, S. T., & Neuberg, S. L. (1990). A continuum of impression formation, from category-based to individuating processes: Influences of information and motivation on attention and interpretation. In M. P. Zanna (Ed.), *Advances in experimental social psychology* (Vol. 23, pp. 1–74). San Diego, CA: Academic Press.

Fiske, S. T., & Pavelchak, M. A. (1986). Category-based and piecemeal-based affective responses: Developments in schema triggered affect. In R. M. Sorrentino

& E. T. Higgins (Eds.), *Handbook of motivation and cognition: Foundations of social behavior* (Vol. 1, pp. 167–203). New York: Guilford Press.

Fowles, D. C. (1980). The three-arousal model: Implications for Gray's two factor learning theory for heart rate, electrodermal activity, and psychopathology. *Psychophysiology, 17,* 87–104.

Fox, R. (1992). Prejudice and the unfinished mind. *Psychological Inquiry, 3,* 137–152.

Gaertner, S. L., & Dovidio, J. F., (1986). The aversive form of racism. In J. F. Dovidio & S. L. Gaertner (Eds.), *Prejudice, racism, and discrimination* (pp. 61–89). New York: Academic Press.

Gilbert, D. T. (1989). Thinking lightly about others: Automatic components of the social inference process. In J. S. Uleman & J. A. Bargh (Eds.), *Unintended thought* (pp. 189–211). New York: Guilford Press.

Gilbert, D. T. (1991). How mental systems believe. *American Psychologist, 46,* 197–119.

Gilbert, D. T., & Hixon, J. G. (1991). The trouble with thinking: Activation and application of stereotypic beliefs. *Journal of Personality and Social Psychology, 60,* 518–517.

Gollwitzer, P. M., & Moskowitz, G. B. (1996). Goal effects on action and cognition. In E. T. Higgins & A. W. Kruglanski (Eds.), *Social psychology: Handbook of basic principles* (pp. 361–399). New York: Guilford Press.

Gray, J. A. (1982). *The neuropsychology of anxiety: An enquiry into the function of the septohippocampal system.* New York: Oxford University Press.

Greenwald, A. G., & Baraji, M. R. (1995). Implicit social cognition. *Psychological Review, 102,* 4–27.

Hamilton, D. L., & Sherman, J. W. (1994). Stereotypes. In R. S. Wyer, Jr., & T. K. Srull (Eds.), *Handbook of social cognition* (2nd ed., Vol. 2, pp. 1–68). Hillsdale, NJ: Erlbaum.

Higgins, E. T., & King, G. (1981). Accessibility of social constructs: Information processing consequences of individual and contextual variability. In N. Cantor & J. F. Kihlstrom (Eds.), *Personality, cognition and social interaction* (pp. 69–121). Hillsdale, NJ: Erlbaum.

Jacoby, L. L., Lindsay, D. S., & Toth, J. P. (1992). Unconscious influences revealed: Attention, awareness, and control. *American Psychologist, 47,* 802–809.

Jamieson, D. W., & Zanna, M. P. (1989). Need for structure in attitude formation and expression. In A. R. Pratkanis, S. J. Breckler, & A. G. Greenwald (Eds.), *Attitude structure and function* (pp. 383–406). Hillsdale, NJ: Erlbaum.

Johnson, M. K., & Hasher, L. (1987). Human learning and memory. *Annual Review of Psychology, 38,* 631–668.

Jones, E. E., Farina, A., Hastorf, A. H., Markus, H., & Scott, R. A. (1984). *Social stigma: The psychology of marked relationships.* New York: Freeman.

Kruglanski, A. W., & Freund, T. (1983). The freezing and unfreezing of lay inferences: Effects on impressional primacy, ethnic stereotyping and numerical anchoring. *Journal of Experimental Social Psychology, 19,* 448–468.

Lepore, L., & Brown, R. (1997). Category and stereotype activation: Is prejudice inevitable? *Journal of Personality and Social Psychology, 72,* 275–287.

Lippman, W. (1922). *Public opinion.* New York: Harcourt & Brace.

Logan, G. D., & Cowan, W. B. (1984). On the ability to inhibit thought and action: A theory of act control. *Psychological Review, 91,* 295–327.

Lombardi, W. J., Higgins, E. T., & Bargh, J. A. (1986). The role of consciousness in priming effects on categorization: Assimilation vs. contrast as a function of awareness of the priming task. *Personality and Social Psychology Bulletin, 13,* 411–429.

Macrae, C. N., Bodenhausen, G. V., & Milne, A. B. (1998). Saying no to unwanted thoughts: Self-focus and the regulation of mental life. *Journal of Personality and Social Psychology, 74,* 578–589.

Macrae, C. N., Bodenhausen, G. V., Milne, A. B., & Jetten, J. (1994). Out of mind but back in sight: Stereotypes on the rebound. *Journal of Personality and Social Psychology, 67,* 808–817.

Macrae, C. N., Milne, A. B., & Bodenhausen, G. V. (1994). Stereotypes as energy-saving devices: A peek inside the cognitive toolbox. *Journal of Personality and Social Psychology, 66,* 37–47.

Macrae, C. N., Bodenhausen, G. V., Milne, A. B., & Wheeler, V. (1996). On resisting the temptation for simplification: Counterintentional effects of stereotype suppression on social memory. *Social Cognition, 14,* 1–20.

Martin, L. L. (1986). Set/reset: Use and disuse of concepts in impression formation. *Journal of Personality and Social Psychology, 51,* 493–504.

Monteith, M. J. (1993). Self-regulation of prejudiced responses: Implications for progress in prejudice reduction efforts. *Journal of Personality and Social Psychology, 65,* 469–485.

Monteith, M. J. (1996a). Affective reactions to prejudice-related discrepant responses: The impact of standard salience. *Personality and Social Psychology Bulletin, 22,* 48–59.

Monteith, M. J. (1996b). Contemporary forms of prejudice-related conflict: In search of a nutshell. *Personality and Social Psychology Bulletin, 5,* 416–473.

Monteith, M. J., Deneen, N. E., & Tooman, G. (1996). The effect of social norm activation on the expression on opinions concerning gay men and blacks. *Basic and Applied Social Psychology, 18,* 267–288.

Monteith, M. J., Devine, P. G., & Zuwerink, J. R. (1993). Self-directed versus other-directed affect as a consequence of prejudice-related discrepancies. *Journal of Personality and Social Psychology, 64,* 198–210.

Monteith, M. J., Sherman, J. W., & Devine, P. G. (1998). Suppression as a stereotype control strategy. *Personality and Social Psychology Review, 2,* 63–82.

Monteith, M. J., Spicer, C. V., & Tooman, G. D. (1998). Consequences of stereotype suppression: Stereotypes on AND not on the rebound. *Journal of Experimental Social Psychology, 34,* 355–377.

Monteith, M. J., & Walters, G. L. (1998). Egalitarianism, moral obligation, and prejudice-related standards. *Personality and Social Psychology Bulletin, 24,* 186–199.

Moskowitz, G. B., Wasel, W., Gollwitzer, P. M., & Schaal, B. (1996). *A model of habitual stereotyping: Stereotype activation and use is silent, efficient, but under volitional control.* Manuscript submitted for publication.

Neely, J. H. (1977). Semantic priming and retrieval from lexical memory: Roles of inhibitionless spreading acti-vation and limited capacity attention. *Journal of Experimental Psychology: General, 106,* 226–254.

Neuberg, S. L. (1989). The goal of forming accurate impressions during social interactions: Attenuating impact of negative expectancies. *Journal of Personality and Social Psychology, 56,* 374–386.

Neuberg, S. L., & Fiske, S. T. (1987). Motivational influences on impression formation: Outcome dependency, accuracy-driven attention, and individuating processes. *Journal of Personality and Social Psychology, 53,* 431–444.

Nisbett, R., & Wilson, D. T. (1977). Telling more than we can know: Verbal reports on mental processes. *Psychological Review, 84,* 231–259.

Patterson, C. M., & Newman, J. P. (1993). Reflectivity and learning from aversive events: Toward a psychological mechanism for the syndromes of disinhibition. *Psychological Review, 100,* 716–736.

Petty, R. E., & Cacioppo, J. T. (1986). The elaboration likelihood model of persuasion. In L. Berkowitz (Ed.), *Advances in experimental social psychology* (Vol. 19, pp. 123–205). San Diego, CA: Academic Press.

Plant, E. A., & Devine, P. G. (1998). Internal and external sources of motivation to respond without prejudice. *Journal of Personality and Social Psychology, 75,* 811–832.

Posner, M. I., & Snyder, C. R. R. (1975). Attention and cognitive control. In R. Solso (Ed.), *Information processing and cognition: The Loyola Symposium* (pp. 55–85). Hillsdale, NJ: Erlbaum.

Pratto, F., & Bargh, J. A. (1991). Stereotyping based on apparently individuating information: Trait and global components of sex stereotypes under attention overload. *Journal of Experimental Social Psychology, 27,* 26–47.

Pressly, S. L., & Devine, P. G. (1992, April). *Sex, sexism, and compunction: Group membership or internalization of standards?* Paper presented at the meeting of the Midwestern Psychological Association, Chicago.

Pressly, S. L., & Devine, P. G. (1997). *Stereotype suppression: When the target group matters.* Unpublished manuscript, University of Wisconsin–Madison.

Purdue, C. W., & Gurtman, M. B. (1990). Evidence for automatic ageism. *Journal of Experimental Social Psychology, 26,* 199–216.

Pyszczynski, T., & Greenberg, J. (1986). Persistent high self-focus after failure and low self-focus after success: The depressive self-focusing style. *Journal of Personality and Social Psychology, 50,* 1039–1044.

Pyszczynski, T., & Greenberg, J. (1987). Self-regulatory perseveration and the depressive self focusing style: A self-awareness theory of reactive depression. *Psychological Bulletin, 102,* 122–138.

Rokeach, M. (1973). *The nature of human values.* New York: Free Press.

Sherman, J. W., Stroessner, S. J., & Azam, O. (1997). *The role of personal attitudes in motivated individuation.* Unpublished manuscript, Northwestern University.

Shiffrin, R. M., & Schnieder, W. (1977). Controlled and automatic human information processing: II. Perceptual learning, automatic attending, and a general theory. *Psychological Review, 84,* 127–190.

Sinclair, L., & Kunda, Z. (1997). *Feedback-dependent evaluation of evaluators: Motivated application and inhibition of stereotypes.* Unpublished manuscript, University of Waterloo.

Smith, E. R. (1994). Procedural knowledge and processing strategies in social cognition. In R. S. Wyer, Jr. & T. K. Srull (Eds.), *Handbook of social cognition* (2nd ed., Vol. 1, pp. 99–151). Hillsdale, NJ: Erlbaum.

Spencer, S. J., Fein, S., Wolfe, C. T., Hodgson, H. L., & Dunn, M. A. (in press). Automatic activation of stereotypes: The role of self-image threat. *Personality and Social Psychology Bulletin.*

Srull, T. K., & Wyer, R. S., Jr. (1979). The role of category accessibility in the interpretation of information about persons: Some determinants and implications. *Journal of Personality and Social Psychology, 37,* 1660–1672.

Tetlock, P. E., & Kim, J. I. (1987). Accountability and judgment processes in a personality prediction task. *Journal of Personality and Social Psychology, 52,* 700–709.

Thompson, E. P., Roman, R. J., Moskowitz, G. B., Chaiken, S., & Bargh, J. A. (1994). Accuracy motivation attenuates covert priming: The systematic reprocessing of social information. *Journal of Personality and Social Psychology, 66,* 474–489.

Trope, Y., & Alfieri, T. (1997). Effortfulness and flexibility of dispositional judgment processes. *Journal of Personality and Social Psychology, 73,* 662–674.

Wegener, D. T., & Petty, R. E. (1997). The flexible correction model: The role of naive theories of bias in bias correction. In M. P. Zanna (Ed.), *Advances in experimental social psychology* (Vol. 29, pp. 141–208). San Diego, CA: Academic Press.

Wegner, D. M. (1994). Ironic processes of mental control. *Psychological Review, 101,* 34–52.

Wegner, D. M., & Erber, R. (1992). The hyperaccessibility of suppressed thoughts. *Journal of Personality and Social Psychology, 63,* 903–912.

Wilson, T. D., & Brekke, N. (1994). Mental contamination and mental correction: Unwanted influences on judgments and evaluations. *Psychological Review, 116,* 117–142.

Wittenbrink, B., Judd, C. M., & Park, B. (1997). Evidence for racial prejudice at the implicit level and its relationship with questionnaire measures. *Journal of Personality and Social Psychology, 72,* 262–274.

Wyer, N. A., Sherman, J. W., & Stroessner, S. J. (1997). *The roles of motivation and ability in controlling the consequences of stereotype suppression.* Manuscript submitted for publication.

Zuwerink, J. R., Devine, P. G., Monteith, M. J., & Cook, D. A. (1996). Prejudice towards blacks: With and without compunction? *Basic and Applied Social Psychology, 18,* 131–150.

18

The Cognitive Monster

THE CASE AGAINST THE CONTROLLABILITY OF AUTOMATIC STEREOTYPE EFFECTS

JOHN A. BARGH

This chapter provides a more or less opinionated history of the standard dual-process model of stereotyping effects on judgment and behavior. It focuses particularly on the fluctuations over the past 30 years in the relative power ascribed to the automatic influences of stereotypes versus the conscious, intentional attempts to control them. The major theme is that the evidence of controllability is weaker and more problematic than we would like to believe.

The Fable of the Cognitive Monster

Once upon a time, in the land of Social Psychology, there lived the Cognitive Miser. This creature was the object of much sympathy and compassion from the good people of Social Psychology, for it was afflicted with the curse of Limited Processing Resources, and therefore could do naught but give scant attention and time to most of the world around it. All agreed that it was necessary and wise for the creature to depend on simplifying modes of thought, in order to conserve its constrained mental capacity for when it was most needed. The people watched and noted how the Cognitive Miser never learned about them as separate individuals, but only reacted

to each of them on the basis of their superficial aspects and the roles they played in daily life. It was unfortunate, but a reasonable strategy for the Miser to pursue, given its limits. And so the people in the land of Social Psychology were (reasonably) content.

But then the people became terribly afraid and anxious. For lo! the Cognitive Miser had become transformed, by the magic of Further Research, into the Cognitive Monster. No longer did the creature use simplifying categories and stereotypes by choice or strategy; their use had become an addiction—uncontrollable, not a matter of choice at all—and the creature's Will was powerless to do anything else.

"We must do something!" cried the people of Social Psychology. "We must slay the Monster!" And so their heroes came forth. They rode to the nearby friendly lands of Awareness and Motivation, and raised a formidable army. Then, cleverly using the very weapons of Further Research that had created the Monster, they turned them against the dreaded foe. The soldiers of Awareness shone their bright lights on the Monster, and thus aided, the people of Motivation lashed and tethered the beast. Victory followed upon victory. The Monster was greatly diminished in power and scope, and the people were no longer afraid. Indeed, soon came the day when they laughed and jeered at the Monster, tethered in chains in the village square.

Unfortunately, monster stories rarely end on such a happy note, as anyone familiar with the tales of King Kong or Frankenstein knows. The chained monster, it turns out in each of these stories, is only temporarily under control. And so, when the populace becomes complacent and lets its guard down, the monster bursts its bonds and rampages again, causing more mayhem than before.

Those classic monster stories were written as allegories for the very real monsters that individuals and societies face (be they dictators or unchecked scientific progress). They were also intended as warnings of the need for constant vigilance against such menaces. My theme in this chapter is similar. It is that in many ways, the field of social cognition has become overly optimistic about the "cognitive monster" of automatic stereotype activation. I contend here that, contrary to what our research is actually showing, the conclusions drawn from the data have overestimated the degree to which automatically activated stereotypes can be controlled through good intentions and effortful thought—and thereby have underestimated the extent to which stereotypes continue today to cause problems in social relations.

META-ASSUMPTIONS ABOUT STEREOTYPE CONTROLLABILITY: A BRIEF HISTORY

"The Fable of the Cognitive Monster" is intended to illustrate the assumptional shifts in social cognition that have taken place since the 1960s concerning the controllability (vs. automaticity) of social perception and judgment. The early attribution models broadly assumed an active and effortful search after meaning, with conscious and deliberate scrutiny of the co-occurrence of effects with their possible causes (e.g., Jones & Davis, 1965; Kelley, 1967; Weiner, 1974). Individuals were assumed to be largely in executive control of their perceptual and judgmental faculties.

The Cognitive Miser

However, the 1970s saw a reaction to this meta-assumption of effortful processing, as Langer (e.g., 1978; Langer & Abelson, 1972) and Taylor and Fiske (e.g., 1978) voiced doubts as to whether people are always so thoughtful and in control. Instead, they argued, people are often "mindless" in their behavior and choice making, following stored scripts based on the routines of social interactions. These authors also described people as lacking the mental and attentional capacity to engage in effortful thought on a moment-to-moment basis. Therefore, people are forced into using mental resources in a sparing or "miserly" fashion—relying on simplifying tactics such as heuristic decision rules and stereotypes (see also Dawes, 1976; Kahneman & Tversky, 1973).

The reliance on simple decision rules and on pigeonholing of individuals into stock characters or categories was viewed mainly as a matter of strategic necessity, or even as an adaptive way of dealing with our mental shortcomings as human beings. A miser, after all, is one who is intentionally and deliberately stingy when doling out money, and who jealously guards existing funds. Because the world is filled with unexpected and potentially dangerous events, and these draw heavily on our limited attention (e.g., Fiske, 1980; Pratto & John, 1993), it would seem to be a reasonable strategy to use attention in this miserly fashion.

As an illustration of how such minimal and noneffortful information processing was viewed at the time as a matter of strategic choice, consider the classic Langer, Blank, and Chanowitz (1978) experiments on mindless behavior. These studies demonstrated how participants would react mindlessly in routine situations, evidently not paying much attention to the content (only to the form) of the social interaction. But at the same time, the experiments also showed that participants quickly became mindful, and engaged in effortful processing, when behaving mindlessly would have had important costs to them. For instance, when a confederate trying to cut ahead in the line to use the copying machine promised the participant that this would cause only a short delay, the quality of the excuse given did not matter to the participant's behavior; however, the quality of the reason *did* matter when the promised delay was longer and thus a real inconvenience.

The Cognitive Monster

It soon became apparent, however, that much of the documented reliance on cognitive shortcuts was not so much a matter of strategic choice as of automatic, unintended processes operating in person perception and social judgment. Automaticity was first raised as a possibility in the closing pages of Taylor and Fiske (1978), and in the 1980s it was applied to and demonstrated for nearly all social-psychological phenomena: trait attributions (e.g., Gilbert, 1989; Gilbert, Pelham, & Krull, 1988; Winter & Uleman, 1984), an attitude's effect on behavior (Fazio, Sanbonmatsu, Powell, & Kardes, 1986), self-judgments (Bargh & Tota, 1988; Paulhus, Graf, & Van Selst, 1989), interpretation of another's behavior (Bargh & Thein, 1985), and of course stereotyping (Brewer, 1988; Deaux & Lewis, 1984; Dovidio, Evans, & Tyler, 1986). The mere perception of easily discernible group features (e.g., skin color, gender, and age-related characteristics) was sufficient in these latter studies to cause the activation of the stereotype associated with the group, which then was shown to influence judgments of a group member in an unintended fashion, outside of a perceiver's awareness (see reviews in Bargh, 1989; Brewer, 1988).

These latter demonstrations were what raised the specter of the cognitive monster of automatic stereotyping. If it were indeed the case, as research appeared to indicate, that stereotyping occurs without an individual's awareness or intention, then the implications for society—specifically, the hope that prejudice and discrimination could eventually be eradicated—were tremendous, as well as tremendously depressing. Most ominously, how could anyone be held responsible, legally or otherwise, for discriminatory or prejudicial behavior when psychological science had shown such effects to occur unintentionally? The legal profession has a term for such a dilemma: the "parade of horribles," in which the appropriate legal cure for an existing unfair or unconstitutional situation itself opens a Pandora's box of still worse evils. Did social psychologists *really* want to go on record as saying that stereotyping and prejudice are uncontrollable?

The "Nightmare Scenario"

More than one social psychologist lost sleep over the implications of these demonstrations of automatic stereotyping, but it was Fiske (1989) who most eloquently captured the essence of the dilemma:

An absence of intent ultimately implies an absence of responsibility for the effects of categorization. . . . It has led me to have the following nightmare: After testifying for the plaintiff in a case of egregious and demonstrable discrimination, a cognitive social psychologist faces the cross-examining attorney. The hostile attorney, who looms taller than Goliath, says, "Tell us, Professor, do people intend to discriminate?" The cognitive social psychologist hedges about not having any hard data with regard to discrimination, being an expert mainly in stereotyping. When pressed, the psychologist admits that stereotypic cognitions are presumed to underlie discriminatory behavior. Pressed still further, the psychologist reluctantly mumbles that, indeed, a common interpretation of the cognitive approach is that people do not stereotype intentionally, whereupon the cross-examining attorney says in a tone of triumph, "No further questions, Your Honor." The plaintiff is led shaking from the courtroom. . . . (Fiske, 1989, p. 265)

Faced with this possibility, Fiske argued that the mind does not work by cognition alone. Although the cognitive miser may shy away from using such effortful control processes, Fiske argued that properly motivated individuals can "make the hard choice" and overcome the influences of automatically activated stereotypes. In her view, this is theoretically possible because of the general ability of conscious or control processes to dominate and inhibit the influence of automatic processes (e.g., Posner & Snyder, 1975); however, it will depend both on the person's being aware of the nonconscious influence in the first place, and then on his or her having the motivation and also the ability (i.e., enough time and attentional resources) to engage in the control process.

There were those who were skeptical about how often all of these conditions can be met in the real world (e.g., Bargh, 1989; Hilton & Darley, 1991), but at the time this was almost beside the point. As the evidence appeared to show that stereotyping and prejudice are inevitable, or at least highly likely, a way out had to be found; the alternative was to give up and go home.

And so, faced with the cognitive monster, the battle cry of social cognition researchers became (to borrow the words of Isaac Bashevis Singer): "We've got to believe in free will—we have no choice!"

A Critique of "Fiske's Dilemma"

Bringing motivation back into stereotyping research transformed what had been seen as a cognitive inevitability (e.g., Billig, 1985; Hamilton, 1979) into a matter of personal choice and goal setting. It was part of a larger trend within social cognition that started around the mid-1980s (e.g., Neuberg & Fiske, 1987; Sorrentino & Higgins, 1986). In another widely cited paper, also appearing in 1989, Devine divided the phenomenon of automatic stereotyping into two distinct components: stereotype activation and stereotype application, with only the first stage being automatic and inevitable. The application and use of the activated stereotype in person perception and judgment were argued to be under motivational control.

The dilemma posed by Fiske (1989) was between the pursuit of scientific insight into how much control an individual does have over prejudicial judgments and behavior on the one hand, and the implications of that knowledge for society on the other. The possibility was clearly and dramatically sketched of a "parade of horribles" if society and the legal system adopted the apparent findings of psychological research as to the unintentional nature of stereotyping. If people cannot help stereotyping, then they cannot be held personally responsible for their actions, and so cannot be sanctioned for any prejudicial actions.

Yet, as participants in a scientific enterprise, we enter upon a very slippery slope when we attempt to tailor our conclusions to fit what we believe to be good for society. We should not be guided, as a field, by a motivation to demonstrate and conclude from our research findings that automatic stereotypes are in fact controllable. No matter how well-meaning and virtuous this intention may be, it can do nothing but compromise our objectivity as psychological scientists.

Societal versus Scientific Concepts of Personal Responsibility

Whether or not personal responsibility over stereotyping and prejudice exists in fact, there is no doubt that society has a powerful interest in presuming that it does. The notion of individual responsibility and culpability for one's own actions is the bedrock of every legal

system, and the "parade of horribles" that would follow from abandonment of this notion would indeed be calamitous. This is one reason why, even if psychologists were someday to prove beyond a shadow of a doubt that free will does not exist, society would nonetheless continue to hold people personally responsible for their actions (see Koestler, 1967, Ch. 1). It would cease to function otherwise.

In a recent essay, Prinz (1996) distinguishes between the *scientific status* and the *moral function* of the concept of "free will." The latter sense of the concept is described as "a social construction aimed toward the societal control of actions." According to this analysis, psychologists focus on the causal explanation of actions, whereas society is much more interested in their evaluation and moral justification than in their causal explanation. But the important point is that the societal and the scientific versions of the concept of personal responsibility can coexist independently of each other. The social utility of the idea of individual responsibility exists, the scientific evidence regarding personal control notwithstanding. Therefore, society's use of the notion of free will is something that can never be dictated to by psychological research findings. At the same time, psychological research into the degree of personal control over stereotyping and prejudice is of enormous theoretical and practical significance. *And so, by the same logic, the conclusions of this research should not be dictated by the agenda of society.*

Prinz (1996) frames the question thus:

> How should we view this? Where is the hen and where is the egg? Should we consider free will to be a basic fact of our psychological make-up that, quite arbitrarily, has desirable social side effects—or as the product of a social construction aimed toward the societal control of actions? Do the psychological facts precede the moral function—or should we at last realize that the moral function elicits psychological facts?

The Monster in Chains

Fiske's (1989) analysis of the interplay between cognitive factors (stereotype activation) and motivational factors (effortful control) in prejudice gave free will and intentionality a chance again. The pendulum was swinging back to a meta-assumption of strategic control over stereotyping, as it had been assumed in the era of the cognitive miser. Note, however, that there was something of a strategic retreat regarding the role of free will in person perception: Whereas the initial deployment and use of categories and stereotypes had been thought to be under the miser's strategic control, now only the subsequent influence of the already activated category or stereotype was believed to be controllable.

Two Stages of Stereotyping

That same year, as noted above, Devine (1989) published a similar analysis of distinct activation and application stages of stereotyping. With the perspective of time, what may well have contributed to the impact and importance of Devine's paper was that it presented, simultaneously, the scariest version of the cognitive monster yet imagined, followed by reasons why and evidence as to how this worst-case scenario was not really the intractable problem we had assumed. This was indeed welcome news: If even the most threatening version of stereotype automaticity could be shown to be ultimately controllable, as Devine argued, then the monster could be fought, and perhaps further diminished in power by additional discoveries.

Devine (1989) found that all of her participants, regardless of their expressed or explicit level of prejudice against African Americans, could accurately report the content of the culture's stereotype of that group. Next—and most chillingly—all of the participants showed evidence of having this stereotype automatically activated by subliminally presented stereotypic features. In her Experiment 2, Devine (1989) showed effects of the primed stereotype on judgments of a target person's degree of hostility, even though in her design the primes did not include "hostile" or a synonym for it. Therefore, the African American stereotype had become active automatically and had affected opinions about a person's hostility in the absence of any information in the experimental situation concerning hostility—exactly the "going beyond the information given" and filling-in-the-blanks function

long associated with stereotyping—yet the experimental participants never intended to stereotype, and low-prejudice individuals showed the effect as much as did high-prejudice individuals.

Therefore, even if a person expressed egalitarian and nonprejudiced beliefs concerning African Americans, he or she nonetheless seemed just as vulnerable to automatic stereotype influences as were prejudiced individuals. Where in these data was there any reason for optimism that a person's values, and egalitarian motives, and good intentions could prevent cultural stereotypes from influencing judgments of minority group members?

Yet there was room for hope. It came from Devine's (1989) theoretical analysis of stereotype automaticity into two components: the activation stage and the application stage. In her view, the activation stage is completely automatic (assuming a stereotype that permeates the culture), in that one cannot help having the stereotype activated by relevant group features. This is what Experiment 2 showed. Experiment 3, on the other hand, concerned the application stage. Assuming an activated stereotype, can an individual consciously control its application to a target individual? In Experiment 3, the participants' level of expressed racism did relate to how stereotypic and prejudicial were thoughts listed about the category "blacks": High-prejudice participants' thoughts were more negative and stereotypic than those of low-prejudice participants.

Further Restrictions on Automatic Stereotype Influences

With the momentum swinging back in the direction of conscious control and away from demonstrations of automaticity, other limits to the phenomenon of automatic stereotyping were documented in short order. Devine (1989) had argued that even though stereotypes become active automatically, their influence on judgment is under motivational control. Neuberg (1989, 1994) showed that the self-fulfilling prophecy effects of negative stereotypic expectancies could be controlled if participants had a conscious goal to form an accurate impression of the target person (see also Fiske & Neuberg, 1990). Gilbert and Hixon (1991) argued that even the stereotype activation stage may not be automatic under all conditions, because it did not happen when participants were busy with a secondary task (holding a series of digits in memory) while a member of a stereotyped group was present. Blair and Banaji (1996) concluded that the initial stage of automatic activation can be prevented through counterstereotypic expectancies. And Jussim (e.g., 1990) argued that if all else fails, and stereotypes are nonconsciously activated and their influence not then controlled, this influence should nonetheless be benign because stereotypes are accurate descriptions of the social group (see also Lee, Jussim, & McCauley, 1995).

Perhaps I'm just a pessimist, but I don't buy any of this. It would be *nice* if stereotypes were found not to be activated automatically. It would be *nice* if, failing that and stereotypes were found to be automatically activated, then it was found that an individual could prevent this activation by having a conscious, counterstereotypic expectancy. It would be *nice* if, even if automatic activation could not be shown to be prevented in this (or any other) way, individuals were found to be indeed cognizant of the possibility of being nonconsciously influenced, and when aware of that influence, to have the motivation and the time to effortfully control it. And it would be *nice* if, even if all these propositions failed and stereotypes were shown to be automatically activated and to affect perceptions of and behavior toward a member of a minority group, this influence was still found to be benign because the group stereotype was a demonstrably accurate portrait of the target individual.

All of this would indeed be nice—if it were true. But the relevant research evidence largely contradicts this rosy picture.

WHAT DOES THE EVIDENCE REALLY SAY ABOUT STEREOTYPE CONTROLLABILITY?

In this section, I first provide a critical appraisal of the evidence as to (1) whether automatic stereotype activation is likely, and, if so, whether such activation is unconditional or depends on the perceiver's current processing goal; (2) whether automatic activation can be eliminated by counterstereotypic expectancies; and (3) whether the influence of a stereotype, once activated, on judgments and behavior is likely to be controlled by the perceiver. Following this review, new evidence supporting a dual-process model of self-fulfilling prophecy effects is described.

Are Stereotypes Always Activated?

The Role of Attentional Resources

Gilbert and Hixon (1991) showed that a load on attentional resources—induced by giving participants a secondary task to perform—disrupted the otherwise automatic activation of the Asian American stereotype. Whereas participants made more stereotypic completions of word stems (e.g., "shy" for "s_ y") when an Asian American woman presented those stems in a video presentation, compared to baseline levels, this effect disappeared if they had to hold a series of digits in memory simultaneously. Thus, at least some stereotypes did not become active upon the mere presence of group features, if the perceiver had been "cognitively busy" at the time.

One question concerning this finding is its generalizability to other stereotypes. Perhaps those for women, African Americans, and the elderly are "stronger" stereotypes (at least in U.S. society), and consequently are more efficiently activated and not prevented from activation by a shortage of attention. Recently, however, Spencer, Fein, Wolfe, Fong, and Dunn (1998) have replicated the Gilbert and Hixon (1991) finding for the African American stereotype, so it does seem that when attention is divided, stereotypes are less likely to become activated.

However, several other studies, beginning with Devine (1989, Experiment 2), show that the African American stereotype is so efficient that it can become activated even with subliminal presentation of group features (see Bargh, Chen, & Burrows, 1996, Experiment 3; Chen & Bargh, 1997; Devine, 1989; Fazio, Jackson, Dunton, & Williams, 1995, Experiment 1), that is, with no conscious attentional processing needed. It therefore seems odd that a shortage of attentional resources would knock out the stereotype activation effect in the Gilbert and Hixon paradigm. This is a clue that the particular manipulation employed may have blocked stereotype activation for a reason other than, or in addition to, the shortage of processing resources it produced.

Macrae, Bodenhausen, Milne, Thorn, and Castelli (1997) have proposed one such alternative explanation for the Gilbert and Hixon (1991) findings. They presented faces of female undergraduates as well as pictures of common household objects to their participants. Some participants were instructed to detect, by means of a key press, whether or not a white dot appeared on each photograph. Others were told merely to press a key upon the presentation of each stimulus photograph on the screen. A third group was directed to process the stimuli in a semantic manner, deciding whether a given photograph was of an animate or an inanimate object. On each trial, following the response to the photograph, a participant was presented a word string and was to indicate, as quickly as possible, whether it was a word or a nonword. Some of the word strings were stereotypic of women, while others were counterstereotypic.

The results showed that on trials on which a photograph of a woman had just been presented, but not on the other trials, responses were faster to the stereotypic word strings than to the counterstereotypic ones in this lexical-decision task. However, as predicted, this effect held only for those participants who had processed the photographs in a semantic fashion; that is, responses were based on the content and meaning of the photograph. Those who had searched each photo for the presence of a white dot, or who had merely pressed a button to indicate the presentation of any stimulus, did not show any evidence of stereotype activation.

This study is reminiscent of earlier work by Uleman and Moskowitz (1994), who studied the goal dependence of spontaneous trait inferences by varying the participants' processing goals during presentation of trait-implying sentences. Across three experiments, Uleman and Moskowitz found that behavioral stimuli automatically activated the trait concept they implied (e.g., "considerate" for "The deliveryman slows down and motions the pedestrians to cross"), as long as the participants processed the behavioral description for meaning in some way—either by indicating (via key press) the gender of the actor, by forming an impression of the actor, by deciding whether they themselves would engage in the given behavior, or by deciding whether they were similar or not to the actor. But in other conditions in which the meaning of the sentence was not relevant to the judgment task, such as detecting the appearance of specific letter combinations, spontaneous trait inferences were reduced or eliminated.

Taken together, these studies suggest that as long as a perceiver is dealing with a target individual as a social being—that is, whenever the perceiver is making judgments about or forming impressions of the target—trait concepts and stereotypes relevant to that target individual will become active automatically. However, if the perceiver is instead dealing with the other person not as a person at all, but as a device that turns cards, or as a stimulus that may or may not contain a white spot, then these social concepts will not be activated.

Beyond the hopeful implication that dermatologists are unlikely to stereotype their patients, what is the "real-world" relevance of studies involving such presemantic processing goals? The results seem to suggest that when we are dealing with minority group members not as people, but as stimuli or devices, the group stereotype will not become active; however, as long as we *are* dealing with them as people (even if it is only to memorize their faces), the stereotype will become active automatically. This may not be a trivial reduction of the scope of automatic stereotyping effects, because we often encounter people, especially functionaries, in whom we have no interest as social beings.

The Role of Processing Goals

In addition, examining the generality of automatic stereotype activation across a variety of processing goals, as Macrae et al. (1997) did, may well turn out to be a promising line of attack on the cognitive monster. The telling evidence is yet to come, however. For instance, people may have many interpersonal goals during social interaction other than impression formation or evaluation (Chaiken, Liberman, & Eagly, 1989; Gollwitzer & Moskowitz, 1996; Hilton & Darley, 1991; Jones & Thibaut, 1958), and some or most of these well may override, prevent, or suppress stereotype activation. Examples include social comparison, having a good time, competing, self-enhancement, self-presentation, having a smooth rather than awkward interaction with the other person, and information seeking, as well as the pursuit of personal goals that involve the other's help or assistance (e.g., a salesperson's advice in making a purchase; negotiation with that same salesperson over the price; working with superiors, subordinates, or equals on a shared task). These are the kind of goals that seem quite relevant to the question of how widespread (vs. goal-dependent) automatic stereotype activation actually is in social life.

One recent study underscores the importance of goals and motivations in automatic stereotyping effects. Spencer et al. (1998) showed that even under the original Gilbert–Hixon conditions that knocked out stereotype activation, the stereotype was nonetheless automatically activated if a participant had just suffered a blow to his or her self-esteem. The moral here is that the impact of motivation on stereotyping is a double-edged sword. Just as motivation *not* to stereotype can possibly overcome the automatic influence, as Devine (1989) and Fiske (1989) argued, so too can there be motivations to *use* stereotypes that can overcome conditions that otherwise successfully block them.

Can Stereotype Activation Be Eliminated by Expectancies?

Blair and Banaji (1996) have approached the cognitive monster from a different direction. Devine (1989) had distinguished between stereotype activation and stereotype application, and argued that only the latter is potentially controllable by the appropriate motivation (i.e., to be egalitarian and nonprejudiced). Blair and Banaji (1996) have gone still further and argued that motivational control is possible even over the first stage of stereotype activation.

In their Experiment 1, participants were faster to classify names as male or female

when those names were immediately preceded (i.e., with a stimulus onset asynchrony [SOA] of 350 milliseconds [ms]) by stereotypic trait and nontrait primes consistent with the gender of the target name (e.g., "aggressive–Mike," "petite–Carol") than when the primes were consistent with the opposite gender stereotype (e.g., "flowers–Tom," "briefcase–Susan"). Previous studies had consistently shown that an SOA of 350 ms or less is too brief for an effect of expectancy or intention on responses (e.g., Fazio et al., 1986; Neely, 1977; see review in Neely, 1991), and so the results of Blair and Banaji's (1996) Experiment 1 were consistent with the hypothesis of automatic activation of gender stereotypes.

In Experiment 3, again with a 350-ms SOA between prime and target on each trial, half of the participants were presented with stereotype-inconsistent primes on most of the trials. That is, male names were usually preceded by primes consistent with the female stereotype, and female names were usually preceded by male stereotypic terms. Participants were explicitly informed, in fact, to expect this combination. The remaining participants were presented most of the time with stereotype-congruent prime–target combinations, and were told to expect that combination.

The startling apparent outcome of the experiment was that for the participants told to expect stereotype-inconsistent prime–target combinations, there was no longer any significant response time advantage for the stereotype-consistent primes, as there had been in Experiment 1 with no expectancies operating. Response times when the stereotypic trait primes matched the target names' gender did not differ significantly from the times when the primes corresponded to the opposite-gender stereotype. The authors conclude that their results "suggest that stereotype activation may not be unconditional and stereotypic cues need not result in a stereotypic response," and moreover that the findings "support proposals . . . that perceivers can control and even eliminate such effects" (Blair & Banaji, 1996, p. 1159).[1]

The present Figure 18.1, however, tells a somewhat different story. It presents the mean response latencies from Experiment 1, from which the authors conclude that the automatic stereotype effect did occur, and from the counterstereotype expectancy (350-ms SOA) condition of Experiment 3, from which they conclude that the automatic stereotype effect did not occur—that is, that the counterstereotypic expectancy successfully controlled and eliminated the automatic stereotype. It is quite evident that the two patterns are nearly identical (if anything, the effect in Experiment 3 was stronger). If one considers the amount of response time facilitation produced by the stereotype-consistent primes compared to the stereotype-inconsistent primes (the difference between the average of the F-F and M-M means and the average of the F-M and M-F means), this facilitation effect was 8 ms in the no-expectancy condition (Experiment 1), but 13 ms under the counterexpectancy conditions (Experiment 3) that were said to have eliminated the effect.

The authors' conclusion that the stereotype activation effect was moderated by counterstereotypic expectations was based on the statistical significance of the Prime × Target interaction in Experiment 1 but not in Experiment 3. However, it should be noted that the Experiment 3 participants were the same people as those who took part in Experiment 1, and that they did so after a 5-minute break (half went into the stereotype expectancy condition and the other half into the counterstereotype expectancy condition of Experiment 3; Blair & Banaji, 1996, p. 1150). Therefore, it would be possible to test whether the expectancy manipulation moderated the size of the Prime × Target interaction, because the same participants experienced both no expectancy in Experiment 1 and the counterstereotypic expectancy in Experiment 3. Blair and Banaji (1996) did not report such a test in the article; I. Blair (personal communication, November 8, 1997) reports that the authors did not consider such a comparison to be valid "because participants reported that the priming tasks made them fatigued, and stereotype effects are more likely when

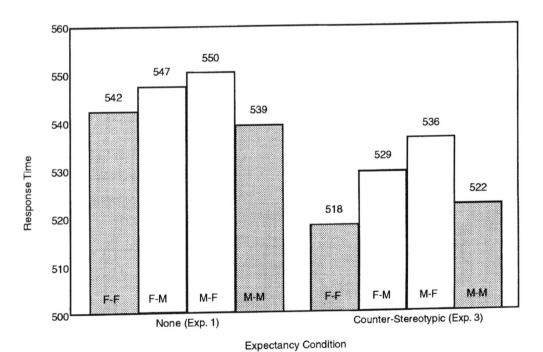

FIGURE 18.1. Mean response latencies to classify common names as male or female, by prime (male vs. female stereotypic trait) and expectancy for prime–target combinations (none vs. counterstereotypic). The first letter on each bar denotes the gender of the prime, and the second denotes the gender of the target stimulus. Shaded bars represent conditions in which prime and target matched in gender. The data are from Blair and Banaji (1996, Experiments 1 and 3, 350-ms SOA conditions).

people are tired." Nonetheless, it appears unlikely, given the results shown in the present Figure 18.1, that such a within-subjects test would reveal that the counterstereotype expectancy conditions had attenuated the effect of prime on target in any way.[2]

Nevertheless, these findings have been cited widely in support of the opposite conclusion: as "demonstrating that perceivers' expectations can impede stereotype activation" (Macrae et al., 1997, p. 474); as showing "that conscious efforts to suppress stereotypically biased reactions can inhibit even the immediate activation of normally automatic associations" (Dovidio, Kawakami, Johnson, Johnson, & Howard, 1997, p. 536); and as demonstrating "that, if perceivers have counterstereotypical replacement thoughts, stereotypes may be inhibited . . . [which is] particularly encouraging in that the effects of the counterstereotypic expectations were revealed within milliseconds, which does not allow enough time for controlled processing" (Monteith, Sherman, & Devine, 1998, p. 71).[3] My own assessment differs; to me, the Blair and Banaji (1996) results are actually the best evidence to date that automatic stereotype activation is *impervious* to cognitive control. That is, even when participants were told that on most trials the gender of the prime name would signal a stereotypic trait associated with the opposite gender, and then encountered a majority of such trials, the automatic stereotype activation effect was unchanged.

Alas, the story gets even bleaker for the possibility of controlling stereotypes through expectancies. The Blair and Banaji (1996) Experiment 3 did find a strikingly powerful effect of expectancies on the size of the automatic stereotype effect—but it was the effect of stereotype-*consistent* expectations, which dramatically *increased* the automatic stereotype effect (see their Figure 4, p. 1152). When participants were notified that stereotype-consistent pairings between prime and target would occur on the majority of the trials, and then experienced these mostly stereotype-consistent trials, the conscious stereotype-consistent expectancy made the automatic stereotype effect even stronger than the automatic effect was by itself, with no expectancy operating, in Experiment 1. When no expectancy was operating (Experiment 1), the average

age stereotype facilitation effect on response latencies was 8 m; by contrast, when participants in Experiment 3 held stereotype-consistent expectancies, the average automatic stereotype effect increased to 96 milliseconds, or *12 times greater*.

The reality is that when people have expectancies about stereotyped groups, those expectancies are for stereotypic—not counterstereotypic—behavior (e.g., Jones, 1990; Neuberg, 1989, 1994). Thus, Blair and Banaji's (1996) findings that expectations either leave the automatic stereotype effect alone if they are inconsistent with the stereotype, or substantially enhance it if they are consistent with the stereotype, are hardly good news about the chances of reducing automatic stereotyping through expectations.

In sum, with enemies like expectancies, the cognitive monster doesn't need friends.

Is Successful Control Following Automatic Activation Likely?

The ability to control a stereotype (given motivation to do so) depends heavily on one's awareness of the possibility of unconscious prejudicial influence, but also on one's theory of how that unconscious prejudice may be manifested and expressed (see Wilson & Brekke, 1994). Devine's (1989) Experiment 3 instructed participants to write down the characteristics of the typical African American, and here people who were not prejudiced (according to an explicit measure of prejudice, the Modern Racism Scale) produced more positive and less stereotypic descriptions. But stereotypic assumptions and beliefs can emerge and be expressed in ways about which a person with egalitarian motives has no theory concerning the unfelt influence. Examples of this phenomenon include the linguistic intergroup bias (Semin & Fiedler, 1988; Maass, Salvi, Arcuri, & Semin, 1989; von Hippel, Sekaquaptewa, & Vargas, 1997), in which the same behavior is described in more abstract, pansituational terms when it confirms a stereotype (e.g., "Ramon was violent") than when it is performed by a member of a nonstereotyped group (e.g., "Bill pushed the reporter away from his car"), or the tendency when completing behavior stem sentences to explain the reasons for counterstereotypic but not stereotype-consistent behavior (von Hippel, Sekaquaptewa, & Vargas, 1995). Stereotype effects emerge in the "tacit inferences" people make when interpreting the meaning of others' behavior; for instance, upon hearing "Some felt that the politician's statements were untrue," people assume that the politician was lying, but do not make this assumption if the actor was a physicist instead (Dunning & Sherman, 1997). Again, these implicit effects are just as likely for those who score low on explicit measures of stereotypic beliefs as for those who score high (Dunning & Sherman, 1997, Study 5).[4]

Stereotype effects appear as well in judgments of fame (Banaji & Greenwald, 1995), in larger priming effects when the primed trait category is stereotype-relevant (Banaji, Hardin, & Rothman, 1993), and also in response latencies to evaluate good and bad adjectives (Dovidio et al., 1997; Fazio et al., 1995). Here again, they are independent of explicit, expressed measures of prejudice. In other words, when a participant does not realize how his or her response can be a sign of stereotyping and prejudice, he or she manifests the stereotype. Even well-meaning attempts at controlling prejudicial influences require knowing what those influences are (Wilson & Brekke, 1994), and for those that are less obvious than overtly describing characteristics of minority groups, the experimental evidence taken as a whole provides scant indications of control being exerted. And if not in psychology experiments, where people know that they are being measured and their behavior scrutinized, why should we expect such control to be exercised elsewhere?

Even if an individual is aware of possibly being prejudiced, and is motivated to engage in control over the stereotype in question, such control attempts often backfire. It is an "ironic" effect of mental control attempts that suppressed thoughts often bounce back, becoming even more accessible than before, when the person's guard is down and there is a letup in control (Wegner, 1994). Consistent with this principle, Macrae, Bodenhausen, Milne, and Jetten (1994) found that participants who had been suppressing stereotypic thoughts about others subsequently responded more negatively to a stereotyped target, compared to those who had not been attempting to control such thoughts. And

Wegner, Erber, Bowman, and Shelton (1997) showed that ongoing control attempts (not to be sexist) backfired under conditions of mental load (time pressure): Participants trying to control their stereotypic assumptions about females actually made more sexist remarks under such conditions than did participants not attempting to control their assumptions. Though attempts at suppression do not always produce such rebound effects (see Monteith et al., 1998), the point is that even in the unlikely event that both of the necessary conditions—awareness of nonconscious stereotype operation and motivation to do something about it—are in place, stereotypic judgments and behavior can nonetheless occur.

Do Behavioral-Confirmation Effects No Longer Exist?

Another avenue of attack on the enormous problem posed by automatic stereotyping has been in the area of self-fulfilling prophecies or behavioral confirmation of stereotypes (e.g., Jussim, 1986; Merton, 1948; Rosenthal & Jacobsen, 1968; Snyder, Tanke, & Berscheid, 1977). The standard model of such effects (for reviews, see Darley & Fazio, 1980; Hamilton, Sherman, & Ruvolo, 1990; Jones, 1990; Olson, Roese, & Zanna, 1996; Snyder, 1984) assumes that activated stereotypes generate negative expectancies concerning the behavior of the minority group member, causing the perceiver to behave toward the other person in such a way as to produce the very stereotype-consistent behavior he or she expects. For instance, a teacher assuming a lack of intelligence or promise from a pupil may spend less time with him or her and in other ways communicate those assumptions, causing the pupil's performance to suffer. This mechanism by which stereotypes perpetuate themselves has also been called into question over the past 10 years.

Accuracy Motivation

Neuberg (1989) manipulated his participants' motivation to produce accurate impressions of a target person by offering a monetary prize for the most accurate judgment, and this did create more positive behavior toward the stereotyped-group member and consequently reduced stereotypic judgments. The behavior in question had to do with the questions asked by participants while interviewing the target person; these were less expectancy-confirming than otherwise (e.g., Snyder & Swann, 1978).

But this is a type of behavior (i.e., verbal) that is under people's cognitive control to a great extent; other forms of behavior in naturalistic social interactions are less controllable (e.g., nonverbal) and provide more possibility for "leakage" from stereotypic assumptions. Fazio and Dunton (1997) conclude that when "the behavior is not easily controllable, the behavior should be less influenced by motivational concerns and more directly and singly influenced by any automatically activated evaluations" (p. 469), and they point to nonverbal behaviors as a good example of such difficult-to-control behaviors (see Dovidio, Brigham, Johnson, & Gaertner, 1996).

Accuracy motivation as a method of reducing stereotyping is not promising for other reasons as well. Even when perceivers are accuracy-motivated, their effortful or systematic processing of person information is influenced by their stereotypes (Chaiken & Maheswaran, 1994; Chen & Chaiken, Chapter 4, this volume; Trope & Alfieri, 1997); for example, stereotypes affect how the target behavior is identified or encoded initially, before the accuracy-driven systematic processing begins (see also Darley & Gross, 1983; Dunning & Sherman, 1997; von Hippel et al., 1995). Furthermore, several recent reviews of expectancy and goal effects have concluded that it is relatively rare in naturally occurring situations for an individual to have the goal of forming an accurate impression (e.g., Hilton & Darley, 1991; Olson et al., 1996).

A Methodological Critique
of Behavioral-Confirmation Studies

Jussim and his colleagues (e.g., Jussim, 1990; Madon, Jussim, & Eccles, 1997, p. 792) have also questioned the existence of behavioral-confirmation effects, on both methodological and theoretical grounds. They point out that experimental demonstrations of self-fulfilling prophecy effects typically induce false expec-

tancies in participants, so that such studies do not address the likelihood that such false beliefs develop on their own, without such interventions on the part of the experimenter. According to Jussim (1990, p. 30), "Despite some grandiose claims to the contrary, there is currently no evidence that naturally occurring expectations lead to huge self-fulfilling prophecy effects or perceptual biases." Jussim's argument is that if the stereotype is *accurate* (Lee et al., 1995), the expectancies it generates in the perceiver are not false, and thus are not factors contributing to the stereotype-consistent behavior of the target person.

A Nonconscious Route
to Behavioral-Confirmation Effects

A recent study (Chen & Bargh, 1997), however, demonstrated that self-fulfilling prophecy effects could be produced experimentally without giving the participants any expectancies at all. Instead, a second, nonconscious route from stereotype activation to the production of confirming behavior in the stereotyped-group member was documented, distinct from the standard route through consciously held expectancies (see Figure 18.2). Building on the long-standing hypothesis in psychology of a direct, "express" link between perception and behavior (see next paragraph), Chen and I argued that automatic stereotype activation can produce a tendency for a perceiver to be the first to act in a stereotype-consistent manner within an interaction with a stereotyped-group member. This may well produce similar behavior in response by the target. However, without awareness of the effect of the stereotype on his or her own behavior, the perceiver will be highly likely to interpret the response of the other as just another confirming instance of the stereotype (cf. Jones & Nisbett, 1971).

The idea that mental activity can directly affect behavior without an intervening act of will was championed by William James (1890) as the principle of "ideomotor action." James argued that merely thinking about a behavior increases its probability of occurrence because of the impulsive nature of consciousness, which does not require an act of "express fiat" or will prior to each behavioral response to the environment. James in

Conscious Route

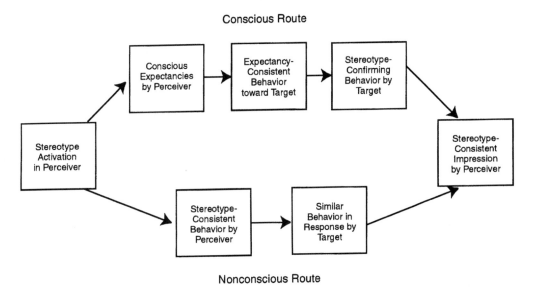

Nonconscious Route

FIGURE 18.2. A dual-process model of behavioral confirmation of stereotypes.

fact argued that such cases of intervention by the will are the exception and not the rule. Later, the Gestalt psychologists endorsed the notion, and Piaget (e.g., 1948) considered it an indispensable mechanism of imitative learning. More recently, Berkowitz (e.g., 1984) and Carver, Ganellen, Froming, and Chambers (1983) argued that an express link between perception and behavior produces passive and unintended media effects on behavior, as well as interpersonal effects.

We (Bargh et al., 1996) combined the idea of a passive perception–behavior link with the evidence of automatic stereotype activation. If stereotypes can be activated automatically, without awareness or intention on the part of the perceiver, then this perceptual activity should activate related behavioral tendencies. That is, we assumed (in line with the common-coding model of Prinz, 1990) that the trait concepts activated in the course of stereotype activation contain within them knowledge not only of how to detect such trait-like behavior in others (e.g., what it means to act honestly or aggressively, etc.) but also of how to produce the same behavior oneself.

In Experiment 2 of the Bargh et al. (1996) study, the stereotype of the elderly was primed through a standard method, the "scrambled-sentence test" (see Bargh & Chartrand, in press; Srull & Wyer, 1979). Words related to the stereotype (e.g., "conservative," "grey," "bingo") were embedded for some participants in a sentence construction task, while the remaining participants received a version of this task with neutral primes. Then participants were thanked for their help and left the experimental room, believing that the experiment was over. However, a confederate posing as the next participant was waiting outside in the hall, and surreptitiously timed how long it took the participants to walk down the hallway on the way to the elevator. The prediction was that because slowness and weakness were components of the elderly stereotype, participants whose stereotype of the elderly had been activated without their awareness would walk more slowly down the hall than the other participants would. Because neither slowness nor weakness (or synonyms of either) appeared as priming stimuli, such an effect could only occur through activation of the elderly stereotype. The prediction was confirmed in two experiments.

The Bargh et al. (1996) Experiment 3 focused on the African American stereotype. First, some participants were subliminally primed with photographs of young black male faces, and others with young white male faces (all participants were white). Then a mild provocation was staged, in which the experimenter requested the participant to do the fairly boring experimental task again because of a computer error in saving the data. A hidden video camera recorded each participant's reaction to this request, and judges who were unaware of the experimental hypotheses rated these tapes later for the degree of hostility shown by the participants. Hostility is a trait component of the African American stereotype (e.g., Devine, 1989). Again as predicted, those whose stereotype of African Americans had been primed subliminally showed greater hostility in response to the provocation than did the other participants, consistent with the hypothesized behavioral effects of the activated stereotype. These stereotype-priming effects on behavior have subsequently been replicated and extended for different stereotypes (e.g., "professor," "soccer hooligan") by Dijksterhuis and van Knippenberg (1998).

The implications of these findings for self-fulfilling prophecies are evident. It has long been established that there are nonverbal modes through which stereotypic affect and beliefs are expressed (e.g., Dovidio et al., 1996; Word, Zanna, & Cooper, 1974), and that nonverbal expressions of affect are difficult to control (e.g., DePaulo, 1992; Ekman & Friesen, 1969; Fazio & Dunton, 1997). Nonverbal expressions of hostility (tone of voice, facial expression, aversion of eye contact, etc.) are also perceived without any difficulty by their target. Thus, it is easily conceivable that activation of the concept of hostility through one's perception of an African American may quickly and nonconsciously cause such nonverbal manifestations in the perceiver, as well as possibly more overt expressions in verbal or behavioral content. The target person may understandably respond in kind with hostility, and this should be perceived by the stereotyper—lacking awareness of his or her own role in producing the interpretation—as occurring without any provocation. Thus, the stereotyper should attribute the hostility to the dispositional characteristics of the target person.

We (Chen & Bargh, 1997) designed a study to test this implication. In essence, the design was a merging of two paradigms—those of automatic stereotype activation and

of behavioral confirmation (as described by Snyder et al., 1977). Pairs of participants played a game of "Catch Phrase"—similar to the old television game show Password—in which one player attempts to get his or her partner to guess each of several target words. The game readily creates mild frustration and sometimes even anger, as one's partner often cannot guess the word, despite what the clue giver often believes to be (biased by his or her knowledge of the word) excellent and obvious hints. In our experimental version of this game, players were in different rooms and communicated via headphones and microphones. We recorded the two players' voices on separate channels of a stereo tape recorder.

Prior to playing the game together, the individual members of a pair performed the priming task alone. This was the same task as in the Bargh et al. (1996) Experiment 3. One member of the pair in each session was randomly assigned the role of "perceiver," and the other the role of "target." During this task, half of the perceiver participants were presented subliminally with black faces, and the other perceiver participants with white faces. All of the target participants were presented with white faces; that is, for none of the target participants was the African American stereotype automatically activated.

Following the game, each participant rated his or her partner on a variety of traits, including hostility. We also had judges who were unaware of the experimental hypotheses listen to the audiotapes in a random order and rate each participant on hostility, as well as on stereotype-irrelevant trait dimensions. The audiotape ratings showed that, as predicted, both the perceiver and the target participants in the stereotype-primed condition were rated as being more hostile than their counterparts in the no-priming condition. Thus, the subliminal priming manipulation increased the hostility of the perceiver participants, and this in turn increased the hostility of the target participants. A path analysis confirmed that the greater the hostility shown by a perceiver participant, the greater was the hostility evidenced by the target participant. Finally, the signature of the behavioral-confirmation effect was also observed: Perceiver participants primed with subliminal black faces rated their interaction partners as being more hostile, compared to nonprimed perceivers' ratings of their partners. That this effect was driven specifically by the activated African American stereotype was further shown by the fact it held only for ratings of hostility and not for the overall negativity of the ratings on stereotype-irrelevant trait dimensions.

This demonstration of self-fulfilling prophecy effects is free from the objections raised concerning the phenomenon by Jussim, Neuberg, and others. The study differed from previous experimental tests in that we did not give our participants any false expectancies; we merely showed them young black male faces outside of awareness. That this presentation evidently activated the stereotype of African Americans, and thus the concept of hostility, had to be because this concept was stored in the memories of the participants—it was not present in their environment.

Furthermore, as to the contention that stereotypes are benign influences on social perception and behavior because they are accurate, note that all of the participants in the Chen and Bargh (1997) study were white and not black. Thus there was no way that the behavior of the target persons could have been actually, or "accurately," more hostile (i.e., because of any presumed "actual" greater hostility of African Americans) to then initiate the greater hostility found in the perceiver–target pairs where the perceivers had been primed with black faces. If the targets had been black, the argument could possibly have been leveled by those who take the position of stereotype accuracy that the targets did behave first with greater hostility because the stereotype is accurate and black people are more hostile. This cannot be raised as an objection to the Chen and Bargh (1997) behavioral-confirmation effects.

In short, the results newly document an insidious way in which stereotypes can be confirmed—unconsciously, because the effect does not depend on consciously held expectancies and their guidance of behavior toward the target person. Although it may be possible for a person with the motivation to behave in a fair and egalitarian manner to be aware of and then control negative, consciously operating stereotypic expectancies, it is less clear how even such motivated individuals will have the opportunity to control the immediate, nonconscious effect of the stereotype on their own behavior (see Fazio & Dunton, 1997, for a similar argument regarding the importance of opportunity conditions).

But perhaps this conclusion is premature, given the currently available evidence. Studies such as ours (Chen & Bargh, 1997) and that of Devine (1989) deliberately did not have participants interact with or read about a member of the focal stereotyped group (i.e., the target person was not African American), in order to rule out conscious or intentional sources of the stereotyping effect. But this also eliminated a potential cue in the situation that might have triggered stereotype suppression or control strategies for at least some participants. In other words, if our white participants had interacted with a black target, perhaps they would have been alerted to the possibility of unintended prejudicial behavior and would have exercised greater care and guidance over their behavior.

Further research is needed on this point, but merely to show that such experimental effects vary with black versus white targets (if indeed they do) is not enough; the question is not how people behave in a psychology experiment setting, in which they are more likely to be on their guard, but how they naturally react to members of stereotyped versus nonstereotyped groups in real life. My feeling is that the Chen and Bargh (1997) findings do generalize to actual encounters between black and white Americans, because these strategic "guards" are often down in both cases, and we are dealing with immediate behavioral reactions for which there exists no lay "theory" of influence (see Wilson & Brekke, 1994). Nonetheless, a well-designed study camouflaging the role that race of target person plays as an independent variable could give us some valuable answers.

IMPLICATIONS FOR ERADICATING PREJUDICE

Some clear prescriptions can be based on the foregoing review. One is not to count too much on a person's ability to control the impact of an automatically activated stereotype. Once it is activated, the horse has left the barn, and shutting the barn door at that point does no good. To be able to control these effects, the person first has to accept the idea of being influenced in ways of which he or she is not aware, and people generally have a difficult time accepting this possibility. The research described above shows that control is especially unlikely for nonobvious manifestations of prejudice, and that stereotypes leak out into nonverbal behavior and evaluations even for those who consciously endorse nonprejudicial values and beliefs.

Should a person accept the possibility of unconscious influence, then he or she must have the motivation and ability to control it. By "ability" here is meant such things as having enough time and attention to engage in the effortful, "hard" choice of individuating information processing. More than that, an individual needs to have a relatively accurate "theory" about the nature of the unfelt influence in order to correct for it, but generally these lay theories are faulty (see Wilson & Brekke, 1994). The odds that all of these necessary conditions will be met in a given situation therefore become vanishingly small.

Can People Break the Habit?

If a "cure" for automatic stereotyping through conscious correction processes is not possible, what are we left with? Clearly, one implication is that efforts would be better spent in "prevention"—that is, finding a way to stop stereotypes from being activated automatically in the first place. Lepore and Brown (1997) and Fazio et al. (1995) have shown that automatic stereotype activation does not occur for everyone, despite a stereotype's permeation of a culture. Although all individuals appear to possess knowledge of the stereotype, there may be individual differences in whether that stereotype is activated upon activation of the group representation. Lepore and Brown (1997) showed this by distinguishing between the representation of the social group (the individual's own knowledge base about the group) and the cultural stereotype associated with that group (see also Pratto & Bargh, 1991). The group representation is automatically activated by distinguishing group features (e.g., skin color), but the group representation may or may not be automatically associated with the group stereotype.

Lepore and Brown (1997) argued that Devine (1989, Experiment 2) showed auto-

matic stereotype activation for all participants, regardless of level of overt racism, because the priming stimuli used were directly relevant to the stereotype (and therefore bypassed the group representation). In an experiment in which the priming stimuli were relevant only to the group representation and not to the stereotype, Lepore and Brown (1997) found automatic stereotype activation to be a function of a participant's degree of overt racism. This result is reminiscent of Gilbert and Hixon's (1991) and Macrae et al.'s (1997) findings of no effect of stereotypes under memory load, despite participants' later ability to recall the race of the target person—except that there was no manipulation of cognitive load in Lepore and Brown's (1997) study. Such dissociations between group representation and stereotype activation suggest that it is possible for individuals not to automatically apply stereotypic conceptions that they do possess, by virtue of the pervasiveness of the beliefs within the culture.

Yet the fact of individual differences in the application of a cultural stereotype is not in itself evidence that stereotypes can be controlled once they become so strong as to be automatically applied. The individual differences in application may exist because the automatic pathway or association has never been developed by some people in the first place. Though this is potentially good news about the degree of pervasiveness of stereotypes, it does not directly address the theme of the present chapter, which is the degree to which automatic stereotype effects can be controlled once they are in place.

Several studies do bear directly on this question. Monteith (1993) provided a potential method for breaking or retraining the stereotype habit. After rating the job suitability of a gay job applicant, participants were informed that their ratings were lower than those given by participants who read and evaluated the identical application, except that the applicant was described as heterosexual. Thus admonished for the prejudice they had shown, those participants who had earlier expressed values for being nonprejudicial reacted to this evident discrepancy between their behavior and their self-concept with an increased effort to be nonprejudicial in subsequent parts of the experimental session (see also Brunstein & Gollwitzer, 1996; Wicklund & Gollwitzer, 1982). Those who did not express such values were not affected by the apparent act of prejudice they had committed.

Therefore, if people can be made aware of committing acts of prejudice, their motivation to be egalitarian (or not to be) may well come into play. But will this motivated engagement in nonstereotypic thought about the target group have any effect on changing the automaticity of the stereotype activation? A recent set of studies by Kawakami (1997) provides some evidence on this score. She found that the link between a group representation and a stereotype could be broken, at least temporarily, by retraining a different set of automatic beliefs about the group. Across a series of 240 trials, participants were instructed to respond by pressing a key labeled "No" whenever a photograph of a skinhead (or elderly person) was presented along with a stereotypic term associated with that group, and to respond "Yes" whenever a term not associated with that group was presented with the photograph. This associative training of different content to the skinhead or elderly group representation was successful in eliminating automatic stereotype activation, as measured by a subsequent Stroop task: The usual effect of greater response interference by stereotype-consistent than by stereotype-inconsistent stimuli was eliminated. Kawakami's procedure of training a different response to the stereotyped group is reminiscent of the approach taken in the cognitive therapy of emotional disorders (Beck, 1976; Beck, Rush, Shaw, & Emery, 1979).

Can an Automatic "Good" Defeat an Automatic "Evil"?

It is too early to tell, but perhaps the greatest hope for stereotype control at the intraindividual level lies in the battle between two different forms of preconscious, automatic processing. If Kawakami's experimental situation can produce at least temporary inhibition or reduction of the automatic stereotyping effect, then perhaps a well-intentioned individual, motivated to be nonprejudicial and egalitarian, can develop chronic inhibition/reduction of the effect over time. That is, repeatedly pursuing egalitarian goals and thoughts when interacting with members of stereotyped

groups may automate that goal (i.e., may make it into an "auto-motive"; Bargh, 1990, 1997), so that the goal operates autonomously when one interacts with such individuals, without needing to be consciously chosen and guided each time. There is already evidence that information-processing as well as behavioral goals can be activated nonconsciously and then operate to produce the same outcomes as when those goals are selected consciously and intentionally (see Bargh, 1997; Bargh & Gollwitzer, 1994; Chartrand & Bargh, 1996).

This reasoning leads to the interesting possibility that both the group stereotype *and* the motivation to be egalitarian can be automatically activated at the same time and in parallel, by the mere features of the stereotyped-group member. How will these two forces interact? Will the automatically activated goal to be fair stifle and defeat the automatic stereotype activation, all in a matter of a few hundred milliseconds or so, before conscious processing has a chance even to notice (if ever) what is going on?

Such a possibility was first raised by Gollwitzer and Moskowitz (1996), and evidence is starting to accrue in its support (Moskowitz, Wasel, Gollwitzer, & Schaal, 1998). This idea of an immediate automatic *inhibition* of stereotypes is also in harmony with the recent theoretical model of Bodenhausen and Macrae (1998), which calls for both automatic facilitative and inhibitional responses in the processing of information about a stereotyped-group member. Indeed, Stangor, Thompson, and Ford (1998) have explicitly linked the idea of an egalitarian "auto-motive" to the Bodenhausen–Macrae model.

If all this sounds too good to be true, well, it may be. How, for example, does the egalitarian motive or goal become automated if not by the individual's chronically pursuing it over time, consciously and intentionally? But doing so, as has been argued above, requires the awareness of possible (nonconscious) bias; knowledge of the effect of the bias on judgments (many of them quite subtle, implicit, and tacit); ability to engage in the effortful processing at the time; and the good intention to be egalitarian—all of which are problematic conditions in real life. Nevertheless, the good news is that if one can get one's egalitarian motivation to the automatic state, it may then routinely win out over the automatic stereotype—a case, if you will, of fighting automatic fire with automatic fire.

CONCLUSIONS

One danger in any critical analysis of a research area is that it can be mistaken for criticism of the goals of the research itself. There is no question that the research described in this chapter has been driven by sincere and laudable goals to discover ways to reduce and ameliorate the social scourge of stereotyping and prejudice, and by optimism that such ways can be found. Such attempts should of course continue. But although the goals and purpose of the research are admirable and optimistic, we must nonetheless accept the findings of that research at face value, and not allow our optimism and hopefulness to color our interpretation of the evidence. In my opinion, the evidence to date concerning people's realistic chances of controlling the influence of their automatically activated stereotypes weighs in heavily on the negative side. The lesson to be learned from the tales of Frankenstein and King Kong is that monsters, once on the loose, cannot be controlled by chains.

Once a stereotype is so entrenched that it becomes activated automatically, there is really little that can be done to control its influence. Even under the scrutiny of a psychology experiment, in which most of the time not only the presented prime–target pairs but the participants' conscious expectations for the targets were counterstereotypic, participants produced the same pattern of means as when no such conscious expectancy existed. Even when a person has egalitarian values and motives, his or her facial expression and tone of voice and reaction to the behavior of a stereotyped-group member can often be a first strike that produces stereotype-confirming behavior and so perpetuates the stereotype. Realistically, there is little that will be done about such nonconscious effects in the real world—mainly because, in the words of Hall of Fame baseball pitcher Bob Feller, "You can't hit what you can't see," and because on those occasions when corrections are attempted, they are often (if not usually) guided by faulty lay theories as to the nature of the bias (Wilson & Brekke, 1994).

Hoping to stop the cognitive monster by trying to control already activated stereotypes is like mowing dandelions; they just sprout back up again. As with dandelions, the only way to kill stereotype effects is to pull them up by their roots—by removing their capability for automatic activation, or (better still) by preventing the seeds from taking root in the first place, through eradication of the cultural stereotype itself. Steele (1997) makes a similar argument in the context of African Americans' rocky road to holding an academic identity. In theory, he points out, one could perform intrapsychic interventions on each affected student in an attempt to counter the panoply of forces that can push them off the academic track, but this is not a realistic strategy. The real solution, Steele concludes, is to eliminate in the first place the culturally shared and transmitted assumption that blacks "can't cut it" academically. Until we find a way to kill the dandelions, reports of the death of the cognitive monster will be greatly exaggerated.

ACKNOWLEDGMENTS

Preparation of this chapter was supported in part by Grant No. SBR-9409448 from the National Science Foundation. Portions were previously presented as the keynote address to the annual meeting of the Netherlands Social Psychology Association, Leiden, December 1996. I am indebted to Mahzarin Banaji, Irene Blair, Galen Bodenhausen, Marilynn Brewer, Patricia Devine, Ap Dijksterhuis, Kimberly Duckworth, Ziva Kunda, Lorella Lepore, Neil Macrae, Bernadette Park, Denise Sekaquaptewa, Charles Stangor, Erik Thompson, and the editors for extensive feedback on an earlier version of the chapter; their generous help should not be taken as implying endorsement of any of the opinions expressed herein.

NOTES

1. Many (see below) have taken this conclusion to express the authors' belief that expectancies can prevent the initial automatic activation of the stereotype, but I. Blair (personal communication, November 11, 1997) considers that the successful elimination of stereotype effects on reaction times in "the 2000 ms SOA condition showed that participants could eliminate stereotype activation with

an expectancy strategy." In other words, the conclusion at the end of the Blair and Banaji (1996) article quoted here apparently referred to the 2,000-ms and not the 350-ms SOA condition results. Perhaps it is just a matter of personal taste, but I consider Devine's'(1989) distinction between the activation of a stereotype and its subsequent use in judgment to be a useful one. That is, 2 seconds is enough time to strategically control the effect of an automatically activated stereotype (Neely, 1977); therefore, a lack of stereotype effects in that condition does not demonstrate the elimination of the stereotype's automatic activation.

2. The experiment × prime × target interaction was in fact not reliable (*F* < 1; Blair, personal communication, November 11, 1997). Although it is my belief that this within-subjects test of the effect of expectancy (none vs. counterstereotypic) on automatic stereotype activation (i.e., the prime x target interaction) is more appropriate than comparing the significance levels of the two separate prime x target interactions (see Keppel, 1973), reasonable people can disagree on this point.

3. Importantly, this is not the position of Blair and Banaji concerning their results: "The position we took in our article and continue to support is that the priming effect was not eliminated under high cognitive constraints" (Blair, personal communication, November 8, 1997).

4. In the great majority of experiments, overt and explicit measures of stereotypic beliefs such as the Modern Racism Scale or the Attitudes Towards Women scale are uncorrelated with these implicit tendencies (for an exception, see Wittenbrink, Judd, & Park, 1997). In an insightful analysis of the role of encoding processes in the persistence of stereotypes, von Hippel et al. (1995) draw a distinction between the content of stereotypes and the way those stereotypes are used to process information about a person, akin to Jacoby's (e.g., Jacoby & Kelley, 1987) distinction between memory as an object and memory as a tool. It is possible, in other words, for the tendency to *process* person information in a way that confirms stereotypes to be somewhat dissociated or independent from the tendency to hold stereotypic *beliefs* (see also Dunning & Sherman, 1997; Trope & Alfieri, 1997).

REFERENCES

Banaji, M. R., & Greenwald, A. G. (1995). Implicit gender stereotyping in judgments of fame. *Journal of Personality and Social Psychology, 68,* 181–198.

Banaji, M. R., Hardin, C., & Rothman, A. J. (1993). Implicit stereotyping in person judgment. *Journal of Personality and Social Psychology, 65,* 272–281.

Bargh, J. A. (1989). Conditional automaticity: Varieties of automatic influence in social perception and cognition. In J. S. Uleman & J. A. Bargh (Eds.), *Unintended thought* (pp. 3–51). New York: Guilford Press.

Bargh, J. A. (1990). Auto-motives: Preconscious determinants of social interaction. In E. T. Higgins & R. M. Sorrentino (Eds.), *Handbook of motivation and cognition: Foundations of social behavior* (Vol. 2, pp. 93–130). New York: Guilford Press.

Bargh, J. A. (1997). The automaticity of everyday life. In R. S. Wyer (Ed.), *Advances in social cognition* (Vol. 10, pp. 1–61). Mahwah, NJ: Erlbaum.

Bargh, J. A., & Chartrand, T. L. (in press). Studying the mind in the middle: A practical guide to priming and automaticity research. In H. Reis & C. Judd (Eds.), *Research methods in the social sciences.* New York: Cambridge University Press.

Bargh, J. A., Chen, M., & Burrows, L. (1996). Automaticity of social behavior: Direct effects of trait construct and stereotype activation on action. *Journal of Personality and Social Psychology, 71,* 230–244.

Bargh, J. A., & Gollwitzer, P. M. (1994). Environmental control over goal-directed action. In W. D. Spaulding (Ed.), *Nebraska Symposium on Motivation: Vol. 41. Integrative views of motivation, cognition, and emotion* (pp. 71–124). Lincoln: University of Nebraska Press.

Bargh, J. A., & Thein, R. D. (1985). Individual construct accessibility, person memory, and the recall–judgment link: The case of information overload. *Journal of Personality and Social Psychology, 49,* 1129–1146.

Bargh, J. A., & Tota, M. E. (1988). Context-dependent automatic processing in depression: Accessibility of negative constructs with regard to self but not others. *Journal of Personality and Social Psychology, 54,* 925–939.

Beck, A. T. (1976). *Cognitive therapy and the emotional disorders.* New York: International Universities Press.

Beck, A. T., Rush, A. J., Shaw, B. F., & Emery, G. (1979). *Cognitive therapy of depression.* New York: Guilford Press.

Berkowitz, L. (1984). Some effects of thought on anti- and prosocial influences of media events: A cognitive-neoassociation analysis. *Psychological Bulletin, 95,* 410–427.

Billig, M. (1985). Prejudice, categorization and particularization: From a perceptual to a rhetorical approach. *European Journal of Social Psychology, 15,* 79–103.

Blair, I., & Banaji, M. (1996). Automatic and controlled processes in stereotype priming. *Journal of Personality and Social Psychology, 70,* 1142–1163.

Bodenhausen, G. V., & Macrae, C. N. (1998). Stereotype activation and inhibition. In R. S. Wyer (Ed.), *Advances in social cognition* (Vol. 11, pp. 1–52). Mahwah, NJ: Erlbaum.

Brewer, M. B. (1988). A dual process model of impression formation. In R. S. Wyer & T. K. Srull (Eds.), *Advances in social cognition* (Vol. 1, pp. 1–36). Hillsdale, NJ: Erlbaum.

Brunstein, J. C., & Gollwitzer, P. M. (1996). Effects of failure on subsequent performance: The importance of self-defining goals. *Journal of Personality and Social Psychology, 70,* 395–407.

Carver, C. S., Ganellen, R. J., Froming, W. J., & Chambers, W. (1983). Modeling: An analysis in terms of category accessibility. *Journal of Experimental Social Psychology, 19,* 403–421.

Chaiken, S., Liberman, A., & Eagly, A. H. (1989). Heuristic and systematic information processing within and beyond the persuasion context. In J. S. Uleman & J. A. Bargh (Eds.), *Unintended thought* (pp. 212–252). New York: Guilford Press.

Chaiken, S., & Maheswaran, D. (1994). Heuristic processing can bias systematic processing: Effects of source credibility, argument ambiguity, and task importance on attitude judgment. *Journal of Personality and Social Psychology, 66,* 460–473.

Chartrand, T. L., & Bargh, J. A. (1996). Automatic activation of social information processing goals: Nonconscious priming reproduces effects of explicit conscious instructions. *Journal of Personality and Social Psychology, 71,* 464–478.

Chen, M., & Bargh, J. A. (1997). Nonconscious behavioral confirmation processes: The self-fulfilling consequences of automatic stereotype activation. *Journal of Experimental Social Psychology, 33,* 541–560.

Darley, J. M., & Fazio, R. (1980). Expectancy confirmation processes arising in the social interaction sequence. *American Psychologist, 35,* 867–881.

Darley, J. M., & Gross, P. H. (1983). A hypothesis-confirming bias in labeling effects. *Journal of Personality and Social Psychology, 44,* 20–33.

Dawes, R. M. (1976). Shallow psychology. In J. S. Carroll & J. W. Payne (Eds.), *Cognition and social behavior.* Hillsdale, NJ: Erlbaum.

Deaux, K., & Lewis, L. L. (1984). Structure of gender stereotypes: Interrelations among components and gender label. *Journal of Personality and Social Psychology, 46,* 991–1004.

DePaolo, B. (1992). Nonverbal behavior and self-presentation. *Psychological Bulletin, 111,* 203–243.

Devine, P. G. (1989). Stereotypes and prejudice: Their automatic and controlled components. *Journal of Personality and Social Psychology, 56,* 680–690.

Dijksterhuis, A., & van Knippenberg, A. (1998). Automatic social behavior or how to win a game of Trivial Pursuit. *Journal of Personality and Social Psychology, 74,* 865–877.

Dovidio, J. F., Brigham, J. C., Johnson, B. T., & Gaertner, S. L. (1996). Stereotyping, prejudice, and discrimination: Another look. In N. Macrae, M. Hewstone, & C. Stangor (Eds.), *Foundations of stereotypes and stereotyping* (pp. 276–319). New York: Guilford Press.

Dovidio, J. F., Evans, N., & Tyler, R. B. (1986). Racial stereotypes: The contents of their cognitive representations. *Journal of Experimental Social Psychology, 22,* 22–37.

Dovidio, J. F., Kawakami, K., Johnson, C., Johnson, B., & Howard, A. (1997). On the nature of prejudice: Automatic and controlled processes. *Journal of Experimental Social Psychology, 33,* 510–540.

Dunning, D., & Sherman, D. A. (1997). Stereotypes and tacit inference. *Journal of Personality and Social Psychology, 73,* 459–471.

Ekman, P., & Friesen, W. V. (1969). Nonverbal leakage and clues to deception. *Psychiatry, 32,* 88–106.

Fazio, R. H., & Dunton, B. C. (1997). Categorization by race: The impact of automatic and controlled components of racial prejudice. *Journal of Experimental Social Psychology, 33,* 451–470.

Fazio, R. H., Jackson, J., Dunton, B., & Williams, C. (1995). Variability in automatic activation as an unobtrusive measure of racial attitudes: A bona fide pipeline? *Journal of Personality and Social Psychology, 69,* 1013–1027.

Fazio, R. H., Sanbonmatsu, D. M., Powell, M. C., & Kardes, F. R. (1986). On the automatic activation of attitudes. *Journal of Personality and Social Psychology, 50,* 229–238.

Fiske, S. T. (1980). Attention and weight in person perception: The impact of negative and extreme behavior. *Journal of Personality and Social Psychology, 38,* 889–906.

Fiske, S. T. (1989). Examining the role of intent: Toward understanding its role in stereotyping and prejudice. In J. S. Uleman & J. A. Bargh (Eds.), *Unintended thought* (pp. 253–283). New York: Guilford Press.

Fiske, S. T., & Neuberg, S. L. (1990). A continuum of impression formation, from category-based to individuating processes: Influences of information and motivation on attention and interpretation. In M. P. Zanna (Ed.), *Advances in experimental social psychology* (Vol. 23, pp. 1–74). San Diego, CA: Academic Press.

Gilbert, D. T. (1989). Thinking lightly about others: Automatic components of the social inference process. In J. S. Uleman & J. A. Bargh (Eds.), *Unintended thought* (pp. 189–211). New York: Guilford Press.

Gilbert, D. T., & Hixon, J. G. (1991). The trouble of thinking: Activation and application of stereotypic beliefs. *Journal of Personality and Social Psychology, 60,* 509–517.

Gilbert, D. T., Pelham, B. W., & Krull, D. S. (1988). On cognitive busyness: When person perceivers meet persons perceived. *Journal of Personality and Social Psychology, 54,* 733–739.

Gollwitzer, P. M., & Moskowitz, G. (1996). Goal effects on thought and behavior. In E. T. Higgins & A. Kruglanski (Eds.), *Social psychology: Handbook of basic principles* (pp. 361–399). New York: Guilford Press.

Hamilton, D. L. (1979). A cognitive-attributional analysis of stereotyping. In L. Berkowitz (Ed.), *Advances in experimental social psychology* (Vol. 12, pp. 53–85). New York: Academic Press.

Hamilton, D. L., Sherman, S. J., & Ruvolo, C. M. (1990). Stereotype-based expectancies: Effects on information processing and social behavior. *Journal of Social Issues, 46*(2), 35–60.

Hilton, J. L., & Darley, J. M. (1991). The effects of interaction goals on person perception. In M. P. Zanna (Ed.), *Advances in experimental social psychology* (Vol. 24, pp. 235–267). San Diego, CA: Academic Press.

Jacoby, L. L., & Kelley, C. M. (1987). Unconscious influences of memory for a prior event. *Personality and Social Psychology Bulletin, 13,* 314–336.

James, W. (1890). *Principles of psychology* (Vol. 2). New York: Holt.

Jones, E. E. (1990). *Interpersonal perception.* New York: Freeman.

Jones, E. E., & Davis, K. E. (1965). From acts to dispositions: The attribution process in person perception. In L. Berkowitz (Ed.), *Advances in experimental social psychology* (Vol. 2, pp. 220–266). New York: Academic Press.

Jones, E. E., & Nisbett, R. E. (1971). The actor and the observer: Divergent perceptions of the causes of behavior. In E. E. Jones, D. E. Kanouse, H. H. Kelley, R. E. Nisbett, S. Valins, & B. Weiner (Eds.), *Attribution:*

Perceiving the causes of behavior (pp. 79–94). Morristown, NJ: General Learning Press.

Jones, E. E., & Thibaut, J. W. (1958). Interaction goals as bases of inference in interpersonal perception. In R. Taguiri & L. Petrullo (Eds.), *Person perception and interpersonal behavior* (pp. 151–178). Stanford, CA: Stanford University Press.

Jussim, L. (1986). Self-fulfilling prophecies: A theoretical and integrative review. *Psychological Review, 93,* 429–445.

Jussim, L. (1990). Social reality and social problems: The role of expectancies. *Journal of Social Issues, 46*(2), 9–34.

Kahneman, D., & Tversky, A. (1973). On the psychology of prediction. *Psychological Review, 80,* 237–251.

Kawakami, K. (1997). *Kicking the habit: The effects of suppression training on stereotype activation.* Unpublished manuscript, University of Nijmegen, The Netherlands.

Kelley, H. H. (1967). Attribution theory in social psychology. In D. Levine (Ed.), *Nebraska Symposium on Motivation* (Vol. 15, pp. 192–241). Lincoln: University of Nebraska Press.

Keppel, G. (1973). *Design and analysis: A researcher's handbook.* Englewood Cliffs, NJ: Prentice-Hall.

Koestler, A. (1967). *The ghost in the machine.* London: Hutchinson.

Langer, E. J. (1978). Rethinking the role of thought in social interaction. In J. H. Harvey, W. J. Ickes, & R. F. Kidd (Eds.), *New directions in attribution research* (Vol. 2, pp. 36–58). Hillsdale, NJ: Erlbaum.

Langer, E. J., & Abelson, R. P. (1972). The semantics of asking a favor: How to succeed in getting help without really dying. *Journal of Personality and Social Psychology, 24,* 26–32.

Langer, E. J., Blank, A., & Chanowitz, B. (1978). The mindlessness of ostensibly thoughtful action: The role of "placebic" information in interpersonal interaction. *Journal of Personality and Social Psychology, 36,* 635–642.

Lee, Y.-T., Jussim, L. J., & McCauley, C. R. (Eds.). (1995). *Stereotype accuracy: Toward appreciating group differences.* Washington, DC: American Psychological Association.

Lepore, L., & Brown, R. (1997). Category and stereotype activation: Is prejudice inevitable? *Journal of Personality and Social Psychology, 72,* 275–287.

Maass, A., Salvi, D., Arcuri, L., & Semin, G. (1989). Language use in intergroup contexts: The linguistic intergroup bias. *Journal of Personality and Social Psychology, 57,* 981–993.

Macrae, C. N., Bodenhausen, G. V., Milne, A. B., & Jetten, J. (1994). Out of mind but back in sight: Stereotypes on the rebound. *Journal of Personality and Social Psychology, 67,* 808–817.

Macrae, C. N., Bodenhausen, G. V., Milne, A. B., Thorn, T. M. J., & Castelli, L. (1997). On the activation of social stereotypes: The moderating role of processing objectives. *Journal of Experimental Social Psychology, 33,* 471–489.

Madon, S., Jussim, L., & Eccles, J. (1997). In search of the powerful self-fulfilling prophecy. *Journal of Personality and Social Psychology, 72,* 791–809.

Merton, R. K. (1948). The self-fulfilling prophecy. *Antioch Review, 8,* 193–210.

Monteith, M. (1993). Self-regulation of prejudiced responses: Implications for progress in prejudice-reduction efforts. *Journal of Personality and Social Psychology, 65,* 469–485.

Monteith, M. J., Sherman, J. W., & Devine, P. G. (1998). Suppression as a stereotype control strategy. *Personality and Social Psychology Review, 2,* 63–82.

Moskowitz, G. B., Wasel, W., Gollwitzer, P. M., & Schaal, B. (1998). *Volitional control of stereotype activation through chronic egalitarian goals.* Unpublished manuscript, Princeton University.

Neely, J. H. (1977). Semantic priming and retrieval from lexical memory: Roles of inhibitionless spreading activation and limited-capacity attention. *Journal of Experimental Psychology: General, 106,* 226–254.

Neely, J. H. (1991). Semantic priming effects in visual word recognition: A selective review of current findings and theories. In D. Besner & G. Humphreys (Eds.), *Basic processes in reading: Visual word recognition* (pp. 264–336). Hillsdale, NJ: Erlbaum.

Neuberg, S. L. (1989). The goal of forming accurate impressions during social interactions: Attenuating the impact of negative expectancies. *Journal of Personality and Social Psychology, 56,* 374–386.

Neuberg, S. L. (1994). Expectancy-confirmation processes in stereotype-tinged social encounters: The moderating role of social goals. In M. P. Zanna & J. M. Olson (Eds.), *The psychology of prejudice: The Ontario Symposium* (Vol. 7, pp. 103–130). Hillsdale, NJ: Erlbaum.

Neuberg, S. L., & Fiske, S. T. (1987). Motivational influences on impression formation: Outcome dependency, accuracy-driven attention, and individuating processes. *Journal of Personality and Social Psychology, 53,* 431–444.

Olson, J. M., Roese, N. J., & Zanna, M. P. (1996). Expectancies. In E. T. Higgins & A. Kruglanski (Eds.), *Social psychology: Handbook of basic principles* (pp. 211–238). New York: Guilford Press.

Paulhus, D. L., Graf, P., & Van Selst, M. (1989). Attentional load increases the positivity of self-presentation. *Social Cognition, 7,* 389–400.

Piaget, J. (1948). *La formation du symbole chez l'enfant.* Paris: Delachaux & Niestlé.

Posner, M. I., & Snyder, C. R. R. (1975). Attention and cognitive control. In R. L. Solso (Ed.), *Information processing and cognition: The Loyola Symposium* (pp. 55–85). Hillsdale, NJ: Erlbaum.

Pratto, F., & Bargh, J. A. (1991). Stereotyping based on apparently individuating information: Trait and global components of sex stereotypes under attention overload. *Journal of Experimental Social Psychology, 27,* 26–47.

Pratto, F., & John, O. P. (1993). Automatic vigilance: The attention-grabbing power of negative social information. *Journal of Personality and Social Psychology, 61,* 380–391.

Prinz, W. (1990). A common coding approach to perception and action. In O. Neumann & W. Prinz (Eds.), *Relationships between perception and action* (pp. 167–201). Berlin: Springer-Verlag.

Prinz, W. (1997). Explaining voluntary action: The role of mental content. In M. Carrier & P. Machamer (Eds.), *Mindscapes: Philosophy, science, and the mind* (pp. 153–175). Konstanz, Germany: Universitaetsverlag.

Rosenthal, R., & Jacobson, L. (1968). *Pygmalion in the classroom*. New York: Holt, Rinehart & Winston.

Semin, G. R., & Fiedler, K. (1988). The cognitive functions of linguistic categories in describing persons: Social cognition and language. *Journal of Personality and Social Psychology, 54,* 557–568.

Snyder, M. (1984). When belief creates reality. In L. Berkowitz (Ed.), *Advances in experimental social psychology* (Vol. 18, pp. 248–305). New York: Academic Press.

Snyder, M., & Swann, W. B., Jr. (1978). Behavioral confirmation in social interaction: From social perception to social reality. *Journal of Experimental Social Psychology, 14,* 148–162.

Snyder, M., Tanke, E. D., & Berscheid, E. (1977). Social perception and interpersonal behavior: On the self-fulfilling nature of social stereotypes. *Journal of Personality and Social Psychology, 35,* 656–666.

Sorrentino, R. M., & Higgins, E. T. (Eds.) (1986). *Handbook of motivation and cognition: Foundations of social behavior* (Vol. 1). New York: Guilford Press.

Spencer, S. J., Fein, S., Wolfe, C. T., Fong, C., & Dunn, M. A. (1998). Automatic activation of stereotypes: The role of self-image threat. *Personality and Social Psychology Bulletin, 24,* 1139–1152.

Srull, T. K., & Wyer, R. S., Jr. (1979). The role of category accessibility in the interpretation of information about persons: Some determinants and implications. *Journal of Personality and Social Psychology, 37,* 1660–1672.

Stangor, C., Thompson, E. P., & Ford, T. E. (1998). An inhibited model of stereotype inhibition. In R. S. Wyer (Ed.), *Advances in social cognition* (Vol. 11, pp. 193–210). Mahwah, NJ: Erlbaum.

Steele, C. M. (1997, October). The rocky road to an academic identity for an African-American. In B. Major (Chair), *The psychological consequences of stigma*. Symposium presented at the annual meeting of the Society for Experimental Social Psychology, Toronto.

Taylor, S. E., & Fiske, S. T. (1978). Salience, attention, and attribution: Top of the head phenomena. In L. Berkowitz (Ed.), *Advances in experimental social psy-* chology (Vol. 11, pp. 249–288). New York: Academic Press.

Trope, Y., & Alfieri, T. (1997). Effortfulness and flexibility of dispositional judgment processes. *Journal of Personality and Social Psychology, 73,* 662–674.

Uleman, J. S., & Moskowitz, G. B. (1994). Unintended effects of goals on unintended inferences. *Journal of Personality and Social Psychology, 66,* 490–501.

von Hippel, W., Sekaquaptewa, D., & Vargas, P. (1995). On the role of encoding processes in stereotype maintenance. In M. P. Zanna (Ed.), *Advances in experimental social psychology* (Vol. 27, pp. 177–254). San Diego, CA: Academic Press.

von Hippel, W., Sekaquaptewa, D., & Vargas, P. (1997). The linguistic intergroup bias as an implicit indicator of prejudice. *Journal of Experimental Social Psychology, 33,* 490–509.

Wegner, D. M. (1994). Ironic processes of mental control. *Psychological Review, 101,* 34–52.

Wegner, D. M., Erber, R., Bowman, R., & Shelton, J. N. (1997). *On trying not to be sexist*. Unpublished manuscript, University of Virginia.

Weiner, B. (1974). *Achievement motivation and attribution theory*. Morristown, NJ: General Learning Press.

Wicklund, R. A., & Gollwitzer, P. M. (1982). *Symbolic self-completion*. Hillsdale, NJ: Erlbaum.

Wilson, T. D., & Brekke, N. (1994). Mental contamination and mental correction: Unwanted influences on judgments and evaluations. *Psychological Bulletin, 116,* 117–142.

Winter, L., & Uleman, J. S. (1984). When are social judgments made? Evidence for the spontaneousness of trait inferences. *Journal of Personality and Social Psychology, 47,* 237–252.

Wittenbrink, B., Judd, C. M., & Park, B. (1997). Evidence for racial prejudice at the implicit level and its relationship with questionnaire measures. *Journal of Personality and Social Psychology, 72,* 262–274.

Word, C. O., Zanna, M. P., & Cooper, J. (1974). The nonverbal mediation of self-fulfilling prophecies in interracial interaction. *Journal of Experimental Social Psychology, 10,* 109–120.

19

The Role of Cognitive Control

EARLY SELECTION VERSUS LATE CORRECTION

LARRY L. JACOBY
COLLEEN M. KELLEY
BRIAN D. McELREE

Marge Schott, owner of the Cincinnati Reds, was in the news in the spring and summer of 1996 because of her inflammatory remarks about minorities. Subsequently, she was removed from control of the Cincinnati Reds and prohibited from attending their games through 1998. During the controversy, she was interviewed for *Sports Illustrated* magazine (Reilly, 1996). We find an exchange recorded in the article written about that interview to be of particular interest. Marge Schott said: "There's what's-his-name, honey." The interviewer responded: "Who?" Schott replied: "The guy I'm paying $3 million a year to sit on his butt" (p. 84). The interviewer then noted that the player in question was a famous pitcher who, because of injury, had not played for any of the 1996 season or for part of the 1995 season. The player was paid $6.15 million a year, not the $3 million a year claimed by Schott.

If she had been asked about this conversation, it seems certain that Marge Schott would have told a different story than did the interviewer. The interviewer used her $3 million mistake, her failure to remember the player's name, and her insensitivity to the injured player to build a case that she was incompetent and out of touch. In contrast, from Schott's perspective, the comment probably simply expressed her frustration over paying an employee a high salary when that employee was not obligated to work.

We offer a third perspective—the perspective of cognitive psychologists whose primary interest is in memory. We find it very interesting that Marge Schott was unable to remember the name of a person to whom she was paying such a high salary. Indeed, she seemed unable to remember anybody's name and so referred to everybody as "honey." Her emotional response also reflected an insensitivity to current norms in baseball salaries. Rather than being uniquely greedy, the pitcher could be seen as an outstanding participant in a system that rewards its members by giving them a fair share of the profits earned, with the absolute levels of salary being extraordinarily high in part because of the effects of inflation. The norm against which Schott compared the salary of the player was in all likelihood a very old one, formed at a much earlier time, when the situation for athletes was different. She was consistent in her use of an antiquated norm: The ticket price for the Reds in 1996 was the lowest in the National League, and its stadium was the only place in the league where one could still buy a hot dog for $1. Later in this chapter, we speculate that there is a relation between Marge Schott's apparent memory deficit and her errors in monitoring. We compare her use of an antiquated norm to a reliance on habit—an automatic basis for responding—and we contrast habit with a consciously controlled basis for responding that can better take the current situation into account.

We are all sometimes guilty of acting on an emotional response or some other automatic process such as habit, rather than relying on reason. Epstein (1994; Epstein & Pacini, Chapter 23, this volume) contrasts an affect-laden experiential system of processing with an effortful, abstract, rational system. To illustrate the two systems, he describes a study in which people said their first thoughts in response to imaginary situations, such as having an accident while backing out of a parking space in which a friend had requested they park. Often people's first thought in this case was to blame the friend, and their first emotion was anger. Their second thought was more rational, accepting responsibility and even feeling guilty for blaming the friend. Chaiken's (1980) work on heuristic and systematic processing of persuasive messages also highlights the prevalence of alternatives to deliberative reasoning. People may be persuaded on the basis of minimal cues such as source credibility or the sheer length of a persuasive message, rather than expending the effort to evaluate the message systematically (see also Chen & Chaiken, Chapter 4, this volume).

AUTOMATIC BASES FOR RESPONDING

We are often reliant on the automatic. Uleman and his colleagues (Newman & Uleman, 1989; Winter & Uleman, 1984; see also Uleman, Chapter 7, this volume) found that people automatically abstract information about traits even when their task is to memorize. John Bargh (1997 and Chapter 18, this volume) vastly extends the realm of priming studies, such that nearly all behavior, affect, and motives appear automatic. Although the selection of higher-level goals has traditionally been viewed as the epitome of conscious control, Bargh argues that even those goals are determined by accessibility effects due to priming and habit. For example, Chartrand and Bargh (cited in Bargh, 1997) primed participants in a supposedly unrelated first phase of an experiment with words related to the goal of forming an impression of someone (words such as "opinion," "personality," "evaluate") or with words related to the goal of memorizing ("absorb," "retain," "remember"). Priming with the former stimuli induced a goal of impression formation when participants later viewed lists of a target's behaviors, as shown by the patterns of greater free recall of behaviors and greater organization according to traits, compared to the patterns of people who were primed with the memory goal terms. Other experiments (Bargh, Gollwitzer, & Barndollar, cited in Bargh, 1997) primed achievement versus affiliation motives and observed corresponding behaviors in a situation where these goals conflicted. Bargh suggests that modern psychology has overemphasized the causal role of conscious choice as a legacy of serial-stage models of cognition. We return to the issue of independent processes versus stage models later in the chapter.

Automaticity in Frontal Lobe Patients

Patients with frontal lobe damage represent the case of a near-total lack of higher-level conscious control. Lhermitte (1983) describes a phenomenon in frontal lobe patients he calls "utilization behavior." If one places an object before a frontal lobe patient, the patient will often pick up and use the object (e.g., make cutting movements with a knife, write with a pen, or light a cigarette lighter). The behavior capture displayed in examples of utilization behavior also occurs at the level of situations and roles. Lhermitte took a man and a woman who were both frontal lobe patients to a reception at a professional conference where neither of the patients had any role. The woman quite inappropriately took on the role of server at the conference. The man, just as inappropriately, took on the role of visiting dignitary. These examples of behavior capture provide a vivid demonstration of the power of context in combination with prior knowledge and experiences to produce automatic influences on behavior. People with fully functioning frontal lobes would be unlikely to assume either of these roles, but instead would clearly acknowledge their roles as outsiders. Perhaps accessibility effects are best thought of as automatic influences that can be opposed by consciously controlled intentions.

Emotional responses are critically important in shaping behavior, and they may also be examples of automatic influences on responding. However, in this case, frontal lobe patients illustrate what can happen when a normally automatic process of emotional responding does not occur. Damasio (1994) has noted that frontal lobe patients often make terrible decisions in real life, even though they perform perfectly normally on laboratory tests of reasoning and decision making. To try to pick up the judgment problems seen in natural situations, Damasio and Bechara (cited in Damasio, 1994) have devised a "gambling" paradigm, in which participants are given play money and seated in front of four decks of cards labeled A, B, C, and D. The object of the game is to increase the money by selecting cards one at a time from the four decks. Most cards have a payoff, but some cards demand that a player pay back money. Nothing else about the game is explained, so the player must learn about the decks by playing. Turning cards in decks A and B generally pays double that of turning cards in decks C and D, but the payback cards are for much higher sums for decks A and B. So, although decks A and B generally pay higher sums, they are accompanied by high risk; and playing them over the long haul will lead to large losses.

Most normal participants sample all four decks at first and are lured into playing decks A and B. However, after about 30 cards they have experienced enough large losses on decks A and B to stop playing them and settle in on decks C and D. In contrast, ventromedial frontal lobe patients are lured into playing decks A and B, but never learn from the high penalties. They stay with decks A and B, even though they go bankrupt halfway through the game and have to borrow money from the experimenter. It is not an intellectual problem for the frontal lobe patients. At the end of the experiment, they can say that decks A and B are dangerous and risky. However, this intellectual understanding of danger

seems unaccompanied by an emotional anticipation as they consider drawing from the decks. In fact, unlike normal participants, who develop a stronger and stronger galvanic skin response (GSR) when they consider drawing from decks A and B, frontal lobe patients show no GSR as they consider those decks. They do show normal GSRs to winning and losing, but lack what Damasio calls a "somatic marker" that would allow them to anticipate the danger in decks A and B.

This dissociation between emotional response and reason is important, because it complements previous findings of dissociations where people show emotional responses in the absence of conscious access to the source of the emotional response. Damasio uses the dissociation findings to argue that reasoning in domains with real consequences is normally inextricably linked to and supported by emotion. We note that the emotional response is typically acquired automatically and serves an important role in shaping behavior.

Dissociations

Dissociations have been critically important for recent theories of memory. Amnesics are the paradigm case: Although they may show little or no ability to consciously recall or recognize events that occur after the onset of their amnesia, they nonetheless reveal the effects of specific past experiences indirectly in their performance on various tasks. These indirect effects of memory include increases in the likelihood of completing word fragments or stems with recently read words. Similar dissociations have been confirmed in people with normally functioning memory, as various independent variables produce dissociative effects on direct memory tests of recall and recognition versus indirect memory tests such as fragment completion (for reviews, see Kelley & Lindsay, 1996; Roediger & McDermott, 1993). As we will discuss later, the ability to consciously recollect events affords much more control over later behavior than do unconscious influences of the past.

Social psychologists have long realized the potential value of indirect tests as a means of measuring attitudes. For example, Gilbert and Hixon (1991) had an Asian American assistant versus a European American assistant hold up cards displaying word fragments, which participants were to complete. Participants' choice of completion words revealed their stereotype of Asians. The word fragment "ri_e" was more likely to be completed with "rice" and the fragment "poli_e" was more likely to be completed with "polite" when an Asian woman was holding up the cards. (Interestingly, the stereotype activation didn't occur when participants were cognitively overloaded by an additional task, which suggests that when the participants were preoccupied, the woman was simply seen as a card holder.) Banaji and Greenwald (1994, 1995) argue for the value of indirect tests as a measure of attitudes. Analogous to projective tests, indirect tests are said to circumvent social desirability to reveal "true" attitudes in a way that direct tests of attitudes cannot.

Among the indirect tests of attitudes discussed by Banaji and Greenwald was our "false-fame" effect. We describe the false-fame effect in this chapter, using it to illustrate the general class of "opposition procedures" that we have employed to show separate effects of automatic and consciously controlled processes. Important advantages can be gained by placing processes in opposition rather than in concert, as is often done for indirect tests. Use of opposition procedures is sufficient to reveal the existence of separate bases for responding. However, we go beyond demonstrating existence to describe procedures that can be used to measure the separate contributions of automatic and consciously controlled processes. By doing so, we provide a different perspective for understanding a type of effect that has been very important to social psychologists—accessibility effects of the sort revealed by Gilbert and Hixon's (1991) experiment.

We argue that effects of category accessibility (e.g., Bruner, 1957) are the same as the memory preserved by amnesics and the automatic form of responding that marks the behavior capture of frontal lobe patients. The automatic basis for responding does not reveal attitudes that are any more "true" than the attitudes revealed by consciously controlled responding as measured by direct tests. Rather, the two types of processes serve as independent bases for responding. The situation is analogous to separating the contributions of knowledge and guessing to performance on

a multiple-choice test. Accessibility effects map onto guessing, whereas consciously controlled processes map onto knowledge. As we will show, "guesses" can be very revealing. However, we argue that guesses have been overinterpreted: The contribution of consciously controlled processing has been relatively neglected by emphasizing situations that rely heavily on accessibility effects.

Much of our recent research has been aimed at age-related deficits in memory. Our goals have been to devise better methods for diagnosing such deficits, along with treatment programs to remedy or diminish age-related differences. The general population is aging, which will lead to a much greater prevalence of Alzheimer's disease (AD) and other diseases that produce tragic reductions in cognitive functioning. In addition, frontal lobe functioning declines with aging (Albert & Kaplin, 1980; Daigneault, Braun, & Whitaker, 1992; West, 1996). We hope that this chapter will help persuade social psychologists to join us in our interest in age-related differences. An important applied problem and test for theorizing can be captured by this question: Can we "rehabilitate" Marge Schott? If she is indeed suffering from some form of cognitive difficulty, she is going to be joined by many others in the near future. We end by speculating about implications of our research for repairing her "deficits."

ADVANTAGE OF OPPOSITION: FAME AND IRONIC EFFECTS OF REPETITION

Baddeley and Wilson (1994) have attempted to rehabilitate the memory performance of people with various forms of neurological damage by building on their intact automatic influences of memory. Our goal is somewhat different, in that we want to measure and train intentional uses of memory. As described later, our hope is that we can return control of memory to the memory-impaired individual, instead of placing the control of memory in the environment.

False Fame

A person can become famous overnight, or even sooner if the audience is not paying attention (Jacoby, Kelley, Brown, & Jasechko, 1989; Jacoby, Woloshyn, & Kelley, 1989). In one series of experiments, automatic influences of memory (familiarity) were placed in opposition to recollection, allowing us to infer recollection deficits through the errors that people commit. Participants read a list of names that they were told were nonfamous, and then took a fame judgment test consisting of old nonfamous names mixed with new famous and new nonfamous names. The prior presentation of nonfamous names increased their familiarity, which made it more likely that the names would be mistakenly judged as famous. However, if participants could remember the source of the name correctly, then any automatic influence of familiarity would be opposed, as they could be certain that the name was nonfamous. In other words, to the extent that participants were able to recollect, they could avoid undesirable effects of the past.

Fame judgment tests were performed immediately after participants read the list of nonfamous names or 24 hours later. Results revealed a "false-fame" effect after a 24-hour delay, in that old nonfamous names were *more* likely to be mistakenly called famous than were new nonfamous names. In contrast, when participants took the fame judgment test immediately after reading the names, the results were the opposite: old nonfamous names were *less* likely to be called famous than were new nonfamous names. This combination of results is akin to a sleeper effect (Hovland & Weiss, 1951). When the test was immediate, participants were able to escape misleading automatic influences of memory by recollecting source information. However, when recollection was reduced by extending the retention interval or by dividing attention at study or test, then the false-fame effect was observed.

Because of a deficit in ability to recollect, individuals with a memory impairment might show a false-fame effect even on an immediate test. Indeed, elderly adults do show a pronounced immediate false-fame effect (Dywan & Jacoby, 1990; Jennings & Jacoby, 1993), as do amnesics (Cermak, Verfaellie, Butler, & Jacoby, 1993; Squire & McKee, 1992) and patients who have sustained a closed head injury (Dywan, Segalowitz, Henderson, & Jacoby, 1993). We have made use of such misleading effects of automatic influences of

memory to diagnose deficits in recollection in elderly adults.

Ironic Effects of Repetition

A friend whose mother is suffering symptoms of AD tells the story of taking her mother to check out a nursing home. The rules and regulations were explained during an orientation lecture, including an explanation of how the dining room operated. The dining hall was described as similar to a restaurant, except that tipping was not required. In fact, the absence of tipping was mentioned frequently during the lecture as an illustration of the quality of care and the advantages of paying in advance. At the end of the meeting, the friend's mother was asked whether she had any questions. She replied that she only had one: "Should I tip?"

Similar to this unwanted effect of repetition, repeated asking of questions is one of the most striking and frustrating symptoms of AD. For the AD patient, each repetition of a question seems to "strengthen" it and paradoxically increases the probability of repeating the question, whereas for people with normally functioning memory, that automatic strengthening is opposed by their ability to recollect earlier asking the question (along with its answer). Repetition may well have two effects, serving both to automatically increase the strength of the question and to increase the probability of recollecting that one already asked it. Because of a deficit in recollection, the AD patient is left only with the increase in strength and so is condemned to repeatedly asking the same question. The result is similar to the false-fame effect in showing automatic influences of memory that are unopposed by recollection.

Jacoby (in press) used an opposition procedure to examine age-related differences in memory and to show that repetition does indeed have two effects. Young and elderly adults read a list of words, with each word being read either one, two, or three times. Next they listened to a list of words that they were told to remember for a later test. At test, participants were instructed to identify words that were heard earlier, and were warned that the test list would include words that were read earlier. They were further told that the earlier-read words were to be excluded, because none of those words were in the list of words that they had heard. Repeatedly reading a word would increase its familiarity and might also increase the likelihood that the word would be mistakenly judged as having been heard, because of a misattribution of the source of the familiarity. However, recollection of having read the word would oppose its familiarity, allowing the word to be excluded, just as in the false-fame experiments.

Because of a deficit in recollection, the performance of elderly participants revealed the strengthening effect of repetition. For elderly participants, repeatedly reading a word *increased* the probability of their mistakenly accepting the word as one that was earlier heard (Table 19.1). The strengthening effect of repetition, unopposed by recollection, may be what underlies AD patients' repetition of questions. Younger participants, in contrast, were better able to use recollection to oppose familiarity. For younger participants, repeatedly reading a word made it more likely that they would later recollect that the word was read, allowing them to be certain it was not heard. For them, repeated reading of a word *decreased* the probability of their mistakenly accepting the word as one that was heard earlier.

The use of recollection is generally slower and more effortful than is reliance on familiarity to make decisions. This difference between the two bases for memory judgments suggests that one could arrange conditions such that young participants would show "ironic" effects of repetition similar to those shown by elderly adults. For example, if young adults were forced to respond rapidly, repeatedly reading a word might have the ironic effect of making it more likely that the word would be mistakenly accepted as heard earlier, just as was found for the elderly participants. Indeed, this was shown to be the case: Forcing young adults to respond rapidly produced effects of repetition that were opposite to those observed when more time was allowed for responding, leading to the same pattern of results produced by the elderly participants. This might suggest that the problem for elderly participants was that they simply did not have enough time to engage in recollection. Because of general slowing (Salthouse, 1991), elderly participants might require more time than younger participants might. However, allowing elderly participants more time to respond was not sufficient to eliminate the ironic effect of repetition. Even when the elderly were allowed more time, repeated reading of a word still increased the probability of its being mistakenly accepted as heard earlier. The ironic repetition effect found for the elderly reflects an age-related deficit in recollection.

We refer to the false-fame effect and to the misleading effect of repetition as "ironic effects," to highlight their similarity to the ironic effects described by Wegner (1994). Wegner has shown that attempts to avoid mental states can have the ironic effect of increasing the probability of their occurrence.

TABLE 19.1. Probability of Identifying Words as Heard Earlier

Response deadline	Read presentations			New	Heard
	1×	2×	3×		
Young					
Long (1,250/750)	.35	.31	.21	.22	.63
Short (750)	.31	.40	.45	.18	.43
Elderly					
Long (1,250/750)	.43	.53	.59	.19	.52
Extra long (1,250/ASAP)	.35	.42	.44	.14	.52

Note. Both for the young and elderly participants, the long (1,250/750) response deadline refers to a 1,250-ms delay before response signal, after which there was a 750-ms response window. The young short (750) response deadline for the young participants refers to a response window of 750 ms (i.e., there was no delay or response signal). The extra long (1,250/ASAP) response deadline for the elderly participants refers to a 1,250-ms delay before response signal, after which they were to respond as soon as possible. Adapted from Jacoby (in press). Copyright 1998 by the American Psychological Association. Reprinted by permission.

For example, as Marge Schott would probably testify, trying to avoid saying things that are sexist or racist can actually increase the probability of making such statements (Wegner, Erber, & Bowman, cited in Wegner, 1994). Attempts to avoid politically incorrect statements increase their accessibility, just as earlier reading of a nonfamous name increases its familiarity, and repetition of a word increases its strength. In all these cases, the result is an automatic influence that can produce an ironic effect if left unopposed by cognitive control.

Reinstating study context can also produce an ironic effect of memory. As a commonplace example, most people have had the experience of telling a joke to the very person from whom they originally heard the joke. In the context of the person who earlier told the joke, the joke comes to mind and is told as one the person might enjoy, left unopposed by recollection of its original telling. The ironic effect seems surprising, because one might expect the presence of the person to serve as a powerful cue for recollection of the earlier telling of the joke. We have evidence to show that reinstating associative context has two effects, just as repetition does. Reinstating associative context decreases the probability of exclusion after divided attention during study, but has the opposite effect after full attention during study (Jacoby, 1996).

In an experiment similar to the one described above, words read in a first list were presented with a context word during study, and that context word was either presented again at test or not. When context was reinstated at test, young participants who had ample time to respond were *less* likely to mistake a read word for one that was heard in a second list than when the context was not reinstated. In contrast, the elderly and the young participants who were forced to respond rapidly were *more* likely to mistakenly accept a read word as a heard word when context was reinstated. Reinstating context thus both increased accessibility and increased the probability of recollection. Similarly, Trope (1986; Trope & Gaunt, Chapter 8, this volume) has shown that context effects on accessibility can alter the interpretation of an ambiguous stimulus, and furthermore that such effects on interpretation are separate from the effects of context on attribution processes. Ironic effects result when the effects of context on accessibility are left unopposed by recollection.

Early Selection versus Late Correction: Process Dissociations

Use of opposition procedures is sufficient to produce results that demonstrate the existence of automatic or unconscious influences of memory, and is useful for diagnosing deficits in recollection—a form of consciously controlled processing. However, our research has been designed to go beyond demonstrations of existence to develop techniques that allow us to measure the separate contributions of consciously controlled and automatic processes. To estimate how much performance is accomplished by unconscious memory requires that we specify the relation between conscious and unconscious memory processes.

In much of our research, participants have been asked to complete word stems or word fragments. The reason for our interest in completion tasks is that even individuals with very dense amnesia show an effect of memory by being more likely to use an earlier-read word as a completion for a stem or fragment (e.g., "bone" as a completion for the fragment "b_n_") than they would be if the word had not been read in the experimental setting. For example, amnesics show near-normal memory for earlier-read words when asked to complete fragments with the first word that comes to mind (an indirect test of memory), although their performance is much poorer than that of people with normally functioning memory when asked to use the fragments as cues for recall of the earlier-studied words (a direct test of memory) (e.g., Graf, Squire, & Mandler, 1984; Jacoby, 1982; Warrington & Weiskrantz, 1982). How do people with normally functioning memory use consciously controlled processing to accomplish cued recall in a way that is different from simply completing a stem with the first word that comes to mind?

One answer to that question is that consciously controlled processes can serve to edit or "correct" potential responses whose accessibility reflect unconscious memory. Jacoby and Hollingshead (1990) advocated an account of this sort by proposing a "generate–

recognize" model to describe recall cued by presentation of word stems. According to this model, earlier reading of a word makes the word later come more readily to mind as a completion for a stem—an automatic influence of memory on the generation of candidate responses for cued recall. Candidate responses are then subjected to a recognition memory test prior to their output. For a test of cued recall, only those words that are recognized as earlier studied are given as a response. Thus, a direct test of cued recall is said to differ from an indirect test of stem completion only in that the direct test involves a recognition memory check. The role of consciously controlled processes is to edit the products of unconscious processes, correcting inappropriate responses so as not to mistakenly output words that were not studied. This is a "late-correction" model of conscious control.

Our alternative is an "early-selection" model of conscious control, whereby conscious memory retrieval starts very early in processing, although it may take longer to complete than an automatic process. This analysis of the relation between automatic and controlled processes in memory tasks is very different from a "response plus correction" model. Conscious memory processes do not always simply follow automatic processes, but can occur in parallel and serve as an independent basis for responding. During attempts to remember, people may rely on conscious recollection of a prior event. In contrast, a response may simply pop into mind because of general knowledge or habit, or because of the sort of unconscious memory that an amnesic exhibits on an indirect memory test. According to the early-selection model, consciously controlled processes tightly constrain what comes to mind, resulting in recollection.

Much of our recent work has been aimed at showing that an early-selection model of conscious memory retrieval sometimes holds. To separately estimate the contributions of conscious recollection versus other bases for responding, we have arranged situations in which only conscious recollection can afford control over responding across experimental situations. Studies using the process-dissociation procedure (Jacoby, 1991; Jacoby, Toth, & Yonelinas, 1993) set up two condi-

tions in which people either tried to or tried not to respond when they could consciously recollect an event. The difference in performance between the two conditions provided an estimate of how much conscious recollection contributed to their performance.

According to the early-selection model, when participants were instructed to consciously remember and to give the first response that comes to mind when they cannot remember (the inclusion condition), their responses should reflect the contributions of both recollection and unconscious memory, $R + U$, minus the overlap of the two processes, UR, or $R + (1 - R)U$. In contrast, when participants were instructed *not* to respond with what they consciously remembered (the exclusion condition), the probability that they would nonetheless inadvertently respond with an item that was studied should be $(1 - R)U$. The performances in the two conditions and the equations that describe them should enable estimates of conscious recollection and unconscious memory to be calculated. In a variety of studies using the process-dissociation procedure, dividing attention or forcing people to respond within a short deadline reduced the estimate of conscious memory, but left the estimate of unconscious memory intact. Those dissociations provided support for the use of the independence assumption in the equations.

The contrast between early-selection and late-correction models is a very general one. Consider the different ways that an exclusion memory task might be accomplished. To return to the task introduced with the "Should I tip?" example, a word that was repeatedly read might seem familiar, and elderly participants' failure to exclude those earlier-read words might reflect a failure to use source memory (Johnson, Hashtroudi, & Lindsay, 1993) to edit or correct familiarity—a relatively automatic influence of memory. Alternatively, one could use the test word as a cue for direct retrieval or recollection.

The same alternatives apply to social monitoring. Why doesn't the average person say obscenities when talking to a nun? According to the late-correction approach, the obscenities may well come to mind while speaking to a nun, but are withheld because they are recognized as being socially inappropriate to say. The early-selection view, in contrast, holds that the person is likely to be sufficiently situated in the "speaking to a nun" context that obscenities never come to mind. That is, cognitive control can take the context into account and operate to determine what comes to mind, rather than only being called forth to serve as an editor for the contents of consciousness.

Although both relations between consciously controlled and automatic processes hold, but in different situations (Jacoby, 1998a), we focus here on an early-selection model, rather than a late-correction model. We do so because the early-selection model has been relatively neglected, due to the greater intuitive appeal and unwarranted general acceptance of a late-correction model.

ACCESSIBILITY BIAS: TOWARD SEPARATING AUTOMATIC AND CONTROLLED PROCESSES

The "New Look" movement in perception (e.g., Bruner, 1957; Greenwald, 1992) argued that perception is influenced by expectancies, values, attitudes, and needs. If perception involves an act of categorization, then it should be influenced by the accessibility of different categories. Social psychology has explored these influences by studying individual differences in the accessibility of particular traits, stereotypes, and attitude categories (Bargh & Pietromonaco, 1982; Fazio, 1986), as well as temporary changes in accessibility due to recent experience that primes a category (e.g., Devine, 1989; Higgins, Rholes, & Jones, 1977; Srull & Wyer, 1980).

The current view in social psychology is that automatic processes provide an early-stage or preliminary analysis that is then "corrected" by more consciously controlled processing (but see Bargh, Chapter 18, this volume). For example, Devine's (1989; Devine & Monteith, Chapter 17, this volume) theory of stereotyping suggests that all members of a culture possess knowledge of various stereotypes—knowledge that is made automatically accessible by priming and so affects judgments of targets. However, people who are not prejudiced strive to counteract these automatic processes by consciously thinking egalitarian thoughts. Similarly, Gilbert and his colleagues (see Gilbert, 1989 for a review)

suggest that perceivers categorize and characterize another person's behavior automatically in terms of personality dispositions, and then, if the perceivers not cognitively overloaded, correct for situational factors.

Although we agree that consciously controlled processes do sometimes serve to correct automatic processes, we believe that cognitive control more often serves an early-selection role, as in the case of obscenities' not coming to mind around a nun. Next, we describe an experiment done to examine effects of a "stereotype" on perception, which illustrates the difference between early-selection and late-correction forms of cognitive control.

The contrast between the two views holds for perception as well as for social monitoring. Perceptual identification has been an important indirect memory test used to show memory dissociations. For example, Jacoby and Dallas (1981) found that reading a word in the experimental setting enhanced its perceptual identification when the word was later briefly flashed, and that this effect on perception did not depend on recognition memory for the word. A recent experiment (Jacoby, 1998b) extended this earlier research to show that prior experience can serve as a basis for guessing during a perceptual task.

Habits of varying strength were created in the first phase of the experiment by having people view words with a fragment of a related word (e.g., "knee–b_n_") on a computer monitor and attempt to predict how those fragments would be completed by the computer program. Immediately after their prediction, one of two possible words was shown that completed the fragment. For some pairs, a biasing habit was created by showing a particular completion 75% of the time during the training phase. For example, 15 out of 20 times when the stimulus "knee–b_n_" was shown, it was completed by the word "bone," and on the remaining 5 trials it was completed by "bend." For other, unbiased pairs, the two completions were presented equally often, and one completion was arbitrarily designated as typical.

The second phase of the experiment was a perceptual task. Words were flashed for a brief duration (28 or 43 milliseconds [ms]), followed by a visual mask. Next the context word and fragment (e.g., "knee–b_n_") were presented; participants were told to complete the fragment with the word that was flashed, or, if they were unable to identify the flashed word, to complete the fragment with the first word that came to mind. The flashed word was either congruent ("bone") or incongruent ("bend") with the habit ("knee–bone") formed in the first phase of the experiment.

This habit can be thought of as akin to a stereotype. As a result of training in the first phase of the experiment, participants learned that "bone" is the sort of a thing that is likely to hang around with "knee." Reliance on that stereotype might serve as a source of errors, resulting in reports of "bone" when "bend" was actually the flashed word. Indeed, there was a high probability of such an error for the incongruent test words (Table 19.2). The probability of "false perception" was much higher in the 75/25 condition than in the unbiased (50/50) condition, and was also higher when the flash duration was short (28 ms). To this point, the results were quite in line with the constructionism spawned by the New Look view of perception. Expectations established during the first phase apparently influenced perception.

However, a different interpretation emerged when the probability of *correct* perception for congruent test items was examined. The probability of correct perception increased with flash duration. Moreover, the improvement in correct perception for the congruent items in the 75/25 condition over the 50/50 condition was accompanied by a nearly equivalent increase in the likelihood of false perception on the incongruent items,

which fit with a bias to produce the habitual response. The bias produced a symmetrical increase in correct responding for congruent items and a decrease in correct responding for incongruent items.

Habit and perception were assumed to make independent contributions to the cued-perception test, as reflected by the equations $P + (1 - P)H$ for correct perception in the congruent cases and $(1 - P)H$ for false perception in the incongruent cases. The independence assumption represented by the equations was confirmed, because different variables produced dissociative effects on the estimates of habit versus perception. The estimate of habit in the perception test mirrored the strength of the habit established in the training phase, but this manipulation of habit strength had no effect on estimates of perception. In contrast, a short flash duration lowered the estimates of perception, but did not affect the estimate of habit.

In sum, these results showed that, contrary to the New Look view, habit or a stereotype did not truly influence perception. That is, habit did not result in an early "bone" percept that had to be corrected to allow the incongruent test word "bend" to be seen. Rather, habit served as a bias, coming into play only when perception failed $(1 - P)$. Note that we have not said that prior experience "just" influenced bias, as was often said by critics of the New Look approach who relied on signal detection theory to analyze their results (e.g., Eriksen, 1960). Our analysis differs from that of signal detection theory in that our dual-process model assumes that perception and habit serve as independent bases

TABLE 19.2. Probabilities of Correct Perception (CP) on Congruent Pairs and of False Perception (FP) on Incongruent Pairs across Training Condition and Mean Estimates of Perception (P) and Habit (H)

Training condition	Probabilities		Estimates	
	Cong. (CP)	Incong. (FP)	P	H
75/25				
Long duration	.81	.43	.37	.67
Short duration	.68	.65	.03	.66
50/50				
Long duration	.69	.32	.37	.51
Short duration	.51	.51	.00	.51

Note. Short duration, 28 ms; long duration, 43 ms. From Jacoby (1998b).

for responding, whereas signal detection theory is a single-process model. In our model, habit is an important process in its own right, as important as perception; it is described as a "bias" only when one focuses on the accuracy of perception.

Habit versus Recollection

One source of automatic responses on a memory test is responding on the basis of habit rather than on the basis of recollection of a particular event. For example, you may habitually leave your keys on your bedroom dresser, but one night you leave them on a table in your entryway. The next morning as you try to remember where you left your keys, you may recollect that you left the keys in the entryway, or you may think of them in their habitual location on the dresser. Hay and Jacoby (1996) used a variant of the process-dissociation procedure to show that habits could serve as a source of bias in cued-recall performance. The habitual response was meant to be analogous to the habit of leaving one's keys in a particular location.

The method of Hay and Jacoby's (1996) experiments paralleled that of the experiment on habit and perception described above. Habitual responses to word fragment combinations such as "knee–b_n_" were established in a first phase. In the second phase of the experiment, participants studied short lists of word pairs and took a cued-recall test. Some of the items on the study list were either congruent with the habit ("knee–bone") or incongruent with the habit ("knee–bend"). The second phase was meant to be analogous to a test of memory for a specific event (e.g., "Where did I leave my keys last night?").

The pattern of results was the same as that described above for the perception experiment. Varying the probability of a particular response during Phase 1 (75/25 vs. 50/50) influenced habit but did not affect the probability of recollecting the response studied in the short list. Other factors, such as the amount of time allowed for study of pairs in the short list, influenced recollection but did not affect habit. Requiring people to respond rapidly, as compared to allowing more time for a response, reduced the probability of recollection but left the estimated contribution of habit unchanged. As described in conjunction

with the "Should I tip?" example, recollection is a slower process than habit, which is an automatic influence of memory. Whether participants were given a test of perception or one of recollection, habit served as a source of guesses, coming into play *only* when perception or recollection failed.

Kelley (1998) recently used a similar paradigm to show that preexisting habits—in this case, general knowledge—also make an independent contribution to memory performance. Participants studied a list of general-knowledge questions paired with what they thought were another student's answers, which were incorrect a certain proportion of the time. Later, they attempted to recall the studied answers when presented with the questions as cues. The estimate of memory in their cued-recall performance was sensitive to manipulations such as time delay, while the use of general knowledge was sensitive to the proportion of correct answers on the studied list. These studies of the interplay of habit and general knowledge with recollection are similar to social-psychological analyses of chronic accessibility effects.

In the studies outlined above, the habit of responding with "knee–bone" whether or not it had been studied can be characterized as an accessibility bias. Similarly, unconscious memory effects can also be characterized as an accessibility bias: Recent experience changes what comes to mind during a task, independently of the likelihood that the person will consciously recollect the experience (see also Jacoby, McElree, & Trainham, in press). However, accessibility bias did not influence perception or remembering, as would be expected from a late-correction model of the sort that has guided theorizing by social psychologists. Rather, accessibility bias served as an alternative source of responses, independent of conscious perception and memory. Similarly, general knowledge is another alternative basis for responding.

Speed–Accuracy Tradeoff

Process-dissociation procedures provide a way of estimating the contribution of underlying processes to a response. In many cases, underlying processes may differ in processing speed. For example, an automatic process may be completed sooner than a slower, consciously controlled process. In cases where there are underlying differences in process speed, one can employ speed–accuracy trade-off (SAT) procedures to precisely track and contrast the time course of component processes underlying a single, overt response.

One such SAT procedure is the response signal procedure. It measures the time-course of responses by tracking changes in accuracy over processing time (e.g., Dosher, 1976, 1979; McElree, 1993, 1996; McElree & Dosher, 1989, 1993; Reed, 1973, 1976; Wickelgren, 1977). Measures of accuracy are derived by requiring participants to judge some key aspect of a test stimulus. Participants are trained to respond within a 100- to 300-ms window marked by the presentation of a response signal such as a tone. Across trials, the response signal is randomly presented at one of six to eight time delays spread throughout the full time course of processing (e.g., from 100 to 3,000 ms after the onset of the test stimulus). In this way, performance is measured across the full extent of processing—from times when performance is at or near chance levels to times when it has reached an asymptotic level. Studies using the response signal methodology reveal three distinct phases: a period of chance-level performance, followed by a period of increasing accuracy, followed by an asymptotic period beyond which further processing does not yield increases in accuracy. Speed of processing is measured by when the function departs from chance levels and how quickly accuracy grows over processing time. Accuracy is measured by the asymptotic level of performance.

When SAT procedures are combined with tasks that place consciously controlled and automatic processes in opposition, it is possible to measure how underlying processes combine over time to form a response. By way of illustration, consider a recent series of recognition experiments (McElree, Jacoby, & Dolan, 1996; McElree, Dolan, & Jacoby, in press). As noted earlier, recognition memory may be mediated by two independent processes: a fast assessment of global familiarity, and a slower recollective process that recovers a specific episodic event from memory. Building on studies described previously (Jacoby, in press), these experiments presented participants with a list of to-be-read items, followed by a list of spoken items. For the read list, half the items were presented once, and half were repeated three times. Following study, participants were presented with test items that were either heard, read (once or three times), or new. They were instructed to respond "yes" to an item only if it was from the heard list, and were explicitly told that if they recalled an item as having being read, they could be assured that it was not in the heard list. The critical tests concerned the once- and thrice-read items. The prediction was that repetition should influence both the familiarity and the recollective process, with thrice-repeated items producing higher familiarity values and also an increased probability of recollection. Note, however, that the experimental design placed these two processes in opposition: Increased familiarity should induce participants to make false alarms (i.e., to mistake a read item as heard), but better recollection of an item as being read should reduce the false-alarm rate. We used SAT procedures to isolate when these two processes influenced "exclusion" judgments.

The first panel (A) of Figure 19.1 shows the SAT functions in d' units when the hit rate for the heard items is scaled against the new, once-read, and thrice-read items (symbols show empirical data, and smooth curves are the best-fitting dual-process model; see McElree et al., in press). We interpret the differences in the speed with which accuracy grows over time as due to the differential impact of the repetition of read items on the two processes. We isolated the impact of the familiarity and recollective processes by a type of pseudo-d' scaling (Dosher, McElree, Hood, & Rosedale, 1989; McElree & Dosher, 1989; McElree & Griffith, 1995). The second panel (B) shows the false-alarm rates for the two types of read items scaled against the false-alarm rate for the new items. Scaled in this manner, higher pseudo-d' values denote poorer performance resulting from higher underlying false-alarm rates in the read conditions. (If the false-alarm rates for the read items equaled the false-alarm rate for the new items, pseudo-d' values would equal zero.)

The important aspect of the curves in the second panel is that both show a clear nonmonotonic shape: There is a peak value at about 800 ms that diminishes with more retrieval time. The early portions of the func-

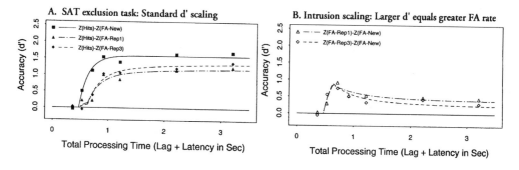

FIGURE 19.1. (A) The speed–accuracy tradeoff (SAT) functions in d' units. (B) The false-alarm (FA) rates. Adapted from McElree, Dolan, and Jacoby (in press). Copyright 1998 by the American Psychological Association. Adapted by permission.

tion (<800 ms) show the fast assessment of familiarity that resulted in high false-alarm rates. The latter portions of the functions show the impact of a recollective process that attenuated (although not perfectly) the misattribution based on high familiarity. We estimated the points in time when the familiarity and recollective processes were operating from the nonmonotonic shape of the pseudo-d' functions (using a two-process growth model as in Dosher et al., 1989; McElree & Dosher, 1989; McElree & Griffith, 1995). Familiarity was operative at 471 ms after the onset of a test probe, whereas the recollective process was operative later, at around 639 ms. Moreover, as hypothesized, both familiarity and recollection were stronger for thrice-repeated than for once-repeated items.

The facts that familiarity and recollection are independent, and that recollection is a slower process than familiarity, mean that recollection can be used to counteract or correct erroneous responses based on familiarity. However, our use of experimental paradigms that place familiarity and recollection in opposition so as to allow their separation should not be misinterpreted as our saying that the only role of conscious recollection is to correct or edit responses based on familiarity. Conscious recollection is not a late stage that relies on the prior stage of computing familiarity. In fact, in nature, it is probably just as likely that familiarity and recollection act in concert as in opposition.

This type of SAT procedure has been profitably used to isolate and examine component processes in several cognitive do-

mains, including language comprehension (e.g., McElree, 1993; McElree & Griffith, 1995; 1998), semantic memory (e.g., Corbett & Wickelgren, 1978), and episodic memory (e.g., Dosher et al., 1989; McElree & Dosher, 1989). Although SAT studies have primarily addressed issues of the architecture of cognitive processing, we believe that similar procedures can be profitably used to examine issues that have been at the forefront of theorizing in social cognition—notably several of the research domains touched upon here, including stereotyping (Devine & Monteith, Chapter 17, this volume), impression formation (e.g., Bargh, 1989; Srull & Wyer, 1979), heuristic and systematic processing (Chen & Chaiken, Chapter 4, this volume), and ironic effects of mental control (Wegner, 1994). The SAT studies and the process-dissociation procedure allow investigators to separate the contributions of several processes to a task, instead of attempting to devise conditions where only a single process might be operating. Much of human behavior is a result of multiple processes rather than "process-pure." These techniques not only look at the processes operating together, but allow very precise assessment of their time course and relative contributions.

EVERYDAY AUTOMATICITY: CONSCIOUSNESS IS NOT A STAGE

Consciousness has returned as a popular topic of discussion for philosophers (e.g., Block, 1995; Dennett, 1991). Dennett argues against the "Cartesian theater" view of consciousness, arguing that there is no one "place" where different processes come together to form a percept that is "viewed." We agree that consciousness is not a theater. Neither is it a stage. Consciousness does not always follow automatic processes at some later stage and enable consciously controlled processing, which can "correct" the errors of automaticity. Rather, consciously controlled processing can provide a basis for responding that is *independent* of that provided by automatic processes.

The often implicit assumption that conscious processes occur at late stages of processing has permeated the thinking of social and cognitive psychologists. As noted earlier, Bargh has argued that the prevalence of serial-stage theories in cognition, with conscious recognition and reasoning following unconscious analysis and preceding behavior, has created a meta-assumption that conscious processes always causally precede behavior. We illustrate the difference between a stage analysis and an analysis that contrasts independent bases for responding by considering Devine's (1989) important research on prejudice. In particular, we consider her research in the context of Jacoby's (1998b) experiments that separated the contributions of habit and perception.

Stages versus Independent Bases for Responding

Devine's research has been very influential in part because the results imply that people are all bigots, although some people do consciously correct their bigotry before it can be expressed in behavior. Devine presented words related to the stereotype of African Americans under conditions meant to allow only unconscious perception. Presenting those words did increase the accessibility of the African American stereotype, as shown by effects on the interpretation of a paragraph which provided an ambiguous description of a racially unspecified person's behavior. Behavior that could be interpreted as either assertive or hostile was interpreted as hostile when the stereotype of African Americans was made accessible, even for those participants who were not prejudiced (according to their responses on a scale that directly assessed their attitude).

Devine's finding is a striking one for those who think of consciousness as a stage. It implies that people automatically view the world in terms of their stereotypes and then act accordingly, unless they consciously correct for their bias. However, we can think of her findings in a somewhat different way by drawing parallels to the research on habit and perception. In that research, habits or stereotypes do not have their effects on an early stage that precedes a second look; rather, they form an alternative basis for responding. The study of perception and habit (Jacoby, 1998b) included cues for perceptual report of items that could not have been perceived because they were not flashed (a blank flash followed by "knee–b_n_"). Responses to those "ambiguous" guessing items showed probability matching to the strength of the habit established in the first phase, just as Devine's ambiguous description revealed increased accessibility of a stereotype. But in the study of perception and habit, perception was independent of bias, as shown by dissociative manipulations. Similarly, consciously controlled individuating processes in impression formation may be independent of stereotype accessibility effects, and not simply follow on the automatic accessibility.

In earlier studies of memory, researchers interested in unconscious memory processes wanted to study "pure cases" and so attempted to arrange situations where participants would not use conscious memory in an implicit memory test. That turned out to be very hard to do in a test of anyone but densely amnesic participants. The process-dissociation procedure moves away from the search for pure cases, and instead tries to gain estimates of conscious and unconscious processes within a single task. Behavior in the "ambiguous" situation, such as recall of the unstudied items in Hay and Jacoby (1996) (cues such as "knee–b_n_" when neither "knee–bone" nor "knee–bend" was on the study list), does not predict behavior in the situation in which consciously controlled processing is also in play unless one takes into account the independence of the two bases for responding. We think that the control afforded by taking an initial set or orientation that constrains what comes to mind will prove to be as powerful in cases of social perception as we have found them to be in the domains of memory and perception.

Does it really matter whether one thinks of consciousness as correcting or as providing an independent basis for responding? To show that it does, we end this chapter by describing different ways of trying to make Marge Schott more sensitive to her situation. When we analyze her behavior from the perspective of the two models, we are led to very different proposals for her "rehabilitation."

"Fixing" Marge Schott

The 1996 controversy surrounding the behavior of Marge Schott was not her first. As a result of an earlier controversy, she was required to participate in "sensitivity training." We know nothing about this sensitivity training, except that it apparently did not work, leaving us free to speculate about how one might design effective training.

Why didn't the sensitivity training work? Schott's difficulty may be similar to that of Damasio's frontal lobe patients who engaged in risky gambles. The patients clearly understood that the gambles were risky and understood the consequences of their behavior. They produced emotional responses after winning and losing. What they lacked was an emotional response when they reached toward the cards in the risky deck. We return to this possibility after considering another possible course of treatment.

The layperson, along with most psychologists, would say that Schott's problem is that she does not think before she speaks. This analysis might be translated to mean that when a thought comes to mind, she should thoroughly inspect it to be certain that it will not be offensive before she says it. According to this account, conscious control is a late stage that allows us to edit thoughts that are generated by an earlier, unconscious, automatic stage. Gilbert (1989) used the metaphor of consciousness as a tailor who alters clothes of all one size to fit the current situation—another late-stage sort of model. The advice to think first seems simple, but may be taxing and miserable to follow. The self-consciousness entailed can be unpleasant (Wicklund, 1986), and the amount of cognitive resources required would be formidable (Macrae, Milne, & Bodenhausen, 1994). Indeed, trying harder to avoid stereotypes can make prejudiced behavior *more* likely—the ironic effect of trying not to be offensive (e.g., Macrae, Boden-

hausen, Milne, & Jetten, 1994). In addition, training a person to "generate, then edit" can even strengthen a habitual pattern of generating stereotypical reactions, as the person repeatedly practices the generation phase.

An alternative approach parallels our attempts to train recollection. In this approach, the attempt is to get people to treat a context word and fragment as cues for recall of the earlier-presented word pair, rather than simply producing the first completion that comes to mind. The difference is in treating memory as an object rather than as a tool (Jacoby & Kelley, 1987). People do not necessarily remember something simply because they are confronted with a stimulus they have seen before. They need to be oriented toward the past or to have a "set" to remember. So—rather than generating the first thoughts that come to mind in a situation, followed by an imperfect and intermittent editing process—the goal is to constrain what comes to mind by maintaining a set for recollection. Similarly, one might train Schott to adopt a set that leads the right thoughts to come to mind in the first place. The analogous treatment for Damasio's frontal lobe patients would be to train them to "see" the deck as a risky gamble even as they reach for a card.

At an abstract level, the set or orienting attitude necessary for recollection might rely on the same sort of cognitive skills required for social monitoring. For both, the problem is to "contextualize" responding by constraining the response that comes to mind, so as to fit the requirements of the past or of a current situation. As an alternative to Gilbert's metaphor, the "clothes" (situations as represented) are different from the outset rather than being altered to fit.

We think that the consciously controlled process of recollection is also necessary for the constancy that represents the self (Singer & Salovey, 1993). Sacks (1995) described a patient who suffered from both amnesia and frontal lobe syndrome and seemed "de-souled," changing identities at a bewildering rate. Without access to the memories that maintained his identity, he was captured by the demands of each new situation. Similarly, Orne and Bauer-Manley (1991) argue that multiple personality disorder is not a problem of having multiple selves, but a problem of memory.[1] Every person has many "selves," in the sense that every person has inconsistent beliefs and behaviors. However, if people recollect rather than repress or dissociate, they incorporate those inconsistencies into one sense of self. Similarly, recollection may be necessary to maintain a constant identity for others across changing situations.

We do not have a "magic bullet" to offer that will miraculously make Marge Schott more sensitive. What we do have to offer are some new procedures for separating automatic and consciously controlled processes, along with a strong prejudice against stage analyses. We hope that social psychologists will join us in thinking about consciousness in different ways. Many of the most exciting problems in psychology are the "property" of social psychologists. We think that an extremely important problem is to better specify the relation between memory and monitoring one's behavior. Much has recently been said about the error(s) of Descartes in describing consciousness (Damasio, 1994). Perhaps Descartes's true error was in saying "I think, therefore I am"; maybe he should have said, "I remember, therefore I am."

ACKNOWLEDGMENTS

The research described in this chapter was supported by grants to Larry L. Jacoby from the National Institute on Aging (No. AG13845-02) and the National Science Foundation (No. SBR-9596209).

NOTE

1. This view may be reflected in the recent renaming of Multiple Personality Disorder (MPD) as Dissociative Identity Disorder (DID) in the fourth edition of the *Diagnostic and Statistical Manual of Mental Disorders* (DSM-IV; American Psychiatric Association, 1994).

REFERENCES

Albert, M. S., & Kaplan, E. (1980). Organic implications of neuropsychological deficits in the elderly. In L. W. Poon, J. Fozard, L. Cermak, D. Arenberg, & L. Thompson (Eds.), *New directions in memory and aging* (pp. 403–432). Hillsdale, NJ: Erlbaum.

American Psychiatric Association. (1994). *Diagnostic and statistical manual of mental disorders* (4th ed.). Washington, DC: Author.

Baddeley, A., & Wilson, B. A. (1994). When implicit learning fails: Amnesia and the problem of error elimination. *Neuropsychologia, 32,* 53–68.

Banaji, M. R., & Greenwald, A. G. (1994). Implicit stereotyping and unconscious prejudice. In M. P. Zanna & J. M. Olson (Eds.), *Psychology of prejudice: The Ontario Symposium* (Vol. 7, pp 55–76). Hillsdale, NJ: Erlbaum.

Banaji, M. R., & Greenwald, A. G. (1995). Implicit gender stereotyping in judgments of fame. *Journal of Personality and Social Psychology, 68,* 181–198.

Bargh, J. A. (1989). Conditional automaticity: Varieties of automatic influences in social perception and cognition. In J. S. Uleman & J. A. Bargh (Eds.), *Unintended thought* (pp. 3–51). New York: Guilford Press.

Bargh, J. A. (1997). The automaticity of everyday life. In R. S. Wyer, Jr. (Ed.), *Advances in social cognition* (Vol. 10, pp. 1–48). Mahwah, NJ: Erlbaum.

Bargh, J. A., & Pietromonaco, P. (1982). Automatic information processing and social perception: The influence of trait information presented outside of conscious awareness on impression formation. *Journal of Personality and Social Psychology, 43,* 437–449.

Block, N. (1995). On a confusion about a function of consciousness. *Behavioral and Brain Sciences, 18,* 227–287.

Bruner, J. S. (1957). On perceptual readiness. *Psychological Review, 64,* 123–152.

Cermak, L. S., Verfaellie, M., Butler, T., & Jacoby, L. L. (1993). Attributions of familiarity in amnesia: Evidence from a fame judgment task. *Neuropsychology, 7,* 510–518.

Chaiken, S. (1980). Heuristic versus systematic information processing and the use of source versus message cues in persuasion. *Journal of Personality and Social Psychology, 39,* 752–766.

Corbett, A., & Wickelgren, W. A. (1978). Semantic memory retrieval: Analysis by speed–accuracy tradeoff functions. *Quarterly Journal of Experimental Psychology, 30,* 1–15.

Daigneault, S., Braun, C. M. J., & Whitaker, H. A. (1992). Early effects of normal aging on perseverative and non-perseverative prefrontal measures. *Developmental Neuropsychology, 8,* 99–114.

Damasio, A. (1994). *Descartes' error: Emotion, reason, and the human brain.* New York: Avon Books.

Dennett, D. C. (1991). *Consciousness explained.* Boston: Little, Brown.

Devine, P. G. (1989). Stereotypes and prejudice: Their automatic and controlled components. *Journal of Personality and Social Psychology, 56,* 5–18.

Dosher, B. A. (1976). The retrieval of sentences from memory: A speed–accuracy study. *Cognitive Psychology, 8,* 291–310.

Dosher, B. A. (1979). Empirical approaches to information processing: Speed–accuracy tradeoff or reaction time. *Acta Psychologica, 43,* 347–359.

Dosher, B. A., McElree, B., Hood, R. M., & Rosedale, G. R. (1989). Retrieval dynamics of priming in recognition memory: Bias and discrimination analysis. *Journal of Experimental Psychology: Learning, Memory, and Cognition, 15,* 868–886.

Dywan, J., & Jacoby, L. L. (1990). Effects of aging on source monitoring: Differences in susceptibility to false fame. *Psychology and Aging, 5,* 379–387.

Dywan, J., Segalowitz, S. J., Henderson, D., & Jacoby, L. L. (1993). Memory for source after traumatic brain injury. *Brain and Cognition, 21,* 20–43.

Epstein, S. (1994). Integration of the cognitive and the

psychodynamic unconscious. *American Psychologist,* 49, 709–724.

Eriksen, C. W. (1960). Discrimination and learning without awareness: A methodological survey and evaluation. *Psychological Review,* 67, 279–300.

Fazio, R. H. (1986). How do attitudes guide behavior? In R. M. Sorrentino & E. T. Higgins (Eds.), *Handbook of motivation and cognition: Foundations of social behavior* (Vol. 1, pp. 204–243). New York: Guilford Press.

Gilbert, D. T. (1989). Thinking lightly about others: Automatic components of the social inference process. In J. S. Uleman & J. A. Bargh (Eds.), *Unintended thought* (pp. 189–211). New York: Guilford Press.

Gilbert, D. T., & Hixon, J. G. (1991). The trouble of thinking: Activation and application of stereotypic beliefs. *Journal of Personality and Social Psychology,* 4, 509–517.

Graf, P., Squire, L. R., & Mandler, G. (1984). The information that amnesic patients do not forget. *Journal of Experimental Psychology: Learning, Memory, and Cognition,* 10, 164–178.

Greenwald, A. G. (1992). New Look 3: Unconscious cognition reclaimed. *American Psychologist,* 47, 766–779.

Hay, J. F., & Jacoby, L. L. (1996). Separating habit and recollection: Memory slips, process dissociations, and probability matching. *Journal of Experimental Psychology: Learning, Memory, and Cognition,* 22, 1323–1335.

Higgins, E. T., Rholes, W. S., & Jones, C. R. (1977). Category accessibility and impression formation. *Journal of Experimental Social Psychology,* 13, 141–154.

Hovland, C. I., & Weiss, W. (1951). The influence of source credibility on communication effectiveness. *Public Opinion Quarterly,* 15, 635–650.

Jacoby, L. L. (1982). Knowing and remembering: Some parallels in the behavior of Korsakoff patients and normals. In L. S. Cermak (Ed.), *Human memory and amnesia* (pp. 97–122). Hillsdale, NJ: Erlbaum.

Jacoby, L. L. (1991). A process dissociation framework: Separating automatic from intentional uses of memory. *Journal of Memory and Language,* 30, 513–541.

Jacoby, L. L. (1996). Dissociating automatic and consciously-controlled effects of study/test compatibility. *Journal of Memory and Language,* 35, 32–52.

Jacoby, L. L. (1998a). Invariance in automatic influences of memory: Toward a user's guide for the process-dissociation procedure. *Journal of Experimental Psychology: Learning, Memory, and Cognition,* 24, 3–26.

Jacoby, L. L. (1998b). *Influence of habit on perception.* Manuscript in preparation.

Jacoby, L. L. (in press). Ironic effects of repetition: Measuring age-related differences in memory. *Journal of Experimental Psychology: Learning, Memory, and Cognition.*

Jacoby, L. L., & Dallas, M. (1981). On the relationship between autobiographical memory and perceptual learning. *Journal of Experimental Psychology: General,* 3, 306–340.

Jacoby, L. L., & Hollingshead, A. (1990). Toward a generate/recognize model of performance on direct and indirect tests of memory. *Journal of Memory, and Language,* 29, 433–454.

Jacoby, L. L., & Kelley, C. M. (1987). Unconscious influ-

ences of memory for a prior event. *Personality and Social Psychology Bulletin,* 13, 314–336.

Jacoby, L. L., Kelley, C. M., Brown, J., & Jasechko, J. (1989). Becoming famous overnight: Limits on the ability to avoid unconscious influences of the past. *Journal of Personality and Social Psychology,* 56, 326–338.

Jacoby, L. L., McElree, B., & Trainham, T. N. (in press). Automatic influences as availability bias in memory and Stroop-like tasks: Toward a formal model. In A. Koriat & D. Gopher (Eds.), *Attention and performance XVII.* Cambridge, MA: MIT Press.

Jacoby, L. L., Toth, J. P., & Yonelinas, A. P. (1993). Separating conscious and unconscious influences of memory: Measuring recollection. *Journal of Experimental Psychology: General,* 122, 139–154.

Jacoby, L. L., Woloshyn, V., & Kelley, C. M. (1989). Becoming famous without being recognized: Unconscious influences of memory produced by dividing attention. *Journal of Experimental Psychology: General,* 118, 115–125.

Jennings, J. M., & Jacoby, L. L. (1993). Automatic versus intentional uses of memory: Aging, attention, and control. *Psychology and Aging,* 8, 283–293.

Johnson, M. K., Hashtroudi, S., & Lindsay, D. S. (1993). Source monitoring. *Psychological Bulletin,* 114, 3–28.

Kelley, C. M. (1998). *Independence of memory and general knowledge in cued recall.* Manuscript submitted for publication.

Kelley, C. M., & Lindsay, D. S. (1996). Conscious and unconscious forms of memory. In E. L. Bjork & R. A. Bjork (Eds.), *Memory* (pp. 31–63). New York: Academic Press.

Lhermitte, F. (1983). 'Utilization behavior' and its relation to lesions of the frontal lobes. *Brain,* 106, 237–255.

Macrae, C. N., Bodenhausen, G. V., Milne, A. B., & Jetten, J. (1994). Out of mind but back in sight: Stereotypes on the rebound. *Journal of Personality and Social Psychology,* 67, 808–817.

Macrae, C. N., Milne, A. B., & Bodenhausen, G. V. (1994). Stereotypes as energy-saving devices: A peek inside the cognitive toolbox. *Journal of Personality and Social Psychology,* 66, 37–47.

McElree, B. (1993). The locus of lexical preference effects in sentence comprehension: A time-course analysis. *Journal of Memory and Language,* 32, 536–571.

McElree, B. (1996). Accessing short-term memory with semantic and phonological information: A time-course analysis. *Memory and Cognition,* 24, 173–187.

McElree, B., & Dosher, B. A. (1989). Serial position and set size in short-term memory: Time course of recognition. *Journal of Experimental Psychology: General,* 118, 346–373.

McElree, B., & Dosher, B. A. (1993). Serial retrieval processes in the recovery of order information. *Journal of Experimental Psychology: General,* 122, 291–315.

McElree, B., & Griffith, T. (1995). Syntactic and thematic processing in sentence comprehension: Evidence for a temporal dissociation. *Journal of Experimental Psychology: Learning, Memory, and Cognition,* 21, 134–157.

McElree, B., & Griffith, T. (1998). Structural and lexical constraints on filling gaps during sentence processing: A time-course analysis. *Journal of Experimental Psy-*

chology: Learning, Memory, and Cognition, 24, 432–460.

McElree, B., Jacoby, L. L., & Dolan, P. O. (1996, November). *Isolating familiarity and recollective retrieval processes: A time-course analysis.* Paper presented at the 37th Annual Meeting of the Psychonomic Society, Chicago.

McElree, B., Dolan, P. O., & Jacoby, L. L. (in press). Isolating the contributions of familiarity and source information to item recognition: A time-course analysis. *Journal of Experimental Psychology: Learning, Memory, and Cognition.*

Newman, L. S., & Uleman, J. S. (1989). Spontaneous trait inference. In J. S. Uleman & J. A. Bargh (Eds.), *Unintended thought* (pp. 155–188). New York: Guilford Press.

Orne, M. T., & Bauer-Manley, N. K. (1991). Disorders of self: Myths, metaphors, and demand characteristics of treatment. In J. Strauss & G. R. Goethals (Eds.), *The self: Interdisciplinary approaches* (pp. 93–106). New York: Springer-Verlag.

Reed, A. V. (1973). Speed–accuracy trade-off in recognition memory. *Science, 181*, 574–576.

Reed, A. V. (1976). The time course of recognition in human memory. *Memory and Cognition, 4*, 16–30.

Reilly, R. (1996, May 20). Heaven help Marge Schott. *Sports Illustrated*, pp. 74–87.

Roediger, H. L., & McDermott, K. B. (1993). Implicit memory in normal human subjects. In H. Spinnler & F. Boller (Eds.), *Handbook of neuropsychology* (Vol. 8, pp. 63–131). Amsterdam: Elsevier.

Sacks, O. (1995). *An anthropologist on Mars.* New York: Knopf.

Salthouse, T. A. (1991). *Theoretical perspectives on cognitive aging.* Hillsdale, NJ: Erlbaum.

Singer, J., & Salovey, P. (1993). *The remembered self: Emotion and memory in personality.* New York: Free Press.

Squire, L. R., & McKee, R. (1992). Influence of prior events on cognitive judgments in amnesia. *Journal of Experimental Psychology: Learning, Memory, and Cognition, 18*, 106–115.

Srull, T. K., & Wyer, R. S. (1979). The role of category accessibility in the interpretation of information about persons: Some determinants and implications. *Journal of Personality and Social Psychology, 37*, 1660–1672.

Srull, T. K., & Wyer, R. S. (1980). Category accessibility and social perception: Some implications for the study of person memory and interpersonal judgments. *Journal of Personality and Social Psychology, 38*, 841–856.

Trope, Y. (1986). Identification and inferential processes in dispositional attribution. *Psychological Review, 93*, 239–257.

Warrington, E. K., & Weiskrantz, L. (1982). Amnesia: A disconnection syndrome? *Neuropsychologia, 20*, 233–248.

Wegner, D. M. (1994). Ironic processes of mental control. *Psychological Review, 101*, 34–52.

West, R. L. (1996). An application of prefrontal cortex function theory to cognitive aging. *Psychological Bulletin, 120*, 272–292.

Wickelgren, W. A. (1977). Speed-accuracy tradeoff and information processing dynamics. *Acta Psychologica, 41*, 67–85.

Wicklund, R. A. (1986). Orientation to the environment versus preoccupation with human potential. In R. M. Sorrentino & E. T. Higgins (Eds.), *Handbook of motivation and cognition: Foundations of social behavior* (Vol. 1, pp. 64–95). New York: Guilford Press.

Winter, L., & Uleman, J. S. (1984). When are social judgments made? Evidence for the spontaneousness of trait inferences. *Journal of Personality and Social Psychology, 47*, 237–252.

IV

Issues of Affect and Self-Regulation in Dual-Process Theories

20

Deliberative versus Implemental Mindsets in the Control of Action

PETER M. GOLLWITZER

UTE BAYER

The distinction between deliberative and implemental mindsets is a dual-process notion in the realm of goal pursuit. It is assumed that the course of goal pursuit entails the distinct tasks of choosing between potential action goals and promoting the implementation of chosen goals. When people get involved in these tasks, different cognitive orientations (deliberative and implemental mindsets) emerge that affect the processing of information and the control of action. In the present chapter, empirical research is reviewed that analyzes the differences in information processing between the two mindsets: the degree of receptiveness to available information, the cognitive tuning toward preferential processing of task-congruent information, the partial versus impartial analysis of desirability-related information, and the realistic versus overly positive illusory analysis of feasibility-related information. Finally, the reported mindset research is related to the debate about realism versus optimism and to the discussion of self-evaluative motives. Moreover, it is pointed out that mindsets affect not only cognition, but also behavior. The deliberative and implemental mindsets are seen as functional to effective goal pursuit, as they provide the cognitive orientations most useful to

solving the tasks of choosing between potential goals and implementing chosen goals, respectively.

THEORIZING ON THE CONTROL OF GOAL-DIRECTED ACTION

According to modern goal theories, whether people meet their goals depends on both how goal content is framed and how people regulate the respective goal-directed activities (Gollwitzer & Moskowitz, 1996). Content theories focus on the thematic and structural properties of set goals and on how these affect the regulation of goal pursuit and actual goal achievement. Such theories attempt to explain differences in goal-directed behaviors in terms of what an individual specifies as the goal, because the content characteristics of the goal are expected to affect the person's successful goal pursuit. Goal content has been considered in terms of both the different needs (e.g., autonomy needs vs. materialistic needs; Deci & Ryan, 1991; Kasser & Ryan, 1994) and the implicit theories (e.g., entity theories vs. incremental theories of ability; Dweck, 1991, 1996) on which it is based. Numerous relevant structural aspects of goal content have also been suggested, such as specific versus abstract (Emmons, 1992; Locke & Latham, 1990), proximal versus distal (Bandura & Schunk, 1981), and positive versus negative outcome focus (Higgins, Roney, Crowe, & Hymes, 1994).

Self-regulation theories of goal striving, on the other hand, focus on the question of how people overcome certain implementational problems. Having set a goal is considered to be just a first step toward goal attainment; it is followed by a host of implementational problems that need to be solved successfully. These problems are manifold, as they pertain to initiating goal-directed actions and bringing them to a successful ending. Various theoretical notions (in parentheses below) have addressed these issues in particular, have delineated useful self-regulatory strategies, and have addressed questions of why and how these strategies are effective. Typical self-regulatory problems of goal pursuit are, for instance, warding off distractions (e.g., action control strategies—Kuhl, 1984; Kuhl & Goschke, 1994), flexibly stepping up efforts in the face of difficulties (e.g., effort mobilization theory—Wright & Brehm, 1989), compensating for failures and shortcomings (e.g., self-regulation of motivation—Bandura, 1991; discrepancy reduction—Carver & Scheier, 1981; symbolic self-completion—Wicklund & Gollwitzer, 1982), and negotiating conflicts between goals (e.g., intelligent pursuit of life tasks—Cantor & Fleeson, 1994).

Both content theories and self-regulation theories start analyzing goal pursuit at the point in time when a goal has been set. They do not concern themselves with the question of how people arrive at setting themselves goals. One approach, however, takes a comprehensive view that extends from a person's wishes and desires to turning them into goals, and to finally realizing these goals. In their model of action phases, Heckhausen and Gollwitzer (1987; Gollwitzer, 1990; Heckhausen, 1991) suggest that successful goal pursuit means solving four consecutive tasks. The first task is setting preferences among a person's wishes and desires by deliberating their desirability and feasibility. As people's motives and needs produce more wishes and desires than can possibly be realized, the individual is forced to choose among

these desires and thus to turn them into goals. Once goals are set, the individual faces the second task, which is getting started with goal-directed behaviors. This may be simple if the necessary goal-directed actions are well practiced and routine, or complex if the individual is still undecided about where and how to act. In such complex cases, the execution of goal-directed action needs to be planned by deciding on when, where, and how to act. The third task is bringing the initiated goal-directed action to a successful ending, and this is best achieved by determined and persistent pursuit of goal completion. Finally, in the fourth task, the individual needs to decide whether the desired goal has indeed been achieved or whether further striving is needed. This problem is solved by evaluating the achieved action outcomes and comparing them to the originally desired outcomes, as well as by deliberating on which further courses of action to take when a discrepancy has been detected.

The model of action phases speaks of people who are solving the four tasks in the described order as traversing consecutive action phases: the "predecisional" phase, the "(postdecisional) preactional" phase, the "actional" phase, and the "postactional" phase. The model postulates that a person's psychological functioning in each of these phases is governed by different principles. Accordingly, theories of motivation, which have traditionally analyzed issues of goal setting (e.g., Atkinson, 1957, 1974; Lewin, Dembo, Festinger, & Sears, 1944), are said to be ill suited to describe and predict the phenomena that occur at the later phases of goal pursuit (i.e., the preactional, actional, and postactional phases), whereas goal theories (see above) are inappropriate to explicate the issues of the predecisional phase.

This radical statement needed empirical support when it was originally made; therefore, Heckhausen and Gollwitzer (1987, Study 2) conducted an early experiment aimed at demonstrating that individuals placed in the predecisional phase evidence different cognitive functioning than individuals placed in the (postdecisional) preactional phase do. Assuming that deliberation of the desirability and feasibility of wishes and desires (the task of the predecisional phase) is cognitively more demanding than committing oneself to a plan that specifies, when, where, and how one wants to initiate goal-directed actions (the task of the preactional phase), Heckhausen and Gollwitzer expected that deliberating persons experience a higher cognitive load than planning persons. They therefore interrupted experimental participants who were either deliberating a choice between two different tests that presumably measured their creative potential or planning how to perform one of the chosen tests, and then asked them to take a short-term memory test (i.e., a noun span test, which presented nouns that were irrelevant to the creativity tests at hand). It was expected that deliberating participants (because of heightened cognitive load) would evidence a reduced noun span, compared to their span as measured at the beginning of the experiment. It was also expected that deliberating participants would evidence a reduced noun span, compared to that of planning participants (because planning was expected to take up less cognitive resources than deliberating). However, the results were just opposite of what had been expected: The deliberating participants showed an *increase* in their short-term memory capacity, compared to both their own earlier span and the span of the planning participants.

In an effort to account for the unexpected finding that the deliberating participants' short-term memory capacity had increased and not decreased, Heckhausen and Gollwitzer (1987) returned to the classic concept of "mindset" as originally advanced at the turn of the century by the German psychologists Külpe (1904), Marbe (1901, 1915), Orth (1903; Mayer & Orth, 1901), and Watt (1905), all members of the Würzburg school. These early cognitive psychologists discovered that becoming intensively involved with solving a given task activates exactly those cognitive procedures that help task completion. The created mindset (i.e., the sum total of the activated cognitive procedures) should consist of the cognitive orientation that is most conductive to successful task performance. This notion allowed Heckhausen and Gollwitzer (1987) to interpret the observed pattern of data as follows: Deliberating between potential action goals creates a cognitive orientation (the deliberative mindset) that facilitates the task at hand.

The same is true for planning the implementation of a chosen goal (the implemental mindset). If it is assumed that deliberating between potential goals requires reflecting on the potential action goals' feasibility and desirability, a heightened receptiveness to all kinds of information (open-mindedness) seems appropriate and functional to task solution. However, as planning demands a more focused and selective orientation to processing information, such heightened receptiveness should be dysfunctional in this situation. This postulated difference in receptiveness between deliberating and planning is expressed in the fact that deliberating experimental participants in the Heckhausen and Gollwitzer study (1987) processed the presented information in the noun span task faster than planning participants (i.e., the deliberating participants demonstrated a broader noun span than that of the planning participants).

THE FEATURES OF DELIBERATIVE AND IMPLEMENTAL MINDSETS

In order to detect the special features of the deliberative as compared to the implemental mindset, one needs to analyze the different demands of the tasks of deliberating in the predecisional phase and of planning in the (postdecisional) preactional phase. The task of deliberating in the predecisional phase is to choose, from among various wishes and desires, those few that one wants to realize (Gollwitzer, 1990). The criteria for selection should be the feasibility and desirability of the wishes and desires at issue. The systematic analysis of the chances of realization as well as the desirability of realization, requires that relevant information be preferentially encoded and retrieved. But the cognitive tuning to this information should not suffice, as feasibility-related information needs to be analyzed objectively (and not in a self-serving manner), and desirability-related information needs to be analyzed in an impartial manner (and not in a biased manner). Only if feasibility-related information is analyzed realistically, and the pros and cons are weighed impartially, can the individual turn those desires into binding goals that can potentially be realized and possess a genuine attractiveness. Moreover, deliberating requires a general open-mindedness (as was demonstrated in the Heckhausen and Gollwitzer [1987] study described above) with respect to available information, as undecided individuals do not know yet in which direction their decision will finally take them.

Once a goal decision has been made, the task of planning is to promote the initiation of goal-directed behaviors. This requires committing oneself to when, where, and how to get started. Accordingly, one needs to discover good opportunities and link them to appropriate goal-directed actions, thus creating plans for action. For this purpose, cognitive tuning toward implementational issues should be beneficial. Feasibility-related and desirability-related issues should no longer matter, and, if forced on the individual, they are avoided by distorting the relevant information in support of the goal decision made: The person sees the feasibility of the chosen goal in an overly optimistic way, and views the desirability of the chosen goal in a partial manner (i.e., pros exceed cons). Finally, processing all of the available information in an open-minded manner should be dysfunctional, as it might derail the individual from the chosen course of action. Accordingly, a reduced open-mindedness (closed-mindedness) favoring the selective processing of information in support of the chosen goal is to be expected.

Given these different features of the cognitive orientations of the deliberative and implemental mindsets, one should not forget that the two different mindsets also possess similar attributes. We assume that the deliberative and implemental mindsets become more pronounced as a person gets mored involved with deliberating between potential goals and with planning chosen goals, respectively. Moreover, neither mindset should immediately vanish when the task activity that produced it is ended; instead, the mindset should show a moment of inertia. This implies that the cognitive orientations associated with the deliberative and implemental mindsets can be detected in their effects on performing temporally subsequent tasks of a different nature.

These ideas have been used to develop a research program aimed at testing the proposed different cognitive features of the deliberative and implemental mindsets. In this research, the following method of inducing the deliberative and implemental mindsets has commonly been used: Experimental participants are asked either to extensively deliberate an unresolved personal problem to be named by the participants (who indicate problems such as "Should I move to another city or not?", "Should I change my major?", "Should I buy a new car?", or "Should I get involved with somebody?") or to plan the implementation of a chosen goal indicated by the participants (projects such as "I will move to another city," "I will change my major," etc., are named). These requests create a deliberative and an implemental mindset, respectively. Deliberating participants are asked to list the short-term and long-term pros and cons of making and not making a decision, in order to get heavily involved with deliberating. Planning participants, on the other hand, are asked to list the five most important steps of implementing the chosen goal, and then to specify when, where, and how they intend to execute each step; all of this serves the purpose of creating an intensive involvement with planning. Thereafter, both the deliberating and the planning participants are asked to perform presumably unrelated tasks (usually presented by a different experimenter in a different situational context), which are designed to measure the very cognitive features hypothesized to differ between the deliberative and implemental mindsets. The manipulations of the deliberative and implemental mindsets are introduced to participants with the cover story that the respective mental exercises are designed to improve people's action control.

Mindsets and Cognitive Tuning

The hypothesis that the deliberative mindset creates cognitive tuning toward information relevant to making goal decisions (information on feasibility and desirability), whereas the implemental mindset tunes a person's cognitions to implementation-related information (information on where, when, and how to act), was tested in the following two ways. The first approach assessed the participants' thoughts while they were either in a deliberative or an implemental mindset. In the second approach, deliberating and planning participants' readiness to encode and retrieve mindset-congruent information was assessed. Following the first approach, Heckhausen and Gollwitzer (1987, Study 1), for instance, asked participants either to deliberate on choosing between potential tasks (i.e., two versions of a creativity test) or to plan to perform the chosen task (i.e., the chosen creativity test), and disrupted participants in the middle of their deliberating or planning. Participants were requested to report on the thoughts they had entertained shortly before the disruption. Content analysis of participants' reported thoughts revealed that deliberating participants were much more concerned with the goal's desirability (e.g., "Reaching the goal is important because . . .") and feasibility (e.g., "I should be able to reach the goal because . . . ") than were planning participants. The latter, on the other hand, reported more implementation-related thoughts (e.g., "I will get started with X and then do Y") than the former.

This study, however, was not all that convincing, as one can argue that participants simply did what they were asked to do (i.e., to deliberate or to plan, respectively); if anything, the working of a task set but not of a mindset was demonstrated. A more convincing demonstration of the cognitive-tuning effects of mindsets on thought production requires the procedure followed by Gollwitzer, Heckhausen, and Steller (1990, Study 1). Participants were placed into either a deliberative or an implemental mindset by having them deliberate on unresolved personal problems or plan chosen goal projects, respectively (the standard procedure described above was used). In a presumably unrelated second part of the experiment, participants were presented with the first few lines of a number of novel fairy tales and were instructed to complete each tale. Even though participants were allowed to continue the stories in any way they liked, deliberating participants had the protagonists of the tales reflect on reasons for choosing or not choosing certain action goals to a greater degree than planning participants did. Thoughts about how to accomplish a chosen goal, however, were more frequently attributed to the protagonists by planning participants than by deliberating participants.

Focusing on the encoding and retrieval of mindset-congruent information, Gollwitzer et al. (1990, Study 2) conducted an experiment in which participants had to recall the presented deliberative and implemental thoughts of others. Participants where placed into either a deliberative or an implemental mindset by having them choose between potential task goals (i.e., two forms of a creativity test) or plan to perform a chosen task. While participants were involved in deliberating or planning, slides were presented that depicted different persons mulling over personal decisions. For example, an elderly lady was thinking of the pros (i.e., "It would be good because . . . ") and cons (i.e., "It would be bad because . . . ") of having her grandchildren spend their summer vacation at her home. For each of these slides, next to the pros and cons of making a decision, potential plans of implementation were also presented. These specified how the person would get started with the particular goal-directed actions (i.e., "If I decide to do it, then I will first . . . and then . . . "; "If I decide to do it, then I won't . . . before . . . "). A cued-recall test of this information was given following a distractor task; it provided participants with the pictures of the persons they had viewed and the stems of the sentences (see above) describing their thoughts. The deliberating participants, who had to view the slides and to recall the information depicted on the slides prior to making a decision about the two types of creativity tests, recalled pros and cons better than they recalled information on the when, where, and how of implementation. The recall performance of the planning participants, who had received and recalled the information after a decision on the creativity tests had been made, showed the reverse pattern.

All of these findings corroborate the cognitive-tuning hypothesis. Still, one wonders how the differential recall performances observed in the last study (Gollwitzer et al., 1990, Study 2) came about. If we assume that individuals' retrieval attempts necessitate constructing descriptions of what they are trying to retrieve (Bobrow & Norman, 1975; Norman & Bobrow, 1976, 1979), it seems possible that mindsets provide perspectives (Bobrow & Winograd, 1977) that allow the easy construction of specific descriptions. The deliberative mindset, for instance, should favor descriptions phrased in terms of pros and cons, benefits and costs, and so forth. In other words, the deliberative mindset supports the ready construction of descriptions that specify desirability-related information, whereas the implemental mindset supports the construction of descriptions that specify implementation-related information. As Norman and Bobrow (1979) point out, quick construction of specific descriptions at the time of retrieval facilitate further successful retrieval. Norman and Bobrow also assume that whenever the description of the information sought matches the elaboration of the information at the time of encoding, recall performance is particularly enhanced. It seems possible, then, that deliberative and implemental mindsets favor congruent recall through both congruent elaboration at the time of encoding and ready construction of congruent descriptions at the time of retrieval.

The cognitive-tuning studies presented remind us of studies that demonstrate the transfer of cognitive procedures activated by a first task to an ostensibly unrelated second task. For instance, Chaiken, Giner-Sorolla, and Chen (1996; Chen, Shechter, & Chaiken, 1996), as a first task, gave their experimental participants a scenario to read in which the target person was portrayed as being concerned either with accurately understanding what was going on or with making a good first impression. In the apparently unrelated second task, participants were given an attitude issue (e.g., gun control) that they would have to discuss with another experimental participant, who was described as holding either a "pro" or a "con" position on that issue. Participants then read an essay containing arguments on both sides, and finally gave their own attitude on the issue. Participants who in the first task had read the scenario describing an impression-managing target person reported attitudes that were closer in line to the anticipated other experimental participant's attitude, compared to the expressed attitudes of participants who had read the scenario describing the target person as concerned with accurately understanding what was going on. Similar to the studies reported above in support of deliberative and implemental mindsets, the Chaiken et al. (1996) study demonstrates that cognitive procedures activated in response to becoming involved in a task are readily transferred to subsequent cognitive tasks. So the effects of prior tasks on the performance of a second task can be used to infer the type of cognitive orientation associated with the first task.

Mindsets and Open-Mindedness

The analysis of the task demands of making a goal decision versus preparing the implementation of a chosen goal reveals that the deliberative mindset should be associated with heightened receptivity for available information, whereas the implemental mindset should be associated with reduced receptivity. As noted above, the study by Heckhausen and Gollwitzer (1987, Study 2) found that deliberating participants showed wider noun spans than planning participants did. Dempster (1985) and others (Case, Kurland, & Goldberg, 1982; Chi, 1976) have pointed out that the noun span task is a good indicator of the speed of processing heeded information. In a typical noun span experiment, participants are read a list of words presented less than 1 second apart. When the experimenter has read the last word of the list, participants are requested to immediately repeat all of the words in the order presented. The faster a person's word identification, the more words can be encoded and thus reproduced correctly.

But heightened receptivity should not only be expressed in a high speed of processing of heeded information; it should also relate to a person's readiness to process peripherally presented information. To explore this idea, a so-called "test of central-incidental memory" was used (Gollwitzer, Bayer, & Wasel, 1998, Study 1). Participants were asked to watch a series of slides that centrally displayed a meaningful sentence and peripherally (in the upper left-hand and lower right-hand corners) displayed isolated unrelated two-syllable nouns. The participants were told to memorize the story that was described by the centrally displayed sentences of these slides. Later on, the participants not only had to recall the centrally presented information, but also had to perform an unexpected recognition test containing the peripherally presented information.

Deliberative and implemental mindsets were created by having participants either make a mock hiring decision (participants were to play the part of a personnel manager, and the problem at hand was to hire one of two applicants for the position of a product manager) or plan the implementation of such a decision. Deliberating participants recognized the incidental information significantly better than planning participants did. In addition, the centrally presented and heeded information was recalled better by deliberating than by planning participants. The latter finding replicated the superior processing of heeded information in the deliberative mindset, as shown in the Heckhausen and Gollwitzer (1987, Study 2) noun span study. However, in the present study an alternative explanation of the deliberating participants' superior recognition of the peripherally presented information was possible. It might not have been caused by the hypothesized heightened readiness to process peripheral information; instead, it might be a simple consequence of the fact that the deliberating participants processed the heeded central information comparatively more effectively (which gave them more time to explore the rest of the slides).

In order to get around this problem, we have started to run mindset experiments that use viewing modified Müller–Lyer figures as the dependent variable (Gollwitzer et al., 1998, Studies 2a/b). In a classic Müller–Lyer figure (see Figure 20.1, left side), shorter illusions are produced by adding wings to a given line and pointing them inward; longer illusions are achieved by pointing the wings outward. The comparison line is presented below or above. We have modified the Müller–Lyer figure by first marking the critical distance and the comparison distance with three dots in a horizontal line. Then we have placed both a set of inward and a set of outward wings on the dot located at the left. Depending on whether one looks at the wings that are pointed inward or the wings that are pointed outward, a shorter or a longer illusion is achieved, respectively (see Figure 20.1, right side).

In the first study (Gollwitzer et al., 1998, Study 2a), participants were placed in either a deliberative or an implemental mindset by use of the standard manipulation. In a presumably independent second task, participants viewed a series of modified Müller–Lyer figures (the angle of the wings and the length of

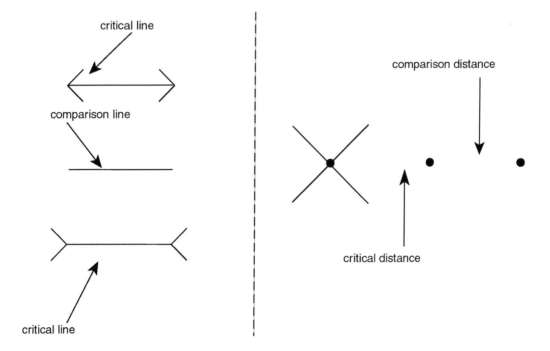

FIGURE 20.1. Classical (left) and modified (right) Müller–Lyer figures. From Gollwitzer, Wasel, and Bayer (1998, Studies 2a/b).

the distances between the dots were varied). For each individual figure, participants had to indicate their perception of how many millimeters shorter or longer the critical distance was than the comparison distance. Prior to each slide presenting a modified Müller–Lyer figure (presentation time was 5 seconds), a focusing slide was presented (for 3 seconds) that showed a cross right in the middle of the slide. The Müller–Lyer figure on the subsequent slide was drawn in such a way that the point separating the critical distance from the comparison distance was placed exactly where the preceding focusing slide had shown the cross. Even though all participants perceived the critical distance as shorter than the comparison distance, the planning participants did so to a significantly greater degree than the deliberating participants; this suggested that the planning participants primarily looked at the center of the modified Müller–Lyer figures, whereas deliberating participants also explored the periphery.

Before replicating this study, we examined (Gollwitzer et al., 1998) whether the strength of shorter illusions was indeed related to a preference for focusing on the center of the presented figures. A new group of participants was asked to perform two tasks: to view the Müller–Lyer figures as our participants had done in the study described above, and to read a large number of presented nouns as fast as possible. For half of the participants, the Müller–Lyer task came first and the fast reading of nouns came second; for the other half, the order was reversed. The nouns were presented in the same way as the Müller–Lyer figures (i.e., a focusing slide preceded each noun). As it turned out, a positive correlation emerged between reading speed and the degree of a person's shorter illusions. This observation supported the assumption that shorter illusions indicated a focus on centrally presented information.

In the replication study (Gollwitzer et al., 1998, Study 2b), we used a within-subjects design and a slightly modified procedure for viewing the Müller–Lyer figures. All participants were placed into both a deliberative and an implemental mindset by means of the standard procedure. Half of the group started with the deliberative mindset and then experienced an implemental mindset; for the other half, this order was reversed. After each

mindset manipulation, participants viewed a series of Müller–Lyer figures. This time the size of the figures was reduced (by about 50%), and the participants had to indicate only whether they perceived the critical distance as either shorter or longer than the comparison distance. When we compared the number of shorter illusions and longer illusions of participants in a deliberative as compared to an implemental mindset, deliberating participants reported more longer illusions and fewer shorter illusions than planning participants (even though, overall, shorter illusions were more frequent than longer illusions). The order of mindset induction did not moderate this pattern of findings.

It appears, then, that the deliberative mindset creates a higher receptiveness for available information—not only by a heightened speed of processing heeded information, but also by an increased readiness to process peripheral information. In the experiments using modified Müller–Lyer figures, the wings pointing outward were located at the periphery of the figure, whereas the wings pointing inward were located at the center. Consequently, deliberating participants experienced fewer and less pronounced shorter illusions than did planning participants, who were characterized by a reduced receptiveness for available information and thus a reduced readiness to process peripheral information.

Mindsets and Biased Inferences

The two types of mindsets are also assumed to differentially affect the way in which feasibility-related and desirability-related information is handled. In a deliberative mindset, information related to desirability should be analyzed impartially; in an implemental mindset, an analysis partial to the chosen goal is expected. Also, feasibility-related information is expected to be analyzed rather accurately in a deliberative mindset, whereas optimistic inferences that overestimate the actual feasibility of the chosen goal are expected in an implemental mindset.

Desirability-Related Information

Female university students were asked to name a personal problem that they wished to solve but for some reason had not solved yet (Gollwitzer & Hammelbeck, 1998, Study 1). Then participants were asked to achieve clarity on whether they wanted to make an affirmative decision or not. This instruction was expected to trigger intensive deliberation and create a deliberative mindset. Participants were also asked to report back to the experimenter when they felt that further deliberation would not achieve greater clarity. At this point participants were handed a thought-sampling questionnaire, which requested them to report on the thoughts they experienced in a way that would reveal the temporal order of the flow of thought.

As it turned out, participants showed a certain pattern of thinking about pros and cons. Deliberation started with reflection on the positive consequences of goal attainment, but turned to reflection on the negative consequences at the end of deliberation. By acting as their own "devil's advocates," participants achieved an impartial analysis of the considered pros and cons. This pattern of impartial deliberation was replicated with male students at a military academy (Gollwitzer & Hammelbeck, 1998, Study 2), who considered quite different unresolved personal problems from those of the female university students. Still, it seems very likely that the sole instruction to report on one's flow of thought creates an impartial analysis of pros and cons.

But a recent study reported by Taylor and Gollwitzer (1995, Study 3) contradicts this objection. Participants were asked to name *either* potential goals *or* chosen goals. Thereafter, they were requested to achieve clarity on the question of whether they should make an affirmative decision or had made the correct decision, respectively. Whereas the predecisional participants reported on positive and negative consequences with the same frequency, postdecisional participants failed to do so. The latter reported about five times more thoughts about pros than about cons, indicating a strong partiality in favor of the chosen goal in postdecisional participants.

Moreover, the counterplea pattern of deliberation (first pros, then cons) observed with predecisional participants in the preceding studies (Gollwitzer & Hammelbeck, 1998, Studies 1 and 2) was replicated by the flow of thought reported by the predecisional participants. This particular course of deliberation apparently ensures an impartial analysis of the positive and negative consequences of making a decision. Whereas postdecisional participants, when asked to find clarity about the correctness of the decision made, started and ended with thinking about positive consequences, predecisional participants experienced thoughts about positive consequences at the beginning and responded to them with thinking about negative consequences at later phases of deliberation.

This readiness to think of cons as a response to thinking about pros may be a highly habitual strategy to prevent the spontaneous making of goal decisions. In a recent study by Gollwitzer and Hammelbeck (1998, Study 4), participants were first asked to name either potential action goals (predecisional participants) or chosen goals (postdecisional participants). Then they were primed outside of awareness in support of either moving ahead (in terms of making a decision or acting on the decision made) or stalling (in terms of refraining from making a decision or acting on the decision made). Participants had to perform a scrambled-sentence task that used such words as "start," "get going," and "set out" (in the "moving-ahead" priming condition) or "hesitate," "wait," and "delay" (in the "stalling" priming condition).

Finally, both predecisional and postdecisional participants were asked to achieve clarity about whether they should make a decision or act on the decision made, respectively, and to report about the thoughts they experienced. Participants' thoughts were classified in terms of whether they favored or hindered making a decision or implementing the chosen project, respectively. A counterplea pattern of thought production was expected with predecisional participants; they should respond to the "moving-ahead" priming with thoughts that hindered the making of a decision, and to the "stalling" priming with thoughts that furthered the making of a decision. For postdecisional participants, on the other hand, simple goal-priming effects were expected, as reported in recent studies by Bargh and Gollwitzer (1994) and Chartrand and Bargh (1996). The "moving-ahead" priming should induce thoughts in favor of acting on the decision, and the "stalling" priming should elicit thoughts against acting on the decision.

Indeed, whereas postdecisional participants' flow of thought evidenced goal-priming effects, the thoughts experienced by predecisional participants closely followed the counterplea principle. We interpret this pattern of results as indicating that the impartial analysis of desirability-related information has habituated in predecisional individuals, in the sense that it occurs without a conscious self-regulatory input. Anything that speaks for making a fast decision is counteracted by engaging in thoughts that hinder the making of a decision, and anything that speaks for postponing the making of a decision is counteracted by engaging in thoughts that favor the making of a decision.

Feasibility-Related Information

The hypothesized accurate analysis of information related to issues of feasibility in the deliberative mindset, and the expected overly optimistic assessment in the implemental mindset, were first demonstrated in experiments by Gollwitzer and Kinney (1989) with the contingency-learning task designed by Alloy and Abramson (1979). In this task, participants are asked to determine to what degree they can influence the onset of a target light (outcome) by choosing to press or not to press a button (alternative actions). Participants commonly go through a series of trials (at least 40); the start of each trial is indicated by a warning light. By observing whether or not the target light comes on after they have pressed or not pressed the button, participants estimate how much control they have over the target light onset. The experimenter varies the actual control by manipulating the frequency of the target light onset associated with each of the two action alternatives (pressing or not pressing). The smaller the difference between these two frequencies, the less objective control participants have over the target light onset.

Nondepressed individuals claim to possess control over target light onset that is noncontingent on their actions, whenever the target light onset occurs frequently (e.g., in the "75/75" problem, where the target light comes on in 75% of pressing and 75% of nonpressing responses; see Alloy & Abramson, 1988). Gollwitzer and Kinney (1989,

Study 2) asked deliberating, planning, and control participants to work on a contingency problem that presented frequent and noncontingent target light onset (i.e., the 75/75 problem). Participants were given the instruction to discover how to produce the target light onset. A set of 40 trials was offered, and participants were then asked to judge how much control they could exert over the target light onset.

Deliberating participants showed the most accurate judgment of control; their judgments of control were lower than those of either the control group or the planning group. The planning participants' judgments of control tended to be even higher than those of the control participants. The mindsets were created via the standard procedure described above. A mindset interpretation of these findings is supported by the additional observation that deliberating participants' judgments of control correlated negatively with the personal importance of the unresolved personal problems these participants were mulling over. Apparently, the more involved participants were in deliberating, the more realistic their subsequent judgments of control. A parallel finding was observed for planning participants, whose judgments of control were positively related to the participants' anticipated frustration in case they should fail to implement their chosen goals.

In an effort to explore how powerful deliberative and implemental mindsets are in affecting people's judgments of control, Wulf (1991) analyzed whether the commonly realistic judgments of depressed persons (i.e., depressive realism; see Alloy & Abramson, 1979, 1982) can be elevated to levels of positive illusion by the implemental mindset. Participants of the study were highly depressed patients (Beck Depression Inventory scores between 15 and 45, with a mean of 28.8) who received treatment at either a hospital or a private practice. The creation of the mindsets and the instructions to work on the contingency-learning task were the same as in the Gollwitzer and Kinney (1989) study. After the depressed patients had been placed in one of the two mindsets, they had to work on the 75/75 problem and then judge their experienced amount of control. Participants in the deliberating and in the control conditions experienced the same low amounts of control. This finding supports the notion of depressive realism. Most interestingly, however, the planning participants reported experiencing extremely high amounts of control, thus showing a strong positive illusion. Apparently the implemental mindset manages to affect the analysis of feasibility-related information in such a way that overly positive judgments are formed, even though depressive patients commonly produce realistic judgments.

In studies reported by Taylor and Gollwitzer (1995, Studies 1 and 2), deliberative and implemental mindsets were also observed to affect people's judgments of the controllability of risks. In the first study, the risks involved being in an automobile accident, becoming divorced, becoming depressed, developing a drinking problem, and being mugged. Participants were college students who had to judge these risks for themselves and for the average college student. Mindsets were induced via the standard procedure just before participants had to judge the named risks. Even though all participants perceived themselves as less vulnerable to these risks than the average college student, deliberating participants did this to a lesser degree than planning participants. This more pronounced illusion of invulnerability in the implemental mindset than in the deliberative mindset was replicated in a second study, in which participants had to rate their vulnerability to risks perceived as controllable (e.g., developing an addiction to prescription drugs, having a drinking problem) versus uncontrollable (e.g., developing diabetes, losing a partner to an early death). For both types of risks, planning participants reported a higher invulnerability as compared to the average college student than deliberating participants did. The fact that mindsets even managed to modify the perceived vulnerability of uncontrollable risks attests again to their enormous influence on the analysis of feasibility-related information.

Summary

Under the assumption that the course of goal pursuit presents itself to the individual as a series of consecutive tasks that need to be solved in order to promote goal attainment, the concept of mindset has been introduced. It has been argued that becoming involved in these tasks leads to characteristic cognitive orientations (mindsets) that are beneficial for solving these tasks effectively, and the features of the cognitive orientations associated with the tasks of choosing between potential action goals (the deliberative mindset) and preparing the implementation of chosen goals (the implemental mindset) have been spelled out. Finally, a number of experiments have been described that tested the postulated characteristics of the deliberative and implemental mindsets. This research has shown that the deliberative mindset is characterized by cognitive tuning toward desirability-related and feasibility-related thoughts and information; by an accurate analysis of feasibility-related information and by an impartial analysis of desirability-related information; and by a heightened general receptivity to available information. The implemental mindset, on the other hand, is characterized by cognitive tuning toward implementational thoughts and information; by an overly positive analysis of feasibility-related information and a partial analysis of desirability-related information; and, finally, by a comparatively reduced receptivity (closed-mindedness) to available information.

MINDSETS AND SELF-EVALUATION

Assessing the feasibility of potential goals in the predecisional action phase not only requires people to assess accurately whether their actions effectively control desired outcomes (see Gollwitzer & Kinney, 1989); they also need to know whether they are in the position to perform these instrumental actions. To answer this question, they have to assess correctly whether they possess the relevant aptitudes and skills. This implies that people in a deliberative mindset should show a relatively accurate evaluation of their personal attributes. People in an implemental mindset, on the other hand, should benefit from relatively positive self-evaluations, as such positive assessments create the optimism needed for the successful and undelayed initiation of goal-directed actions. Following this line of thought, Steller, Malzacher, and Gollwitzer (1990) asked deliberating and planning participants to agree or disagree with a list of various self-descriptive statements that claimed the possession of talents relevant to professional or interpersonal success (e.g., "I possess great potential as a leader" or "I can be very sensitive to the feelings of others," respectively). As it turned out, planning participants claimed to possess these attributes to a higher degree than deliberating participants did.

In a study by Taylor and Gollwitzer (1995, Study 2), deliberating and planning participants were also asked to rate themselves on 21 qualities and skills (e.g., cheerfulness, athletic ability, writing ability, popularity, artistic ability) in comparison to the average college student of the same age and gender. Even though all participants perceived themselves as more capable than the average college student, planning participants did so to a higher degree than deliberating participants did. The mindset manipulations also affected the participants' mood, so that the implemental mindset was associated with a more positive mood than the deliberative mindset was. However, the observed differences in self-perception were not mediated by these differences in mood, as the effect of mindset on self-perception remained intact when mood was covaried out.

Mindset Effects on Positive Illusions: Implications for the Debate about Optimism versus Realism

Taylor and Brown (1988) proposed that mentally healthy people are *not* characterized by accurate assessments of their personal qualities, realistic estimates of personal control, and a realistic outlook on the future; instead, they maintain overly positive, self-aggrandizing perceptions of the self, the world, and the future. More specifically, mentally healthy people are said to be characterized by unrealistically positive self-perceptions, an illusion of a high degree of personal control, and unrealistic optimism about the future. Instead of being maladaptive, these positively distorted perceptions foster the criteria normally associated with mental health: positive self-regard, the ability to care for and about other people, the capacity for creative and productive work, and the ability to manage stress effectively (Taylor, 1989; Taylor & Brown, 1994).

Despite empirical support for the model, this portrait raises a disturbing question: If

normal people's perceptions are marked by positive biases, how do they effectively identify and make use of negative feedback they may encounter in the world? If people are capable of explaining away, compartmentalizing, or otherwise dismissing or minimizing negative feedback, as Taylor and Brown (1988) suggest, these self-serving illusions that bolster self-esteem and produce a positive mood in the short run may ultimately set people up for long-term disappointment and failure. This is because they fail to incorporate negative feedback into their goal setting and planning (Colvin & Block, 1994; Weinstein, 1984).

One potential resolution, already offered by Taylor and Brown (1988), is the possibility that there may be times when people are more frank and honest with themselves. Such "time outs" from positive illusions are obviously provided by the deliberative mindset that originates from the consideration of potential goals. People in a deliberative mindset become more modest and realistic in their self-perceptions (e.g., their perceived leadership potential, social intelligence, artistic ability, writing ability); they show reduced illusions of control (e.g., in the contingency-learning task used by Gollwitzer & Kinney, 1989); and they exhibit less unrealistic optimism about the future (e.g., with respect to developing a heart disease, being mugged). Relatively realistic thinking seems to be highly functional when it comes to making decisions about important potential goals (e.g., whether or not to go to graduate school, to get married, to have children). Such decisions deeply affect a person's day-to-day conduct, as well as long-term strivings and aspirations. If positive illusions were in ascendancy during deliberations, they could lead to decisions that are prone to frustrations: People would commit themselves to pursue goals that were too difficult for them and that might lead to outcomes they did not enjoy.

One should not forget, however, that once a course of action has been selected and is being or about to be implemented, an implemental mindset that favors positive illusions prevails. Positively distorting one's resources, one's chances for success, and the given conditions of the environment seems to be beneficial for postdecisional individuals, as it should enable people to strive longer and harder to reach their goals, thus bringing about a self-fulfilling prophecy. Moreover, unbroken persistence is vital if implementation is to be successful, especially in the face of hindrances and barriers. It is highly functional, then, that people who are in the process of implementing an intended project do not reflect on its feasibility and desirability in a realistic manner (see Taylor & Gollwitzer, 1995, Study 3). Such deliberation would only undermine their illusions and thus hinder efficient goal achievement.

Accordingly, mindset theory offers the following insights to the debate about positive illusions versus realism. First, neither realism nor positive illusions are adaptive in general to a person's psychological functioning. Realistic thinking is functional when it comes to making goal decisions, whereas positive illusions are functional when the chosen goals are to be implemented. Second, people can easily open the window to realism provided by the deliberative mindset. People do not have to go through the effortful mental exercises we have used to create a deliberative mindset; simply trying to achieve clarity in regard to an unresolved personal problem will trigger an intensive deliberation of pros and cons (see Taylor & Gollwitzer, 1995, Study 3). Postdecisional participants, on the other hand, are protected from such deliberation and thus can profit from the enhanced optimism that is associated with starting to implement, or being in the process of implementing, goal-directed actions. It appears, then, that the individual's cognitive apparatus readily adjusts to the various demands of the control of action: Choosing between action goals leads to realism, and implementing chosen goals leads to positive illusions.

Mindsets and Self-Evaluative Motives

Current theorizing on self-evaluation (Sedikides, 1993; Sedikides & Strube, 1995, 1997; Taylor, Wayment, & Carrillo, 1995; Wood, 1996) agrees on the following three self-evaluative motives: a need for self-enhancement, a need for accurate self-assessment, and a need for self-verification. Modern approaches to self-evaluation focus on the question of when the individual serves one of these needs over the other. According to the model of action phases, different self-evaluative motives should become activated in the predecisional versus postdecisional action phases. Efficient acting requires accurate self-assessment in the predecisional phase and self-enhancement in the postdecisional phase. Accordingly, we hypothesized that the deliberative mindset should promote the need for accurate self-assessments, whereas the implemental mindset should promote the need for self-enhancement; the need for self-verification was expected to be so strongly affected by a person's sense of certainty–uncertainty of possessing a given self-attribute that it should stay unaffected by the deliberative and implemental mindsets.

In order to test these assumptions, we (Bayer & Gollwitzer, 1995) conducted an experiment that analyzed participants' seeking of information about the self. Participants started the experiment with filling out a self-concept scale, which (among many other self-perceptions) assessed whether participants claimed to possess the general ability to make up their minds and come to decisions in everyday life. We deemed this ability to be equally important for deliberating and planning individuals; predecisional persons need to decide which goals they want to pursue, and postdecisional persons need to decide on when, where, and how to get started on the chosen goal.

Thereafter, participants worked on a test that was said to assess various different abilities and skills. After participants had taken this test, the deliberative and implemental mindsets were induced via the standard procedure. Finally, participants were allowed to seek information on their ability to make decisions. The experimenter offered a list of questions, to which she claimed to have prepared answers based on participants' performance on the preceding extensive ability and skill testing. Altogether, 16 questions were offered; 8 were related to the strengths of having the critical ability (e.g., persuasiveness in group discussions), and 8 were related to weaknesses associated with not possessing the critical ability (e.g., nervousness prior to the act of making a decision). Half of the questions were worded in a diagnostic fashion (e.g., "What is the amount of my persuasiveness when it comes to making decisions in groups?"), whereas the other half were worded in a nondiagnostic manner (e.g., "How do I show my nervousness prior to the act of making a decision?"). Whereas the diagnostic questions aimed at answers that described the exact degree of possessing the critical attribute, the nondiagnostic questions aimed at answers that were silent about the exact degree of the attribute and thus allowed for confirmatory answers. This way of constructing questions allows investigators to assess the need for self-enhancement and the need for accurate self-assessment independently (see Devine, Hirt, & Gehrke, 1990).

From the pool of 16 questions, participants were requested to select those 5 questions they felt most interested in. As a first step, we analyzed the choices of questions of all participants. It was observed that planning participants selected more questions on strengths than on weaknesses related to possessing the ability to make decisions, whereas deliberating participants showed an evenhanded pattern of selection. This interaction effect was in line with the hypothesis that self-enhancement needs would be stronger in the implemental mindset than in the deliberative mindset. The diagnosticity of the questions did not produce a main effect on participants' choice of questions, and neither an interaction of diagnosticity with mindset nor a three-way interaction (diagnosticity × strengths–weaknesses × mindset) was observed.

We wondered why deliberating participants did not show a stronger preference for diagnostic questions over nondiagnostic questions than planning participants did. Therefore, as a second step, we analyzed the data separately for participants who were certain about possessing the ability to make decisions (positive self-concept) versus not possessing this ability (negative self-concept). Among participants with a positive self-concept, we observed that deliberating participants preferred diagnostic questions to nondiagnostic questions, and this was true for strengths and weaknesses alike. By contrast, planning participants showed a strong preference for questions about strengths as compared to weaknesses, and this was even more pronounced for nondiagnostic questions than for diagnostic questions. This pattern of results clearly indicates that deliberating participants with a positive self-concept focused on an accurate analysis of their strengths and weaknesses,

whereas planning participants with a positive self-concept were oriented toward self-enhancement.

But what about participants with a negative self-concept? In both the deliberating and planning conditions, more questions on weaknesses than on strengths were chosen, and this was true for diagnostic and nondiagnostic questions alike. When we looked at questions related to strengths only, the deliberating participants preferred nondiagnostic questions to diagnostic questions, whereas the planning participants preferred diagnostic questions to nondiagnostic questions. The seeking of information about the self by persons with a negative self-concept thus seems highly dysfunctional in both the deliberative and implemental mindsets.

Instead of focusing on diagnostic information about strengths and weaknesses in an evenhanded manner, our deliberating participants sought more diagnostic as well as nondiagnostic information on weaknesses than on strengths; with respect to seeking information on strengths, a preference for nondiagnostic information was observed. Given that the task of deliberating persons is to assess their potential accurately in order to choose goals that can be successfully implemented, avoiding diagnostic information on one's strengths should lead to refraining from goal decisions even when chances are high that a goal can be successfully implemented. Moreover, soliciting nondiagnostic information on one's weaknesses may hinder any pragmatic self-assessment aimed at improving future goal choice (see Trope, 1986).

Instead of focusing on information on their strengths and on nondiagnostic information, our planning participants preferred both diagnostic and nondiagnostic information on weaknesses over information on strengths, and the information solicited about strengths was diagnostic. Given that the task of planning persons is to promote goal attainment, this way of soliciting information about the self is also highly dysfunctional, as it precludes overly positive self-perceptions that should promote goal attainment (see the research on positive illusions presented above).

In summary, people with a negative self-concept adhere to a style of soliciting information about the self that does not allow effective goal choice and goal implementation, and thus prevents the experiences needed to revise a negative self-concept. People with a positive self-concept, on the other hand, solicit information about the self in a manner that leads to effective control of their actions, which will in turn verify their positive self-concepts. This pattern of data is in clear support of Swann's (1990, 1997) theorizing that seeking of information about the self is strongly affected by people's consistency needs. From the perspective of mindset theory, this pattern of data suggests that even though deliberative and implemental mindsets lead to seeking different types of information about the self, these differences are modified by whether people possess a positive or a negative self-concept. In other words, it is only individuals with a positive self-concept who solicit information about the self as predicted by mindset theory. This suggests that the effects of mindsets on soliciting information about the self can be modified by personal attributes such as a negative or positive self-concept. Other potentially relevant personal attributes (e.g., implicit theories about the variability or lack of variability of personal abilities—Dweck, 1996; perceived degree of competence—Harter, 1985) still need to be explored.

MINDSET EFFECTS ON BEHAVIOR

In the research on deliberative and implemental mindsets, the focus has been on analyzing the features of the associated cognitive orientations. A first indication that deliberative and implemental mindsets may also affect behavior came from a study (Bayer & Gollwitzer, 1996) that asked deliberating and planning participants to evaluate another person on attributes related to behavioral energization (e.g., "persistent," "strong," "activated"). More specifically, participants who had been placed into either a deliberative or an implemental mindset by a female experimenter who applied the standard procedure were asked to fill out a so-called "experimenter evaluation sheet" before they departed. The implemental mindset favored more extreme descriptions of the experimenter on aspects related to behavioral energization than the deliberative mindset,

suggesting that the implemental mindset is associated with the determined pursuit of goal-directed actions.

Immediacy of Action Initiation

Recent studies have begun to analyze the behavioral energization generated by mindsets more systematically. If one assumes that the implemental mindset serves the function of getting started with goal-directed actions, situations in which swift action initiation is hindered should benefit greatly from an implemental mindset. Situations that make action initiation difficult are commonly characterized by either one of the following two problems: People do not know whether they should act now or later, or whether they should perform one action or another. In such conflict situations, a person in an implemental mindset should, because of the associated reduced open-mindedness, have less of a problem in initiating actions than a person in a deliberative mindset should.

Following this line of thought, Pösl (1994) conducted an experiment in which participants were asked by a first experimenter to list a number of personal projects they had failed to get started on until now. From this list, participants were requested to select two projects that could easily be initiated by writing a letter to somebody. Finally, they were asked to compose such letters by beginning to put down the names and addresses of the two persons they wanted to write to on two separate sheets of paper. Immediately thereafter, participants were disrupted and moved on to a second experimenter in a different room, who induced either the deliberative or the implemental mindset via the standard procedure. Control participants were asked to perform simple arithmetic tasks during this time.

Finally, all participants were sent back to the first experimenter's room to continue the disrupted experiment. Here, participants found either one or both of their incomplete letters sitting on the desk. Through a one-way mirror, the experimenter watched from an adjacent experimental room when the participants started to write again. It was expected that the implemental mindset would help participants to deal effectively with the difficult action initiation problem associated with the two-letters situation. Through the one-way mirror, the experimenter observed that control participants took much longer to start writing when they were facing two letters as compared to one letter, and the same effect was observed with the deliberating participants. On the other hand, the planning participants started to write even faster when two letters were sitting on the desk as compared to one. If one only considers participants' resumption of writing in the two-letters condition, the planning participants started significantly faster than either the control or the deliberating participants. In the one-letter condition, however, no significant differences were observed between groups.

Pösl wondered whether the observed pattern of data was caused by planning participants' unwillingness to deliberate the pros and cons of turning to one or the other letter first or by their general closed-mindedness (i.e., effectively ignoring the nonchosen letter while writing on the chosen letter). Additional observations favored the second possibility. While observing when the participants started to write, the experimenter also took notice of when the participants grabbed one of the letters in the two-letter condition, because this was thought to indicate how long it took participants to make up their minds about which of the two letters they wanted to answer first. However, no differences were observed between conditions on this variable. This implies that the differences in getting started with writing had to do with the participants' ability to shield action control with respect to the chosen letter from distractions stemming from the nonchosen letter. Apparently the closed-mindedness associated with the implemental mindset served this purpose well. The fact that the implemental mindset did not facilitate participants' getting started with writing in the one-letter condition is also in line with the general hypothesis that the implemental mindset facilitates the initiation of goal-directed action via the associated closed-mindedness.

Persistence in Goal-Directed Action

Because the implemental mindset creates positive illusions with respect to people's self-perceptions, their perceptions of control over behavioral outcomes, and their expectations about future events (see above), and because positive illusions foster the successful execution of complex behaviors (e.g., to care for and about other people, to perform creative and productive work, and to manage stress effectively; Taylor, 1989; Taylor & Brown, 1994), one would expect the implemental mindset to promote the determined execution of goal-directed behaviors. Accordingly, Brandstätter and Frank (1997) handed an intricate geometrical puzzle to deliberating and planning participants that, unknown to them, was unsolvable. Brandstätter and Frank predicted a higher persistence in working on this puzzle for planning than for deliberating participants. Indeed, the planning participants did persist longer than the deliberating participants did, and this persistence was mediated by the enhanced perceived desirability of solving the puzzle produced by the implemental mindset.

In a follow-up study, it was discovered that the differences between the deliberative and implemental mindsets in their effects on task persistence were particularly pronounced when the perceived desirability and feasibility of task completion pointed in different directions. When perceived desirability and feasibility were both low, and thus little activity engagement was strongly suggested, the mindset effects on persistence were weak; the same was true when perceived desirability and feasibility were both high, and thus intensive activity engagement was strongly suggested. Only when perceived desirability was low and perceived feasibility was high or vice versa did strong mindset effects emerge, in the sense that the implemental mindset led to more persistence than the deliberative mindset.

We take this observation to mean that the implemental mindset has its positive effects on persistence via the associated positive illusions only when the individual is in doubt on whether to persist or not. This reminds us of the mindset effects observed on action initiation (see Pösl, 1994): The beneficial effects of the implemental mindset could only be observed when participants had the option of resuming one or the other of two disrupted courses of action first (i.e., writing one or the other letter first). Apparently, activated mindsets, like activated semantic concepts (Higgins, 1996), are applicable to certain situations only. Whereas activated semantic concepts are most applicable to ambiguous information, activated deliberative and implemental mindsets seem most applicable to behavioral conflict situations.

GENERAL SUMMARY AND CONCLUSION

Deliberating potential action goals induces a general cognitive orientation (the deliberative mindset) that favors the effective choice of goals. People in a deliberative mindset are found to be open-minded with respect to available information, to be tuned toward feasibility-related and desirability-related information, to analyze feasibility-related information accurately, and to analyze desirability-related information impartially. The deliberative mindset provides a window to realism, as it can reduce people's pervasive positive illusions, and it serves the accuracy motive when people evaluate themselves. Finally, it hampers action initiation and persistence in behavioral conflict situations.

Planning the implementation of chosen goals induces a general cognitive orientation (the implemental mindset) that favors the effective implementation of goals. People in an implemental mindset are found to be closed-minded to available information, to be tuned toward implementation-related information, to analyze feasibility-related information in an overly positive manner, and to analyze desirability-related information in a partial manner. The implemental mindset enhances people's pervasive positive illusions, and it serves the self-enhancement motive when people evaluate themselves. Finally, it furthers immediate action initiation and strengthens persistence in behavioral conflict situations.

The ideas and research originating within the framework of the notion of deliberative and implemental mindsets constitute a dual-process theory in the realm of goal pursuit. The approach taken is to juxtapose a cognitive orientation that is functional to choosing goals with a cognitive orientation that is functional to the implementation of chosen goals. In other words, the ideal information-processing styles for solving two different tasks that serve one end (i.e., the effective control of action) are analyzed in contrast to each other. This is different from those dual-process models that compare two different styles of information processing in the service

of one and the same task, such as perceiving another person (Bargh, 1984; Brewer, 1988; Fiske & Neuberg, 1990), making attributions (Gilbert, 1989; Gilbert & Malone, 1995; Trope & Gaunt, Chapter 8, this volume), or forming attitudes (Chaiken, Liberman, & Eagly, 1989; Fazio, 1990). The approach taken in those models is to analyze how the two forms of information processing delineated differ in meeting the task at hand.

At the same time, the notion of deliberative versus implemental mindsets seems to be a stage model, like some other dual-process theories (e.g., Gilbert & Malone, 1995). People in everyday life should experience deliberative mindsets, prior to implemental mindsets as people mostly prefer to make plans on how to achieve a goal only after they have made a binding goal choice. In this temporal sense, therefore, the mindset model qualifies as a stage model. This is not true, however, with respect to the quality of cognitive processes associated with the two mindsets. For instance, in the two-step model of the attribution process—a stage model suggested by Gilbert (1989; Gilbert & Malone, 1995)—the first step is simple and automatic (i.e., a quick personal attribution), whereas the second step requires attention, thought, and effort (i.e., adjusting that inference to account for situational influences). The notion of deliberative versus implemental mindsets, however, does *not* assume that the deliberative mindset is associated with more rudimentary cognitive processes than the implemental mindset (or vice versa). In both the deliberative mindset and the implemental mindset, highly complex cognitive procedures are activated that determine the individual's cognitive and behavioral functioning. Moreover, in both mindsets these procedures can but do not need to reach consciousness to unfold their effects (because they can become habitual; see the Gollwitzer & Hammelbeck, 1998), and their effects can but do not have to be detected by the individual (e.g., the illusion of control in the implemental mindset).

Mindset theory sees the deliberative and implemental mindsets as distinct and independent of each other. Whereas it is assumed in some dual-process theories (e.g., Chaiken et al., 1989) that the postulated modes of information processing can operate at the same time, the deliberative and implemental mindsets are assumed to preclude each other. This is because the strength with which the cognitive procedures associated with the deliberative mindset are activated is positively related to the degree of involvement with the task of choosing between potential goals, whereas the strength with which the cognitive procedures associated with the implemental mindset are activated is positively related to the degree of involvement with the task of planning the implementation of a chosen goal. Because a person cannot become intensely involved in both of these tasks at one and the same time, but only successively, pronounced deliberative and implemental mindsets cannot coexist. They also do not affect each other in the sense that a preceding strong deliberative mindset makes for a strong succeeding implemental mindset (see the description of the studies using the modified Müller–Lyer figures, above); it all depends on how intensely people become involved with solving the task of choosing between potential goals and with planning the implementation of a chosen goal, respectively.

Finally, the effects of the deliberative and implemental mindsets are rather general, in the sense that the processing of all kinds of informational inputs is affected. The deliberative and implemental mindsets can influence control judgments in a contingency-learning task, perceptual illusions, recall of desirability-related information, recall of implementation-related information, speed of processing of heeded information, a person's self-perception, the perceived controllability of risks, and so forth. Even though the mindsets are created via becoming involved in deliberating a specific goal choice or planning the implementation of a specific chosen goal, the activated cognitive procedures affect the processing of all kinds of different informational inputs. The only limit seems to be that these cognitive procedures are applicable to the informational input at hand (see Pösl, 1994).

REFERENCES

Alloy, L. B., & Abramson, L. Y. (1979). Judgment of contingency in depressed and nondepressed students: Sadder but wiser? *Journal of Experimental Psychology: General, 108,* 441–485.

Alloy, L. B., & Abramson, L. Y. (1982). Learned helplessness, depression, and the illusion of control. *Journal of Personality and Social Psychology, 42,* 1114–1126.

Alloy, L. B., & Abramson, L. Y. (1988). Depressive realism: Four theoretical perspectives. In L. B. Alloy (Ed.), *Cognitive processes in depression* (pp. 223–265). New York: Guilford Press.

Atkinson, J. W. (1957). Motivational determinants of risk-taking behavior. *Psychological Review, 64,* 359–372.

Atkinson, J. W. (1974). Strength of motivation and efficiency of performance. In J. W. Atkinson & J. O. Raynor (Eds.), *Motivation and achievement* (pp. 193–218). Washington, DC: V. H. Winston.

Bandura, A. (1991). Self-regulation of motivation through anticipatory and self-reactive mechanisms. In R. A. Dienstbier (Ed.), *Nebraska Symposium on Motivation: Vol. 38. Perspectives on motivation: Current theory and research in motivation* (pp. 69–164). Lincoln: University of Nebraska Press.

Bandura, A., & Schunk, D. H. (1981). Cultivating competence, self-efficacy, and intrinsic interest through proximal self-motivation. *Journal of Personality and Social Psychology, 41,* 586–598.

Bargh, J. A. (1984). Automatic and conscious processing of social information. In R. S. Wyer, Jr., & T. K. Srull (Eds.), *Handbook of social cognition* (Vol. 3, pp. 1–43). Hillsdale, NJ: Erlbaum.

Bargh, J. A., & Gollwitzer, P. M. (1994). Environmental control of goal-directed action: Automatic and strategic contingencies between situations and behavior. In W. Spaulding (Ed.), *Nebraska Symposium on Motivation: Vol. 41. Integrative views of motivation, cognition, and emotion* (pp. 71–124). Lincoln: University of Nebraska Press.

Bayer, U., & Gollwitzer, P. M. (1995). *Informationssuche zur Einschätzung der eigenen Fähigkeiten und Fertigkeiten* [Mindset effects on the assessment of one's own aptitudes and skills]. Paper presented at the 37th Tagung experimentell arbeitender Psychologen (TeaP), Bochum, Germany.

Bayer, U., & Gollwitzer, P. M. (1996). *Der Einfluß der Bewußtseinslagen auf die soziale Urteilsbildung* [Mindset effects on social judgments]. Paper presented at the 40th Kongreß der Deutschen Gesellschaft für Psychologie, München.

Bobrow, D. G., & Norman, D. A. (1975). Some principles of memory schemata. In D. G. Bobrow & A. Collins (Ed.), *Representation and understanding* (pp. 131–149). New York: Academic Press.

Bobrow, D. G., & Winograd, T. (1977). An overview of KRL, a knowledge representation language. *Cognitive Science, 1,* 3–46.

Brandstätter, V., & Frank, E. (1997). *Bewußtseinslageneffekte auf das Handeln* [Mindset effects on acting]. Paper presented at the 6th Tagung der Fachgruppe Sozialpsychologie, Konstanz, Germany.

Brewer, M. B. (1988). A dual process model of impression formation. In T. K. Srull & R. S. Wyer (Eds.), *Advances in social cognition* (Vol. 1, pp. 1–36). Hillsdale, NJ: Erlbaum.

Cantor, N., & Fleeson, W. (1994). Social intelligence and intelligent goal pursuit: A cognitive slice of motivation. In W. D. Spaulding (Ed.), *Nebraska Symposium on Motivation: Vol. 41. Integrative views of motivation, cognition, and emotion* (pp. 125–179). Lincoln: University of Nebraska Press.

Carver, C. S., & Scheier, M. G. (1981). *Attention and self-regulation: A control-theory approach to human behavior.* New York: Springer-Verlag.

Case, R., Kurland, D. M., & Goldberg, J. (1982). Operational efficiency and the growth of short-term memory span. *Journal of Experimental Child Psychology, 33,* 386–404.

Chaiken, S., Giner-Sorolla, R., & Chen, S. (1996). Beyond accuracy: Defense and impression motives in heuristic and systematic information processing. In P. M. Gollwitzer & J. A. Bargh (Eds.), *The psychology of action: Linking cognition and motivation to behavior* (pp. 553–578). New York: Guilford Press.

Chaiken, S., Liberman, A., & Eagly, A. H. (1989). Heuristic and systematic information processing within and beyond the persuasion context. In J. S. Uleman & J. A. Bargh (Eds.), *Unintended thought* (pp. 212–252). New York: Guilford Press.

Chartrand, T. L., & Bargh, J. A. (1996). Automatic activation of social information processing goals: Nonconscious priming reproduces effects of explicit conscious instructions. *Journal of Personality and Social Psychology, 71,* 464–478.

Chen, S., Shechter, D., & Chaiken, S. (1996). Getting at the truth or getting along: Accuracy-versus impression-motivated heuristic and systematic processing. *Journal of Personality and Social Psychology, 71,* 262–275.

Chi, M. T. (1976). Short-term memory limitations in children: Capacity or processing deficits? *Memory and Cognition, 4,* 559–572.

Colvin, C. R., & Block, J. (1994). Do positive illusions foster mental health?: An examination of the Taylor and Brown formulation. *Psychological Bulletin, 116,* 3–20.

Deci, E. L., & Ryan, R. M. (1991). A motivational approach to self: Integration in personality. In R. A. Dienstbier (Ed.), *Nebraska Symposium on Motivation: Vol. 38. Perspectives on motivation: Current theory and research in motivation* (pp. 237–288). Lincoln: University of Nebraska Press.

Dempster, F. N. (1985). Short-term memory development in childhood and adolescence. In C. J. Brainerd (Ed.), *Basic processes in memory development* (pp. 209–248). New York: Springer-Verlag.

Devine, P. G., Hirt, E. R., & Gehrke, E. M. (1990). Diagnostic and confirmation strategies in trait hypothesis testing. *Journal of Personality and Social Psychology, 58,* 952–963.

Dweck, C. S. (1991). Self-theories and goals: Their role in motivation, personality, and development. In R. A. Dienstbier (Ed.), *Nebraska Symposium on Motivation: Vol. 38. Perspectives on motivation: Current theory and research in motivation* (pp. 199–235). Lincoln: University of Nebraska Press.

Dweck, C. S. (1996). Implicit theories as organizers of goals and behavior. In P. M. Gollwitzer & J. A. Bargh (Eds.), *The psychology of action: Linking cognition and motivation to behavior* (pp. 69–90). New York: Guilford Press.

Emmons, R. A. (1992). Abstract versus concrete goals: Personal striving level, physical illness, and psychological well-being. *Journal of Personality and Social Psychology, 62,* 292–300.

Fazio, R. H. (1990). Multiple processes by which attitudes guide behavior: The MODE model as an integrative framework. In M. P. Zanna (Ed.), *Advances in experimental social psychology* (Vol. 23, pp. 75–109). San Diego, CA: Academic Press.

Fiske, S. T., & Neuberg, S. L. (1990). A continuum of impression formation, from category-based to individuating processes: Influences of information and motivation on attention and interpretation. In M. P. Zanna (Ed.), *Advances in experimental social psychology* (Vol. 23, pp. 1–73). San Diego, CA: Academic Press.

Gilbert, D. T. (1989). Thinking lightly about others: Automatic components of the social inference process. In J. S. Uleman & J. A. Bargh (Eds.), *Unintended thought* (pp. 189–211). New York: Guilford Press.

Gilbert, D. T., & Malone, P. S. (1995). The correspondence bias. *Psychological Bulletin, 117,* 21–38.

Gollwitzer, P. M. (1990). Action phases and mind-sets. In T. E. Higgins & R. M. Sorrentino (Eds.), *Handbook of motivation and cognition: Foundations of social behavior* (Vol. 2, pp. 53–92). New York: Guilford Press.

Gollwitzer, P. M., & Hammelbeck, H.-J.-P. (1998). *Impartiality in the deliberative mindset: The counterplea heuristic.* Unpublished manuscript, Universität Konstanz, Konstanz, Germany.

Gollwitzer, P. M., Heckhausen, H., & Steller, B. (1990). Deliberative and implemental mind-sets: Cognitive tuning toward congruous thoughts and information. *Journal of Personality and Social Psychology, 59,* 1119–1127.

Gollwitzer, P. M., & Kinney, R. F. (1989). Effects of deliberative and implemental mind-sets on illusion of control. *Journal of Personality and Social Psychology, 56,* 531–542.

Gollwitzer, P. M., & Moskowitz, G. B. (1996). Goal effects on action and cognition. In E. T. Higgins & A. W. Kruglanski (Eds.), *Social psychology: Handbook of basic principles* (pp. 361–399). New York: Guilford Press.

Gollwitzer, P. M., Bayer, U., & Wasel, W., (1998). *Deliberative versus implemental mindsets: The issue of openmindedness.* Unpublished manuscript, Universität Konstanz, Konstanz, Germany.

Harter, S. (1985). Competence as a dimension of self-evaluation: Toward a comprehensive model of self-worth. In R. L. Leary (Ed.), *The development of the self* (pp. 55–121). New York: Academic Press.

Heckhausen, H. (1991). *Motivation and action.* New York: Springer-Verlag.

Heckhausen, H., & Gollwitzer, P. M. (1987). Thought contents and cognitive functioning in motivational versus volitional states of mind. *Motivation and Emotion, 11,* 101–120.

Higgins, E. T. (1996). Knowledge activation: Accessibility, applicability, and salience. In E. T. Higgins & A. W. Kruglanski (Eds.), *Social psychology: Handbook of basic principles* (pp. 133–168). New York: Guilford Press.

Higgins, E. T., Roney, C. J. R., Crowe, E., & Hymes, C. (1994). Ideal versus ought predilections for approach and avoidance distinct self-regulatory systems. *Journal of Personality and Social Psychology, 66,* 276–286.

Kasser, T., & Ryan, R. M. (1993). A dark side of the American dream: Correlates of financial success as a central life aspiration. *Journal of Personality and Social Psychology, 65,* 410–422.

Kuhl, J. (1984). Volitional aspects of achievement motivation and learned helplessness: Toward a comprehensive theory of action control. In B. A. Maher & W. A. Maher (Eds.), *Progress in experimental personality re-*

search (Vol. 13, pp. 99–171). New York: Academic Press.

Kuhl, J., & Goschke, T. (1994). A theory of action control: Mental subsystems, modes of control, and volitional conflict-resolution strategies. In J. Kuhl & J. Beckmann (Eds.), *Volition and personality: Action versus state orientation* (pp. 93–124). Seattle: Hogrefe & Huber.

Külpe, O. (1904). Versuche über Abstraktion [Experiments on abstraction]. *Bericht über den 1. Kongreß für experimentelle Psychologie* (pp. 56–68). Leipzig: Barth.

Lewin, K., Dembo, T., Festinger, L. A., & Sears, P. S. (1944). Level of aspiration. In J. M. Hunt (Ed.), *Personality and the behavior disorders* (pp. 333–378). New York: Ronald Press

Locke, E. A., & Latham, G. P. (1990). *A theory of goal setting and task performance*. Engelwood Cliffs, NJ: Prentice-Hall.

Marbe, K. (1901). *Experimentell-Psychologische Untersuchung über das Urteil* [Experimental psychological studies on judgment]. Leibzig: Wilhelm Engelmann.

Marbe, K. (1915). Zur Psychologie des Denkens [The psychology of thinking]. *Fortschritte der Psychologie und ihre Anwendungen, 3*, 1–42.

Mayer, A., & Orth, J. (1901). Zur qualitativen Untersuchung der Association [A qualitative analysis of associations]. *Zeitschrift für Psychologie, 26*, 1–13.

Norman, D. A., & Bobrow, D. G. (1976). On the role of active memory processes in perception and cognition. In C. N. Coffer (Ed.), *The structure of human memory* (pp. 114–132). San Francisco: W. H. Freeman.

Norman, D. A., & Bobrow, D. G. (1979). Descriptions: An intermediate stage in memory retrieval. *Cognitive Psychology, 11*, 107–123.

Orth, J. (1903). Gefühl und Bewußtseinslage: Eine kritisch-experimentelle Studie [Feelings and mindsets: An experimental study]. In T. Ziegler & T. Ziehen (Eds.), *Sammlung von Abhandlungen aus dem Gebiet der Pädagogischen Psychologie und Physiologie* (Vol. 4, pp. 225–353). Berlin: Verlag von Reuter & Reichard.

Pösl, I. (1994). *Wiederaufnahme unterbrochener Handlungen: Effekte der Bewußtseinslagen des Abwägens und Planens* [Mindset effects on the resumption of disrupted activities]. Unpublished MA thesis, LMU München, München, Germany.

Sedikides, C. (1993). Assessment, enhancement, and verification determinants of the self-evaluation process. *Journal of Personality and Social Psychology, 65*, 317–338.

Sedikides, C., & Strube, M. J. (1995). The multiply motivated self. *Personality and Social Psychology Bulletin, 21*, 1330–1335.

Sedikides, C., & Strube, M. J. (1997). Self-evaluation: To thine own self be good, to thine own self be sure, to thine own self be true, and to thine own self be better.

In M. P. Zanna (Ed.), *Advances in experimental social psychology* (Vol. 29, pp. 209–269). San Diego, CA: Academic Press.

Steller, B., Malzacher, J., & Gollwitzer, P. M. (1990). *Wann sind wir besser als die anderen?: Der Einfluß verschiedener Bewußtseinslagen auf das Selbstbild* [Mindsets and positive illusory self-concepts]. Paper presented at the 32nd Tagung experimentell arbeitender Psychologen (TeaP), Regensburg, Germany.

Swann, W. B., Jr. (1990). To be adored or to be known?: The interplay of self-enhancement and self-verification. In E. T. Higgins & R. M. Sorrentino (Eds.), *Handbook of motivation and cognition: Foundations of social behavior* (Vol. 2, pp. 408–450). New York: Guilford Press.

Swann, W. B., Jr. (1997). The trouble with change: Self-verification and allegiance to the self. *Psychological Science, 8*, 177–183.

Taylor, S. E. (1989). *Positive illusions*. New York: Basic Books.

Taylor, S. E., & Brown, J. D. (1988). Illusion and well-being: A social psychological perspective on mental health. *Psychological Bulletin, 103*, 193–210.

Taylor, S. E., & Brown, J. D. (1994). Positive illusions and well-being revisited: Separating fact from fiction. *Psychological Bulletin, 116*, 21–27.

Taylor, S. E., & Gollwitzer, P. M. (1995). The effects of mindsets on positive illusions. *Journal of Personality and Social Psychology, 69*, 213–226.

Taylor, S. E., Wayment, H. A., & Carrillo, M. (1995). Social comparison, self-regulation, and motivation. In R. M. Sorrentino & E. T. Higgins (Eds.), *Handbook of motivation and cognition: Vol. 3. The interpersonal context* (pp. 3–27). New York: Guilford Press.

Trope, Y. (1986). Self-enhancement and self-assessment in achievement behavior. In R. M. Sorrentino & E. T. Higgins (Eds.), *Handbook of motivation and cognition: Foundations of social behavior* (Vol. 1, pp. 350–378). New York: Guilford Press.

Watt, H. J. (1905). Experimentelle Beiträge zu einer Theorie des Denkens. *Archiv für die gesamte Psychologie, 4*, 289–436.

Weinstein, N. D. (1984). Why it won't happen to me: Perceptions of risk factors and susceptibility. *Health Psychology, 3*, 431–457.

Wicklund, R. A., & Gollwitzer, P. M. (1982). *Symbolic self-completion*. Hillsdale, NJ: Erlbaum.

Wood, J. V. (1996). What is social comparison and how should we study it? *Personality and Social Psychology Bulletin, 22*, 520–537.

Wright, R. A., & Brehm, J. W. (1989). Energizing and goal attractiveness. In L. A. Pervin (Ed.), *Goal concepts in personality and social psychology* (pp. 169–210). Hillsdale, NJ: Erlbaum.

Wulf, H. (1991). *Der depressive Realismus als motivationale Bewußtseinslage* [Mindsets and depressive realism]. Unpublished MA thesis, Universität Gießen, Gießen, Germany.

21

Sufficient and Necessary Conditions in Dual-Process Models

THE CASE OF MOOD AND INFORMATION PROCESSING

HERBERT BLESS
NORBERT SCHWARZ

The question of how much people think about social situations has played a major role in social-psychological theorizing. On the one hand, it has been suggested that individuals act as lay scientists (cf. Fiske & Taylor, 1991), often investing considerable effort in examining information specific to a situation, and in systematically analyzing social situations before making a judgment. On the other hand, it has been proposed that individuals often act as "cognitive misers" (Taylor, 1981; cf. Fiske & Taylor, 1991), processing social information in a rather unsystematic way by relying on rules of thumb and general-knowledge structures, such as heuristics, stereotypes, or schemas. In the domains of persuasion (Chaiken, 1980, 1987; Chen & Chaiken, Chapter 4, this volume; Petty & Cacioppo, 1986; Petty & Wegener, Chapter 3, this volume) and person perception (Brewer, 1988; Brewer & Harasty; Chapter 12, this volume; Fiske, Lin, & Neuberg, Chapter 11, this volume; Fiske & Neuberg, 1990), dual-process models have been proposed to bridge the gap between these two positions. These models specify conditions under which indi-

viduals are likely to act as lay scientists or as cognitive misers. In general, it is argued that systematic processing requires sufficient processing motivation and processing capacity. In contrast, heuristic processing is more likely if either processing motivation or processing capacity is low.

One obvious advantage of these models is their ability to integrate rather diverse and seemingly inconsistent findings. In addition to their integrative character, dual-process models can be applied to investigate how given specific variables influence the cognitive processes involved in persuasion or person perception. From these investigations, it is concluded that the variables of interest increase processing motivation or processing capacity when the patterns of results suggest systematic elaboration of the information, and that the variables of interest decrease processing motivation or processing capacity when the patterns of results suggest reliance on heuristics or stereotypes.

In the present chapter, we highlight some problems associated with this research strategy by emphasizing the importance of distinguishing between *sufficient* and *necessary* conditions of systematic and heuristic processing. Specifically, dual-processing models propose sufficient conditions in the form of "if *P*, then *Q*" (e.g., if processing motivation or capacity is low, than the impact of heuristic cues increases). Manipulations of processing motivation or capacity provide the appropriate test of this hypothesis. However, the reverse logic has sometimes been applied when the impact of a specific variable is of interest (we elaborate on this reverse logic focusing on our own work on mood and processing styles). Following the logic that "if *Q*, then *P*", researchers infer, for example, that an observed increase in the impact of heuristic cues must indicate that processing motivation or capacity is deficient. The crucial difference is that the former inference ("if *P*, then *Q*") implies that reductions in processing motivation or capacity are *sufficient* conditions for heuristic processing, whereas the latter inference ("if *Q*, then *P*") requires that reductions in processing motivation or capacity are necessary conditions for heuristic processing. To the extent that other variables, unrelated to processing capacity or motivation, may foster heuristic processing (see Chen & Chaiken, Chapter 4, this volume), the inference from heuristic processing to deficient capacity or motivation may be unwarranted. Note that this line of argument does not imply that the "if *Q*, then *P*" logic is necessarily inherent to dual-process models. In fact, researchers proposing dual-process models have criticized the "if *Q*, then *P*" logic themselves (see Eagly & Chaiken, 1993). Yet theoretical models are not always applied as intended—and we have inadvertently followed the "if *Q*, then *P*" logic in some of our own work, discussed below. We address this general issue in the context of a specific domain of research—namely, the influence of mood states on processing strategies.

We first review empirical research into the interplay of affect and cognition, drawing on examples from persuasion and person perception. This research indicates that being in a happy mood fosters heuristic processing, whereas being in a sad mood fosters systematic processing. Next we address how these findings have been used to infer decreased processing motivation or decreased processing capacity in the context of dual-process models. Specifically, we focus on empirical and conceptual inconsistencies that raise doubts about the assumption that increased heuristic processing reflects decreased motivation or resources. Finally, we suggest an alternative account—namely, that affective influences on the use of heuristic strategies may be independent of processing motivation or capacity—and present some relevant data, before we address general theoretical and methodological implications for dual-process models.

INVESTIGATING THE ROLE OF AFFECT WITHIN DUAL-PROCESS MODELS

Although dual-process models have been suggested for a variety of different domains in social psychology (see various chapters of this volume), the role of affective states has primarily been investigated in persuasion, person perception, and stereotyping. We first outline the general assumptions of this research and then review selected data.

Mood and Persuasion

Dual-process models in the persuasion domain assume that recipients of a persuasive communication may arrive at an attitude judgment in one (Petty & Cacioppo, 1986) or both (Chaiken, Liberman, & Eagly, 1989; Chaiken, Giner-Sorolla, & Chen, 1996, Chen & Chaiken, Chapter 4, this volume) of two ways. On the one hand, they may carefully consider the content of the message, paying close attention to the implications of the presented arguments. On the other hand, they may not engage in a thorough consideration of message content, but may rely on heuristic cues (e.g., the communicator's expertise or likability, or the sheer length of a message). The former, content-oriented processing strategy is known as "systematic processing" (Chaiken, 1980, 1987) or the "central route to persuasion" (Petty & Cacioppo, 1986); the latter strategy is known as "heuristic processing" or the "peripheral route to persuasion." Which processing strategy is more likely to be chosen depends on recipients' processing motivation and capacity. If the recipient is sufficiently motivated and able to process the content of the message, systematic processing is likely to predominate. Heuristic processing, on the other hand, is more likely if motivation, ability, or both are low.

If the message is processed systematically, the resulting attitude change is a function of recipients' cognitive responses to the message. Accordingly, messages that present strong arguments, which elicit agreeing thoughts, are more effective than messages that present weak or flawed arguments, which elicit counterarguing. The quality of the message affects attitude change less, however, if recipients engage in heuristic processing. Accordingly, comparisons of the impact of strong and weak arguments have been treated as key criteria in distinguishing between systematic and heuristic processing.

Researchers interested in the interplay of affect and cognition have applied this general methodological paradigm to their domain. In a number of studies, participants in different affective states were presented with either strong or weak persuasive messages. In a study typical of this line of research we (Bless,

Bohner, Schwarz, & Strack, 1990) induced a happy or a sad mood by asking participants to provide a vivid report of either a pleasant or an unpleasant life event. As part of a purportedly independent second study, participants were subsequently exposed to a tape recorded communication that presented either strong or weak arguments in favor of an increase in fees for student services. After participants listened to the message, their attitudes toward an increase in these fees were assessed. As shown in Figure 21.1, participants in a sad mood reported more favorable attitudes toward an increase in fees for student services when they were exposed to strong arguments than when they were exposed to weak arguments. Participants in a happy mood, on the other hand, were equally persuaded by strong *and* by weak arguments, and showed moderately positive attitude change under both conditions.

This pattern of findings has been replicated in a number of studies with a range of different mood inductions and persuasive

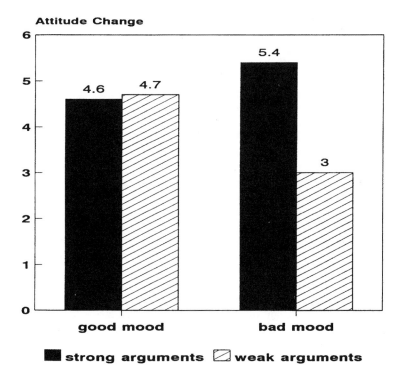

FIGURE 21.1. Attitude change as a function of participants' mood and the quality of the arguments. Data from Bless, Bohner, Schwarz, and Strack (1990).

messages about different attitudinal issues (for examples, see Bless et al., 1990; Bless, Mackie, & Schwarz, 1992; Bohner, Crow, Erb, & Schwarz, 1992; Innes & Ahrens, 1991; Mackie & Worth, 1989; Sinclair, Mark, & Clore, 1994; Worth & Mackie, 1987; for overviews, see Bohner, Moskowitz, & Chaiken, 1995; Schwarz, Bless, & Bohner, 1991). In sum, these studies suggest that recipients' processing of persuasive communications depends on their affective state. Whereas recipients in a neutral or negative mood are persuaded by strong but not by weak messages, recipients in a positive mood are about equally persuaded by both. For the purposes of the present discussion, we focus on this interaction of recipients' mood and message quality. We note, however, that moods may influence attitude judgments in multiple ways (see Petty & Wegener, Chapter 3, this volume; Wegener & Petty, 1994; Wegener, Petty, & Smith, 1995)—an issue that is of secondary concern for the present discussion.

Mood and Stereotyping

The development of dual-process models in persuasion has been paralleled by the development of models addressing cognitive processes in person perception and stereotyping. Again, these models distinguish between two different processing strategies (Brewer, 1988; Fiske & Neuberg, 1990). On the one hand, judgments may be primarily based on the implications of a target person's category membership. In this case, judgments reflect the perceiver's general knowledge about the category to which the target is assigned (i.e., the implications of the stereotype). On the other hand, judgments may be primarily based on available individuating information about a specific target person. In this case, the impact of category membership information is attenuated. Again, the key assumptions hold that judgments based on category membership information are more likely if processing capacity, motivation, or both are low, whereas judgments based on individuating information are more likely if both components are sufficiently high (see Fiske & Neuberg, 1990; Kruglanski, 1989).

Investigating the role of affect within such frameworks, a number of studies have explored the impact of moods on individuals' reliance on stereotypes in impression formation. For example, Bodenhausen, Kramer, and Süsser (1994; see also Bodenhausen, 1993) presented participants in different mood states with descriptions of a student's alleged misconduct and asked participants to determine the target's guilt. Happy participants rated the offender as more guilty when he was identified as a member of a group stereotypically associated with the described offense than when this was not the case. This impact of the stereotype, however, was not observed for participants in a sad mood.[1] Similarly, Edwards and Weary (1993) reported converging evidence based on naturally depressed moods. Nondepressed participants were more likely to rely on category membership information than were depressed participants, who were more strongly influenced by individuating information about the target.

If we equate reliance on category membership information with reliance on peripheral cues, and reliance on individuating information with reliance on the presented arguments, these findings converge with the findings obtained in the persuasion domain. In combination, these findings suggest that individuals in a happy mood are more likely to rely on heuristics or stereotypes, whereas individuals in a sad mood are more likely to attend to the specific information provided.

Interpretations

Two different explanations have been offered for these findings. The two accounts share the notion that happy moods reduce the amount of processing, but they differ in emphasizing either capacity deficits or motivational deficits as the likely cause. On the one hand, it has been argued that being in a good mood limits processing capacity, due to the activation of a large amount of interconnected positive material stored in memory (e.g., Isen, 1987; Mackie & Worth, 1989). Hence individuals in a good mood may not have the cognitive resources required by systematic strategies of processing, and may therefore default to less taxing heuristic strategies.

On the other hand, it has been suggested that the impact of mood on processing style reflects the informative function of affective states (Schwarz, 1990; Schwarz & Bless,

1991). According to this account, being in a bad mood signals that the environment poses a problem, whereas being in a good mood signals that the environment is safe and benign. As a result, individuals in a bad mood are more motivated to engage in detail-oriented systematic processing, which is typically adaptive in handling problematic situations. In contrast, individuals in a good mood may see little reason to engage spontaneously in effortful processing, unless this is called for by other goals (see Schwarz, 1990, and Schwarz & Clore, 1996, for more detailed discussions). Consistent with the assumption that mood states signal processing requirements, Sinclair et al. (1994) observed that the otherwise obtained impact of moods on processing style was eliminated when recipients attributed their mood to the weather, thus rendering it uninformative.

Both of these explanations may account for the decreased impact of message quality and the increased impact of stereotypes during happy moods, and several studies have attempted to disentangle the two potential causes. In this respect, Mackie and Worth (1989) reported empirical support for the reduced-capacity assumption. In their studies, attitudes of happy participants again failed to reflect the quality of a persuasive message, whereas attitudes of participants in a neutral mood showed differential effects of exposure to strong or weak arguments. Happy participants did, however, differentiate between strong and weak arguments when they were encouraged to take as much time as they wanted for reading the message. Mackie and Worth concluded that the extra processing time provided to participants eliminated the capacity deficits of happy participants, resulting in the observed differential impact of strong and weak arguments.

However, there is also evidence supporting the assumption that happy moods reduce processing motivation. In the study described above, we (Bless et al., 1990) observed that happy participants differentiated between strong and weak arguments when they were instructed to pay attention to argument quality. If participants in a good mood were severely restricted in their processing capacity, simply instructing them to pay attention to the quality of the arguments should have been unlikely to overcome these constraints. Accordingly, we considered these findings to support the motivational hypothesis, rather than the capacity hypothesis. As noted elsehwere Schwarz et al., 1991), both of these studies are open to reinterpretations: Whereas the Mackie and Worth (1989) instructions to take as much time as needed may also have affected subjects' processing motivation, the Bless et al. (1990) instruction to attend to argument quality may also have reduced the capacity required for processing the persuasive message by providing a more focused task. In the latter respect, it is conceivable that recipients who were told to evaluate the arguments paid less attention to other aspects of the message (e.g., style, use of terms, etc.) than they might otherwise have done.

Similarly, in the stereotyping domain, Bodenhausen, Kramer, and Süsser (1994) explicitly contrasted the reduced-capacity hypothesis and the reduced-processing-motivation hypothesis. To reduce the likelihood that the mood manipulation would tax participants' cognitive capacity, they selected mood manipulations that were unlikely to drain cognitive resources (smells or facial feedback manipulations). Since these nontaxing mood inductions replicated the previously observed increased impact of stereotypes for happy participants, the authors concluded that the cognitive-capacity approach cannot account for their findings. Moreover, increasing participants' processing motivation with an accountability manipulation (Tetlock, 1983) eliminated the differential impact of stereotypes on happy versus neutral-mood participants. These findings suggest that the increased impact of stereotypes during happy moods is not due to pronounced reductions in processing capacity: Whatever capacity constraints may be induced by being in a happy mood, they cannot be very severe if they can be easily overridden by motivational manipulations.

In sum, considerable effort has been invested in trying to distinguish the two accounts. Yet most of the conclusions are open to reinterpretations of the procedures used (see Schwarz et al., 1991). More importantly, the debate over mood-induced differences in motivation versus capacity has overlooked the possibility that the observed findings may be due to processes that are unrelated to motivation or capacity to begin with. Throughout, the absence of systematic processing has been treated as a strong indicator for processing constraints: It has been concluded that, given the observed impact of heuristic cues and stereotypes under a happy mood, a happy mood must have constrained processing motivation or processing capacity. As noted above, this logic treats reductions in motivation or capacity as a *necessary*, rather than merely a *sufficient*, prerequisite of increased heuristic and decreased systematic processing. In fact, this logic has seemed so compelling that the basic premise of the motivational account as well as the capacity account has typically not been directly tested—namely, that being in a positive mood really reduces the amount of processing.

Although several researchers have attempted to assess mediating variables, including cognitive-response measures, argument recall, and latencies (e.g., Bohner et al., 1992; Bohner, Chaiken, & Hunyadi, 1994; Wegener et al., 1995; Mackie & Worth, 1989), the implications of these measures are sometimes ambiguous. For example, in our own research we initially concluded that the obtained pattern of cognitive responses supported our hypothesis that happy mood reduces processing motivation (Bless et al., 1990). The very same cognitive-response data, however, have led other researchers to conclude that happy individuals are more likely "to think critically about the message and to process it analytically" than sad individuals are (see Wyer & Srull, 1989, p. 403). Similar ambiguities may arise from measuring how much time recipients spend on reading a message. If recipients take longer to read the message, this may imply either that individuals are more motivated to process the message carefully or that they require more time because of capacity constraints. As these examples illustrate, the interpretation of process measures is often theory-dependent. We return to other measures, such as argument recall and assessments of argument strength, below.

In sum, research on mood and processing style has provided little direct evidence that being in a good mood actually reduces processing motivation and/or processing capacity. This is particularly surprising, in light of the fact that the evidence cited in support of motivation or capacity constraints is less

conclusive than it is often assumed to be. We address these inconsistencies in the next section.

SOME PROBLEMS FOR THE REDUCED-PROCESSING ASSUMPTION

Although the available evidence strongly suggests more heuristic processing under happy moods, the findings are less conclusive with regard to the premise that being in a happy mood reduces the amount of processing effort people invest (because of either motivational or capacity deficits). As already noted, the crucial mediating variable, amount of processing, has rarely been directly *assessed*. In most cases, the degree of processing has only been inferred from individuals' judgments by applying the logic of "if Q, then P"; that is, if the judgments indicate heuristic processing, than there must be processing constraints. In addition, a closer look at the available evidence reveals some rarely addressed problems.

First, in the persuasion domain, it has been argued that happy participants do not elaborate on the content of the message and miss differences in message quality. Yet the number of cognitive responses reported by happy and sad subjects has typically been the same (e.g., Bless et al., 1990), although the valence of these responses—and the attitude judgments—reflect message quality for sad recipients, but not for happy recipients. More importantly, the very same happy recipients have been found to differentiate between strong and weak messages (as much as neutral-mood or sad participants) when explicitly asked to rate the quality of the message (e.g., Bless et al., 1990; Worth & Mackie, 1987). Hence, they process message content in sufficient detail to notice differences in message quality, but apparently do not draw on these differences in forming a judgment.

Second, participants in happy, neutral, and sad moods did not differ in their ability to recall the content of a persuasive message in several studies (e.g., Bless et al., 1990), despite the usual differences in attitude judgments. Similarly, happy and sad participants' recall for stereotype-consistent and stereotype-inconsistent individuating information did not differ, although happy participants showed increased reliance on stereotypes in their judgments (Bless, Schwarz, & Wieland, 1996). If being in a happy mood decreases the amount of processing, however, we should also expect it to affect the amount and quality of recall.

Third, the conclusion of reduced processing under happy moods seems at odds with available evidence from other domains. For example, happy participants outperform participants in a neutral or sad mood on creativity and problem-solving tasks (for an overview, see Isen, 1987). In a related vein, Martin, Ward, Achee, and Wyer (1993) found that good mood could decrease as well as increase participants' willingness to elaborate on a task, depending on how they interpreted their mood.

Fourth, a specific problem associated with inferring decreased processing motivation or capacity from a decreased impact of message quality is highlighted by the Bless et al. (1992) findings. In these studies, happy participants were less influenced by message quality when mood was induced prior to the encoding of the message. However, when mood was induced after encoding but prior to the judgment, happy participants' attitudes reflected message quality *more* strongly than sad participants' attitudes did. Thus, the same variable resulted in more or less differentiation between strong and weak arguments, depending on the processing stage it affected. Although we initially tried to reconcile both findings with the notion that happy moods lead to simplified processing, this pattern points to the problem that increases or decreases in the differential impact of message quality do not necessarily imply parallel changes in the amount of processing.

In sum, happy individuals' increased reliance on heuristic strategies appears to be a robust finding. The conclusion that this pattern reflects deficits in processing motivation or capacity, however, lacks direct support and faces challenging inconsistencies in the available data. Next we consider the possibility that happy moods may increase reliance on heuristics without necessarily decreasing either processing motivation or processing capacity.

HEURISTIC PROCESSING'S POSSIBLE INDEPENDENCE OF PROCESSING CONSTRAINTS

Based on the analyses above, we propose that heuristic processing may sometimes result from causes other than reduced motivation or capacity for processing. We first present a conceptual rationale for why this may be the case and subsequently review relevant data.

The Mood-and-General-Knowledge Assumption

We have recently proposed an approach that accounts for increased heuristic processing under happy moods without making assumptions about the amount of processing (Bless, 1994; Bless, Clore, et al., 1996). Building on our previous theorizing (Schwarz, 1990; Schwarz & Bless, 1991), we assume that positive affective states inform an individual that his or her current situation is safe and benign, whereas negative affective states signal a problematic situation. This basic-informative-functions assumption has received considerable support. According to this assumption, mood effects on processing style should only be observed when the informational value of one's current mood is not called into question. When individuals attribute their current feelings to an influence that is unrelated to the task at hand, mood effects on processing style should be eliminated. Consistent with this prediction, Sinclair et al. (1994) observed that moods did not influence the processing of a persuasive message when recipients attributed their mood to the weather, much as Schwarz and Clore (1983) had observed that moods did not influence evaluative judgments under these conditions (see Schwarz, 1990, and Schwarz & Clore, 1996, for reviews). The emergence of these discounting effects is not predicted by models of capacity constraint and indicates that the impact of moods is indeed mediated by their informational value.

What, however, are the processes that mediate between the information provided by one's mood and the observed effects on processing style? In our initial theorizing (Schwarz, 1990; Schwarz & Bless, 1991; Schwarz et al., 1991), we proposed that the key effect of these different signals is *motiva-*

tional: Individuals in a positive mood see no reason to invest major processing effort, unless this is called for by a current goal. Hence they do not spontaneously engage in systematic processing, unless this is required by task instructions or similar variables. In contrast, individuals in a negative mood are motivated to pay attention to the specifics of the situation, which is usually adaptive in addressing problems. Hence they spontaneously engage in systematic processing. Yet this motivational assumption runs into the problems discussed above.

As an alternative, we (Bless, 1994; Bless, Clore, et al., 1996) have proposed that the crucial difference may be related to individuals' reliance on preexisting *general-knowledge structures*. If being in a positive mood informs people that the present situation poses no particular problem, this "business-as-usual" signal may increase the likelihood that they will rely on general-knowledge structures, which usually serve them well. In contrast, if being in a negative mood signals a problematic situation, reliance on defaults and general-knowledge structures may not be adaptive, and people may be more likely to attend to the specifics of the information at hand. As a result, being in a positive mood should foster top-down processing, whereas being in a negative mood should foster bottom-up processing. Note that this position departs from our previous theorizing, as we now refrain from making assumptions about the influence of mood on individuals' processing motivation. This mood-and-general-knowledge assumption is compatible with much of the available evidence. If we consider heuristic processing as the application of general-knowledge structures to specific information (Nisbett & Ross,

1980; see also Chen & Chaiken, Chapter 4, this volume), then heuristics may be viewed as one variant in a larger set of general-knowledge representations including schemas, scripts, stereotypes, and global categories.

How does this account differ from the assumption that happy moods decrease either processing capacity or processing motivation? Conceptually, the key issue is (A) if mood affects processing motivation or capacity, and these deficits in turn increase reliance on general-knowledge structures, or (B) if mood affects reliance on general-knowledge structures in a way that is not mediated by deficits in processing motivation and/or capacity. Figure 21.2 shows these two alternatives. In the former case (Alternative A), reliance on general-knowledge structures is a *consequence* of reduced elaboration under happy moods: Given deficits in motivation or capacity, happy individuals do not elaborate on the details and hence need to rely on general-knowledge structures when making a judgment. In the latter case (Alternative B), reliance on general-knowledge structures is an *antecedent* of reduced elaboration under happy moods: Given a "business-as-usual" signal, happy individuals rely on general-knowledge structures and hence do not need to elaborate on the details (unless those details fly in the face of a general-knowledge structure, as we shall see below).

Obviously, both process assumptions lead to the prediction that general-knowledge structures will have more impact during a positive mood than during a negative mood. Hence, they cannot be distinguished by assessing the impact of general-knowledge structures per se. They do, however, lead to different additional predictions, which allow

Alternative A:

Happy -> Reduces processing motivation -> Increased reliance on
mood   or processing capacity   general-knowledge structures

Alternative B:

Happy -> Increases reliance on -> Simplified processing
mood   general-knowledge structures

FIGURE 21.2. Two alternative processes mediating the impact of mood on the use of general-knowledge structures.

empirical testing. One of these predictions pertains to performance on a secondary task: If happy moods reduce processing motivation or capacity, they should impair not only performance on the primary task, but also performance on a secondary task. In contrast, if happy moods elicit reliance on general-knowledge structures pertaining to the primary task, the primary task should be less taxing, and performance on a secondary task should improve. A second prediction pertains to the impact of information that is inconsistent with the implications of the general-knowledge structure: If happy moods reduce processing motivation or capacity, any inconsistencies should be less likely to be noted, and the judgment should be based on the general-knowledge structure. In contrast, if happy moods elicit reliance on general-knowledge structures, inconsistent information should be particularly salient and should receive special weight in judgment formation. In the next two sections, we address these predictions in more detail and report relevant data.

Mood, Scripts, and the Advantages of a Dual-Task Paradigm

One way to test the two competing accounts described above is to assess the cognitive effort individuals are willing or able to spend in a dual-task paradigm (see Navon & Gopher, 1979). In this paradigm, participants work simultaneously on two tasks, with one often being designated as the primary and the other as the secondary task. We are familiar with these situations from everyday life (e.g., reading the newspaper while watching television). It is assumed that efficient processing of one task enables individuals to allocate more resources to the other task, resulting in improved performance on that task. For example, Macrae, Milne, and Bodenhausen (1994) asked participants to form an impression of a person based on a list of trait adjectives. While performing this task, half of the participants were working on a secondary task. Prior activation of a category label resulted in improved recall of adjectives that were consistent with the label, but had no impact on the recall of inconsistent or irrelevant adjectives. More important, the activation of the category label

resulted in *better* performance on the secondary task. This presumably indicated that the category label allowed access to a general-knowledge structure (a stereotype), which in turn made it easier for participants to process the stereotype-consistent items, thus enabling them to allocate additional resources to the secondary task.

We applied this logic to happy individuals' reliance on scripts, another form of general-knowledge structures (Bless, Clore, et al., 1996). Our general approach was to present participants in different affective states with information about well-known activities (e.g., "going out for dinner"), for which they were likely to have well-developed scripts (Abelson, 1981; Graesser, Gordon, & Sawyer, 1979). Some of this information was script-typical ("The hostess placed the menus on the table"), whereas other information was script-atypical ("He put away his tennis racket"). While encoding this information, participants had to work on a secondary task—namely, a concentration test that allowed us to assess how much effort participants were able and willing to allocate to it. After a short delay, participants received a surprise recognition test, assessing their memory for the information about daily activities that had been presented to them.

This approach allowed us to address two issues. First, would happy and sad moods affect participants' reliance on a script? If so, this should be reflected in their recognition performance. Second, would happy or sad moods affect the amount of effort that participants were willing or able to invest? If so, this should be reflected in their performance on the secondary task. Moreover, the covariation of performance on both measures provided additional information, as discussed below.

Recognition

We predicted that if being in a happy mood fosters reliance on general-knowledge structures, our happy participants would be more likely to "recognize" script-typical items, regardless of whether these were actually presented or not. This would indicate that reliance on a script allowed participants to infer script-typical behaviors, resulting in good recognition of typical behaviors that were actually presented, as well as in erroneous recognition of script-typical behaviors that were not ("intrusion errors"; see Graesser et al., 1979; Snyder & Uranowitz, 1978; cf. Fiske & Taylor, 1991). The data confirmed these predictions.

Specifically, happy participants were more likely than sad participants to recognize typical information as having been presented. However, they were also more likely to erroneously recognize typical behaviors that were not presented, resulting in a higher rate of intrusion errors. As expected, these mood effects were not obtained for atypical information, reflecting that this information could not be inferred from the script. Note that this differential pattern for typical and atypical information ruled out an alternative explanation, based on the possibility that different moods may elicit different response tendencies.

Secondary Task

Although the recognition data suggested that happy individuals are more likely to rely on general-knowledge structures, such as scripts, our participants' performance on the secondary task allowed us to tackle the underlying processes. The two approaches outlined above (Alternatives A and B) enabled us to make different predictions with respect to secondary-task performance. If happy individuals' reliance on general-knowledge structures is due to motivational or capacity constraints (Alternative A), we predicted that these constraints should also influence performance on the secondary task. Thus happy participants should show poorer performance than sad participants.

We based a different prediction on the mood-and-general-knowledge assumption, which makes no assumption about mood-dependent differences in processing motivation or processing capacity. In general, reliance on a script simplifies the processing of script-related information, thus making the primary task less taxing (e.g., Macrae et al., 1994). If so, our happy participants—who could be assumed to rely on the script, given their recognition data—should have more resources available to allocate to the secondary task. Accordingly, they should perform better

on this task than sad participants, in contrast to the prediction based on reduced-processing assumptions.

Again, the results confirmed this latter prediction. Most importantly, happy participants showed *better* performance on the secondary task than either sad or neutral-mood participants. If happy participants' reliance on the script were due to reduced motivation or capacity for processing, the respective deficit should also have impaired their secondary-task performance, which was not the case. Instead, the findings suggested that happy participants relied more on top-down, script-based processing for the primary task, thus enabling them to allocate additional resources to the secondary task, and resulting in improved performance.[2]

Further supporting this conclusion, happy participants' secondary-task performance depended on the amount of script-inconsistent information presented as part of the primary task. Specifically, increasing the amount of script-atypical information decreased happy participants' advantage on the secondary task (Bless, Clore, et al., 1996, Experiment 3). This indicated that increasing the amount of atypical information decreased the resources that could be set free by relying on the script.

The results obtained in control conditions further indicated that these findings were unlikely to be reflecting a direct impact of mood on secondary-task performance. Specifically, control group participants were working on the secondary task as their only task. Under this condition, their mood did *not* affect their performance. In addition to bearing on our interpretation of the results obtained under dual-task conditions, this latter finding is itself remarkable. As the secondary task was designed to measure cognitive capacity and processing motivation (Brickenkamp, 1975), the investigation of mood effects on this task is one of the few attempts to date at directly assessing the hypothesis that mood affects the amount of processing. The absence of any impact is hardly compatible with the notion that happy moods reduce the amount of processing, due to either capacity or motivational deficits (although the latter may have been mitigated by the explicit task instructions).

In sum, these findings suggest that happy

moods increase individuals' reliance on general-knowledge structures. Although this general conclusion is consistent with previous theorizing, the presented findings also indicate that increased reliance on general-knowledge structures is not *necessarily* caused by deficits in processing motivation or processing capacity. Instead, the results indicate that reduced motivation, capacity, or both may be *sufficient* but not *necessary* causes of heuristic processing. This conclusion is further supported by research into the impact of moods on stereotyping, to which we turn next.

Mood, Stereotyping, and the Impact of Inconsistent Information

Like to heuristics and scripts, stereotypes are another form of general-knowledge structures. As discussed above, stereotypes have a stronger impact on happy than on sad individuals in impression formation tasks (Bodenhausen, Kramer, & Süsser, 1994). Again, happy individuals' increased reliance on stereotypes may either be due to happy moods' impact on processing motivation or capacity (Alternative A) or to happy moods' impact on individuals' reliance on general-knowledge structures (Alternative B). Again, the two approaches lead to similar predictions under most circumstances. They differ, however, in their predictions pertaining to the impact of individuating information that is inconsistent with the stereotype. Hence, we have treated the impact of inconsistent individuating information as an indicator for the underlying processes, similar to secondary-task performance in the script studies reviewed above.

If happy individuals are less likely to engage in extensive processing (either due to limited capacity or limited motivation—Alternative A), they may use the stereotype simply as a peripheral cue that simplifies their task. If so, specific information about the target is less likely to be elaborated. As a consequence, judgments should be independent of whether stereotype-consistent or stereotype-inconsistent individuating information is provided. In the case of inconsistent information, happy individuals either may not detect or may simply ignore the discrepancy, due to their reduced processing motivation or capacity. Hence,

their judgments should only reflect category membership information, but not individuating information.

In contrast, different predictions result from the mood-and-general-knowledge assumption. If the increased impact of stereotypes on happy individuals is mediated by happy individuals' reliance on general-knowledge structures in processing new information, specific individuating information is unlikely to go unnoticed. In this case, individuals' encoding of new individuating information should be guided by the activated stereotype. As long as the individuating information is consistent with the implications of the stereotype, the two sources of information have the same implications for evaluative judgments. As a consequence, the "peripheral-cue" and the "guided-encoding" mechanisms cannot be distinguished on the basis of individuals' judgments if the individuating information is consistent with the stereotype (as has been the case in all studies reported in the literature, except the ones to be reviewed below). In contrast, individuating information that is inconsistent with the implications of the stereotype should strongly affect the obtained judgments. This requires, however, that the inconsistency is noticed in the first place. According to the mood-and-general-knowledge assumption, this should be more likely when individuals are in a happy mood (and hence more likely to rely on stereotypes) than when they are in a sad mood (and hence unlikely to draw on the stereotype to begin with). Accordingly, the mood-and-general-knowledge assumption leads to the prediction that stereotype-inconsistent information should receive more weight in judgment formation under happy than under sad moods. Note, however, that dealing with stereotype-inconsistent information requires considerable cognitive resources (e.g., Macrae, Hewstone, & Griffiths, 1993; Stangor & Duan, 1991; see also Fiske & Taylor, 1991; Srull & Wyer, 1989). Thus, observing a more pronounced impact of stereotype-inconsistent information under happy-mood rather than sad-mood conditions should again argue against the assumption that being in a happy mood reduces processing capacity or processing motivation.

Finally, both accounts hold that individuals in a sad mood should be less likely to stereotype. This may indicate either that a sad mood is less likely than a good mood to reduce processing capacity (a controversial assumption—see Clore, Schwarz, & Conway, 1994, for a discussion); that a sad mood increases processing motivation (Schwarz, 1990); or that a sad mood discourages reliance on general-knowledge structures (Bless, 1994; Bless, Clore, et al., 1996). In either case, sad individuals' judgments should reflect the implications of the individuating information, rather than the implications of the target's category membership.

We tested these considerations by exploring the impact of moods under conditions where the individuating information was either consistent or inconsistent with the implications of the stereotype (see Bless, Schwarz, & Wieland, 1996). In these studies, participants in a happy, neutral, or sad mood listened to descriptions of a target person, and later evaluated the target along various dimensions. The target person was described as a member of either a positively or a negatively evaluated group (category membership information) performing either positive or negative behaviors (individuating information). Given the orthogonal manipulation of the valence of the categorical and individuating information, the implications of the stereotype were either consistent or inconsistent with the implications of the target's specific behaviors. This design allowed us to test (1) whether happy individuals were more likely to rely on category membership information than sad individuals, and (2) whether this reliance was mediated by an impact of happy moods on the amount of processing.

Under conditions where the individuating information was *consistent* with the implications of the stereotype, our results replicated previous findings (see Bless, Schwarz, & Wieland, 1996, for details). Specifically, happy participants provided stereotypical judgments, whereas sad participants did not, indicating that the former relied on the stereotype and the latter on the individuating information. These findings are compatible with either of the mediating mechanisms of interest. The findings obtained under conditions where the individuating information was *inconsistent* with the implications of the stereotype, however, are diagnostic for our current purposes. Importantly, these findings showed

that happy participants evaluated the target most negatively when the target was described as a member of a positive group engaging in negative behaviors. Moreover, this pronounced impact of stereotype-inconsistent information on happy participants was only observed when the behavioral information was perceived as diagnostic (for a more extended discussion of this aspect, see Bless, Schwarz, & Wieland, 1996, Experiment 2). In contrast, sad individuals again relied solely on the implications of the individuating information, without weighing it differentially as a function of its consistency or inconsistency with the stereotype.

Thus, we observed an *increased* impact of stereotype-inconsistent individuating information during happy moods. If happy participants had simply relied on the stereotype as a peripheral cue, as predicted by reduced-processing assumptions, a member of a positively evaluated group should have been evaluated more favorably than a member of a negatively evaluated group, regardless of the individuating information. Instead, the inconsistent individuating information received particular weight. Note, however, that this required happy participants (1) to process the individuating information in the first place, (2) to relate it to the implications of the script, (3) to notice the inconsistency, and (4) to draw on its implications in forming a judgment. Such steps require considerable processing effort, as indicated by previous research into the processing of expectancy-inconsistent information (Macrae et al., 1993; Stangor & Duan, 1991; for meta-analyses on the role of inconsistent information, see Rojahn & Pettigrew, 1992; Stangor & McMillan, 1992). Hence, the obtained findings are again difficult to reconcile with the assumption that our happy moods cause motivational or capacity deficits. Instead, they indicate that happy participants processed the individuating information *and* elaborated on the relationship between both sources of information, whereas our sad participants did not rely on the category information to begin with, but focused solely on the behavioral information.

Further supporting the notion that happy participants processed the individuating information in light of the category information, we did obtain the described pattern only when the category membership information was introduced *prior* to the individuating information, but not when the category information was presented *after* the individuating information (Bless, Schwarz, & Wieland, 1996, Experiment 4). Moreover, we observed that instructing neutral-mood participants to focus on the *relation* between the individuating and the categorical information resulted in the same pattern that we obtained for happy participants without this instruction. In contrast, instructing neutral-mood participants to focus on the individuating information resulted in the same pattern that we obtained for sad participants without this instruction (Bless, Schwarz, & Wieland, 1996, Experiment 3). This suggests that being in a happy mood is functionally equivalent with instructions that evoke top-down processing of incoming information, whereas being in a sad mood is functionally equivalent with instructions that evoke bottom-up processing of incoming information.

Summary and Theoretical Implications

In combination, the reviewed findings indicate that individuals in a happy mood are more likely to rely on general-knowledge structures, such as scripts and stereotypes, than sad individuals are. These findings are generally consistent with a growing body of literature that indicates increased heuristic processing during happy moods and increased systematic processing during sad moods (see Clore et al., 1994, and Schwarz & Clore, 1996, for recent reviews; see Bohner et al., 1995, for evidence that individuals in a sad mood may combine message content and heuristic cues in arriving at a judgment). Previous theorizing has attributed these differences to general influences of moods on processing motivation (e.g., Schwarz, 1990; Schwarz et al., 1991) or processing capacity (e.g., Mackie & Worth, 1989). The findings reviewed in the present chapter are difficult to reconcile with the core assumption of these approaches—namely, that being in a happy mood results in reduced processing. Specifically, we observed that happy individuals outperformed sad and neutral-mood individuals on a secondary task, and that they were more likely to consider and integrate stereotype-inconsistent information in forming an impression—perfor-

mances that require considerable processing effort.

These findings are, however, consistent with the mood-and-general-knowledge assumption that generated the relevant predictions (Bless, 1994; Bless, Clore, et al., 1996; Bless, Schwarz, & Wieland, 1996; for additional evidence, see Bless & Fiedler, 1995). Extending our previous theorizing (Schwarz, 1990; Schwarz & Bless, 1991), we propose that positive affective states signal that the current situation is benign, allowing individuals to rely on their general-knowledge structures, which usually serve them well. Hence, happy individuals engage in top-down processing, unless they encounter material that calls the applicability of the general-knowledge structure into question (as we have seen in the stereotyping studies). Moreover, reliance on general-knowledge structures reduces the demands on processing capacity, allowing the allocation of resources to other tasks (as we have seen in the dual-task studies). In contrast, negative affective states signal a problematic situation, which may require attention to specifics. Hence, relying on general-knowledge structures may not seem wise, resulting in bottom-up processing with considerable attention to detail. As a result, inconsistencies between the input information and the general-knowledge structures are more likely to be missed, reflecting that the general-knowledge structures are less likely to be used in the first place (as seen in the stereotyping studies). Moreover, bottom-up processing requires more resources, thus reducing the resources that can be allocated to other tasks (as seen in the dual-task studies). Importantly, however, reliance on heuristics and schemas will only be less taxing than bottom-up processing when the specific information is not inconsistent with the implications of the general-knowledge structures. If inconsistent information is encountered, individuals who engage in top-down processing need to expend as much processing effort as individuals who engage in bottom-up processing do, if not more (cf. Maheswaran & Chaiken, 1991).

Note that this proposal departs from our previous theorizing, as we now refrain from making general assumptions about mood effects on individuals' global processing motivation. As noted earlier, direct measures of processing capacity and processing motivation have rarely been assessed in previous research. Instead, motivation or capacity deficits have been inferred from the obtained judgment data—a conclusion that is only warranted when we assume that the respective deficit is a necessary, rather than only a sufficient, condition of heuristic processing. Indeed, the dual-task data reviewed above argue against such general deficits. These data indicated that performance on the concentration test was unaffected by mood in the absence of a primary task. Moreover, happy individuals outperformed sad and neutral-mood individuals in the presence of a primary task to which they could apply general-knowledge structures.

Does this imply that motivation plays no role in eliciting heuristic processing? Obviously not. Numerous studies have demonstrated that decreased processing motivation (as well as decreased processing capacity) is *sufficient* to elicit heuristic processing; however, the present data suggest that they are not *necessary*. We also hasten to add that we assume that increasing happy individuals' processing motivation is likely to override their otherwise observed reliance on general-knowledge structures, in line with the generally observed impact of accuracy motivation on the choice of processing strategies (see Fiske & Neuberg, 1990, and Kruglanski, 1989, for overviews). Hence manipulations of processing motivation or capacity may have a rather strong impact, relative to the presumably more subtle impact of affective states (see Bless et al., 1990; Bodenhausen, Kramer, & Süsser, 1994; Mackie & Worth, 1989).

Finally, we emphasize that our present theorizing does not imply that moods are generally unlikely to influence processing motivation under any condition. However, the underlying process may be less general than we have previously assumed. As an example, consider a series of experiments reported by Martin et al. (1993), who drew on previous research into the impact of moods on evaluative judgments. This research suggested that individuals may arrive at evaluative judgments by relying on their current feelings as information, essentially asking themselves, "How do I feel about this?" (see Schwarz & Clore, 1983; Schwarz, 1990). Applying this logic to processing motivation, Martin et al. (1993) asked participants to generate a list of birds from memory. Some participants were instructed to ask themselves how satisfied they were with their performance and to stop when they felt that this was a good time to stop. Under this performance-oriented decision rule, sad participants spent more time listing birds, and listed more birds, than happy participants did. This presumably indicated that sad participants inferred from their feelings that they were not very happy with their performance, and hence kept going. In contrast, happy participants presumably inferred that they were satisfied with their performance, and hence stopped. Supporting this interpretation, a different pattern of results was obtained when participants were told to stop "when [they] no longer enjoy[ed] the task." Under this enjoyment-related decision rule, sad participants spent less time on the task, and listed fewer birds, than happy subjects did, presumably indicating that they were more likely to infer that they no longer enjoyed the task. Finally, subjects who were not given an explicit decision rule also spent more time on the task, and listed more birds, when they were in a sad rather than in a happy mood, suggesting that they spontaneously adopted a task-oriented decision rule. Hirt, Melton, McDonald, and Harackiewicz (1996) reported a conceptual replication of this interactive impact of mood and decision rule on task performance, using a different task and a different mood induction.

These findings clearly indicate that moods *can* influence processing motivation when they are brought to bear on assessments of one's task performance or task enjoyment (for a more extensive discussion of this issue, see Schwarz & Bohner, 1996), and that their specific impact depends on the decision rule for which they serve as input. Hence, the findings reviewed in the present chapter do not put the assumption that moods may influence processing motivation to rest. They do, however, indicate that mood states may influence processing strategies for reasons other than their impact on motivation. In fact, it is conceivable that framing manipulations of the kind used by Martin et al. (1993) may evoke mood effects on individuals' motivation that may interact with mood effects on the use of general-knowledge structures. Exploring these possibilities will provide a challenging avenue for future research.

CONCLUSIONS

In sum, mood researchers have concluded that being in a good mood reduces either processing capacity (e.g., Mackie & Worth, 1989) or processing motivation (e.g., Schwarz, 1990). This conclusion has been based on observations that being in a good mood fosters heuristic processing across a range of domains. Given that numerous studies demonstrated that deficits in motivation or capacity (for overviews, see Eagly & Chaiken, 1993; Fiske & Neuberg, 1990; Kruglanski, 1989; Petty & Cacioppo, 1986) do indeed elicit heuristic processing, this conclusion has seemed straightforward. Yet it requires the assumption that these deficits are *necessary*, rather than merely *sufficient*, conditions for the emergence of heuristic processing. Although processing motivation and capacity do influence the choice of processing strategies (Eagly & Chaiken, 1993; Fiske & Neuberg, 1990; Petty & Cacioppo, 1986), the reverse conclusion—namely, that a heuristic strategy indicates the presence of a deficit—is (1) not implied by the underlying models, and (2) fraught with uncertainty (for an explicit discussion of conditions that elicit stronger impact of heuristics under conditions of high processing motivation, see Chen & Chaiken, Chapter 4, this volume). If we entertain the possibility that motivation and capacity are not the only determinants of heuristic processing, as the data reviewed in the present chapter would suggest, we have to refrain from equating increased heuristic processing with decreased processing motivation or capacity. We emphasize that this equation is *not* logically entailed in dual-processing models; yet as our own and others' research on mood and processing style (and its ready acceptance) illustrates, this unwarranted leap is tempting.

On the empirical side, the present discussion indicates that we need to pay more attention to direct measures of motivation and capacity. In the domain of persuasion, for example, sufficient motivation and capacity are sometimes inferred from an impact of message strength manipulations or the absence of cue effects, whereas insufficient motivation or capacity are inferred from the presence of cue effects and the absence of message strength effects. What, however, determines whether something is considered an argument or a peripheral cue? In some cases, the same information may be considered an argument when it exerts an influence under conditions of high motivation or capacity, and a cue when it does so under conditions of low motivation or capacity, thus playing multiple roles (see Petty & Cacioppo, 1986; Petty, Cacioppo, & Kasmer, 1988). We do not deny the possibility that the same piece of information may serve as a peripheral cue or as an argument. But if we infer sufficient processing motivation and capacity from the impact of argument strength on the one hand, and conclude that some information should be considered an argument because it has an impact under high-elaboration conditions on the other hand, we run the risk of circular definitions. We acknowledge that researchers proposing dual-processing models are well aware of the potential problems associated with inferring processing motivation and capacity from the impact of message quality (for a critical discussion, see Eagly & Chaiken, 1993, ch. 7). Moreover, some dual-process models explicitly emphasize the possibility of increased reliance on heuristic processes under conditions of high processing motivation (see Chaiken, 1987; Chen & Chaiken, Chapter 4, this volume). Yet, again, 10 years of research into mood and processing style illustrate how easily these problems are overlooked.

Obviously, how much of a problem it is depends on which variable is examined. Some operationalizations of processing motivation (e.g., personal relevance, accountability, or need for cognition) or processing capacity (e.g., time pressure, distraction) are sufficiently straightforward to render independent assessments of motivation or capacity unnecessary. This is not the case, however, when dual-processing paradigms are used to determine *whether* a specific variable of interest influences processing motivation or capacity— as we have done in our own research into mood and persuasion (Schwarz et al., 1991). In these cases, the distinction between sufficient and necessary conditions is particularly crucial, as seen in the results reviewed in the present chapter.

On the theoretical side, the impact of heuristics is often traced to reduced motivation or capacity. In many situations, however, people may well rely on heuristics not because of processing deficits, but because they capture general knowledge across a large number of experiences. The fact that reliance on heuristics may also be observed under conditions of high elaboration likelihood is explicitly addressed in the heuristic–systematic model (Chaiken, 1980, 1987; Chen & Chaiken, Chapter 4, this volume), which entails the possibility that highly motivated and capable respondents may simultaneously draw on argument strength and heuristic cues (e.g., expertise) to arrive at judgments of high subjective certainty. Moreover, Maheswaran and Chaiken (1994) observed increased processing under conditions where participants processed a message heuristically and encountered information that was inconsistent with their heuristics. These findings again indicate that heuristic processing is not necessarily a consequence of reduced capacity or motivation. Instead, it may seem the most plausible strategy, given the circumstances.

To summarize, we propose that applications of dual-process models need to pay closer attention to the distinction between necessary and sufficient conditions. Most important, we cannot unambiguously infer deficits in processing capacity or motivation when we observe heuristic rather than systematic processing. As the reviewed research indicates, individuals may rely on general-knowledge structures and heuristic processing under conditions where the capacity and motivation required for systematic processing are available. Once stated, this point does not seem not surprising; however, it has often been overlooked by researchers—including ourselves.

ACKNOWLEDGMENT

The research reported here was supported by Grant No. B1 289/5 from the Deutsche Forschungsgemeinschaft to Herert Bless, Norbert Schwarz, and M. Wanke.

NOTES

1. It is important to add that Bodenhausen, Sheppard, and Kramer (1994) also observed that not all negative affective states are alike, and that only sadness, not anger, decreased stereotyping.

2. The mood-and-general-knowledge assumption was indirectly also supported by the recognition data. Specifically, we observed a rather high accuracy for atypical information, *independent of participants' mood*. If happy mood reduced cognitive resources or motivation, we should have observed poor recognition performance on the atypical and unrelated items, as their recognition requires cognitive effort. The mood-independent high accuracy suggests that happy participants allocated resources on these items that were not important or essential for understanding the story. Again, this finding seems more in line with the mood-and-general-knowledge assumption than with the notion of reduced processing during happy moods.

REFERENCES

Abelson, R. P. (1981). The psychological status of the script concept. *American Psychologist, 36,* 715–729.

Bless, H. (1994). *Stimmung und die Nutzung allgemeiner Wissensstrukturen: Ein Modell zum Einfluß von Stimmungen auf Denkprozesse* [Mood and the use of general-knowledge structures]. Habilitationsschrift, Universität Heidelberg.

Bless, H., Bohner, G., Schwarz, N., & Strack, F. (1990). Mood and persuasion: A cognitive response analysis. *Personality and Social Psychology Bulletin, 16,* 331–345.

Bless, H., Clore, G. L, Schwarz, N., Golisano, V., Rabe, C., & Wölk, M. (1996). Mood and the use of scripts: Does happy mood make people really mindless? *Journal of Personality and Social Psychology, 63,* 585–595.

Bless, H., & Fiedler, K. (1995). Affective states and the influence of activated general knowledge. *Personality and Social Psychology Bulletin, 21,* 766–778.

Bless, H., Mackie, D. M., & Schwarz, N. (1992). Mood effects on encoding and judgmental processes in persuasion. *Journal of Personality and Social Psychology, 63,* 585–595.

Bless, H., Schwarz, N., & Wieland, R. (1996). Mood and stereotyping: The impact of category and individuating information. *European Journal of Social Psychology, 26,* 935–959.

Bodenhausen, G. V. (1993). Emotions, arousal, and stereotype-based discrimination: A heuristic model of affect and stereotyping. In D. M. Mackie & D. L. Hamilton (Eds.), *Affect, cognition, and stereotyping: Interactive processes in group perception* (pp. 13–35). San Diego, CA: Academic Press.

Bodenhausen, G. V., Kramer, G. P., & Süsser, K. (1994). Happiness and stereotypic thinking in social judgment. *Journal of Personality and Social Psychology*, 66, 621–632.

Bodenhausen, G. V., Sheppard, L. A., & Kramer, G. P. (1994). Negative affect and social judgment: The differential impact of anger and sadness. *European Journal of Social Psychology*, 24, 45–62.

Bohner, G., Crow, K., Erb, H.-P., & Schwarz, N. (1992). Affect and persuasion: Mood effects on the processing of message content and context cues. *European Journal of Social Psychology*, 22, 511–530.

Bohner, G., Chaiken, S., & Hunyadi, P. (1994). The role of mood and message ambiguity in the interplay of heuristic and systematic processing. *European Journal of Social Psychology*, 24, 207–221.

Bohner, G., Moskowitz, G. B., & Chaiken, S. (1995). The interplay of heuristic and systematic processing of social information. In W. Stroebe & M. Hewstone (Eds.), *European review of social psychology* (Vol. 6, pp. 33–68). Chichester, England: Wiley.

Brewer, M. A. (1988). A dual-process model of impression formation. In T. K. Srull & R. S. Wyer, Jr. (Eds.), *Advances in social cognition* (Vol. 1, pp. 1–36). Hillsdale, NJ: Erlbaum.

Brickenkamp, R. (1975). *Handbuch psychologischer Tests*. Göttingen, Germany: Hogrefe.

Chaiken, S. (1980). Heuristic versus systematic information processing and the use of source versus message cues in persuasion. *Journal of Personality and Social Psychology*, 39, 752–766.

Chaiken, S. (1987). The heuristic model of persuasion. In M. P. Zanna, J. M. Olson, & C. P. Herman (Eds.), *Social influence: The Ontario Symposium* (Vol. 5, pp. 3–39). Hillsdale, NJ: Erlbaum.

Chaiken, S., Giner-Sorolla, R., & Chen, S. (1996). Beyond accuracy: Defense and impression motives in heuristic and systematic information processing. In P. M. Gollwitzer & J. A. Bargh (Eds.), *The psychology of action: Linking cognition and motivation to behavior* (pp. 553–578). New York: Guilford Press.

Chaiken, S., Liberman, A., & Eagly, A. H. (1989). Heuristic and systematic information processing within and beyond the persuasion context. In J. S. Uleman & J. A. Bargh (Eds.), *Unintended thought* (pp. 212–252). New York: Guilford Press.

Clore, G. L., Schwarz, N., & Conway, M. (1994). Affective causes and consequences of emotion. In R. S. Wyer, Jr. & T. K. Srull (Eds.), *Handbook of social cognition* (2nd ed., Vol. 1, pp. 323–417). Hillsdale, NJ: Erlbaum.

Eagly, A. H., & Chaiken, S. (1993). *The psychology of attitudes*. Fort Worth, TX: Harcourt Brace Jovanovich.

Edwards, J. A., & Weary, G. (1993). Depression and the impression-formation continuum: Piecemeal processing despite the availability of category information. *Journal of Personality and Social Psychology*, 64, 636–645.

Fiske, S. T., & Neuberg, S. L. (1990). A continuum of impression formation, from category-based to individuating processing: Influences of information and motivation on attention and interpretation. In M. P. Zanna (Ed.), *Advances in experimental social psychology* (Vol. 23, pp. 1–74). San Diego, CA: Academic Press.

Fiske, S. T., & Taylor, S. E. (1991). *Social cognition* (2nd ed.). New York: McGraw-Hill.

Graesser, A. C., Gordon, S. E., & Sawyer, J. D. (1979). Memory for typical and atypical actions in scripted activities: Test of a script pointer + tag hypothesis. *Journal of Verbal Learning and Behavior*, 18, 319–332.

Hirt, E. R., Melton, R. J., McDonald, H. E., & Harackiewicz, J. M. (1996). Processing goals, task interest, and the mood-performance relationship: A mediational analysis. *Journal of Personality and Social Psychology*, 71, 245–261.

Innes, J. M., & Ahrens, C. R. (1991). Positive mood, processing goals, and the effects of information on evaluative judgment. In J. Forgas (Ed.), *Emotion and social judgment* (pp. 221–239). Oxford: Pergamon Press.

Isen, A. M. (1987). Positive affect, cognitive processes, and social behavior. In L. Berkowitz (Ed.), *Advances in Experimental social psychology* (Vol. 20, pp. 203–253). San Diego, CA: Academic Press.

Kruglanski, A. W. (1989). The psychology of being "right": On the problem of accuracy in social perception and cognition. *Psychological Bulletin*, 106, 395–409.

Mackie, D. M., & Worth, L. T. (1989). Cognitive deficits and the mediation of positive affect in persuasion. *Journal of Personality and Social Psychology*, 57, 27–40.

Macrae, C. N., Hewstone, M., & Griffiths, R. J. (1993). Processing load and memory for stereotype-based information. *European Journal of Social Psychology*, 23, 77–87.

Macrae, C. N., Milne, A. B., & Bodenhausen, G. V. (1994). Stereotypes as energy-saving devices: A peek inside the cognitive toolbox. *Journal of Personality and Social Psychology*, 66, 37–47.

Maheswaran, D., & Chaiken, S. (1991). Promoting systematic processing in low-motivation settings: Effects of incongruent information on processing and judgment. *Journal of Personality and Social Psychology*, 61, 13–25.

Martin, L. M., Ward, D. W., Achee, J. W., & Wyer, R. S., Jr. (1993). Mood as input: People have to interpret the motivational implications of their moods. *Journal of Personality and Social Psychology*, 64, 317–326.

Navon, D., & Gopher, D. (1979). On the economy of human processing systems. *Psychological Review*, 86, 214–255.

Nisbett, R., & Ross, L. (1980). *Human inference: Strategies and shortcomings in social judgment*. Englewood Cliffs, NJ: Prentice-Hall.

Petty, R. E., & Cacioppo, J. T. (1986). The elaboration likelihood model of persuasion. In L. Berkowitz (Ed.), *Advances in experimental social psychology* (Vol. 19, pp. 124–203). New York: Academic Press.

Petty, R. E., Cacioppo, J. T., & Kasmer, J. A. (1988). The role of affect in the elaboration likelihood model of persuasion. In L. Donohue, H. E. Sypher, & E. T. Higgins (Eds.), *Communication, social cognition, and affect* (pp. 117–146). Hillsdale, NJ: Erlbaum.

Rojahn, K., & Pettigrew, T. F. (1992). Memory for schema-relevant information: A meta-analytic resolution. *British Journal of Social Psychology*, 31, 81–110.

Schwarz, N. (1990). Feelings as information: Informational and motivational functions of affective states. In E. T. Higgins & R. M. Sorrentino (Eds.), *Handbook of* motivation and cognition: Foundations of social behavior (Vol. 2, pp. 527–561). New York: Guilford Press.

Schwarz, N., & Bless, H. (1991). Happy and mindless, but sad and smart?: The impact of affective states on analytic reasoning. In J. Forgas (Ed.), Emotion and social judgment (pp. 55–71). Oxford: Pergamon Press.

Schwarz, N., Bless, H., & Bohner, G. (1991). Mood and persuasion: Affective states influence the processing of persuasive communications. In M. Zanna (Ed.), Advances in experimental social psychology (Vol. 24, pp. 161–197). San Diego, CA: Academic Press.

Schwarz, N., & Bohner, G. (1996). Feelings and their motivational implactions: Mood and the action sequence. In P. M. Gollwitzer & J. A. Bargh, (Eds.), The psychology of action: Linking cognition and motivation to behavior (pp. 119–145). New York: Guilford Press.

Schwarz, N., & Clore, G. L. (1983). Mood, misattribution, and judgments of well-being: Informative and directive functions of affective states. Journal of Personality and Social Psychology, 45, 513–523.

Schwarz, N., & Clore, G. L. (1996). Feelings and phenomenal experiences. In E. T. Higgins & A. Kruglanski (Eds.), Social psychology: Handbook of basic principles (pp. 433–465). New York: Guilford Press.

Sinclair, R. C., Mark, M. M., & Clore, G. L. (1994). Mood-related persuasion depends on misattributions. Social Cognition, 12, 309–326.

Snyder, M., & Uranowitz, S. W. (1978). Reconstructing the past: Some cognitive consequences of person perception. Journal of Personality and Social Psychology, 36, 941–950.

Srull, T. K., & Wyer, R. S., Jr. (1989). Person memory and judgment. Psychological Review, 96, 58–83.

Stangor, C., & Duan, C. (1991). Effects of multiple task demands upon memory for information about social groups. Journal of Experimental Social Psychology, 27, 357–378.

Stangor, C., & McMillan, D. (1992). Memory for expectancy-congruent and expectancy-incongruent information: A review of the social and social developmental literatures. Psychological Bulletin, 111, 42–61.

Taylor, S. E. (1981). The interface of cognitive and social psychology. In J. Harvey (Ed.), Cognition, social behavior, and the environment (pp. 189–211). Hillsdale, NJ: Erlbaum.

Tetlock, P. E. (1983). Accountability and complexity of thought. Journal of Personality and Social Psychology, 45, 74–83.

Wegener, D. T., & Petty, R. E. (1994). Mood management across affective states: The hedonic contingency hypothesis. Journal of Personality and Social Psychology, 66, 1034–1048.

Wegener, D. T., Petty, R. E., & Smith, S.M. (1995). Positive mood can increase or decrease message scrunity: The hedonic contingency view of mood and message processing. Journal of Personality and Social Psychology, 69, 5–15.

Worth, L. T., & Mackie, D. M. (1987). Cognitive mediation of positive affect in persuasion. Social Cognition, 5, 76–94.

Wyer, R. S., Jr., & Srull, T. K. (1989). Memory and cognition in its social context. Hillsdale, NJ: Erlbaum.

22

Affect in Attitude

IMMEDIATE AND DELIBERATIVE PERSPECTIVES

ROGER GINER-SOROLLA

I have, I said, heard a story which I believe, that Leontius, the son of Aglaion, as he came up from the Piraeus on the outside of the northern wall, saw the executioner with some corpses lying near him. Leontius felt a strong desire to look at them, but at the same time he was disgusted and turned away. For a time he struggled with himself and covered his face, but then, overcome by his desire, pushing his eyes wide open and rushing toward the corpses: "Look for yourselves," he said, "you evil things, get your fill of the beautiful sight!"—I've heard that story myself.

It certainly proves, I said, that anger sometimes wars against the appetites as one thing against another.—It does.

Besides, I said, we often see this elsewhere, when his appetites are forcing a man to act contrary to reason, and he rails at himself and is angry with that within himself which is compelling him to do so; of the two civic factions at odds, as it were, the spirited part becomes the ally of reason . . .

—PLATO, *Republic, IV* (ca. 370–360 B.C./1974, pp. 103–104)

This passage occurs in the midst of one of the earliest and most influential schemes in Western psychological thought—Plato's three-part classification of psychological functions in the *Republic*. The example of Leontius expands the *Republic*'s model of the psyche beyond pre-Socratic concepts of the struggle between reason and appetite, and even beyond Plato's previous metaphor of the soul in the *Phaedrus*—a chariot whose driver must discipline the unruly black horse of desire, and favor the obedient white horse of reason. Now Plato acknowledges a third, "spirited" part of the soul, alike in kind to the other two, but having a special hybrid nature: emotional in its expression, yet always responsive to the dictates of reason.

McGuire (1969) has identified the three parts of Plato's scheme as a distant relation of modern concepts of attitude as a tripartite construct made up of affective, cognitive, and behavioral components. Although this identification is a reasonable one, I would like to use Plato's scheme in a different way—to make a point about the single category of "affect" as it is used in psychology, and particularly in the psychology of attitudes. Specifically, just as Plato identifies two different kinds of emotional process at war within Leonidas, I believe that various theorists and researchers have used the term "affect" to refer to two different kinds of material within the attitude, and the term "affective attitude" to refer to two different kinds of phenomena that can yield an evaluative judgment.

Dual-process theories of social cognition

441

typically stress the distinction between relatively easy and thoughtless cognitive processes on the one hand, and relatively difficult and thoughtful cognitive processes on the other (e.g., Chaiken, Giner-Sorolla, & Chen, 1996; Epstein, 1994; Langer, 1989; Petty & Cacioppo, 1986; Trope, 1986). I hope to draw a similar distinction between two affective processes in the area of attitudes. One of these can be characterized as *"immediate affect"*—feelings and emotions that are activated rapidly and effortlessly upon identification of the attitude object. The other can be characterized as *"deliberative affect."* This includes feelings and emotions that are activated later on, in response to other objects associated with the attitude object; it also includes emotions activated slowly and intentionally, as part of a self-regulatory process that has not yet been fully automatized.

The individual components of an attitude do usually tend toward evaluative consistency (Rosenberg & Hovland, 1960; Zanna & Rempel, 1988). But at the same time, the conceptual value of any scheme of attitude components rests most crucially upon those cases in which the valence of one component conflicts with that of the others. We can speak of separate cognitive and behavioral components of an attitude, rather than of cognitive and behavioral expressions of a single attitude, because we sometimes find ourselves thinking one thing but doing another. Statistically, too, empirical validations of the tripartite model of attitudes (e.g., Breckler, 1984; Kothandapani, 1971; Ostrom, 1969) have typically rested on finding evaluative differences and similarities among measures of each proposed attitude component.[1] Although in many cases immediate and deliberative affect will lead to similar evaluative outcomes, there are also objects and situations that will be likely to pit deliberative affect against immediate affect.

PRELIMINARY NOTES ON TERMINOLOGY

Both historically and today, there have been considerable differences in psychologists' use of such basic terms as "emotion," "attitude," "cognition," and "evaluation." Because of this, several terms that appear in my analysis

of affect and attitudes require some clarification against a backdrop of historical and current usage. The last and most important of these terms is "affect" itself. In particular, I argue that the use of "affect" to refer to both deliberative and immediate affective processes has clouded the distinction between the two.

"Attitude"

Two characteristics of "attitude" have remained fairly constant across 20th-century definitions, and these characteristics are useful in specifying what constitutes affect within attitude. First, an attitude is organized around responses to a real or imagined *object* (e.g., Allport, 1935; Eagly & Chaiken, 1993; McGuire, 1969; Thurstone, 1931). This excludes the use of the term "affective attitude" in psychology to refer to a global, objectless mood, although it is certainly true that such affect has a pervasive and complex influence upon more specific attitudes (Forgas, 1992; Schwarz, 1990).

Second, an attitude is *evaluative* in nature—that is, organized around the basic categories of "good" and "bad." Some theorists have questioned the unconditional equation of attitude with evaluation. Allport (1935), for one, doubted the wisdom of entirely reducing attitude to a "for–against" distinction, and his skepticism was later echoed by McGuire (1969). Contemporaneously, Thurstone (1931) took pains to separate the attitude itself from the evaluatively relevant beliefs and emotions that might underlie it; later, Katz and Stotland (1959) would specifically exclude unconscious evaluative associations from consideration as attitudes. More recently, Cacioppo and Petty (1993) have made a distinction between affect, which is conceived as a transitory feeling state, and the attitude itself, which is conceived as a more stable, propositionally represented general evaluation.

However, others have widened the attitude concept to include virtually all mental phenomena with positive or negative implications for a given object: beliefs, emotions, feelings, conditioned responses, behavioral intentions, and the influence of past behaviors (Eagly & Chaiken, 1993; Greenwald, 1968). In such views, the attitude is a potentially vast memory network with several distinct components, each of which consists of evaluatively relevant associations to a specific object. Qualitative distinctions within the attitude are accounted for as differences among the evaluative valence, strength, and accessibility of the attitude system's separate components. A cognitively based attitude, for example, is one in which the object is associated with many beliefs, but relatively fewer feelings or behavioral memories. It is this broader definition of "attitude" that I use, so that this treatment of affect within attitude can include processes both unconscious and conscious—primitive affective associations, as well as complex, emotionally laden opinions.

"Evaluation"

The term "evaluation" itself needs to be handled with care, because of recent attempts to establish a separate evaluative component within the attitude. Zanna and Rempel (1988) have proposed that an attitude is a "summary evaluation" based on evaluative information such as beliefs, feelings, and behaviors—information that, in the broader definition of attitude, is part of the attitude itself. A summary evaluation may be measured by a general opinion question concerning the object. In another context, Breckler and Wiggins (1989, 1991) have drawn a theoretical and empirical distinction between evaluation, as measured by semantic-differential questions with stems implying objective judgment (e.g., "Legalized abortion *is* . . . good/bad"), and affect, as measured by responses to the same questions subjectively worded (e.g., "Legalized abortion *makes me feel* . . . good/bad").

Nonetheless, I apply the term "evaluation" more generally, to refer not only to a conscious, objective decision about an object's value, but to any mental process associating a valence with an object. Thus the overall evaluation of an object, thought still important, needs to be referred to specifically as the "summary evaluation," to distinguish it from the evaluation implicit in beliefs, feelings, behaviors, and other components and expressions of attitude. Specifically, the term "evaluation" as proposed by Breckler and Wiggins (1989) may need to be qualified as "summary evaluation" within my terminology; both "affect" and "evaluation" are evaluative dimensions, insofar as they are organized around the distinction between positive and negative.

"Cognitive"

Psychologists have been accustomed to use the term "cognitive" to refer to processes involving deliberate, conscious, propositional thought, often in contrast to variously defined "affective" processes. Attitude researchers, in particular, typically measure the "cognitive" component of attitudes by asking people to report upon their beliefs about the objective attributes or consequences of an object (e.g., Crites, Fabrigar, & Petty, 1994; Millar & Tesser, 1989; Rosenberg, 1956, 1960). A more general use of "cognition," though, refers to "anything that is said to be mentally represented" (Mandler, 1982, p. 6). In this latter sense, cognition necessarily encompasses very quick, automatic processes, including what has been called the "cognitive unconscious" (Kihlstrom, 1987). Such a disagreement over the term "cognitive" has been a point of contention in the debate over whether emotions and affect are cognitively mediated, given that they can be activated immediately and automatically (Lazarus, 1982, 1984; Mandler, 1982; Zajonc, 1984).

Nevertheless, there has been considerable agreement in both theory and measurement that the cognitive component of an attitude refers not to all mental representations, but specifically to *beliefs* about an attitude object (Chaiken, Pomerantz, & Giner-Sorolla, 1995; Greenwald, 1968; Krech & Crutchfield, 1948; Rosenberg & Hovland, 1960; Smith, 1947). In these schemes, beliefs can be characterized as associations between the object (e.g., "cake") and another concept (e.g., "has calories") that is not itself an evaluation or emotion, but whose evaluation may color the evaluation of the attitude object (cf. Insko & Schopler, 1967). In line with traditional methods of measurement, I define the cognitive component of attitude as consisting of propositional beliefs about the object that can be expressed explicitly and deliberatively. All the same, the demonstrated existence of implicit and automatic beliefs, such as trait schemas, other schemas, and unconsciously activated stereotype categories (Andersen & Cole, 1990; Bargh & Pietromonaco, 1982; Devine, 1989; Greenwald & Banaji, 1995; Wyer &

Srull, 1981), presents a special problem for this view of the cognitive component. It may remain for a future treatment of attitude structure to arrange the cognitive component along an immediate–deliberative continuum, in the way I propose to analyze the affective component.

"Affect"

Affect as Evaluation

Early attitude theorists used the term "affect" almost exclusively to indicate an attitude's evaluative sign, without implying it to be emotional or arousing in nature (e.g., Allport, 1935; Smith, 1947; Katz & Stotland, 1959; Insko & Schopler, 1967). Even when an author suggested that measures of physiological arousal may indicate attitudinal affect (Rosenberg & Hovland, 1960; McGuire, 1969), the overall definition of the term remained an evaluative one. But more recently, attitude theorists have used "affect" to refer to processes more specific than evaluation; for example, Rosenberg's (1956) construct of "affective–cognitive consistency" has had to be renamed "evaluative–cognitive consistency" to avoid confusion with more restrictive uses of "affect" (Chaiken et al., 1995).

In some areas of study, though, the former use of "affect" to signify "evaluation" still holds. Thus, some recent studies on priming contrast "affective," or evaluative, judgment against other kinds of categorization (e.g., Kitayama, 1990), and Fiske and Pavelchak's (1986) model of category-based and piecemeal "affect" is essentially a model of how evaluations of people are formed. In a view of "attitude" that already encompasses most evaluative phenomena, using "affect" in this way would be redundant. But in examining the psychological literature for more specific usages of "affect," I have found that it has been used to refer to two potentially distinct types of evaluative phenomena: on the one hand, those that are quick and immediate; and on the other, those that are associated with emotional experience.

Affect as Immediate Evaluation

Greenwald (1968), in analyzing the tripartite model of attitudes, provided one of the earliest points of departure in attitude research from the equation of affect with evaluative sign. In Greenwald's model, the affective component is a separate subsystem within the attitude, with its origins to be found in processes of classical conditioning. Later reviews, too, have classified the conditioning of attitudes—in which stimuli or responses acquire the valence of other stimuli through mere association—as an "affective" process (e.g., Eagly & Chaiken, 1993). Although some studies demonstrating classical conditioning have included emotion words among the unconditioned stimuli (Staats & Staats, 1958; de Houwer, Baeyens, & Eelen, 1994), others have used less obviously emotional unconditioned stimuli, such as food names and attitude statements (Staats, Minke, Martin, & Higa, 1972; Byrne & Clore, 1970). Conditioning appears to be implicated as a purely affective process, not because it always involves the emotions, but because it represents the transfer of evaluative meaning from one concept to another without conscious thought—that is, "immediate" in the etymological sense of "not mediated" by deliberative cognition.

Zajonc's (1980) influential arguments for "affective primacy" have also fostered the view of "affect" as an evaluative system that is immediately activated. Affect, in Zajonc's view, is to be understood primarily as evaluative preference: "This article is confined to those aspects of affect and feeling that are generally involved in preferences. . . . Thus, for the present purposes, other emotions such as surprise, anger, guilt, or shame . . . are ignored" (p. 152). Consistent with this definition, Zajonc takes the subliminal "mere-exposure" effect as evidence of the rapid workings of affect. In this phenomenon, previous exposure to abstract shapes increases liking for them, even when the shapes are presented tachistoscopically at exposure durations that are too brief to allow conscious recognition (Kunst-Wilson & Zajonc, 1980). It is unlikely that these irregular octagons evoke actual emotions. Instead, Zajonc is arguing for the rapid and unconscious operation of the association of positive and negative value with an object—preference, but not necessarily passion.

More recently, the rapidity of affective processes has been implicated in experiments showing that positive or negative facial expressions influence, or "prime," the evaluation of neutral targets only at very rapid, suboptimal presentation times (e.g., 4 milliseconds [ms]). By contrast, cognitive categorizations such as gender and symmetry are only primed at longer exposure durations (Murphy, Monahan, & Zajonc, 1995; Murphy & Zajonc, 1993; see also Edwards, 1991; Krosnick, Betz, Jussim, Lynn, & Stephens, 1992). Again, the rapid activation of evaluative meaning is taken as evidence that affect is often accessed without effortful cognitive mediation. Even though the priming stimuli are facial expressions carrying emotional meaning, these studies have mainly concerned themselves with the transfer of positive and negative evaluation to fairly unemotional stimuli, such as Chinese ideograms.[2]

Converging evidence that evaluation can be very rapid comes from recent experiments demonstrating evaluative priming in a different paradigm (Bargh, Chaiken, Govender, & Pratto, 1992; Bargh, Chaiken, Raymond, & Hymes, 1996; Fazio, Sanbonmatsu, Powell, & Kardes, 1986; Giner-Sorolla, Garcia, & Bargh, in press; Hermans, de Houwer, & Eelen, 1996). These experiments have used a longer prime presentation interval, typically 250 ms with a 50-ms blank interval before the target stimulus is presented. The target is a word of clear evaluative meaning, and the participant's task is either to judge the word as positive or negative, or merely to pronounce the word. The prime can be consciously recognized, but its presentation interval is still too fast to allow for deliberate processing; yet the presentation of the prime tends to speed responses to same-valence targets, relative to different-valence ones. This work is usually characterized as dealing with evaluation or attitude rather than with affect, but it demonstrates a similar phenomenon: the mind can respond on the basis of an evaluative category before deliberative thought can take place.

These perspectives, then, suggest one possible way to differentiate affect from evaluation in general—by assigning the term "affect" only to evaluative processes that occur without necessarily involving deliberative thought, in a manner similar to Greenwald and Banaji's (1995) use of the term "implicit attitude." This seems to be the intent, for example, behind Edwards's (1990) use of the term "affective" to characterize attitude formation and change based on suboptimal con-

ditioning and odor association, as opposed to "cognitive" attitude change and formation based on persuasive messages. Murphy and Zajonc (1993), in contrast, specify that "affect" can refer not only to cognitively unmediated evaluative processes, such as the suboptimal priming effect of a face's emotional expression, but also to evaluative processes that are mediated by slower appraisals. However, this perspective apparently equates affect with all evaluative processes, whereas the notion that "affect" refers only to immediate evaluation uses the term in a more specific way.

Affect as Emotional Response

In attitude psychology, a quite different point of departure from the older idea of affect as evaluative sign can also be traced to Greenwald (1968): specifically, the assertion that although the affective component of attitude is formed primarily through conditioning, it is expressed primarily through *emotional* responses. In fact, clinical psychologists had previously used the term "affect" to connote processes of emotion and arousal, rather than mere evaluation. To give a notable example, Jung (1922/1923) characterized the mental function of "feeling" as an immediate evaluative appraisal, but went on to specify that "affect" is "a state of feeling accompanied by appreciable bodily innervations" (p. 544). A similar idea began to make itself known in social psychology subsequent to Greenwald's model, as attempts to validate the tripartite model of attitude (e.g., Bagozzi, 1978; Breckler, 1984; Kothandapani, 1971; Ostrom, 1969) used questions about specific emotional responses to the object as a distinctive measure of the affective component.

More recently, many researchers have used explicit self-report measures of object-associated emotions to operationalize the affective component of attitude (e.g., Abelson, Kinder, Peters, & Fiske, 1982; Millar & Millar, 1990; Edwards & von Hippel, 1995; Chaiken et al., 1995). In a particularly well-defined and validated study of the affective and cognitive components of attitude, Crites et al. (1994) define the affective component as consisting of "discrete, qualitatively different emotions" (p. 621) with clear evaluative implications. This definition of affective attitude is not far from those of other recent theoretical perspectives on attitude structure (e.g., Chaiken & Stangor, 1987; Zanna & Rempel, 1988). It seems, then, that much work on affect in attitudes has been carried out under a definition of "affect" as explicitly expressable emotions, rather than as a simple evaluation that can be formed rapidly and activated automatically.

IMMEDIATE EVALUATION AND EMOTIONS

These two views of affect in attitudes are based on different definitions—one emphasizing immediacy, the other emphasizing emotional content. But do they refer to different processes? That is, can the valence of immediate evaluations of an object always be expected to correspond to the summed valence of all emotional responses to the object?

The question of how closely emotions are linked to immediate processes, rather than more deliberative ones, has hung over two of psychology's most famous controversies over the nature of emotions. The James–Lange theory of emotions (James, 1890; Lange, 1922) argued that the experience of emotion is derived from the perception of visceral changes in a situation, rather than from the situation itself. A similar controversy attended the views of Schachter and Singer (1962), who interpreted emotional experience as a cognitive attribution of arousal. In contrast to these views, which both characterize emotional experience as a mediated process, other investigators of emotion have argued that many emotional experiences occur spontaneously upon the perception of relevant stimuli, without introspection or self-perception (e.g., Cannon, 1927; Plutchik & Ax, 1969).

Appraisal theories of emotion have provided one possible resolution by proposing that emotions can arise from rapid cognitive appraisals of features of the environment, accounting for the often immediate nature of emotions (e.g., Arnold, 1960; Lazarus, 1991; Ortony, Clore, & Collins, 1988; Smith & Ellsworth, 1985). In addition, most appraisal theories place the evaluation of a situation as positive or negative early in the sequence of appraisal, leading to the distinction between pleasant and unpleasant emotions. Assuming

in the first place that all emotions are caused by immediate appraisals of an object, and in the second place that all immediately evaluated objects arouse emotions, one might expect the valence of emotions to correspond closely to the valence of immediate evaluation.

There are reasons to doubt both of these assumptions. Not all emotions are likely to arise immediately on perceiving an object; in fact, most appraisal theories of emotion specify that appraisals are cognitive categorizations, which may be made immediately or slowly, and which may be modified by subsequent thought. Late-arriving cognitive interpretations can heighten an emotional experience, as when I retrospectively magnify an insult of little consequence into a cause for hatred; can subdue it, as when I try to mitigate the impact of losing a friend by thinking of all the friends I still have; or can change its qualitative nature, as when the realization of my own responsibility for a misdeed turns anger to guilt. Cognitive theories of coping (Lazarus, 1966) and anger (Berkowitz & Heimer, 1989), as well as the cognitive therapy of emotional disorders (Beck, 1976), rely on the ability of deliberation to produce a more positive emotional state both among people under stress and among depressive people, for whom negative emotions are often immediately, automatically activated (cf. Bargh & Tota, 1988).

Other theorists (e.g., Arieti, 1970) have also remarked that emotions can respond both to immediate stimuli such as physical sensations and images, and to potentially deliberative forms of thought and symbolic representation. More recently, Leventhal (1984) has offered a perceptual–motor theory of emotion, synthesizing three major perspectives on emotion into a single model. According to Leventhal, three mutually reinforcing systems contribute to the experience of emotion: expressive–motor, schematic, and conceptual. The expressive–motor system mainly includes facial expressions of emotion, and may be activated by the other systems or in turn may activate them—such as when a person "puts on a smile" and consequently feels happy. The schematic system is an automatic memory system in which emotions are associated directly with specific stimuli; for example, an individual's phobia of a caged snake can largely be attributed to schematic activation. The conceptual system is a more sophisticated system in which rules guide the interpretation and generation of emotional experiences; for example, a phobic individual undergoing desensitization therapy may have to use the conceptual system to reduce the fear of a harmless snake in a cage, by realizing that the fear is inappropriate.

These theoretical perspectives suggest that although emotions can be evoked immediately, via automatic appraisals or primitive associations, they are also capable of being evoked or controlled through more deliberative processes of appraisal and thought. A definition of the affective component of attitude that encompasses the evaluative consequences of *all* emotions aroused by the attitude object, then, may potentially include emotions whose evaluative consequences are different from those of immediately activated evaluation. To update Plato's example slightly, a driver's immediate reaction upon seeing the empty wrecks of six cars piled on the shoulder of the Interstate may be one of slightly positive interest, or even fascination. But, upon thinking of the consequences of this spectacle to the cars' drivers, and especially upon imagining himself or herself in the driver's seat of one of the wrecked cars, the driver may well experience more negative emotions of anxiety. Self-regulation, too, may bring up negative emotions of guilt in connection with the wreck, as the driver berates himself or herself for initially reacting with morbid interest instead of with horror and compassion.

Just as object-related emotions may arise after an immediate evaluation has been made, so immediate evaluations may arise in the absence of any emotional response. To give a concrete example, consider the University of Virginia football stadium. I may acquire an unconscious preference for this edifice via mere exposure, because I pass it on the way to the office every day; however, it is unlikely that my liking will manifest itself in felt and expressed emotion, as opposed to unemotional evaluation. Some support for this possibility comes from recent evaluative-priming experiments indicating that the immediate evaluation is accessed within 300 ms even for weakly and presumably unemotionally evaluated stimuli, such as the words "tree" and

"tuna" (Bargh et al., 1995), and from others demonstrating that novel nonsense words have evaluative-priming effects as a consequence of their phonetic characteristics (Garcia & Bargh, 1994).

Immediate evaluation and emotions in an attitude, then, will have the same valence if all associated emotions are evoked immediately upon perceiving or imagining the attitude object, or if emotions that are not evoked immediately are still consistent with the initial evaluation of the object. However, if the attitude object does not evoke any emotions in a person, or if it evokes differently valenced emotions after the person thinks about it deliberatively, then the emotional implications of the object are likely to be different from the immediate evaluation of the object.

The affect associated with an object, then, can be characterized along a continuum ranging from immediate to deliberative. The most immediate affective reactions are basic evaluative associations and emotions that are activated rapidly and without conscious intervention; deliberative affect consists of those emotions that come into play more slowly, as a result of conscious thought about the attitude object. An object can evoke both immediate and deliberative affective responses, and like any two elements in an attitude system, these responses will often have a similar valence. However, under certain circumstances, rapidly accessed feelings and emotions will have different evaluative implications for an object, when compared to feelings and emotions that are less quickly accessible. In such cases, the extent to which deliberative feelings actually influence behavior and judgment may depend on the amount of time, ability, and motivation a person can call upon to bring them forth.

IMMEDIATE AND DELIBERATIVE AFFECT

Automaticity of Immediate and Deliberative Affect

The distinction I wish to draw between immediate and deliberative affect bears a marked resemblance to the distinctions typically drawn between "automatic" and "controlled" processes in the study of affect and elsewhere (LaBerge, 1981; Spielman, Pratto, & Bargh, 1988). Recently, though, several distinct criteria of automaticity have been identified (Bargh, 1989; Neumann, 1984). The most prototypical automatic process, perhaps, is that which requires minimal effort, occurs outside of awareness, is not under conscious control, and operates spontaneously rather than intentionally; yet many processes that have been labeled as "automatic" fit some of these four criteria, but not others (Bargh, 1994). Which criteria, then, are most relevant to the immediate–deliberative distinction?

In my view, deliberative affect depends upon the ability to think consciously and reflectively about the attitude object, either through verbal reasoning or through a more image-based memory search. This process takes time and cognitive capacity. For this reason, I see effortlessness as the criterion of automaticity that best captures the nature of immediate affect. Because it occurs effortlessly upon perceiving or imagining the attitude object, immediate affect has several advantages over deliberative affect. It is more accessible, arriving earlier in the time course of processing when attention is fixed on the object; it can be activated when the object appears only momentarily; and it may possibly occur even when attention is disrupted by cognitive load, by competing tasks, or by masking of the stimulus (see Greenwald, Klinger, & Liu, 1989).

Of course, this analysis suggests a continuum of greater and lesser degrees of accessibility, so that a reaction obtained at a stimulus exposure time of 200 ms is more immediate than one that needs 1,000 ms in which to show itself, yet less immediate than one that needs only 5 ms. Pending further investigation, a reasonable place to fix a boundary between automatic and controlled processes on the immediate–deliberative continuum might be at 500–750 ms of required processing time. Evaluative priming experiments typically find an immediate, automatic effect of prime valence upon judgments at prime exposures ranging from 3 to 500 ms, and no such effect at prime exposures greater than 1,000 ms (Fazio et al., 1986; Hermans et al., 1996; Murphy & Zajonc, 1993). Presumably, at longer exposure times, more deliberative processes attenuate the immediate impact

of evaluative priming (Bornstein, 1989; Kihlstrom, 1987). The proposed boundary is also consistent with experiments using nonevaluative stimuli, which suggest that automatic spreading activation, rather than a more controlled process of facilitation and inhibition, characterizes stimulus effects in the first 500 ms of processing time (Neely, 1977; Posner & Snyder, 1975).

Because we humans have to be aware of a thing before we can reflect on it, I consider it unlikely that deliberative affect can be evoked by something presented outside of consciousness. Nevertheless, immediate affect does not always occur in response to stimuli perceived outside of consciousness. A smiling face, for example, is certainly able to evoke a rapid positive response even if we know we have seen it. A more interesting question is whether immediate affect typically occurs without awareness of the *process* of evaluation, even when the stimulus is perceived clearly (cf. Bargh, 1992).

Most likely, the basic process of immediate evaluation occurs without our being aware of it, and without necessarily having an explicit goal to evaluate the object. Bargh et al. (1995, Experiment 3) found a strong evaluative-priming effect upon response times even when none of the stimuli were explicitly evaluative in nature, and when the participants' task was merely to pronounce, rather than evaluate, the target word. Fazio, Jackson, Dunton, and Williams (1995), too, found evaluative-priming effects; they used an elaborate cover story for the paradigm, which employed picture primes representing members of different ethnic groups. As anticipated, most participants were not aware that their evaluations of the pictures were being studied.[3] Most recently, Winkielman, Zajonc, and Schwarz (1997) found that the effects of happy and unhappy facial expressions presented at subliminal durations upon evaluation of subsequently presented Chinese ideograms were not accompanied by any consciously reported awareness of positive or negative feelings. These subliminal effects also resisted misattribution manipulations, in which participants were told (correctly) that any feelings they might have about the ideograms were due to the presentation of subliminal stimuli.

Finally, what role does intentional control play in immediate and deliberative affect? Generally speaking, because immediate affect occurs rapidly and effortlessly, and often outside awareness, we might expect control processes to be fairly ineffectual in regulating its initial influence (Fiske, 1989). Work on the controlled suppression of emotional reactions, for example, suggests that although such an effort may reduce self-reports of affective experience, it will have little effect upon, and perhaps will even increase, objective indicators of emotional arousal such as galvanic skin response (Koriat, Melkman, Averill, & Lazarus, 1972). Little is known, however, of the effectiveness of control upon the basic, immediate evaluation of objects—for example, when people not only are made aware of evaluative primes (as in Winkielman et al., 1997), but are also told to consciously try to nullify their influence. Certainly, people's best efforts may allow them to alter their controlled judgments so as to nullify the effects of priming (Fiske, 1989; Wegener & Petty, 1995). But it is less clear whether controlled processes may intervene in an automatic expression of attitude, as they may intervene to quell automatic expression of gender stereotypes (Blair & Banaji, 1996).

It is equally unclear whether deliberative affect always responds to conscious control. Because deliberative emotions can arise from intentional thought processes, it is possible to activate them as part of a process of self-control or self-regulation (Carver & Scheier, 1990; Clark & Isen, 1982; Higgins, 1991). The activation of deliberative emotions in a process of self-control occurs in many important personal situations, as when a dieter confronting a cheesecake thinks about extreme obesity to arouse disgust, or when a filmgoer watching a disturbing scene thinks of happier things. It should be noted that what is under control in these instances is not the emotion itself, which arises spontaneously, but the thoughts evoking that particular emotion.

Despite these examples, I do not see all deliberative affect as consequent upon controlled thinking. Deliberative emotions may also arise as a result of an undirected process of association. For example, the image of a masked surgeon may provoke in me an immediate dread of sickness and invasive medical procedures. However, as I think more about the situation, emotions arising from more distantly associated concepts—trust in the medical profession, vicarious pride in a friend who is an MD, fear of *not* being able to get medical treatment—may arise and mitigate the initial negative reaction. Alternatively, my deliberative thoughts about surgery may dwell even more obsessively on images of blood, organs, surgical instruments left inside the patient, and the like; in this case, the deliberate affect accompanying these ruminative thoughts may transform an immediate mild shudder into a full-blown panic attack (cf. Martin & Tesser, 1989). In either case, my deliberative emotions do not necessarily follow an explicit self-regulatory goal. Rather, they are evoked in the course of free association, along the lines of James's (1890) notion of the "stream of consciousness."

In addition, processes of self-regulation themselves often become automatized so that they need not depend on intent (Carver & Scheier, 1990; Kuhl & Kraska, 1993). An experienced dieter, for example, may feel deliberative emotions of guilt following the immediate desire for the fattening cheesecake, but without the explicit intention of making himself or herself feel guilty; a new dieter, however, may very well need to intentionally remind or himself herself of dieting goals in order to feel the same emotions. Because they depend on conscious control, the inexperienced dieter's self-conscious emotions may be even more "deliberative" than the experienced dieter's, taking more time to be activated and occurring less predictably.

To go one step further, the process of self-control may become so efficiently automatized that self-regulating affect becomes immediate, rather than deliberative, and outside intentional control. The social learning of the emotion of disgust is a good example of a self-regulatory process that becomes automatized (Elias, 1939/1978; Rozin & Fallon, 1987). As an example, very young children will unhesitatingly pick up and eat food that has fallen on the ground. If a child's elders see this appalling behavior, reprimands quickly ensue: "That's gross!" "Don't pick it up, it's dirty." Eventually, the taboo against fallen food becomes an immediate affective reaction, and many of us would have qualms about eating a piece of cake directly off a section of kitchen floor that had been sterilized more thoroughly than any plate (see also

Rozin & Nemeroff, 1990). In fact, in situations where immediate, uncontrolled self-regulatory responses are recognized as inappropriate, we may have to enlist later-activated emotions against them—as when shame and compassion encourage a person to overcome irrational beliefs about contagion and hug an acquaintance who has been diagnosed with AIDS.

MEASURES AND MANIPULATIONS OF AFFECTIVE ATTITUDE

In light of this theoretical distinction between the immediate and the deliberative affective attitude, it is instructive to review existing research methodologies that have been characterized as tapping the affective attitude, and to classify each measure and manipulation as dealing primarily with immediate or deliberative aspects of affect. As a general principle to guide this taxonomy, I propose that procedures requiring little deliberation or awareness will be more likely to access immediate affect, whereas those that require active introspection about feelings and emotions will be more likely to access deliberative affect.

Measures of Affective Attitude

Many measures of affective attitude ask the respondent to report the feelings and emotions typically aroused by an object. These measures, because they potentially include all conscious emotional associations with the object, are most likely to reflect primarily the deliberative affective attitude. In addition, as the measure becomes more specific in naming emotional experiences that may be associated with the attitude object, it will become more likely to reflect deliberative rather than immediate emotions. In effect, a list of specific emotions in an affective-attitude questionnaire is a recognition memory task, asking the respondent to reflect upon his or her attitude and to think about whether each emotion is ever associated with that object. As such, it is more likely to reflect the sum of all available emotional associations, rather than to reflect only those that are accessible and immediate.

Researchers seeking to measure attitudinal affect often provide a list of specific emotions such as "fear" and "love," and ask respondents to characterize the extent to which the attitude object evokes each emotion. Abelson et al. (1982) have used this method to study affective attitude toward political candidates; Stangor, Sullivan, and Ford (1991), and Eagly, Mladinic, and Otto (1994), to study the affective bases of prejudiced attitudes; and Zuwerink and Devine (1996), to study affective reactions to persuasive messages about gays in the military. Specific-emotion checklists or scales have also appeared in multimeasure validations of the concept of affective attitude, such as those by Ostrom (1969), Breckler (1984), and Breckler and Wiggins (1989). Finally, recent attempts to establish a standardized measure of the affective component of attitude across attitude objects (Chaiken et al., 1995; Crites et al., 1994) have relied on bipolar scales anchored by one positive-emotion and one negative-emotion term. All of these explicit measures, because they encourage an active search of memory for specific emotions associated with the attitude object, are most likely to be associated with deliberative affect.

Thought listing is an alternate measure of affective attitude, used either in its own right or to validate manipulations of affective attitude. The participant can be instructed either to write down all feelings and emotions he or she feels toward the attitude object (e.g., Millar & Millar, 1990; Millar & Tesser, 1989), or simply to write down all thoughts evoked by the attitude object, which are then coded according to whether they represent a feeling or emotion (e.g., Zuwerink & Devine, 1996). The valence of thoughts is assessed by having the respondent or an independent coder rate each statement. Although the thought-listing method does not explicitly provide a list of emotions, it still appears quite likely to capture emotions that are deliberatively associated with the attitude object—especially when the respondent is given a relatively long time (e.g., 3 minutes, as in Millar & Millar, 1990) and is told specifically to list affective states.

Implicit measures of attitude (Greenwald & Banaji, 1995), on the other hand, are most likely to tap immediate affect. Like implicit measures of memory (Roediger & McDermott, 1993), implicit measures of attitude do not engage deliberative processes in responding. The automatic-evaluative-priming paradigm (Fazio et al., 1986) has already been used as an implicit measure of attitudes toward pictures of people of diverse races; investigators calculate whether a given picture, when used as a prime, tends to facilitate responding to positive or negative targets (Fazio et al., 1995). This measure shows quite low correlations with explicit measures of prejudice, but greater correlations with implicit behavioral indicators, such as perceived friendliness in a cross-race interaction.

Fazio et al.'s (1995) implicit measure has been presented mainly as a way of bypassing self-presentational bias, and of getting to the "real attitude" rather than to any specific component of the attitude. All the same, it is also possible that the implicit measure primarily measures immediate affect in the attitude, and that other, equally genuine affective components of the attitude might surface if deliberative affect were to be measured. For example, persons with immediately negative reactions to different-race faces may still experience deliberative feelings with more positive evaluative consequences for other races: positive emotions based on ideals of equality (Katz & Hass, 1988), or feelings of guilt and compunction based on antiprejudice ideals (Devine, Monteith, Zuwerink, & Elliot, 1991). In any event, evaluative priming appears to be the most promising technique available to measure the immediate affective attitude.

Manipulations of Affective Attitude

Some studies have sought to manipulate, rather than merely to measure, the affective or cognitive nature of an attitude, by creating attitudes that are based primarily on affective or cognitive material. As in the measures just discussed, some manipulations of affective attitude use deliberative means to establish an affective attitude; that is, participants are asked to think actively about the emotions and feelings associated with the attitude object. Other manipulations can be said to engage more immediate processes; that is, the attitude object is associated with positive or negative stimuli without the participants' knowledge.

To instill an affective attitude, some experiments have used a focus procedure, in which participants are told to think about their feelings toward the object for a period of time. By contrast, to instill a cognitive attitude, participants are told to engage in introspection about the reasons for their attitude, or why they feel the way they do about the object. These manipulations of affective attitude are influential in several ways: They increase the predominance of feelings versus beliefs in free thought listings (Millar & Tesser, 1986, 1989; Millar & Millar, 1990; Wilson & Dunn, 1986); and they also increase self-reported emotionality (Edwards & von Hippel, 1995). Almost by definition, focus manipulations can be said to strengthen the availability and accessibility of the deliberative affective attitude, since they involve actively thinking about the feelings and emotions that the attitude object arouses.

Another explicit manipulation of affective attitude, perhaps used more in politics and advertising than in laboratory research, is the use of rhetoric and imagery to link the attitude object to emotions. One classic study on the effectiveness of fear appeals (e.g., Janis & Feshbach, 1953) contrasted vivid accounts of the consequences of poor dental hygiene with more abstract messages, to demonstrate the sometimes paradoxical influence of strong emotions upon persuasion. More recently, Edwards and von Hippel (1995), in addition to the thought-focusing manipulation previously described, used the relative primacy of sentimental and unsentimental autobiographical narratives to manipulate the affective or cognitive basis of attitudes toward a person. However, neither study explicitly measured the extent to which these manipulations actually created an attitude with affective or cognitive content.

Even if such emotion-arousing rhetoric is assumed to be effective in creating primarily affect-based attitudes, whether it creates deliberative or immediate affective attitudes may depend on the depth to which the message can be, and is, processed (cf. Petty & Cacioppo, 1986). If the message only influences attitudes by pairing a concept associatively with a valenced reaction, as when ominous music plays behind the black-framed picture of a rival candidate in a political advertisement, it seems that immediate affect should be most directly manipulated. However, if the message explicitly encourages emotional reactions based on attributes of the object, as when the political opponent is described as a "sleazy politician," it can be classified as a more deliberative process.

Immediate affective attitudes have also been established and manipulated implicitly. Edwards (1990, Experiment 1) used very rapidly presented pictures of positive and negative facial expressions as an affective method of creating and altering attitudes toward novel Chinese ideograms, in contrast to a cognitive method that involved reading written esthetic descriptions of the ideograms. The relative ordering of these two manipulations constituted the manipulation of attitude basis; when the affective method came first, affectively based attitudes were assumed to result. We may also tentatively consider the numerous experimental demonstrations of classical-conditioning and "mere-exposure" effects upon liking as examples of implicit manipulations of affective attitude. However, we should bear in mind that some doubt exists over whether these effects actually depend on cognitive processes: awareness of the contingency of pairings, in the case of classical conditioning (Fishbein & Ajzen, 1975), and misattribution of perceptual fluency to liking, in the case of mere exposure (Bornstein, 1992).

In all these implicit manipulations, the processes leading to the establishment of a new attitude can certainly be described as "immediate" as I have defined the term. But a more vexing set of questions remains. Do immediate manipulations of affect mainly influence rapid and effortless expressions of immediate affect, as opposed to more deliberative expressions? And, in turn, do deliberative manipulations most effectively influence deliberative rather than immediate expressions?

The answer to a stronger form of this question—whether immediate manipulations influence *only* the immediate affective attitude—is clearly "no." The manipulations of immediate affect that I have reviewed were all validated by their ability to influence explicit, deliberative measures of liking and attitude. But does immediately formed affect have a privileged influence upon immediately *expressed* affect? To answer this question, we need to consider how people come to acquire immediate and deliberative affective attitudes in the first place.

ANTECEDENTS OF IMMEDIATE AND DELIBERATIVE AFFECT

Immediate affective responses to an object probably have a variety of origins, according to their intensity and nature. Given the apparent ubiquity of the basic immediate evaluative response across both strong and weak attitude objects (Bargh et al., 1995), this tendency is unlikely to arise only from well-established or emotionally significant experience with an attitude object. Rather, the immediate evaluation seems to be a reflection of any and all evaluative associations with the attitude object in memory, potentially including those associations arising from the most superficial features of the stimulus itself (Garcia & Bargh, 1994), although it is not clear exactly which associations are most influential when the attitude consists of evaluatively conflicted material (Giner-Sorolla, 1996).

When a specific emotion arises from an immediate appraisal of an object or situation, its positive or negative character is likely to be determined by just such an automatic evaluative response. Yet not all automatic evaluations lead to emotions, or our everyday lives would be a histrionic inferno of constantly triggered passions. Cognitive theories of emotion that place the appraisal of valence early in the time course of processing (e.g., Lazarus, 1991; Smith & Ellsworth, 1985) also recognize that at about the same time, an appraisal of self-relevance is needed in order to determine whether or not an emotional reaction is warranted. This suggests that a specific emotion can arise immediately from the perception of a novel object, to the extent that features of that object immediately activate all of the following: (1) representations associated in memory with positive or negative valence; (2) a judgment of self-relevance; and (3) other appraisals (e.g., agency, certainty) that lead to the experience of the specific emotion in question.

At the same time, other perspectives indicate that emotions may be associated with objects directly in memory, through classical-conditioning processes (Greenwald, 1968) or, more specifically, through emotionally significant past experiences with the object (Epstein, 1994). The schematic system in Leventhal's (1984) perceptual–motor model of emotion also implies a direct associative process, in which emotional experiences are encoded in conjunction with images or more abstract representations. LeDoux (1995), reviewing investigations of the neurological underpinnings of fear learning, argues that the conditioning of emotional responses can proceed without any cortical processing, via a direct association from the stimulus representation in the sensory thalamus to the emotion-arousing amygdala.

Immediate but explicitly emotional affect elicited by an object, then, may arise because the object's attributes are appraised automatically, or because the object itself cues an emotional memory. Although the latter process is likely to remain fairly unresponsive to the context in which the object appears (e.g., a phobic individual's immediate reaction to a picture of a snake), the former process of appraisal, because it depends on an assessment of the motivational relevance of the object, should be more sensitive to context effects (e.g., whether a snake is merely pictured, or alive and curled around the individual's leg). The cueing of the memory may itself be more immediate than the appraisal of context. As described by LeDoux (1996), cortically unmediated emotional learning is very fast but responds only to crude surface features. However, alternate emotion-learning routes, mediated by the sensory and frontal cortex, can respond to more complex stimuli, integrated memories, and cognitive interpretations.

In any event, immediate object-related affect can have several potential antecedents. One possibility, which appears most relevant to basic automatic evaluative responses, is that an immediate response need not be the product of lengthy, well-practiced, or emotionally significant involvement with the object, but is a simple tag summing up the most accessible evaluation of the object. The other possibility, which appears more relevant to "hot" responses that involve actual emotional experience, is that immediate responses are learned from past emotional experiences, or are produced in response to current situations that are deemed self-relevant. To the extent that manipulations of immediate affective attitude occur for relatively short periods of time in the laboratory, then, they may be expected to have more of an influence upon the more fickle and labile automatic evaluation,

and relatively little influence upon actual emotional responses that are rooted in a substantial history with the object. This prediction parallels recent theory and research showing that subliminal priming and classical conditioning of evaluative material have the greatest effect upon relatively novel stimuli (Cacioppo, Marshall-Goodell, Tassinary, & Petty, 1992; Kihlstrom, 1987; Kitayama, 1990). Still, when immediate emotions are generated by appraising a novel, self-relevant object, manipulations of immediate affect may be able to push the nascent emotion in one direction or another. For example, having been primed to like or dislike a stranger who lends a hand in a critical self-relevant task may have consequences for emotional reactions to this person as a godsend or as an annoyance.

Deliberative affect is no less complex in the variety of ways in which it may be established. First of all, a minimal perspective on deliberative affect would regard it merely as the attitude object's borrowing of emotions from other concepts that are associatively linked with it. Thus, although the concept of capital punishment may immediately arouse positive emotions in a person, other concepts or images that do carry specific, immediate emotional baggage—racist sentencing, innocent people going to the electric chair—may arise upon reflection about the issue. The particular set of emotionally charged concepts that ultimately determines the deliberative affective attitude, under this spreading-activation view, will include less well-established associations to recently learned or infrequently thought-of concepts (cf. Wilson, 1995).

A less passive view of deliberative affect, however, would characterize the activation of specifically deliberative emotions not just as the product of a random walk through the synapses, but as a consequence of self-awareness, planning, and motivation in certain situations. In the familiar dilemmas analyzed by Cross and Guyer (1980) under the rubric of "traps" and "countertraps," an object may have short-term benefits but long-term drawbacks (e.g., a luscious but fattening cake), or the reverse may be true (e.g., an inconvenient prophylactic may reduce the risk of catching a sexually transmitted disease). When self-control depends on choosing the long-term view over the short-term one, as it so often does, deliberative thoughts and associated emotions are often pitted against the more immediate affect associated with short-term rewards. Guilt and self-disgust may induce the dieter to pass up that cake; fear may propel the would-be Casanova to practice safer sex.

A recent study (Giner-Sorolla, 1997a) shows the qualitative and quantitative differences in affect associated with the various aspects of such dilemmas. Thirty undergraduates at the University of Virginia were each asked to give four examples of self-relevant activities: two with short-term benefits and long-term disadvantages for themselves (which I refer to as "guilty pleasures"); and two with short-term disadvantages and long-term benefits (which I refer to as "grim necessities"). To give some idea of the kind of activities nominated, most "guilty pleasures" fell into the broad categories of food (nominated at least once by 40% of participants), drinking (40%), and sexual activity (30%); most "grim necessities" had to do with schoolwork (70%), exercise (43%), and employment (13%).

Participants were also asked to write down up to 10 short statements of "things that came to mind" when thinking about each activity in terms of its short-term consequences, and 10 similar statements with respect to each activity's long-term consequences. The Johnson-Laird and Oatley (1989) lexicon of 590 words denoting emotion was taken as a basis for coding, with the addition of the terms "fun" and the various "feel"-plus adjective phrases (e.g., "feel good"). These listings were then coded for affective content by counting the proportion of statements that contained at least one affect word referring to the respondent's own psychological state.

In both kinds of dilemma, affective terms were significantly more prevalent in associations to short-term consequences than in those to long-term consequences. Nonetheless, an appreciable proportion of the associations to long-term consequences were affective. Moreover, the affective terms most frequently associated with long-term consequences were, for the most part, qualitatively different from those associated with short-term consequences. The feelings most fre-quently associated with long-term positive consequences were "confidence" and "respect," whereas those most frequently associated with short-term positive consequences were "fun" and "relaxation." Among negative terms, "guilt" and "regret" were the most frequent associations to negative long-term consequences, but "boredom" and "stress" were the most frequent associations to negative short-term consequences.

Comparable findings emerged from a different study (Giner-Sorolla, 1997b) exploring the role of self-conscious affect in attitudes toward food items. Twenty-eight undergraduates at the University of Virginia rated 16 pictures of food objects likely to evoke opposed affective and cognitive attitudes (e.g., an appealing but rich cake, a bunch of uncooked asparagus) on modified versions of the Crites et al. (1994) affect, cognition, and evaluation scales. Specifically, the affect scale was modified to include two additional items about self-conscious emotions: "proud/regretful" and "at ease/guilty." An exploratory factor analysis of responses revealed three factors: one consisting of evaluative items and most of the affective items; another consisting of all the cognitive items; and an additional factor composed of "at ease/guilty," "proud/regretful," "relaxed/angry," and "calm/tense." As in the free-listing study, this qualitatively distinct affective factor was most strongly characterized by the "guilt" and "regret" constructs, as opposed to the main affect factor, which mostly contained items dealing with happiness, disgust, and excitement.

It seems, then, that qualitatively distinct emotions of a more self-conscious nature form a separate affective factor in some attitudes, and that these are associated with long-term (as opposed to short-term) consequences of behavior. One question that remains, though, is whether this partitioning into self-conscious and non-self-conscious feelings always coincides with the deliberative–immediate distinction. That is, do considerations of feelings such as happiness arrive sooner than consideration of feelings such as guilt when a dieter thinks of eating a 300-calorie piece of cheesecake? And, when a person actually confronts such an activity, does the actual experienced happiness precede the actual experienced guilt? Although this is often the case, it may also be true that processes of self-control can potentially become automatized through practice. In this case, the emotions that are originally activated as a product of conscious reflection may become spontaneous, if late-arriving, associations. These in turn, through long experience, can eventually come to characterize the immediate response to the object, so that a highly experienced and motivated dieter will feel guilt and aversion to the cake at the same time that, or even before, he or she feels a desire for it.

A second study of self-control dilemmas (Giner-Sorolla, 1997a) examined the relative accessibility of the affect terms typically associated with short- and long-term consequences in the first study. As before, participants nominated their own dilemmas, which were entered into a computer program. The computer then presented each participant with 31 affect questions about each dilemma (e.g., *"eating candy* makes me feel *guilty"*) and measured how much time it took for the participant to make a yes–no response. Overall, the affective judgments typically associated with long-term consequences were significantly slower than those typically associated with short-term consequences. This effect remained significant even when the influence of other factors (e.g., affect word length, affect word frequency, and proportion of yes vs. no responses) on response time was statistically controlled for.

More intriguingly, this accessibility difference was significantly smaller among people who reported high self-control for each dilemma, as opposed to those who reported low self-control. This finding provides some basis for identifying self-conscious affective associations to an object (e.g., "guilt") as more deliberative in nature than the more hedonic affective associations (e.g., "relaxation") that may oppose them. It also indicates that high self-control is associated with more immediate self-conscious affect; that is, people who can effectively control their behavior in a dilemma need to deliberate less in order to bring such affect to mind. More generally, while self-conscious affect in attitude tends to be more deliberative overall, this is probably because people generally have little practice in associating it with the object, not because self-conscious affect is intrinsically brought up from memory more slowly.

CONCLUSION

Apart from the preliminary efforts mentioned above, most research in the area of attitudinal affect has focused on discriminating affect (however this is defined) from other processes such as cognition and evaluation, rather than on examining different processes within affect. Nonetheless, the immediate–deliberative distinction is an important and potentially interesting one to make. In the first place, it provides a framework for speaking more clearly about affect and emotions within attitude theory, and for more clearly implementing the various concepts of affect in research. This area is fraught with confusing terminology; in Berscheid's (1982) picturesque words, "that door in psychology's corridor entitled 'The Psychology of Emotion' carries a skull-and-crossbone warning for many psychologists that says 'Enter at Your Own Risk'" (p. 47). Positioning our concepts of "affect" on an immediate–deliberative continuum will, I hope, help to open the door and lay down the welcome mat for research in this complex and interesting area.

More specifically, the categories of deliberative and immediate affect can be fruitfully applied to the existing literature on affect and persuasion. For example, when deliberatively expressed emotions support a person's attitude system, resistance to persuasion has been shown to increase (Chaiken et al., 1995; Zuwerink & Devine, 1996). Nevertheless, it is not clear whether resistance in these cases always involves deliberative use of affective thoughts in a sort of emotional counter-arguing, or whether feelings are sometimes mobilized more immediately and reflexively. Also unclear is the role of immediate and deliberative defensive processes in dealing with persuasive attempts having different kinds of affective content (cf. Cacioppo & Petty, 1993; Edwards, 1990; Edwards & von Hippel, 1995; Millar & Millar, 1990). Are subliminal persuasive attempts more likely to manifest themselves in explicit emotional reactions than in cognitive beliefs? Are attitudes formed through emotion-laden rhetoric more immediately accessible than those formed by cold reasoning? Drawing a distinction between two types of affect will allow us to ask these questions, and to answer them in future research.

One area that seems especially receptive to analysis in terms of immediate and deliberative affect is the social-cognitive study of prejudice. Recently, as I have mentioned, research on prejudice seems to be emphasizing both the immediate evaluation of group members (Fazio et al., 1995) and the deliberative emotional consequences of trying to control prejudiced reactions (Devine et al., 1991), though not always within the same framework. Although bona fide attempts at deliberative self-control of prejudice may be difficult to empirically distinguish from intentional dissimulation of prejudice, existing results suggest an interesting partition of affective influences on behavior. As might be expected, immediate affect, as expressed in automatic-evaluative-priming results, is associated with implicit, uncontrolled behaviors such as perceived friendliness (Fazio et al., 1995); deliberative, self-conscious affect, as expressed in self-reports of guilt and compunction, is associated with awareness of one's prejudice and with motivation to control it (Devine et al., 1991; Monteith, 1996).

More generally, the same logic can be applied to the psychology of other social dilemmas requiring self-control. Every day, most people are confronted with some activity that pits the immediate perspective of gratification and frustration against long-term personal or social consequences. Smoking, drinking, overeating, exercise, work performance, and unsafe sex are just some of the problems that have been studied from the perspective of psychological self-control (Baumeister, Heatherton, & Tice, 1994). Recent work in neurology suggests that some emotional deficits resulting from brain lesions are associated with a syndrome of impairment in self-regulation and planning, showing that emotion plays a part not only in impulsivity (as commonly thought), but in self-control as well (Damasio, 1994). Moreover, the studies reported earlier (Giner-Sorolla, 1997a) did find that self-conscious affect was associated with long-term perspectives, and was more easily called to mind among people with high self-control.

Effective self-mastery, then, may depend on bringing to mind the self-conscious affect associated with long-term consequences (guilt, regret, pride, self-esteem, etc.) *before* confronting an activity demanding self-control. In attitude psychology, the well-known findings of Millar and Tesser (1986, 1989), who used puzzle tasks as attitude objects, demonstrate that affectively based attitudes are better predictors of behavior focused on short-term consummatory consequences, whereas cognitively based attitudes are better predictors of behavior that focuses on long-term instrumental consequences. But within an attitude that represents a conflict between construing a single activity in consummatory terms or in instrumental terms, self-conscious affect may counteract more impulsive feelings and thus help in self-control—provided that the self-conscious affect makes its presence known before the act.

If self-conscious affect proves to be largely deliberative in nature, at least among people who have not fully mastered self-control, then such people should be vulnerable to breakdowns in self-control when they are under cognitive load. This should be so not only because such load impedes the rational consideration of long-term consequences of an activity, but because it also impedes the activation of motivating affect such as guilt or self-confidence. Factors such as alcoholic intoxication have already been shown to reduce self-focus and self-control (Steele & Southwick, 1985). Possibly drunkenness creates impulsivity because it acts as a cognitive load, interfering with the kind of deliberative processing that some people may need to carry out in order to remind themselves of the guilt and regret that will follow their actions.

Some perspectives on self-control, especially within the dieting literature (e.g., Herman & Polivy, 1975; Polivy, Heatherton, & Herman, 1988; Baumeister et al., 1994) indicate that negative self-focused emotions can be a potential setback. This may be an explanation for the "snowballing" binges often observed in conflicted people who fail an initial test of restraint. After having one toaster pastry, for example, the problem eater may choose to finish off the whole box rather than face the guilt that would follow an admission of failure in self-regulation. In contrast, I see negative self-conscious emotions such as guilt and regret as potentially helpful to self-control when memories or anticipations of these emotions are associated with the object as part of the attitude. The more the bar, the bartender, and the beer mug *remind* the problem drinker of drinking-related guilt, the more he or she should show restraint in drinking. And, at least in research on drinking, an initial failure in self-control has not been shown to lend to subsequently less restraint (Bensley, Kuna, & Steele, 1990). Rather, restraint seems to accompany negative self-focused affect (Collins, Lapp, & Izzo, 1994). A distinction, then, may be drawn between the constructive role of an emotional memory before temptation, and the destructive role of guilt feelings that are inappropriately dealt with after temptation.

With this distinction in mind, the stage may be set for a more effective theory guiding self-help and educational interventions. Instead of pitting naked reason against immediate feelings and emotions, perhaps a social persuader can enlist Plato's "spirited part"—deliberative emotional reactions—in the struggle of reason against desire. At the same time, an overly strong focus on self-evaluative emotions may lead people to focus more on alleviating emotional distress than on taking effective action in self-control dilemmas, as in the areas of interpersonal helping (Batson et al., 1989)and relationships (Tangney, 1995). When self-evaluation has destructive effects on self-control, cognitive load or distractions may reduce the severity of the binge reaction, by impeding the self-focused appraisals that lead to lowered mood and negative self-esteem. At the same time, distracting a person away from guilt and regret may prove counterproductive in the long term, because the activity will end up being affectively associated with positive hedonic feelings rather than negative emotions.

Clearly, more empirical work remains to be done in the extremely complicated area of affect and self-regulation. The distinction between immediate and deliberative affect, in fact, is only one of several distinctions—between the live emotion and the emotional memory, between self-conscious and hedonic emotions—that will ultimately have to be made before the role of feelings and emotions in psychology is completely understood. One thing is evident, though: What we have been calling "affect" in social psychology is actually a cluster of diverse phenomena that demands a clear, well-organized nomenclature, rather than a vague blanket term. The immediate–deliberative distinction in affect is one possible starting point for such a system—a distinction that, as with many of the two-stage models presented in this volume, contrasts the fast, crude, and easy with the slower, more sophisticated, and more difficult.

ACKNOWLEDGMENTS

The writing of this chapter was supported by National Institute of Mental Health National Research Service Award Postdoctoral Grant No. 5-21550. I would like to thank John Bargh, Shelly Chaiken, and Tim Wilson for their comments on an earlier version of the chapter.

NOTES

1. Plato may be the originator of this method of testing attitude structure, as suggested in the *Republic, X*: "That part of the soul which gives an opinion contrary to the measurements could not be the same as the part of which the opinion is in accordance with them" (ca. 370–360 B.C./1974, p. 247).

2. Contrast this emphasis with that of Niedenthal (1990), who has used a similar paradigm to demonstrate the transfer of specific emotional meanings from subliminally presented facial expressions to neutral cartoon figures.

3. Presumably, when an object provokes an actual emotional state in a person, he or she will be more likely to notice the emotion consciously and to interpret it as an evaluative reaction. Even so, awareness of the emotion is likely to be a relatively slow reaction, compared to the rapidity with which the evaluative appraisal itself appears.

REFERENCES

Abelson, R. P., Kinder, D. R., Peters, M. D., & Fiske, S. T. (1982). Affective and semantic components in political person perception. *Journal of Personality and Social Psychology, 42,* 619–630.

Allport, G. W. (1935). Attitudes. In C. Murchison (Ed.), *Handbook of social psychology* (pp. 798–844). Worcester, MA: Clark University Press.

Andersen, S. M., & Cole, S. W. (1990). "Do I know you?": The role of significant others in general social perception. *Journal of Personality and Social Psychology, 59,* 384–399.

Arieti, S. (1970). Cognition and feeling. In M. B. Arnold (Ed.), *Feelings and emotions: The Loyola Symposium* (pp. 135–143). New York: Academic Press.

Arnold, M. B. (1960). *Emotion and personality.* New York: Columbia University Press.

Bagozzi, R. P. (1978). The construct validity of the affective, behavioral, and cognitive components of attitude by analysis of covariance structures. *Multivariate Behavior Research, 13,* 9–31.

Bargh, J. A. (1989). Conditional automaticity: Varieties of automatic influence in social perception and cognition. In J. S. Uleman & J. A. Bargh (Eds.), *Unintended thought* (pp. 3–51). New York: Guilford Press.

Bargh, J. A. (1992). Does subliminality matter to social psychology?: Awareness of the stimulus versus awareness of its influence. In R. Bornstein & T. Pittman (Eds.), *Perception without awareness: Cognitive, clinical, and social perspectives* (pp. 236–255). New York: Guilford Press.

Bargh, J. A. (1994). The four horsemen of automaticity: Awareness, intention, efficiency and control in social cognition. In R. S. Wyer, Jr., & T. K. Srull (Eds.), *Handbook of social cognition* (2nd ed., Vol. 1, pp. 1–40). Hillsdale, NJ: Erlbaum.

Bargh, J. A., Chaiken, S., Govender, R., & Pratto, F. (1992). The generality of the automatic evaluation effect. *Journal of Personality and Social Psychology, 62,* 893–912.

Bargh, J. A., Chaiken, S. C., Raymond, P., & Hymes, C. (1996). The automatic evaluation effect: Unconditional automatic activation of attitudes with a pronunciation task. *Journal of Experimental Social Psychology, 32,* 104–128.

Bargh, J. A., & Pietromonaco, P. (1982). Automatic information processing and social perception: The influence of trait information presented outside of conscious awareness on impression formation. *Journal of Personality and Social Psychology, 43,* 437–449.

Bargh, J. A., & Tota, M. E. (1988). Context-dependent automatic processing in depression: Accessibility of negative constructs with regard to self but not others. *Journal of Personality and Social Psychology, 54,* 925–939.

Batson, C. D., Batson, J. G., Griffitt, C. A., Barrientos, S., Brandt, J. R., Sprenglemeyer, P., & Bayly, M. J. (1989). Negative-state relief and the empathy–altruism hypothesis. *Journal of Personality and Social Psychology, 56,* 922–933.

Baumeister, R. F., Heatherton, T. F., & Tice, D. M. (1994). *Losing control: How and why people fail at self-regulation.* San Diego, CA: Academic Press.

Beck, A. T. (1976). *Cognitive therapy and the emotional disorders.* New York: International Universities Press.

Bensley, L. S., Kuna, P. H., & Steele, C. M. (1990). The role of drinking restraint success in subsequent alcohol consumption. *Addictive Behaviors, 15,* 491–496.

Berkowitz, L., & Heimer, K. (1989). On the construction of the anger experience: Aversive events and negative priming in the formation of feelings. In L. Berkowitz (Ed.), *Advances in experimental social psychology* (Vol. 22, pp. 1–37). San Diego, CA: Academic Press.

Berscheid, E. (1982). Attraction and emotion in interpersonal relationships. In M. S. Clark & S. T. Fiske (Eds.), *Affect and cognition: The Seventh Annual Carnegie Symposium on Cognition* (pp. 37–54). Hillsdale, NJ: Erlbaum.

Blair, I. V., & Banaji, M. R. (1996). Automatic and controlled processes in stereotype priming. *Journal of Personality and Social Psychology, 70,* 1142–1163.

Bornstein, R. F. (1989). Exposure and affect: Overview and meta-analysis of research, 1968–1987. *Psychological Bulletin, 106,* 265–289.

Bornstein, R. F. (1992). Subliminal mere exposure effects. In R. F. Bornstein & T. S. Pittman (Eds.), *Perception without awareness: Cognitive, clinical, and social perspectives* (pp. 191–210). New York: Guilford Press.

Breckler, S. J. (1984). Empirical validation of affect, behavior and cognition as distinct components of attitude. *Journal of Personality and Social Psychology, 47,* 1191–1205.

Breckler, S. J., & Wiggins, E. C. (1989). Affect versus evaluation in the structure of attitudes. *Journal of Experimental Social Psychology, 25,* 253–271.

Breckler, S. J., & Wiggins, E. C. (1991). Cognitive responses in persuasion: Affective and evaluative determinants. *Journal of Experimental Social Psychology, 52,* 384–389.

Byrne, D. E., & Clore, G. L. (1970). A reinforcement model of evaluative responses. *Personality: An International Journal, 12,* 193–196.

Cacioppo, J. T., Marshall-Goodell, B. S., Tassinary, L. G., & Petty, R. E. (1992). Rudimentary determinants of attitudes: Classical conditioning is more effective when prior knowledge about the attitude stimulus is low rather than high. *Journal of Experimental Social Psychology, 28,* 207–233.

Cacioppo, J. T., & Petty, R. E. (1993). The elaboration likelihood model: The role of affect and affect-laden information processing in persuasion. In P. Cafferata & A. Tybout (Eds.), *Cognitive and affective responses in advertising* (pp. 69–89). Lexington, MA: Lexington Books.

Cannon, W. B. (1927). The James–Lange theory of emotion: A critical examination and alternate theory. *American Journal of Psychology, 34,* 106–124.

Carver, C. S., & Scheier, M. F. (1990). Principles of self-regulation: Action and emotion. In E. T. Higgins & R. M. Sorrentino (Eds.), *Handbook of motivation and cognition: Foundations of social behavior* (Vol. 2, pp. 3–52). New York: Guilford Press.

Chaiken, S., Giner-Sorolla, R., & Chen, S. (1996). Beyond accuracy: Defense and impression motives in heuristic and systematic information processing. In P. M. Gollwitzer & J. A. Bargh (Eds.), *The psychology of action: Linking motivation and cognition to behavior* (pp. 553–578). New York: Guilford Press.

Chaiken, S., Pomerantz, E. M., & Giner-Sorolla, R. (1995). Structural consistency and attitude strength. In R. E. Petty & J. A. Krosnick (Eds.), *Attitude strength: Antecedents and consequences* (pp. 387–412). Hillsdale, NJ: Erlbaum.

Chaiken, S., & Stangor, C. (1987). Attitudes and attitude change. *Annual Review of Psychology, 38,* 575–630.

Clark, M. S., & Isen, A. M. (1982). Toward understanding the relationship between feeling states and social behavior. In A. H. Hastorf & A. M. Isen (Eds.), *Cognitive social psychology* (pp. 73–108). New York: Elsevier/North-Holland.

Collins, R. L., Lapp, W. M., & Izzo, C. V. (1994). Affective and behavioral reactions to the violation of limits on alcohol consumption. *Journal of Studies on Alcohol, 55,* 475–486.

Crites, S. L., Fabrigar, L., & Petty, R. E. (1994). Measuring the affective and cognitive properties of attitudes: Conceptual and methodological issues. *Personality and Social Psychology Bulletin, 20,* 619–634.

Cross, J. G., & Guyer, M. J. (1980). *Social traps.* Ann Arbor: University of Michigan Press.

Damasio, A. R. (1994). *Descartes' error: Emotion, reason, and the human brain.* New York: Putnam.

de Houwer, J., Baeyens, F., & Eelen, P. (1994). Verbal evaluative conditioning with undetected US presentation. *Behaviour Research and Therapy, 32*, 629–633.

Devine, P. G. (1989). Stereotypes: Their automatic and controlled components. *Journal of Personality and Social Psychology, 56*, 5–18.

Devine, P. G., Monteith, M. J., Zuwerink, J. R., & Elliot, A. J. (1991). Prejudice with and without compunction. *Journal of Personality and Social Psychology, 60*, 817–830.

Eagly, A. H., & Chaiken, S. (1993). *The psychology of attitudes*. Fort Worth, TX: Harcourt Brace Jovanovich.

Eagly, A. H., Mladinic, A., & Otto, S. (1994). Cognitive and affective bases of attitudes toward social groups and social policies. *Journal of Experimental Social Psychology, 30*, 113–137.

Edwards, K. (1990). The interplay of affect and cognition in attitude formation and change. *Journal of Personality and Social Psychology, 59*, 202–216.

Edwards, K., & von Hippel, W. (1995). Hearts and minds: The priority of affective versus cognitive factors in person perception. *Personality and Social Psychology Bulletin, 21*, 996–1011.

Elias, N. (1978). *The history of manners: Vol. 1. The civilizing process* (E. Jephcott, Trans.). New York: Pantheon Books. (Original work published 1939)

Epstein, S. (1994). Integration of the cognitive and the psychodynamic unconscious. *American Psychologist, 49*, 709–724.

Fazio, R. H., Jackson, J. R., Dunton, B. C., & Williams, C. J. (1995). Variability in automatic activation as an unobtrusive measure of racial attitudes: A bona fide pipeline? *Journal of Personality and Social Psychology, 69*, 1013–1027.

Fazio, R. H., Sanbonmatsu, D. M., Powell, M. C., & Kardes, F. R. (1986). On the automatic activation of attitudes. *Journal of Personality and Social Psychology, 50*, 229–238.

Fishbein, M., & Ajzen, I. (1975). *Belief, attitude, intention, and behavior: An introduction to theory and research*. Reading, MA: Addison-Wesley.

Fiske, S. T. (1989). Examining the role of intent: Towards understanding its role in stereotyping and prejudice. In J. S. Uleman & J. A. Bargh (Eds.), *Unintended thought* (pp. 253–286). New York: Guilford Press.

Fiske, S. T., & Pavelchak, M. A. (1986). Category-based versus piecemeal-based affective responses: Developments in schema-triggered affect. In R. M. Sorrentino & E. T. Higgins (Eds.), *Handbook of motivation and cognition: Foundations of social behavior* (Vol. 1, pp. 167–203). New York: Guilford Press.

Forgas, J. P. (1992). Affect and social perception: Research evidence and an integrative theory. In W. Stroebe & M. Hewstone (Eds.), *European review of social psychology* (Vol. 3, pp. 182–223). Chichester, England: Wiley.

Garcia, M. T., & Bargh, J.A. (1994). [Automatic evaluation of nonsense words based on phonetic symbolism]. Unpublished raw data.

Giner-Sorolla, R. (1996). *Affective and cognitive influences on the immediate expression of attitudes: Are feelings really first?* Unpublished doctoral dissertation, New York University.

Giner-Sorolla, R. (1997a). *Guilty pleasures and grim necessities: Immediate and deliberative affective attitudes in dilemmas of self-control*. Unpublished manuscript, University of Virginia.

Giner-Sorolla, R. (1997b). [Affective and cognitive responses to food objects: A pretest]. Unpublished raw data, University of Virginia.

Giner-Sorolla, R., Garcia, M., & Bargh, J. A. (1998). The automatic evaluation of pictures. *Social Cognition*.

Greenwald, A. G. (1968). Cognitive learning, cognitive response to persuasion, and attitude change. In A. G. Greenwald, T. C. Brock, & T. M. Ostrom (Eds.), *Psychological foundations of attitudes* (pp. 147–170). New York: Academic Press.

Greenwald, A. G., & Banaji, M. (1995). Implicit social cognition: Attitudes, self-esteem, and stereotypes. *Psychological Review, 102*, 4–27.

Greenwald, A. G., Klinger, M. R., & Liu, T. J. (1989). Unconscious processing of dichoptically masked words. *Memory and Cognition, 7*, 35–47.

Herman, C. P., & Polivy, J. (1975). Anxiety, restraint and eating behavior. *Journal of Abnormal Psychology, 84*, 666–672.

Hermans, D., de Houwer, J., & Eelen, P. (1996). The affective priming effect: Automatic activation of evaluative information in memory. *Cognition and Emotion, 8*, 515–533.

Higgins, E. T. (1991). Development of self-regulatory and self-evaluative processes: Costs, benefits, and trade-offs. In M. R. Gunnar & L. A. Sroufe (Eds.), *Self processes and development: The Minnesota Symposia on Child Development* (Vol. 23, pp. 125–165). Minneapolis: University of Minnesota Press.

Insko, C. A., & Schopler, J. (1967). Triadic consistency: A statement of affective–cognitive–conative consistency. *Psychological Review, 74*, 361–376.

James, W. (1890). *The principles of psychology*. New York: Holt.

Janis, I. L., & Feshbach, S. (1953). Effects of fear-arousing communications. *Journal of Abnormal and Social Psychology, 48*, 78–92.

Johnson-Laird, P. N., & Oatley, K. (1989). The language of emotions: An analysis of a semantic field. *Cognition and Emotion, 3*, 81–123.

Jung, C. G. (1923). *Psychological types or the psychology of individuation*. New York: Harcourt, Brace. (Original work published 1922)

Katz, D., & Stotland, E. (1959). A preliminary statement to a theory of attitude structure and change. In S. Koch (Ed.), *Psychology: A study of a science* (Vol. 3, pp. 423–475). New York: McGraw-Hill.

Katz, I., & Hass, R. G. (1988). Racial ambivalence and American value conflict: Correlational and priming studies of dual cognitive structures. *Journal of Personality and Social Psychology, 55*, 893–905.

Kihlstrom, J. F. (1987). The cognitive unconscious. *Science, 237*, 1445–1452.

Kitayama, S. (1990). Interaction between affect and cognition in word processing. *Journal of Personality and Social Psychology, 58*, 209–217.

Koriat, A., Melkman, R., Averill, J. A., & Lazarus, R. S. (1972). The self-control of emotional reactions to a stressful film. *Journal of Personality, 40*, 601–619.

Kothandapani, V. (1971). Validation of feeling, belief, and intention to act as three components of attitude and their contribution to prediction of contraceptive behavior. *Journal of Personality and Social Psychology, 19*, 321–333.

Krech, D., & Crutchfield, R. S. (1948). *Theory and problems of social psychology.* New York: McGraw-Hill.

Krosnick, J. A., Betz, A. L., Jussim, L. J., Lynn, A. R., & Stephens, L. (1992). Subliminal conditioning of attitudes. *Personality and Social Psychology Bulletin, 18,* 152–162.

Kuhl, J., & Kraska, K. (1989). Self-regulation and metamotivation: Computational mechanisms, development, and assessment. In R. Kanfer, P. L. Ackerman, & R. Cudeck (Eds.), *Abilities, motivation, and methodology: The Minnesota Symposium on Learning and Individual Differences* (pp. 343–374). Hillsdale, NJ: Erlbaum.

Kunst-Wilson, W. R., & Zajonc, R. B. (1980). Affective discrimination of stimuli that cannot be recognized. *Science, 207,* 557–558.

LaBerge, D. (1981). Automatic information processing: A review. In J. Long & A. Baddeley (Eds.), *Attention and performance IX* (pp. 173–186). Hillsdale, NJ: Erlbaum.

Lange, C. (1922). *The emotions.* Baltimore: Williams & Wilkins.

Langer, E. J. (1989). Minding matters: The consequences of mindfulness–mindlessness. In L. Berkowitz (Ed.), *Advances in experimental social psychology* (Vol. 22, pp. 137–173). San Diego, CA: Academic Press.

Lazarus, R. M. (1966). *Psychological stress and the coping process.* New York: McGraw-Hill.

Lazarus, R. S. (1982). Thoughts on the relations between emotion and cognition. *American Psychologist, 37,* 1019–1024.

Lazarus, R. S. (1984). On the primacy of cognition. *American Psychologist, 39,* 124–139.

Lazarus, R. S. (1991). *Emotion and adaptation.* New York: Oxford University Press.

LeDoux, J. E. (1995). Emotion: Clues from the brain. *Annual Review of Psychology, 46,* 209–235.

LeDoux, J. E. (1996). *The emotional brain: The mysterious underpinnings of emotional life.* New York: Simon & Schuster.

Leventhal, H. (1984). A perceptual–motor theory of emotion. In L. Berkowitz (Ed.), *Advances in experimental social psychology* (Vol. 17, pp. 117–183). San Diego, CA: Academic Press.

Mandler, G. (1982). The structure of value: Accounting for taste. In M. S. Clark & S. T. Fiske (Eds.), *Affect and cognition: The Seventh Annual Carnegie Symposium on Cognition* (pp. 3–36). Hillsdale, NJ: Erlbaum.

Martin, L. L., & Tesser, A. (1989). Toward a motivational and structural theory of ruminative thought. In J. S. Uleman & J. A. Bargh (Eds.), *Unintended thought* (pp. 306–326). New York: Guilford Press.

McGuire, W. J. (1969). The nature of attitudes and attitude change. In G. Lindzey & E. Aronson (Eds.), *Handbook of social psychology* (2nd ed., Vol. 3, pp. 136–314). Reading, MA: Addison-Wesley.

Millar, M. J., & Millar, K. U. (1990). Attitude change as a function of attitude type and argument type. *Journal of Personality and Social Psychology, 59,* 217–228.

Millar, M. J., & Tesser, A. (1986). Effects of affective and cognitive focus on the attitude–behavior relation. *Journal of Personality and Social Psychology, 51,* 270–276.

Millar, M. J., & Tesser, A. (1989). The effects of affective–cognitive consistency and thought on the attitude–behavior relation. *Journal of Experimental Social Psychology, 51,* 189–202.

Monteith, M. J. (1996). Affective reactions to prejudice-related discrepant responses: The impact of standard salience. *Personality and Social Psychology Bulletin, 22,* 48–59.

Murphy, S. T., Monahan, J. L., & Zajonc, R B. (1995). Additivity of nonconscious affect: Combined effects of priming and exposure. *Journal of Personality and Social Psychology, 69,* 589–602.

Murphy, S. T., & Zajonc, R. B. (1993). Affect, cognition and awareness: Affective priming with optimal and suboptimal stimulus exposures. *Journal of Personality and Social Psychology, 64,* 723–739.

Neely, J. H. (1977). Semantic priming and retrieval from lexical memory: Roles of inhibitionless spreading activation and limited-capacity attention. *Journal of Experimental Psychology: General, 106,* 226–254.

Neumann, O. (1984). Automatic processing: A review of recent findings and a plea for an old theory. In W. Prinz & A. F. Sanders (Eds.), *Cognition and motor processes* (pp. 255–293). Berlin: Springer-Verlag.

Niedenthal, P. M. (1990). Implicit perception of affective information. *Journal of Experimental Social Psychology, 26,* 505–527.

Ortony, A., Clore, G. L., & Collins, A. (1988). *The cognitive structure of emotions.* New York: Cambridge University Press.

Ostrom, T. M. (1969). The relationship between the affective, behavioral and cognitive components of attitude. *Journal of Experimental Social Psychology, 5,* 12–30.

Petty, R. E., & Cacioppo, J. A. (1986). *Communication and persuasion: Central and peripheral routes to attitude change.* New York: Springer-Verlag.

Plato. (1974). *The republic* (G. M. A. Grube, Trans.). New York: Hackett. (Original work written ca. 370–360 B.C.)

Plutchik, R., & Ax, A. F. (1969). A critique of "Determinants of emotional state" by Schachter and Singer (1962). *Psychophysiology, 4,* 79–82.

Polivy, J., Heatherton, T. F., & Herman, C. P. (1988). Self-esteem, restraint, and eating behavior. *Journal of Abnormal Psychology, 97,* 354–356.

Posner, M. I., & Snyder, C. R. R. (1975). Attention and cognitive control. In R. L. Solso (Ed.), *Information processing and cognition: The Loyola Symposium* (pp. 55–85). Hillsdale, NJ: Erlbaum.

Roediger, H. L., III, & McDermott, K. B. (1993). Implicit memory in normal human subjects. In F. Boller & J. Graufman (Eds.), *Handbook of neuropsychology* (Vol. 8, pp. 63–132). New York: Elsevier.

Rosenberg, M. J. (1956). Cognitive structure and attitudinal affect. *Journal of Abnormal and Social Psychology, 53,* 367–372.

Rosenberg, M. J. (1960). An analysis of affective–cognitive consistency. In C. I. Hovland & M. J. Rosenberg (Eds.), *Attitude organization and change: An analysis of consistency among attitude components* (pp. 15–64). New Haven, CT: Yale University Press.

Rosenberg, M. J., & Hovland, C. I. (1960). Cognitive, affective, and behavioral components of attitudes. In C. I. Hovland & M. J. Rosenberg (Eds.), *Attitude organization and change: An analysis of consistency among attitude components* (pp. 1–14). New Haven, CT: Yale University Press.

Rozin, P., & Fallon, A. E. (1987). A perspective on disgust. *Psychological Review, 94,* 23–41.

Rozin, P., & Nemeroff, C. J. (1990). The laws of sympathetic magic: A psychological analysis of similarity and contagion. In J. Stigler, G. Herdt, & R. A. Shweder (Eds.), *Cultural psychology: Essays on comparative human development* (pp. 205–232). Cambridge, England: Cambridge University Press.

Schachter, S., & Singer, J. E. (1962). Cognitive, social and physiological determinants of emotional state. *Psychological Review, 69,* 379–399.

Schwarz, N. (1990). Feelings as information: Informational and motivational functions of affective states. In E. T. Higgins & R. M. Sorrentino (Eds.), *Handbook of motivation and cognition: Foundations of social behavior* (Vol. 2, pp. 527–561). New York: Guilford Press.

Smith, C. A., & Ellsworth, P. C. (1985). Patterns of cognitive appraisal in emotion. *Journal of Personality and Social Psychology, 52,* 475–488.

Smith, M. B. (1947). The personal setting of public opinions: A study of attitudes toward Russia. *Public Opinion Quarterly, 11,* 507–523.

Spielman, L. A., Pratto, F., & Bargh, J. A. (1988). Automatic affect: Are one's moods, attitudes, evaluations and emotions out of control? *American Behavioral Scientist, 31,* 296–311.

Staats, A. W., & Staats, C. K. (1958). Attitudes established by classical conditioning. *Journal of Abnormal and Social Psychology, 57,* 37–40.

Staats, A. W., Minke, K. A., Martin, C. H., & Higa, W. R. (1972). Deprivation-satiation and strength of attitude conditioning: A test of attitude-reinforcer-discriminative theory. *Journal of Personality and Social Psychology, 24,* 178–185.

Stangor, C., Sullivan, L. A., & Ford, T. L. (1991). Affective and cognitive determinants of prejudice. *Social Cognition, 9,* 359–380.

Steele, C. M., & Southwick, L. (1985). Alcohol and social behavior: I. The psychology of drunken excess. *Journal of Personality and Social Psychology, 48,* 18–34.

Tangney, J. P. (1995). Shame and guilt in interpersonal relationships. In J. P. Tangney & K. W. Fischer (Eds.), *Self-conscious emotions: The psychology of shame, guilt, embarrassment, and pride* (pp. 114–139). New York: Guilford Press.

Thurstone, L. L. (1931). The measurement of social attitudes. *Journal of Abnormal and Social Psychology, 26,* 249–269.

Trope, Y. (1986). Identification and inferential processes in dispositional attribution. *Psychological Review, 93,* 239–257.

Wegener, D. T., & Petty, R. E. (1995). Flexible correction processes in social judgment: The role of naive theories in corrections for perceived bias. *Journal of Personality and Social Psychology, 68,* 36–51.

Wilson, T. D. (1995). *Predispositions and attitude construction processes.* Unpublished manuscript (National Science Foundation grant proposal).

Wilson, T. D., & Dunn, D. S. (1986). Effects of introspection on attitude-behavior consistency: Analyzing reasons versus focusing on feelings. *Journal of Experimental Social Psychology, 22,* 249–263.

Winkielman, P., Zajonc, R. B., & Schwarz, N. (1997). Subliminal affective priming resists attributional interventions. *Cognition and Emotion, 11,* 433–465.

Wyer, R. S., Jr., & Srull, T. K. (1981). Category accessibility: Some theoretical and empirical issues concerning the processing of social stimulus input. In E. T. Higgins, C. P. Herman, & M. P. Zanna (Eds.), *Social cognition: The Ontario Symposium* (Vol. 1, pp. 161–197). Hillsdale, NJ: Erlbaum.

Zajonc, R. B. (1980). Feeling and thinking: Preferences need no inferences. *American Psychologist, 35,* 151–175.

Zajonc, R. B. (1984). On the primacy of affect. *American Psychologist, 39,* 117–123.

Zanna, M. P., & Rempel, J. K. (1988). Attitudes: A new look at an old concept. In D. Bar-Tal & A. W. Kruglanski (Eds.), *The social psychology of knowledge* (pp. 315–334). Cambridge, England: Cambridge University Press.

Zuwerink, J. R., & Devine, P. G. (1996). Attitude importance and resistance to persuasion: It's not just the thought that counts. *Journal of Personality and Social Psychology, 70,* 931–944.

23

Some Basic Issues Regarding Dual-Process Theories from the Perspective of Cognitive–Experiential Self-Theory

SEYMOUR EPSTEIN
ROSEMARY PACINI

In this chapter, we discuss some fundamental issues concerning dual-process theories. First, we consider the evidence for two processing systems that operate by different rules. Although most of the authors of chapters in the present volume believe that there are two different modes of information processing, this view is not universally shared by others. Second, we examine whether there is any basis for choosing among the various contrasting modes that have been proposed, which include verbal versus nonverbal, controlled versus automatic, central versus peripheral, and rational versus experiential (among others), and, relatedly, whether there is one that can subsume the others. Agreement on a common designation not only would simplify communication, but could foster integration and the development of more sophisticated theory. Third, we review the principles by which the two systems operate. We concentrate on those proposed by cognitive–experiential self-theory (CEST; Epstein, 1994), as it includes an encompassing set of principles. Fourth, we consider whether the proposed processing modes interact—and, if so, whether their interaction is sequential, simultaneous, or both, and what

the broader implications of such interactions are. Fifth, we discuss the development of the two systems. Although we approach these issues from the perspective of CEST, the discussion and the research we report are not limited by their relevance to CEST, but extend to all dual-process theories.

Before we proceed further, it will be helpful to present a brief summary of the more relevant aspects of CEST.

COGNITIVE–EXPERIENTIAL SELF-THEORY

According to CEST, people adapt to their environments by means of two information-processing systems: a preconscious experiential system and a primarily conscious rational system. The two systems operate in parallel and are interactive. The rational system operates through a person's understanding of logical rules of inference. The experiential system operates according to heuristic principles, and despite the limitations of such operation, it has the advantage of being far more rapid and efficient than the rational system for coping with events in everyday life. Table 23.1 provides a detailed comparison of the characteristics of the two systems.

As Table 23.1 shows, the rational system is a deliberative, analytical system that operates primarily in the medium of language and is relatively affect-free. It is capable of high levels of abstraction and long-term delay of gratification, but it is inefficient for reacting to everyday events. It has a relatively brief evolutionary history, and its long-term adaptability from an evolutionary perspective remains to be demonstrated. In this last respect, it is important to consider that although it has certain adaptive advantages, it also can be the source of great destructiveness, as demonstrated by the development of modern weaponry.

In contrast, the experiential system encodes information in a concrete, holistic, primarily nonverbal form; is intimately associated with affect; and is inherently highly compelling. Although it represents events concretely, the experiential system is capable of abstraction through the use of generalization, prototypes, metaphors, and narratives. The experiential system has a very long evolutionary history and is the same system through which nonhuman, higher-order animals adapt to their environments, but it is more complex in humans because of the greater development of their cerebral cortex. At its lower reaches, it is a relatively crude, albeit efficient, system for automatically, rapidly, and effortlessly processing information while placing minimal demands on cognitive resources. At its higher reaches, and particularly in interaction with the rational system, the experiential system can be a source of intuitive wisdom and creativity.

The operation of the experiential system is assumed to be intimately associated with the experience of affect, including "vibes," a term referring to subtle feelings of which people are often unaware. When a person responds to an emotionally significant event, the sequence of reactions is assumed to be as follows: The experiential system automatically searches its memory for related events and their emotional accompaniments. The recalled feelings influence the course of further processing and reactions, which in nonhuman animals are actions, and in humans are conscious and unconscious thoughts as well as actions. If the activated feelings associated with the memories are pleasant, they motivate

TABLE 23.1. Comparison of the Experiential and Rational Systems

Experiential system	Rational system
1. Holistic responding	1. Analytic responding
2. Automatic, effortless processing	2. Intentional, effortful processing
3. Affective processing: Pleasure- or pain-oriented (what feels good or bad)	3. Logical processing: Reason-oriented (what is rational)
4. Associative connections	4. Logical connections
5. Encoding of reality in concrete images, metaphors, and narratives	5. Encoding of reality in abstract symbols, words, and numbers
6. More rapid processing: Oriented toward immediate action	6. Slower processing: Oriented toward delayed action
7. Slower, more difficult changes: Changes with repetitive or intense experience	7. More rapid, easier changes: Changes with strength of argument and new evidence
8. More crudely differentiated constructs: Broad generalization gradient, stereotypical thinking	8. More highly differentiated constructs
9. More crudely integrated and less coherent networks: Dissociative, emotional complexes; context-specific processing	9. More highly integrated and coherent networks: Context-general principles
10. Passive and preconscious experience of events: We are seized by our emotions	10. Active and conscious experience of events: We are in control of our thoughts
11. Self-evident validity: "Experiencing is believing"	11. Need for justification via logic and evidence

Note. Adapted from Epstein (1991b). Copyright 1991 by The Guilford Press. Adapted by permission.

actions and thoughts anticipated to reproduce the previous outcomes and feelings. If the feelings are unpleasant, they motivate actions and thoughts anticipated to avoid the previous outcomes and feelings.

Although CEST is consistent with modern cognitive psychology in many ways, it differs in one important way, which is that information processing in the experiential system is assumed to be emotionally driven. This assumption allows CEST to integrate the irrational, conflictual, psychodynamic aspects of human behavior that are emphasized in psychoanalytic theory with the "kinder, gentler" conceptualization of the cognitive unconscious of modern cognitive theory (Epstein, 1994). The result is that the unconscious of CEST is more emotional and irrational than the cognitive unconscious as conceived by modern cognitive psychologists. At the same time, it is also more adaptive, realistic, and defensible from an evolutionary perspective than the Freudian unconscious.

Unlike most personality theories, which assume the existence of a single fundamental need, CEST assumes that there are four basic needs, each of which has been considered central in some major personality theories and ignored in others. The basic needs are (1) to maximize pleasure and minimize pain (corresponding to the pleasure principle in psychoanalytic theory and the reinforcement principle in learning theory); (2) to maintain a stable, coherent conceptual system for organizing the data of experience (emphasized in phenomenological theories, such as those by Kelly, 1955; Lecky, 1961; and Rogers, 1959); (3) to maintain relatedness to others (emphasized in object-relations theories, such as those by Bowlby, 1988, and Fairbairn, 1954); and (4) to maintain a favorable level of self-esteem (emphasized by Adler, 1954; Allport, 1961; and Kohut, 1971). Behavior is assumed to be influenced by the simultaneous influence of all of the basic activated needs. Two interesting implications follow from this assumption. One is that behavior often represents a compromise among needs (see Epstein & Morling, 1995; Morling & Epstein, 1998). The other is that the needs serve as checks and balances against each other; when one need is fulfilled at the expense of the other needs, the other needs become more insistent,

which normally serves to moderate the influence of the first need.

People have beliefs in both the rational and experiential systems about themselves, the world, and the connections between them, which constitute their implicit and explicit theories of reality. We refer to beliefs in the rational system as "explicit beliefs," or just "beliefs," and those in the experiential system as "schemas" or "implicit beliefs." Our emphasis is on the schemas in the experiential system, as, according to CEST, this system has more influence on everyday behavior. The cognitions and affects associated with fulfilling (or not fulfilling) the basic needs provide the basis for the formation of four corresponding basic beliefs. According to CEST, every individual's personal theory of reality includes intuitive assessments of the degree to which (1) the world is benign versus malevolent; (2) the world is meaningful (including predictable, controllable, and just) versus chaotic (including unpredictable, uncontrollable, and unjust); (3) relationships with others are supportive versus threatening; and (4) the self is worthy (including competent, good, and lovable) versus unworthy (including incompetent, bad, and unlovable). Basic beliefs are so fundamental that a change in any one of them will have a major effect on the overall conceptual system. The Basic Beliefs Inventory (Catlin & Epstein, 1992) has been developed to measure the four basic beliefs.

The schemas in the experiential system consist primarily of generalizations derived from emotionally significant experiences. There are two fundamental kinds of experiential schemas: descriptive and motivational. Descriptive schemas are generalizations about what the self and the world are like, and include the four basic beliefs. Examples are "Authority figures are untrustworthy," and "I am a worthy person." Motivational schemas are implicit beliefs about means-end relations. Examples are "The best way to deal with authority figures is to placate them," and "If I work hard enough, I can succeed in anything I undertake." Motivational schemas are not sufficient by themselves to promote action. Rather, action in the experiential system is motivated by the affect that is anticipated from the association of action and outcomes as determined by past experience (whether direct or indirect) in similar situations. Believing that hard work will ultimately result in success will motivate hard work in the experiential system only if the belief is accompanied by the anticipation of positive affect or a decrease in negative affect. It follows that a person's desire for success in the rational system may or may not be accompanied by a corresponding affect-driven motive in the experiential system.

Because the experiential and rational systems operate in parallel and are interactive, each can influence the other with respect to both content and process. Of particular interest is the influence of the experiential system on the rational system, as it identifies a means by which unconscious information processing can bias conscious reasoning. In common with psychoanalytic theory, CEST assumes that thought and imagery outside of awareness have a ubiquitous influence on conscious thinking and behavior. In most situations, the automatic processing of the experiential system is the major determinant of behavior, because it is more rapid, less effortful, and accordingly more efficient than the rational system. Moreover, because its operation is usually accompanied by affect, it is likely to be experienced as more compelling than dispassionate analytical thinking is. Finally, because the influence of the experiential system is normally outside of awareness, the rational system often fails to control processing in the experiential system, because the person does not know that there is anything to control. The advantage of insight is that it permits rational control to be exercised. Thus, relative to psychoanalysis, CEST does not diminish the importance of the unconscious in human behavior; rather, it emphasizes a different source of unconscious influence.

Additional information about CEST is available elsewhere. (For reviews of the overall theory, see Epstein, 1973, 1980, 1991b, 1993b, 1994; for in-depth discussions of particular aspects of the theory and examples of supportive research, see Denes-Raj & Epstein, 1994; Epstein, 1976, 1983, 1984, 1985, 1987, 1990, 1991a, 1991c, 1993a, 1993b; Epstein & Erskine, 1983; Epstein & Katz, 1992; Epstein, Lipson, Holstein, & Huh, 1992; Epstein & Meier, 1989; Epstein, Pacini, Denes-Raj, & Heier, 1996; Katz & Epstein, 1991; Kirkpatrick & Epstein, 1992; Pacini, Muir, & Epstein, 1998.)

SOME BASIC ISSUES CONCERNING DUAL-PROCESS THEORIES

Two Systems or One?

Cognitive psychologists are divided on whether people are parallel information processors who operate by associative connections, or whether they operate according to a more deliberative, rule-based, sequential mode of information processing. Noting that there is impressive evidence on both sides of the issue, Sloman (1996) has suggested a resolution based on the assumption that people operate both ways. As support for his recommendation, he cites informal and indirect evidence from studies not explicitly designed to test his proposed solution. In order to provide more direct evidence, Epstein and his colleagues have conducted a series of studies explicitly designed to demonstrate the existence of two systems, and also to verify their principles of operation as proposed by CEST.

Research Support for Two Systems of Information Processing

In a series of investigations of judgmental heuristics that used modifications of procedures introduced by Tversky, Kahneman, and other cognitive psychologists (e.g., Kahneman, Slovic, & Tversky, 1982), Epstein and associates (Denes-Raj, Epstein, & Cole, 1995; Epstein, 1994; Epstein, Donovan, & Denes-Raj, in press; Epstein et al., 1992; Epstein, Pacini, et al., 1996) asked participants to respond to vignettes from three perspectives: how they believe most people would behave in the situations described, how they themselves would behave, and how a logical person would behave. In all of these studies, the majority of participants indicated that although they were well aware of how a logical person would behave, they believed that neither they nor most people would behave that way. The ratings from the perspective of how most people, including themselves, would behave followed the principles of the experiential system, whereas the ratings from the perspective of how a logical person would behave followed the principles of the rational system.

Similar results with other experimental paradigms in which people reported both their emotion-based and more intellectual solutions to problems have been reported by Sappington and his associates (Sappington & Russell, 1978; Sappington, Russell, Triplett, & Goodwin, 1980). Employing an experimental paradigm in which participants responded from different perspectives relevant to experiential and rational processing, Zukier and Pepitone (1984) and Schwarz, Strack, Hilton, and Nadderer (1991) also obtained similar results. Thus, the evidence from a variety of studies that examined how people believe they and others would behave from different perspectives indicates that most are aware of two modes of reasoning that correspond to the rational and experiential systems of CEST, and that although people "know better" (from a logical perspective), they report that they, like others, would behave in everyday life according to the principles of the experiential system.

Yet more impressive evidence of simultaneous processing in two different modes is provided by a series of studies of the "ratio bias" (RB) phenomenon (Denes-Raj & Epstein, 1994; Denes-Raj et al., 1995; Kirkpatrick & Epstein, 1992; Pacini & Epstein, in press; Pacini, Muir, & Epstein, 1998). The RB phenomenon refers to the judgment of low-probability events as having a lower subjective probability when represented by equivalent ratios of smaller numbers (e.g., 1 in 10) than of larger numbers (e.g., 10 in 100). In a typical RB experiment (e.g., Denes-Raj & Epstein, 1994), participants are given an opportunity to win money by blindly drawing a red jelly bean from one of two bowls that contain a designated percentage of red and white jelly beans. A small bowl always contains 1 in 10 (10%) red jelly beans, and a large bowl always contains 100 jelly beans, with the percentage of red jelly beans varying from 5% to 10%. We have found that most participants choose to draw from the 9% (large) rather than from the 10% (small) bowl, and that a surprisingly high number (nearly a quarter) even prefer to draw from the 5% (large) bowl (Denes-Raj & Epstein, 1994). When queried, participants say they know their behavior is irrational, but they feel they have a better chance of getting a red jelly bean when there are more of them. One participant informed us that she knew the correct answer and would give it in a statistics class, but that in real life it is better to go with the bowl that offers more absolute chances to win.

The RB experimental paradigm has been of particular interest to us because it presents a conflict between the appeal of numerosity in the experiential system (an extremely fundamental heuristic present in very young children and nonhuman animals; Gallistel & Gelman, 1992) and formal knowledge of ratios in the rational system. The series of studies of the RB phenomenon has demonstrated with both behavioral measures and self-reports that people in certain situations experience a conflict between rational and experiential reasoning, and that their responses often reflect a compromise between the two.

Other evidence for two systems is provided by our research on individual differences. If it is assumed that there are two fundamental adaptive systems, experiential and rational, then there should be two kinds of corresponding intelligence. The intelligence of the rational system is measurable with standard intelligence tests. Because no comparable instrument for measuring the intelligence of the experiential mode was available, Epstein and Meier (1989) constructed one, the Constructive Thinking Inventory (CTI). The CTI is a self-report test that measures the frequency of certain adaptive and maladaptive automatic thoughts and ways of construing events. The inventory provides scores on a global scale and six main scales, most of which have several subscales or facets. The six main scales are Emotional Coping, Behavioral Coping, Categorical Thinking, Esoteric Thinking, Personal Superstitious Thinking, and Naive Optimism. In line with the CEST assumption of independence between the two systems, Global Constructive Thinking and IQ are independent (Epstein & Meier, 1989). CTI scores are associated with a wide variety of measures of success in living, including work success, social success, and mental and physical well-being (Epstein, 1990, 1992a; Epstein with Brodsky, 1993; Epstein & Katz, 1992; Epstein & Meier, 1989; Katz & Epstein, 1991).

In another line of research involving individual differences in degree, rather than quality, of experiential and rational processing, we constructed the Rational-Experiential Inventory (REI; Epstein, Pacini, et al., 1996). To measure degree of processing in the rational mode, we used a modification of Cacioppo and Petty's (1982) Need for Cognition (NFC) scale. An example of an NFC item is "I would rather do something that requires little thought than something that is sure to challenge my thinking abilities." To measure degree of processing in the experiential mode, we constructed the Faith in Intuition (FI) scale. An example of an FI item is "I believe in trusting my hunches." Scores on the two scales are independent, and are coherently and differentially related to a wide variety of variables (Epstein, Pacini, et al., 1996). In general, NFC scores are more strongly directly associated with good adjustment (e.g., low depression, high self-esteem), and FI scores are more strongly directly associated with the ability to establish relationships, as well as with esoteric and superstitious beliefs.

We have also examined individual differences in the degree and quality of information processing in the two modes in reference to psychopathological states, such as depression. In one study (Pacini et al., 1998), we found that subclinically depressed college students reported engaging in less rational processing (as measured by the REI) and in more maladaptive experiential processing (as measured by the CTI) than did nondepressed controls. The results suggest that subclinically depressed students are unable to control their maladaptive experiential processing because of their insufficient rational processing, resulting in uncontrollable negative thoughts and feelings (see also Wenzlaff, Wegner, & Roper, 1988).

In summary, the findings from these individual-differences studies are consistent with the CEST assumption that there are two independent processing modes corresponding to the rational and experiential systems, and that although everyone employs both, there are important individual differences in the quantity and quality of their use. Other laboratory evidence in support of two systems of information processing is provided by studies examining the differences between the operating principles of the experiential and the rational systems—a topic discussed later.

Support from Everyday Life for Two Systems of Information Processing

Evidence for two independent systems that operate in parallel is prevalent in everyday behavior. An example is the maintenance of irrational fears in spite of awareness that the fears are unrealistic. Thus many people fear riding in airplanes but not in automobiles, despite knowing that the likelihood of a fatal accident is much greater in the latter case; similarly, many adults are terrorized by harmless mice, despite recognizing the absurdity of their fear. It has long been observed that intellectual intelligence (in the rational system) often fails to coincide with practical intelligence (in the experiential system). Insight derived directly from experience in or out of psychotherapy is widely recognized by therapists as more influential in changing behavior than intellectual knowledge obtained from books and lectures.

Superstitious beliefs are also very common in human thinking, despite people's capacity for complex intellectual thinking. Moreover, instead of being displaced by rational thinking as a function of maturity (which would be expected if there were only a single system of information processing), superstitious thinking and rational competence both increase with age (Epstein, 1994). In a study of superstitious thinking during the game of bingo (Epstein, 1998), many people reported that they did not believe that their magic charms or rituals actually worked, but nevertheless they felt compelled to continue with these practices. They added that they would not continue to play the game if they could not do so. Perhaps the strongest evidence for the operation of two systems that operate by different rules is provided by the ubiquity of religion across time and cultures. Many people find that religion provides them with more satisfactory explanations and guides for living than does science. The reason for this, according to CEST, is that religion directly appeals to the experiential system through the use of narrative, metaphor, emotionally engaging messages, music, and social relatedness, whereas science primarily appeals to intellect.

(For a more thorough discussion of real-life evidence for two independent modes of information processing, see Epstein, 1994.)

It may thus be concluded, based on the overall evidence from research and everyday behavior, that there is compelling evidence for the existence of two independent modes of information processing that operate in parallel by different rules.

How Are the Two Modes of Processing Best Conceived?

During the past two decades, many dual-process theories have been proposed (both in and out of the domain of social cognition) that include divisions somewhat similar to the experiential and rational modes of information processing proposed by CEST (Epstein, 1994). Several in the social-cognitive domain are represented in the present volume. Following is a sample of dual-process theories outside of the social-cognitive domain: Paivio's (1986, 1991) and Bucci's (1985) verbal and nonverbal modes; Anderson's (1976, 1982) and Winograd's (1975) declarative knowledge and procedural knowledge; Reber's (1993), Schacter's (1987), Broadbent, FitsGerald, and Broadbent's (1986), and Nissen, Willingham, and Hartman's (1989) tacit/implicit and explicit knowledge and memory systems; Tversky and Kahneman's (1983) extensional and heuristic reasoning; Labouvie-Vief's (1989, 1990) logos and mythos; Bruner's (1986) propositional and narrative modes; McClelland, Koestner, and Weinberger's (1989) implicit and self-attributed motives; Leventhal's (1982, 1984) schematic and conceptual modes; Buck's (1985, 1991) learning and logical modes; and Brewin's (1989) subconscious/automatic and conscious/deliberative modes (for brief summaries of these positions, see Epstein, 1994).

The very existence of so many divisions within and outside the social-cognitive domain raises the question of which of them is most useful and valid. The answer is that it depends on the theorist's purpose and the level of analysis of interest. Thus, domain-specific divisions may be suitable for the restricted domain that they are meant to encompass, but may not be suited for other domains or for more general conceptualizations. At the most general level, we believe

that a strong case can be made for the experiential-rational division proposed by CEST, in common with similar divisions by Buck (1985, 1991) and Leventhal (1982, 1984). First, it is the most inclusive division and can subsume the other approaches (Epstein, 1994). Second, it makes sense from an evolutionary perspective, as learning directly from experience is basic to adaptation in nonhuman and human animals, and the use of language (and, relatedly, symbolic thinking) is a later development that is unique to humans.

Simply identifying two systems is obviously just a beginning. Of greater importance is validating the principles by which they are assumed to operate—the topic to which we turn next.

What Are the Operating Principles of the Two Systems?

What support is there for the differential rules of experiential and rational processing outlined in Table 23.1? In this section, we briefly review the logical and empirical support for each of the principles.

Holistic versus Analytic Processing

According to CEST, the experiential system responds to the overall context of situations rather than to isolated, abstracted elements, which requires analytical thinking and is in the domain of the rational system. This is illustrated in our studies of conjunction problems, including the notorious "Linda" problem (Donovan & Epstein, 1992; Epstein, Denes-Raj, & Pacini, 1995). Linda is described as a bright 31-year-old woman who majored in philosophy and was active in antinuclear demonstrations. Participants are asked to rank the likelihood that she is a feminist, a bank teller, and both a feminist and a bank teller. In repeated studies, a majority of respondents rank "Linda is both" as more likely than "Linda is a bank teller," thereby violating the conjunction rule, according to which two events cannot be more likely than one (Tversky & Kahneman, 1983). These studies have shown that the major reason why people make conjunction errors is that even when they are instructed to treat the problem as a statistical problem and ignore irrelevant information, most are unable or unwilling to do so (Donovan & Epstein, 1997). That is, they are unable or unwilling to disregard the overall context in which the problem is presented. When asked to explain their rankings, many participants construct a narrative based on an interpretation of the overall situation (Epstein et al., 1995). For example, they say that Linda is more likely to be a bank teller and a feminist than just a feminist, because she has to make a living. When asked to select the correct statistical principle from among several that are presented, many change the principles to match their holistic impressions of the situations, instead of applying the principles consistently across relevant situations as an analytical approach would require (Donovan & Epstein, 1997).

Other research has found a strong tendency for people to judge others in holistic ways when they respond from an experiential but not from a rational perspective. More specifically, they obtain a broadly general impression of a person (e.g., the person is good or bad, or a winner or a loser), based on limited, arbitrary information, when they respond from an experiential but not from a rational perspective. For example, in one study, one version of a vignette described a situation in which a rich benefactor offered three friends $100 each if they each threw heads in a coin toss (reported in Epstein, 1994). The first two people threw heads, but the third, Smith, threw tails. The benefactor gave them another chance, only to have the same events occur. Participants were asked to rate the emotions of the three friends, and to judge the likelihood that the other two would invite Smith on a gambling trip to Las Vegas in which they would share wins and losses. Most reported that Smith would feel guilty, that the others would feel angry, and that they would not invite Smith because "he is a loser." Although the participants reported knowing that these reactions were irrational, many felt that this is the way most people, including themselves, would react in real life.

Using a different experimental paradigm, Gilbert and Malone (1995) found that under time constraints and other conditions of reduced cognitive resources (conducive to experiential processing), people tended to make holistic judgments about personality characteristics; under conditions of less constraint (conducive to rational processing), they qualified their judgments by taking into account situational influences.

Automatic, Effortless versus Intentional, Effortful Processing

The experiential system is assumed to be a highly efficient, automatic system that is effortless and makes minimal demands on cognitive resources. The difference between the two systems in this respect is immediately apparent in many examples in everyday life, such as the ease and speed with which pictures can be perused compared to reading about the same material. It is also evident in the sequential processing of information. Initial reactions, including perception and initial impressions occur automatically. They then may be followed by more deliberate thinking, which may correct impulsive, inappropriate interpretations. In a study we conducted on the sequential processing of information (reported in Epstein, 1994) participants recorded their initial and following reactions to a variety of events described in vignettes. The initial reactions tended to operate according to the principles of the experiential system and the later reactions according to the principles of the rational system. Gilbert and Malone (1995), using a different procedure, reported similar observations. Research by others on unconscious priming effects (see review in Bargh, 1989), as well as our own studies on priming (Epstein, 1994; Epstein et al., 1992) support the automatic operation of experiential processing, and indicates something of additional considerable importance, namely, its ability to influence rational processing in the absence of awareness of the influence.

Affect-Related versus Affect-Free Processing

CEST assumes that the experiential system is emotionally driven and intimately associated with the experience of affect, whereas the rational system is relatively affect-free. This is not meant to deny that people can react with emotion and even passion to intellectual matters, but to suggest that when this occurs it is the result of a contribution by the experiential system. It will be recalled that all human behavior, according to CEST, is assumed to be a joint function of both modes of processing.

An example of the affective processing of the experiential system is provided by a vignette study of counterfactual thinking in which the emotional intensity of outcomes was systematically varied (Epstein et al., 1992). It was found that experiential processing, in the form of nonrational, associative responses, was more prevalent under conditions of higher than of lower emotional intensity. For example, one vignette depicted two characters whose behavior differed according to whether it was constrained or unconstrained in selecting a parking space. In the constrained condition, Robert parked his new car in the only available spot in the lot. In the unconstrained condition, Tom parked his new car in a half-empty lot. In both conditions, as the protagonist backed out of his space, the car parked opposite also backed out, resulting in either minor or major damage to the new cars. Most people rated Tom (in the unconstrained condition) as feeling more foolish than Robert (in the constrained condition) when they responded from an experiential but not from a rational perspective. The effect was heightened when the damage to the car was described as major rather than minor. In the vignette study described earlier in which a rich benefactor offered money ($1 or $100) for getting three heads in a coin toss, participants were more likely to make negative judgments of Smith as "a loser" in the $100 than in the $1 condition (reported in Epstein, 1994).

Associative versus Logical Connections

According to CEST, the experiential system makes connections through association, whereas the rational system does so through logical considerations. In a vignette study of counterfactual thinking, many responses from an experiential but not from a rational orientation were associative (Epstein et al., 1992). For example, one vignette described a situation in which a protagonist arrived at the airport late because of being tied-up in traffic. In the "far-miss" version of the vignette, the flight left on time, and the protagonist missed it by 30 minutes. In the "near-miss" version,

the flight was delayed, and the protagonist missed it by 5 minutes. Participants were asked to choose in which scenario the protagonist would feel more foolish for having dawdled at home for 10 minutes before departing for the airport. Experiential responses were expected to follow associative connections, such as that dawdling was a more significant factor in the near-miss than in the far-miss version, whereas rational responses were expected to reflect the awareness that the association of dawdling and lateness was no more significant in one situation than in the other. In line with prediction, significantly more participants selected the near-miss situation when responding from an experiential perspective (how most people would respond in real life) than when responding from a rational perspective (how a completely logical person would respond). From the latter perspective but not the former, most selected a "no-difference" option.

Of particular interest was an RB study in which participants chose, in a game of chance, between alternatives that differed in absolute number of winners but offered equivalent odds (e.g., 1 in 10 vs. 10 in 100) that were varied along a probability dimension (e.g., from 10% to 90%; Pacini et al., 1998). Earlier research showed that most people select the larger numerator when asked to select between 1 in 10 and 10 in 100 chances of winning (Kirkpatrick & Epstein, 1992), in accordance with experiential, heuristic numerosity. Consistent with past findings, participants in the probability continuum study rarely gave the logical response of "no difference" between the equivalent alternatives, except in one condition. The exception occurred when both alternatives offered 50% odds, in which case the no-difference response was given with surprising frequency (Pacini & Epstein, 1998a). This finding was explained by the consideration that 50% indicates an equivalent likelihood, which made available the association of "no difference."

Concretive, Imagistic versus Abstract, Verbal Processing

The experiential system is assumed to be primarily a nonverbal, imagistic system. This is not to deny that in humans, the experiential system can react to language in the same manner as to any other event or stimulus. It does suggest that the most basic rules of operation of the experiential system were developed to be applicable to nonverbal information processing.

The experiential system encodes information in the form of concrete exemplars, images, and narratives; consequently, it is more responsive to concrete than to abstract representations. In contrast, the rational system encodes information in abstract symbols, and is therefore better equipped to deal with abstractions and delay of gratification. Our studies of the RB effect have repeatedly demonstrated the concretive processing of the experiential system. Smaller numbers, because they are easier to visualize (Paivio, 1991), are more concrete than larger numbers, and absolute numbers are more concrete than ratios because ratios refer to a relation between numbers. As such, the experiential system should be better able to comprehend smaller rather than large numbers, absolute numbers rather than ratios, and ratios expressed in smaller rather than larger numbers. In support of these assumptions, we have repeatedly found that a majority of our participants perform as if they believe that a tray with 1 in 10 red jelly beans offers a lower probability of obtaining a red jelly bean than a tray with 10 in 100 red jelly beans, despite acknowledging that they know the probabilities are identical (Kirkpatrick & Epstein, 1992; Denes-Raj & Epstein, 1994; Pacini & Epstein, 1998a; Pacini, et al., 1998). In their explanations, they attribute this preference to the higher number of red jelly beans in the larger tray and the lower number in the smaller tray. Even when the trays offer unequal ratios (e.g., 1 in 10 vs. 9 in 100), a majority prefer to draw from the probability-disadvantaged tray that has more target items.

According to CEST, the experiential system represents events primarily in the form of concrete images, and therefore tends to respond similarly to real and imagined objects and events. If this is true, reactions to a visualized situation can be expected to mimic those observed in a real situation. We tested this hypothesis in an RB study in which one group vividly imagined the jelly bean trays and another simply read a description of them. We found that the former group be-

haved in a manner similar to what we have observed in a real situation (in which most people respond heuristically), whereas the nonvisualizing group behaved more rationally (Pacini & Epstein, 1998). The reaction of the experiential system to imagined experience may explain why visualization is a useful technique in training athletes and in treating phobias with systematic desensitization.

An important facet of the concretive principle of experiential processing is the affirmative-representation principle (Pacini & Epstein, 1998a). According to this principle, people understand direct, affirmative information (i.e., what is) better than they do negative information (i.e., what is not), because the latter is too abstract to be directly represented in the experiential system. In an RB study with a condition in which red jelly beans were desirable and with another condition in which they were undesirable, we (Pacini & Epstein, 1998) found that participants tended to reformulate the avoidance task (i.e., not to select a red bean) into an approach task (i.e., to select a white bean).

Another concretive operation is narrative processing. This operation is exhibited in the tendency of the experiential system to integrate information in the form of concrete stories rather than abstract principles (Epstein et al., 1995; Epstein, Donovan, & Denes-Raj, in press). As previously noted, several investigators (e.g., Epstein et al., 1995; Tversky & Kahneman, 1983; Yates & Carlson, 1986) have expressed surprise at the degree to which people spontaneously produce narratives in their responses to the "Linda" conjunction problem.

Although concrete representations often facilitate performance (Gilhooly & Falconer, 1974; Johnson-Laird & Wason, 1977), this is clearly not the case with conjunction problems like the Linda problem, which is couched in concrete personality information about Linda. As noted earlier, a majority do not interpret the Linda problem as a conjunction problem, but rather as one that requires matching personality attributes to behavior. Our research that has simultaneously varied the dimensions of abstract versus concrete and natural versus unnatural in conjunction problems has suggested the following general principle: Concrete representations facilitate performance in natural problems and interfere with performance in unnatural problems, with "natural" independently defined as the customary way in which a problem is interpreted based on past experience with similar problems (Epstein et al., 1995; Epstein, Donovan, & Denes-Raj, in press; Donovan & Epstein, 1997; see also Nisbett, Krantz, Jepson & Kunda, 1983). For example, the natural solution to a statistical problem presented in abstract form is to apply statistical principles. Concrete representations engage experiential processing, which results in natural responding—a source of error when the correct solution requires an unnatural response. Because of the Linda problem's concrete attributes, nearly everyone responds with a natural solution, which is the prediction of behavior from personality attributes, rather than responding with an unnatural solution in terms of abstract statistical principles.

Rapid, Immediate versus
Delayed, Reflective Processing

The experiential system is a rapid, preconscious system for responding efficiently to daily events, whereas the rational system is a slower, deliberative system better suited for delayed action and solving abstract problems. Support for this position has been provided by a series of studies in which people reported their immediate and delayed responses to a sample of situations described in vignette form (described in Epstein, 1993b; Epstein & Morling, 1995; Morling & Epstein, 1997). First thoughts or "gut-level" reactions were often associative and nonrational, in the manner of the experiential system, whereas later thoughts were more often logical, in the manner of the rational system. For example, when participants put themselves in the place of a protagonist who had an accident when backing out his car from a space that his friend had selected, many reported that their first thought was that the accident was the friend's fault, and that they would feel anger. "It's his fault. Except for him, I wouldn't have had the accident." By their third thought, their thinking had become more rational. They accepted the responsibility as their own, and they reported a corresponding change in emotion from anger to guilt. Similar results were reported by Gilbert and Malone (1995) with a different experimental paradigm.

Slow Changes with Accumulating Experience
versus Rapid Changes
with the Speed of Thought

We have not yet conducted research on the principle of how the two systems change. However, it necessarily follows that if experiential processing involves learning from cumulative experience, then it takes time for such learning to occur. Changes in the rational system, on the other hand, can occur immediately and permanently with simply the presentation of new information. If a person mistakenly believes that fractions should be added by separately adding the numerators and denominators and is informed that the denominators have to be first converted to a common base, after which only the numerators should be added, the person can make the adjustment immediately and permanently. Contrast this with what it would take to change the experientially derived belief that people are untrustworthy.

More Crudely versus More Highly
Differentiated Operations

The experiential system operates according to heuristic rules of thumb that are often sources of overgeneralization. In contrast, the rational system is more prone to make distinctions. This has been well illustrated in our studies of reactions to arbitrary outcomes (e.g., Epstein, 1994; Epstein et al., 1992), where participants fail to distinguish between intended and arbitrary outcomes when responding from an experiential but not from a rational perspective. In a vignette study in which a protagonist was described as having an unfortunate, arbitrary outcome, participants were quick to label the protagonist as "a loser," and to indicate that they would not trust his luck in other situations when they responded from an experiential but not from a rational perspective. The same principle is supported in studies demonstrating that people are prone to make broad generalizations on the basis of irrelevant characteristics, such as skin color and surname (see review in Fiske & Taylor, 1991).

More Crudely versus More Highly
Integrated Operations

The experiential system is assumed to operate on the basis of context-specific schemas derived from emotionally significant and/or repetitive experience, whereas the rational system operates to a greater extent according to context-general, abstract principles. Certain rules, such as the conjunction rule, are obviously supposed to hold across all situations. However, we have found that when people respond in the experiential mode, they apply different rules according to the context in which the same basic problem is presented (Donovan & Epstein, 1997). That is, rather than apply the same rule across all situations, they modify the rule according to the context in which the problem is embedded. For example, in certain situations they endorse the correct principle that two independent events are less likely than one, and in others they endorse the false principle that two events are more likely than one. This does not occur when they are presented with context-free representations, such as abstract versions of the same problem.

Other evidence that there is less integration in the experiential than in the rational system is that when people respond to a variety of vignettes, the internal-consistency reliability coefficient of their responses across vignettes from an experiential perspective is lower than when they respond from a rational perspective (Denes-Raj & Epstein, 1994; Epstein, Pacini, et al., 1996). This indicates that they perceive less integration in situations when responding from an experiential than from a rational perspective.

Passive, Automatic, and Preconscious versus Active, Deliberate, and Conscious Experience of Processing

The experiential system operates automatically and effortlessly by heuristic rules and is experienced passively, whereas the rational system operates consciously and effortfully by people's understanding of logical rules, and is experienced as consciously controlled. This is most clearly exhibited in people's experience of emotions. People feel that they are seized by their emotions, but are in control of their conscious thoughts. They fail to realize that the emotions themselves are almost invariably produced by preconscious interpretations of events in their experiential system. People, of course, react not to situations as objectively defined, but to their interpretations of situations. As they are not aware of their preconscious thoughts, they are unable to control them, and, in fact, do not realize there is anything that can be controlled.

Other evidence of the uncontrollable, passive experience of thoughts in the experiential system is provided by intrusive thoughts (Wegner & Schneider, 1989), subliminal processing (see review in Bargh, 1989), and unconscious priming effects (e.g., Lombardi, Higgins, & Bargh, 1987; Newman & Uleman, 1990; also see review in Fiske & Taylor, 1991), which are discussed later.

Self-Evident Validity versus Need for Justification via Logic and Evidence

In the experiential system, experience, either direct or vicarious, is the only reality. The rational system, on the other hand, bases its concepts of truth and reality on logic and evidence. Experientially, the earth is flat, very large, and stable, and the sun is a small round ball that rises above and sinks below the horizon. Rationally, the picture people have is very different. Members of technologically advanced societies have been taught to give their rational understanding priority over their experiential impressions. However, as our research has shown, people do not always do this; not infrequently they give their subjective experience priority over their intellectual knowledge.

In the series of RB studies, many people have reported that they find their experiential processing more compelling than their rational thinking, and act "against their better judgment" (Kirkpatrick & Epstein, 1992; Denes-Raj & Epstein, 1994; Denes-Raj et al., 1995; Donovan & Epstein, 1997; Epstein, Pacini, et al., 1996). Similar reactions were observed in our studies of arbitrary outcomes, in which people said they subjectively experienced certain outcomes as more unfortunate than others, although they knew that on a logical basis that there was no difference.

Conclusion

Taken together, our research as well as the research of others provides strong evidence for two independent systems of information processing that operate according to the rules of the experiential and rational systems, as proposed in CEST.

How Do the Two Systems Interact?

According to CEST, the experiential and rational modes of processing are interactive, with both modes contributing to all behavior. This raises the following two questions: Does the interaction occur sequentially, simultaneously, or both: And what determines the degree of influence of each mode in an interaction? Our research has indicated that rational and experiential interactions can be sequential or simultaneous, and that the form of the interaction can be influenced both by the situation and individual differences.

Sequential Interaction:
Evidence and Implications

The influence of the experiential on the rational system is of particular interest in CEST, because it describes a means by which unconscious, automatic processing routinely influences conscious reasoning. There is ample evidence attesting to the operation of such a process. For example, innumerable studies demonstrate that priming the experiential system by presenting stimuli at subthreshold levels influences subsequent responses in the rational system (see review in Bargh, 1989). Other evidence indicates that the form, independent of the content, of processing in the rational system can also be influenced by priming the experiential system. When processing in the experiential mode is followed by attempts to process information in the rational mode, the rational mode itself may be compromised by intrusions of heuristic reasoning principles (e.g., Chaiken & Maheswaran, 1994; Denes-Raj et al., 1995; Edwards, 1990; Epstein et al., 1992). Thus people often believe that they are operating purely in a rational mode when their rational processing is distorted by processing in the experiential mode (Epstein et al., 1992).

Does the influence also occur in the opposite direction? That is, does thinking in the rational mode influence subsequent processing in the experiential mode? There are several ways in which this can occur. First, because the experiential system is an associative system, a thought that occurs in the rational mode can trigger an association in the experiential system. An example is someone working on a problem in reasoning for which the content is meant to be arbitrary but happens to be personally meaningful. The result is a string of associations in the experiential system, and attendant emotions, that can bias or otherwise distort logical reasoning. This example is an illustration of the rational system's influence on the experiential system, which in turn can influence the rational system, in a chain of reciprocal interactions.

Second, the slower-reacting rational system can respond in a corrective way to the more rapid, "impulsive" experiential system. This commonly occurs when people identify an automatic thought as unreasonable and replace it with a more adaptive thought. Such a process was documented in a study in which we had college students keep daily records of the most stressful event of the day for 30 days. They were asked to report their initial construal of the stressful event, and then to record the emotional, mental, and behavioral reactions that followed (Epstein & Pacini, 1998). The students frequently reported initially inappropriate construals that they subsequently corrected through more deliberate rational reasoning. The same process was observed in a vignette study of sequential processing (reported in Epstein, 1994).

Similar results have been reported by Gilbert (1989) and his associates, who used a different experimental paradigm. They examined people's inferences about whether the behavior that was described in others was revealing about the others' traits or could be attributed to situational factors. They found that dispositional inferences tended to occur rapidly, effortlessly, and unconsciously, signifying processing in the experiential system. Inferences about situational influences, on the other hand, required more deliberative reasoning, thereby implicating the rational system. These delayed thoughts were often used to correct initial unwarranted trait inferences.

Another possibility is that, once instigated, rational processing can interfere with attempts to think experientially. In an experiment in which individuals were instructed to respond first from the perspective of one mode and then from the other, with order counterbalanced, each mode was found to strongly influence processing in the subsequent mode, that is, there were very strong priming effects in both directions (Epstein, Donovan, & Denes-Raj, in press; Epstein et al., 1992). Rational responding decreased after experiential responding, and experiential responding decreased after rational responding. However, unlike the consistent finding of a direct influence of experiential on rational processing, we have found that the influence of the rational on the experiential mode is inconsistent. Sometimes it produces a direct effect (Epstein, Donovan, & Denes-Raj, in press), sometimes a contrast effect (Epstein et al., 1992), and sometimes no effect at all (Epstein et al., 1995). The reason why we have uniformly found a direct influence of the experiential on the rational system, but not the reverse, may be that the former effect is more likely to occur outside of awareness. It has been found in research by others that direct priming effects tend to be exhibited when participants are unaware of the influence of the prime, whereas when they are aware of it, they overcompensate and produce a contrast effect (Petty & Jarvis, 1996).

It may be concluded that the influence of one system on the other proceeds in both directions (i.e., the experiential and the rational systems mutually influence each other). There is an important difference, however: The influence of the experiential on the rational system seems thus far to be always direct, suggesting that people often rationalize their experiential processing, whereas the reverse effect is more variable, possibly because automatic processing in the experiential system often occurs outside of awareness.

Simultaneous Interaction: Evidence and Implications

So far, we have discussed the sequential interaction of the two systems. There is also evidence that the two modes interact simultaneously. This is particularly important to CEST, because it is the basis of the view that all behavior represents a compromise between the two modes of information processing.

The simultaneous operation of the two modes is most clearly indicated by our research on the RB phenomenon. In this research, simultaneous operation of the two modes is indicated by the direct report of conflict ("My reason tells me to go with the ratios, but my feelings tell me to select the tray with more winners"), and by compromises, as

indicated by the preference, in most participants, for the tray that offers a numerosity advantage over the one that offers a slight, but not greater, probability advantage. We found in one study that individual differences in degree of rational processing, as determined by the REI (Epstein, Pacini, et al., 1996), were directly associated with degree of optimal (rational) responding in the RB paradigm (Pacini & Epstein, 1998).

In an RB study of particular interest with respect to individual differences (Yanko et al., 1998) adults, with a well-consolidated understanding of ratios, produced compromises that were only slightly short of optimal responses (nearly half preferred 9 in 100 over 1 in 10), and children with a newly acquired understanding of ratios produced compromises that were more nonoptimal, preferring to draw from a bowl that offered 5 in 100, but not one that offered 3 in 100 winners in comparison to one that offered 1 in 10 winners. This study, like the other RB studies, indicates that people compromise between the appeal of numerosity in the experiential system and their knowledge of ratios in the rational system. However, it goes further by indicating a shift toward a greater weighting of the rational component as a function of increasing age, suggesting that there is an increasing appreciation that a higher priority should be accorded to rational than to experiential processing with maturity.

How Do the Two Systems Develop?

It is beyond the scope of this chapter to review developmental issues thoroughly from the perspective of CEST. For present purposes, a brief discussion of the more general implications of the theory will have to suffice. Other sources can be consulted for further information on the developmental implications of CEST (Epstein, 1973, 1991c, 1993b; Epstein & Erskine, 1983).

It follows from CEST that development should be examined along three different avenues: development of the experiential system, development of the rational system, and development of the relation and interaction between the two systems. It is interesting, in this respect, to compare the developmental views of CEST to those of Freud and Piaget. The systems in Freud's theory that most resemble the experiential and rational systems of CEST are the id and the ego. Freud assumed that the ego develops with experience, but the id remains unchanged as a primitive reservoir of psychic energy and instinctual impulse. Mature development consists of appropriately controlling the id and constructively channeling its energy through a process referred to as "sublimation." The id, if it were not regulated by the ego, would be a totally maladaptive system and would not be sufficient for survival. This is in sharp contrast to the position of CEST, in which the experiential and rational systems are both considered to be adaptive and to develop over time.

Piaget assumed that lower, more primitive stages of cognition are replaced as children mature by increasingly sophisticated stages, terminating in a stage of "formal operations," in which people think in a logical manner. It is acknowledged in Piaget's system that there is overlap between the stages, and that individuals at higher stages sometimes regress to functioning at lower levels, but the basic assumption is that more advanced stages generally replace more primitive ones along a continuum of nonrational to increasingly rational information processing. This differs from the position of CEST, in which the rational and experiential systems function in parallel at all stages of development. Thus, according to CEST, rational thinking never replaces experiential thinking. Both systems develop, albeit from different kinds of experiences, and they interact throughout the life span.

CEST has little new to say about the development of the rational system. It is obvious that people's ability to think rationally improves with maturity and training. CEST simply accepts what has been learned through research about the rational thinking ability of individuals across the life span. The one unique contribution that CEST has to make with respect to an understanding of rational thinking is that it is far more influenced by experiential processing than has been recognized. What poses as rational, objective thinking, according to CEST, is often, to a considerable extent, a rationalization of experientially derived impressions.

The development of the experiential system involves changes in both process and content. Differences in thinking style between younger and older children illustrate changes in process. For example, younger children confuse fantasy with reality and tend to overgeneralize grossly, whereas older children think in ways that are more realistic and differentiated. As for content in the experiential system, it will be recalled that according to CEST, all individuals acquire schemas that are generalizations from emotionally significant and repetitive experience. These generalizations, in the normal course of development, become increasingly differentiated and integrative. Included are the preconscious cognitions that mediate emotions, which in the process become increasingly acculturated. The result is that the emotions themselves become socialized. For example, a young child who becomes angry following any injury, accidental or otherwise, becomes an older child who forgives unintended injuries but becomes angry at perceived malevolent intentions, whether or not they materialize.

An initial set of schemas develops around emotions, which are viewed in CEST as preprogrammed tendencies to react in certain ways to critical life events of evolutionary significance. Examples are feeling fear and being motivated to escape or seek support when confronted with a threatening stimulus, and feeling anger and being motivated to attack when restrained or otherwise thwarted. These cognitive-affective schemas provide the foundation for the development of more differentiated and integrative networks of schemas with increasing experience. The important point is that there is an initial disposition for certain kinds of schematic networks to develop on the basis of biological structures, but that the networks become increasingly "psychologized" through interactions with the environment.

As already noted, important cognitive networks develop in relation to the fulfillment and frustration of four basic needs. For example, as a result of the need to maximize well-being, individuals automatically attend to events that are associated with pain and pleasure. With increasing experience, they develop an increasingly differentiated and integrative network of descriptive and motivational schemas concerning the world and the self as sources of pleasure and pain and ways to cope with it.

The four basic needs have their own developmental trajectory. The most biologically based one, and therefore the first to exert an influence on the infant's emerging comprehension of the world and the self, is the need to achieve pleasure and to avoid pain. Objects associated with pleasure or pain are automatically attended to and internalized as mental constructs, thereby becoming the earliest schematic representations. Once a construct of an object is formed, its recognition as well as that of similar objects becomes a source of pleasure, and deviations from it beyond a certain point become a source of distress. Here we see in primitive form the emergence of the need to maintain a stable coherent conceptual system, the second most basic need. The need for relationship, the third most basic need, is assumed to develop as a result of the consequences of relationships for infants with respect to both pleasure–pain and familiarity considerations. The fourth most basic need, the need to enhance self-esteem, is assumed in CEST to be derived at its most rudimentary level from the need for relationship. Initially, a child's feeling of being loved by significant others is critically important for the child's emotional well-being. With the development of a self-concept, the view of the self to be loved becomes internalized, and the need for self-love then becomes equivalent to being loved by significant others (for a more thorough development of this position, see Epstein, 1980; Epstein & Erskine, 1983). It is important to recognize that once the four basic needs have developed, they are considered to be equally important in influencing behavior. As for having once had a higher biological priority than others, it is of no consequence, because any one need can override any of the others, depending on the individual and circumstances. As an example, consider the case of someone enduring torture in order to maintain self-esteem or to protect the life of a loved one.

In common with Bowlby's theory, CEST assumes that people's models of relationships are derived from their past emotionally significant relationships, and that the models importantly influence how they relate to others. The theories differ, however, in that Bowlby confined his discussion of models to relationships, whereas CEST also includes schemas about the impersonal world (e.g., whether it is viewed as harsh or benign, predictable or chaotic). A second important difference is that CEST emphasizes the existence of two conceptual systems, whereas Bowlby did not concern himself with this issue, but described phenomena corresponding to CEST's view of the operation of the experiential system.

To turn to the developmental course of the relative influence of the experiential on the rational system, CEST assumes that the infant, before acquiring language, can only respond in the experiential mode. The rational system develops in relation to the acquisition of language. Language permits a higher level of abstract reasoning and a distancing from immediate experience. Not only is the older child able to respond with a wider array of rational reactions as a result of maturation, the acquisition of language, and of training, but the older child also learns about the priority that is expected to be accorded to rational processing under most circumstances. This view is supported by the study of probability decisions in children and adults (Yanko et al., 1998), described earlier.

Although the balance of influence between the two systems shifts in the direction of rational processing with age and training, the degree of this shift varies with situations and individuals. Moreover, the shift is always less than complete, as the experiential system continues to influence the rational system no matter how much a person attempts to be completely rational. Even if it were possible for a person to be completely rational, it would not be desirable, for the person would lose the advantages gained from appropriate experiential processing. According to CEST, an ideal state of development would involve a high level of functioning in both systems, with the rational system being in touch with the experiential system, and the person being able to weigh the relative advantages of each when making decisions.

A brief word is in order about the development of individual differences in experiential processing. At this point, we have conducted only preliminary research on this issue; what we can offer, therefore, are only logical considerations and hypotheses to be tested. According to CEST, emotions are intimately associated with the experiential system. It follows that people who are more emotional by temperament than others should be prone to develop a style of information processing that is highly influenced by the experiential mode. In an initial study with a narrow, preliminary measure of experiential processing, we failed to find a relation between individual differences in emotional reactivity and experiential processing (Epstein, Pacini, et al., 1996). However, more recently we have found a direct relationship between a broader measure of experientiality and emotional expressiveness (Pacini & Epstein, in press). In other research, Norris and Epstein (1998) have found that the relation between self-reported emotionality and other facets of experiential processing is strong enough to warrant incorporating it in a more broadly conceptualized scale of experiential processing.

We also have some tentative evidence suggesting that high levels of rationality may be associated with adverse childhood experiences, at least within limits. In preliminary research, participants who obtained high rationality scores on the REI reported a greater incidence of distressing events in childhood than others (Epstein, Pacini, et al., 1996). It remains to be seen whether this result is replicable, and in particular whether it can be confirmed in prospective studies. If so, a possible explanation is that facing some degree of adversity may provide an impetus to developing a more thoughtful rather than a spontaneous, intuitive approach to life. Expressed otherwise, people may tend not to take life seriously unless they have to.

It is possible that the particular kind of aversive experience an individual is exposed to is no less important than its intensity and duration with respect to its influence on thinking style. Following some kinds of aversive experience, people may fail to develop a normal interest in rational, analytical thinking. In a study of subclinically depressed students, the depressed group reported less interest and less engagement in rational, analytical thinking than the control group did (Pacini et al., 1998). Our data say nothing about why this should occur. One possibility is that under extreme circumstances, such as the death of a loved one, a child may feel helpless and find that thinking about the situation simply adds to negative feelings. Such a child may develop a tendency to avoid thinking deeply in general. A somewhat similar alternative hypothesis is that if a child's thinking about a loved one leads to negative thoughts about that person, such as that the loved one is bad and the child is good and undeserving of being treated badly, the child may avoid thinking deeply because of its negative implications for maintaining the hope of eventually securing love through good behavior (Epstein, 1992b; Sullivan, 1953). Another hypothesis, not incompatible with the others, is that strong emotions at critical stages of development may directly interfere with thinking in the rational mode.

Having separately considered temperamental and situational factors, one might question how they interact developmentally. A person who is temperamentally highly emotional can be expected to be more strongly affected by negative events than someone who is less emotional. Thus, the same kind of negative events that foster avoidance of thinking in one person may stimulate the development of another thinking style in another.

Admittedly, much of what we have said about the development of thinking styles is highly speculative. There is obviously much work that remains to be done on this issue.

BROADER IMPLICATIONS

The most important implication of our findings is that they provide support for a more defensible psychodynamic theory of personality than the model provided by classical psychoanalysis (Epstein, 1994). Given the nature of the interaction between the two systems proposed by CEST, including the influence of experiential on subsequent rational processing and compromises between the two processes as a result of their simultaneous operation, attempts at rational thinking are often compromised by automatic information processing in the experiential system. It follows that the only way people can hope to be reasonably objective and rational is to compensate for their experiential processing, which means that they must be aware of it. Relatedly, it follows that to deny the experiential system is to be controlled by it. Lest it appear that the experiential system is primarily a source of distortion and otherwise maladaptive thinking, it is important to recognize that the experiential system is a highly efficient system for coping with the events of everyday life, and that it is intimately associated with affect and therefore with motivation. It may be difficult to live with the experiential system, but it would be impossible to live without it.

IN DEFENSE OF BROAD THEORY

A word is in order in defense of a broad personality theory, such as CEST, as contrasted with the more domain-specific dual-process theories that have typically been proposed by social-cognitive theorists.

It is evident that many of the principles proposed by CEST are not new. The finding that processing under limited resources and motivation tends to be more superficial than under the opposite conditions has been well established and explained by other theories. There is also nothing new about the finding that information processing in certain circumstances tends to be associative, and that problem solving is often facilitated by concrete representations. It might therefore be argued that CEST is unnecessary because the phenomena it explains can be satisfactorily explained by other theories. This argument can be rejected for two reasons. One is that CEST has uncovered several new phenomena, such as the independence of individual differences in degree of heuristic and analytical processing (Epstein, Pacini, et al., 1996), the greater compellingness of the outcome of heuristic than of rational processing in circumstances where the two are equally accessible (Denes-Raj & Epstein, 1994; Donovan & Epstein, 1997; Epstein, Pacini, et al., 1996; Kirkpatrick & Epstein, 1992; Pacini et al., 1998), compromises between processing in the experiential and rational modes (Denes-Raj & Epstein, 1994; Kirkpatrick & Epstein, 1992; Pacini et al., 1998), compromises between basic needs within the experiential system (Morling & Epstein, 1997), and the greater degree of nonrationality in human information processing than there was reason to suspect from previous research (Donovan & Epstein, 1997; Epstein et al., 1995; Epstein, Pacini, et al., 1996). The principles of experiential processing have also led to detecting the invalidity of previous explanations of certain phenomena, such as the norm theory explanation (Kahneman & Miller, 1986) of counterfactual thinking as applied to what Epstein and colleagues subsequently labeled the RB phenomenon. Kahneman and Miller argued that the phenomenon is the result of postoutcome counterfactual thinking and cannot be attributed to subjective probability. Based on the concretive and experiential principles of CEST, Kirkpatrick and Epstein (1992) hypothesized that it can be attributed to subjective probability and does not require postoutcome processing, and a series of studies demonstrated this position to be correct (Denes-Raj & Epstein, 1994; Denes-Raj et al., 1995; Kirkpatrick & Epstein, 1992).

The second reason to reject the argument that CEST is unnecessary is that a single theory that can account for a wide variety of phenomena with a coherent, limited set of principles provides an important advantage over multiple theories, each of which can account for only some of the phenomena. Apart from the parsimony of a single set of postulates that can account for a wide variety of phenomena, validity is enhanced by a network of interconnected relations within a single theory. Broad theories provide a triangulation or convergence that is absent in narrower theories. The result is that broad theories can provide a perspective that permits the detection of limitations in the generalizations endorsed by narrower theories. For example, it is tempting to conclude from research on impression formation that when the outcomes of heuristic and analytical processing are both accessible, people will invariably find the latter more compelling and behave accordingly. Yet a basic assumption in CEST makes this doubtful as a broad generalization, and has stimulated research demonstrating that the outcomes of heuristic processing in certain situations are more compelling than the equally accessible outcomes of rational processing (e.g., Denes-Raj & Epstein, 1994; Donovan & Epstein, 1997; Epstein, Pacini, et al., 1996). Another example is provided by the interpretation of the finding that normal individuals are unrealistic self-enhancers as implying that reality awareness is not a useful criterion of mental adjustment (see review in Taylor & Brown, 1988). From the perspective of CEST, the same data can be reinterpreted as simply indicating that reality awareness is an important criterion of good adjustment, but not the only one. Reality awareness and the need to enhance self-esteem (or to view the world positively) interact in a manner that produces compromises, with each variable constraining the influence of the other (Morling & Epstein, 1997). The result is that normal individuals interpret events in a way that is unrealistically self-serving only to a limited degree, and when the cost of doing so is more than minimal, they cease doing it (Pacini et al., 1998).

To place the issue of the importance of broader relative to narrower theories in brief historical perspective, there was a period when broad theories of personality offered great promise and were highly influential. Before long, it became apparent that the theories promised more than they could deliver. This was understandably followed by a period of disillusionment. The result was a proliferation of minitheories (often little more than broad hypotheses) and of domain-specific research that tested the minitheories. It is important to recognize that in the absence of more integrative theory, there is the danger that narrowly focused theory and equally narrow experimental paradigms will contribute little to the development of a cumulative science. Research interest fads will come and go, and will not build on each other. It is just possible that the pendulum has swung too far in the direction of studying limited phenomena in depth, and that a correction of a previous overcorrection is now in order.

REFERENCES

Adler, A. (1954). *Understanding human nature.* New York: Fawcett.

Allport, G. W. (1961). *Pattern and growth in personality.* New York: Holt, Rinehart & Winston.

Anderson, J. R. (1976). *Language, memory, and thought.* Hillsdale, NJ: Erlbaum.

Anderson, J. R. (1982). Acquisition of cognitive skill. *Psychological Review, 89,* 369–406.

Bargh, J. A. (1989). Conditional automaticity: Varieties of automatic influence in social perception and cognition. In J. S. Uleman & J. A. Bargh (Eds.), *Unintended thought* (pp. 3–51). New York: Guilford Press.

Bowlby, J. (1988). *A secure base.* New York: Basic Books.

Brewin, C. R. (1989). Cognitive change processes in psychotherapy. *Psychological Review, 96,* 379–394.

Broadbent, D. E., FitsGerald, P., & Broadbent, M. H. P. (1986). Implicit and explicit knowledge in the control of complex systems. *British Journal of Psychology, 77,* 33–50.

Bruner, J. S. (1986). *Actual minds, possible worlds.* Cambridge, MA: Harvard University Press.

Bucci, W. (1985). Dual coding: A cognitive model for psychoanalytic research. *Journal of the American Psychoanalytic Association, 33,* 571–607.

Buck, R. (1985). Prime theory: An integrated view of motivation and emotion. *Psychological Review, 92,* 389–413.

Buck, R. (1991).Motivation, emotion, and cognition: A developmental-interactionist view. In K. T. Strongman (Ed.), *International review of studies on emotion* (Vol. 1, pp. 101–142). New York: Wiley.

Cacioppo, J. T., & Petty, R. E. (1982). The need for cognition. *Journal of Personality and Social Psychology, 42,* 116–131.

Catlin, G., & Epstein, S. (1992). Unforgettable experiences: The relation of life events to basic beliefs about the self and world. *Social Cognition, 10,* 189–209.

Chaiken, S., & Maheswaran, D. (1994). Heuristic processing can bias systematic processing: Effects of source credibility, argument ambiguity, and task importance on attitude judgment. *Journal of Personality and Social Psychology, 66,* 460–473.

Denes-Raj, V., & Epstein, S. (1994). Conflict between experiential and rational processing: When people behave against their better judgment. *Journal of Personality and Social Psychology, 66,* 819–829.

Denes-Raj, V., Epstein, S., & Cole, J. (1995). The generality of the ratio-bias phenomenon. *Personality and Social Psychology Bulletin, 21,* 1083–1092.

Donovan, S., & Epstein, S. (1997). The difficulty of the Linda conjunction problem can be attributed to its simultaneous concrete and unnatural representation, and not to conversational implicature. *Journal of Experimental Social Psychology, 33,* 1–20.

Edwards, K. (1990). The interplay of affect and cognition in attitude formation and change. *Journal of Personality and Social Psychology, 59,* 202–216.

Epstein, S. (1973). The self-concept revisited, or a theory of a theory. *American Psychologist, 28,* 404–416.

Epstein, S. (1976). Anxiety, arousal, and the self-concept. In I. G. Sarason & C. D. Spielberger (Eds.), *Stress and anxiety* (pp. 183–224). Washington, DC: Hemisphere.

Epstein, S. (1980). The self-concept: A review and proposal of an integrated theory of personality. In E. Staub (Ed.), *Personality: Basic issues and current research* (pp. 82–132). Englewood Cliffs, NJ: Prentice-Hall.

Epstein, S. (1983). The unconscious, the preconscious and the self-concept. In J. Suls & A. Greenwald (Eds.), *Psychological perspectives on the self* (Vol. 2, pp. 219–247). Hillsdale, NJ: Erlbaum.

Epstein, S. (1984). Controversial issues in emotion theory. In P. Shaver (Ed.), *Annual review of research in personality and social psychology* (pp. 64–87). Beverly Hills, CA: Sage.

Epstein, S. (1985). The implications of cognitive–experiential self-theory for research in social psychology and personality. *Journal for the Theory of Social Behaviour, 15,* 283–310.

Epstein, S. (1987). Implications of cognitive self-theory for psychopathology and psychotherapy. In N. Cheshire & H. Thomae (Eds.), *Self, symptoms, and psychotherapy* (pp. 43–58). New York: Wiley.

Epstein, S. (1990). Cognitive–experiential self-theory. In L. Pervin (Ed.), *Handbook of personality: Theory and research* (pp. 165–192). New York: Guilford Press.

Epstein, S. (1991a). The self-concept, the traumatic neurosis, and the structure of personality. In D. Ozer, J. M. Healy, Jr., & A. J. Stewart (Eds.), *Perspectives in personality* (Vol. 3A, pp. 63–98). London: Jessica Kingsley.

Epstein, S. (1991b). Cognitive–experiential self-theory: An integrative theory of personality. In R. C. Curtis (Ed.), *The relational self: Theoretical convergences of psychoanalysis and social psychology* (pp. 111–137). New York: Guilford Press.

Epstein, S. (1991c). Cognitive–experiential self theory: Implications for developmental psychology. In M. R. Gunnar & L. A. Sroufe (Eds.), *Self process and development* (Vol. 23, pp. 79–123). Hillsdale, NJ: Erlbaum.

Epstein, S. (1992a). Constructive thinking and mental and physical well-being. In L. Montada, S. H. Filipp, & M. J. Lerner (Eds.), *Life crises and experiences of loss in adulthood* (pp. 385–409). Hillsdale, NJ: Erlbaum.

Epstein, S. (1992b). Coping ability, negative self-evaluation, and overgeneralization: Experiment and theory. *Journal of Personality and Social Psychology, 62*, 826–836.

Epstein, S. (1993a). Emotion and self-theory. In M. Lewis & J. Haviland (Eds.), *Handbook of emotions* (pp. 313–326). New York: Guilford Press.

Epstein, S. (1993b). Implications of cognitive–experiential self-theory for personality and developmental psychology. In D. Funder, R. Parke, C. Tomlinson-Keasey, & K. Widaman (Eds.), *Studying lives through time: Personality and development* (pp. 399–438). Washington, DC: American Psychological Association.

Epstein, S. (1994). Integration of the cognitive and the psychodynamic unconscious. *American Psychologist, 49*, 709–724.

Epstein, S. (1998). [Superstitious thinking during the game of bingo]. Unpublished raw data.

Epstein, S., with Brodsky, A. (1993). *You're smarter than you think: How to develop your practical intelligence for success in living.* New York: Simon & Schuster.

Epstein, S., Denes-Raj, V., & Pacini, R. (1995). The Linda problem revisited from the perspective of cognitive–experiential self-theory. *Personality and Social Psychology Bulletin, 21*, 1124–1138.

Epstein, S., Donovan, S., & Denes-Raj, V. (in press). The missing link in the paradox of the Linda conjunction problem: Beyond knowing and thinking of the conjunction rule, the intrinsic appeal of heuristic processing. *Personality and Social Psychology Bulletin.*

Epstein, S., & Erskine, N. (1983). The development of personal theories of reality. In D. Magnusson & V. Allen (Eds.), *Human development: An interactional perspective* (pp. 133–147). New York: Academic Press.

Epstein, S., & Katz, L. (1992). Coping ability, stress, productive load, and symptoms. *Journal of Personality and Social Psychology, 62*, 813–825.

Epstein, S., Lipson, A., Holstein, C., & Huh, E. (1992). Irrational reactions to negative outcomes: Evidence for two conceptual systems. *Journal of Personality and Social Psychology, 62*, 328–339.

Epstein, S., & Meier, P. (1989). Constructive thinking: A broad coping variable with specific components. *Journal of Personality and Social Psychology, 57*, 332–349.

Epstein, S., & Morling, B. (1995). Is the self motivated to do more than enhance and verify itself? In M. H.

Kernis (Ed.), *Efficacy, agency, and self-esteem* (pp. 9–29). New York: Plenum Press.

Epstein, S., & Pacini, R. (1998). *Coping with stress in everyday life.* Unpublished raw data.

Epstein, S., Pacini, R., Denes-Raj, V., & Heier, H. (1996). Individual differences in intuitive–experiential and analytical–rational thinking styles. *Journal of Personality and Social Psychology, 71*, 390–405.

Fairbairn, W. R. D. (1954). *An object relations theory of the personality.* New York: Basic Books.

Fiske, S. T., & Taylor, S. E. (1991). *Social cognition* (2nd ed.). New York: McGraw-Hill.

Gallistel, C. R., & Gelman, R. (1992). Preverbal and verbal counting and computation. *Cognition, 44*, 43–74.

Gilbert, D. T. (1989). Thinking lightly about others: Automatic components of the social inference process. In J. S. Uleman & J. A. Bargh (Eds.), *Unintended thought* (pp. 189–211). New York: Guilford Press.

Gilbert, D. T., & Malone, P. S. (1995). The correspondence bias. *Psychological Bulletin, 117*, 21–38.

Gilhooly, K. J., & Falconer, W. A. (1974). Concrete and abstract terms and relations in testing a rule. *Quarterly Journal of Experimental Psychology, 26*, 355–359.

Johnson-Laird, P. N. (1983). *Mental models.* Cambridge, England: Cambridge University Press.

Kahneman, D., & Miller, D. T. (1986). Norm theory: Comparing reality to its alternatives. *Psychological Review, 93*, 136–153.

Kahneman, D., Slovic, P., & Tversky, A. (1982). *Judgment under uncertainty: Heuristics and biases.* New York: Cambridge University Press.

Katz, L., & Epstein, S. (1991). Constructive thinking and coping with laboratory-induced stress. *Journal of Personality and Social Psychology, 61*, 789–800.

Kelly, G. A. (1955). *The psychology of personal constructs* (2 vols.). New York: Norton.

Kirkpatrick, L. A., & Epstein, S. (1992). Cognitive–experiential self-theory and subjective probability: Further evidence for two conceptual systems. *Journal of Personality and Social Psychology, 63*, 534–544.

Kohut, H. (1971). *The analysis of the self.* New York: International Universities Press.

Labouvie-Vief, G. (1989). Modes of knowledge and the organization of development. In M. L. Commons, J. D. Sinnott, F. A. Richards, & C. Armon (Eds.), *Adult development* (Vol. 2, pp. 43–62). New York: Praeger.

Labouvie-Vief, G. (1990). Wisdom as integrated thought: Historical and developmental perspectives. In R. J. Sternberg (Ed.), *Wisdom: Its nature, origins, and development* (pp. 52–83). New York: Cambridge University Press.

Lecky, P. (1961). *Self-consistency: A theory of personality.* Hamden, CT: Shoe String Press.

Leventhal, H. (1982). The integration of emotion and cognition: A view from the perceptual-motor theory of emotion. In M. S. Clark & S. T. Fiske (Eds.), *Affect and cognition: The Seventeenth Annual Carnegie Symposium on Cognition* (pp. 121–156). Hillsdale, NJ: Erlbaum.

Leventhal, H. (1984). A perceptual-motor theory of emotion. In L. Berkowitz (Ed.), *Advances in experimental social psychology* (Vol. 17, pp. 117–182). New York: Academic Press.

Lombardi, W. J., Higgins, E. T., & Bargh, J. A. (1987). The role of consciousness in priming effects on categorization: Assimilation versus contrast as a function of awareness of the priming task. *Personality and Social Psychology Bulletin, 13,* 411–429.

McClelland, D. C., Koestner, R., & Weinberger, J. (1989). How do self-attributed and implicit motives differ? *Psychological Review, 96,* 690–702.

Morling, B., & Epstein, S. (1997). Compromises produced by the dialectic between self-verification and self-enhancement. *Journal of Personality and Social Psychology, 73,* 1268–1283.

Newman, L. S., & Uleman, J.S. (1990). Assimilation and contrast effects in spontaneous trait inference. *Personality and Social Psychology Bulletin, 16,* 224–240.

Nisbett, R. E., Krantz, D. H., Jepson, C., & Kunda, Z. (1983). The use of statistical heuristics in everyday inductive reasoning. *Psychological Review, 90,* 339–363.

Nissen, M. J., Willingham, D., & Hartman, M. (1989). Explicit and implicit remembering: When is learning preserved in amnesia? *Neuropsychologie, 27,* 341–352.

Norris, P., & Epstein, S. (1998). *Correlates of a broader measure of experiential processing.* Unpublished manuscript, University of Massachusetts at Amherst.

Pacini, R., & Epstein, S. (in press). The relation of rational and experiential information-processing styles to personality, basic beliefs, and the ratio–bias phenomenon. *Journal of Personality and Social Psychology.*

Pacini, R., & Epstein, S. (1998a). *The interaction of three facets of concrete thinking in a game of chance.* Manuscript submitted for publication.

Pacini, R., & Epstein, S. (1998b). *The influence of visualization on intuitive–experiential information processing.* Unpublished manuscript, University of Massachusetts at Amherst.

Pacini, R., Muir, F., & Epstein, S. (1998). Depressive realism from the perspective of cognitive–experiential self-theory. *Journal of Personality and Social Psychology, 74,* 1056–1068.

Paivio, A. (1986). *Mental representations: A dual-coding approach.* New York: Oxford University Press.

Paivio, A. (1991). Dual-coding theory: Retrospect and current status. *Canadian Journal of Psychology, 45,* 225–287.

Petty, R. E., & Jarvis, B. G. (1996). An individual difference perspective on assessing cognitive processes. In N. Schwarz & S. Sudman (Eds.), *Answering questions: Methodology for determining cognitive and communicative processes in survey research* (pp. 221–257). San Francisco: Jossey-Bass.

Reber, C. R. (1993). *Implicit learning and tacit knowledge.* New York: Oxford University Press.

Rogers, C. R. (1959). A theory of therapy, personality, and interpersonal relationship, as developed in the client-centered framework. In S. Koch (Ed.), *Psychology: A study of a science* (Vol. 3, pp. 184–256). New York: McGraw-Hill.

Sappington, A. A., & Russell, J. C. (1978). Self-efficacy and meaning: Candidates for a uniform theory of behavior. *Personality and Social Psychology Bulletin, 2,* 327.

Sappington, A. A., Russell, J. C., Triplett, V., & Goodwin, J. (1980). Self-efficacy expectancies, response-outcome expectancies, emotionally-based expectancies, and their relationship to avoidance behavior. *Journal of Clinical Psychology, 37,* 737–744.

Schacter, D. L. (1987). Implicit memory: History and current status. *Journal of Experimental Psychology: Learning, Memory, and Cognition, 13,* 501–518.

Schwarz, N., Strack, F., Hilton, D., & Nadderer, G. (1991). Base rates, representativeness, and the logic of conversation: The contextual relevance of "irrelevant" information. *Social Cognition, 9,* 67–84.

Sloman, S. (1996). The empirical case for two systems of reasoning. *Psychological Review, 119,* 3–22.

Sullivan, H. S. (1953). *The interpersonal theory of psychiatry.* New York: Norton.

Taylor, S. E., & Brown, J. D. (1988). Illusions and well-being: A social-psychological perspective on mental health. *Psychological Bulletin, 103,* 193–210.

Tversky, A., & Kahneman, D. (1983). Extensional versus intuitive reasoning. The conjunction fallacy in probability judgment. *Psychological Review, 90,* 293–315.

Wegner, D. M., & Schneider, D. J. (1989). Mental control: The war of the ghosts in the machine. In J. S. Uleman & J. A. Bargh (Eds.), *Unintended thought* (pp. 287–305). New York: Guilford Press.

Wenzlaff, R. M., Wegner, D. M., & Roper, D. W. (1988). Depression and mental control: The resurgence of unwanted negative thoughts. *Journal of Personality and Social Psychology, 55,* 882–892.

Winograd, T. (1975). Frame representation and the declarative–procedural controversy. In D. G. Bobrow & A. M. Collins (Eds.), *Representation and understanding: Studies in cognitive science* (pp. 185–210). New York: Academic Press.

Yanko, J., Epstein, S., Pacini, R., & Barrows, P. (1998). [Compromises between intuitive and rational processing as a function of age]. Unpublished raw data.

Yates, J. F., & Carlson, B. W. (1986). Conjunction errors: Evidence for multiple judgment procedures, including "signed summation." *Organizationl Behavior and Human Decision Processes, 37,* 230–253.

Zukier, H., & Pepitone, A. (1984). Social roles and strategies in prediction: Some determinant of the use of base-rate information. *Journal of Personality and Social Psychology, 47,* 349–360.

24

Processes Underlying Metacognitive Judgments

INFORMATION-BASED AND EXPERIENCE-BASED MONITORING OF ONE'S OWN KNOWLEDGE

ASHER KORIAT

RAVIT LEVY-SADOT

There has been extensive work in recent years on a variety of metacognitive operations that supervise and control different aspects of cognitive processing and behavior (see Koriat, 1998b; Metcalfe & Shimamura, 1994; Nelson & Narens, 1990; Reder, 1996; Schwartz, 1994). This work has been motivated by both theoretical and practical considerations. Metacognitive operations take place at different stages of learning and remembering. For example, when studying new material, students normally monitor the likelihood of remembering different pieces of this material and control the allocation of learning resources accordingly. Of course, whether they ultimately succeed in remembering the material depends not only on their memory, but also on their "metamemory"—that is, on the extent to which they can monitor the state of their knowledge and regulate their time and effort accordingly. Similarly, people can often feel whether a solicited piece of information is available or unavailable in memory, and on the basis of their "feeling of knowing," they may decide either to spend time and effort

searching for it or simply to pass. Finally, a person on a witness stand generally exercises some censorship over what he or she reports, withholding information about which he or she is not sure. Here too, the accuracy of the report depends not only on the accuracy of the person's memory, but also on the extent to which the person can discriminate between correct and incorrect pieces of information and control his or her reporting correspondingly.

In this chapter we propose a dual-process framework for the analysis of metacognitive monitoring, focusing on the question of how people know that they know. We make a distinction between metacognitive *feelings*, based on nonanalytic processes, and metacognitive *judgments*, based on analytic processes. Metacognitive feelings have much in common with certain forms of affective responses. In fact, they represent a blend between affective and cognitive processes, as implied by such terms as "knowing feelings" (see Clore, 1992) and "feelings of knowing" (Koriat, 1993; Nelson & Narens, 1990).

Metacognitive judgments, on the other hand, are more purely cognitive or informational in nature. We begin by drawing an analogy between metacognitive processes and certain forms of affective responses. This analogy helps bring to the fore the unique function of metacognitive and affective feelings in mediating judgments and behavior (see also Clore, 1992; Schwarz & Clore, 1996); it also elucidates the distinction between experience-based and information-based processes in general.

AFFECTIVE EXPERIENCE AS A BASIS OF BEHAVIOR: AN EXAMPLE

Consider the following example of affect-based behavior, taken from Asher Koriat's student days (Koriat is the "I" in what follows). One of the fortunate jobs that I held during my days as an undergraduate student at the Hebrew University was that of an elevator boy in the administration building of the university. There was actually little work involved. In fact, there were two elevators, one of which was automatic; the other had to be operated manually. Usually I would spend my time sitting on a chair reading, unless an elderly lady insisted on riding with me, or unless the other elevator was busy and the person was in a hurry. Then, I would stop reading, leave my book on the chair, take the person to whichever floor he or she wanted, and then go back to my own business. In most cases, however, people did not want to disturb me; they simply took the stairs or waited for the other elevator.

During my work I saw many new people, most of whom I could not remember. However, I had an interesting experience that repeated itself several times. A person who looked like a complete stranger to me would walk to my elevator. I would drop my book, enter the elevator, and close the door; before the person had a chance to indicate his or her destination, I would push the "1" button for the first floor. Typically, the person would express surprise: "How do you know?" or "How do you remember?" In fact, I too would be quite surprised, because I usually did not have the faintest memory that I had seen that person before. However, I was quite confident that he or she was heading for the first floor.

After some reflection and introspection, I realized what was going on. Because people could generally manage without my help, I was normally annoyed when someone insisted on using my service, stopping me in the middle of my reading, and having me go through my routine (closing my book, getting into the elevator, closing the door, pushing the button, etc.). However, I was particularly annoyed when after this ordeal, the person announced, "First floor, please." After all, the stairs were nearby. Apparently, then, after one or more such experiences with such a person, I developed a sort of conditioned emotional response that was associated with that person. So next time, when the person walked toward me, the negative feeling tone that he or she evoked served as a sufficiently potent cue that this individual was going to say "First floor" again.

I have not done any systematic experimentation on the subject, but I suspect that such an affective association would not have been formed if the need to use the elevator to the first floor had somehow been justified. Thus, perhaps if the person in question had been an elderly lady, such an affectively mediated memory would not have occurred, and I would not have been spared the need to ask for the desired floor. Possibly the same would have been true if the person had gone to the fifth floor.

We may tentatively propose that the process underlying my reaction can be expressed as follows: Cognitive content → Affective feeling → Inference. The first component of this process is the cognitive or informational content that gives rise to the feeling tone. In my case, this was the correlation between the person's appearance and the fact that he or she wanted to go to the first floor. This correlation could be expressed in a propositional form: "The person who looks so-and-so goes to the first floor."

The second component is the affective association. In my case, a negative feeling tone was attached to the person's look because of the reasons described above.

The third component is again cognitive. In my case, my affective response to the person served as a mnemonic cue that the person apparently wanted to get to the first floor.

One obvious question that arises is this: Why are subjective feelings necessary for mediating between one cognitive content and another? Why doesn't the first cognitive content feed directly into behavior? We propose that affective reactions can code limited, shallow aspects of the information in the environment, and can be formed unconsciously without (or before) a full articulation of the specific informational content on which they are based. Therefore, although the content of the information that originally gave rise to the feeling tone is not available to consciousness, the subjective feeling itself can serve as a basis for judgment and behavior, and can even help reconstruct certain aspects of the original content.

DISTINGUISHING BETWEEN AFFECT-BASED AND INFORMATION-BASED JUDGMENTS

A second question that we wish to address involves the difference between the affect-based process described above and the more common process in which the decision relies directly on informational content (see, e.g., Epstein & Pacini, Chapter 23, this volume, and Strack, 1992, for similar distinctions). Clearly, after repeated encounters with a particular person who used the elevator, I could simply have remembered that that person generally went to the first floor. Or else, if I knew what the person's job was, I could easily have inferred that his or her office was on the first floor. If that person walked into my elevator, I might still have experienced negative affect toward him or her, but that affect would not have served as the basis for pressing the first-floor button. Rather, the basis for my action would have been an explicit cognitive content. Affective mediation, then, apparently circumvents the need to rely explicitly on such associated informational-associative content.

What, then, are the differences between the affect-based and information-based processes? There are three differences that we wish to stress, because they also apply to the difference between experience-based and information-based metacognitive judgments.

1. *Mediation.* The information-based process is uniform: The informational content in explicit memory feeds into judgment and behavior (though it may also give rise to an affective reaction). That is, explicit beliefs and explicit knowledge retrieved from memory serve to guide behavior. The affect-centered process, in contrast, is composed of two qualitatively different processes whose junction lies at the experiential, feeling state. The process that gives rise to the affective reaction is essentially implicit and unconscious, whereas the process that uses this reaction as a source of information is part and parcel of explicit and controlled modes of thought. Hence, affective feelings are seen to serve a crossover function, mediating between implicit/automatic and explicit/controlled modes of operation (see Koriat, 1998b).

2. *Content.* In the information-based process, the basis of the judgment lies in domain-specific content retrieved from memory. In contrast, in the affect-centered process, the content of the information underlying the feeling is not available to consciousness. All that is available to consciousness is a feeling state.

3. *Phenomenal quality.* In the information-based process, an aware mode of operation is maintained throughout: A person retrieves a certain belief and behaves accordingly in a controlled, deliberate manner. In the affect-mediated process, in contrast, the decision or judgment has an intuitive quality; it comes as a "hunch." In part, this distinction parallels that between "know" and "remember" responses (Gardiner & Java, 1993): In the affect-mediated process, the effect of stored information has the quality of a "know" response, whereas in the information-based process, it has a quality more like that of "remember." The distinction also parallels in part that between "familiarity" and "recollection" (Jacoby, 1991; Jacoby, Lindsay, & Toth, 1992).

Koriat, Edry, and De Marcas (1998) noted a similar phenomenological distinction between the retrieval of a complete entry from memory (e.g., recalling the word "love") and the retrieval of partial information about it (e.g., judging that the nonrecalled word has a positive emotional tone). It was proposed that access to partial information shares certain features with implicit memory: It has the quality of an intuitive guess; it elicits more "know" than "remember" states of awareness (see Gardiner & Java, 1993); and it is less sensitive to manipulations of attention and retention interval.

Our distinction between affect-based and information-based processes also overlaps with that of Smith and DeCoster (Chapter 16, this volume; see also Sloman, 1996) between automatic associative processing and rule-based processing. They propose that the products of associative processing are experienced as intuitive and affective responses, whereas those of rule-based processing are regarded as the derivatives of logical reasoning.

As will be further clarified later, our distinction accords particularly well with that of Epstein and Pacini (Chapter 23, this volume; see also Epstein, 1994; Epstein, Lipson, Holstein, & Huh, 1992) between an experiential system and a rational system. Consistent with our analysis of the elevator example, Epstein and Pacini propose that connections in the experiential system are made through associations, whereas those in the rational system are made through logical inference. Importantly, they maintain that whereas processing in the rational system is affect-free, the experiential system is emotionally driven and is intimately associated with the experience of affect.

Let us now turn to metacognitive judgments. We begin our analysis with the feeling of knowing that accompanies retrieval failure, and use this analysis to illustrate some of the basic issues concerning metacognitive judgments in general. Then we examine these issues with regard to judgments of learning elicited during study and subjective confidence in the correctness of one's answer. Finally, we point out some of the similarities between affective and "noetic" (knowing) feelings.

PROCESSES UNDERLYING THE FEELING OF KNOWING

A common experience in everyday life is that we fail to retrieve some piece of information from memory—for example, the name of an acquaintance—and yet we are absolutely sure that we know the name and that we can immediately recognize it when it is presented to us, or can even retrieve it at some later time. Such episodes have attracted the interest of memory researchers because they seem to suggest that people can monitor the information stored in memory even when they fail to recall it.

In studies on the feeling of knowing, participants are typically presented with vocabulary or general-information questions asking for a particular name or a particular term (e.g., "What is the name of the architect who designed Brasilia?"). When they fail to recall the answer, they are asked to judge how likely they are to recognize the solicited memory target when it is presented among distractors, and are then given a recognition memory test. In most studies a positive correlation has been found between feeling-of-knowing judgments and recognition performance, suggesting that people can accurately monitor memory.

Our focus in the present chapter is not on the accuracy of metacognitive judgments, but on the basis of these judgments. How do people know that they know? We propose that a feeling-of-knowing judgment may be based on two sources of information: first, domain-specific knowledge retrieved from memory; and, second, a sheer subjective experience. In the former case, the process is more like that of a probability judgment: A person engages in an effortful retrieval and evaluation of relevant information to reach an educated assessment of the likelihood that he or she may possess the solicited name or term. This information-based process leads to what might be better described as "judgment of knowing" than as "feeling of knowing" (Koriat, 1993). In some cases the person may in fact prefer to phrase the judgment as "I ought to know the answer," rather than "I feel that I know the answer" (see Costermans, Lories, & Ansay, 1992).

The second process, in contrast, is mediated by a subjective feeling. The person may have the experience of directly detecting the presence of the solicited target and its imminent recall (see Brown & McNeill, 1966). This feeling may sometimes be so strong as to be accompanied by a feeling of tension and frustration. The feeling-of-knowing judgment in this case is based on an effortless, direct readout of that noetic feeling.

What is the mechanism responsible for feelings of knowing as opposed to judgments of knowing? Current theoretical discussions generally distinguish between two classes of mechanisms for the feeling of knowing: inferential/analytic mechanisms on the one hand, and trace access mechanisms on the other (Nelson, Gerler, & Narens, 1984; see also Krinsky & Nelson, 1985). Inferential mechanisms are those in which the person analyzes different types of information in order to deduce the likelihood that the solicited target is indeed available in memory. Trace access mechanisms, on the other hand, are based on the direct detection of the presence of the solicited target in store. A simple hypothesis, then, is that inferential mechanisms give rise to "judgments" of knowing, whereas unmediated "feelings" of knowing are based on trace access mechanisms.

The idea that a trace access mechanism underlies feelings of knowing has been most explicitly argued by Hart (1965, 1967a, 1967b). According to Hart, the feeling of knowing is based on a special memory-monitoring module that has privileged access to memory traces and can directly monitor their availability in memory. This mechanism can help to ascertain that a solicited target is indeed stored in memory before a retrieval attempt is initiated. A similar trace access mechanism has been also implied to underlie judgments of learning—that is, judgments that a studied item has been committed to memory and will be remembered in the future (e.g., Cohen, Sandler, & Keglevich, 1991; see Koriat, 1997). The assumption is that people can directly read out the strength of the memory trace that is formed following study, and can also assess on-line the increase in trace strength that occurs as more time is spent studying an item.

Trace access mechanisms would seem to be best suited to explain feeling-based judgments. They capture the phenomenal quality that is sometimes associated with the "tip-of-the-tongue" state—the feeling that one directly monitors the presence of the elusive target in memory and its emergence into consciousness (James, 1890). This phenomenal quality, together with the observation that metacognitive judgments are generally predictive of actual memory performance, lends credence to the idea that feeling-based metacognitive judgments rest on direct access to memory traces, as opposed to information-based judgments, which may rely on inferential processes.

The view advocated in this chapter, in contrast, denies the possibility of direct trace monitoring. Rather, it is proposed that metacognitive judgments, both feeling-based and information-based, are inferential in nature (see Benjamin & Bjork, 1996). The difference between them lies in the nature of the inferential process: Whereas information-based judgments rely on analytic inferences, feeling-based judgments rest on nonanalytic inferences. This is true for feeling-of-knowing judgments, as well as for other types of metacognitive judgments that are discussed below. Let us examine this idea more closely.

ANALYTIC AND NONANALYTIC DETERMINANTS OF METACOGNITIVE JUDGMENTS

The distinction between analytic and nonanalytic processes was first proposed by Jacoby and Brooks (1984). These terms are borrowed here to distinguish between two different bases of metacognitive judgments, although they do not capture all aspects of the distinction (but see Brown & Siegler, 1993; Jacoby & Kelley, 1987; Kelley & Jacoby, 1996a; Koriat, 1994, 1997; Smith & DeCoster, Chapter 16, this volume). Analytic/inferential bases entail the conscious, deliberate utilization of specific beliefs and information to form an educated guess about one's own knowledge. Nonanalytic bases, in contrast, entail the implicit application of some global, general-purpose heuristics to reach a metacognitive judgment. Although these heuristics are inferential in nature, they operate unconsciously and automatically to influence and shape subjective experience. Hence they can explain precisely the type of noetic feelings for which trace access mechanisms have appeared to provide the most suitable account.

Several nonanalytic heuristics have been invoked in explaining feelings of knowing, judgments of learning, and subjective confidence, and it is not entirely clear whether they imply the same or different mechanisms. All of them involve reliance on mnemonic cues—internal, experiential cues that accompany thought and retrieval (see, e.g., Schwarz & Clore, 1996; Strack, 1992). Among these are the mere accessibility of pertinent information (Dunlosky & Nelson, 1992; Koriat, 1993; Morris, 1990), the ease with which information comes to mind (Kelley & Lindsay, 1993; Koriat, 1993; Mazzoni & Nelson, 1995), the familiarity of the cue that serves to prompt retrieval (Metcalfe, Schwartz, & Joaquim,

1993; Reder, 1987; Reder & Schunn, 1996), and the fluency of processing (Begg, Duft, Lalonde, Melnick, & Sanvito, 1989; Benjamin & Bjork, 1996; Kelley & Jacoby, 1996b). Each of these internal cues can serve as the basis for a noetic feeling.

Unlike analytic inferences, nonanalytic heuristics are used unconsciously, and their effects are automatic. These effects are often experienced as intuitive feelings rather than as logical deductions, and their validity is generally taken for granted by the person. Epstein and Pacini (Chapter 23, this volume) make a similar point: Distinguishing between the experiential and rational systems, they note the self-evident quality of the experiential system, in contrast to the logical justification that characterizes the rational system. Thus, we propose that the nonanalytic basis of noetic feelings is responsible for their direct, unmediated quality and for their perceived validity.

HEURISTIC-DRIVEN FEELINGS OF KNOWING

Let us now return to feeling-of-knowing judgments, focusing on two candidate heuristics that have received experimental attention in recent years as potential determinants of the feeling of knowing: cue familiarity and accessibility. According to the cue familiarity hypothesis (e.g., Metcalfe, 1993; Reder, 1987), feeling-of-knowing judgments are based on the overall familiarity of the stimulus that is designed to cue the memory target. Thus, when a person is presented with a question, a rapid feeling of knowing is computed, based on the overall familiarity of the question rather than on the retrievability of the answer.

Support for the cue familiarity hypothesis comes from studies indicating that the feeling of knowing associated with a cue is enhanced by advance priming of that cue or of elements thereof. This occurs even when cue priming does not improve actual memory performance. Thus, in Reder's (1987, 1988) studies, advance priming of some of the words of a general-information question was found to enhance the feeling of knowing associated with that question, without affecting subsequent recall or recognition of the answer. Similarly, Schwartz and Metcalfe

(1992), using a paired-associates task, found that feeling-of-knowing judgments were enhanced by advance cue priming but not by advance target priming. Metcalfe et al. (1993) found that repetition of the cue word across two lists of paired associates increased feeling-of-knowing judgments, whereas repetition of the response word did not.

In other studies by Reder and her associates (Reder & Ritter, 1992; Schunn, Reder, Nhouyvanisvong, Richards, & Stroffolino, 1997), participants were presented with arithmetic problems, and were asked to judge rapidly whether they knew the answer to each and could produce it without having to compute it. As would be expected, the probability of "know" responses increased with repetition of a problem. However, it also increased when only some of the components of the problem were repeated, and even when participants were given little opportunity to solve the problem. Thus feeling-of-knowing judgments are affected by the mere familiarity with the question.

A second heuristic that has received experimental attention is the accessibility heuristic. Koriat (1993) proposed that feeling-of-knowing judgments are based on the overall accessibility of partial information pertaining to the target. When recall fails, many partial clues often come to mind. Some of these may stem from the target itself and hence represent correct partial clues, whereas others may derive from irrelevant activations (such as those emanating from neighboring targets or from priming), and constitute wrong partial clues. Because participants cannot monitor the accuracy of the information that comes to mind, both correct and wrong partial clues contribute to the enhancement of feeling-of-knowing judgments. Nevertheless, these judgments tend by and large to be accurate, because of the high output-bound accuracy of memory (Koriat & Goldsmith, 1994, 1996): Information that comes to mind is much more likely to be correct than wrong. For example, the probability of providing an answer to a certain memory question may be quite low, but given that a person does retrieve an answer, the probability is quite high that the answer provided is correct. The implication is that there is no need to postulate a trace access mechanism to explain the accuracy of the feeling of knowing. Rather, the accuracy of metamemory simply stems from the general accuracy of memory itself.

Support for the accessibility account of the feeling of knowing came from a study (Koriat, 1993) in which participants memorized a letter string on each trial, and were then asked to recall it or to report as many letters as they could remember. Feeling-of-knowing judgments about the future recognition of the target increased systematically with the overall number of letters reported, regardless of the accuracy of these letters. Thus, both number of correct letters recalled and number of wrong letters recalled were positively and strongly correlated with feeling-of-knowing judgments. Nevertheless, feeling-of-knowing judgments were accurate in predicting subsequent recognition memory, simply because the reported letters had a .90 probability of being correct. Additional findings indicated that feeling-of-knowing judgments also increased with the ease with which partial clues came to mind: When the number of letters reported was controlled, feeling-of-knowing judgments increased with decreasing retrieval latency. In parallel, ease of access was also predictive of the correctness of the partial information retrieved, as well as the success of subsequent target recognition. These results suggest that the accuracy of feeling-of-knowing judgments in predicting actual memory performance derives from the implicit utilization of cues that are generally valid, rather than from privileged access to stored traces.

Because the validity of feeling-of-knowing judgments depends on the validity of the cues on which these judgments rest, it should be possible to find dissociations between knowing and the feeling of knowing. Such dissociations should occur when the overall amount of information that comes to mind is not diagnostic of the availability of the correct target. Indeed, Koriat (1995) obtained results indicating that the accuracy of feeling-of-knowing judgments in predicting subsequent recognition of the target varied strongly with the quality of the partial clues precipitated. When these clues were predominantly correct, which is true of typical memory questions, feeling-of-knowing judgments were valid in predicting actual recognition performance. However, when deceptive questions were used (Fischhoff, Slovic, &

Lichtenstein, 1977), which tend to bring to mind more incorrect than correct answers, a dissociation was found between feeling-of-knowing judgments and actual memory performance. First, feeling-of-knowing judgments following recall failure were inflated considerably relative to actual recognition memory performance, thus evidencing a strong illusion of knowing stemming from the heightened accessibility of wrong partial clues (see Koriat, 1998a). Second, the correlation between feeling-of-knowing judgments and subsequent recognition memory performance was *negative*: The higher one's feeling of knowing, the greater the likelihood that one's answer in the recognition test was wrong.

In sum, the recent work on feelings of knowing suggests that these feelings and their accuracy can be explained in terms of nonanalytic heuristics that utilize certain mnemonic cues. These cues have a certain degree of predictive validity. For example, because questions and answers generally occur together in our experience (e.g., "The capital of Argentina is Buenos Aires"), familiarity with the question ("What is the capital of Argentina?") is predictive of the familiarity of the answer (see Metcalfe, 1996). Indeed, Kelley and Jacoby (1996b) observed that familiarity with a cue term was predictive of the probability of recognizing the corresponding response term in a paired-associates task. In a similar manner, the number of partial clues retrieved in response to a question, and the ease with which they come to mind, are generally predictive of the recallability of the correct target.

HEURISTIC-DRIVEN JUDGMENTS OF LEARNING

Let us now turn to "judgments of learning"— that is, judgments made by a person during the encoding of information about the likelihood of remembering the encoded material in the future. As noted earlier, these judgments are important because they generally mediate the allocation of time and effort. For example, when making a note to oneself about a prospective action (e.g., to call the doctor, to return a book to the library, to take a cake out of the oven), one must also assess the likelihood that one will remember to perform the planned action at the appropriate time. On the basis of that assessment, one may decide to take some special measures so as not to forget to perform the act (see Brandimonte & Ellis, 1996).

In a typical experiment on judgments of learning, participants study a list of paired associates, and after studying each pair they are asked to assess its future recallability—that is, to assess the chances that they will be able to provide the second word of the word pair (target word) when presented with the first word (cue word) in a later phase of the experiment. Research findings indicate that judgments of learning are generally accurate in predicting memory performance (e.g., Dunlosky & Nelson, 1994; Lovelace, 1984; Mazzoni & Nelson, 1995), and that under self-paced learning conditions participants allocate study time in accordance with their judgments of learning, spending more time studying those items that are associated with lower judgments (Mazzoni & Cornoldi, 1993; Nelson & Leonesio, 1988).

What is the basis of judgments of learning? How do people assess their competence during study? As noted earlier, a simple hypothesis about judgments of learning is that they are based on the direct readout of the strength of the applicable memory traces. If participants can monitor an item's memory trace on-line, they should be able to allocate more study time to the item until a desirable strength is reached. Such a trace-monitoring account can readily explain the predictive validity of judgments of learning.

In contrast, a cue utilization approach assumes that these judgments are inferential in nature, rather than being based on a direct readout of the strength of memory traces (see, e.g., Begg et al., 1989; Koriat, 1997). According to this view, judgments of learning utilize a variety of cues, and apply different heuristics and beliefs to infer the future recallability of the studied information. One mnemonic cue that has been proposed to underlie judgments of learning is ease or fluency of processing (Begg et al., 1989; Benjamin & Bjork, 1996; Bjork, 1998). This cue is generally diagnostic of the future recallability of the studied item, because easily processed items have a better chance to be recalled or recognized in the future. However, in some cases ease of processing may be invalid, resulting in dissociations between judgments of learning and memory performance. Thus, Begg et al. (1989) observed that whereas concrete words yielded both higher judgments of learning and better recognition memory than abstract words, common words yielded higher judgments of learning but poorer recognition memory than rare words. Their explanation is that both concrete words and common words are easier to process, and therefore produce relatively high judgments of learning. Indeed, in their study concrete and common words were rated as easier to imagine, easier to pronounce, and easier to understand than abstract and rare words. The implication, then, is that variables that make similar contributions to ease of processing (at the time of making judgments of learning) and to eventual memory performance should enhance the validity of judgments of learning. In contrast, those that affect these variables differentially (e.g., word frequency) should impair the validity of judgments of learning.

Dissociations between judgments of learning and memory performance have also been reported by others. Narens, Jameson, and Lee (1994) found that a subthreshold presentation of the target in a paired-associates task increased judgments of learning without affecting final recall. Perhaps advance priming facilitated the processing of the target without affecting its subsequent recall. In Zechmeister and Shaughnessy's (1980) study, words presented twice produced higher judgments of learning when their presentation was massed than when it was distributed, although the reverse pattern was observed for recall. Perhaps massed repetition of a word enhances its ease of processing more than its distributed repetition does.

Benjamin and Bjork (1996) have distinguished between perceptual fluency and retrieval fluency as two possible bases of metacognitive judgments. "Perceptual fluency," like Begg et al.'s "ease of processing," refers to the ease with which the stimulus is perceived and the sense of familiarity it evokes. "Retrieval fluency," on the other hand, refers to the ease with which information comes to mind, as indicated, for example, by the latency of retrieving responses to a certain cue, the persistence with which the cue tends to elicit the same response, and the amount of information accessed. Both perceptual fluency and retrieval fluency are influenced by a variety of factors that also affect memory performance, thus contributing to the validity of fluency-driven metacognitive judgments. For example, information that is well learned, or that has been frequently or recently accessed, tends to lead to fluent retrieval. However, fluent retrieval may sometimes misinform metacognitive judgments, as nicely demonstrated by Benjamin, Bjork, and Schwartz (1998). In one experiment, they capitalized on the finding that the more difficult the generation of an answer is, the higher the probability that the answer will be recalled in a later free-recall test (Gardiner, Craik, & Bleasdale, 1973). Accordingly, they had participants answer general-information questions and make judgments of learning about the likelihood of recalling the answer in a later free-recall test. Whereas the probability of eventual recall increased with the latency of retrieving the answer, judgments of learning actually decreased with retrieval latency. Thus retrieval fluency can sometimes be counterdiagnostic.

In a second experiment, participants studied a series of six lists of words, recalled each list immediately after study, and then recalled the words from all six lists in a final free-recall test. In addition, after recalling each word in the immediate test, participants indicated their judgments of learning regarding its future retrievability in the final test. Judgments of learning were higher for items recalled in the first part of the recall output in immediate recall, but these items were in fact less likely to be recalled in the final test than those that occurred in later output positions. Thus retrieval fluency as indexed by output position in immediate recall seems to enhance judgments of learning while reducing the probability of final recall.

THE ROLE OF THEORY-BASED AND EXPERIENCE-BASED PROCESSES IN JUDGMENTS OF LEARNING

Koriat (1997), elaborating a cue utilization approach to judgments of learning, has proposed a model that distinguishes three classes of cues (intrinsic, extrinsic, and mnemonic) and two types of inferential processes (theory-based and experience-based) (see also Jacoby

& Kelley, 1987). Intrinsic cues pertain to inherent characteristics of the study items that disclose their *a priori* ease or difficulty of learning or remembering (e.g., word frequency, associative relatedness between paired associates). Extrinsic cues, in contrast, pertain to the conditions of learning (e.g., number of presentations) or to the encoding operations applied by the learner (e.g., level of processing). Koriat has proposed that both intrinsic and extrinsic factors can affect judgments of learning directly, through the explicit application of a particular rule or theory. For example, a person may believe that memory performance in a paired-associate task should be better for associatively related pairs than for unrelated pairs (an intrinsic factor), or that it should be better when a pair is presented three times than when it is presented only once (an extrinsic factor). However, both intrinsic and extrinsic cues may also influence judgments of learning indirectly, through their effects on the third class of cues—mnemonic cues.

Mnemonic cues are internal, subjective indicators that may signal to the person the extent to which an item has been mastered. These may include any of the cues discussed earlier, such as perceptual fluency and retrieval fluency. An important advantage of mnemonic cues as predictors of memory performance is that they are generally sensitive to both intrinsic and extrinsic factors that affect degree of learning. Thus, for example, Jacoby and his associates have provided evidence suggesting that fluency of processing and experienced familiarity are enhanced by a previous exposure to a stimulus (Jacoby & Kelley, 1987; Whittlesea, Jacoby, & Girard, 1990).

The direct and mediated effects of intrinsic and extrinsic cues are assumed to involve an analytic and a nonanalytic process, respectively. The direct effects involve an analytic inference based on the person's *a priori* theory about the memory-related consequences of various factors. The mediated effects, in contrast, rest on the implicit use of a nonanalytic inference rather than on a logical, conscious deduction. They are based on the utilization of mnemonic cues that provide an experiential basis for judgments of learning.

Koriat has proposed that the relative weight of different cues in determining judgments of learning may differ from one condition to another, and may also change with practice studying the same list of items. A series of experiments using paired-associates learning has supported the following two propositions. First, judgments of learning focus on the relative recallability of different items within a list, and are less sensitive to factors that affect overall performance (see Shaw & Craik, 1989). Therefore they tend to discount the effects of extrinsic factors relative to those of intrinsic factors (see also Carroll, Nelson, & Kirwan, 1997). Second, and more pertinent to the focus of the present chapter, is that with repeated practice studying a list of items, the basis of judgments of learning changes from a theory-based analytic inference toward greater reliance on heuristic-driven subjective experience. Thus the direct contribution of intrinsic cues to judgments of learning diminishes with practice studying the same set of items, whereas that of mnemonic cues increases.

For example, in one experiment (Experiment 2), a list of paired associates was shown for four study–test presentations, and during study participants indicated their judgments of learning for each item. The results yielded divergent effects of practice on calibration and resolution. On the one hand, practice impaired calibration by increasing underconfidence. This impairment resulted from the tendency to discount the extrinsic cue of number of presentations. At the same time, it increased resolution (i.e., the discrimination between items that were likely to be recalled and those that were not). This improvement apparently reflected a shift from theory-based to experience-based judgments. Thus, during initial study, the judgments of learning associated with different items reflected primarily the direct assessment of their preexperimental difficulty on the basis of some preconception about the memory-related consequences of different stimulus attributes. With increased practice learning these items, participants became increasingly sensitive to internal cues that disclose their relative memorability.

Whereas theory-based judgments of learning tend to rely on commonly shared beliefs about the possible memory-related consequences of different factors, mnemonic cues tend to be idiosyncratic, reflecting the person's unique processing of the items. The result is that participants tend to make similar judgments of learning to the same items during their initial study, but with increased practice they tend to diverge.

In sum, the study of judgments of learning also suggests a distinction between two different underlying processes: an analytic, theory-based process that involves a deliberate inference, and a nonanalytic, experience-based process that is mediated by the application of global heuristics.

PROCESSES AFFECTING SUBJECTIVE CONFIDENCE

Subjective confidence in the correctness of a proposition or an answer represents yet another kind of metacognitive judgment. Confidence judgments are generally elicited retrospectively, after participants have produced or chosen an answer to a question or after they have reached some decision. Although a large amount of work has been carried out on subjective probabilities and confidence judgments (see Wright & Ayton, 1994), only a small part of this work has any bearing on the distinction addressed in the present chapter between information-based (or theory-based) and experience-based judgments. In fact, much of the work on confidence judgments conducted in the area of decision making has centered on the calibration of confidence judgments, rather than on the processes underlying subjective confidence as such. The most widely documented phenomenon is that of overconfidence, as reflected, for example, in the tendency of people to overestimate the correctness of their answers (Keren, 1991; McClelland & Bolger, 1994).

Nevertheless, it may be noticed in the work on subjective confidence that whereas some researchers imply that confidence judgments are based on an analytic process, others imply that they rest on experiential-mnemonic cues. For example, a study by Koriat, Lichtenstein, and Fischhoff (1980) addressed the question of why people are overconfident in the correctness of their knowledge. It was proposed that the assessment of subjective confidence is generally biased by attempts to justify the decision: When answering forced-choice two-alternative questions, participants initially interrogate their memories for pertinent considerations (i.e., considerations that speak for and against each of the alternatives) and evaluate the implications of these considerations until a decision is reached. Once a decision is made, the evidence is reviewed to assess the likelihood that the answer is correct. This retrospective review tends to be biased by the decision already reached: It tends to focus on evidence that is consistent with that decision and to disregard evidence contradicting it, thereby resulting in overconfidence in the decision. Thus subjective confidence rests on a process of self-justification.

This account of overconfidence implies that subjective confidence is based on an analytic process that considers the information retrieved from memory to reach a reasonable assessment of the probability that the answer is correct. A similar view seems to underlie the theoretical framework proposed by Gigerenzer, Hoffrage and Kleinbölting (1991). In this framework, confidence judgments represent the outcome of a well-structured inductive inference. When participants encounter a problem such as "Which city has more inhabitants, Heidelberg or Bonn?," they will assign a 100% confidence to their answer if they can retrieve the number of inhabitants in each city. Otherwise they form a probabilistic mental model, which puts the specific task into a larger context and enables its solution by inductive inference. This model contains a reference class (all cities in Germany), a target variable (number of inhabitants), and several probability cues with their respective cue validities (e.g., the perceived probability that one city has more inhabitants than the other, given that it is the only city of the two that has a soccer team in the German Bundesliga). People base their answer on the probability cue, and their confidence on the respective cue validity.

In contrast to the view of confidence judgments as being determined by information-based inference, other work emphasizes the contribution of mnemonic cues, such as perceptual fluency and retrieval fluency. As for retrieval fluency, Nelson and Narens (1990) found that people express stronger confidence in the answers that they retrieve more quickly, whether those answers are correct or incorrect. Similarly, in a study by Kelley and Lindsay (1993), retrieval fluency was manipulated through priming. Partici-

pants were asked to answer general-information questions and to express their confidence in the correctness of their answers. Prior to this task, participants were asked to read a series of words, some of which were correct and some of which were plausible but incorrect answers to the questions. This prior exposure was found to increase the speed and probability with which the answers were provided in the recall test, and, in parallel, to enhance the confidence in the correctness of these answers. Importantly, these effects were observed for both correct and incorrect answers. These results support the view that retrospective confidence is based on a simple heuristic: Answers that come to mind easily are more likely to be correct than those that take longer to retrieve.

Processing fluency also seems to underlie an interesting effect observed by Chandler (1994). In her experiments participants were presented with a series of target and nontarget stimuli, each consisting of a scenic nature picture. In a subsequent recognition memory test for the targets, two opposing effects were found: Targets for which there existed a similar stimulus in the nontarget series (e.g., both depicted a lake) (1) were recognized less often, and (2) were endorsed with stronger confidence than targets for which no similar nontarget counterpart was included. Thus seeing a related target impaired participants' memory accuracy. However, it increased their confidence in the correctness of their choices, presumably because it enhanced fluent processing of the stimulus. Chandler's effect is analogous to one noted by Koriat and Lieblich (1977) with regard to feeling-of-knowing judgments: When people fail to retrieve a word that fits a certain definition, their feeling of knowing about the future recognition of that word is inflated by the presence in memory of "close neighbors"—that is, incorrect answers that partly fit the definition (see Koriat, 1998a).

The results of an experiment by Busey, Tunnicliff, Loftus, and Loftus (1995) may also point to the role of perceptual fluency in confidence judgments. Their participants studied a series of faces. Each face was seen under one of five luminance conditions, and its recognition was tested under a bright or a dim condition. When a face was studied in a dim condition, its testing in a bright condition reduced recognition accuracy but increased confidence. Possibly the fluent perceptual processing of the faces in the bright condition inflated participants' confidence judgments.

Postevent questioning, in which participants are asked to think about each of their responses in a memory test, has also been found to increase subsequent confidence ratings for these responses (Shaw, 1996; Wells, Ferguson, & Lindsay, 1981). In Shaw's study, this was found to be the case for incorrect answers made to misleading questions (questions referring to objects not presented) as well as those made to nonmisleading questions. Shaw has proposed that the retrieval attempt induced by postevent questioning increases subsequent retrieval fluency, which in turn results in enhanced confidence.

The imagination inflation phenomenon is probably yet another manifestation of the effects of retrieval fluency on confidence judgments. "Imagination inflation" refers to the observation that the mere act of imagining a past event increases one's confidence that the event did happen in the past. Garry, Manning, Loftus, and Sherman (1996) pretested their participants on how confident they were that a number of childhood events had happened, asked them to imagine some of those events, and then gathered new confidence judgments. Imagination instructions inflated confidence that an event had occurred in childhood. Moreover, merely asking about an event twice (on pretest and posttest) without instructing participants to imagine it led to an increase in subjective confidence, although not as large as the one produced by the act of imagination. Probably imagination of an event or even the mere attempt to recall it increases its retrieval fluency, which in turn contributes to the confidence that the event has occurred. Gregory, Burroughs, and Ainslie (1985; see also Gregory, Cialdini, & Carpenter, 1982; Sherman, Cialdini, Schwartzman, & Reynolds, 1985) have reported a similar effect of imagination on prospective probabilities (i.e., the perceived likelihood of future events).

Hastie, Landsman, and Loftus (1978) also found that repeated questioning about an imagined detail of a story increased confidence in that detail, and Turtle and Yuille (1994, Experiment 1) observed an increase in subjective confidence from one to two recall occasions (but see Ryan & Geiselman, 1991).

In sum, the work on confidence judgments suggests the possibility that these judgments may be mediated both by an analytic, knowledge-based inference that takes into account domain-specific considerations retrieved from memory, and by a nonanalytic, experience-based process that relies on the application of general-purpose heuristics. Little is known about the relative contribution of these processes. Perhaps knowledge-based assessment is more strongly activated when the task is defined as involving the "assessment of probabilities" than when it is defined as that of reporting one's unmediated "subjective confidence."

NOETIC FEELINGS AND NOETIC JUDGMENTS COMPARED

The foregoing review has examined the processes underlying metacognitive judgments elicited at different stages of learning and remembering—during the encoding of a piece of information, during the attempt to retrieve it from memory, and following recall or recognition of the item. Theories and findings on all three types of metacognitive judgments would seem to concur in suggesting two general propositions. First, metacognitive judgments are often based on the implicit application of general-purpose heuristics that make use of mnemonic cues. These heuristics give rise to an unmediated noetic feeling. The phenomenal immediacy of this feeling sometimes creates the sense of direct trace monitoring, as well as an illusion of validity.

Second, in addition to metacognitive judgments that are based on direct noetic feelings, we must recognize that such judgments may also be based on an analytic, deliberate inference that takes into account a variety of cognitive considerations. This type of judgment has been variously termed "theory-based" or "information-based," depending on the specific research context (e.g., Jacoby & Kelley, 1987; Kelley & Jacoby, 1996a; Koriat, 1997; Strack, 1992). Unlike noetic feelings, noetic judgments rest on domain-specific, content-specific information, including theories and beliefs, semantic memory, recollected episodes, and so on.

In order to appreciate the important difference between the two types of metacognitive judgments, it is necessary to examine the role of these judgments in guiding behavior. A commonly held assumption among students of metacognition is that metacognitive judgments exert a causal role in governing behavior (see Barnes, Nelson, Dunlosky, Mazzoni, & Narens, 1998; Nelson, 1996). As noted earlier, judgments of learning seem to affect the amount of time spent studying a certain item in self-paced learning (e.g., Mazzoni & Cornoldi, 1993; Nelson & Leonesio, 1988). Feeling-of-knowing judgments associated with a question seem to guide the choice of a question-answering strategy, as well as the amount of time spent searching for the answer before giving up (e.g., Costermans et al., 1992; Gruneberg & Monks, 1974; Reder, 1987). Finally, confidence judgments in a piece of information that comes to mind appears to determine whether that information is volunteered or withheld under conditions that place a premium on accurate reporting (Koriat & Goldsmith, 1994, 1996). It is important to stress that the effects of metacognitive judgments on behavior occur whether these judgments are experience-based or information-based, and whether these judgments are accurate or inaccurate.

Koriat (1998b) has proposed a crude distinction between two modes of operation that can underlie behavior. The first is the explicit/controlled mode of operation: When a goal has to be reached, various considerations are consciously examined in an analytic fashion, and these come to govern controlled behavior. We associate this mode of operation with what is sometimes referred to as "rational behavior." Clearly, noetic judgments constitute an integral part of this mode of operation. For example, a student who is asked to answer one of two questions of his or her choice in a final exam may begin by assessing the probability that he or she can provide a correct and complete answer to each question, and then may choose to answer the question that has the higher assessed probability (see Koriat & Goldsmith, 1998).

In the implicit/automatic mode of operation, in contrast, unconscious activations may automatically affect and guide behavior. For example, stimuli registered below full consciousness may influence behavior directly and automatically without the mediation of conscious control. This mode of operation has been amply documented by social psychologists (see Bargh, 1997; Bargh, Chen, & Burrows, 1996). Clearly, the implicit/automatic mode of operation does not implicate metacognitive monitoring at all.

Where do noetic feelings belong, then? According to Koriat (1998b), noetic feelings occupy a unique role in mediating between the implicit/automatic mode of operation and the explicit/controlled mode of operation: They are implicit and unconscious as far as their antecedents are concerned, but explicit and controlled as far as their consequences are concerned. As argued throughout this chapter, noetic feelings (as distinct from noetic judgments) are the outcome of the implicit application of nonanalytic heuristics that rely on mnemonic cues. These heuristics may operate below full consciousness. However, once such heuristics give rise to conscious, noetic feelings, these feelings can serve to guide and motivate controlled behavior. For example, spurious priming of the terms of a question may unconsciously inflate the feeling of knowing associated with that question. The enhanced feeling of knowing, in turn, may result in spending more time trying to search for the answer before giving up (see Reder, 1987).

Using this general framework, we can now summarize the differences between the modes of operation involved when behavior is controlled by noetic feelings and when it is mediated by noetic judgments. These differences parallel those mentioned in our discussion of affective states between affect-based and information-based processes.

1. Mediation. The analytic process incorporating noetic judgments is a uniform process that operates in the explicit/controlled mode of operation throughout: Analytic, conscious considerations result in a noetic judgment, which can then affect choice and behavior in a "rational" manner. In contrast, when noetic feelings are implicated, these feelings serve to mediate between two qualitatively different processes, an implicit, nonanalytic process that operates below full awareness to shape subjective experience, and a controlled, largely conscious process that guides self-controlled behavior.

2. *Content.* A second difference is that the analytic determination of noetic judgments entails inspection of the content of domain-specific knowledge—theories, beliefs, and semantic and episodic memories. In contrast, in the nonanalytic process underlying noetic feelings, the content of the information does not enter into consideration (Koriat, 1993). Rather, the cues for feelings of knowing, judgments of learning, or subjective confidence lie in structural aspects of the information-processing system. This system, so to speak, engages in a self-reflective inspection of its own operation and uses the ensuing information as a basis for metacognitive judgments. This is precisely the process assumed to underlie the use of the availability heuristic for estimating frequencies (Tversky & Kahneman, 1973): People judge frequencies by the ease with which instances come to mind. Thus, all of the mnemonic cues mentioned as possible determinants of noetic feelings—cue familiarity, accessibility, and fluency—are indifferent to the content of the information.

3. *Phenomenal quality.* Finally, as stressed throughout this chapter, the phenomenal quality of monitoring processes differs when these processes entail an analytic inference and when they are based on a nonanalytic heuristic. Analytic inferences lead to a cognitive, intellectual judgment, whereas nonanalytic processes tend to lead to a feeling tone, an impression, or an intuition, without a clear awareness of the basis of this feeling. In this case, as Strack (1992) noted, the immediacy of the phenomenal experience seems to be transferred automatically to the judgment.

THE RELATION BETWEEN ANALYTIC AND NONANALYTIC PROCESSES IN METACOGNITIVE JUDGMENTS

Although in our discussion we have drawn a sharp distinction between the analytic and nonanalytic processes underlying metacognitive judgments, the two types of processes presumably operate together in determining metacognitive judgments (see Kelley & Jacoby, 1996a, 1996b). Thus analytic and nonanalytic processes may act in concert to influence behavior. Often, however, their combined effect is far from being additive. For example, Glucksberg and McCloskey (1981) found that participants could reach a "don't know" decision very quickly when presented with some questions (e.g., "Does Margaret Thatcher use an electric toothbrush?"). However, when they were informed beforehand that the answers to these questions were not known (e.g., "It is not known whether Margaret Thatcher uses an electric toothbrush"), this information actually slowed down "don't know" judgments, possibly because now the judgments tended to be based on retrieved information rather than on sheer subjective experience. Furthermore, it has been amply documented that awareness of the spurious source of subjective feelings may sometimes prevent their effects on judgments and behavior. For example, Jacoby and Whitehouse (1989) showed that an unaware presentation of a word just before its presentation for a recognition test misled participants into judging that word as "old." Supposedly, the increased processing fluency of the word (resulting from its prior presentation) was unconsciously misattributed to the word's presentation in the study phase. In contrast, a longer and aware presentation of the word prior to the recognition test yielded the opposite effect: It decreased the probability of judging the word as "old."

Similarly, it has been observed that a bad mood resulting from bad weather reduces participants' judgments of their happiness and satisfaction with their life as a whole. However, participants tend to correct for the effects of a bad mood when their attention is drawn to the rainy weather in an opening remark (Schwarz & Clore, 1983; see also Murphy & Zajonc, 1993; Murphy, Monahan, & Zajonc, 1995).

In fact, the rich social-psychological literature on assimilation and contrast effects (e.g., Higgins, Bargh, & Lombardi, 1985; Higgins, Rholes, & Jones, 1977; Lombardi, Higgins, & Bargh, 1987; Martin, Seta, & Crelia, 1990; Strack, Erber, & Wicklund, 1982; Strack & Hannover, 1996; Strack, Schwarz, Bless, Kübler, & Wänke, 1993) offers a good demonstration of how awareness of an irrelevant activation of a certain concept enables analytic processes to correct (and even overcorrect) for the biased effects of nonanalytic processes on judgment. For example, Strack et al. (1993) had participants judge the likability of a target character whose behavior was ambiguous. They were found to give relatively high likability ratings when primed with positive adjectives in a previous, seemingly irrelevant task, and relatively low ratings when primed with negative adjectives (assimilation effect). However, when participants were reminded of the priming task, the opposite pattern emerged (contrast effect). (For other demonstrations of the operation of effortful and automatic processes in opposition, see also Jacoby, Kelley, Brown, & Jasechko, 1989; Jacoby, Kelley & McErlee, Chapter 19, this volume; Kelley & Jacoby, 1996a; Trope, 1986; Trope & Gaunt, Chapter 8, this volume.)

We believe that in a similar manner, analytic processes can circumvent the effects of nonanalytic processes on metacognitive judgments. Thus, under those conditions in which irrelevant episodic events inflate metacognitive judgments by enhancing fluent processing, the explicit recollection of these irrelevant events should prevent the effects of processing fluency on metacognitive judgments (see Kelley & Jacoby, 1996a, 1996b).

AFFECTIVE FEELINGS REVISITED

Our analysis of the role of metacognitive judgments in terms of the distinction between an explicit/controlled mode, an implicit/automatic mode, and a crossover mode of operation may have implications beyond the realm of metacognitive judgments. We illustrate some of these implications with regard to the analysis of affective feelings.

In discussions of affective responses, there has been a debate concerning the possibility of nonconscious affect. Whereas some believe that emotions are by definition conscious, subjectively experienced states of awareness (e.g., Clore, 1994; LeDoux, 1994), others argue for the possibility that emotions may be apparent in behavior and physiology with no experiential component (e.g., Lang, 1988). For example, Zajonc (1980, 1994) and Epstein and Pacini (Chapter 23, this volume) argued that behavior can sometimes be mediated by gross, diffuse affective reactions of which the person is not aware (see, e.g.,

Murphy et al., 1995). In fact, a similar proposal has been recently voiced in the area of metacognition: Reder and Schunn (1996) have argued that metacognitive monitoring and control processes, such as those involved in the feeling of knowing, also operate automatically and without awareness.

However, as detailed above, the position advocated in Koriat (1998b) and adopted in the present chapter suggests that stimuli that have a positive or negative valence may affect approach–avoidance behavior directly and automatically, without the mediation of consciousness or subjective experience. Such automatic effects are like those discussed by Bargh (1997) and need not invoke the notion of nonconscious affect. These effects are part of the implicit/automatic mode of operation, in which unconscious processes find their way automatically into behavior. A similar argument may be raised with regard to some of the observations cited by Reder and Schunn (1996): Various events may implicitly affect strategies of information processing, without any mediation of conscious metacognitive monitoring and control.

However, in the same way that unconscious processes can influence behavior directly and automatically, they may also influence and shape affective feelings. For example, a person may feel cheerful or depressed without knowing why, or may experience a disgust toward a particular food with no particular explanation (see Rozin, Millman, & Nemeroff, 1986; Spielman, Pratto, & Bargh, 1988). In such a case we are not talking about unconscious affect, because the feeling itself, like the feeling of knowing, is clearly conscious. The important point to stress, however, is that once unconscious influences give rise to a subjective feeling state, that state can now guide and direct behavior in a controlled, conscious manner. Thus, like noetic feelings, affective feelings may serve a crossover function, mediating between implicit and explicit modes of operation.

In addition, affective feelings may result from an explicit analysis of information. For example, a person who does not like fish may feel some repulsion toward a salad offered in a buffet when he or she learns (or suspects) that it contains tuna fish. On the basis of that information, the person may consciously and deliberately choose to avoid that salad. This kind of avoidance behavior may emanate directly from the pertinent information, or may be mediated by the affective reactions that ensue from that information.

It is important to stress that even when affective reactions are information-based, people may still rely on their immediate feelings in guiding their behavior, rather than on the information on which these feelings are based. This may occur, for example, under time constraints or competing task demands that make it difficult to retrieve or reassess the pertinent information (see Clore, Schwarz, & Conway, 1994; Schwarz, 1990; Strack, 1992). Of course, when the informational basis of affective reactions is not available to consciousness, people have no choice but to base their judgment and behavior on the affective feelings.

Extending our analysis of noetic processes to affective processes, we can make the following two propositions: First, the phenomenal quality of a feeling state should be different when the person is aware of the source of the feeling and when he or she is not (see Murphy et al., 1995). This proposal was in fact advanced by Freud (1917/1963) in his discussion of free-floating anxiety. For example, when a feeling of disgust associated with a particular salad is based on the knowledge that the salad contains tuna fish, this should differ from disgust associated with the same salad but based on an unexplained gut sensation. As noted earlier, the distinction between the qualities of explained and unexplained affective states parallels the distinction between types of noetic states—for example, the distinction between "knowing" and "just knowing" (Block, 1995), or between recollection-based and familiarity-based processes (e.g., Jacoby & Brooks, 1984).

Second, our review of the work on noetic feelings indicates that these feelings can be contaminated by a variety of factors of which a person is not aware. Possibly the same is true of affective feelings (Spielman et al., 1988). When this occurs, the person's feelings may be judged to be "inappropriate" or "invalid" (Schwarz & Clore, 1996). What is important to stress is that people act on the basis of their gut feelings, whether or not these feeling are "founded," "justified," or "adequate." A person who feels disgust toward some food will tend to avoid it, whether the feeling of disgust indeed reflects some undesirable property of the food or reflects some irrelevant property, such as the circumstances in which that food has been previously encountered (see Rozin et al., 1986). A similar pattern has been found with regard to metacognitive judgments: When people decide whether to report an answer to a question, they base their decision heavily on their confidence in the answer, and they do so even when their confidence judgments are not diagnostic of the accuracy of their answer (see Koriat & Goldsmith, 1996). Thus, the importance of both noetic and affective feelings is that they play a critical role in governing behavior, regardless of their basis or of the extent to which they are "accurate" or "appropriate."

In sum, in this chapter we have outlined a conceptual framework that emerges from the study of metacognitive judgments, and have also shown how it can be extended to the analysis of emotional feelings and behavior. Our distinction between analytic and nonanalytic processes and between experience-based and information-based reactions accords well with current views in cognitive and social psychology that distinguish between two different modes of information processing. In the present analysis, however, we have stressed the distinction between two processes: one that is explicit and controlled throughout, and one that entails a transition from an implicit/automatic mode of operation to a mode of operation that is more explicit and controlled. The important feature of the latter, crossover process lies in the unique role played by subjective feelings, noetic or affective, in mediating between unconscious influences and conscious, controlled behavior.

ACKNOWLEDGMENTS

The preparation of this chapter was supported by Grant No. 40/96 from the Israel Foundations Trustees to Asher Koriat, and by the Max-Wertheimer Minerva Center for Cognitive Processes and Human Performance. The chapter was completed while the first author was a visiting professor at the Max-Planck Institute for Psychological Research, Munich, Germany.

REFERENCES

Bargh, J. A. (1997). The automaticity of everyday life. In R. S. Wyer, Jr. (Ed.), *Advances in social cognition* (Vol. 10, pp. 1–61). Mahwah, NJ: Erlbaum.

Bargh, J. A., Chen, M., & Burrows, L. (1996). Automaticity of social behavior: Direct effects of trait construct and stereotype activation on action. *Journal of Personality and Social Psychology, 71*, 230–244.

Barnes, A. E., Nelson, T. O., Dunlosky, J., Mazzoni, G., & Narens, L. (1998). An integrative system of metamemory components involved in retrieval. In D. Gopher & A. Koriat (Eds.), *Cognitive regulation of performance: Interaction of theory and application* (pp. 287–313). Cambridge, MA: MIT Press.

Begg, I., Duft, S., Lalonde, P., Melnick, R., & Sanvito, J. (1989). Memory predictions are based on ease of processing. *Journal of Memory and Language, 28*, 610–632.

Benjamin, A. S., & Bjork, R. A. (1996). Retrieval fluency as a metacognitive index. In L. M. Reder (Ed.), *Implicit memory and metacognition* (pp. 309–338). Hillsdale, NJ: Erlbaum.

Benjamin, A. S., Bjork, R. A., & Schwartz, B. L. (1998). The mismeasure of memory: When retrieval fluency is misleading. *Journal of Experimental Psychology: General, 127*, 55–68.

Bjork, R. A. (1998). Assessing our own competence: Heuristics and illusions. In D. Gopher & A. Koriat (Eds.), *Cognitive regulation of performance: Interaction of theory and application* (pp. 435–459). Cambridge, MA: MIT Press.

Block, N. (1995). On a confusion about a function of consciousness. *Behavioral and Brain Sciences, 18*, 227–287.

Brandimonte, M., & Ellis, J. (1996). *Prospective memory*. Mahwah, NJ: Erlbaum.

Brown, N. R., & Siegler, R. S. (1993). Metrics and mappings: A framework for understanding real-world quantitative estimation. *Psychological Review, 100*, 511–534.

Brown, R., & McNeill, D. (1966). The "tip of the tongue" phenomenon. *Journal of Verbal Learning and Verbal Behavior, 5*, 325–337.

Busey, T. A., Tunnicliff, J. L., Loftus, G. R., & Loftus, E. F.(1995, November). *Predicting picture memory performance: Not all confidence judgments are equal.* Paper presented at the 36th Annual Meeting of the Psychonomic Society, Los Angeles.

Carroll, M., Nelson, T. O., & Kirwan, A. (1997). Trade-off of semantic relatedness and degree of overlearning: Differential effects on metamemory and on long-term retention. *Acta Psychologica, 95*, 239–253.

Chandler, C. C. (1994). Studying related pictures can reduce accuracy, but increase confidence, in a modified recognition test. *Memory & Cognition, 22*, 273–280.

Clore, G. L. (1992). Cognitive phenomenology: Feelings and the construction of judgment. In L. L. Martin & A. Tesser (Eds.), *The construction of social judgments* (pp. 133–164). Hillsdale, NJ: Erlbaum.

Clore, G. L. (1994). Why emotions are never unconscious. In P. Ekman & R. J. Davidson (Eds.), *The nature of emotion: Fundamental questions* (pp. 285–290). New York: Oxford University Press.

Clore, G. L., Schwarz, N., & Conway, M. (1994). Affective causes and consequences of social information processing. In R. S. Wyer, Jr., & T. K. Srull (Eds.), *Handbook of social cognition* (2nd ed., Vol. 1, pp. 323–418). Hillsdale, NJ: Erlbaum.

Cohen, R. L., Sandler, S. P., & Keglevich, L. (1991). The failure of memory monitoring in a free recall task. *Canadian Journal of Psychology, 45*, 523–538.

Costermans, J., Lories, G., & Ansay, C. (1992). Confidence level and feeling of knowing in question answering: The weight of inferential processes. *Journal of Experimental Psychology: Learning, Memory, and Cognition, 18*, 142–150.

Dunlosky, J., & Nelson, T. O. (1992). Importance of the kind of cue for judgments of learning (JOLs) and the delayed-JOL effect. *Memory & Cognition, 20*, 373–380.

Dunlosky, J., & Nelson, T. O. (1994). Does the sensitivity of judgments of learning (JOLs) to the effects of various study activities depend on when the JOLs occur? *Journal of Memory and Language, 33*, 545–565.

Epstein, S. (1994). Integration of the cognitive and psychodynamic unconscious. *American Psychologist, 49*, 709–724.

Epstein, S., Lipson, A., Holstein, C., & Huh, E. (1992). Irrational reactions to negative outcomes: Evidence for two conceptual systems. *Journal of Personality and Social Psychology, 62*, 328–339.

Fischhoff, B., Slovic, P., & Lichtenstein, S. (1977). Knowing with certainty: The appropriateness of extreme confidence. *Journal of Experimental Psychology: Human Perception and Performance, 3*, 552–564.

Freud, S. (1963). *A general introduction to psychoanalysis* (J. Riviere, Trans.). New York: Liveright. (Original work published 1917)

Gardiner, J. M., Craik, F. I. M., & Bleasdale, F. A. (1973). Retrieval difficulty and subsequent recall. *Memory & Cognition, 1*, 213–216.

Gardiner, J. M., & Java, R. I. (1993). Recognizing and remembering. In A. F. Collins, S. E. Gathercole, M. A. Conway, & P. E. Morris (Eds.), *Theories of memory* (pp. 163–188). Hove, England: Erlbaum.

Garry, M., Manning, C. G., Loftus, E. F., & Sherman, S. J. (1996). Imagination inflation: Imagining a childhood event inflates confidence that it occurred. *Psychonomic Bulletin and Review, 3*, 208–214.

Gigerenzer, G., Hoffrage, U., & Kleinbölting, H. (1991). Probabilistic mental models: A Brunswikian theory of confidence. *Psychological Review, 98*, 506–528.

Glucksberg, S., & McCloskey, M. (1981). Decisions about ignorance. *Journal of Experimental Psychology: Human Learning and Memory, 7*, 311–325.

Gregory, W. L., Burroughs, W. J., & Ainslie, F. M. (1985). Self-relevant scenarios as an indirect means of attitude change. *Personality and Social Psychology Bulletin, 11*, 435–444.

Gregory, W. L., Cialdini, R. B., & Carpenter, K. M. (1982). Self-relevant scenarios as mediators of likelihood estimates and compliance: Does imagining make it so? *Journal of Personality and Social Psychology, 43*, 89–99.

Gruneberg, M. M., & Monks, J. (1974). "Feeling of

knowing" and cued recall. *Acta Psychologica*, 38, 257–265.

Hart, J. T. (1965). Memory and the feeling-of-knowing experience. *Journal of Educational Psychology*, 56, 208–216.

Hart, J. T. (1967a). Memory and the memory-monitoring process. *Journal of Verbal Learning and Verbal Behavior*, 6, 685–691.

Hart, J. T. (1967b). Second-try recall, recognition and the memory-monitoring process. *Journal of Educational Psychology*, 58, 193–197.

Hastie, R., Landsman, R., & Loftus, E. F. (1978). Eyewitness testimony: The dangers of guessing. *Jurimetrics Journal*, 19, 1–8.

Higgins, E. T., Bargh, J. A., & Lombardi, W. (1985). The nature of priming effects on categorization. *Journal of Experimental Psychology: Human Learning and Memory*, 11, 59–69.

Higgins, E. T., Rholes, W. S., & Jones, C. R. (1977). Category accessibility and impression formation. *Journal of Experimental Social Psychology*, 13, 141–154.

Jacoby, L. L. (1991). A process dissociation framework: Separating automatic from intentional uses of memory. *Journal of Memory and Language*, 30, 513–541.

Jacoby, L. L., & Brooks, L. R. (1984). Nonanalytic cognition: Memory, perception and concept learning. In G. Bower (Ed.), *The psychology of learning and motivation: Advances in research and theory* (Vol. 18, pp. 1–47). Orlando, Florida: Academic Press.

Jacoby, L. L., & Kelley, C. M. (1987). Unconscious influences of memory for a prior event. *Personality and Social Psychology Bulletin*, 13, 314–336.

Jacoby, L. L., Kelley, C. M., Brown, J., & Jasechko, J. (1989). Becoming famous overnight: Limits on the ability to avoid unconscious influences of the past. *Journal of Personality and Social Psychology*, 56, 326–338.

Jacoby, L. L., Lindsay, S. D., & Toth, J. P. (1992). Unconscious influences revealed: Attention, awareness, and control. *American Psychologist*, 47, 802–809.

Jacoby, L. L., & Whitehouse, K. (1989). An illusion of memory: False recognition influenced by unconscious perception. *Journal of Experimental Psychology: General*, 118, 126–135.

James, W. (1890). *The principles of psychology* (Vol. 1). New York: Holt.

Kelley, C. M., & Jacoby, L. L. (1996a). Adult egocentrism: Subjective experience versus analytic bases for judgment. *Journal of Memory and Language*, 35, 157–175.

Kelley, C. M., & Jacoby, L. L. (1996b). Memory attributions: Remembering, knowing, and feeling of knowing. In L. M. Reder (Ed.), *Implicit memory and metacognition* (pp. 287–307). Hillsdale, NJ: Erlbaum.

Kelley, C. M., & Lindsay, D. S. (1993). Remembering mistaken for knowing: Ease of retrieval as a basis for confidence in answers to general knowledge questions. *Journal of Memory and Language*, 32, 124.

Keren, G. (1991). Calibration and probability judgments: Conceptual and methodological issues. *Acta Psychologica*, 77, 217–273.

Koriat, A. (1993). How do we know that we know? The accessibility model of the feeling of knowing. *Psychological Review*, 100, 609–639.

Koriat, A. (1994). Memory's knowledge of its own knowledge: The accessibility account of the feeling of knowing. In J. Metcalfe & P. Shimamura (Eds.), *Metacognition: Knowing about knowing* (pp. 115–135). Cambridge, MA: MIT Press.

Koriat, A. (1995). Dissociating knowing and the feeling of knowing: Further evidence for the accessibility model. *Journal of Experimental Psychology: General*, 124, 311–333.

Koriat, A. (1997). Monitoring one's own knowledge during study: A cue-utilization approach to judgments of learning. *Journal of Experimental Psychology: General*, 126, 349–370.

Koriat, A. (1998a). Illusions of knowing: The link between knowledge and metaknowledge. In V. Y. Yzerbyt, G. Lories, & B. Dardenne (Eds.), *Metacognition: Cognitive and social dimensions* (pp. 16–34). London, England: Sage.

Koriat, A. (1998b). Metamemory: The feeling of knowing and its vagaries. In M. Sabourin, F. I. M. Craik, & M. Robert (Eds.), *Advances in Psychological Science: Biological and cognitive aspects* (Vol. 2, pp. 461–479). Hove, England: Psychology Press.

Koriat, A., Edry, E., & de Marcas, G. (1998). *What do we know about what we cannot remember? Accessing the semantic attributes of words that cannot be recalled*. Manuscript in preparation.

Koriat, A., & Goldsmith, M. (1994). Memory in naturalistic and laboratory contexts: Distinguishing the accuracy-oriented and quantity-oriented approaches to memory assessment. *Journal of Experimental Psychology: General*, 123, 297–315.

Koriat, A., & Goldsmith, M. (1996). Monitoring and control processes in the strategic regulation of memory accuracy. *Psychological Review*, 103, 490–517.

Koriat, A., & Goldsmith, M. (1998). The role of metacognitive processes in the regulation of memory accuracy. In G. Mazzoni & T. Nelson (Eds.), *Metacognition and cognitive neuropsychology: Monitoring and control processes* (pp. 97–118). Mahwah, NJ: Erlbaum.

Koriat, A., Lichtenstein, S., & Fischhoff, B. (1980). Reasons for confidence. *Journal of Experimental Psychology: Human Learning and Memory*, 6, 107–118.

Koriat, A., & Lieblich, I. (1977). A study of memory pointers. *Acta Psychologica*, 41, 151–164.

Krinsky, R., & Nelson, T. O. (1985). The feeling of knowing for different types of retrieval failure. *Acta Psychologica*, 58, 141–158.

Lang, P. J. (1988). What are the data of emotion? In V. Hamilton, G. Bower, & N. Frijda (Eds.), *Cognitive science perspectives on emotion and motivation* (pp. 173–194). Amsterdam: Martinus Nijhoff.

LeDoux, J. E. (1994). Emotional processing but not emotions can occur unconsciously. In P. Ekman & R. J. Davidson (Eds.), *The nature of emotion: Fundamental questions* (pp. 291–292). New York: Oxford University Press.

Lombardi, W. J., Higgins, E. T., & Bargh, J. A. (1987). The role of consciousness in priming effects on categorization: Assimilation versus contrast as a function of awareness of a priming task. *Personality and Social Psychology Bulletin*, 13, 411–429.

Lovelace, E. A. (1984). Metamemory: Monitoring future recallability during study. *Journal of Experimental Psychology: Learning, Memory, and Cognition*, 10, 756–766.

Martin, L. L., Seta, J. J., & Crelia, R. (1990). Assimilation and contrast as a function of people's willingness and ability to expend effort in forming an impression. *Journal of Personality and Social Psychology, 59,* 27–37.

Mazzoni, G., & Cornoldi, C. (1993). Strategies in study time allocation: Why is study time sometimes not effective? *Journal of Experimental Psychology: General, 122,* 47–60.

Mazzoni, G., & Nelson, T. O. (1995). Judgments of learning are affected by the kind of encoding in ways that cannot be attributed to the level of recall. *Journal of Experimental Psychology: Learning, Memory, and Cognition, 21,* 1263–1274.

McClelland, A. G. R., & Bolger, F. (1994). The calibration of subjective probabilities: Theories and models 1980–1994. In G. Wright & P. Ayton (Eds.), *Subjective probability* (pp. 453–482). Chichester, England: Wiley.

Metcalfe, J. (1993). Novelty monitoring, metacognition and control in a composite holographic associative recall model: Implications for Korsakoff amnesia. *Psychological Review, 100,* 322.

Metcalfe, J. (1996). Metacognitive processes. In E. L. Bjork & R. A. Bjork (Eds.), *Memory* (pp. 381–407). San Diego, CA: Academic Press.

Metcalfe, J., Schwartz, B. L., & Joaquim, S. G. (1993). The cue-familiarity heuristic in metacognition. *Journal of Experimental Psychology: Learning, Memory, and Cognition, 19,* 851–861.

Metcalfe, J., & Shimamura, A. P. (1994). *Metacognition: Knowing about knowing.* Cambridge, MA: MIT Press.

Morris, C. C. (1990). Retrieval processes underlying confidence in comprehension judgments. *Journal of Experimental Psychology: Learning, Memory, and Cognition, 16,* 223–232.

Murphy, S. T., Monahan, J. L., & Zajonc, R. B. (1995). Additivity of nonconscious affect: Combined effects of priming and exposure. *Journal of Personality and Social Psychology, 69,* 589–602.

Murphy, S. T., & Zajonc, R. B. (1993). Affect, cognition, and awareness: Affective priming with subliminal and optimal stimulus. *Journal of Personality and Social Psychology, 64,* 723–739.

Narens, L., Jameson, K. A., & Lee, V. A. (1994). Subthreshold priming and memory monitoring. In J. Metcalfe & P. Shimamura (Eds.), *Metacognition: Knowing about knowing* (pp. 71–92). Cambridge, MA: MIT Press.

Nelson, T. O. (1996). Consciousness and metacognition. *American Psychologist, 51,* 102–116.

Nelson, T. O., Gerler, D., & Narens, L. (1984). Accuracy of feeling-of-knowing judgment for predicting perceptual identification and relearning. *Journal of Experimental Psychology: General, 113,* 282–300.

Nelson, T. O., & Leonesio, R. J. (1988). Allocation of self-paced study time and the "labor-in-vain effect." *Journal of Experimental Psychology: Learning, Memory, and Cognition, 14,* 676–686.

Nelson, T. O., & Narens, L. (1990). Metamemory: A theoretical framework and new findings. In G. Bower (Ed.), *The psychology of learning and motivation: Advances in research and theory* (Vol. 26, pp. 125–123). San Diego, CA: Academic Press.

Reder, L. M. (1987). Strategy selection in question answering. *Cognitive Psychology, 19,* 90–138.

Reder, L. M. (1988). Strategic control of retrieval strate-gies. In G. Bower (Ed.), *The psychology of learning and motivation* (Vol. 22, pp. 227–259). San Diego, CA: Academic Press.

Reder, L. M. (Ed.). (1996). *Implicit memory and metacognition.* Hillsdale, NJ: Erlbaum.

Reder, L. M., & Ritter, F. E. (1992). What determines initial feeling of knowing? Familiarity with question terms, not with the answer. *Journal of Experimental Psychology: Learning, Memory, and Cognition, 18,* 435–451.

Reder, L. M., & Schunn, C. D. (1996). Metacognition does not imply awareness: Strategy choice is governed by implicit learning and memory. In L. M. Reder (Ed.), *Implicit memory and metacognition* (pp. 45–78). Hillsdale, NJ: Erlbaum.

Rozin, P., Millman, L., & Nemeroff, C. (1986). Operation of the laws of sympathetic magic in disgust and other domains. *Journal of Personality and Social Psychology, 50,* 703–712.

Ryan, R. H., & Geiselman, R. E. (1991). Effects of biased information on the relationship between eyewitness confidence and accuracy. *Bulletin of the Psychonomic Society, 29,* 79.

Schunn, C. D., Reder, L. M., Nhouyvanisvong, A., Richards, D. R., & Stroffolino, P. J. (1997). To calculate or not to calculate: A source activation confusion (SAC) model of problem-familiarity's role in strategy selection. *Journal of Experimental Psychology: Learning, Memory, and Cognition, 23,* 329.

Schwartz, B. L. (1994). Sources of information in metamemory: Judgments of learning and feeling of knowing. *Psychonomic Bulletin and Review, 1,* 357–375.

Schwartz, B. L., & Metcalfe, J. (1992). Cue familiarity but not target retrievability enhances feeling-of-knowing judgment. *Journal of Experimental Psychology: Learning, Memory, and Cognition, 18,* 1074–1083.

Schwarz, N. (1990). Feelings as information: Informational and motivational functions of affective states. In E. T. Higgins & R. M. Sorrentino (Eds.), *Handbook of motivation and cognition: Foundations of social behavior* (Vol. 2, pp. 528–561). New York: Guilford Press.

Schwarz, N., & Clore, G. L. (1983). Mood, misattribution, and judgments of well-being: Informative and directive functions of affective states. *Journal of Personality and Social Psychology, 45,* 513–523.

Schwarz, N., & Clore, G. L. (1996). Feelings of phenomenal experiences. In E. T. Higgins & A. W. Kruglanski (Eds.), *Social psychology: Handbook of basic principles* (pp. 433–465). New York: Guilford Press.

Shaw, J. S., III (1996). Increases in eyewitness confidence resulting from postevent questioning. *Journal of Experimental Psychology: Applied, 2,* 126–146.

Shaw, R. J., & Craik, F. I. M. (1989). Age differences in predictions and performance on a cued recall task. *Psychology and Aging, 4,* 133–135.

Sherman, S. J., Cialdini, R. B., Schwartzman, D. F., & Reynolds, K. D. (1985). Imagining can heighten or lower the perceived likelihood of contracting a disease: The mediating effect of ease of imagery. *Personality and Social Psychology Bulletin, 11,* 118–127.

Sloman, S. (1996). The empirical case for two systems of reasoning. *Psychological Bulletin, 119,* 322.

Spielman, L. A., Pratto, F., & Bargh, J. (1988). Automatic affect: Are one's moods, attitudes, evaluations, and emotions out of control? *American Behavioral Scientist, 31,* 296–311.

Strack, F. (1992). The different routes to social judgments: Experimental versus informational strategies. In I. I. Martin & A. Tesser (Eds.), *The construction of social judgments* (pp. 249–275). Hillsdale, NJ: Erlbaum.

Strack, F., Erber, R., & Wicklund, R. (1982). Effects of salience and time pressure on ratings of social causality. *Journal of Experimental Social Psychology, 18,* 581–594.

Strack, F., & Hannover, B. (1996). Awareness of influence as a precondition for implementing correctional goals. In P. Gollwitzer & J. Bargh (Eds.), *The psychology of action: Linking cognition and motivation to behavior* (pp. 579–596). New York: Guilford Press.

Strack, F., Schwarz, N., Bless, H., Kübler, A., & Wänke, M. (1993). Awareness of the influence as a determinant of assimilation versus contrast. *European Journal of Social Psychology, 23,* 53–62.

Turtle, J., & Yuille, J. C. (1994). Lost but not forgotten details: Repeated eyewitness recall leads to reminiscence but not hypermnesia. *Journal of Applied Psychology, 79,* 260–271.

Trope, Y. (1986). Identification and inferential processes in dispositional attribution. *Psychological Review, 93,* 239–257.

Tversky, A., & Kahneman, D. (1973). Availability: A heuristic for judging frequency and probability. *Cognitive Psychology, 4,* 207–232.

Wells, G. L., Ferguson, T. J., & Lindsay, R. C. L. (1981). The tractability of eyewitness confidence and its implications for triers of fact. *Journal of Applied Psychology, 66,* 688–696.

Whittlesea, B. W. A., Jacoby, L. L., & Girard, K. (1990). Illusions of immediate memory: Evidence of an attributional basis of feelings of familiarity and perceptual quality. *Journal of Memory and Language, 29,* 716–732.

Wright, G., & Ayton, P. (Eds.). (1994). *Subjective probability.* Chichester, England: Wiley.

Zajonc, R. B. (1980). Feeling and thinking: Preferences need no inferences. *American Psychologist, 35,* 151–175.

Zajonc, R. B. (1994). Evidence for nonconscious emotions. In P. Ekman & R. J. Davidson (Eds.), *The nature of emotion: Fundamental questions* (pp. 293–297). New York: Oxford University Press.

Zechmeister, E. B., & Shaughnessy, J. J. (1980). When you know that you know and when you think that you know but you don't. *Bulletin of the Psychonomic Society, 15,* 41–44.

25

Promotion and Prevention as a Motivational Duality

IMPLICATIONS FOR EVALUATIVE PROCESSES

E. TORY HIGGINS

Following their love for "cognitive-consistency" models in the 1950s and 1960s (see Abelson et al., 1968), social psychologists fell in love with "dual-process" models in the 1980s and 1990s. Although any love can have its blind spots, it also inspires imagination and great works. This has been true of both cognitive-consistency and dual-process models. These two types of models are alike in other ways as well. Both types are concerned with the interface of motivation and cognition. More important, both are concerned specifically with the motivational significance of cognitive properties.

Consistency models, such as balance theory (Heider, 1958) and cognitive-dissonance theory (Festinger, 1957), typically distinguish between two cognitive states in which cognitive elements have different relations to one another. The state with the greater motivational significance is the one involving cognitively inconsistent relations. In Festinger's (1957) cognitive-dissonance theory, for example, the relation between two cognitive elements, X and Y, constitutes an inconsistent or dissonant state when not-X follows from Y. In Heider's (1958) balance theory, the interrelations involving two or three

cognitive elements constitute an inconsistent state or state of imbalance when multiplying across all the positive or negative signs of the relations yields a negative product. Consistency models propose that there is a strong motivation to change one or more cognitive elements when the state of their interrelations is inconsistent.

One might characterize such consistency models as "dual-state" models. To do so highlights an important similarity (as well as a difference) between these earlier models and current "dual-process" models. Both kinds of models are concerned with the motivational significance of a distinction between two cognitive properties. The two cognitive properties are interrelational states in cognitive-consistency models and information-processing modes in dual-process models.

Dual-process models distinguish between two types of information processing, one of which is relatively more effortful and extensive than the other. Several of the most influential dual-process models are concerned with the implications of this processing difference for evaluative processes. Two early and now classic dual-process models concerned with evaluative processes are Petty and Cacioppo's elaboration likelihood model (see Petty & Cacioppo, 1981, 1986; see also Petty & Wegener, Chapter 3, this volume) and Chaiken's heuristic–systematic model (see Chaiken, 1980, 1987, and Chaiken, Liberman, & Eagly, 1989; see also Chen & Chaiken, Chapter 4, this volume). These models consider how different kinds of information processing influence attitudinal reactions to a persuasive message. Both models distinguish between less and more effortful and extensive processing of messages, which relate to less and more scrutiny (and impact) of the quality of the message arguments, respectively.

Fiske's model of category-based versus piecemeal-based evaluations (see Fiske & Neuberg, 1990; Fiske & Pavelchak, 1986; see also Fiske, Lin, & Neuberg, Chapter 11, this volume) and Fazio's MODE model of how attitudinal evaluations guide behavior (see Fazio, 1990; see also Fazio & Towles-Schwen, Chapter 5, this volume) also distinguish between less and more effortful and extensive processing of information. Fiske's model distinguishes between impressions formed relatively easily on the basis of a target person's category membership and its associated evaluation on the one hand, and impressions formed more effortfully and extensively by integrating evaluations of the target's individual attributes on the other (cf. Brewer & Harasty, Chapter 12, this volume). Similarly, Fazio's model distinguishes between behaviors guided relatively easily on the basis of a highly accessible association between an attitude object category and its evaluation on the one hand, and behaviors guided more effortfully and extensively by integrating likelihoods and evaluations of the behavioral outcomes related to the attitude object on the other.

Whether the evaluative reaction concerns message persuasion, impression formation, or the guiding of behaviors, these and other dual-process models of evaluative reactions all distinguish between relatively more and relatively less effortful and extensive processing of information. Although the duality in each case has motivational significance, the duality itself concerns cognitive-processing properties. The role of motivation as an independent variable in these models is to influence the likelihood of the alternative types of processing, where higher accuracy motivation is said to increase the likelihood that the more

effortful and extensive processing will occur (see, e.g., Chaiken et al., 1989; Fazio, 1990; Fiske & Neuberg, 1990; Petty & Cacioppo, 1986; see also Brewer & Harasty, Chapter 12, this volume; Chen & Chaiken, Chapter 4, this volume; Fazio & Towles-Schwen, Chapter 5, this volume; Fiske et al., Chapter 11, this volume; Petty & Wegener, Chapter 3, this volume).

It is notable that, as in earlier cognitive-consistency models, a *cognitive* duality once again is proposed as underlying evaluative reactions when evaluative reactions might, if anything, be considered more a motivational than a cognitive variable. After all, approach and avoidance underlie evaluation, and movement is the core meaning of motivation. I am not claiming that evaluative reactions are motivational rather than cognitive responses; clearly, they are both (Sorrentino & Higgins, 1986). But given this, it should be useful to consider evaluative reactions in terms of motivational distinctions as well. This is the purpose of the present chapter.

The chapter begins by introducing "regulatory focus" as a distinct motivational principle. Regulatory focus constitutes a motivational duality concerning two types of self-regulation: self-regulation with a "promotion focus" and self-regulation with a "prevention focus." Evidence is then presented to show how regulatory focus, both as an individual-difference variable and as a situational variable, influences people's affective reactions to events. Next, the impact of regulatory focus on the processes underlying evaluative judgments and decisions is discussed. The chapter ends with a discussion of some implications of promotion and prevention for understanding the evaluative processes underlying attitudes and impressions, as well as the effects of these processes on interpersonal relationships, attitude–behavior relations, and persuasion.

THE MOTIVATIONAL DUALITY OF PROMOTION AND PREVENTION

The hedonic principle that people approach pleasure and avoid pain underlies motivational models across all levels of analysis in psychology, from the biological to the social. Biological models have distinguished between the appetitive system, involving approach, and the defensive or aversive system, involving avoidance (e.g., Gray, 1982; Konorski, 1967; Lang, 1995); social/personality models have distinguished between the motive to move toward desired end states and the motive to move away from undesired end states (e.g., Atkinson, 1964; Bandura, 1986; Cacioppo & Berntson, 1994; Carver & Scheier, 1981, 1990; Lewin, 1935, 1951; McClelland, Atkinson, Clark, & Lowell, 1953; Roseman, 1984; Roseman, Spindel, & Jose, 1990). Certainly people are motivated to approach pleasure and avoid pain. But is the hedonic principle sufficient for an understanding of the approach and avoidance tendencies that are so central to conceptualizations of evaluative reactions?

The perspective taken in this chapter is analogous to that taken by the influential dual-process models described earlier. A basic motivation underlying communication and persuasion, for example, is the desire for accuracy and truth. People prefer to hold accurate rather than inaccurate opinions, and this influences the impact of persuasive messages on them. But recent dual-process models have shown that it is not enough to know that an accuracy motive underlies people's processing of persuasive messages. It is also critical to know *how* the information is processed—whether it is processed systematically or heuristically (e.g., Chaiken, 1987), or centrally or peripherally (see Petty & Cacioppo, 1986). As another example, a basic motivation underlying impression formation is the need for evaluation. People want to determine whether some other person is good or bad. But once again, it is not enough to know that an evaluation motive underlies people's processing of information about a target person. It is also critical to know *how* the information is processed—whether the processing is piecemeal-based or category-based (see Fiske & Pavelchak, 1986).

I believe that it is also not enough to know that people approach pleasure and avoid pain. It is critical to know *how* people deal with their world to make this happen. The concept of regulatory focus concerns two basic ways of regulating pleasure and pain: one with a promotion focus and the other with a prevention focus. These different ways of regulating pleasure and pain have a major impact on people's feelings, thoughts, and actions that is independent of the hedonic principle per se (see Higgins, 1997, 1998). Indeed, there is evidence suggesting that regulatory focus might influence strategic motivation as much as the hedonic principle itself (see Crowe & Higgins, 1997). The present chapter is concerned with regulatory-focus effects on evaluative processes. Before I discuss these specific effects, however, I describe the nature of regulatory focus as a general motivational principle.

In distinguishing regulatory focus from the hedonic principle, it is especially important to distinguish regulatory focus from regulatory reference. Inspired by earlier work on cybernetics and control processes (e.g., Miller, Galanter, & Pribram, 1960; Powers, 1973; Wiener, 1948), Carver and Scheier (1981, 1990) distinguish between self-regulatory systems that have positive and negative reference values. A self-regulatory system with a positive reference value has a desired end state as the reference point. The system is discrepancy-reducing and involves attempts to move one's own (represented) current state as close as possible to the desired end state. In contrast, a self-regulatory system with a negative reference value has an undesired end state as the reference point. This system is discrepancy-amplifying and involves attempts to move one's own current state as far away as possible from the undesired end state.

It should be noted that Carver and Scheier (1981, 1990) suggest that self-regulation with a negative reference value is inherently unstable and relatively rare. Their research therefore emphasized self-regulation with a positive reference value. Positive reference values were also emphasized in Miller et al.'s (1960) famous TOTE model, which involved the execution of operations to reduce existing incongruities or discrepancies to positive reference values. Because most theories and research concern movement toward goals, which are positive reference values, this emphasis is evident throughout the self-regulatory literature (see, e.g., Gollwitzer & Bargh, 1996; Pervin, 1989).

Another reason why self-regulation with a negative reference value has received less attention is that several models describe it in terms of behavioral inhibition rather than behavioral production (e.g., Atkinson, 1964;

Gray, 1982). That is, these models propose that self-regulation in relation to desired end states will be reflected in taking action, whereas self-regulation in relation to undesired end states will be reflected in behavioral suppression. Thus, if one is interested in why people act the way they do, positive reference values will naturally be emphasized. In the classic learning literature as well, behavioral production associated with positive end states received greater emphasis than behavioral suppression associated with negative end states (e.g., Estes, 1944; Skinner, 1953; Thorndike, 1935).

This chapter also emphasizes movement toward positive reference values or desired end states. According to the literature, the critical characteristic of such movement is its overall direction—approach. Consistent with the basic hedonic principle, animal learning/biological models (e.g., Gray, 1982; Hull, 1952; Konorski, 1967; Lang, 1995; Miller, 1944; Mowrer, 1960), cybernetic-control models (e.g., Carver & Scheier, 1990; Powers, 1973), and dynamic models (e.g., Atkinson, 1964; Lewin, 1935; McClelland et al., 1953) all highlight the basic distinction between approaching desired end states and avoiding undesired end states. No distinction is made, however, between different means for approaching the desired end states or between different types of desired end states that might be associated with different means of approach. As one example, Gray (1982) explicitly treats approaching "reward" and "nonpunishment" as equivalent. Regulatory focus, in contrast, distinguishes between types of approaching desired end states (as well as between types of avoiding undesired end states).

If the hedonic principle of approaching pleasure and avoiding pain is truly basic to motivation, one would expect that this principle would operate in more than one way. In particular, one would expect that the principle would operate differently when it serves fundamentally different needs, such as the distinct survival needs of nurturance and security. Human survival requires adaptation to the surrounding environment, especially the social environment (see Buss, 1996). To obtain the nurturance and security they need to survive, children must establish and maintain relationships with caretakers who fulfill these needs by supporting and encouraging them

and by protecting and defending them (see Bowlby, 1969, 1973).

Sometimes caretakers respond to children in ways that are pleasurable to the children, and at other times they respond in ways that are painful to the children. As the hedonic principle suggests, children must learn how to behave in order to approach pleasure and avoid pain. They must learn how their behaviors influence caretakers' responses to them as objects in the world (see Bowlby, 1969; Cooley, 1902/1964; Mead, 1934; Sullivan, 1953). But what is learned about regulating pleasure and pain can be different for nurturance and security needs. I propose that nurturance-related regulation and security-related regulation differ in regulatory focus: Nurturance-related regulation involves a promotion focus, whereas security-related regulation involves a prevention focus.

Earlier publications on self-discrepancy theory have described how certain modes of caretaker–child interaction increase the likelihood that children will acquire strong desired end states (e.g., Higgins, 1987, 1989a). These desired end states represent either their own or significant others' hopes, wishes, and aspirations for them (strong "ideals") or their own or significant others' beliefs about their duties, obligations, and responsibilities (strong "oughts"). Regulatory-focus theory proposes that self-regulation in relation to strong ideals versus strong oughts differs in regulatory focus: Ideal self-regulation involves a promotion focus, whereas ought self-regulation involves a prevention focus. To illustrate the difference between these two types of regulatory focus, let us briefly consider how children's experiences of pleasure and pain and what they learn about self-regulation vary when their interactions with caretakers involve a promotion versus a prevention focus (see also Higgins & Loeb, in press).

Consider first caretaker–child interactions that involve a promotion focus. A child experiences the pleasure of the presence of positive outcomes when caretakers, for example, hug and kiss the child for behaving in a desired manner, encourage the child to overcome difficulties, or set up opportunities for the child to engage in rewarding activities. A child experiences the pain of the absence of positive outcomes when caretakers, for example, end a meal when the child throws food, take away a toy when the child refuses to share it, stop a story when the child is not paying attention, or act disappointed when the child fails to fulfill their hopes for them. The pleasure and pain resulting from these interactions are experienced as the presence and absence of positive outcomes, respectively. The caretaker's message to the child in both cases is that what matters is attaining accomplishments or fulfilling hopes and aspirations, but it is communicated in reference to a state of the child that does or does not attain the desired end state—either "This is what I would *ideally* like you to do" or "This is not what I would *ideally* like you to do." The regulatory focus is one of promotion—a concern with advancement, growth, and accomplishment.

Consider next caretaker–child interactions that involve a prevention focus. The child experiences the pleasure of the absence of negative outcomes when caretakers, for example, "child-proof" the house, train the child to behave safely, or teach the child to "mind your manners." The child experiences the pain of the presence of negative outcomes when caretakers, for example, behave roughly with the child to get his or her attention, yell at the child when he or she doesn't listen, criticize the child when he or she makes a mistake, or punish the child for being irresponsible. The pleasure and pain resulting from these interactions are experienced as the absence and presence of negative outcomes, respectively. The caretaker's message to the child in both cases is that what matters is ensuring safety, being responsible, or meeting obligations, but it is communicated in reference to a state of the child that does or does not attain the desired end state— either "This is what I believe you *ought* to do" or "This is not what I believe you *ought* to do." The regulatory focus is one of prevention—a concern with protection, safety, and responsibility.

These socialization differences illustrate how children learn in interacting with caretakers as significant others to regulate themselves in relation to a promotion focus (ideals) or a prevention focus (oughts) (see Higgins & Loeb, in press). Significant others in later phases of life can be friends, spouses, teachers, coworkers, or employers rather than care-

takers. Momentary situations are also capable of temporarily inducing either a promotion focus or a prevention focus. Just as the responses of caretakers to their children's actions communicate information to the children about how to attain desired end states, feedback from a boss to an employee or from a teacher to a student is a situation that can communicate gain–nongain information (promotion-related outcomes) or nonloss–loss information (prevention-related outcomes). Task instructions that present task contingency or "if–then" rules concerning which actions produce which consequences can also communicate either gain–nongain (promotion) or nonloss–loss (prevention) information. Thus the concept of regulatory focus is broader than just socialization of strong ideals (promotion focus) or oughts (prevention focus). Regulatory focus can also be induced temporarily in momentary situations.

People are motivated to approach desired end states, which can be either aspirations and accomplishments (promotion focus) or responsibilities and safety (prevention focus). But within this general approach toward desired end states, regulatory focus can induce either approach or avoidance strategic inclinations. Because a promotion focus involves a sensitivity to positive outcomes (their presence and absence), an inclination to approach matches to desired end states is the natural strategy for promotion self-regulation. In contrast, because a prevention focus involves a sensitivity to negative outcomes (their absence and presence), an inclination to avoid mismatches to desired end states is the natural strategy for prevention self-regulation (see Higgins, Roney, Crowe, & Hymes, 1994).

Figure 25.1 summarizes the different sets of psychological variables discussed thus far that have distinct relations to promotion focus and prevention focus (as well as some variables to be discussed later). On the input side (left side of Figure 25.1), nurturance needs, strong ideals, and situations involving gain–nongain induce a promotion focus, whereas security needs, strong oughts, and situations involving nonloss–loss induce a prevention focus. On the output side (right side of Figure 25.1), a promotion focus yields sensitivity to the presence or absence of positive outcomes and approach as strate-

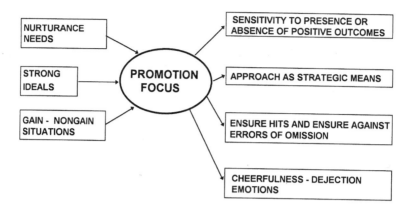

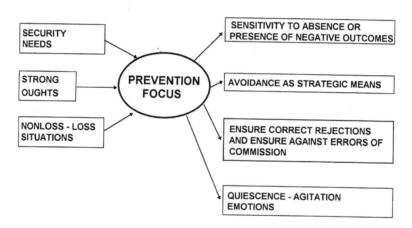

FIGURE 25.1. Psychological variables with distinct relations to promotion focus and prevention focus.

gic means, whereas a prevention focus yields sensitivity to the absence or presence of negative outcomes and avoidance as strategic means.

Regulatory focus distinguishes between two different kinds of desired end states: (1) aspirations and accomplishments, and (2) responsibilities and safety. People are motivated to approach both kinds of desired end states, but regulatory-focus theory proposes that the pleasurable experience of approach working or the painful experience of approach not working will be different for these two kinds of desired end states. The next section reviews evidence that because of this difference, people have distinct affective reactions to events in their lives.

REGULATORY FOCUS AND AFFECTIVE REACTIONS

Ideal self-regulation involves a promotion focus, whereas ought self-regulation involves a prevention focus. Self-discrepancy theory (Higgins, 1987, 1989a) was developed specifically to consider how affective reactions to discrepancies between ideals and oughts may be different. Let us now briefly review the predictions of this theory.

Self-Discrepancies, Regulatory Focus, and Affective Reactions

The distinction between ideal and ought self-regulation in self-discrepancy theory was initially described in terms of differences in the psychological situations represented by discrepancies and congruencies involving ideal versus ought self-guides (see Higgins, 1989a, 1989b). Actual self-congruencies to hopes, wishes, or aspirations represent the presence of positive outcomes, whereas discrepancies represent the absence of positive outcomes. Thus the psychological situations involved in ideal self-regulation are the presence and absence of positive outcomes.

Whereas the hopes, wishes, and aspirations represented in ideal self-guides function like maximal goals, the duties, obligations, and responsibilities represented in ought self-guides function more like minimal goals that a person must attain (see Brendl & Higgins, 1996). Discrepancies to such minimal goals represent the presence of negative outcomes, whereas congruencies represent the absence of negative outcomes (see Gould, 1939; Rotter, 1982). Thus, the psychological situations involved in ought self-regulation are the absence and presence of negative outcomes.

Attaining a goal with a promotion focus reflects the presence of positive outcomes underlying cheerfulness-related emotions (e.g., feeling happy or satisfied), whereas not attaining a goal with a promotion focus reflects the absence of positive outcomes underlying dejection-related emotions (e.g., feeling disappointed or discouraged). In contrast, attaining a goal with a prevention focus reflects the absence of negative outcomes underlying quiescence-related emotions (e.g., feeling calm or relaxed), whereas not attaining a goal with a prevention focus reflects the presence of negative outcomes underlying agitation-related emotions (e.g., feeling tense or uneasy) (see Figure 25.1).

My colleagues and I have conducted several studies to test whether self-regulation in relation to ideals versus oughts as desired end states produces such distinct affective reactions. Both studies relating chronic discrepancies to chronic affective reactions and studies relating momentary activation of discrepancies to momentary affective reactions have been conducted. In addition, we have investigated whether affective reactions from self-regulation in relation to ideals and oughts vary, depending on the strength of individuals' promotion and prevention focus. Finally, we have also examined how situational manipulations of regulatory focus, independent of self-discrepancies, influence affective reactions. Elsewhere (Higgins, Grant, & Shah, in press), we provide an extensive review of this research program and its implications for understanding emotional experiences. The present chapter reviews only some illustrative studies that are particularly relevant to the issue of evaluative reactions. The effects of regulatory focus as an individual-difference variable on affective reactions to chronic goal attainment are considered first.

Affective Reactions and Regulatory Focus as an Individual-Difference Variable

Participants in our studies typically fill out a Selves Questionnaire, which is included in a general battery of measures handed out 6–8 weeks before the dependent measures are collected. The Selves Questionnaire asks respondents to list up to 8–10 attributes for each of a number of different self-states. It is administered in two sections, the first involving the respondent's own standpoint and the second involving the standpoints of the respondent's significant others (e.g., mother, father, best friend). The magnitude of self-discrepancy between any two self-states is calculated by summing the total number of mismatches and subtracting the total number of matches.

In an early study (Higgins, Bond, Klein, & Strauman, 1986, Study 1) that examined affective reactions to imagined events, undergraduate participants filled out the Selves Questionnaire several weeks before the experimental session. Individuals varying in their magnitudes of actual–ideal and actual–ought discrepancies were selected for the study. It was predicted that when the participants imagined a negative event happening to them, both the quality and the intensity of their affective reactions would vary, depending on the type and magnitude of their self-discrepancies.

When they arrived for the experiment, participants in one condition were asked to imagine a negative event happening to them (e.g., receiving a grade of D in a course that was necessary for obtaining an important job, or being turned down for a date by another student). Participants' dejection-related affect (e.g., feeling discouraged) and agitation-related affect (e.g., feeling tense) were measured both before and after their imagining of the negative event. Our analysis of the relation between each type of self-discrepancy (as measured weeks before) and each type of postimagining affect statistically controlled for the alternative type of self-discrepancy, the alternative type of affect, and affect at the beginning of the session prior to imagining the negative event. This analysis revealed the unique relations between the magnitude of each type of self-discrepancy and the intensity of each type of affective reaction to imagining a negative event. The study found that as predicted, both the intensity *and* the quality of participants' affective reactions to imagining a negative event varied, depending on the magnitude and type of self-discrepancy they possessed. Individuals with greater actual–ideal discrepancies had stronger dejection-related affective reactions to failing to attain academic or social goals, whereas individuals with greater actual–ought discrepancies had stronger agitation-related reactions.

The psychological literature has suggested that goal strength conceptualized as goal accessibility (e.g., Clore, 1994) may moderate the relation between goal attainment and affective reactions (see Clore, 1994; Frijda, 1996; Frijda, Ortony, Sonnemans, & Clore, 1992). Although there has been little direct support for this hypothesis, evidence that attitude accessibility moderates the relation between attitudes and behavior (Fazio, 1986, 1995) prompted us (Higgins, Shah, & Friedman, 1997) to test the possibility that strength of regulatory focus may moderate the relation between chronic goal attainment and affective reactions. As discussed earlier, ideal goals involve a promotion focus, and ought goals involve a prevention focus. Thus strength of promotion focus increases as strength of ideal goals increases, and strength of prevention focus increases as strength of ought goals increases. Consistent with previous work on attitude accessibility (see Bassili, 1995, 1996; Fazio, 1986, 1995), the strength of ideals and oughts was conceptualized and operationalized in terms of their accessibility, and accessibility was measured via individuals' response times to inquiries about their ideal and ought attributes.

Accessibility is activation potential, and knowledge units with higher activation potentials should produce faster responses to

knowledge-related inputs (see Higgins, 1996). A computer measure of actual, ideal, and ought attributes was developed that was similar to the original Selves Questionnaire. Ideal and ought strength was measured by response latencies in listing ideal and ought attributes and giving extent ratings. Actual–ideal and actual–ought discrepancies were measured by comparing the extent rating of each ideal or ought attribute, respectively, with the extent rating of the actual self for that attribute (see Higgins, Shah, & Friedman, 1997).

We hypothesized the following relations among participants' ideal and ought strength, ideal and ought discrepancies, and type of affective reaction: (1) an interaction of ideal strength and actual–ideal discrepancy, such that the correlation between actual–ideal discrepancy and feeling dejected (or actual–ideal congruency and feeling cheerful) would increase as the accessibility of ideals increased; and (2) an interaction of ought strength and actual–ought discrepancy, such that the correlation between actual–ought discrepancy and feeling agitated (or actual/ought congruency and feeling quiescent) would increase as the accessibility of oughts increased. It should be noted that these predictions presume that strength of ideals and oughts as measured by accessibility is relatively independent of magnitude of discrepancies (or congruencies) to ideal and oughts as measured by actual self mismatches and matches. Indeed, we (Higgins, Shah, & Friedman, 1997) found in each study that these two measures were uncorrelated.

We conducted three correlational studies. Two studies with undergraduate participants tested the relation between self-discrepancies (or congruencies) and the frequency of different kinds of affective reactions during the previous week. A third study with undergraduate participants tested the relation between self-discrepancies (or congruencies) and the intensity of different kinds of affective reactions before beginning a performance task. All three studies supported the predictions.

These studies support the proposal that strength of regulatory focus, as a motivational variable independent of magnitude of self-discrepancy, moderates the relation between chronic goal attainment and affective reactions. More generally, they demonstrate how self-regulation in relation to ideals and oughts as desired end states produces distinct affective reactions. Ideal self-regulation involves a promotion focus; the stronger this focus is, the stronger are the cheerfulness-related affective reactions when promotion is working, and the stronger are the dejection-related affective reactions when promotion is not working. In contrast, ought self-regulation involves a prevention focus; the stronger this focus is, the stronger are the quiescence-related affective reactions when prevention is working, and the stronger are the agitation-related affective reactions when prevention is not working.

The studies just described (Higgins, Shah, & Friedman, 1997) demonstrate that stronger promotion or prevention focus as an individual-difference variable influences the relation between chronic goal attainment and affective reactions. The relation between regulatory focus and affective reactions for momentary goal attainments and situationally induced focus is considered next.

Affective Reactions and Regulatory Focus as a Situational Variable

I have described earlier how prolonged caretaker–child interactions that occur over long periods can communicate information to the child about his or her contingencies in the world. The different messages can engender ideal self-regulation involving a promotion focus concerned with advancement, growth, and accomplishment, or ought self-regulation involving a prevention focus concerned with protection, safety, and responsibility. But regulatory focus is not limited to such chronic individual differences. After all, momentary situations are also capable of temporarily inducing either a promotion focus or a prevention focus. Just as the responses of caretakers to their children's actions provide feedback to the children about how to attain desired (rather than undesired) end states, feedback from another person can communicate to someone how he or she can attain desired end states in the current situation. And feedback is not the only situational variable that is capable of inducing different types of regulatory focus. Again as in caretaker–child interactions, it is possible to induce a regulatory focus with instructions that present a task contingency concerning which actions

produce which consequences (i.e., contingency information about how to attain desired end states).

We (Higgins, Shah, & Friedman, 1997) hypothesized that effects of regulatory focus on affective reactions similar to those found for chronic regulatory focus and chronic goal attainment would also be found for momentary goal attainments and situationally induced regulatory focus. We used a framing technique to manipulate regulatory focus in a manner that kept constant both the actual consequences of attaining or not attaining the goal and the criterion of success and failure. Only the regulatory focus of the instructions varied.

The task involved memorizing trigrams. For the promotion focus, the participants began with $5, and the instructions were about gains and nongains: "If you score above the 70th percentile—that is, if you remember a lot of letter strings—then you will gain a dollar. However, if you don't score above the 70th percentile—that is, if you don't remember a lot of letter strings—then you will not gain a dollar." For the prevention focus, the participants began with $6, and the instructions were about losses and nonlosses: "If you score above the 70th percentile—that is, if you don't forget a lot of letter strings—then you won't lose a dollar. However, if you don't score above the the 70th percentile—that is, if you do forget a lot of letter strings—then you will lose a dollar." Following performance of the task, the participants were given false feedback that they had either succeeded or failed on the task.

It was predicted that feedback-consistent affective reactions (i.e., increasing positive and decreasing negative emotions following success, and decreasing positive and increasing negative emotions following failure) would be different in the promotion-framing versus prevention-framing conditions. Specifically, we predicted that feedback-consistent change on the cheerfulness–dejection dimension would be greater for participants in the promotion-framing than in the prevention-framing condition, whereas feedback-consistent change on the quiescence–agitation dimension would be greater for participants in the prevention-framing than in the promotion-framing condition. The results of the study supported both predictions.

Roney, Higgins, and Shah (1995) also found evidence that situational variability in regulatory focus can influence affective reactions. Undergraduate participants in the first study were told that they would perform two tasks. For everyone, the first task was an anagrams task that included both easy anagrams pretested to be solvable by everyone and unsolvable anagrams. The number of easy anagrams included in the task ensured that the participants would ultimately succeed in attaining the assigned goal. All of the participants were told that the second task would be either a computer simulation of the popular *Wheel of Fortune* game show or a task called "unvaried repetition" and described so as to appear very boring.

Although the performance contingency for playing the fun game rather than the boring game as the second task was the same for everyone, the framing of the contingency was experimentally varied. Half of the participants were given a promotion focus, in which they were told that if they solved 22 (or more) of the 25 anagrams, they would get to play the *Wheel of Fortune* game; otherwise, they would do the "unvaried repetition" task. The other half of the participants were given a prevention focus, in which they were told that if they got 4 (or more) of the 25 anagrams wrong, they would do the "unvaried repetition" task; otherwise, they would play the *Wheel of Fortune* game. As mentioned earlier, all participants succeeded on the task. The study found that participants with a promotion focus felt more cheerful than participants with a prevention focus after attaining the goal, whereas the latter felt more quiescent.

Undergraduate participants in the second study worked on a set of anagrams that included both solvable anagrams and unsolvable anagrams. Success or failure feedback was given on each trial. Half of the participants received feedback with a promotion focus, such as "Right, you got that one" when they solved an anagram, or "You didn't get that one right" when they did not solve an anagram. The other half of the participants received feedback with a prevention focus, such as "You didn't miss that one" when they solved an anagram, and "No, you missed that one" when they did not solve an angram. The number of unsolvable anagrams included in the task ensured that all participants ultimately failed to attain the assigned goal. The study found that participants with a promotion focus felt more dejected than participants with a prevention focus after failing to achieve the goal, whereas the latter felt more agitated.

Taken together, the studies reviewed in this section clearly indicate that regulatory focus influences how people react affectively to success or failure at attaining their goals. The next section reviews some studies that demonstrate how regulatory focus can also influence evaluative judgments and decisions.

REGULATORY FOCUS AND EVALUATIVE JUDGMENTS AND DECISIONS

The studies reviewed in the preceding section examined people's affective reactions to events in their lives. An interesting question is this: How do observers evaluate another person's affective reaction to an event in his or her life? This question was addressed by Houston (1990) as part of reconsidering the nature of empathy. Undergraduate participants were selected who were high or low in actual–ideal discrepancy and high or low in actual–ought discrepancy. During the experimental session, these participants read a transcript of an interview with a target person who described a recent specific incident when his or her shyness caused him or her distress. The target person either described his or her goal in terms of something he or she hoped or wanted to be and behaved in a dejected manner, or described his or her goal in terms of something he or she ought to be and behaved in an agitated manner.

Houston (1990) found that participants' own dejected reactions to the target experiencing dejection were greater for those possessing high actual–ideal discrepancies than for those with high actual–ought discrepancies, whereas participants' own agitated reactions to the target experiencing agitation were greater for those possessing high actual–ought discrepancies than for those with high actual–ideal discrepancies. The participants also evaluated the appropriateness of the target's emotional reaction to his or her situation. For the dejected target, predominantly ideal-discrepant participants (i.e., high ideal discrepancy and low ought discrepancy) evaluated the target's reaction as more appropriate than did predominantly ought-discrepant participants (i.e., high ought discrepancy and low ideal discrepancy). For the agitated target on the other hand, predominantly ought-discrepant participants evaluated the target's reaction as more appropriate than did predominantly ideal-discrepant participants. Thus evaluative judgments of the appropriateness of another person's affective reaction depend on the relation between the regulatory focus of observer and target, with matches yielding evaluations of greater appropriateness than mismatches.

The results of this study and those in the preceding section demonstrate that regulatory focus influences the kinds of evaluative reactions people have to target objects. But does regulatory focus only influence which kinds of positive or negative evaluative reactions will occur? Might not regulatory focus also influence evaluative efficiency? This possibility is considered next.

Regulatory Focus and Evaluative Efficiency

The kinds of emotional dimensions that are significant for people's evaluative responses to themselves and other attitude objects vary as a function of regulatory focus. The cheerfulness–dejection dimension is especially significant for promotion self-regulation, whereas the quiescence–agitation dimension is especially significant for prevention self-regulation. The significance of a particular emotional dimension for evaluation is independent of the extent to which pleasant versus painful emotions have been experienced. Consider two persons who both have a strong promotion focus. They may differ in their history of successes or failures, with one having primarily successes and cheerfulness-related experiences, and the other having primarily failures and dejection-related experiences. Although their specific emotional experiences differ, for *both* of these persons the emotional significance of their performance involves the cheerfulness–dejection dimension. Their concern when they are evaluating themselves is with the cheerfulness–dejection significance of their personal qualities. Similarly, when they are evaluating another attitude object, their concern is with the cheerfulness–dejection significance of that object (e.g., "How happy or sad does this object make me?"). In contrast, persons with a strong prevention focus are concerned with the quiescence–agitation significance of their personal qualities or the qualities of some other attitude object.

If one considers a dimension like cheerfulness–dejection as a bipolar construct, then this dimension is one way to construe the world of objects and events (see Kelly, 1955). Indeed, Kelly (1955) pointed out that similarity and contrast are inherent in the same construct. A cheerful response is similar to other cheerful responses and contrasts with dejected responses, and a dejected response is similar to other dejected responses and contrasts with cheerful responses. Thus, when objects and events are evaluated in terms of their cheerfulness–dejection significance, both cheerfulness and dejection are relevant to the construal even when the emotional experience is just feeling cheerful or just feeling dejected. Because of this, the cheerfulness–dejection dimension can have special significance for two different persons with a strong promotion focus, despite their having different histories of feeling cheerful or dejected. Similarly, the quiescence–agitation dimension of appraisal can have special significance for two different persons with a strong prevention focus, despite their having different histories of feeling quiescent or agitated.

Kelly (1955) also proposed that the ways of construing the world that are significant for a person increase that person's efficiency in evaluating objects and events in relation to the construct. Similarly, we (Shah, Higgins, Idson, & Liberman, 1998) proposed that the more a particular emotional dimension was significant for a participant in our research, the more efficient that person would be in evaluating objects or events along that dimension. Such efficiency would be revealed in faster reaction times when the participant was reporting emotional experiences along that dimension. The specific predictions were these: (1) As ideal strength increased (i.e., stronger promotion focus), emotional evaluations related to both cheerfulness and dejection would be faster; and (2) as ought strength increased (i.e., stronger prevention focus), emotional evaluations related to both quiescence and agitation would be faster.

Because strength of regulatory focus also influences the frequency and intensity of experiencing different kinds of emotions, as discussed earlier, it was important in testing these predictions to control for the magnitude of different individuals' experience with each emotion. Otherwise, for example, relatively fast reaction times of strong-promotion-focus participants reporting dejection evaluations could occur because the dejection experiences of these individuals were stronger, rather than because these individuals were more concerned with the cheerfulness–dejection dimension of evaluation. In all of our studies, therefore, the analyses of reaction times statistically controlled for participants' extent ratings of each emotional experience (Shah, Higgins, Idson, & Liberman, 1998).

The predictions above were tested in a series of studies (Shah, Higgins, Idson, & Liberman, 1998). The participants in every study made emotional appraisals on cheerfulness-related scales, dejection-related scales, quiescence-related scales, and agitation-related scales. Two studies involved participants' reporting on how much they experienced each emotion, either during the last week or currently during an experimental session. Two other studies involved participants' appraising positive or negative objects like those previously used by Fazio, Sanbonmatsu, Powell, and Kardes (1986) and by Bargh, Chaiken, Govender, and Pratto (1992) in studying automatic attitude activation.

All four studies strongly supported the predictions. In one study, for example, undergraduate participants were asked to rate how each word describing a positive object (e.g., "music") or a negative object (e.g., "guns") made them feel. The object words were rated in relation to both the cheerfulness–dejection dimension and the quiescence–agitation dimension. Half of the positive object words were rated in relation to "happy" (or "satisfying") and the other half in relation to "relaxed." Half of the negative object words were rated in relation to "sad" (or "depressing") and the other half in relation to "tense" (or "agitating"). (Across the participants, each object word was rated on each emotional dimension an equal number of times.) The study found that ideal strength was significantly positively related to speed of appraising the object words in relation to the cheerfulness–dejection dimension, and was, if anything, slightly negatively related to speed of appraising these words in relation to the quiescence–agitation dimension. In contrast, ought strength was significantly positively related to speed of appraising the object words in relation to the quiescence–agitation dimension, and was, if anything, slightly negatively related to speed of appraising these words in relation to the cheerfulness–dejection dimension.

This study and the others in this series Shah, Higgins, Idson, & Liberman, 1998) indicate that strength of regulatory focus also influences people's efficiency in emotionally evaluating self and others as attitude objects. Individuals with a strong promotion focus are more efficient in evaluating attitude objects along the cheerfulness–dejection dimension, whereas individuals with a strong prevention focus are more efficieitn in evaluating attitude objects along the quiescence–agitation dimension; this differential efficiency (reflected in speed of responding) is independent of magnitude of evaluation (reflected in the extent ratings). The results of these studies suggest not only that positive and negative evaluative processes are separable (see Cacioppo & Berntson, 1994), but that promotion and prevention evaluative processes are separable as well. That is, efficiency in evaluating attitude objects along the quiescence–agitation dimension is independent of efficiency in evaluating them along the cheerfulness–dejection dimension.

The studies reviewed thus far all involved affective or evaluative judgments of target objects, whether the object was self, another person, or a nonsocial object. But evaluative processes are not restricted to such judgments. Indeed, psychologists and other social scientists have been especially interested in the evaluative processes that underlie people's decisions and choices. The relation of regulatory focus to decision making is considered next.

Regulatory Focus and Decision Making

Historically, the most influential models regarding the evaluative processes underlying people's decisions and choices have been expectancy–value models. A basic assumption of expectancy–value models of motivation has been that both expectancy and value have an impact on goal commitment, and that in addition to their main effects, they combine multiplicatively (Lewin, Dembo, Festinger, & Sears, 1944; Tolman, 1955; Vroom, 1964; for a review, see Feather, 1982). The multiplicative assumption is that as either expectancy or value increases, the impact of the other variable on commitment increases. For example, it is assumed that the effect on goal commitment of a high versus a low likelihood of attaining the goal is greater when the goal is highly valued than when the goal has little value. This assumption reflects the notion that the goal commitment involves a motivation to maximize the product of value and expectancy.

Not all studies, however, have found the predicted positive interactive effect of value and expectancy. We (Shah & Higgins, 1997) proposed that the inconsistencies in the literature might be due to differences in the regulatory focus of decision makers. We suggested that making a decision with a promotion focus might be more likely to involve the motivation to maximize the product of value and expectancy. A promotion focus on goals as accomplishments might induce a strategic inclination to "approach matches"—that is, to pursue highly valued goals with the highest expected utility, which would maximize value × expectancy. Thus, we predicted that the positive interactive effect of value and expectancy assumed by classic expectancy–value models would increase as strength of promotion focus increased.

But what about a prevention focus? A prevention focus on goals as security or safety might induce a strategic inclination to "avoid mismatches"—that is, to avoid all unnecessary risks by striving to meet only responsibilities that are either clearly necessary (i.e., high value prevention goals) *or* safely attainable (i.e., high expectancy of attainment). This strategic inclination would create a different interactive relation between value and expectancy. As the value of a prevention goal increases, the goal becomes a necessity, like the Ten Commandments or the safety of one's child. When a goal becomes a necessity, one *must* do whatever one can to attain it, regardless of the ease or likelihood of goal attainment. That is, expectancy information becomes less relevant as a prevention goal becomes more like a necessity. Thus, we (Shah

& Higgins, 1997) predicted that as strength of prevention focus increased, the interactive effect of value and expectancy would become *negative*.

Strength of promotion focus and prevention focus were again measured in terms of the strength of participants' ideals and oughts, respectively. Ideal strength and ought strength were measured by response latencies in listing ideal and ought attributes and giving extent ratings. Using this new measure of promotion and prevention strength to study both performance and decision making, we (Shah & Higgins, 1997) tested the predictions (1) that as strength of promotion focus increased, the positive interactive effect of value and expectancy would increase; and (2) that as strength of prevention focus increased, the interactive effect of value and expectancy would decrease.

The performance study involved solving anagrams. The participants varied in ideal strength and in ought strength. Measures were obtained of their subjective estimate of the value of getting an extra dollar for succeeding at the task and their subjective estimate of the likelihood that they would succeed. Both predictions were confirmed. As participants' ideal strength (i.e., promotion focus) increased, the interactive effect of value and expectancy on performance was more positive. In contrast, as participants' ought strength (i.e., prevention focus) increased, the interactive effect of value and expectancy on performance was more negative.

In work more germane to the present chapter, we (Shah & Higgins, in press) also tested our predictions in three additional studies on making decisions to take a class in one's major or to take an entrance exam for graduate school. One study obtained measures of the participants' subjective estimates of value and expectancy, and the other two studies experimentally manipulated high and low levels of value and expectancy. One study involved comparing individuals who differed chronically in regulatory focus, and the other two studies experimentally manipulated regulatory focus, using a framing procedure that emphasized "approaching matches" for the promotion focus and "avoiding mismatches" for the prevention focus. Together these studies found (as predicted) that the interactive effect of value and expectancy was more positive when promotion focus was stronger, but was more negative when prevention focus was stronger.

As an example, one study asked participants to evaluate the likelihood that they would take a course in their major for which the value of doing well and the expectancy of doing well in the course were experimentally manipulated, and participants' strength of regulatory focus was measured. High versus low value was established in terms of 95% versus 51% of previous majors' being accepted into their honor society when they received a grade of B or higher in the course. High versus low expectancy was established in terms of 75% versus 25% of previous majors' receiving a grade of B or higher in the course. The study found that (as predicted) the contrast representing the expectancy × value effect on the decision to take the course was positive for individuals with a strong promotion focus (i.e., high ideal strength), but was negative for individuals with a strong prevention focus (i.e., high ought strength).

The results of the Shah and Higgins (1997) studies clearly indicate that a strong promotion focus and a strong prevention focus can influence the evaluative processes underlying decision making. Other research (Safer & Higgins, 1998) tested whether regulatory focus also influenced people's preference choices. Participants' strength of promotion focus and strength of prevention focus were measured as in the previous studies. In the experimental session, participants were given information about either two cars or two apartments. For each pair, the participants were asked to form their impressions of each alternative and then to make a choice between the two, without considering the cost of each alternative. The information consisted of attributes that in pretesting had received either high luxury ratings and neutral security/reliability ratings (e.g., plush, soft leather seats and a premium music sound system as car attributes; grand, 12-foot-high ceilings and elegant, intricate wall moldings as apartment attributes) or high security/reliability ratings and neutral luxury ratings (e.g., reliable battery backup for cold days and antilock brakes as car attributes; secure, solid-steel safety locks on the front door and reliable smoke detectors as apartment attributes).

For each pair of products, the overall desirability of the alternatives were equal, but one alternative was described primarily with luxury attributes (the promotion alternative), whereas the other alternative was described primarily with security/reliability attributes (the prevention alternative). The results of the study were the same for the two cars and the two apartments. As the strength of participants' promotion focus increased (i.e., higher ideal strength), the likelihood of choosing the luxurious alternative increased; as the strength of participants' prevention focus increased (i.e., higher ought strength), the likelihood of choosing the secure/reliable alternative increased.

An additional analysis was conducted on participants' ratings of the luxuriousness and the security/reliability of each alternative product. As one would expect, the more the luxurious alternative received a higher luxury rating than the secure/reliable alternative, the more likely it was to be chosen. But this effect was moderated by strength of regulatory focus, such that differences in luxury ratings had significantly more impact on participants with stronger promotion focus (i.e., higher ideal strength). As one would also expect, the more the secure/reliable alternative received a higher security/reliability rating than the luxurious alternative, the more likely it was to be chosen. But again this effect was moderated by strength of regulatory focus, such that differences in security or reliability ratings had significantly more impact on participants with stronger prevention focus (i.e., higher ought strength).

Thus participants' evaluative reactions as reflected in their consumer choices varied as a function of the strength of their promotion or prevention focus and the relevance of different kinds of product information to the concerns of each focus. Information about the luxuriousness of each alternative influenced choices more for individuals with a strong promotion focus, whereas information about security/reliability influenced choices more for individuals with a strong prevention focus. It is notable that the self-system attributes used to measure strength of promotion and prevention focus had no content overlap whatsoever with the information about the alternative products. They were only related at the abstract level of reflecting promotion versus prevention concerns.

An additional part of the Safer and Higgins (1998) study provided further evidence of how regulatory focus can influence evaluative processes underlying decision making. Following their choices between cars and between apartments, the participants were told to imagine that they wanted to purchase a computer (with cost again not an issue). They were provided with a list of 24 questions about a computer, and were asked to read all of them and then select those 10 questions that they believed would be most helpful in making their purchase decision. Which kinds of information would the participants seek out? Of the 24 questions, 8 concerned promotion attributes of the computer (e.g., how advanced it was), 8 were about prevention attributes of the computer (e.g., its ability to prevent system crashes or other problems), and 8 were neutral features (e.g., total weight of the unit). The study found that participants with a stronger promotion focus (i.e., higher ideal strength) were more likely to seek information about the promotion attributes, whereas participants with a stronger prevention focus (i.e., higher ought strength) were more likely to seek information about the prevention attributes.

The results of these studies indicate that strength of regulatory focus influences both which kind of information about alternatives is sought out prior to decision making *and* which kind of given information is used in making a decision. Does regulatory focus also influence the effectiveness of persuasive messages in motivating recipients to take action? Some research examining this final issue is considered next.

Regulatory Focus and the Effectiveness of Persuasive Messages

Much of the research on how framing influences message effectiveness, and especially research on health-related actions (see, e.g., Meyerowitz & Chaiken, 1987; Rothman & Salovey, 1997), has been concerned with whether persuasive messages are more effective when they are positive (i.e., emphasizing benefits or gains) or when they are negative (i.e., emphasizing costs or losses). Our research on the motivational effects of regulatory focus, however, suggests that what might be critical is not message valence or prospect

per se, but the relation between the action advocated in the message and the regulatory focus of the message. Specifically, we (Grant & Higgins, 1997) proposed that motivation to act as advocated would increase when an action was represented as a strategic means for goal attainment and was compatible with the strategic inclination of the regulatory focus activated by the message framing.

The action advocated for all of the undergraduate participants in this study was to eat (more) fruits and vegetables. The regulatory focus of the message was manipulated by framing this action as a means of achieving either an accomplishment goal of intellectual and interpersonal success (the promotion focus) or a safety goal of fortifying the immune system and preventing sickness (the prevention focus). In both the promotion-framing and prevention-framing conditions, the advocated action as a means of goal attainment was framed either as approaching a match to the goal (e.g., "Eat fruits and vegetables and feel accomplished!"; "Eat fruits and vegetables and enjoy the safety of good health!") or as avoiding a mismatch to the goal (e.g., "Neglect to eat fruits and vegetables, and you won't feel accomplished!"; "Neglect to eat fruits and vegetables, and you'll miss the safety of good health!").

There is considerable evidence that the strategic inclination for self-regulation with a promotion focus is to make progress by approaching matches to the desired goal, whereas the strategic inclination for self-regulation with a prevention focus is to be prudent, be cautious, and avoid mismatches to the desired goal (e.g., Higgins et al.,1994; for reviews, see Higgins, 1997, 1998). Given this, we (Grant & Higgins, 1997) predicted that the promotion-framed message would be more effective in motivating the advocated action when the action as a means of goal attainment was framed as approaching a match rather than as avoiding a mismatch, whereas the prevention-framed message would be more effective in motivating the same action when the action was framed as avoiding a mismatch rather than as approaching a match. This predicted interaction was significant. The participants' servings of fruits and vegetables over 6 days, as recorded by their daily diaries, were greater in the promotion goal condition when the framed means was approaching a match ($M = 8.4$) than when it was avoiding a mismatch ($M = 7.1$), and was greater in the prevention goal condition when the framed means was avoiding a mismatch ($M = 8.8$) than when it was approaching a match ($M = 6.2$).

The results of this study indicate that motivation to act as advocated in a persuasive message is enhanced when the action as a strategic means for attaining the goal is compatible with the strategic inclination of the regulatory focus framed in the goal. We (Shah, Higgins, & Friedman, 1998) recently found a similar effect for performance: Performance on an anagrams task was enhanced when the strategic means for goal attainment was compatible with the strategic inclination of the performer's regulatory focus. Does matching the regulatory focus of the advocated behavior with the actor's regulatory focus always enhance motivation? One study (Tykocinski, Higgins, & Chaiken, 1994) suggests that it does not. In this study, eating more breakfasts was advocated; we found that participants with predominant actual–ideal discrepancies responded more negatively to a persuasive message (as reflected in intentions, feelings, and thoughts) when the message was framed with a promotion than with a prevention focus, and that participants with predominant actual–ought discrepancies responded more negatively when the message was framed with a prevention than with a promotion focus.

The results of the Tykocinski et al. (1994) study suggest that it may be critical for the goal that the advocated behavior is a means of attaining to be already established. As we mentioned in that paper, it is unlikely that eating more breakfasts was a preestablished goal for our participants. The participants might have resisted establishing a new goal whose regulatory focus was the same as their chronically problematic goals (as reflected in their ideal or ought self-discrepancies). In contrast, the goal in the Shah et al. (1996) study was explicitly established by the experimental task, and moreover was probably already part of the participants' well-established achievement goal. In the Grant and Higgins (1997) study as well, both the goal of health maintenance and the goal of achievement were probably well-established goals of the participants. Thus

matching the regulatory focus of the advocated behavior with an actor's regulatory focus may increase motivation when the goal is already well established, but may decrease motivation when the goal is not yet established and has a regulatory focus that has been problematic for the actor.

The difference in the effect of regulatory focus on message effectiveness between the Grant and Higgins (1997) study and the Tykocinski et al. (1994) study has an intriguing implication beyond regulatory focus per se. Both of these studies involved a persuasive message attempting to motivate recipients to act in a certain way for a particular reason. Both studies advocated similar actions (i.e., to eat fruits and vegetables in the Grant and Higgins [1997] study, and to eat breakfast in the Tykocinski et al. [1994] study), and both studies gave similar reasons for these actions (i.e., achievement or health reasons in the Grant and Higgins [1997] study, and achievement reasons in the Tykocinski et al. [1994] study). The *framed relation* between the action and the reasons was different in the two studies, however. In the Grant and Higgins (1997) study, the action (eating fruits and vegetables) was described as the strategic means, and the reason for this action (achievement or health) was represented as the goal. In contrast, the action (eating breakfast) in the Tykocinski et al. (1994) study was represented as the goal, and the reason to perform this action (achievement) was described as a consequence of attaining this goal. These results suggest, then, that a persuasive message attempting to motivate recipients to act in a specific way for a specific reason can vary in effectiveness, depending on how the relation between the action and the reason is framed. The effects of such variation in framing motivational contingencies may be well worth examining in future research.

IMPLICATIONS OF REGULATORY FOCUS FOR EVALUATIVE PROCESSES

This chapter has reviewed several studies investigating how promotion and prevention as a motivational duality influence evaluative processes. These studies demonstrate the following effects:

1. The affective evaluations of chronic successes and failures in goal attainment involve feelings of cheerfulness and dejection, respectively, for individuals with a chronically strong promotion focus, and involve feelings of quiescence and agitation, respectively, for individuals with a chronically strong prevention focus.

2. The affective evaluations of momentary successes and failures in goal attainment involve feelings of cheerfulness and dejection, respectively, when a promotion focus is situationally induced, and involve feelings of quiescence and agitation, respectively, when a prevention focus is situationally induced.

3. Evaluative judgments of the appropriateness of another person's affective reaction depend on the relation between the regulatory focus of observer and target, with matches yielding evaluations of greater appropriateness than mismatches.

4. Individuals with a strong promotion focus are more efficient in evaluating attitude objects along the cheerfulness–dejection dimension, whereas individuals with a strong prevention focus are more efficient in evaluating attitude objects along the quiescence–agitation dimension; this differential efficiency (reflected in speed of responding) is independent of magnitude of evaluation (reflected in extent ratings).

5. The interactive motivational effect of value and expectancy on performance and decision making is more positive when promotion focus is stronger, but is more negative when prevention focus is stronger.

6. Regulatory focus influences both which kinds of information about alternatives are sought out prior to decision making and which kinds of given information are used in making the decision.

7. Regulatory focus influences the effectiveness of persuasive messages in motivating recipients' to take action, such as increasing message effectiveness when the advocated strategic action is compatible with the strategic inclination of the message's regulatory focus.

These effects of regulatory focus on evaluative reactions have several implications for understanding the evaluative processes underlying attitudes and impressions, as well as the effects of these processes on attitude–behavior relations and interpersonal relationships. Let us briefly consider some of these implications.

Both attitude formation and impression formation involve acquiring an evaluative reaction—a positive or negative response—to the attitude object or target person (see Eagly & Chaiken, 1993; Tesser & Martin, 1996). But what kind of positive or negative response is acquired, beyond just "good" or "bad" and "like" or "dislike"? Models of attitude formation and impression formation are generally silent on this issue. Contemporary research on attitude structure has gone beyond simply distinguishing between positive and negative attitudes by recognizing that attitudes can be based primarily on cognitions, primarily on affects, or on some blend of the two (see Eagly & Chaiken, 1998). Distinctions between types of positive affects and types of negative affects have received relatively little attention, however. Regulatory focus, whether as an individual-difference variable or a situational variable, can influence whether the positive response is likely to be a cheerfulness-related feeling (promotion) or a quiescence-related feeling (prevention) and whether the negative response is likely to be a dejection-related feeling (promotion) or an agitated-related feeling (prevention). Beyond specifying particular types of positive and negative responses, what are some implications of these distinct responses?

The affective appraisal of a person or other attitude object is only one aspect of the overall self-regulatory reaction. The self-regulatory reaction also includes strategic responses. As mentioned earlier (see also Higgins, 1997, 1998), there is considerable evidence that the strategic inclination for self-regulation with a promotion focus is to make progress by approaching matches to the desired goal, whereas the strategic inclination for self-regulation with a prevention focus is to be prudent, be cautious, and avoid mismatches to the desired goal. In a study of people's strategic preferences for maintaining their friendships, for example, we (Higgins et al., 1994) found that individuals with a promotion focus preferred strategies such as "Be supportive to your friends. Be emotionally supportive," whereas individuals with a prevention focus preferred strategies such as "Stay in touch. Don't lose contact with friends."

Self-regulation with a promotion focus versus a prevention focus differ strategically in other ways as well. People with a promotion focus are in a self-regulatory state of *eagerness* to attain advancement and gains, whereas people with a prevention focus are in a self-regulatory state of *vigilance* to assure safety and nonlosses. In signal detection terms (e.g., Tanner & Swets, 1954; see also Trope & Liberman, 1996), individuals in a state of eagerness from a promotion focus should want especially to accomplish "hits" and to avoid errors of omission (i.e., failures to accomplish). In contrast, individuals in a state of vigilance from a prevention focus should want especially to attain "correct rejections" and to avoid errors of commission (i.e., making mistakes). To use Bruner, Goodnow, and Austin's (1956) terms for describing strategies, regulation with a promotion focus involves a strategic inclination to ensure hits and ensure against errors of omission, whereas regulation with a prevention focus involves a strategic inclination to ensure correct rejections and ensure against errors of commission (see Figure 25.1).

We (Crowe & Higgins, 1997) found that these strategic differences between promotion and prevention focus influenced performance on a wide variety of problem-solving tasks, which can be summarized as follows: (1) When individuals worked on a difficult task or had just experienced failure, those with a promotion focus performed better, and those with a prevention focus quit more readily; (2) when individuals worked on a task where generating any number of alternatives was correct, those with a promotion focus generated more distinct alternatives, and those with a prevention focus were more repetitive; and (3) when individuals had to decide whether they did or did not detect a signal, those with a promotion focus had a "risky" response bias, and those with a prevention focus had a "conservative" response bias and took more time to respond.

Thus it is not simply that regulatory focus influences which kind of positive or which kind of negative appraisal of a person or other attitude object is likely to occur. Regulatory focus is also likely to influence the strategic response to the target person or attitude object. For example, as suggested earlier, two persons varying in regulatory focus may both

have very positive, liking responses to their best friend but may still differ in their behavior toward that friend, with the promotion-focused person being more emotionally supportive and the prevention-focused person staying more in contact. The Crowe and Higgins (1997) findings suggest other potential differences as well. Over an extended period of their relationship, the promotion-focused person may propose more varied activities to do together, whereas the prevention-focused person may be more repetitive. And when difficulties arise in the relationship, the promotion-focused person may try harder to find a solution, whereas the prevention-focused person may quit problem-solving more readily.

Such differences may also influence how people discriminate between their ingroup and an outgroup. Imagine two persons varying in regulatory focus who both like ingroup members better than outgroup members. The promotion-focused person may respond to this attitudinal difference by making an effort to be with ingroup members as much as possible, thereby approaching a match to the goal of being closer to ingroup than to outgroup members. The prevention-focused person, in contrast, may respond to this attitudinal difference by making an effort to avoid outgroup members as much as possible, thereby avoiding a mismatch to the goal of being closer to ingroup than to outgroup members. Thus, the actual behaviors of these two persons may be very different, such as hosting social gatherings of ingroup members versus vetoing decisions to admit outgroup members to ingroup organizations, respectively. With respect to resource allocation, a promotion-focused person may choose to reward ingroup members, whereas a prevention-focused person may choose to punish outgroup members.

Not only may regulatory focus influence strategic behavioral responses when attitudes and impressions have been acquired; it may also influence the formation of the attitudes and impressions to begin with. The evidence reviewed earlier that regulatory focus influences information seeking and evaluative efficiency is consistent with this possibility. Two persons varying in regulatory focus, whether chronically or situationally induced, may observe instances of the same person or type of object and may develop a concept of that person or type of object. Moreover, the two persons may have the same name for the target person or object, apply the name to the same instances (i.e., extension agreement), and have the same intensity of either positive or negative response to the target. Even with all this held constant, however, regulatory focus may still influence how the target is represented and evaluatively tagged. Analogous to the Safer and Higgins (1997) research described earlier, promotion focus and prevention focus may differentially represent the target's promotion attributes (e.g., status or accomplishment attributes, supportive attributes) and prevention attributes (e.g., responsible or reliability attributes), with each representation containing sufficient attributes (including common neutral attributes) for correct identification of instances.

In addition to skewing the representation of the target attributes itself toward promotion or prevention attributes, regulatory focus may also cause the evaluative tag to vary. Most models of evaluative tagging of person or object representations describe tagging as involving "good" or "bad" tags, "positive" or "negative" tags, "like" or "dislike" tags, and so on (e.g., Fazio, 1986; Fiske & Pavelchak, 1986). But rather than a "good" tag, there may be a "winner" tag for the promotion-represented target and a "safe" tag for the prevention-represented target. And rather than a "bad" tag, there may be a "loser" tag for the promotion-represented target and a "dangerous" tag for the prevention-represented target. Having such distinct promotion tags or prevention tags for both liked and disliked targets should have important effects, because, as discussed earlier, the strategic inclinations associated with the two "good" tags should be different, as should the strategic inclinations associated with the two "bad" tags. Taking such distinct promotion tags or prevention tags into account may improve our understanding of attitude–behavior relations.

Because persons or other objects can be experienced with either a promotion or a prevention focus, it is also possible for the same target to be experienced in two different ways by the same observer, depending on the observer's regulatory focus at each time. Thus, it is possible for a target's representation to have both a promotion tag and a prevention tag (or even all four tags connected to distinct contin-

gencies). Depending on which tag is activated in a particular circumstance, the observer may behave quite differently in relation to the target. And such varied behavioral responses may occur even though the extent to which the observer likes or dislikes the target varies little across time. Once again, taking such multiple tags into account may improve our understanding of how attitude–behavior relations can vary across situations.

Another possibility is also worth considering. In Fiske's model of category-based versus piecemeal-based evaluations (see Fiske & Neuberg, 1990; Fiske & Pavelchak, 1986; see also Fiske et al., Chapter 11, this volume), the representation of a social category contains attributes associated with the category. These attributes can include both promotion attributes and prevention attributes. Again let us consider the case where the valence of a category's promotion and prevention attributes is the same (i.e., all attributes are positive or all are negative). A situationally induced promotion focus while one is observing a target category member (e.g., a "wealthy" person) may activate more promotion attributes (e.g., luxury/status attributes) than prevention attributes (e.g., power/security attributes), whereas a situationally induced prevention focus may do the reverse. The activated attributes should become a basis for making inferences about the target category member, and these inferences in turn should influence behavioral responses to the target. Thus, once again different behaviors toward the same target may occur because of the regulatory focus of the observer, despite the observer's liking or disliking of the target remaining basically the same.

Some potential effects of regulatory focus on the evaluative processes involved in persuasion should also be briefly noted. The Tykocinski et al. (1994) and Grant and Higgins (1997) research demonstrates that the persuasive impact of a message is influenced by its regulatory focus (as well as its relation to the recipient's regulatory focus), and that taking into account the different strategic inclinations associated with a promotion versus a prevention focus when framing a persuasive message can enhance its effectiveness. In light of these findings, researchers might reconsider when "prestige" messages (promotion focus) and "fear" appeals (prevention focus) are likely to be most effective. Perhaps even more importantly, researchers might consider the possibility that "prestige" messages are just one kind of message related to a promotion focus and "fear" appeals are just one kind of message related to a prevention focus. A message linked to accomplishment need not concern prestige to have a promotion focus. Likewise, a message linked to responsibility need not activate fear to have a prevention focus. It may be the regulatory focus of prestige and fear messages that underlies their reported effects, and perhaps similar effects would be obtained without the prestige or fear content per se. In any case, the regulatory focus of message and recipient may be an important variable underlying the effectiveness of persuasive messages.

It is also possible that regulatory focus influences the information-processing variables described in Petty and Cacioppo's elaboration likelihood model (see Petty & Cacioppo, 1981, 1986; see also Petty & Wegener, Chapter 3, this volume) and in Chaiken's heuristic–systematic model (see Chaiken, 1980, 1987; Chaiken et al., 1989; see also Chen & Chaiken, Chapter 4, this volume). As mentioned earlier, both of these models distinguish between less and more effortful and extensive processing of messages, which relates to less and more scrutiny (and impact) of the quality of the message arguments, respectively. These models propose that more effortful and extensive processing of messages will occur when recipients have high (versus low) information-processing capacity and high (versus low) accuracy motivation. Both of these variables might be reconsidered in light of regulatory focus.

Recipients are more highly motivated when they perceive the message as personally relevant. Personal relevance is usually described in terms of the importance of the issue or topic and its consequences to the recipient (see Eagly & Chaiken, 1993). As our own research indicates, however, a message on the same issue with the same consequences can be framed or processed with either a promotion focus or a prevention focus. It may be that a message is experienced as more personally relevant when the regulatory focus of the issue and/or of the advocated action is compatible with the regulatory focus of the recipient. Regulatory focus, then, may be a motiva-

tional variable influencing message effectiveness through its effect on perceived personal relevance.

Beyond influencing perceived personal relevance, regulatory focus may also influence the actual nature of message recipients' motivation. Chaiken et al. (1989; see also Chen & Chaiken, Chapter 4, this volume) proposed that message recipients can be motivated by a defense motivation rather than an accuracy motivation. Individuals with a prevention focus, whether chronically or situationally induced, may be more likely than individuals with a promotion focus to have a defense motivation when a message is threatening. A defense motivation for a threatening message may be especially likely among individuals who have had a history of ineffective prevention. This is not to say that individuals with a prevention focus are generally less likely to have an accuracy motivation. Indeed, individuals with a prevention focus should generally be vigilant to ensure against making mistakes. With respect to the classic "speed–accuracy" or "quantity–quality" tradeoff, individuals with a prevention focus are more likely than individuals with a promotion focus to emphasize accuracy or quality over speed or quantity.

Finally, regulatory focus may have implications for the variable of information-processing capacity. A popular technique for experimentally manipulating capacity is to vary the difficulty of processing and/or responding to the input, such as varying the speed of input presentation, setting a time limit on input responses, or introducing other capacity-draining features to the task ("high-load" conditions). Such manipulations are conceptualized as capacity-reducing procedures. It is possible, however, that these procedures also influence motivation by manipulating regulatory focus as well. For example, the likelihood of making a mistake increases when there is little time to process input or when other tasks interfere with the processing. This situation may increase individuals' concern with making mistakes, thereby inducing a prevention focus. And this may be especially true of those who are predisposed to a prevention focus. A prevention focus under these circumstances should motivate simplification of the task (see Crowe & Higgins, 1997), which should reduce systematic or elaborated processing. Indeed, an unintended induction of prevention focus may have contributed to the findings of past persuasion studies that intended to manipulate reduced capacity alone. It may be useful in future studies to manipulate capacity and regulatory focus independently. More generally, it may be useful to consider how regulatory focus as a motivational duality can be wedded to dual-process models. Who knows what "blessings" might come from such a marriage?

REFERENCES

Abelson, R. P., Aronson, E., McGuire, W. J., Newcomb, T. M., Rosenberg, M. J., & Tannenbaum, P. H. (Eds.) (1968). *Theories of cognitive consistency: A sourcebook*. Chicago: Rand McNally.

Atkinson, J. W. (1964). *An introduction to motivation*. Princeton, NJ: Van Nostrand.

Bandura, A. (1986). *Social foundations of thought and action: A social cognitive theory*. Englewood Cliffs, NJ: Prentice-Hall.

Bargh, J. A., Chaiken, S., Govender, R., & Pratto, F. (1992). The generality of the automatic attitude activation effect. *Journal of Personality and Social Psychology, 62*, 893–912.

Bassili, J. N. (1995). Response latency and the accessibility of voting intentions: What contributes to accessibility and how it affects vote choice. *Personality and Social Psychology Bulletin, 21*, 686–695.

Bassili, J. N. (1996). Meta-judgmental versus operative indices of psychological attributes: The case of measures of attitude strength. *Journal of Personality and Social Psychology, 71*, 637–653.

Bowlby, J. (1969). *Attachment and loss: Vol. 1. Attachment*. New York: Basic Books.

Bowlby, J. (1973). *Attachment and loss: Vol. 2. Separation: Anxiety and anger*. New York: Basic Books.

Brendl, C. M., & Higgins, E. T. (1996). Principles of judging valence: What makes events positive or negative? In M. P. Zanna (Ed.), *Advances in experimental social psychology* (Vol. 28, pp. 95–160). San Diego, CA: Academic Press.

Bruner, J. S., Goodnow, J. J., & Austin, G. A. (1956). *A study of thinking*. New York: Wiley.

Buss, D. (1996). The evolutionary psychology of human social strategies. In E. T. Higgins & A. W. Kruglanski (Eds.), *Social psychology: Handbook of basic principles* (pp. 3–38). New York: Guilford Press.

Cacioppo, J. T., & Berntson, G. G. (1994). Relationship between attitudes and evaluative space: A critical review, with emphasis on the separability of positive and negative substrates. *Psychological Bulletin, 115*, 401–423.

Carver, C. S., & Scheier, M. F. (1981). *Attention and self-regulation: A control-theory approach to human behavior*. New York: Springer-Verlag.

Carver, C. S., & Scheier, M. F. (1990). Principles of self-regulation: Action and emotion. In E. T. Higgins & R. M. Sorrentino (Eds.), *Handbook of motivation and*

cognition: *Foundations of social behavior* (Vol. 2, pp. 3–52). New York: Guilford Press.

Chaiken, S. (1980). Heuristic versus systematic information processing and the use of source versus message cues in persuasion. *Journal of Personality and Social Psychology, 39*, 752–766.

Chaiken, S. (1987). The heuristic model of persuasion. In M. P. Zanna, J. M. Olson, & C. P. Herman (Eds.), *Social influence: The Ontario Symposium* (Vol. 5, pp. 3–39). Hillsdale, NJ: Erlbaum.

Chaiken, S., Liberman, A., & Eagly, A. H. (1989). Heuristic and systematic information processing within and beyond the persuasion context. In J. S. Uleman & J. A. Bargh (Eds.), *Unintended thought* (pp. 212–252). New York: Guilford Press.

Clore, G. L. (1994). Why emotions vary in intensity. In P. Ekman & R. J. Davison (Eds.), *The nature of emotion: Fundamental questions* (pp. 386–393). Oxford: Oxford University Press.

Cooley, C. H. (1964). *Human nature and the social order*. New York: Schocken Books. (Original work published 1902)

Crowe, E., & Higgins, E. T. (1997). Regulatory focus and strategic inclinations: Promotion and prevention in decision-making. *Organizational Behavior and Human Decision Processes, 69*, 117–132.

Eagly, A. H., & Chaiken, S. (1993). *The psychology of attitudes*. Fort Worth, TX: Harcourt Brace Jovanovich.

Eagly, A. H., & Chaiken, S. (1998). Attitude structure and function. In D. T. Gilbert, S. T. Fiske, & G. Lindzey (Eds.), *Handbook of social psychology* (4th ed., pp. 269–322). New York: McGraw-Hill.

Estes, W. K. (1944). An experimental study of punishment. *Psychological Monographs, 57*(No. 263).

Fazio, R. H. (1986). How do attitudes guide behavior? In R. M. Sorrentino & E. T. Higgins (Eds.), *Handbook of motivation and cognition: Foundations of social behavior* (Vol. 1, pp. 204–243). New York: Guilford Press.

Fazio, R. H. (1990). Multiple processes by which attitudes guide behavior: The MODE model as an integrative framework. In M. P. Zanna (Ed.), *Advances in experimental social psychology* (Vol. 23, pp. 75–109). San Diego, CA: Academic Press.

Fazio, R. H. (1995). Attitudes as object–evaluation associations: Determinants, consequences, and correlates of attitude accessibility. In R. E. Petty & J. A. Krosnick (Eds.), *Attitude strength: Antecedents and consequences* (pp. 247–282). Hillsdale, NJ: Erlbaum.

Fazio, R. H., Sanbonmatsu, D. M., Powell, M. C., & Kardes, F. R. (1986). On the automatic activation of attitudes. *Journal of Personality and Social Psychology, 50*, 229–238.

Feather, N. T. (1982). Actions in relation to expected consequences: An overview of a research program. In N. T. Feather (Ed.), *Expectations and actions: Expectancy-value models in psychology* (pp. 53–95). Hillsdale, NJ: Erlbaum.

Festinger, L. (1957). *A theory of cognitive dissonance*. Evanston, IL: Row, Peterson.

Fiske, S. T., & Neuberg, S. L. (1990). A continuum of impression formation, from category-based to individuating processes: Influences of information and motivation on attention and interpretation. In M. P. Zanna

(Ed.), *Advances in experimental social psychology* (Vol. 23. pp. 1–74). San Diego, CA: Academic Press.

Fiske, S. T., & Pavelchak, M. A. (1986). Category-based versus piecemeal-based affective responses: Developments in schema-triggered affect. In R. M. Sorrentino & E. T. Higgins (Eds.), *Handbook of motivation and cognition: Foundations of social behavior* (Vol. 1, pp. 167–203). New York: Guilford Press.

Frijda, N. H. (1996). Passions: Emotion and socially consequential behavior. In R. D. Kavanaugh, B. Zimmerberg, & S. Fein (Eds.), *Emotion: Interdisciplinary perspectives* (pp. 1–27). Mahwah, NJ: Erlbaum.

Frijda, N. H., Ortony, A., Sonnemans, J., & Clore, G. (1992). The complexity of intensity. In M. Clark (Ed.), *Review of personality and social psychology: Vol. 13. Emotion* (pp. 60–89). Newbury Park, CA: Sage.

Gollwitzer, P. M., & Bargh, J. A. (Eds.). (1996). *The psychology of action: Linking cognition and motivation to behavior.* New York: Guilford Press.

Gould, R. (1939). An experimental analysis of "level of aspiration." *Genetic Psychology Monographs, 21,* 3–115.

Grant, H., & Higgins, E. T. (1997). *Are positive or negative messages more persuasive?: Regulatory focus as moderator.* Unpublished manuscript, Columbia University.

Gray, J. A. (1982). *The neuropsychology of anxiety: An enquiry into the functions of the septo-hippocampal system.* New York: Oxford University Press.

Heider, F. (1958). *The psychology of interpersonal relations.* New York: Wiley.

Higgins, E. T. (1987). Self-discrepancy: A theory relating self and affect. *Psychological Review, 94,* 319–340.

Higgins, E. T. (1989a). Self-discrepancy theory: What patterns of self-beliefs cause people to suffer? In L. Berkowitz (Ed.), *Advances in experimental social psychology* (Vol. 22, pp. 93–136). San Diego, CA: Academic Press.

Higgins, E. T. (1989b). Continuities and discontinuities n self-regulatory and self-evaluative processes: A developmental theory relating self and affect. *Journal of Personality, 57,* 407–444.

Higgins, E. T. (1996). Knowledge activation: Accessibility, applicability, and salience. In E. T. Higgins & A. W. Kruglanski (Eds.), *Social psychology: Handbook of basic principles* (pp. 133–168). New York: Guilford Press.

Higgins, E. T. (1997). Beyond pleasure and pain. *American Psychologist, 52,* 1280–1300.

Higgins, E. T. (1998). Promotion and prevention: Regulatory focus as a motivational principle. In M. P. Zanna (Ed.), *Advances in experimental social psychology* (Vol. 30, pp. 1–46). San Diego, CA: Academic Press.

Higgins, E. T., Bond, R. N., Klein, R., & Strauman, T. (1986). Self-discrepancies and emotional vulnerability: How magnitude, accessibility, and type of discrepancy influence affect. *Journal of Personality and Social Psychology, 51,* 5–15.

Higgins, E. T., Grant, H., & Shah, J. (in press). Self-regulation and quality of life: Emotional and nonemotional life experiences. In D. Kahneman, E. Deiner, & N. Schwarz (Eds.), *Understanding quality of life: Scientific perspectives on enjoyment and suffering.* New York: Russell Sage.

Higgins, E. T., & Loeb, I. (in press). Development of regulatory focus: Promotion and prevention as ways of living. In J. Heckhausen & C. S. Dweck (Eds.), *Motivation and self-regulation across the life span.* New York: Cambridge University Press.

Higgins, E. T., Roney, C., Crowe, E., & Hymes, C. (1994). Ideal versus ought predilections for approach and avoidance: Distinct self-regulatory systems. *Journal of Personality and Social Psychology, 66,* 276–286.

Higgins, E. T., Shah, J., & Friedman, R. (1997). Emotional responses to goal attainment: Strength of regulatory focus as moderator. *Journal of Personality and Social Psychology, 72,* 515–525.

Houston, D. A. (1990). Empathy and the self: Cognitive and emotional influences on the evaluation of negative affect in others. *Journal of Personality and Social Psychology, 59,* 859–868.

Hull, C. L. (1952). *A behavior system: An introduction to behavior theory concerning the individual organism.* New Haven, CT: Yale University Press.

Kelly, G. A. (1955). *The psychology of personal constructs.* New York: W. W. Norton.

Konorski, J. (1967). *Integrative activity of the brain: An interdisciplinary approach.* Chicago: University of Chicago Press.

Lang, P. J. (1995). The emotion probe: Studies of motivation and attention. *American Psychologist, 50,* 372–385.

Lewin, K. (1935). *A dynamic theory of personality.* New York: McGraw-Hill.

Lewin, K. (1951). *Field theory in social science.* New York: Harper.

Lewin, K., Dembo, T., Festinger, L., & Sears, P. S. (1944). Level of aspiration. In J. McHunt (Ed.), *Personality and the behavior disorders* (Vol. 1, pp. 333–378). New York: Ronald Press.

McClelland, D. C., Atkinson, J. W., Clark, R. A., & Lowell, E. L. (1953). *The achievement motive.* New York: Appleton-Century-Crofts.

Mead, G. H. (1934). *Mind, self, and society.* Chicago: University of Chicago Press.

Meyerowitz, B. E., & Chaiken, S. (1987). The effect of message framing on breast self-examination attitudes, intentions, and behavior. *Journal of Personality and Social Psychology, 52,* 500–510.

Miller, G. A., Galanter, E., & Pribram, K. H. (1960). *Plans and the structure of behavior.* New York: Holt, Rinehart & Winston.

Miller, N. E. (1944). Experimental studies of conflict. In J. M. Hunt (Ed.), *Personality and the behavior disorders* (Vol. 1, pp. 431–465). New York: Ronald Press.

Mowrer, O. H. (1960). *Learning theory and behavior.* New York: Wiley.

Petty, R. E., & Cacioppo, J. T. (1981). *Attitudes and persuasion: Classic and contemporary approaches.* Dubuque, IA: William C. Brown.

Petty, R. E., & Cacioppo, J. T. (1986). *Communication and persuasion: Central and peripheral routes to attitude change.* New York: Springer-Verlag.

Pervin, L. A. (Ed.). (1989). *Goal concepts in personality and social psychology.* Hillsdale, NJ: Erlbaum.

Powers, W. T. (1973). *Behavior: The control of perception.* Chicago: Aldine.

Roney, C. J. R., Higgins, E. T., & Shah, J. (1995). Goals and framing: How outcome focus influences motivation and emotion. *Personality and Social Psychology Bulletin, 21,* 1151–1160.

Roseman, I. J. (1984). Cognitive determinants of emotion: A structural theory. *Review of Personality and Social Psychology, 5,* 11–36.

Roseman, I. J., Spindel, M. S., & Jose, P. E. (1990). Appraisals of emotion-eliciting events: Testing a theory of discrete emotions. *Journal of Personality and Social Psychology, 59,* 899–915.

Rothman, A. J., & Salovey, P. (1997). Shaping perceptions to motivate healthy behavior: The role of message framing. *Psychological Bulletin, 121,* 3–19.

Rotter, J. B. (1982). Some implications of a social learning theory for the practice of psychotherapy. In J. B. Rotter (Ed.), *The development and applications of social learning theory* (pp. 237–262). New York: CBS Educational and Professional.

Safer, D., & Higgins, E. T. (1998). *How do personal concerns influence preferences?: The case of promotion and prevention concerns.* Unpublished manuscript.

Shah, J., & Higgins, E. T. (1997). Expectancy × value effects: Regulatory focus as a determinant of magnitude and direction. *Journal of Personality and Social Psychology, 73,* 447–458.

Shah, J., Higgins, E. T., & Friedman, R. (1998). Performance incentives and means: How regulatory focus influences goal attainment. *Journal of Personality and Social Psychology, 74,* 285–293.

Shah, J., Higgins, E. T., Idson, L. C., & Liberman, N. (1998). *Promotion and prevention appraisals: How functional relevance increases efficiency.* Unpublished manuscript, Columbia University.

Skinner, B. F. (1953). *Science and human behavior.* New York: Macmillan.

Sorrentino, R. M., & Higgins, E. T. (1986). Motivation and cognition: Warming up to synergism. In R. M. Sorrentino & E. T. Higgins (Eds.), *Handbook of motivation and cognition: Foundations of social behavior* (Vol. 1, pp. 3–19). New York: Guilford Press.

Sullivan, H. S. (1953). *The collected works of Harry Stack Sullivan: Vol. 1. The interpersonal theory of psychiatry* (H. S. Perry & M. L. Gawel, Eds.). New York: Norton.

Tanner, W. P., Jr., & Swets, J. A. (1954). A decision-making theory of visual detection. *Psychological Review, 61,* 401–409.

Tesser, A., & Martin, L. (1996). The psychology of evaluation. In E. T. Higgins & A. W. Kruglanski (Eds.), *Social psychology: Handbook of basic principles* (pp. 400–432). New York: Guilford Press.

Thorndike, E. L. (1935). *The psychology of wants, interests, and attitudes.* New York: Appleton-Century-Crofts.

Tolman, E. C. (1955). Principles of performance. *Psychological Review, 62,* 315–326.

Trope, Y., & Liberman, A. (1996). Social hypothesis testing: Cognitive and motivational mechanisms. In E. T. Higgins & A. W. Kruglanski (Eds.), *Social psychology: Handbook of basic principles* (pp. 239–270). New York: Guilford Press.

Tykocinski, O., Higgins, E. T., & Chaiken, S. (1994). Message framing, self-discrepancies, and yielding to persuasive messages: The motivational significance of psychological situations. *Personality and Social Psychology Bulletin, 20,* 107–115.

Vroom, V. H. (1964). *Work and motivation.* New York: Wiley.

Wiener, N. (1948). *Cybernetics: Control and communication in the animal and the machine.* Cambridge, MA: MIT Press.

V

Applications and Extensions of Dual-Process Theorizing

26

Exploring the Boundary between Fiction and Reality

DEBORAH A. PRENTICE
RICHARD J. GERRIG

The relation of fictional information to real-world knowledge and beliefs presents us with something of a paradox. On the one hand, the information contained in works of fiction is defined explicitly as unreliable: Authors of fictions are free to invent people, places, and events as needed to facilitate their plot development. The standard to which they are held is aesthetic, not veridical. Every reader (or listener or viewer) knows that.[1] On the other hand, fictional information does influence beliefs about the real world. Readers can use works of fiction to gain access to distant people, places, and events that fall outside of their ordinary, everyday experience. Fiction can provide insight into human nature and the opportunity to explore possible worlds, varieties of characters, events that might occur. Most readers know that as well. So the question then becomes this: How do readers reconcile the competing normative and experiential claims of fictional information on their beliefs about reality?

In an attempt to answer this question, philosophers and literary theorists have developed models of human information processing that include special mental operations designed to deal with fiction. Most of these models elaborate in some way or another on

Samuel Taylor Coleridge's notion of a "willing suspension of disbelief" that must be invoked when readers partake of a work of fiction (see Gerrig, 1993, for a review). That is, they assume that because a fictional narrative is not strictly true, readers experience an initial hesitancy, or even inability, to participate in it; this inclination to doubt is the major hurdle that readers of fiction must overcome. Consistent with this assumption, they propose various processes that enable readers to overcome the hurdle of default disbelief. For example, some propose a theoretical set of conventions that suspend the normal operation of rules relating claims about the world to reality (Searle, 1975); others argue for the complete compartmentalization of information contained in works of fiction from real-world knowledge (Adams, 1985). Although these models differ considerably in their particulars, what all of them share is the premise that the distinction between fiction and nonfiction is primary in the human information-processing system. They assume that fictional information makes unique demands on people's cognitive capabilities and therefore necessitates the use of special mental processes.

In contrast to these models, which have been developed specifically to explain the ex-

529

perience of fiction, contemporary psychological models of belief and attitude formation suggest a very different set of assumptions about how human information processing works. In particular, these models call into serious question the notion that information is ever greeted with default disbelief (see especially Gilbert, 1991). Instead, they point to people's inherent credulity—their tendency to allow any information, reliable or unreliable, to gain entry into their store of knowledge and to influence their beliefs about the world. Given that these so-called "dual-process" models have a considerable data base to support their assertions, we take them as our point of departure. In this chapter, we consider their implications for our understanding of the impact of fictional information on real-world beliefs and attitudes. In so doing, we start with the assumption that there is nothing unique about the experience of fiction, and no need to invoke special mental processes to account for it. Instead, we can use what we know about ordinary information processing to predict and explain the fate of information presented in fiction.

In our empirical work thus far, we have invoked dual-process models more in the way of explanation than of prediction. We make this confession up front because it helps to explain the somewhat uncertain relation between theory and experimental design that characterizes this program of research. We began our data collection efforts with predictions derived not from psychology but from formal theory and phenomenological experience; it is only as these investigations have proceeded that we have realized the utility of models of belief and attitude formation for understanding our findings. As a result, our research does not stand as a test of these models, nor does it speak directly to the differences between them. Instead, it provides a measure of their general utility—the extent to which existing models can account for phenomena that they were not explicitly developed to explain. We believe that this type of investigation is timely: The accumulated research evidence makes it clear that each of these models provides an adequate account for an existing body of literature, and that each can be used to generate testable predictions that are typically sustained in the laboratory. What is less clear is the breadth of the models—the extent of their applicability to

new domains. Our research provides one test of this applicability.

In this chapter, we begin by outlining what we know, from phenomenological experience, common sense, and existing data, about the psychology of fiction. Next we describe several models of the processes underlying belief and attitude formation. We rely on several models rather than just one, because each was developed to explain different phenomena, all of which bear some relation to the experience of fiction. We then use these models to develop some initial ideas about how fictional information might influence real-world beliefs and attitudes, and to test out those ideas with the empirical evidence we have accumulated to date. Finally, we consider the implications of this theory and research for our understanding of fictional experience, for the evaluation of existing psychological models, and for future empirical research.

THE EXPERIENCE OF FICTION

As an illustration of the uncertain relation between fiction and reality, consider the following excerpt from Thomas Pynchon's novel *Gravity's Rainbow* (see also Gerrig & Prentice, 1991):

> Gustav is a composer. For months he has been carrying on a raging debate with Säure over who is better, Beethoven or Rossini. . . . "I'm not so much for Beethoven qua Beethoven," Gustav argues, "but as he represents the German dialectic, the incorporation of more and more notes into the scale, culminating with dodecaphonic democracy, where all notes get an equal hearing. . . . While Rossini was retiring at the age of 36, womanizing and getting fat, Beethoven was living a life filled with tragedy and grandeur."
>
> "So?" is Säure's customary answer to that one. "Which would you rather do? The point is . . . a person feels *good* listening to Rossini. All you feel like listening to Beethoven is going out and invading Poland. Ode to Joy indeed." (Pynchon, 1973, p. 440.)

The difficulty here is apparent: On the one hand, the reader has no reason to trust this information about Beethoven and Rossini; its proximal source is two fictional characters, and its distal source is Thomas

Pynchon, whose knowledge and opinions about music are unknown. On the other hand, the arguments are consistent with general preexisting knowledge about Beethoven and Rossini and are quite persuasive. Is the reader of *Gravity's Rainbow* influenced by these claims? And what of the case in which a particular viewpoint is expressed not just by a snippet of dialogue, but by the setting, characters, and events of a narrative? Are readers compelled by the real-world implications of these fictional worlds?

Both anecdotal and empirical evidence suggest that the answer to these general, descriptive questions is often "yes." On the anecdotal side, history provides us with many cases of (apparent) persuasion by fiction. For example, Harriet Beecher Stowe's novel *Uncle Tom's Cabin* has long been given credit for helping to foment antislavery sentiment that eventuated in the Civil War. Similarly, Upton Sinclair's novel *The Jungle* is considered to have been a major force leading to changes in labor practices. More recently, fictional movies have also served as persuasive vehicles: The movie *Jaws* offered such vivid and compelling evidence for the dangers of shark attacks that it kept many vacationers out of the water, despite the fact that shark attacks are highly improbable in the real world. And the movie *JFK* had sufficient impact on beliefs about the assassination of President Kennedy to inspire new inquiries into the case. On the empirical side, the mass-communication literature contains many findings of attitude change resulting from exposure to fiction. For example, numerous studies have shown that media portrayals of sex-role and ethnic stereotypes affect children's attitudes toward women and members of minority groups (see Christenson & Roberts, 1983, for a review). In one of the earliest studies, Peterson and Thurstone (1933) found that a single exposure to a feature film produced significant attitude change (e.g., viewing *The Birth of a Nation* affected attitudes toward blacks). In the television age, Gerbner and his colleagues have demonstrated a correlation between television viewing and beliefs about violence in the real world (e.g., Gerbner & Gross, 1976; Gerbner, Gross, Morgan, & Signorielli, 1980). These findings are consistent with the contention that fiction often influences real-world judgments.

Why are readers vulnerable to influence from fictional sources? We trace their vulnerability to the assumptions they make about what authors of fiction seek to accomplish. We contend that in many or perhaps most of their experiences with fiction, readers assume that authors are attempting to represent real life. The plot of the story may be fictional, and the characters and events may be fabricated, but basic facts about the world should remain true. Thus readers may be vulnerable to fictional information because they have (misplaced) faith in the truth standard to which authors subscribe. Even though a novel is fictional, they may assume that there is no reason to doubt its general assertions about the world. Of course, not all works of fiction adhere to this truth standard, and readers are aware of that fact. If there is some reason to doubt that a fictional work is intended to represent real life—as in the case of a fantasy or science fiction novel, for example—readers will be more skeptical of its assertions. But in the absence of obvious cues to doubt, they will approach information in fiction with the assumption that it applies to the real world.

The vulnerability induced by this trusting attitude may be exacerbated by the unfamiliarity of most fictional worlds. Readers of fiction will often find themselves acquiring information about times and places that are quite outside their own knowledge and experience. Indeed, numerous writers have argued that one of the primary functions of fiction is to broaden people's experiences beyond ordinarily accessible spheres (see Lewis, 1983; Rockwell, 1974; Walsh, 1969). As a result, readers may often find themselves not only disinclined but also ill equipped to question the contents of a fictional story. Again, in the absence of any obvious reason to be skeptical, they will tend to assume that the story information is true.

To validate these intuitions regarding readers' assumptions about fiction, we asked 29 Yale undergraduates to rate their agreement (on 7-point scales) with each of the following statements:

1. Information presented in fictional works (for example, novels or movies) can make me change my beliefs about the real world.
2. Information encountered in fictional works should not be assumed to be true of the real world.

3. Authors of fiction often invent facts that are inconsistent with the real world to fulfill the requirements of their plots.
4. Information present in fiction is invented by the author of the fictional work.

Our informants agreed that fictional information can change their beliefs about the real world ($M = 5.24$) and that authors often invent information to facilitate their plots ($M = 5.07$; both ratings were significantly higher than a neutral rating of 4). However, they were agnostic with respect to the questions of whether information encountered in fictional works should not be assumed to be true ($M = 4.38$) and whether information present in fiction is invented by the author of the fictional work ($M = 3.69$; neither rating was significantly different from neutral). Clearly, they were hesitant to endorse broad-based statements about fiction's unreliability. Their responses suggest that readers are aware that some of the information contained in fictional works is untrue, especially information directly connected to the development of the plot. But other information—background details and general assertions about the world—they assume to be true. Moreover, readers (unlike theorists) are well aware that they are influenced by fictional information, and they seem to see no reason to protect themselves from this influence.

We can summarize this discussion in the language of analyses of informational influence. Concerns about the unreliability of fictional information and normative claims for excluding it from real-world knowledge rest on the assumption that fictional sources have low credibility. This assumption in turn derives from the simple fact that authors of fiction are explicitly licensed to make up information. Clearly, there is considerable potential to be misinformed by a work of fiction. But readers are less concerned with potential than with practice, and in practice, they believe that authors do adhere to a reasonable standard of truth whenever they can (i.e., except in cases where their plots requires fabrication)—a belief that is sustained by their experiences with fiction. In fact, readers invest authors with a moderate degree of credibility. As a result, they approach works of fiction with credulity, not with disbelief they must willingly suspend.

MODELS OF BELIEF AND ATTITUDE FORMATION

In light of this evidence against the claims of normative models on readers' everyday experiences with fiction, we now turn to a consideration of descriptive models. In particular, we focus on recent models of the psychological processes underlying belief and attitude formation. Our purpose in doing so is to bring the study of fiction into the mainstream of social-cognitive theory and research. Indeed, once we abandon the notion that fiction is a unique category of information requiring special mental processes, then we can use what we know about ordinary information processing to analyze it. Because our interest is in the ways in which fictional information affects real-world beliefs and attitudes, we restrict our consideration to models of these processes.

In recent years, researchers across many different areas of psychology have converged on the idea that the human information-processing system operates in multiple modes, each invoked by particular circumstances and with distinct consequences for the representation and use of information. The present volume is a testimony to the growing popularity of these multiprocess models. Among those that focus specifically on beliefs and attitudes, there is consensus on the existence of two separable processes: a systematic process that operates according to principles of logic and rationality, and a second process that operates according to different principles (see, e.g., Brewer & Harasty, Chapter 12, this volume; Chen & Chaiken, Chapter 4, this volume; Fiske, Lin, & Neuberg, Chapter 11, this volume; Petty & Wegener, Chapter 3, this volume). These models also agree that the systematic process requires effort; one must have both motivation and capacity to engage in it. But that is the extent of their common ground. The models diverge sharply in their specifications of the nonsystematic process—in the principles by which it operates, the level of analysis at which it is described, and the phenomena that it is invoked to explain.

Of course, it is in the specification of the

nonsystematic process that the models become interesting from our point of view, for if there is any conclusion to be drawn from the foregoing analysis, it is that fictional information is not processed systematically. Two lines of reasoning support this conclusion. First, fictional works are not created to withstand critical scrutiny. Typically, fictional arguments are not well drawn, and both their sources and their evidentiary bases are unknown. It is difficult to believe that readers would be influenced by fiction (or that they would derive much pleasure from a fictional work, for that matter) if they did a systematic analysis of its contents. Second, there is no reason to think that readers have the motivation and capacity necessary to engage in systematic processing of fictional information. As we have noted earlier, readers do not approach works of fiction concerned about being misled by their contents, or equipped with the knowledge that would be necessary to evaluate them. Therefore, it seems unlikely that they can or do put in the effort to engage in systematic processing.

If fictional information is not processed systematically, how is it processed? The following are the alternatives to rational, systematic processing that seem to us most useful for characterizing the processing of fiction. These various models are not independent of one another; each represents an attempt to describe the processes underlying a particular set of phenomena that involve departures from strict logic or rationality. All of these modes of processing are treated in considerable detail in other chapters of this volume, so we describe them only briefly here.

Mere Comprehension

The simplest view of the nonsystematic process comes from Gilbert (1991), who has proposed, in line with the theorizing of 17th-century Dutch philosopher Baruch Spinoza, that the very process of comprehension carries with it acceptance (see also Gilbert, Chapter 1, this volume). According to Gilbert, belief is an automatic concomitant of simple understanding; disbelief can be achieved only through effort, after information is initially accepted as true. This view stands in sharp contrast to most existing models of the human belief system, which

have adopted René Descartes's distinction between a passive process of comprehension and an active process of evaluation. That is, most models have assumed that the belief system remains agnostic as to the truth or falsity of a proposition until it has assessed the validity of the information. Instead, according to Gilbert's model and now a considerable amount of data (Gilbert, Krull, & Malone, 1990; see also Gilbert, 1991, for a review), the belief system is never impartial. Truth is assumed unless falsity is proven.

In this view, fictional information may gain acceptance by default. Readers may accept fictional assertions, like factual assertions, as they comprehend them. Because they lack the motivation and capacity to carry out a thorough evaluation of these assertions, the information then remains in their belief system as true. If this characterization of the processing of fiction is valid, then we should expect belief in fiction to be moderated by any factor that increases or decreases readers' motivation and ability to evaluate it. Acceptance of fictional propositions should depend primarily on readers' *not* engaging in an active evaluation process.

Heuristics

A second view of nonsystematic processing is that it is governed by cognitive heuristics that serve to simplify otherwise taxing judgmental tasks. The idea behind heuristic processing is that in the absence of the motivation or resources necessary to engage in a thorough, systematic evaluation of the information relevant to a particular judgment or decision, people focus more narrowly on information that readily comes to mind, and use relatively simple cognitive structures to process it. The best-known demonstrations of heuristic processing come from Tversky and Kahneman (1974), who showed how use of the "availability" and "representativeness" heuristics influences judgments of frequency and category membership. When asked to make a judgment of the relative frequencies of two categories of events, for example, Tversky and Kahneman's participants did not adopt a systematic research strategy or formal algorithm to make the judgment, but instead relied on the ease with which instances of the two categories came to mind. Similarly, when asked to indicate to which of two categories a particular instance belongs, they did not use Bayesian logic to estimate the relative probabilities of category membership, but instead relied on the similarity of the instance to the prototype of each category. Thus, when confronted with a question they lack the motivation or resources to answer (e.g., "Are there more *A*'s or *B*'s in the population?"), people appear to respond by answering a simpler question, one that approximates the original (e.g., "Can I think of more *A*'s or *B*'s?"). Chaiken and her colleagues (Chaiken, 1987; Chaiken, Liberman, & Eagly, 1989) have applied this notion of heuristic processing to the persuasion context; they have shown how people use simple decision rules such as "Experts' statements can be trusted," and "Length implies strength," to judge the validity of persuasive messages (see Chen & Chaiken, Chapter 4, this volume, for a review).

In the case of fiction, heuristics may enhance the impact of fictional information on real-world beliefs and judgments in at least two ways. First, there may be heuristics specific to the processing of fiction that validate its contents. For example, readers may use credence-giving heuristics such as "Authors of fiction don't just make things up," or "Authors of fiction have insight into the human condition," when processing story information. Second, fictional information may be exploited by the various heuristics that operate when readers make real-world judgments. For example, the vividness and concreteness of fictional information may enhance its availability in memory; fictional narratives may provide some striking instances of representativeness (as when good things happen to good people and bad deeds never go unpunished); fictional circumstances may serve as an anchor from which people fail to adjust sufficiently when making judgments about reality (see Kahneman & Tversky, 1973); and works of fiction may guide readers through the simulation of counterfactual alternatives to reality, which then serve as standards to which they compare the existing state of affairs (see Kahneman & Miller, 1986; Miller & Prentice, 1996). If these are in fact routes through which fiction exerts its influence, then we should expect belief in fiction to be moderated both by factors that influence readers'

motivation and ability to process systematically and by the accessibility and reliability of relevant judgmental heuristics (see Chen & Chaiken, Chapter 4, this volume, for a discussion). The absence of systematic evaluation is a necessary, but not a sufficient, condition for heuristic processing to occur; it additionally requires access to principles according to which fictional information is valid.

Peripheral Cues

A third view of nonsystematic processing is proposed by Petty and Cacioppo (1986) in their elaboration likelihood model (see also Petty & Wegener, Chapter 3, this volume). One of the central tenets of this model is that when motivation and ability to elaborate persuasive arguments (i.e., to engage in systematic processing) are low, people form and change attitudes through any of a number of mechanisms that are triggered by the presence of peripheral cues. These cues include variations in the source, length, and context of the persuasive message (see also Johnson, Hashtroudi, & Lindsay, 1993, and Ross & Newby, 1996, on the use of these sorts of cues to distinguish false from true memories). Thus, for example, when motivation and ability to process systematically are low, high-credibility sources produce more persuasion than low-credibility sources; highly attractive sources produce more persuasion than unattractive sources; long messages produce more persuasion than short messages; overhearing a positive audience response to a message produces more persuasion than overhearing a negative audience response; information that other people were persuaded produces more persuasion than no such information; and so on (see Eagly & Chaiken, 1993, for a review). When motivation and ability to process systematically are high, none of these peripheral cues influences persuasion.

If fictional information is processed via the peripheral route, then belief in fiction should depend on the peripheral cues that authors embed in their narratives. For example, authors can put words they wish readers to believe into the mouths of intelligent, attractive characters with whom readers closely identify; they can put words they wish readers to dismiss into the mouths of foolish or unsavory characters. They can depict a sensitive and discerning character being persuaded by, or alternatively rejecting, another's arguments. They can manipulate the setting and tone of their work so as to increase or decrease the likelihood that readers will see a link between the events of the story and the real world. In short, authors can use peripheral cues to their advantage to ensure that their stories have the real-world effects they wish them to have. If this characterization of the processing of fictional information is valid, then we should expect belief in fiction to be moderated both by factors that influence readers' motivation and ability to process systematically and by the implications of the peripheral cues in the story. Belief will be most likely in the absence of systematic processing and in the presence of confidence-inspiring peripheral cues.

Experience

Finally, a number of other theorists have proposed alternatives to systematic processing that highlight some aspect of moment-to-moment experience. These proposals include nonverbal processing (Paivio, 1986), narrative processing (Bruner, 1986; McAdams, 1985; Schank & Abelson, 1977), automatic processing (Bargh, 1996), intuitive processing (Buck, 1985), and many others. Epstein (1994; see also Epstein & Pacini, Chapter 23, this volume) has reviewed these proposals and argued that they, along with heuristic processing and peripheral-route processing, all reflect the workings of an "experiential" system, which is distinguished from the so-called "rational" system in that it is affect-laden, encodes information in the form of concrete exemplars and narratives, and operates according to its own inferential rules and principles. In support of this model, Epstein and his colleagues have provided evidence that people's judgments and actions under conditions of uncertainty differ sharply, depending on the set they adopt (responding as ordinary vs. rational persons), the nature of the information they are given (concrete vs. abstract), the emotional consequences of their actions, and their relative effectiveness at using rational versus experiential modes of thought (all reviewed in Epstein, 1994). Whether all of these phenomena are best conceived as the products of one information-processing system or sev-

eral is a matter of some debate, but they all illustrate the fact that people react to information not just rationally but also intuitively, affectively, and viscerally, with consequences for their subsequent judgments and actions.

At a descriptive level, the application of these experiential modes to the processing of fictional information is quite compelling. They seem to capture very well the phenomenology of fictional experience. It is difficult, however, to use them as a basis for predicting when fictional information will influence beliefs about the real world. One clear prediction is that this influence will be greatest when readers are responding in the experiential rather than the rational mode. In addition, fiction may exert a greater influence on intuitive than on rational beliefs, and may be more influential for readers who favor the experiential over the rational mode of thinking, though these latter two predictions are less straightforward.

THE PROCESSING OF FICTIONAL INFORMATION

Taken together, dual-process models in social and personality psychology provide a useful starting point for a theory of the processing of fictional information. They concur on the existence of two separable processes—one systematic and deliberative and the other not—and they concur that the operation of the latter depends on the absence of motivation or ability to perform the former. If, as we expect, the influence of fiction on real-world beliefs depends on its being processed through this latter route, then all models converge on the prediction that belief in fictional information will be moderated by factors that influence the motivation and ability to process systematically. Several of our empirical studies indirectly test this claim.[2]

Where the models diverge is in the additional conditions, besides the absence of motivation or ability for systematic processing, that must be met in order for information to be processed via the nonsystematic route. Some of the models specify no additional conditions (e.g., Epstein, 1994; Gilbert, 1991); others maintain that the accessibility of relevant knowledge structures and the presence of peripheral cues are also necessary (e.g., Chaiken, 1987; Petty & Cacioppo, 1986). Our empirical studies do not address these different views, though several of them do speak generally to the ubiquity of fictional influence.

EMPIRICAL EVIDENCE

Representation of Fictional Information

We began our empirical investigations of the impact of fiction on reality with the question of how fictional information is represented in memory. This initial focus on representation was suggested by the competing hypotheses of normative and experiential models that we described at the beginning of this chapter. In particular, normative models presuppose that fictional information is compartmentalized from real-world knowledge, such that the information about Beethoven and Rossini contained in *Gravity's Rainbow*, for example, is kept completely separate from real-world knowledge about the two composers. This separation is necessary from a normative standpoint, to ensure that readers are not misled by unreliable fictional assertions. However, the evidence for real-world effects of fictional information strongly suggests at least some degree of incorporation of this information into real-world knowledge structures. Our first two experiments tested these competing models, with response time paradigms designed to assess the relative degree of incorporation versus compartmentalization of a body of text (Gerrig & Prentice, 1991).

In the first experiment, we used a simple verification task to demonstrate that fictional information is incorporated into real-world knowledge, and to begin to assess the conditions under which incorporation occurs. In particular, one factor that we thought might moderate the degree of incorporation was the potential real-world utility of the fictional information. Thus, we wrote two versions of a fictional short story, in which we embedded different types of information that varied in their potential utility. One type consisted of "context details"—features of the story setting that were specific to that particular fictional world. For example, our stories contained information about the identity of the

president and vice-president of the United States, the national speed limit, and the city and time of year in which the story was taking place. A second type of information consisted of "context-free assertions"—general statements that were not conditioned upon particular features of the fictional world. For example, our stories included arguments about the beneficial versus detrimental health consequences of penicillin and aerobic exercise, the contagiousness of mental illness, and the effects of legacy status on college admissions (see Gerrig & Prentice, 1991, for examples of context details and context-free assertions). We reasoned that if our readers were sensitive to the real-world utility of fictional information, then we should find more evidence of incorporation for context-free assertions than for context details.

The experimental stories themselves shared a plot in which a group of college students woke up one morning and read that a professor at their institution had been kidnapped. Along the way to uncovering the perpetrator of this apparent crime, the characters discussed 32 topics, 16 of which concerned context details and 16 of which concerned context-free assertions. Within each of these types of discussions, half presented information consistent with the real world (e.g, aerobic exercise has beneficial health consequences; mental illness is not contagious) and half presented information inconsistent with the real world (e.g., aerobic exercise has detrimental health consequences; mental illness is contagious). The arguments were casual and embedded in the ongoing dialogue between characters; importantly, none of them included enough supporting information to withstand critical scrutiny. Topics that were consistent with the real world in one story were inconsistent in the other, and vice versa. Each story version was about 20 single-spaced pages long and took 20–25 minutes to read.

Participants began the experiment by reading one of the two experimental stories or a control story of comparable length and tone that contained no information relevant to the 32 experimental topics. Then they were asked to verify true and false statements about these 32 topics and 32 others. We compared the judgment times for target statements of participants who read the experimental stories with those of control participants. Interference, as indicated by longer judgment times, would suggest that the fictional information had been incorporated into real-world knowledge.

The design of this experiment enabled us to test a range of hypotheses about the incorporation versus compartmentalization of fictional information. At one extreme, the simplest compartmentalization model would predict that neither context details nor context-free assertions would interfere with real-world judgments. At the other extreme, the simplest incorporation model would suggest that both of these types of fictional information would interfere with real-world judgments. But if, as we expected, our readers were sensitive to the potential utility of the information they encountered in fictional works, then we would find evidence for interference only by information appearing to have general applicability beyond the boundaries of any particular fictional setting. Thus, we predicted that fictional information would have a stronger interference effect on judgments for context-free assertions than for context details.

The results supported our prediction: There was significantly stronger evidence of interference for context-free assertions than for context details. This effect was driven entirely by participants' responses to false test statements after they had read arguments in the story supporting a counterfactual position. That is, when participants had read in the story that mental illness is contagious, for example, they took much longer (approximately 600 milliseconds [ms] longer) to reject that statement as false than did control participants. Thus it appeared that the counterfactual context-free assertions retained some substance in memory. Although they did not replace what was already present, they were incorporated as competitive alternatives. Context details, by contrast, did not become established in memory. We believe that this result supports the claim that readers process fictional information with an eye to its potential real-world utility.

The finding of selective incorporation in our first experiment clearly invalidates a pure compartmentalization model. However, it does not invalidate the notion of compartmentalization altogether. Perhaps fictional in-

formation retains some features of a compartmentalized representation, but with links to real-world knowledge. Some initial evidence in support of this view was provided by Potts, St. John, and Kirson (1989). In their experiments, participants read stories that introduced information about novel topics, such as a bird called a "takahe." They then verified relevant statements in two different contexts. In "story contexts," statements such as "Takahe is a bird" appeared in blocks of trials that were composed almost entirely of facts also presented in the original story. In "nonstory contexts," the same statements appeared in blocks of trials that were composed almost entirely of facts absent from the story. Potts et al. reasoned that compartmentalization would facilitate responding in the story contexts, whereas incorporation would facilitate responding in nonstory contexts. A relative advantage of story over nonstory contexts, then, would constitute evidence of at least some degree of compartmentalization. Of particular relevance to our research, Potts et al. found a greater degree of compartmentalization by this measure when participants were led to believe that the information they were reading was fictional than when they believed that it was factual. We sought to extend this result to fictional information bearing on familiar real-world topics.

In the second experiment, we adapted Potts et al.'s (1989) paradigm to assess the compartmentalization of our story information. Participants read only one version of the story from the first experiment, which was updated somewhat to reflect changes in real-world context details. For the verification phase of the experiment, they made true–false judgments for 16 blocks of 20 statements each, 8 of which were story blocks and 8 of which were nonstory blocks. Half of each of these types of blocks were composed entirely of context details, and the other half were composed entirely of context-free assertions. Once again, we had a control group of participants who performed the verification task without reading the original story.

The results provided clear evidence of compartmentalization: Participants verified both types of information more quickly in the context of other statements from the story. The advantage of story blocks over nonstory blocks was 365 ms for context details and

565 ms for context-free assertions. The story context advantage was especially great for the first block of trials. Participants who began with a story block verified the target statements 719 ms faster than control participants, whereas those who began with a nonstory block verified the target statements 409 ms slower than the controls. These results provide strong support for the claim that fictional information is stored in a coherent form in memory.

Taken together, the results of these two experiments suggest a hybrid representation for fictional information. Potts et al. (1989) argued on the basis of their results that when readers encounter information about a bird called a "takahe" in a fictional story, they create a new "bird" node to encode this story information. Similarly, we would argue that when our readers encountered information about mental illness in our experimental stories, they created a new "mental illness" node to encode this information. The evidence we found for incorporation can then be explained if we assume that a link was formed between the fictional and preexisting mental illness nodes. Such a link would have caused our readers to access fictional information when making real-world judgments, to the extent that the link was sufficiently strong. To account for the selective incorporation found in the first experiment, therefore, we would posit a weak link between aspects of the fictional and real-world contexts, but a stronger link between the more general properties of the fictional and real worlds. The results of our second experiment follow directly from the assumption of story-specific concept nodes.

With respect to their implications for models of the processing of fictional information, the results of these two experiments enable us to draw several conclusions. On the one hand, the evidence for incorporation in our first experiment suggests that story information was not processed thoroughly enough for our readers to reject it. If it had been, the weak and unsupported story assertions would easily have been dismissed. As it was, the counterfactual assertions retained at least enough substance in memory to hinder access to the existing state of affairs. Therefore, it seems safe to assume that participants did not process the story information systematically;

however, they did not process it mindlessly either. The selective incorporation of context-free assertions, but not context details, suggests that participants did not believe everything they comprehended. Rather, they were sensitive to the potential real-world utility of different types of story information. If we assume that some nonsystematic form of processing was responsible for this pattern of results, then that form of processing must include some mechanism to account for this sensitivity.

Belief in Fiction

In our next set of experiments, we sought additional evidence for the conditions of belief in fiction, with hypotheses derived more directly from dual-process models. In particular, we tested the prediction (made by all dual-process models) that belief in fictional information should be moderated by factors that influence the motivation and ability to process systematically. We manipulated the likelihood of systematic processing in two ways: by varying readers' familiarity with the setting of a fictional work, and by labeling the stories as either fictional or factual.

Familiarity with the Fictional Setting

In the next two experiments, we tested the hypothesis that the influence of fictional information on real-world beliefs would vary with readers' familiarity with the fictional story setting (Prentice, Gerrig, & Bailis, 1997). Our choice of setting familiarity as a potential moderator of belief in fiction was based on the premise that both motivation and ability to evaluate story information would vary inversely with the distance of the fictional world from real-world experience. Suppose, for example, a fictional story includes the claim that most forms of mental illness are contagious. Readers know that mental illness is not contagious in their experience and can reject the assertion out of hand if it is applied to their real world. But how are they to evaluate the contagiousness of mental illness in a fictional world? And why, for that matter, should they undertake such an evaluation? We predicted that when the fictional world of a story was distant and unfamiliar to readers (as is typically the case in works of fiction), they would lack the ability and the motivation to process the information systematically; as a result, they would be inclined to accept even weak and unsupported story assertions. Substantial overlap between the fictional world and the real world, on the other hand, would promote systematic processing and thereby eliminate the influence of unsupported fictional claims. This prediction had considerable precedent in the persuasion literature: Numerous experiments have shown that both prior knowledge (Wood, 1982) and personal relevance (Petty & Cacioppo, 1984) enhance people's motivation and ability to process what they believe to be factual information (see Petty & Cacioppo, 1986, and Eagly & Chaiken, 1993, for reviews). We expected these variables to operate similarly in a fictional context.

We revised the stories used in our first experiment for use in these experiments. Specifically, we changed the context details so that one version of the story was set at Yale University, the other version was set at Princeton University, and all context information was accurate for those settings. Each story still contained eight context-free assertions that were consistent with the real world and eight that were inconsistent with the real world. The two experiments differed only in their participant populations: One used a sample of Yale undergraduates, and the other used a sample of Princeton undergraduates. In both experiments, participants read one of the two experimental stories or the control story that we had used previously; then, after completing a few filler tasks, they rated their agreement with 32 statements about the real world, 16 of which were relevant to the assertions they had read in the stories.

We expected that Yale participants would be influenced by the fictional assertions if they read the story set at Princeton, but not if they read the story set at Yale. Conversely, we expected that Princeton participants would be influenced by the fictional assertions if they read the story set at Yale, but not if they read the story set at Princeton. The results were consistent with these predictions. If we combine the agreement ratings to produce a simple measure of yielding to story assertions,[3] we find that Yale students who read the Princeton story were persuaded by its assertions ($M = .55$), whereas Yale students who read the Yale story were not persuaded ($M = .07$). By contrast, Princeton students who read the Yale story were persuaded by its assertions ($M = .50$), whereas Princeton students who read the Princeton story showed evidence of reactance ($M = -.31$). Clearly, the relation of reader to text determined the extent of fictional influence. Students at both schools were more persuaded by the assertions embedded in the away-school story than by those embedded in the home-school story. We take these results as evidence for our processing account: Students were less likely to process systematically, and therefore more likely to believe, weak and unsupported assertions when they were embedded in an unfamiliar fictional context.

Fiction versus Fact

Our second manipulation of the likelihood of systematic processing involved labeling the same material as either fiction or fact (Prentice & Bailis, 1995). The logic of this manipulation was straightforward: Fictional information is taken to be motivated by aesthetic considerations, low in persuasive intent, and of indirect relevance to real-world concerns; factual information is taken to be motivated by a desire to inform, or perhaps even to persuade, and of direct relevance to real-world concerns. Therefore, everything else being equal, readers should feel more strongly encouraged to engage in systematic processing of factual than of fictional information.

We again modified our experimental stories for use in this experiment. Specifically, we set both stories at a school unfamiliar to our participants, since that was the condition in which we had found an influence of fictional assertions in the Yale–Princeton experiments. In all other respects, the experimental stories and dependent measures were identical to those used in the Yale–Princeton experiments. The procedure was also the same, except that before reading a story, each participant was given one of two sets of instructions. In the fact condition, participants were told that they would be evaluating a description by a journalist of events that took place several months prior; in the fiction condition, they were told that they would be evaluating a fictional short story. Control participants read no story in this experiment.

We expected the story assertions to influence real-world beliefs when the story was presented as fiction, but not when it was presented as fact. The results were consistent with this prediction. If we again combine the agreement ratings to produce a measure of yielding to story assertions, we find that participants who read the story presented as fiction were persuaded by its assertions ($M =$ .50), whereas participants who read the story presented as fact were not ($M = .11$).[4] We interpret these results, like those of the previous two experiments, as reflecting differences in the processing of the two types of information. Because participants processed story information less systematically when it was labeled as fiction than when it was labeled as fact, they were more vulnerable to influence from its weak and unsupported assertions.

Evidence for Process

Our account of the differential patterns of belief in fiction demonstrated in this set of experiments would be strengthened considerably by direct evidence of how participants processed the story information across conditions. For example, if participants listed more message-relevant thoughts in response to home-school stories than to away-school stories, if distraction eliminated the difference between the fact and fiction conditions in the last experiment, and if participants low in need for cognition showed stronger effects than those high in need for cognition across all of these experiments, then we would have a more direct link between our empirical results and our processing assumptions (see Eagly & Chaiken, 1993, for a full discussion of these process measures). Although we did not include direct measures of processing in any of our experiments, other investigators have conducted similar experiments that included such measures and have obtained encouraging results. In particular, Wheeler, Green, and Brock (in press) conducted a replication of the Yale–Princeton experiments, replacing Princeton with Ohio State as one of the two story settings and using only Ohio State participants. They succeeded in replicating our results, but only for participants low in need for cognition. This qualification to our general conclusions regarding the effects of setting familiarity is completely consistent with the processing account that we are developing. It is precisely those participants low in motivation for systematic processing who should be most influenced by fictional information.

Biased Assimilation of Fictional Information

In our most recent research, we have moved away from the persuasion context to examine judgments of fictional and factual information that has obvious relevance to strongly held attitudes. Considerable previous research has shown that when a story raises an issue toward which readers have a strong attitude, they will interpret the story information as supportive of their position (Lord, Ross, & Lepper, 1979). In one especially nice demonstration of this biased assimilation effect, Vidmar and Rokeach (1974) conducted a survey of television viewers' opinions of the program *All in the Family*. The unprecedented candor with which this very popular show addressed issues of race and ethnicity prompted controversy over its potential to promote bigotry. Vidmar and Rokeach's survey revealed that these concerns were well founded: Viewers high and low in racial prejudice were equally able to interpret the show as supporting their point of view. Low-prejudiced viewers saw the show as a satire on Archie Bunker's racist beliefs; high-prejudice viewers saw Archie as the hero of the show. Low-prejudice viewers saw Archie's liberal son-in-law, Mike, as winning most of his arguments with Archie; high-prejudice viewers saw Mike as the butt of all the jokes.

Our next experiment was motivated by the intuition that the biased-assimilation effect would be stronger in response to fictional stories than to factual stories. This intuition was stimulated in part by a letter to *Newsweek* magazine that appeared in the March 6, 1989, issue. The author, Edward F. Roberts, was writing to challenge a recent article in the magazine that had characterized the celebration surrounding the execution of serial murderer Ted Bundy as unseemly:

As a child, I remember going to see "Peter Pan" and cheering, along with everyone else, when the crocodile ate the evil Captain Hook. I also cheered when the Wicked Witch melted away in "The Wizard of Oz." . . . So would the all-seeing, all-knowing *Newsweek* please tell me why I should feel guilty for cheering the long-awaited demise of Theodore Robert Bundy? Sometimes I really don't understand how you people think. (Quoted in Gerrig, 1991, p. 166)

We were compelled by Roberts's observations. Indeed, we too remember cheering the fates of Captain Hook and the Wicked Witch of the West. And yet we were not persuaded by the claim that these reactions should have served as the appropriate normative or psychological model for reactions to the execution of Ted Bundy. Fictional events are unlike real-world events in that they have no consequences and no implications. One can cheer the melting of the Wicked Witch, unfettered by concerns with the historical, moral, or societal significance of the event; one can allow oneself to be transported by the narrative (Gerrig, 1993).[5] The same was not true of the execution of Ted Bundy, which was firmly grounded in real-world concerns. Therefore, our intuition was that attitudes and emotions would exert a stronger influence in fictional contexts than in factual ones.

The research literature also provides a basis for this prediction: Systematic studies of the biased-assimilation effect have shown that it occurs most strongly when prior attitudes are extreme and highly accessible or routinely activated, and when situational inducements to consider alternative constructions of the information are minimal (Houston & Fazio, 1989; Lord, Lepper, & Preston, 1984; Miller, McHoskey, Bane, & Dowd, 1993; Pomerantz, Chaiken, & Tordesillas, 1995). It is this latter condition that most sharply distinguishes fiction from fact. In fiction, there is little inducement to consider alternative constructions of the information; if anything, the enjoyment of a fictional work requires one not to. Considering alternative constructions of information would require readers to engage in systematic processing—precisely what we are claiming they do not do when reading a fictional story. Thus, theory, research, and intuition all converge on the prediction that sta-

tus of the information as fiction or fact will moderate the biased-assimilation effect.

In this experiment (Prentice & Bailis, 1995), we used a real fictional story— Flannery O'Connor's short story "A Good Man Is Hard to Find," in which a vacationing family is murdered by a group of outlaws led by the Misfit. We presented this story either as fiction or as a police reconstruction of events that actually took place. The story was suitable for our purposes in at least two respects: First, its style makes it a plausible instance of either realistic fiction or dramatized fact. Second, it ends immediately after the killings, and thus gives no indication of whether the outlaws will ever be punished for their misdeeds. We left that decision up to our readers.

We selected as participants students who had extreme attitudes either in favor of or against capital punishment, as indicated on a screening questionnaire. These students read the story, presented either as fact or as fiction, and then answered a series of questions about it. The critical dependent measures were three questions regarding what should happen to the killers: how severely they should be punished, whether or not capital punishment should be applied in this case, and how strongly participants would recommend capital punishment.

We expected participants to give more extreme answers to these questions, in line with their prior attitudes, when they read the story as fiction than when they read it as fact. The results supported this prediction. In response to the question of whether capital punishment should be applied, for example, 100% of pro-capital-punishment participants and 0% of anti-capital-punishment participants recommended capital punishment in the fiction condition, whereas the comparable percentages were 86% and 9% in the fact condition. Responses to the questions regarding the strength of their capital punishment recommendations and the appropriate severity of punishment for the murderers showed the same pattern.[6] When participants believed that they were reading fiction, they gave free rein to their prior attitudes; when they believed that they were reading fact, they moderated their judgments.

These results provide still further evidence consistent with the differential processing of fictional and factual information. Dan Bailis has conducted several replications of this experiment in which he has tested the processing assumption more directly. In several studies using different prior attitudes and different experimental stories, he has found that the fact–fiction difference in extremitization occurs only for readers who are low in need for cognition, and that it is eliminated when readers of fact are distracted by performing a competing task (Bailis, 1995; Bailis & Strong, 1997). Again, these qualifications add support to our contention that the effects found for fictional information occur at least in part because the information is processed nonsystematically.

DISCUSSION

These experiments have shown that readers resolve the competing normative and experiential claims of fiction in complex and sophisticated ways. They do incorporate fictional information into their real-world knowledge structures, but selectively, with an eye to its potential value for expanding their knowledge base. Compared to fact, fiction seems to be approached with greater credulity and greater abandon, but also with greater selectivity. Although this processing strategy is by no means foolproof (as we have demonstrated), it appears to be well designed to maximize the potential for intellectual and emotional gain from fiction, while minimizing the potential for being misled.

The results of these experiments can all be accommodated by dual-process models of belief and attitude formation. In particular, they are consistent with the notion that fictional information is persuasive because it is processed via some nonsystematic route. We have already argued for the nonsystematic processing of fiction on both logical and phenomenological grounds. Now we can add empirical evidence to the argument. Belief in fiction is determined not by a critical analysis of the strength of its arguments, but instead by the absence of motivation or ability to perform such an analysis. As a result, the persuasiveness of fiction depends less on its substance and more on rhetorical features of the narrative context and the expectations readers bring to it.

On the whole, our experiments have only mildly exploited the repertory of rhetorical devices available to creators of fictions to enhance the persuasive impact of their works. We offer some less conservative possibilities:

1. Because they are not subject to reality constraints, authors of fictions can overcome some limitations on the magnitude of variables that have been shown to influence persuasion via the peripheral route. Researchers have found, for example, that physical attractiveness can enhance the impact of a persuasive message (see Chaiken, 1986, for a review). In a written work of fiction, an author can describe (or assert) a degree of beauty in a character that can rarely be achieved in a research assistant.

2. Authors can set their works in future times, when knowledge will have accumulated to prove current convictions wrong. For example, one of the most memorable moments in Woody Allen's movie *Sleeper* comes when one doctor asks another why Allen's character has shown no interest in "deep fat . . . steak, or cream pies, or hot fudge." The second doctor's reply: "These were thought [in the past] to be unhealthy. Precisely the opposite of what we now know to be true."

3. Authors can exploit our emotional responses so that we find ourselves advocating courses of action that we would normally find reprehensible. At the end of the movie *Lethal Weapon II*, for example, many viewers find themselves fervently rooting for the police officer (played by Danny Glover) to take the law into his own hands and kill the chief criminal (played by Joss Ackland) even though they would strongly disapprove of any real-life police officer's doing the same (see Gerrig & Prentice, 1996).

We can be sanguine about the potential of fiction to influence real-world beliefs and attitudes as long as we have faith (as readers seem to) that authors of fictions adhere to a reasonable truth standard and are benign in their persuasive intentions. Experiences with fiction leave us doubtful on both of these fronts. Consider, for example, the comment that Don DeLillo appended to the end of his novel *Libra*, a fictional account of the assassination of John F. Kennedy:

This is a work of imagination. While drawing from the historical record, I've made no attempt to furnish factual answers to any questions raised by the assassination. Any novel about a major unresolved event would aspire to fill some of the blank spaces in the known record. To do this, I've altered and embellished reality, extended real people into imagined space and time, invented incidents, dialogues, and characters. (DeLillo, 1988)

DeLillo makes his expectations clear: It is up to the reader to keep straight the fictional and historical circumstances surrounding Kennedy's assassination. The interpretation of authors' persuasive intentions can present a similar challenge. For example, authors often deliver their messages in ironic form (see Booth, 1974). We can wonder, in a classic case, whether Jonathan Swift's essay "A Modest Proposal" convinced anyone that the English should consume Irish babies—clearly not what Swift had in mind. But because the essay is ironic, the text does not state what Swift did have in mind. Readers of "A Modest Proposal" are left to their own devices to infer his meaning.

Largely absent from our account thus far is a characterization of how readers actually process fictional information. Our experimental evidence suggests very strongly that they do not process it systematically, but the data do not reveal the nature of the nonsystematic alternative. Earlier in this chapter, we described several models of nonsystematic processing that may be useful for characterizing the way readers process fiction. In particular, models of heuristic processing (Chaiken, 1987) and peripheral-route processing (Petty & Cacioppo, 1986) seem especially fruitful for generating testable predictions about the conditions under which fictional information will be influential. We have been hesitant to embrace either of these models, however, because neither of them seems to capture the phenomenological experience of reading (or hearing or viewing) a work of fiction.

Instead, we have begun to develop our own account of the processing of fiction—one that takes phenomenological experience as its starting point. More specifically, our account focuses on the role that active participation plays in experiences with fiction. Readers contribute actively to the construction of nar-

rative worlds in a variety of ways: They use their own knowledge of the world to fill gaps in the text; they interpret story events in light of their own experiences and emotions; and they imbue characters with complex mental and emotional lives. In short, they are active participants in their own experience of a fictional story, and we believe that any model of the processing of fiction must take their active participation into account. Thus, we have coined the term "participatory responses" (or "p-respones" for short; Albritton & Gerrig, 1991; Gerrig, 1993) to describe the family of voluntary, noninferential responses readers emit, given a particular perspective on a text. These responses can reflect hopes and fears for the characters in a story, warnings or advice one would like to give them, comments on the ongoing narrative, elaborations of the characters' thoughts and statements, and any other thoughts or emotions that arise in the moment-to-moment experience of a narrative (see Gerrig, 1993, and Gerrig & Prentice, 1996, for examples). We maintain that p-responses play the same mediating role in the narrative context that cognitive responses play in the persuasion context (Petty, Ostrom, & Brock, 1981); that is, they adjust the real-world impact of information from fictional stories.

What remains to be specified is the mechanism underlying this mediation. Because p-responses are highly heterogeneous and the process through which they operate is nonsystematic, it is difficult to give a precise description of how they function. But we can offer three general ideas about the link between p-responses and belief in fiction:

1. Like cognitive responses, p-responses may direct fiction's influence through inferential and quasi-inferential processes. Accepting thoughts and feelings about the arguments ("Gee, I never thought of that"), characters ("I hope everything turns out all right for her"), and events ("I wonder if that shark will eat anyone else") of a story may translate into incorporation of that information; nonaccepting thoughts may translate into compartmentalization. The important feature of p-responses, in this view, is their content.

2. It is also possible that p-responses serve as a source of interference with systematic processing. When readers are busy react-

ing to an ongoing narrative, they do not have available to them the cognitive resources necessary to generate disbelief (Gilbert, 1991). Therefore, the more actively they participate in the narrative, the more inclined they will be to believe its assertions. The important features of p-responses, in this view, are their frequency and intensity.

3. Participation may function as a form of role playing (see Eagly & Chaiken, 1993, pp. 500–505). To the extent that readers identify closely with one or more characters and experience the events of a story as they unfold, they are likely to come away feeling that those people and events could have been real. The more vividly they experience the story, and the more strongly they react to it cognitively and emotionally, the more inclined they will be to believe it. Therefore, in this view, the important feature of p-responses, is the extent to which they reflect an internal rather than an external perspective on the characters and events in the text.

These ideas about participation remain largely untested. Our goal in future experiments will be to obtain direct empirical evidence for the processes through which p-responses mediate belief in fiction.

CONCLUSION

Dual-process models have proven to be extremely productive in our research on the real-world impact of fictional information. Perhaps their greatest contribution has been to overturn the notion that the processing of fiction is characterized by special mental operations. Instead, they have pointed us toward an analysis of the aesthetic and rhetorical qualities of fictional narratives as the key to their influence. Indeed, the persuasive power of these properties of fiction has been discovered by authors of nonfiction. As Wolfe (1973) put it, through the 1960s "journalists began to discover the devices that gave the realistic novel its unique power, variously known as its 'immediacy,' its 'concrete reality,' its 'emotional involvement,' its 'gripping' or 'absorbing' quality" (p. 31). Journalists have come to exploit these devices regularly. It would be ironic if nonfiction, which is anchored largely in truth, becomes more persuasive as it becomes more similar to fiction—

which is anchored largely in an author's imagination.

ACKNOWLEDGMENTS

We appreciate the comments of Dan Bailis, Shelly Chaiken, Tanya Fudyk, Dale Miller, Jesse Preston, Brian Strong, Yaacov Trope, and Mark Zanna on an earlier version of this chapter.

NOTES

1. People experience fiction in many different forms: They read stories and novels; listen to radio broadcasts; watch television, movies, and live performances; and so on. In this chapter, we use "readers" to stand in for all consumers of fiction, for two reasons: first, because the materials we use in our experiments are written narratives; and second, because it is simpler and more convenient than the alternatives.

2. Of course, fiction is not a category of information completely distinct from fact. All fictional works include some factual information, and certain genres of fiction (e.g., historical fiction) rely quite heavily on factual characters and circumstances. According to dual-process logic, the impact of this factual content on belief in fiction should depend on the extent to which it triggers systematic processing of the text, and several of our own studies have provided support for this claim (see Prentice, Gerrig, & Bailis, 1997).

3. We calculated the measure of yielding to story assertions by first subtracting the average agreement rating given by participants who read the control story from the agreement rating of each of the experimental participants for each item, reversing the sign of the difference scores for the eight items for which the story assertion and test statement did not match (i.e., the four items with true story assertions and false test statements and the four items with false story assertions and true test statements) and then averaging the difference scores across the 16 items for each participant. The means presented in the text are averages of this index across participants from each school who read each story. See Prentice et al. (1997) for a full description of the results of these experiments.

4. Inferential analyses revealed that the effect of story assertions was significant in the fiction condition and nonsignificant in the fact condition, though the two conditions did not differ significantly from each other.

5. Note that the fantasy elements in children's stories like *Peter Pan* and *The Wizard of Oz* increase their distance from real-world concerns, even relative to other forms of fiction, and thus liberate viewers to indulge their emotional responses fully. We expect that animation functions similarly.

6. Inferential analyses on responses to the latter two questions revealed that the prior attitude × story label interaction was significant for the strength-of-recommendation measure and marginally significant ($p < .06$) for the severity-of-punishment measures.

REFERENCES

Adams, J. K. (1985). *Pragmatics and fiction.* Amsterdam: John Benjamins.

Albritton, D. W., & Gerrig, R. J. (1991). Participatory responses in prose understanding. *Journal of Memory and Language, 30,* 603–626.

Bailis, D. S. (1995). *The influence of existing attitudes on judgments of fictional and factual narratives.* Unpublished doctoral dissertation, Princeton University.

Bailis, D. S., & Strong, B. N. (1997, August). *What we bring and leave behind when we travel to fictional worlds.* Paper presented at the annual conference of the American Psychological Association, Chicago.

Bargh, J. A. (1996). Automaticity in social psychology. In E. T. Higgins & A. W. Kruglanski (Eds.), *Social psychology: Handbook of basic principles* (pp. 169–183). New York: Guilford Press.

Booth, W. C. (1974). *A rhetoric of irony.* Chicago: University of Chicago Press.

Bruner, J. (1986). *Actual minds, possible worlds.* Cambridge, MA: Harvard University Press.

Buck, R. (1985). Prime theory: An integrated view of motivation and emotion. *Psychological Review, 92,* 389–413.

Chaiken, S. (1986). Physical appearance and social influence. In C. P. Herman, M. P. Zanna, & E. T. Higgins (Eds.), *Physical appearance, stigma, and social behavior: The Ontario Symposium* (Vol. 3, pp. 143–177). Hillsdale, NJ: Erlbaum.

Chaiken, S. (1987). The heuristic model of persuasion. In M. P. Zanna, J. M. Olson, & C. P. Herman (Eds.), *Social influence: The Ontario Symposium* (Vol. 5, pp. 3–39). Hillsdale, NJ: Erlbaum.

Chaiken, S., Liberman, A., & Eagly, A. E. (1989). Heuristic and systematic processing within and beyond the persuasion context. In J. S. Uleman & J. A. Bargh (Eds.), *Unintended thought* (pp. 212–252). New York: Guilford Press.

Christenson, P. G., & Roberts, D. F. (1983). The role of television in the formation of children's social attitudes. In M. J. A. Howe (Ed.), *Learning from television: Psychological and educational research* (pp. 79–99). London: Academic Press.

DeLillo, D. (1988). *Libra.* New York: Viking.

Eagly, A. H., & Chaiken, S. (1993). *The psychology of attitudes.* Fort Worth, TX: Harcourt Brace Jovanovich.

Epstein, S. (1994). Integration of the cognitive and the psychodynamic unconscious. *American Psychologist, 49,* 709–724.

Gerbner, G., & Gross, L. (1976). Living with television (Violence Profile). *Journal of Communication, 26,* 173–199.

Gerbner, G., Gross, L., Morgan, M., & Signorelli, N. (1980). The "mainstreaming" of America (Violence Profile no. 11). *Journal of Communication, 30,* 10–29.

Gerrig, R. J. (1991). Moral and aesthetic respones to narratives. *American Psychologist, 46,* 165–166.

Gerrig, R. J. (1993). *Experiencing narrative worlds.* New Haven, CT: Yale University Press.

Gerrig, R. J., & Prentice, D. A. (1991). The representation of fictional information. *Psychological Science, 2,* 336–340.

Gerrig, R. J., & Prentice, D. A. (1996). Notes on audience response. In N. Carroll & D. Bordwell (Eds.), *Post-theory: Reconstructing film studies* (pp. 388–403). Madison: University of Wisconsin Press.

Gilbert, D. T. (1991). How mental systems believe. *American Psychologist, 46,* 107–119.

Gilbert, D. T., Krull, D. S., & Malone, P. S. (1990). Unbelieving the unbelievable: Some problems in the rejection of false information. *Journal of Personality and Social Psychology, 59,* 601–613.

Houston, D. A., & Fazio, R. H. (1989). Biased processing as a function of attitude accessibility: Making objective judgments subjectively. *Social Cognition, 7,* 51–66.

Johnson, M. K. Hashtroudi, S., & Lindsay, D. S. (1993). Source monitoring. *Psychological Bulletin, 114,* 3–28.

Kahneman, D., & Miller, D. T. (1986). Norm theory: Comparing reality to its alternatives. *Psychological Review, 93,* 136–153.

Kahneman, D., & Tversky, A. (1973). On the psychology of prediction. *Psychological Review, 80,* 237–251.

Lewis, D. (1983). Postscripts to "truth in fiction." In D. Lewis (Ed.), *Philosophical papers* (Vol. 1, pp. 276–280). New York: Oxford University Press.

Lord, C. G., Lepper, M. R., & Preston, E. (1984). Considering the opposite: A corrective strategy for social judgment. *Journal of Personality and Social Psychology, 47,* 1231–1243.

Lord, C. G., Ross, L., & Lepper, M. R. (1979). Biased assimilation and attitude polarization: The effects of prior theories on subsequently considered evidence. *Journal of Personality and Social Psychology, 37,* 2098–2109.

McAdams, D. (1985). *Power, intimacy, and the life story.* Homewood, IL: Dorsey Press.

Miller, A. G., McHoskey, J. W., Bane, C. M., & Dowd, T. G. (1993). The attitude polarization phenomenon: Role of response measure, attitude extremity, and behavioral consequences of reported attitude change. *Journal of Personality and Social Psychology, 64,* 561–574.

Miller, D. T., & Prentice, D. A. (1996). The construction of social norms and standards. In E. T. Higgins & A. W. Kruglanski (Eds.), *Social psychology: Handbook of basic principles* (pp. 799–829). New York: Guilford Press.

Paivio, A. (1986). *Mental representations: A dual-coding approach.* New York: Oxford University Press.

Peterson, R. C., & Thurstone, L. L. (1933). *Motion pictures and the social attitudes of children.* New York: Macmillan.

Petty, R. E., & Cacioppo, J. T. (1984). The effects of involvement on responses to argument quantity and quality: Central and peripheral routes to persuasion. *Journal of Personality and Social Psychology, 46,* 69–81.

Petty, R. E., & Cacioppo, J. T. (1986). The elaboration likelihood model of persuasion. In L. Berkowitz (Ed.), *Advances in experimental social psychology* (Vol. 19, pp. 123–205). New York: Academic Press.

Petty, R. E., Ostrom, T. M., & Brock, T. C. (Eds.). (1981). *Cognitive responses in persuasion*. Hillsdale, NJ: Erlbaum.

Pomerantz, E., Chaiken, S., & Tordesillas, R. (1995). Attitude strength and resistance processes. *Journal of Personality and Social Psychology, 69*, 408–419.

Potts, G. R., St. John, M. F., & Kirson, D. (1989). Incorporating new information into existing world knowledge. *Cognitive Psychology, 21*, 303–333.

Prentice, D. A., & Bailis, D. S. (1995, June). *How does fictional information influence real-world judgments?* Paper presented at the annual conference of the American Psychological Society, New York.

Prentice, D. A., Gerrig, R. J., & Bailis, D. S. (1997). What readers bring to the processing of fictional texts. *Psychonomic Bulletin and Review, 4*, 416–420.

Pynchon, T. (1973). *Gravity's rainbow*. New York: Viking.

Rockwell, J. (1974). *Fact in fiction*. London: Routledge & Kegan Paul.

Ross, M., & Newby, I. R. (1996). Distinguishing memory from fantasy. *Psychological Inquiry, 7*, 173–177.

Schank, R. C., & Abelson, R. P. (1977). *Scripts, plans, goals, and understanding*. Hillsdale, NJ: Erlbaum.

Searle, J. R. (1975). The logical status of fictional discourse. *New Literary History, 6*, 319–332.

Tversky, A., & Kahneman, D. (1974). Judgment under uncertainty: Heuristics and biases. *Science, 185*, 1124–1131.

Vidmar, N., & Rokeach, M. (1974). Archie Bunker's bigotry: A study in selective perception and exposure. *Journal of Communication, 24*, 36–47.

Walsh, D. (1969). *Literature and knowledge*. Middletown, CT: Wesleyan University Press.

Wheeler, S. C., Green, M. C., & Brock, T. C. (in press). Fictional narratives change beliefs: Replications of Prentice, Gerrig, & Bailisi (1997) with mixed corroboration. *Psychonomic Bulletin and Review*.

Wolfe, T. (1973). *The new journalism*. New York: Harper & Row.

Wood, W. (1982). Retrieval of attitude-relevant information from memory: Effects on susceptibility to persuasion and on intrinsic motivation. *Journal of Personality and Social Psychology, 42*, 798–810.

27

Motives and Modes of Processing in the Social Influence of Groups

WENDY WOOD

Influence in everyday life occurs in social contexts marked by group memberships and group identities. This is an obvious point in mass persuasion; for example, in politics, an electorate identified by political party membership or ideology (e.g., conservative, libertarian) receives information from elected representatives in government and other party officials, who similarly belong to or represent political groups. This point holds also in dyadic influence in close relationships. For example, married couples and family members may exert influence through reminders of relationship norms and standards (e.g., when children are told, "We don't use that kind of language in this house"). Even nonpartisan news coverage of current events is often grounded in discussion of the implications for international relations and the domestic groups likely to suffer or benefit.

The present chapter considers how acceptance of influence from others is regulated by social groups. In particular, the chapter considers how the social group identity of the source of an appeal and that of the recipient affect the influence process. I will argue that social group identity is important to the extent that it establishes particular motivations for recipients to agree or disagree with the source.

TYPES OF GROUPS AND TYPES OF SOCIAL INFLUENCE

Social groups have wide-ranging impact, extending beyond those people holding formal group membership. Hyman (1942, 1960) proposed the idea of reference groups to represent this broad impact—specifically, to explain how the values and standards of other people and of reference groups are, through evaluation and through self-appraisal processes, adopted as a comparative frame of reference.

Reference groups proved useful in early studies of group attitudes, especially explanations of soldiers' attitudes during World War II. Soldiers apparently relied on a variety of reference groups as personal standards of comparison when interpreting their experiences (Merton, 1957), including "actual groups" (defined as those who interact with each other in accord with established patterns, who label themselves as a group, and who are labeled as such by others), "collectivities" (defined as "people who have a sense of solidarity by virtue of sharing common values and who have acquired an attendant sense of moral obligation to fulfill role-expectations," p. 299), and "social categories" (defined as "aggregates of social statuses, the occupants of which are not in social interaction," p. 299). For example, ambitious soldiers appeared to reject the values and attitudes of those of similar rank (i.e., their current membership group) in favor of the standards advocated by the social category of senior officers. Following Newcomb (1950), Merton (1957) did not limit his discussion to positively valued groups, but also included as reference groups those negatively viewed, derogated groups that motivate rejection and development of counternorms (e.g., the prototypic adolescent rebellion).

Reference groups exert influence because they provide comparison standards for self-evaluation and because they provide valued outcomes (e.g., group acceptance). These motives for agreement were formalized in Kelley's (1952) distinction between the "social comparison" function of reference groups, in which group members' responses provide an informational standard or comparison for evaluating people's own attitudes and behavior, and the "normative" function, in which group members' responses represent social norms with which people comply in order to gain or maintain group acceptance.

Comparative and normative motives for agreeing or disagreeing with groups reflect Deutsch and Gerard's (1955) more general distinction between "informational" needs and "normative" needs. People who are influenced for informational reasons are motivated by validity concerns and accept information obtained from others as evidence about reality (Deutsch & Gerard, 1955). Informational influence is independent of the target's social relationship to the source and derives solely from the validity of the information communicated, such as the logic of the arguments in the appeal. People who are influenced for normative reasons are motivated to conform with the positive expectations of another (Deutsch & Gerard, 1955). The other can be a group, another person, or the self. Supposedly, fulfilling others' positive expectations leads to positive rather than negative feelings and to solidarity rather than alienation. When conforming to self-expectations, people feel self-esteem and self-approval, and avoid feeling anxiety and guilt. Thus Deutsch and Gerard's definition of normative pressures specifies a broadly conceived set of social motives and goals that excludes only informational reasons for agreement. (See similar distinctions proposed in Festinger's [1950] motive to evaluate social reality vs. the motive to promote group locomotion toward a goal, Jones and Gerard's [1967] information dependence vs. effect dependence, and Abrams and Hogg's [1990] reasons to agree vs. pressures to comply.)

The usefulness of Deutsch and Gerard's (1955) distinction between normative and informational motives is apparent in its having provided an organizing framework for the field for the past 40 years. This perspective has been adapted to explain social influence phenomena ranging from individuals' agreement with groups, as in minority group influence (Moscovici, 1985a), to group-level shifts in attitude, as in group polarization (Isenberg, 1986). Across these various lines of investigation, Deutsch and Gerard's dual-motive view is typically interpreted as specifying not only separate goals or motives for influence, but also unique influence outcomes tied to these motives.

In general, social influence researchers have assumed that agreement with others for informational, validity-seeking reasons generates enduring change that is apparent in publicly as well as privately expressed attitudes. In the typical social influence experiment, enduring change is demonstrated through shifts in recipients' attitudes that are maintained in private assessment settings, outside the social context in which the appeal was delivered. Enduring change is also captured on "indirect" measures of agreement—measures that are not, from the recipients' perspective, directly linked to the position advocated by the source.[1] The processes through which this change is produced involve informational mechanisms, including attention to and evaluation of the content of the appeal and other information about the issue or object under consideration. In contrast, agreement for normative reasons is thought to generate superficial (public but not private) conformity that is relatively unstable across time and context, and that arises from people's analysis of the social implications of their attitudes. In the typical social influence experiment, this transitory change is demonstrated by comparing recipients' attitude statements in public settings, usually under surveillance of the source of the appeal, with their subsequent attitude judgments in private settings. Attitude shifts toward the appeal that are apparent in public but not private settings are interpreted as evidence of normatively based influence. The processes that underlie normatively based judgment change have been more clearly defined in terms of what they are *not* than in terms of what they are: Normative influence is presumed to involve minimal processing of the content of the appeal or information related to the attitude object itself. As a consequence, normatively based attitude judgments supposedly are bolstered by minimal issue-relevant information in memory (i.e., supporting affective reactions, cognitions, behaviors) and are not maintained across social contexts.

There is good reason, however, to question whether informational motives produce both public and private judgment change, whereas normative motives yield public, overt shifts but not private judgment change. As Levine and Russo (1987) note, because social influence research has rarely obtained direct measures of the instigating motives (or, I add, the mechanisms through which agreement is generated), the link between motive and influence outcome is "better viewed as an hypothesis than as a fact" (p. 20). Indeed, this hypothesis has been challenged by the extensive empirical findings of message-based persuasion studies, indicating that people are highly flexible and use multiple strategies to meet their goals (see, e.g., Chaiken, 1980; Petty & Cacioppo, 1986). The predominant goals investigated in persuasion research are informational ones. It appears that validity-seeking recipients, when motivated and able, engage in extensive, systematic, issue-relevant thought and evaluation that yields relatively stable attitudes. When less motivated or able, validity-seeking recipients appear to use relatively efficient peripheral and heuristic strategies that yield more transitory shifts in judgment.

This chapter considers whether recipients motivated by normative and informational concerns associated with group membership are similarly flexible in meeting their processing goals. The analysis draws heavily on research in the area of minority and majority group influence; this work provides an especially complete representation of the range of social and informational goals that can direct

agreement with social groups. Furthermore, the theoretical model of influence outlined in this chapter was originally developed to explain the findings in this research literature (Wood, Lundgren, Ouellette, Busceme, & Blackstone, 1994; Wood, Pool, Leck, & Purvis, 1996).

It is important to note that researchers' definitions of normative motivations have varied somewhat over the years, beginning with Deutsch and Gerard's (1955) highly inclusive construct covering a wide range of outcomes associated with self and other. Normative motives are now often limited to concern with evaluation by others or with the outcomes provided by others (e.g., group acceptance, rejection); self-definitional aspects of social pressures, especially the motive to align one's attitudes with valued reference groups, are excluded (e.g., Abrams & Hogg, 1990; Turner, 1991). Self-related motives are excluded in part because these pressures supposedly direct influence through unique processes that differ from those instigated by impression-related goals. In the present chapter, I revert to Deutsch and Gerard's (1955) inclusive definition, in which normative motivations arise from (1) the outcomes provided by others, including both the influence source and those who have surveillance over the opinion expressed by recipients; and (2) the implications of agreement or disagreement for recipients' own self-evaluation and self-integrity. The resulting tripartite model of goals in social influence contexts thus differentiates among normative motives grounded in concern for self, normative motives stemming from concern with others, and informational motives reflecting concern for the stimulus object or issue (see similar distinctions by Chaiken, Giner-Sorolla, & Chen, 1996; Johnson & Eagly, 1989).

The idea that a general set of needs or motives energizes and directs attitudinal functioning has been a central component of classic theories of attitude functions. The present set of motives overlaps to some extent with these earlier schemes. For example, many important outcomes provided by others have been considered in terms of the social adjustment function of attitudes (Smith, Bruner, & White, 1956) and, in Greenwald and Breckler's (1985) self-concept theory, as the public facet of the self. Self-defining reasons for holding attitudes have been included in ego-defensive functions (Katz, 1960) and are part of the collective facet of the self (Greenwald & Breckler, 1985). Validity seeking incorporates aspects of knowledge (Katz, 1960) and object appraisal functions (Smith et al., 1956) of attitudes, and it overlaps with the private facet of the self (Greenwald & Breckler, 1985). I do not claim that the present tripartite model represents a comprehensive list of potential motives. It does, however, identify three aspects of social influence that are likely to be made salient by group identity in a wide variety of settings.

NORMATIVE MOTIVES TO AGREE OR DISAGREE WITH MINORITY AND MAJORITY GROUPS

A "majority" source group has typically been defined as one that advocates the numerically most frequent or consensual position within a larger group. A "minority" source group is one proposing a low-frequency, nonconsensual position, and may also be a nonmainstream social group (e.g., for environmental issues, a minority group may consist of Greenpeace members). Minority sources have also been defined more broadly in terms of their legitimacy to influence others (Perez, Papastamou, & Mugny, 1995). In this view, minority influence occurs when recipients of an appeal are in an ascendant relation to the appeal's source: They possess the legitimate right to exert influence over the source, but instead are influenced by the source's position.

Moscovici's (1980, 1985a, 1985b) theory of minority influence can be understood in terms of the distinction between normative and informational motives. He argued that majorities exert influence through a "comparison" process. That is, people publicly agree with opinion majorities for normative reasons stemming from the outcomes they can provide (attaining social position and other rewards, and avoiding rejection and other punishments). However, Moscovici maintained that agreement with majorities is not reflected in private assessments, because people wish to maintain their personal integrity and sense of control. From the present perspective, the lack of private agreement also emerges from normative pressures. The wish to maintain

one's individuality represents a self-defensive motive to differentiate from the source. In contrast, minorities that advocate deviant positions consistently without compromise are thought to instigate conflict and a "validation" process (Moscovici, 1985a). Similar to the processes involved in informational influence, people evaluate the minority view to determine how the source could advocate such a deviant idea; they reevaluate the bases for their own position; and they change their judgments on private and on indirect measures that appear to them to be unrelated to the appeal. Agreement with minorities is not apparent on public, direct measures. From the present perspective, this resistance occurs because of the negative normative motivations associated with the source's deviant identity; people do not want to be aligned with a minority source group.

A meta-analytic synthesis (Wood et al., 1994) of past research on minority influence revealed distinct patterns of influence associated with minority and majority source groups. However, little support emerged for the idea that majorities exert influence primarily on public measures of agreement and minorities on private measures. Instead, majorities had greater influence than minorities on public measures as well as private measures that directly tapped agreement with the issue in the appeal.

Even more troubling for Moscovici's perspective is the equivocal support that emerged for the prediction that minority sources foster a validation process that generates change in people's underlying beliefs and attitudes. This informationally based change should have been reflected in private, indirect agreement. However, we (Wood et al., 1994) found that minorities were not overall more influential than majorities on indirect measures. Minorities' indirect influence emerged only inconsistently.

It appears, then, that responses to minority appeals are more typically directed by normative motives than by validation. The negative normative motives established by the source's deviant identity inhibit influence. When we (Wood et al., 1994) compared the impact of minority sources to that of no-message control conditions, minority sources generated less influence on public and private direct measures than on private, indirect measures, on which recipients were unaware that agreement aligned them with the minority source. This pattern suggests that recipients suppressed agreement with minority sources on direct measures in order to differentiate themselves from the deviant source group. To account for these patterns of influence effects associated with opinion majority and minority groups, it is useful to consider in detail the normative and informational motives established by group membership.

NORMATIVE MOTIVES: OUTCOMES PROVIDED BY OTHERS

The idea that influence is regulated by the reward and punishment outcomes provided by others was an important component of early typologies of social influence (Kelman, 1958; French & Raven, 1959; French, 1956). Social groups were thought to exert influence through their control over such outcomes: People align their attitudes with groups in order to receive rewards and avoid punishments. Even social norms such as reciprocity may direct influence through instrumental means, so that people tend to express greater agreement with those who have agreed with them in the past than with those who have resisted their past influence attempts (Cialdini, Green, & Rusch, 1992).

Being influenced by valued groups also yields less tangible, more affective outcomes, such as being accepted as a group member and avoiding social rejection. Although these goals are typically associated with an alternate form of normative pressure, involving personal identification with the source (i.e., Kelman's [1958] "identification" and French and Raven's [1959] "referent power"), acceptance and approval outcomes may function like other instrumental reasons for agreement with reference groups. Hogg and Turner (1987) take this position, suggesting that "since reference groups are implicitly defined in terms of emotional attachment on the basis of liking and admiration," people comply with such groups for instrumental reasons, such as "avoidance of punishment, censure, or rejection for deviation, or in order to cultivate social approval and acceptance" (p. 142).

To what extent do the outcomes provided by others motivate direct agreement with majority and minority sources? My colleagues and I (Wood et al., 1994) suggested that this can be detected by comparing recipients' stated attitudes in public settings, in which a source can potentially deliver rewards and punishments, with attitudes given in private settings, in which interpersonal consequences should be less apparent. Because in the meta-analytic synthesis the influence of majority sources proved comparable across public and private direct measures of agreement, as did the influence of minority sources, we (Wood et al., 1994) concluded that recipients' attitude judgments in this research paradigm were not simply a function of the rewards and punishments present in the immediate influence setting. These findings, then, contradict Moscovici's (1980) argument that majority advocacy yields public agreement designed to attain immediate social rewards, and that this agreement does not extend to private measures.

The general idea that influence can be controlled by the specific interpersonal outcomes of fear of others' rejection and desire for others' approval has formed the basis for theories of impression motivation (Schlenker, 1980; Tetlock & Manstead, 1985). Impression-motivated recipients wish to convey particular impressions to the source of the influence attempt or to others, who may have surveillance over their responses (Chaiken, Giner-Sorolla, & Chen, 1996; see also Fiske, Lin, & Neuberg, Chapter 11, this volume). This desire to project a particular impression orients people to consider the social consequences of their attitude judgments. Recipients are likely to adopt the source's position to the extent that by so doing, they can convey the desired social identity.

The outcomes provided by others motivate agreement by focusing recipients on the positive and negative consequences of their opinion judgments. When other-provided outcomes are not highly important, recipients are likely to use efficient strategies to determine the best position to take. They may rely, for example, on the heuristic rule "Go along to get along" and align their opinions with those of others in a relatively superficial manner. Considerable empirical evidence suggests that outcomes provided by others can instigate limited processing and transitory shifts in attitudes while recipients are under surveillance and their judgments can yield the desired rewards and prevent punishments. For example, forewarning participants that their attitudes will be challenged by a discussion partner has been found to generate strategic shifts toward midrange positions that are easily defended and unlikely to offend the partner. When participants are then informed that the discussion is canceled, they revert to their original position, suggesting that the original judgment change represented an "elastic shift" (Cialdini & Petty, 1981; Babcock & Wood, 1998).

When other-provided outcomes are important and people are highly motivated to acquire them, they are likely to conduct a careful, systematic analysis of the relevant information when deciding what position to take, and this analysis is likely to yield relatively enduring change in opinion. For example, Higgins's (1992) research on the "communication game" suggests that communicators are influenced by their own statements as they try to achieve a shared understanding with their audience. In this research, people's goal of conveying an interpretable reasonable position affected their understanding of the issue under discussion. The impression motivations instigated in forewarning paradigms can also yield systematic processing and enduring change in attitudes. For example, Chen, Schechter, and Chaiken (1996, Study 2) had some participants read passages that primed the need to tailor thought and behavior to social demands. When subsequently informed of the opinions of their partners in an impending discussion, these participants evaluated a set of persuasive arguments on the topic in a direction congruent with their partners' position and shifted their attitudes to be more consistent with their partners' views. Further suggesting that impression goals colored recipients' thoughtful, careful analysis of the issue, these attitude shifts were maintained across a span of several weeks (see Chen & Chaiken, Chapter 4, this volume).

Given that the outcomes provided by others can motivate not only superficial change in people's attitudes that is apparent primarily in the influence context, but also more enduring change that is apparent across contexts, comparisons between publicly and privately expressed attitudes may

not be a reliable strategy to identify these motives for agreement. That is, recipients' concern for other-provided outcomes could yield superficial processing of relevant information and attitude change observable primarily when they are under others' surveillance, or more extensive analyses and enduring attitude judgments that emerge in both public and private contexts. Baldwin and Holmes (1987) nicely demonstrated the effects of others' approval and disapproval on attitudes expressed privately. In this study, female college students read a sexually explicit passage after they had engaged in a directed-imagery procedure in which they imagined their elderly relatives or their campus friends. Ratings of how much they liked the passage conformed to what would be acceptable to the previously imagined group; those who thought about older people rated it as significantly less enjoyable than those who thought about peers.

The often-used strategy, then, of comparing attitude change in public contexts under others' surveillance with attitude change expressed privately, can identify certain kinds of other-related motives—ones made salient by others' surveillance. The strategy is less useful, however, for detecting the effects of other-related motives that do not depend on surveillance. For example, some issues (e.g., caffeine consumption) can chronically elicit other-related motives (i.e., for Mormons, concerns about Church disapproval). In the domain of minority and majority influence, then, the comparable source impact across public and private measures (Wood et al., 1994) provides suggestive but not definitive evidence that participants in the original studies were not highly motivated by other-related goals. As I explain in the next section, clearer evidence of the kind of normative motives directing influence in these studies emerged in Wood et al.'s (1994) analyses that considered the extent to which the minority source was socially deviant.

NORMATIVE MOTIVES: SELF AND IDENTITY

The idea that influence can arise from a motivation to align the self with personally valued reference groups and to defend the self against alliance with derogated groups is analogous to a central assumption of social identity theory (Tajfel, 1978, 1981, 1982) and self-categorization theory (Turner, 1991; Turner & Oakes, 1989). Tajfel argued that people are driven by the need for a positive identity, which can be met through social comparison with other individuals or with relevant reference groups. When a social group or category is evaluated favorably or unfavorably, people engage in social comparison on relevant dimensions and achieve a positive identity through alignment with positively valued ingroups or categories and differentiation from negatively valued outgroups.

In general, the motives to align with positive groups and to differentiate from negative ones can be considered manifestations of a defensive orientation that emerges from the desire to achieve a valued, coherent self-identity (Chaiken, Giner-Sorolla, & Chen, 1996; Chaiken, Wood, & Eagly, 1996). Most experimental tests of this idea have examined the effects of group membership on the evaluative components of people's self-images (Tajfel, 1978; Tesser, 1988). However, self-related goals in addition to self-esteem may direct agreement with groups, including the desire for an optimally distinctive identity (Brewer, 1991), and consistency-related motives in which people strive to be true to themselves, achieve a coherent self-view, and reduce uncertainty about the world (Abrams & Hogg, 1988; Hogg & Abrams, 1993; Swann, 1990).

Direct evidence of the role of recipients' self-esteem in group influence was provided in a recent experiment (Pool, Wood, & Leck, 1998). In this work, social groups exerted normative pressure by advocating positions that threatened recipients' self-definitions. In an initial session of the study, participants rated their self-esteem on Rosenberg's (1965) self-esteem scale. In the experimental session, participants indicated their attitudes on a social issue, learned the attitudes supposedly held by a social group, and then rated their self-esteem a second time. For some participants, the social group represented a majority (either students at their university or residents of their state), and the attitudes supposedly held by the group on the target social issue differed from participants' own. For other

participants, the social group was a minority (either a gay and lesbian student organization or a lesbian feminist group), and the position advocated was similar to participants' own. It was predicted that participants' self-esteem would be threatened when the valued majority group held a contrasting position to their own or the derogated minority held a position similar to their own.

To determine the extent to which the target group was self-relevant and thus likely to exert normative pressure, we had participants complete a questionnaire that assessed the extent to which they defined themselves as being similar to (for a majority) or dissimilar from (for a minority) the group. On the basis of their responses, participants were categorized as those for whom the group was highly relevant and those for whom it was less relevant. As anticipated, self-esteem decreased from the initial session to the experiment only for those participants rating groups as highly self-relevant. This decrease was approximately equal in magnitude for disagreement with majority groups and agreement with minority groups.

To further clarify the type of normative threat posed by the group's attitude, we evaluated whether the decrease in self-esteem occurred when participants' attitudes were displayed publicly versus privately. In the public condition, participants were led to believe that others present in the experimental session would receive information on the group position and the participants' attitude (i.e., their disagreement with the majority or their agreement with the minority). In the private condition, only a participant was informed of his or her own and the group's attitude. Self-definitional motives should be present in both public and private contexts; they emerge from failures to conform to self-standards (Deutsch & Gerard, 1955) and are not necessarily tied to surveillance by others and the rewards or punishments they can provide (e.g., rejection for deviant positions). Indeed, the decrease in self-esteem was uniform across public and private conditions (Pool et al., 1998).

Influence and Self-Relevant Normative Pressures

The idea that personally relevant social groups can motivate influence emerged early in the history of communication and persuasion research, and was evident in the program of Hovland and his coworkers at Yale (Hovland, Janis, & Kelley, 1953). Groups were found to regulate attitudes to the extent that a group was personally important and salient. For example, Boy Scouts who reported valuing their troop membership were more resistant to a message criticizing woodcraft activities than Scouts who placed little value on the troop (Kelley & Volkart, 1952). Similarly, Catholic high school students who had been reminded about their religious identity proved more resistant to anti-Catholic positions (e.g., involving censorship of books and movies) than students who were not reminded of their Catholic identity (Kelley, 1955).

The influence of minority and majority source groups can also be understood in terms of their implications for recipients' personal identities. In the Wood et al. (1994) review, recipients' motivation to align themselves in judgment with the consensus represented by majority sources was apparent in the greater impact of majorities than of minorities on recipients' public and private direct agreement. In addition, recipients' desire to differentiate themselves from the deviant views of minorities was apparent in the greater agreement that emerged on private, indirect measures of attitudes (on which recipients were not aware that their judgments had implications for agreement with the appeal) than on direct public or private measures of attitudes. Additional evidence that identity-related normative motives inhibited agreement with minorities was obtained in analyses that compared minority sources who had a deviant social identity (e.g., members of a radical political group) to those who that lacked a clear social identity and were instead identified through, for example, a statistical designation (e.g., the "minority" position supposedly had been endorsed by 12% of prior subjects). Specifically, the characteristic pattern of minority influence, represented by less public and private direct agreement and greater private, indirect change, appeared only with minority sources that had a deviant social group identity; other types of minorities did not generate any clear pattern of agreement. In sum, it appears that normative pressures to adopt majority views and to disown minority views regulated both public and private measures of agreement in our (Wood et al., 1994) review.

Normative Motives and Information Processing

In general, self-relevant groups motivate influence by focusing people on the implications of their attitudes for adopting positively valued group identities and rejecting negatively valued identities. When people are highly motivated to align with or to differentiate from a source group, they are likely to conduct a careful, systematic analysis of the relevant information when deciding what position to take. When group identities are less important or people are unable to conduct a detailed analysis (e.g., they are distracted), they are likely to use more efficient strategies, relying on peripheral or heuristic rules to identify the position they should hold (e.g., for political issues, "Vote the party line").

These various information-processing strategies instigated by self-related normative pressures are apparent in earlier research findings, although it should be kept in mind that these studies were not designed to be interpreted from this perspective. For example, in the hostile-media phenomenon, partisan group members have been found to judge "balanced" media presentations in a directed manner, perceiving them as biased in favor of the opposing side (Vallone, Ross, & Lepper, 1985). Process-oriented research has found that judgments of bias arise from heuristic processing in which people base their evaluations of a specific presentation on their general beliefs that the media is biased against their group (Giner-Sorolla & Chaiken, 1994). In addition, simple perceptual processes were suggested by social judgment theory's accounts of group membership effects. In this research paradigm, membership in a self-defining group was sometimes used as an indicator of ego involvement (Sherif & Hovland, 1961). Ego-involved persons are supposedly more resistant to counterattitudinal messages than less involved ones, because involvement widens their latitude of rejection (i.e., the range of unacceptable positions) and narrows their latitude of acceptance (i.e., the range of acceptable positions). Indeed, Sherif and Hovland (1953) found black participants more likely than whites to reject so-called "moderate" attitude statements on the issue of "the social position of Negroes." Black participants evaluated these moderate positions from their own favorable stance and grouped them with "anti-Negro" positions. White participants, presumably because of their lower ego involvement in the issue, judged these statements as representing relatively neutral positions.

Turner's (1982, 1991) model of group influence (developed from Tajfel's [1978, 1982] social identity theory) also suggests a relatively efficient, heuristic-like process of attitude judgment. Group identity is thought to affect people's attitudes as part of a cognitive categorization process. When people define themselves as members of a social group, they supposedly infer attitudes and opinions from the available exemplars or prototypes of the social group category and assign these to all members including themselves. Those whom people categorize as similar to themselves are expected to agree; agreement indicates that people's own judgments or attitudes are valid responses to objective reality. Especially for issues that are centrally related to group membership, the group position is adopted with certainty and confidence because it possesses high subjective validity (McGarty, Turner, Oakes, & Haslam, 1993; Mackie & Skelly, 1994). When similar others disagree, people experience uncertainty because their evaluation cannot be unambiguously attributed to reality, and they may engage in mutual influence to produce the expected agreement. Ingroups that are especially effective at reducing subjective uncertainty—those that are distinctive, consistent, and consensual—should be especially influential (Turner, 1991; Turner, Oakes, Haslam, & McGarty, 1994).

Turner's (1982) self-categorization analysis of influence (initially called "referent informational influence") derives from Kelman's (1961) idea that influence can arise from identification with socially valued sources, and from French and Raven's (1959) argument that a source's power to influence others can derive from his or her value as a social referent. Consistent with these perspectives, self-categorization based agreement is supposed to be apparent on both public and private judgments. Change is maintained as long as the source group remains salient and re-

tains its positive or negative value. It is important to note, however, that Turner (1982) conceived of this mode of influence as an alternative to normative bases for agreement (which he defined narrowly as involving other-provided social outcomes; see also Abrams & Hogg, 1990; Hogg & Abrams, 1993) and not, as I am treating it here, as a type of normative motive.

In addition to the relatively efficient process in self-categorization theory, evaluation of information on issues related to group membership can also arise from a relatively thoughtful, cognitively demanding analysis of information. For example, Asch's (1940, 1948) Gestalt approach to social influence suggested that influence appeals do not directly affect recipients' attitudes, but instead change their interpretations of the object or issue referenced in the appeal. In one of Asch's (1940) experiments, participants exposed to others' favorable evaluations of the attitude object, "politicians," appeared to assume that this referred to "statesmen"; because of this interpretation, participants reported relatively favorable views themselves. In contrast, participants exposed to others' unfavorable judgments apparently inferred that "politician" referred to the "more offensive forms" of the political animal (meaning, back then, Tammany Hall, low politics, underlings), and they expressed relatively negative evaluations. Apparently, the positions "imputed to congenial groups produced changes in the meaning of the objects of judgment" (Asch, 1940, p. 462). Similar ideas emerged, although in slightly different form, in other theoretical analyses within the Gestalt tradition (Festinger, 1957; Heider, 1958). More recently, Allen and Wilder (1980) extended Asch's ideas into a multistage process of meaning change, in which (1) recipients modify their interpretation of an issue in light of the position advocated by a majority group; (2) this new interpretation of the issue makes the source's position seem reasonable and acceptable; and (3) recipients then agree with their (new) interpretation of the advocated position.

My colleagues and I conducted process-oriented research to test whether self-defining normative motives can generate shifts in interpretation of positions held by minority and majority groups (Wood et al., 1996). Participants were informed of the positions held by social groups on attitude issues, which were phrased so as to be ambiguous and open to multiple interpretations. For example, one issue was whether sex of employees should be considered in promotion. Pretesting suggested that the phrase "should be considered" could be given a qualified interpretation, meaning that the best person should be promoted (regardless of sex) unless a job requires certain physical skills such as strength, or that it could be given a more extreme interpretation involving sex discrimination—in other words, that sex of employees should *determine* who gets promoted. At the beginning of the study, most participants believed that it meant discrimination and thus were strongly opposed to the statement.

In the first study in our research (Wood et al., 1996), participants were told that a majority group, composed of students at their university, had indicated in an earlier poll a counterattitudinal position on the issue. Given this normative pressure, the phrase "should be considered" was construed in the relatively congenial terms of disregarding sex unless the job required certain physical skills. This interpretation rendered the source's position that sex should be considered in promotion reasonable and acceptable, and recipients who adopted this interpretation could then align their attitudes with the majority and endorse the statement themselves.

However, the shifts in interpretation and attitudes were not shown by all participants. On a separate questionnaire, participants had rated the extent to which their self-definition was tied to their student identity. On the basis of these ratings, participants were divided into two groups: those for whom the student identity was highly self-relevant, and those for whom it was not especially relevant (i.e., participants who were indifferent but not opposed to the group). Only those participants judging the majority source group as highly self-relevant experienced normative pressure and shifted interpretation and attitudes to align with majority opinion. Those judging it as less self-relevant were not influenced.

Our second experiment (Wood et al., 1996) examined whether the normative pressures instigated by (negatively) self-relevant minority groups similarly affect influence through directed interpretation of appeals.

The source group in this second study was presented as holding a position that recipients endorsed. Aligning source and recipient allowed us to examine the extent to which recipients shifted their own positions away from that of the minority group. Conceptually, this effect parallels the negative normative pressures that appeared to attenuate direct (vs. indirect) agreement with minority source groups in the Wood et al. (1994) review.

Participants in this second study were thus told that a derogated minority group (e.g., the Ku Klux Klan) agreed with them about an ambiguously phrased attitude issue, such as "In the United States, anyone who is willing and able to work hard has a good chance of succeeding." Pretesting had established that the attitude statements were open to multiple interpretations: The phrase "anyone who is willing and able" could be interpreted in absolute terms, suggesting that success is attainable by anyone, regardless of race or sex; or it could be given the more qualified interpretation that although most people can succeed if they work hard, women and minorities have it tougher than others because of discrimination.

As predicted, the negative normative pressure to differentiate from the minority group affected recipients' interpretations and attitudes. When faced with agreement from the Klan, for example, participants adopted a qualified interpretation of the attitude statement, recognizing the barriers for women and minorities, and as a result were able to shift their attitudes away from the minority group's position. Again, however, not all subjects evidenced this shift. Only those who indicated on a separate questionnaire that the Ku Klux Klan was negatively self-relevant (i.e., they defined themselves as not being members of this group) experienced the normative pressure to differentiate their attitudes from the group position. Other students who indicated that the Klan had minimal relevance for their self-definitions (i.e., they were indifferent to the group but did not support it) did not shift interpretations and did not change their attitudes.

In addition, to ensure that the interpretation shift mediated change and was not an after-the-fact justification for change (Buehler & Griffin, 1994), the order in which participants completed the questionnaires was varied in our research; participants either indicated their attitudes first and then rated their interpretations or rated their interpretations before attitudes. Supporting the interpretation-then-attitude-change causal ordering, recipients judging the source group as high in personal relevance shifted their attitudes toward the majority group's views and away from those of the minority group only when they had been given an initial opportunity to rate the meaning of the issue in the appeal, and thus to reinterpret it to support their desired identity of being a good university student or not being a Klan member. When rating attitudes first, they were apparently unable or not sufficiently motivated to construct a biased interpretation of the appeal themselves, and as a result did not shift their attitudes.

In general, constructing an interpretation that is congruent with a desired attitude position is likely to be cognitively demanding and effortful. My colleagues and I suspect that people do not often face this challenging task in everyday life; one of the functions of social groups is to provide these interpretations for members. Thus, for example, members of prolife groups interpret abortion as "murder," whereas members of prochoice groups label it a "woman's right to choose." Reference groups, then, do not just provide guides for the stance to take on an issue; they also suggest what the issue means. Indeed, investigations of attitude structure have indicated that people who endorse opposing attitudes on a social issue accord different meaning to the issue. For example, Kerlinger's (1984) investigation of political ideology revealed that liberals favor social equality, tolerance, and constructive social change and are relatively indifferent to conservative values, whereas conservatives endorse social stability, morality, and individualism and are indifferent to liberal values. Thus liberals and conservatives may hold divergent positions on political issues in part because they are invoking different value systems to interpret the issues (see also Tourangeau, Rasinski, & D'Andrade, 1991).

When groups do not provide congenial interpretations, people may be able to achieve their processing goals with strategies that are less effortful than generating their own interpretation of an attitude position (see Abelson, 1959 for the extensive variety of strategies people use to achieve cognitive consistency). One possibility is to reassess the self-relevance of the source group, reducing normative pressure by judging that the group is not especially important for their self-definition. However, in our research (Wood et al., 1996), this strategy was not used by high-relevance participants; their ratings of the negative self-relevance of the minority sources remained high from pre- to postappeal (unfortunately, change in relevance ratings was not assessed in the study of majority influence).

Instead, it appears that in this paradigm, participants who experience high levels of self-definitional normative pressure but are not sufficiently motivated or able to reinterpret the advocated position simply misrecall the group view. We (Pool, Wood, & Leck, 1997), using a paradigm similar to that used in the Wood et al. (1996) research, informed participants that a majority social group (e.g., residents of their state) had taken a position on an issue that diverged from participants' own. However, half of their participants were not given the cue about how to reinterpret the group's position (by completing the interpretation rating scales). After participants had engaged in a 20-minute interpolated task, their recall of the advocated position was assessed. Participants who had earlier indicated that the group was highly self-relevant demonstrated the greatest error in recall; they misremembered the valued majority group as advocating a position closer to their own than the group actually had. In addition, we administered the interpretation measures to the remaining participants and, after 20 minutes, assessed their recall of the group position. In this condition, participants who indicated that the group was highly self-relevant reinterpreted the source position to be congenial with their own and revealed minimal recall errors. Thus, misrecall appears to be an alternative processing strategy to reinterpretation; the negative correlation between misrecall and reinterpretation in this condition suggested that participants misrecalled the message position (i.e., remembering valued majority positions as similar to their own and derogated minority positions as divergent from their own) to the extent that they had not initially reinterpreted the source group position when given the opportunity on the interpretation scales.

In general, our findings (Pool et al., 1997) suggest that normative pressures instigated by self-relevant minority groups have a variety of effects on recipients' processing of influence appeals. Reinterpretation of the advocated position to be congenial with participants' own appears to be a relatively effortful strategy that recipients are unable or unwilling to implement without a structured guide in the form of the interpretation rating scales. Distortions in recall appear to be a less effortful strategy that research participants spontaneously adopt to meet the normative goals of aligning with valued majorities and differentiating from derogated minorities.

One striking finding from this research paradigm is that the negative and positive self-definitional normative pressures exerted by social groups appear to be mirror images of each other; the motivation to align with positively self-relevant majorities differed only in direction from the motivation to differentiate from negatively self-relevant minorities. However, positive and negative normative pressures may not mirror each other in all respects. The effects for the majority source in the Wood et al. (1996) research proved to be slightly larger in magnitude than those for the minority source, despite our attempts to identify minority groups that were strongly self-relevant for at least some participants. It may be that negative normative pressures are typically less strong than positive pressures.

Supporting the idea of asymmetry in self-relevant normative pressures, research on the self-concept has found that people are more likely to focus on attributes that they possess and groups they belong to (e.g., "I am a Texan") than on attributes that they lack (e.g., "I am not a New Yorker"; see McGuire & McGuire's [1992, 1996] cognitive-positivity bias). Indeed, affirmations of personal attributes plausibly hold more information value than negations of attributes and should more effectively meet the self-relevant goals of a coherent identity (e.g., Swann, 1990) and a positive self-view (e.g., Tesser, 1988). An important exception to this generalization occurs when groups are in conflict with each other; self-definitions of "not the adversary group" may be highly salient and meaningful for members of rival groups. However, in nonconflict situations, people may experience pressures to align with positively valued self-relevant groups more often and perhaps more intensely than pressures to differentiate from negatively valued self-relevant groups.

INFORMATIONAL MOTIVES ESTABLISHED BY GROUP IDENTITY

When motivated by informational concerns, people wish to adopt the most valid, correct position on an attitude issue (Chaiken, Giner-Sorolla, & Chen, 1996; Petty & Cacioppo, 1986). Research on message-based persuasion has typically established validity-seeking motives by highlighting the personal relevance of message topics for recipients (however, see Liberman & Chaiken, 1996). When recipients are highly motivated to identify an accurate, valid position on a topic, they carefully consider persuasive arguments and other issue-relevant information. When they are only moderately motivated by such concerns or are limited in their ability to evaluate information critically, recipients are likely to rely on heuristic cues and other less cognitively demanding strategies; an example is agreeing more with majorities than with minorities, using the heuristic "Consensus is correct" (see Petty & Wegener, Chapter 3, this volume).

Informationally based agreement was a central feature of Moscovici's (1985a, 1985b) account of minority group influence. As I have noted in the introductory section of this chapter, minorities that consistently advocate a counterattitudinal position were thought to instigate a validation process. Recipients do not experience the normative pressures to comply that constrain their responses to majority groups, and instead experience informational conflict as they try to understand why a minority is advocating such a deviant position. However, our review (Wood et al., 1994) did not find an overall pattern suggestive of minority informational influence. That is, in the overall analysis, minority sources were not more influential than majorities on indirect or private measures; given that recipients did not wish to align directly with a deviant minority, attitude measures that were indirect and did not appear to be linked to the influence appeal should have been more likely to reveal shifts toward the source position than public or direct measures. A greater informational impact of minority than of majority sources did emerge, however, in certain selected analyses in the review, and we concluded that the effect was "fragile and easily muted by a number of not well-understood moderating factors" (Wood et al., 1994, p. 336).

One possible explanation for this inconsistency is that minorities in past research have not presented uniformly strong, valid appeals, and people who are highly motivated to identify an accurate position are unlikely to shift their attitudes in the absence of cogent evidence. In the conformity paradigm in which most research on minority influence has been conducted, appeals typically consist of only a stated position, and people motivated to engage in critical evaluation of such a message need to generate their own interpretation of the message position and reasons for supporting it or opposing it. If the advocated position appears arbitrary or is not easily understood, it may, like "weak" messages in research on message-based persuasion, fail to be influential for informationally motivated people.

It is also possible that minority group identity alone is not sufficient to motivate validity seeking. In the information-rich environment provided by modern communication technology, people are likely to be exposed to divergent views from a variety of groups on a daily basis. Even consistently advocated minority group positions may not be sufficient to engage validity seeking (see a similar point by De Vries, De Dreu, Gordijn, & Schuurman, 1996). Indeed, process-oriented research evaluating the extent to which minorities instigate careful analysis of persuasive messages has yielded inconsistent effects: Although minority messages have been found to attract more attention than majority ones (Tesser, Campbell, & Mickler, 1983), majority messages have sometimes been found to elicit greater thought from recipients than minority messages (e.g., Mackie, 1987), and still other studies suggest no overall difference in amount of cognitive response to majority versus minority sources (e.g., Martin, 1996; Maass & Clark, 1983; Trost, Maass, & Kenrick, 1992).

Minority group identity probably combines with other factors to instigate informational motives. In particular, more extensive processing is elicited by unexpected positions. Given that people expect their attitudes to be shared by a majority of others, majorities that violate this expectation and advocate counter-attitudinal positions may evoke careful, extensive thought (Mackie, 1987). Incongruity between source group and message position can also explain instances of minority influence. Baker and Petty (1994) presented participants with expected source–position pairings, in which majority sources advocated consensual positions and minorities deviant ones, or with unexpected pairings, in which majorities advocated deviant positions and minorities consensual ones. Unexpected pairings were surprising and evoked curiosity; consequently, recipients were more likely to systematically process unexpected (vs. expected) appeals, and were more likely to be influenced by (unexpected) appeals supported by cogent than by specious arguments. Expected pairings of source and message were processed at a more superficial level and suggested use of a consensus heuristic, in which majorities' positions were more influential than minorities'.

Instead of informational motives, minority influence may sometimes stem from the normative motivations associated with pressures to innovate. When social norms support innovation, people are likely to favorably evaluate unique, creative ideas (Moscovici, 1985b). Especially in decision-making contexts, minority task solutions and strategies are likely to appear innovative and to pose minimal threat to recipients' understanding of social reality or to valued social identities. Similarly, in social influence contexts in which people expect a range and diversity of opinions, being in the minority may be evaluated positively, as with exclusive tastes in clothing or the arts (Maass, Volpato, & Mucchi-Faina, 1996). These innovative contexts, in which minorities possess a positive identity, can be contrasted to the standard social influence experiment, in which recipients appear to be concerned with validating their views and minority positions seem deviant and unacceptable (Wood et al., 1994).

The idea that minorities can stimulate innovation formed the basis for Nemeth's (1986) work on group decision making and judgment. Exposure to consistent, unusual solutions from minorities in decision-making groups apparently inspires other members to generate more creative, high-quality task solutions than does exposure to these same solutions from majorities (Nemeth, 1986; Nemeth, Mayseless, Sherman, & Brown, 1990). These findings are typically explained by the absence of normative pressure with minority advocacy; recipients are not pressured to converge on the majority view, and instead engage in divergent thought and consider the full range of possible solutions and perspectives on the focal issue (Martin, 1996; Nemeth & Rogers, 1996; Smith, Tindale, & Dugoni, 1996). However, given that divergent thought, like other forms of systematic analysis, requires substantial effort, it seems unlikely to be instigated simply through the absence of pressure toward uniformity. Instead, I suggest that minorities exert their own unique normative pressure in problem-solving contexts.

Minorities are likely to instigate creative analysis and problem generation to the extent that they model "courage" and innovation in problem solution (Crano, 1991; Nemeth & Chiles, 1988). Innovative-appearing minorities are especially likely to increase consideration of a wide range of positions and perspectives, although they may have little effect on the overall level of message-relevant thought (Maass, West, & Cialdini, 1987; Nemeth, 1986). Whether innovative-appearing minorities generate shifts toward the advocated position is less clear. Moscovici and Lage (1978) provided participants with (false) feedback indicating that they were creative, thereby presumably enhancing the extent to which they valued innovation; as a result, participants demonstrated significant direct agreement with minority sources. However, to the extent that recipients are motivated to be innovative and creative in their own judgments, judgment shifts will not necessarily be in the direction of the minority position. Instead, recipients may generate new, divergent perspectives not represented in the minority appeal (Nemeth, 1986).

Certain of the normative pressures associated with minority advocacy may work in conjunction with informational motives to generate Moscovici's (1985a) predicted pattern of stronger indirect than direct minority influence. When ingroup members advocate a minority stance, the shared group identity may motivate recipients to adopt a lenient, live-and-let-live orientation (Alvaro & Crano, 1996, 1997; see also Mucchi-Fahina, Maass, & Volpato, 1991). Although the minority's position is not necessarily accepted, it is also not actively disparaged. Because the minority identity is not really favorable, however, most people will not want to align with the minority on direct measures of agreement. The informational component emerges because the minority position is distinctive and unexpected. Ingroup minorities attract attention, and people are likely to be motivated to process their appeals carefully. This informational analysis should, when the minority advocates a reasonable position, yield change on indirect measures of agreement. Indeed, in an elegant series of studies, Alvaro and Crano (1996, 1997) found that ingroup minority positions, although they had little direct impact, were recalled as well as majority positions, were not actively counterargued, and (most importantly) exerted influence on issues indirectly related to the topic of the appeal. This pattern of influence results, in which normative pressures stemming from negative source identity inhibit agreement on measures directly but not indirectly related to an appeal, is reminiscent of the "sleeper" effect. In persuasion contexts, low-credibility sources have been found to gain influence over time as the negative source cue is forgotten or becomes dissociated from the message, and as recipients' attitudes continue to be influenced by strong, cogent message arguments (Cook, Gruder, Hennigan, & Flay, 1979).

In summary, there appears to be little evidence that the minority group identity by itself instigates informational pressures to evaluate the content of an influence appeal. Instead, careful processing of an appeal appears to be instigated when any sources, including minorities, advocate unexpected, distinctive positions. Minorities can, however, instigate relatively favorable normative motives. People are unlikely to discount a minority view when the person advocating this view is an ingroup member. They may even be motivated to evaluate such an appeal carefully, yet with a favorable orientation, when a minority appears creative and unique and recipients wish to be innovative themselves.

Some group identities do appear to be linked to informational motives. In task-performing groups, in which members are motivated to achieve group goals, influence may be regulated by members' beliefs about how to achieve the best group-level outcomes. This idea has been used to explain Bales's (1953) research findings on participation rates and influence in small ad hoc discussion groups. Bales noted that even though his groups were composed of highly similar members, stable status hierarchies emerged, with some members reliably contributing to the group task and influencing others at an especially high rate. These status hierarchies are thought to develop from the performance expectations members form about their own and others' likely value to the group, based on initial task contributions, presentational style, and personal attributes (Berger, Fisek, Norman, & Zelditch, 1977; Ridgeway, 1984; Webster & Foschi, 1988).

Although normative goals such as acquisition of personal status may also regulate influence in task groups (e.g., Ridgeway & Diekema, 1989), it is thought to be in the rational self-interest of each member to defer to others on the basis of relative expectations for performance, so that the group may generate higher rewards for all members through greater success at the task (Berger et al., 1977). As a result, the task contributions of high-expectations group members receive more careful consideration and attention from others, are evaluated more favorably, and are more influential than the ideas of less competent members.[2]

I suspect that the processes through which influence occurs in task groups vary with the extent to which members adopt validity-seeking motives. In real-world group interactions, a large amount of information is available about other group members, interaction procedures, and possible task solutions. When group members are only moderately motivated by group goals, or when the task is especially ambiguous or difficult, the members will not be motivated or able to verify the accuracy of solutions. They are then likely to rely on relatively efficient strategies, using others' and their own performance expectations as a guide to accepting influence. However, when group members are highly motivated to achieve the best performance

outcome, and when solution accuracy can be verified, the members will probably be willing to conduct more effortful, cognitively demanding analyses of relevant information in order to identify the best solution. Highly motivated recipients, then, should be more likely than less motivated ones to recognize valid suggestions and ideas proposed by low-expectations members. Similarly, if they themselves possess low expectations, they should be more willing to counter others' views and advocate solutions they believe to be accurate.

Empirical evidence of the effects of accuracy motivation on social influence was recently provided by Baron, Vandello, and Brunsman's (1996) adaptation of Asch's (1955) classic line-judging conformity paradigm. Although Baron et al. (1996) manipulated individual and not group accuracy motivation, their study provides insight into the effects of validity seeking in group contexts. Participants estimated the length of a series of lines after hearing other participants, who were actually experimental confederates, give wrong answers to the task. Participants' accuracy motivation was increased in some conditions by stressing the importance of the task and offering monetary incentives to participants for correct answers. The results replicated those of Asch's earlier research: Participants who were not highly motivated to perform well were moderately influenced by confederates' incorrect estimates, regardless of whether participants had the opportunity to inspect the lines and determine the correct answer themselves. In contrast, participants who were strongly motivated to be accurate processed others' responses more carefully. When they had an extensive opportunity to view the stimuli and could verify the correct solution, they were relatively unaffected by others' judgments; when the stimuli were presented too briefly for them to identify the correct answer clearly, they conformed markedly to others' suggestions. In most real-world task groups, members cannot easily verify the quality of suggestions. Consequently, when others' judgments are the only source of valid information, they are likely to have a strong impact even when the group task is highly important. Thus high motivation to achieve the correct answer should encourage group members to rely on all available information about solution validity, including others' suggestions and their own analysis of the issue, to decide whether to accept or reject the solutions others propose.

INFORMATIONAL VERSUS NORMATIVE MOTIVATIONS ESTABLISHED BY GROUP IDENTITY

According to social identity theory, informational and normative motives instigated by group identity are not separable, but are inextricably linked aspects of the search for a valid understanding of reality congruent with one's social identity (Abrams & Hogg, 1990; Tajfel, 1978; Turner, 1991; Turner et al., 1994). In this view, people use the normative standards of relevant reference groups to determine the validity and cogency of information. Consequently, validity-seeking and normative motives are interdependent. In a strong statement of this position, Turner (1991) argued that for self-categorization theory, "the distinction between normative and informational influence is replaced by the idea that the basic influence process is one where the normative position of people categorized as similar to self tends to be subjectively accepted as valid" (p. 171).

It would be difficult to argue with the conclusion that assessments of the validity of information ultimately rest on social consensus. This valuable insight has often been overlooked in research on message-based persuasion, which has treated validity as an intrinsic attribute of information that can be evaluated outside of social norms (see a related criticism by Moscovici, 1980). The social identity perspective, in conjunction with theories of individual information processing, provides a useful framework for identifying the social determinants of validity. Specifically, assertions supported by consensus are more likely to be perceived as valid to the extent that (1) people value the relevant social group or collectivity yielding consensus; (2) the consensus was established through the convergence of independent rather than dependent views; and (3) the consensual position is validated by an individual's own cognitive processing (Mackie & Skelly, 1994). Asch (1952) similarly stressed individual information processing in his analysis of the contingencies under

which consensus suggests validity (see Levine, 1996). In his words, a consensual response is valid only if "each individual asserts his own relation to facts and retains his individuality" (Asch, 1952, p. 494).

From the perspective of predicting and understanding social influence, however, there is good reason to maintain the distinction between informational and normative goals. Quite simply, in everyday influence contexts, people's responses vary when they are motivated by social groups to achieve the informational goal of a valid opinion or the normative goals of receiving a valued outcome or establishing a desired identity. To the extent that groups instigate these different motives, theories of social influence must also differentiate between these orientations.

PUBLIC AND PRIVATE INFLUENCE

The present perspective counters the popular assumption in social influence research that normative motives yield relatively transitory shifts in attitudes that are apparent primarily on public measures of change, and that informational motives yield more enduring shifts that are apparent on both public and private measures. Indeed, one of the striking findings from the literature on minority influence is that the normative motivations to agree with positively valued majorities and to disagree with negatively valued minorities affect both public attitude statements and private attitude judgments (Wood et al., 1994). Uniformity across public and private measures of agreement is also anticipated by self-categorization approaches to social influence (Turner, 1991).

Maintenance of attitude judgments across settings and types of attitude measures is most likely to emerge when recipients are sufficiently motivated to conduct a careful, thoughtful analysis of the (self-, other-, or issue-related) information relevant to the motivational goal, and when the goal continues to hold value across settings and measures. Stability in attitude judgments across public and private settings also can emerge from a variety of other processes, including people's after-the-fact interpretation of their publicly expressed attitudes. For example, people may internalize and privately adopt their publicly stated views through self-perception (Bem,

1972) and through cognitive-dissonance processes (Festinger, 1957). However, after-the-fact interpretations can also lead people to question the veracity of their attitude statements and can yield unstable, transitory judgments. For example, publicly expressed attitudes that are attributed to salient contextual forces, and are considered strategic pronouncements or interpersonal tactics, are unlikely to be internalized as private opinions (Cialdini et al., 1992). Thus, in attribution analyses to determine the cause of people's public attitude statements, contextual forces can serve as discounting cues that reduce the plausibility of intrinsic belief in the attitude position.

In general, then, I suggest that the distinction between public and private agreement is not a reliable indicator of the motives underlying participants' responses in social influence research. Consider Sherif's (1936/1966) classic finding that participants judging the movement of lights in the presence of others in a darkened room converged in judgment and developed seemingly arbitrary "group" norms, which were maintained when individuals later gave their judgments privately. This conformity in the "autokinetic" paradigm is commonly interpreted as an example of informational influence because of the continuity in participants' responses across public and private settings. The present review suggests, in contrast, that participants' processing goals are difficult to infer from the form of their agreement response. Although participants may have relied on others' judgments for informational reasons (i.e., they wished to attain an accurate estimate but were unable to achieve a clear assessment themselves), they also may have conformed because of normative goals (i.e., they wished to obtain favorable outcomes, such as appearing reasonable and likable to the other participants). Both of these motives can elicit enduring change.

The conformity evident in Asch's (1955, 1956) classic line-judging experiments, by contrast, is typically attributed to normative pressures. In this paradigm, participants publicly stated their own estimates of the length of a series of lines after hearing several experimental confederates provide obviously incorrect answers. The standard interpretation of participants' conformity centers on the dis-

continuity between public and private responding evident from Asch's postexperimental interviews with participants; when adopting others' judgments, most did not report believing the positions they publicly endorsed. In addition, normative pressures are suggested by the unambiguous physical stimulus, which should have obviated any need for subjects to rely on one another for information about physical reality. Because participants had to contradict objective reality in order to conform, this paradigm opposes social outcome concerns with motives to respond accurately. It is interesting to note that Asch himself did not emphasize normative factors, preferring to focus on the two-thirds of the trials in which participants resisted others' influence rather than the one-third in which they conformed (cf. Levine, 1996). Evidence suggesting the conflicting social and informational motives was provided by Bond and Smith's (1996) meta-analytic synthesis of 133 experiments that used an Asch-type conformity paradigm. Conformity increased with increasing normative pressures based on others' responses (i.e., when the majority was composed of ingroup rather than outgroup members, when the majority was larger in size) and with limits on participants' ability to meet validity-seeking goals (i.e., when the majority's incorrect answer was not easy to distinguish from the correct one). Similarly, in related research paradigms, conformity has been found to decrease when validity-seeking motives are strong—at least when people can conduct their own evaluations of the task (e.g., monetary incentives are offered for accuracy; Baron et al., 1996) and when normatively based pressures are reduced (e.g., experimental payoff schemes that apply to other group members but not participants; Ross, Bierbrauer, & Hoffman, 1976).

MOTIVATIONS AND INFORMATION PROCESSING

The overarching theme of this chapter is that a variety of motivations can be instigated by social groups to direct attitude processes. The group identities of sources and recipients direct influence by motivating recipients to be concerned with the outcomes provided by others; with their own self-definitions; and with the adoption of accurate, valid positions. People hold other-motivated attitudes because these judgments help them achieve desired interpersonal outcomes in a given social context. They hold self-defining attitudes because these views are congruent with material self-interests or with important aspects of their self-definition. People hold accuracy-motivated attitudes because these judgments reflect the "objective" truth on an issue or the most valid approach to a problem.

Understanding the motivations instigated by social groups is important because it provides insight into the manner in which people process relevant information. When people are only moderately motivated by one of these goals, their processing strategies are likely to be governed by efficiency concerns, and they may use heuristic rules or other economical strategies to evaluate the influence appeal (Chaiken, Wood, & Eagly, 1996; Chaiken, Giner-Sorolla, & Chen, 1996). As a result, the expressed attitudes are likely to be transitory and tied to specific contexts, interaction partners, or short-term social identities. To the extent that any motivation increases the desired levels of judgmental confidence or decreases actual judgmental confidence, it should increase the extensiveness of information processing (Chaiken et al., 1989). When desired confidence is especially high, people presumably conduct a more careful, thoughtful analysis of the relevant information. Moreover, any shifts in judgment are likely to be relatively stable, reflecting enduring change. Note that these various types of processing are not necessarily mutually exclusive; when individuals are motivated to conduct a careful, thoughtful analysis, they are also likely to simultaneously pursue more efficient strategies, such as heuristic rules. The conclusions reached through one analysis may augment or detract from the conclusions reached through other analyses, or they may have no impact on each other (Chaiken et al., 1989).

In addition, understanding the motives instigated by groups is important because people's motivations focus their processing on goal-relevant thoughts, feelings, and behaviors. People motivated to attain positive and avoid negative outcomes provided by others are likely to consider the social consequences of their attitudes and to adopt positions most likely to yield the desired result (e.g., more favorably evaluating positions yielding reward than yielding punishment). People motivated by self-related concerns to identify with positively valued social groups and to differentiate themselves from derogated groups are likely to process information in a manner that allows them to achieve these normative goals (e.g., more favorably evaluating positions taken by valued than by derogated groups). People motivated by validity seeking are likely to process information in a way that they believe will yield an accurate judgment (e.g., more favorably evaluating cogent than specious positions).

I speculate also that normative and informational motivations affect how judgments are represented in memory. When normative concerns based on interpersonal outcomes are salient, and attitudes are generated in response to the rewards and punishments that a group can deliver, attitudes are likely to be represented in memory as part of achieving interpersonal goals and to be endorsed as long as these outcomes remain salient and retain their value. When self-related normative concerns are salient, and attitudes are generated in response to the implications of social group positions for recipients' identity, attitudes are likely to be represented in memory as part of the self-concept and to be endorsed as long as this self-view is salient and valued. In contrast, when a validity-seeking motivation is primary, and attitudes are generated in response to the cogency of information, attitudes are more likely to be embedded in cognitive structures related to the attitude object itself or the broader values tied to it, and maintenance of the relevant attitude will depend on the accessibility of these structures.

Echabe, Guede, and Castro's (1994) investigation of beliefs about smoking provides preliminary support for the idea that attitude structure is related to function, at least with respect to self-related attitudes. In the study, smokers' beliefs proved to be organized around their self-identification with the group, so that those who identified with it also endorsed favorable beliefs about smoking. Nonsmokers' beliefs, in contrast, were organized around negative personal attributes of smokers; to the extent that they believed in this stereotype, they also endorsed other negative beliefs. Echabe et al. (1994) suggest that smokers, like other stigmatized groups, organize group-related information in a defensive manner, and link attitudes and beliefs together in terms of judged relevance for their self-concept.

RESEARCHING MOTIVES IN PERSUASION AND SOCIAL INFLUENCE PARADIGMS

The single motivational theme of accuracy seeking has predominated in the history of message-based persuasion research. Persuasion researchers have devised a variety of measures to identify the extent to which participants are motivated by accuracy concerns, and they have elegantly documented the effects of this motive on information processing (Eagly & Chaiken, 1993; Petty & Cacioppo, 1986). Social influence paradigms have the advantage of considering a broader range of possible motivations, including (self- and other-related) normative concerns along with validity seeking. Unfortunately, the research methods in social influence paradigms typically have not matched the sophistication of this dual-motive scheme. The central variables of interest have usually not been assessed directly; only rarely have researchers assessed the motives instigated in the influence setting or the information-processing mechanisms through which these motives yield influence and resistance.

A call for measures to distinguish among the variety of motives established by source group identity may seem like yet another tired reminder of the need for manipulation checks in experimental research. The lack of standard procedures to assess the meaning of source group identity is, however, a real problem that hinders cumulative integration of social influence research findings (see also Levine & Russo, 1987). Indeed, to explain the outcomes of a number of studies, I have often been forced in the present review to speculate about the likely motivation established by source groups.

It may be argued that measures of the goals established by source group identity are not always necessary to predict influence and other group behaviors. In Tajfel's minimal-group paradigm, for example, a generic perception of oneself-as-group-member emerges

with the categorization processes involved in differentiating people into groups. In this research, ingroup and outgroup identities can be formed from merely dividing people into groups based on trivial criteria or random assignment (Billig & Tajfel, 1973; Tajfel & Billig, 1974; Rabbie & Horwitz, 1969). Tajfel (1982) maintained, however, that group identity involves more than simple categorization. Supposedly it depends on personal identification with the group (i.e., knowledge of group membership, along with the value and emotional significance of that membership) and on the external, social definition of the group or category. In support, research that has obtained participants' ratings of their identification with a group has revealed the usefulness of such ratings, demonstrating, for example, that discrimination toward outgroups occurs primarily among participants who personally identify with their ingroup (e.g., Gagnon & Bourhis, 1996).

In research on minority influence, the assumption that a source's minority status elicits a standard cognitive representation for recipients has similarly discouraged checks on the motivations established by the minority identity. Moskowitz (1996) makes a similar point, arguing that the standard definition of a "minority" in numerical terms (e.g., the percentage of a population that holds a deviant opinion) has led researchers to ignore the prior expectancies, attributional biases, and needs for a positive social identity that guide processing of appeals from minority social groups. Whatever the reason for disregarding the nature of minority identity, it is now clear that "minority" refers to a heterogeneous category. Indeed, the Wood et al. (1994) review revealed that different types of minorities yielded characteristically different influence effects. Studies in which the source was a member of a minority social group (e.g., civil libertarians) appeared to generate the standard pattern of greater indirect than direct agreement, presumably because recipients were motivated to differentiate themselves from the source on direct measures. However, studies in which the minority source held positions endorsed by a small percentage of the population appeared to yield no systematic influence effects, presumably because this source identity established no clear motivation for recipients.

A variety of strategies can be used to assess group-related motivations, although most of these have been tailored to evaluate the extent of self-related normative motives established by groups. Ratings of the extent to which respondents identify with a group have proved to be effective measures of a group's self-related importance (e.g., Crocker & Luhtanen, 1990; Hogg & Hains, 1996; Pool et al., 1998; Wood et al., 1996). The self-related impact of a group potentially can also be assessed through more objective measures, such as the frequency with which participants engage in group activities. Similarly, in research on other-related motives, assessments of the extent to which participants are concerned about attaining positive outcomes and avoiding negative outcomes should be useful in predicting the extent to which the groups that deliver these outcomes are likely to exert influence. Direct assessment or manipulation of the group attributes that instigate these motives may also be useful, such as the actual ability of the group to deliver rewards and punishments (e.g., group resources and immediacy). It is unlikely, however, that validity-seeking motives instigated by groups can be assessed through self-report measures of the importance of achieving a valid, accurate judgment. Most people believe that their judgments are valid, regardless of the extent to which they are motivated by validity seeking (or other concerns), and such ratings may be uniformly high. Instead, researchers may want to manipulate a feature of the group that instigates validity motives, and to assess perceptions of that feature. For example, validity-seeking motives may be enhanced through incentives for accurate group performance.

CONCLUSION

The approach to social influence taken in this chapter builds on the informational mechanisms identified in dual-process models of persuasion (Chaiken, Liberman, & Eagly, 1989; Petty & Cacioppo, 1986) and includes the broad range of informational and social motives instigated by group identity (Kelley, 1952). When motivated by normative concerns, people try to obtain favorable outcomes provided by others and to avoid unfa-

vorable ones, and they try to maintain and bolster a coherent, positive self-view. When motivated to achieve informational goals, people try to identify a valid, accurate position. These motives affect people's judgments by directing the way they process information about the source and the influence appeal. Motives direct attention to relevant information, instigate favorable evaluation of information that meets people's goals, and direct the organization and retrieval of judgment-relevant information in memory.

Given that the content of the appeal in social influence paradigms is typically less rich and provides less information than that in persuasion studies, information processing has unique features in influence contexts. In addition to attention, evaluation, organization, and retrieval, groups direct interpretation of attitude issues. In daily life, the interpretative framework provided by valued groups determines, for example, whether abortion is murder or a woman's right to choose, and whether capital punishment represents justified retribution, an effective crime deterrent, or inhumane treatment. The other-provided outcomes, social identity concerns, or informational goals that motivate people to adopt or reject a group's position work by guiding how people think about the issue, including the way they interpret what the issue means.

ACKNOWLEDGMENT

Preparation of this chapter was supported by Grant No. SBR-9514537 from the National Science Foundation.

NOTES

1. Indirect measures assess change in attitudes without recipients' awareness that their responses indicate acceptance or rejection of the advocated position. For example, the source may advocate that corporations are primarily responsible for pollution, and an indirect measure of acceptance of this position may be recipients' disagreement with the idea that individuals are primarily responsible for pollution.

2. Presumably, members accorded higher performance expectations typically provide better-quality, more accurate suggestions than lower expectation members, and for this reason expectations serve as a reliable heuristic cue to the relative

validity of each member's contributions. However, performance expectations are no guarantee of the quality of any given suggestion or of any member's ideas. For example, expectations that are based on general social attributes that are not tied to actual task competence (e.g., social stereotypes that value men's performance at many tasks above women's) are likely to be poor indicators of members' actual task contributions, and reliance on such expectations will not maximize group performance.

REFERENCES

Abelson, R. P. (1959). Modes of resolution of belief dilemmas. *Journal of Conflict Resolution, 3,* 343–352.

Abrams, D., & Hogg, M. A. (1988). Comments on the motivational status of self-esteem in social identity and intergroup discrimination. *European Journal of Social Psychology, 18,* 317–334.

Abrams, D., & Hogg, M. A. (1990). Social identification, self-categorization, and social influence. In W. Stroebe & M. Hewston (Eds.), *European review of social psychology* (Vol. 1, pp. 195–228). Chichester, England: Wiley.

Allen, V. L., & Wilder, D. A. (1980). Impact of group consensus and social support on stimulus meaning: Mediation of conformity by cognitive restructuring. *Journal of Personality and Social Psychology, 39,* 1116–1124.

Alvaro, E. M., & Crano, W. D. (1996). Cognitive responses to minority- or majority-based communications: Factors that underlie minority influence. *British Journal of Social Psychology, 35,* 105–121.

Alvaro, E. M., & Crano, W. D. (1997). Indirect minority influence: Evidence for leniency in source evaluation and counterargumentation. *Journal of Personality and Social Psychology, 72,* 949–964.

Asch, S. E. (1940). Studies in the principles of judgments and attitudes: II. Determination of judgments by groups and ego standards. *Journal of Social Psychology, 41,* 258–290.

Asch, S. E. (1948). The doctrine of suggestion, prestige, and imitation in social psychology. *Psychological Review, 55,* 250–276.

Asch, S. E. (1952). *Social psychology.* New York: Prentice-Hall.

Asch, S. E. (1955). Opinions and social pressure. *Scientific American, 193,* 31–35.

Asch, S. E. (1956). Studies of independence and conformity: I. A minority of one against a unanimous majority. *Psychological Monographs: General and Applied, 70*(Whole No. 416), 1–70.

Babcock, D., & Wood, W. (1998). *When is forewarned fore-armed?: A meta-analytic synthesis of forewarnings of influence appeals.* Unpublished manuscript, Texas A&M University.

Baker, S. M., & Petty, R. E. (1994). Majority and minority influence: Source–position imbalance as a determinant of message scrutiny. *Journal of Personality and Social Psychology, 67,* 5–19.

Baldwin, M. W., & Holmes, J. G. (1987). Salient private audiences and awareness of the self. *Journal of Personality and Social Psychology, 52,* 1087–1098.

Bales, R. F. (1953). The equilibrium problem in small groups. In T. Parsons, R. F. Bales, & E. A. Shills (Eds.), *Working papers in the theory of action* (pp. 111–161). Glencoe, IL: Free Press.

Baron, R. S., Vandello, J. A., & Brunsman, B. (1996). The forgotten variable in conformity research: Impact of task importance on social influence. *Journal of Personality and Social Psychology, 71,* 915–927.

Bem, D. J. (1972) Self-perception theory. In L. Berkowitz (Ed.), *Advances in experimental social psychology* (Vol. 6, pp. 1–62). New York: Academic Press.

Berger, J., Fisek, M. H., Norman, R. Z., & Zelditch, M., Jr. (1977). *Status characteristics and social interaction.* New York: Elsevier.

Billig, M. G., & Tajfel, H. (1973). Social categorization and similarity in intergroup behavior. *European Journal of Social Psychology, 3,* 27–51.

Bond, R., & Smith, P. B. (1996). Culture and conformity: A meta-analysis of studies using Asch's (1952, 1956) line judgment task. *Psychological Bulletin, 119,* 111–137.

Brewer, M. B. (1991). The social self: On being the same and different at the same time. *Personality and Social Psychology Bulletin, 17,* 475–582.

Buehler, R., & Griffin, D. (1994). Change-of-meaning effects in conformity and dissent: Observing construal processes over time. *Journal of Personality and Social Psychology, 67,* 984–996.

Chaiken, S. (1980). Heuristic versus systematic information processing and the use of source versus message cues in persuasion. *Journal of Personality and Social Psychology, 39,* 752–766.

Chaiken, S., Giner-Sorolla, R., & Chen, S. (1996). Beyond accuracy: Defense and impression motives in heuristic and systematic information processing. In P. M. Gollwitzer & J. A. Bargh (Eds.), *The psychology of action: Linking motivation and cognition to behavior* (pp. 553–578). New York: Guilford Press.

Chaiken, S., Liberman, A., & Eagly, A. H. (1989). Heuristic and systematic information processing within and beyond the persuasion context. In J. S. Uleman & J. A. Bargh (Eds.), *Unintended thought* (pp. 212–252). New York: Guilford Press.

Chaiken, S., Wood, W., & Eagly, A. H. (1996). Principles of persuasion. In E. T. Higgins & A. Kruglanski (Eds.), *Social psychology: Handbook of basic principles* (pp. 702–742). New York: Guilford Press.

Chen, S., Schechter, D., & Chaiken, S. (1996). Getting at the truth or getting along: Accuracy- versus impression-motivated heuristic and systematic processing. *Journal of Personality and Social Psychology, 71,* 262–275.

Cialdini, R. B., Green, B. L., & Rusch, A. J. (1992). When tactical pronouncements of change become real change: The case of reciprocal persuasion. *Journal of Personality and Social Psychology, 63,* 30–40.

Cialdini, R. B., & Petty, R. E. (1981). Anticipatory opinion effects. In R. E. Petty, T. M. Ostrom, & T. C. Brock (Eds.), *Cognitive responses in persuasion* (pp. 217–235). Hillsdale, NJ: Erlbaum.

Cook, T. D., Gruder, C. L., Hennigan, K. M., & Flay, B. R. (1979). History of the sleeper effect: Some logical pitfalls in accepting the null hypothesis. *Psychological Bulletin, 86,* 662–679.

Crano, W. D. (1991, October). *Minority and majority influence: Prescriptions for future research.* Paper presented at the annual meeting of the Society for Experimental Social Psychology, Columbus, OH.

Crocker, J., & Luhtanen, R. (1990). Collective self-esteem and ingroup bias. *Journal of Personality and Social Psychology, 58,* 60–67.

Deutsch, M., & Gerard, H. B. (1955). A study of normative and informational social influences upon individual judgment. *Journal of Abnormal and Social Psychology, 51,* 629–636.

De Vries, N. K., De Dreu, C. K. W., Gordijn, E., & Schuurman, M. (1996). Majority and minority influence: A dual role interpretation. In W. Stroebe & M. Hewstone (Eds.), *European review of social psychology* (Vol. 7, pp. 145–172). Chichester, England: Wiley.

Eagly, A. H., & Chaiken, S. (1993). *The psychology of attitudes.* Orlando, FL: Harcourt, Brace, Jovanovich.

Echabe, E. A., Guede, E. F., & Castro, J. L. G. (1994). Social representations and intergroup conflicts: Who's smoking here? *European Journal of Social Psychology, 24,* 339–355.

Festinger, L. (1950). Informal social communication. *Psychological Review, 57,* 271–282.

Festinger, L. (1957). *A theory of cognitive dissonance.* Evanston, IL: Row Peterson.

French, J. R. P., Jr. (1956). A formal theory of social power. *Psychological Review, 63,* 181–194.

French, J. R. P., Jr., & Raven, B. (1959). The bases of social power. In D. Cartwright (Ed.), *Studies in social power* (pp. 150–167). Ann Arbor: University of Michigan Press.

Gagnon, A., & Bourhis, R. Y. (1996). Discrimination in the minimal group paradigm: Social identity or self-interest? *Personality and Social Psychology Bulletin, 22,* 1289–1301.

Giner-Sorolla, R., & Chaiken, S. (1994). The causes of hostile media judgments. *Journal of Experimental Social Psychology, 30,* 165–180.

Greenwald, A. G., & Breckler, S. J. (1985). To whom is the self presented? In B. R. Schlenker (Eds.), *The self and social life* (pp. 126–145). New York: McGraw-Hill.

Heider, F. (1958). *The psychology of interpersonal relations.* New York: Wiley.

Higgins, E. T. (1992). Achieving 'shared reality' in the communication game: A social action that creates meaning. *Journal of Language and Social Psychology, 11,* 107–131.

Hogg, M., & Abrams, D. (1993). Towards a single-process uncertainty-reduction model of social motivation in groups. In M. A. Hogg & D. Abrams (Eds.), *Group motivation: Social psychological perspectives* (pp. 173–190). London: Harvester Wheatsheaf.

Hogg, M. A., & Hains, S. C. (1996). Intergroup relations and group solidarity: Effects of group identification and social beliefs on depersonalized attraction. *Journal of Personality and Social Psychology, 70,* 295–309.

Hogg, M. A., & Turner, J. C. (1987). Social identity and conformity: A theory of referent informational influence. In W. Doise & S. Moscovici (Eds.), *Current issues in European social psychology* (Vol. 2, pp. 139–182). Cambridge, England: Cambridge University Press.

Hovland, C. I., Janis, I. L., & Kelley, H. H. (1953). *Communication and persuasion: Psychological studies of opinion change.* New Haven, CT: Yale University Press.

Hyman, H. H. (1942). *The psychology of status.* New York: Archives of Psychology, No. 269.

Hyman, H. H. (1960). Reflections on reference groups. *Public Opinion Quarterly, 24,* 383–396.

Isenberg, D. J. (1986). Group polarization: A critical review and meta-analysis. *Journal of Personality and Social Psychology, 50,* 1141–1151.

Johnson, B. T., & Eagly, A. H. (1989). The effects of involvement on persuasion: A meta-analysis. *Psychological Bulletin, 106,* 290–314.

Jones, E. E., & Gerard, H. B. (1967). *Foundations of social psychology.* New York: Wiley.

Katz, D. (1960). The functional approach to the study of attitudes. *Public Opinion Quarterly, 24,* 163–204.

Kelley, H. H. (1952). Two functions of reference groups. In G. E. Swanson, T. M. Newcomb, & E. L. Hartley (Eds.), *Readings in social psychology* (2nd ed., pp. 410–414). New York: Holt.

Kelley, H. H. (1955). Salience of membership and resistance to change of group-anchored attitudes. *Human Relations, 8,* 275–289.

Kelley, H. H., & Volkart, E. H. (1952). The resistance to change of group anchored attitudes. *American Sociological Review, 17,* 453–465.

Kelman, H. C. (1958). Compliance, identification, and internalization: Three processes of attitude change. *Journal of Conflict Resolution, 2,* 51–60.

Kelman, H. C. (1961). Processes of opinion change. *Public Opinion Quarterly, 25,* 57–78.

Kerlinger, F. N. (1984). *Liberalism and conservatism: The nature and structure of social attitudes.* Hillsdale, NJ: Erlbaum.

Levine, J. M. (1996, October). *Solomon Asch's legacy for group research.* Paper presented at the annual meeting of the Society for Experimental Social Psychology, Sturbridge, MA.

Levine, J. M., & Russo, E. M. (1987). Majority and minority influence. In C. Hendrick (Ed.), *Review of personality and social psychology: Vol. 8. Group processes* (pp. 13–54). Newbury Park, CA: Sage.

Liberman, A., & Chaiken, S. (1996). The direct effect of personal relevance on attitudes. *Personality and Social Psychology Bulletin, 22,* 269–279.

Maass, A., & Clark, R. D., III. (1983). Internalization versus compliance: Differential processes underlying minority influence and conformity. *European Journal of Social Psychology, 13,* 197–215.

Maass, A., Volpato, C., & Mucchi-Faina, A. (1996). Social influence and the verifiability of the issue under discussion: Attitudinal versus objective items. *British Journal of Social Psychology, 35,* 15–26.

Maass, A., West, S. G., & Cialdini, R. B. (1987). Minority influence and conversion. In C. Hendrick (Ed.), *Review of personality and social psychology: Vol. 8. Group processes* (pp. 55–79). Beverly Hills, CA: Sage.

Mackie, D. M. (1987). Systematic and nonsystematic processing of majority and minority persuasive communications. *Journal of Personality and Social Psychology, 53,* 41–52.

Mackie, D. M., & Skelly, J. (1994). The social cognition analysis of social influence: Contributions to the understanding of persuasion and conformity. In P. Devine, D. Hamilton, & T. Ostrom (Eds.), *Social cog-*

nition: Impact on social psychology (pp. 259–289). San Diego, CA: Academic Press.

Martin, R. (1996). Minority influence and argument generation. *British Journal of Social Psychology, 35,* 91–104.

McGarty, C., Turner, J. C., Oakes, P. J., & Haslam, S. A. (1993). The creation of uncertainty in the influence process: The roles of stimulus information and disagreement with similar others. *European Journal of Social Psychology, 23,* 17–38.

McGuire, W. J., & McGuire, C. V. (1992). Cognitive-versus-affective positivity asymmetries in thought systems. *European Journal of Social Psychology, 22,* 571–591.

McGuire, W. J., & McGuire, C. V. (1996). Enhancing self-esteem by direct-thinking tasks: Cognitive and affective positivity asymmetries. *Journal of Personality and Social Psychology, 70,* 1117–1125.

Merton, R. K. (1957). Continuities in the theory of reference groups and social structure. In R. K. Merton (Ed.), *Social theory and social structure* (rev. ed., pp. 281–386). Glencoe, IL: Free Press.

Moscovici, S. (1980). Toward a theory of conversion behavior. In L. Berkowitz (Ed.), *Advances in experimental social psychology* (Vol. 13, pp. 209–239). New York: Academic Press.

Moscovici, S. (1985a). Innovation and minority influence. In S. Moscovici, G. Mugny, & E. Van Avermaet (Eds.), *Perspectives on minority influence* (pp. 9–52). Cambridge, England: Cambridge University Press.

Moscovici, S. (1985b). Social influence and conformity. In G. Lindzey & E. Aronson (Eds.), *Handbook of social psychology* (3rd ed., Vol. 2, pp. 347–412). New York: Random House.

Moscovici, S., & Lage, E. (1978). Studies in social influence IV: Minority influence in the context of original judgements. *European Journal of Social Psychology, 8,* 349–365.

Moskowitz, G. B. (1996). The mediational effects of attributions and information processing in minority social influence. *British Journal of Social Psychology, 35,* 47–66.

Mucchi-Faina, A., Maass, A., & Volpato, C. (1991). Social influence: The role of originality. *European Journal of Social Psychology, 21,* 183–197.

Nemeth, C. J. (1986). Differential contributions of majority and minority influence. *Psychological Review, 93,* 23–32.

Nemeth, C. J., & Chiles, C. (1988). Modelling courage: The role of dissent in fostering independence. *European Journal of Social Psychology, 18,* 275–280.

Nemeth, C. J., Mayseless, O., Sherman, J., & Brown, Y. (1990). Exposure to dissent and recall of information. *Journal of Personality and Social Psychology, 58,* 429–437.

Nemeth, C. J., & Rogers, J. (1996). Dissent and the search for information. *British Journal of Social Psychology, 35,* 67–76.

Newcomb, T. M. (1950). *Social psychology.* New York: Dryden.

Perez, J. A., Papastamou, S., & Mugny, G. (1995). 'Zeitgeist' and minority influence—where is the causality: A comment on Clark (1990). *European Journal of Social Psychology, 25,* 703–710.

Petty, R. E., & Cacioppo, J. T. (1986). The elaboration likelihood model of persuasion. In L. Berkowitz (Ed.),

Advances in experimental social psychology (Vol. 19, pp. 123–205). Orlando, FL: Academic Press.

Pool, G., Wood, W., & Leck, K. (1998). The self-esteem motive in social influence: Agreement with valued majorities and disagreement with derogated minorities. *Journal of Personality and Social Psychology, 75,* 967–975.

Pool, G., Wood, W., & Leck, K. (1997). [Misrecall of group positions]. Unpublished raw data, Texas A&M University.

Rabbie, J. M., & Horwitz, M. (1969). The arousal of ingroup and outgroup bias by a chance to win or lose. *Journal of Personality and Social Psychology, 69,* 223–228.

Ridgeway, C. L. (1984). Dominance, performance, and status in groups. In E. J. Lawler (Ed.), *Advances in group processes* (Vol. 1, pp 59–93). Greenwich, CT: JAI Press.

Ridgeway, C. L., & Diekema, D. (1989). Dominance and collective hierarchy formation in male and female task groups. *American Sociological Review, 54,* 79–93.

Rosenberg, M. (1965). *Society and the adolescent self-image.* Princeton, NJ: Princeton University Press.

Ross, L., Bierbrauer, G., & Hoffman, S. (1976). The role of attribution processes in conformity and dissent: Revisiting the Asch situation. *American Psychologist, 31,* 148–157.

Schlenker, B. R. (1980). *Impression management: The self-concept, social identity, and interpersonal relations.* Monterey, CA: Brooks/Cole.

Sherif, M. (1966). *The psychology of social norms.* New York: Harper & Row. (Original work published 1936)

Sherif, M., & Hovland, C. I. (1953). Judgmental phenomena and scales of attitude measurement: Placement of items with individual choice of number of categories. *Journal of Abnormal and Social Psychology, 48,* 135–141.

Sherif, M., & Hovland, C. I. (1961). *Social judgment: Assimilation and contrast effects in communication and attitude change.* New Haven, CT: Yale University Press.

Smith, C. M., Tindale, R. S., & Dugoni, B. L. (1996). Minority and majority influence in freely interacting groups: Qualitative versus quantitative differences. *British Journal of Social Psychology, 35,* 137–150.

Smith, M. B., Bruner, J. S., & White, R. W. (1956). *Opinions and personality.* New York: Wiley.

Swann, W. B., Jr. (1990). To be adored or to be known?: The interplay of self-enhancement and self-verification. In E. T. Higgins & R. M. Sorrentino (Eds.), *Handbook of motivation and cognition: Foundations of social behavior* (Vol. 2, pp. 408–448). New York: Guilford Press.

Tajfel, H. (1978). *Differentiation between social groups: Studies in the social psychology of intergroup relations.* London: Academic Press.

Tajfel, H. (1981). *Human groups and social categories: Studies in social psychology.* Cambridge, England: Cambridge University Press.

Tajfel, H. (1982). Social psychology of intergroup relations. *Annual Review of Psychology, 33,* 1–39.

Tajfel, H., & Billig, M. (1974). Familiarity and categorization in intergroup behavior. *Journal of Experimental Social Psychology, 10,* 159–170.

Tesser, A. (1988). Toward a self-evaluation maintenance model of social behavior. In L. Berkowitz (Ed.), *Ad-*

vances in experimental social psychology (Vol. 21, pp. 181–227). New York: Academic Press.

Tesser, A., Campbell, J. A., & Mickler, S. (1983). The role of social pressure, attention to the stimulus, and self-doubt in conformity. European Journal of Social Psychology, 13, 217–234.

Tetlock, P. E., & Manstead, A. S. R. (1985). Impression management versus intrapsychic explanations in social psychology: A useful dichotomy? Psychological Review, 92, 59–77.

Tourangeau, R., Rasinski, K. A., & D'Andrade, R. (1991). Attitude structure and belief accessibility. Journal of Experimental Social Psychology, 27, 48–75.

Trost, M. R., Maass, A., & Kenrick, D. T. (1992). Minority influence: Personal relevance biases cognitive processes and reverses private acceptance. Journal of Experimental Social Psychology, 28, 234–254.

Turner, J. C. (1982). Towards a cognitive redefinition of the social group. In H. Tajfel (Ed.), Social identity and intergroup relations (pp. 15–40). Cambridge, England: Cambridge University Press.

Turner, J. C. (1991). Social influence. Pacific Grove, CA: Brooks/Cole.

Turner, J. C., & Oakes, P. J. (1989). Self-categorization theory and social influence. In P. B. Paulus (Ed.), The psychology of group influence (2nd ed., pp. 233–275). Hillsdale, NJ: Erlbaum.

Turner, J. C., Oakes, P. J., Haslam, S. A., & McGarty, C. (1994). Self and collective: Cognition and social context. Personality and Social Psychology Bulletin, 20, 454–463.

Vallone, R. P., Ross, L., & Lepper, M. R. (1985). The hostile media phenomenon: Biased perceptions of media bias in coverage of the Beirut massacre. Journal of Personality and Social Psychology, 49, 577–585.

Webster, M. Jr., & Foschi, M. (1988). Status generalization: New theory and research. Stanford, CA: Stanford University Press.

Wood, W., Lundgren, S., Ouellette, J., Busceme, S., & Blackstone, T. (1994). Minority influence: A meta-analytic review of social influence processes. Psychological Bulletin, 115, 323–345.

Wood, W., Pool, G., Leck, K., & Purvis, D. (1996). Self-definition, defensive processing, and influence: The normative impact of majority and minority groups. Journal of Personality and Social Psychology, 71, 1181–1193.

28

The Social Contingency Model

IDENTIFYING EMPIRICAL AND NORMATIVE
BOUNDARY CONDITIONS ON THE ERROR-AND-BIAS
PORTRAIT OF HUMAN NATURE

PHILIP E. TETLOCK
JENNIFER S. LERNER

About 20 years ago, the first author of this chapter began his first study of accountability—although he did not categorize it as such at the time. Levi and Tetlock (1980) were interested in constructing cognitive maps of the Japanese decision to go to war with the United States in 1941. They quite accidentally discovered that the cognitive maps of Japanese decision making looked different, depending on whether they constructed those maps from the verbatim deliberations of the Liaison conferences (at which military leaders actually made policy decisions) or from the Imperial conferences (at which those same leaders justified their decisions before the Emperor and his advisors). By the fall of 1941, there was relatively little tolerance in the Liaison conferences for dissenters who wanted to avoid military confrontation with the United States; there was accordingly little need to anticipate such objections and to incorporate them into the group's shared assessment of Japan's geopolitical predicament. The Emperor and his key advisors, however, were known to be skeptical about the wisdom of attacking a country with a vastly larger economy. When

the military leaders came before this high-status audience, they went to considerable lengths to demonstrate that they had thought through all the alternatives, weighed the pertinent tradeoffs, and worked through the necessary contingency plans. As a result, the cognitive maps in the Imperial conferences were considerably more complex—with more references to interactive causation and trade-offs—than were the cognitive maps derived from the Liaison conferences. In the spirit of this volume, we might say that a dual-process model fits these two levels of the Japanese decision-making process.

This chapter examines the evolution of research on the impact of accountability on judgment and choice over the last 20 years. The story to be told is one of progressive "complexification," in which temptingly parsimonious hypotheses have been repeatedly confounded by recalcitrantly complex patterns of evidence. One example is the pure-impression-management model of how people cope with accountability. This model gained empirical sustenance from findings that people often respond to pressures to justify their views via the low-effort expedient of simply shifting their views toward those of the anticipated audience (Cialdini, Levy, Herman, Kozlowski, & Petty, 1976; Jones & Wortman, 1973). Moreover, some people apparently do not internalize these public presentations, and as soon as it is convenient, they "snap back" in elastic-band fashion to their original position.

Using a variety of methodological strategies, later work demonstrated, however, that accountability effects are not strictly confined to public posturing. There are conditions under which people cope with accountability by resorting to more complex, self-critical, and effort-demanding strategies of information processing (Tetlock, 1992; Lerner & Tetlock, in press). Accountability can affect not only what people say they think, but also how they actually do think. Although it was a valuable corrective to a purely impression-management model, this line of research encouraged a second misconception of the "It is nothing but . . . " type: the tendency to treat accountability manipulations as simply generic motivators of cognitive effort that can be subsumed under the same category as financial incentives (Stone & Ziebart, 1995), personal involvement (Petty & Cacioppo, 1986), outcome dependency (Fiske & Neuberg, 1990), decision importance (McAllister, Mitchell, & Beach, 1979), and market competition (Camerer, 1995). One problem with lumping these diverse constructs and manipulations into the same equivalence class is that different types of accountability can have very different effects on the content and character of thought. As we shall soon see, much depends on whether the views of the prospective audience are known or unknown; on whether people learn of being accountable before or after exposure to the evidence on which they are asked to base their judgments; on whether people learn of being accountable before or after making a difficult-to-reverse public commitment; and on a host of other particular details that define the ground rules of the accountability relationship.

It is also tempting, but equally misleading, to posit that those forms of accountability that do encourage self-critical thinking automatically enhance the quality of judgment and choice. It is tempting because several experiments have revealed the power of certain types of accountability to induce more self-critical patterns of thinking, which in turn attenuate response tendencies widely considered to be inferential biases and shortcomings (Chaiken, 1980; Hagafors & Brehmer, 1983; Kassin, Castillo, & Rigby, 1991; Lerner, Golberg, & Tetlock, 1996; Rozelle & Baxter, 1981; Tetlock, 1992). It is misleading because a substantial body of work also highlights when these same types of accountability amplify response tendencies widely considered to be errors and biases, such as the tendency to dilute one's confidence in predictions in reaction to nondiagnostic evidence (Tetlock & Boettger, 1989; Tetlock, Lerner, & Boettger, 1996), the tendency for the choice process to be swayed by the introduction of irrelevant (dominated) alternatives in choice tasks (Simonson, 1989), and the tendency to stick with the status quo when changing social policy requires imposing losses on identifiable subgroups (notwithstanding that the net benefit to society as a whole would be substantial; Tetlock & Boettger, 1994). These results should remind us that although cognitive effort triggered by accountability can be channeled in the direction of thoughtful self-criticism that checks biases rooted in overreliance on easy-to-execute heuristics, it can also be channeled in a host of potentially maladaptive directions. Decision makers can become paralyzed in self-doubt; they may be so anxious to avoid criticism that they take obsessive precautions against worst-case scenarios and are easily distracted in environments with unfavorable signal-to-noise ratios (Tetlock, 1992). Or decision makers can become mired in self-justification; they may be so anxious to defend past commitments that the majority of their mental effort is devoted to generating reasons why they are right and their would-be critics are wrong (Brockner & Rubin, 1985; Staw, 1980; Tetlock, Skitka, & Boettger, 1989). Or decision makers may devote cognitive effort to thinking of ways to beat the system—to exploiting loopholes in the accountability ground rules that organizations inevitably create (Tetlock, 1998b). Which of these directions cognitive effort takes hinges on the cognitive style of the decision maker, on the character of the relationship between decision maker and audience(s), and on the content of the internalized dialogue triggered by the expectation of justifying one's opinions and actions.

There is also a final layer of complexity. Accountability research entails more than the identification of social-contextual moderator variables that amplify or attenuate already well-replicated judgmental tendencies. It also requires careful analysis of whether we are justified—and in whose eyes—in labeling these tendencies "errors" or "biases" once we consider the social and political (as well as cognitive) functions served by processing information in certain ways and by expressing conclusions in certain ways. Judgmental tendencies that look flawed if we assume that people are striving to be good intuitive scientists or economists (trying to understand the world or to maximize expected utility) often look quite reasonable if we view them through an alternative set of functionalist lenses and posit people to be intuitive politicians striving to protect their social identities in the eyes of key constituencies (Tetlock, 1992, 1998a, 1998c). For most of this chapter, we work with the prevailing practice that an effect is an error or bias if it deviates from a normative model anchored in a functionalist model that portrays people as intuitive scientists or intuitive economists. If people are trying to explain and predict the surrounding world, then response tendencies such as overattribution, overconfidence, and dilution are indeed maladaptive; if people are trying to maximize expected utility, then they should not be influenced by irrelevant information such as dominated alternatives, sunk costs, and the nature of the status quo, and they should be influenced by relevant information such as opportunity costs. But these same effects that look dysfunctional within these "cognitivist" frameworks that treat an individual in isolation from his or her social environment often look highly adaptive within a functionalist framework that imbeds the individual within complex networks of accountability relationships and stresses the individual's goal of preserving and enhancing those relationships. Savvy politicians appreciate the importance of appearing to be attentive to conversational partners (even if that sometimes means diluting their predictions in response to "nondiagnostic cues"), of defending their reputations as rational decision makers (even if that means trying to recoup sunk costs), of holding others strictly responsible for their actions (even if that means "overattributing" to dispositional causes), and of giving preference to easily justified response options (even if that means being swayed by dominated options that make one option "look better" for specious but persuasive reasons).

THE SOCIAL CONTINGENCY MODEL

Accountability is a potentially vast topic. It can be studied experimentally (the focus of this chapter), but it can also be studied in a wide range of institutional settings in which debates over who should be answerable to whom, and under what ground rules, are central to the political contest for power (March & Olson, 1995). It is easy to get lost without some kind of theoretical road map. Our preferred map is the social contingency model of (SCM) accountability. Here we sketch the SCM's key assumptions about motives and coping strategies.

1. The universality of accountability. People do some things alone, but it is difficult to escape the evaluative scrutiny of others in a complex, interdependent society. Escape arguably becomes impossible if we count self-accountability—the obligation that most human beings (excluding psychopaths) feel to internalized mental representations of significant others who keep conscientious watch over them when no one else is looking (Mead, 1934; Schlenker, 1980, 1985). In this most abstract sense, accountability is the missing link in the seemingly perpetual level-of-analysis controversy; it is the connection between individual decision makers and the collectivities within which they live and work. Accountability serves as a linkage construct by continually reminding people of the need to (a) act in accord with prevailing norms, and (b) advance compelling justifications or excuses for conduct that deviates from those norms.[1]

2. The motive to seek audience approval. It is useful to think of people as intuitive politicians who seek the approval of the constituencies to whom they feel accountable. People do so for combinations of intrinsic and extrinsic reasons. Evidence for an intrinsic ap-

proval motive comes from laboratory studies that point to a propensity that appears early in human development to respond automatically and viscerally to signs of censure (frowns, angry words, contemptuous looks). One can interpret this robust finding (Baumeister & Leary, 1995) in either a social learning framework (over the course of a lifetime, other people become incredibly potent secondary reinforcers by virtue of their association with primary drive reduction) or in an evolutionary framework (people have been naturally and sexually selected to be extraordinarily sensitive to signs of social disapproval because the survival of early hominids hinged on their maintaining the goodwill of their companions). Evidence for an extrinsic motive comes largely from the exchange theory tradition (Blau, 1964; Kelley & Thibaut, 1978; Rusbult, Insko, Lin, & Smith, 1990), in which social approval is a means to other ends and should be especially potent under conditions of asymmetric resource dependency (in ordinary language, when others control resources that people value to a greater degree than people control resources that others value).

3. *Competition among motives.* Although social approval is a major driving force for intuitive politicians, the SCM does not reify it as the sovereign motive for human conduct. Social psychology has already had too many disappointing flirtations with monistic theories that have promised to identify master motives (Allport, 1985). Drawing on major strands of past work, the SCM identifies four additional, potentially conflicting motives: the goals (a) of achieving cognitive mastery of causal structure (the goal of the "intuitive scientist" of classic attribution theory—Heider, 1958; Kelley, 1967); (b) of minimizing mental effort and achieving rapid cognitive closure (the goal of the "cognitive miser" of more recent social cognitive lineage—Fiske & Taylor, 1991; Kruglanski, 1990); (c) of maximizing benefits and minimizing the costs of relationships (the goal of the "intuitive economist" of exchange theory—Blau, 1964); and (d) of asserting one's autonomy and personal identity by remaining true to one's innermost convictions (a key theme of theories of ego and moral development [Loevinger, 1976] as well as reactance theory and self-affirmation variants of disso-

nance theory [Aronson, 1976; Schlenker, 1982, 1985; Steele, Spencer, & Lynch, 1993]). For additional discussion of motives in dual-process theorizing, see Chen & Chaiken, Chapter 4, this volume) and Fiske, Lin, and Neuberg (Chapter 11, this volume).

4. *Linking motives to coping strategies.* The final component of the SCM links broad motivational assumptions to particular coping strategies by specifying how each of the five core motives can be amplified or attenuated by the interpersonal and institutional context. We propose a two-step conceptual formula for generating predictions from the model, which requires identifying situational and dispositional factors that either increase or decrease (a) the perceived importance of a given core motive, and (b) the perceived feasibility of achieving a given motivational objective in a given context.

Let's focus on how we might use the schematic formula just described to identify the optimal preconditions for activating each of four coping strategies that have received considerable experimental attention: strategic attitude shifting, preemptive self-criticism, defensive bolstering, and the decision evasion tactics of buckpassing and procrastination. It is worth noting, however, that the SCM makes predictions about a much wider array of coping strategies likely to be activated in actual organizational and political networks of accountability—in particular, strategies of resisting illegitimate accountability demands (e.g., identifying and exploiting loopholes in performance standards, exercising the "voice option" of protesting against unfair standards or offering accounts for performance shortfalls, and exercising the "exit option" of leaving the accountability relationship; see Tetlock, 1998b, 1998c). This chapter concentrates on the experimental literature and its implications for contingency theories of judgment and choice that depict people as relatively flexible "meta-level decision makers," endowed with the capacity to shift from one style of information processing to another in response to situational demands.

1. *Strategic attitude shifting.* Decision makers are especially likely to adjust their public attitudes toward the views of the anticipated audience to the degree that the social

approval motive is strong. That is, the audience should be perceived to be powerful (it should control resources that the decision makers value, but the decision makers should control little that the audience values—a condition of asymmetric resource dependency), and the audience should be seen as both firmly committed to its position and intolerant of other positions (a further incentive for accommodation). Strategic attitude shifting is, however, a feasible strategy for gaining social approval only to the degree that decision makers think they know the views of the anticipated audience. And attitude shifting becomes a psychologically costly strategy to the degree that it requires compromising basic convictions and principles (creating dissonance with decision makers' self-concept) or backtracking on past commitments (making decision makers look duplicitous, hypocritical, or sycophantic). But when these obstacles have been removed and the facilitative conditions are present, attitude shifting represents a cognitively efficient, politically expedient strategy that does not undermine decision makers' self-concept as moral and principled beings or their reputation for integrity in the wider social arena.

2. *Preemptive self-criticism.* Decision makers are especially likely to engage in flexible perspective taking, in which they try to anticipate objections that reasonable critics might raise, when they are accountable either to an audience with unknown views or to multiple audiences with conflicting views. To maximize the likelihood of preemptive self-criticism, the evaluative audience should be perceived to be well informed (so that it cannot easily be tricked) and powerful (so that decision makers want its approval), and the decision makers should not feel constrained by prior commitments that it would be now embarrassing to reverse. In the case of accountability to two (or more) audiences, it is also important that the two audiences be approximately equally powerful (otherwise, the low-cognitive-effort and politically expedient option is for decision makers to align themselves with the more powerful audience); that the two audiences recognize each other's legitimacy (otherwise, decision makers will see the search for complex integrative solutions as futile); and that there be no institutional precedents for escaping responsibility (otherwise,

many decision makers will adopt decision evasion tactics, such as buckpassing, procrastination, or obfuscation).

3. *Defensive bolstering.* Decision makers are especially likely to engage in self-justifying patterns of thinking (in which they try to demonstrate that they are right and would-be critics are wrong) when they feel accountable to a skeptical or even hostile audience for past actions that it is now impossible to reverse and implausible to deny. The evaluative audience should ideally be coercive and contemptuous (stimulating reactance and autonomy motives), but not so powerful that decision makers are simply intimidated into capitulating. And the decision makers should ideally have rigid cognitive styles and high needs for closure, feel strongly that the prior stands they have taken are justifiable, and have ready mental access to arguments that they can deploy in defense of these positions.

4. *Decision evasion.* Decision makers are especially likely to resort to one of the trilogy of decision-evasion tactics—buckpassing, procrastination, and obfuscation—when they feel accountable to two audiences that not only hold conflicting views about what should be done but also hold each other in contempt. (A paradigmatic example is the abortion debate in the late 20th-century United States.) As a result, each evaluative audience does not recognize the legitimacy of the accountability demands that the other audience places on the decision makers, thereby rendering the prospects of either a logrolling solution or an integratively complex compromise hopeless. The audiences should also be approximately equal in power, thereby reducing the attractiveness for decision makers of aligning themselves with one or the other camp. And there should be widely accepted normative or institutional precedents for engaging in decision evasion (i.e., no "The buck stops here" norm). Finally, decision makers should have weak personal convictions and be highly motivated to maintain good relations with both of the affected parties.

TESTING PREDICTIONS ABOUT COPING STRATEGIES

It is fair to say that existing research has yet to test—in a comprehensive design—the optimal preconditions for activating any of these four coping strategies. Several studies have, however, manipulated subsets of the hypothesized antecedents of the various coping strategies. This work has yielded a number of replicable results.

For example, when people are unencumbered by past commitments or strongly held views and are asked to justify their opinions to an evaluative audience whose own views are known, they tend to engage in conformity, ingratiation, and attitude shifting, in which their expressed opinions move perceptibly toward those of the anticipated audience (Hare, 1976; Jones & Wortman, 1973; Tetlock, 1983a; Tetlock et al., 1989). Although some people do internalize these public attitudes (Chen, Schechter, & Chaiken, 1996), many "snap back" (in elastic-band fashion) to their original position (Cialdini et al., 1976). It would be wrong to suppose, however, that all attitude shifting is self-conscious or duplicitous; people often seem unaware of what they are doing. And it would be wrong to label this coping strategy "maladaptive" at either an individual level of analysis (attitude shifting can be critical for sustaining a positive social identity in the eyes of key constituencies) or a group level of analysis (effective functioning requires coming to agreement, once group deliberations have reached the point of diminishing marginal returns). To be sure, however, the coping strategy can be maladaptive: Individuals may overuse attitude shifting and come to be seen as spineless or duplicitous, and groups that consist only of attitude shifters will be highly vulnerable to polarization and groupthink effects.

In addition, when people are not encumbered by past public commitments or strongly held private views and are held accountable to an audience whose own views are difficult to decipher, they often engage in preemptive self-criticism, in which they attempt to anticipate plausible objections of potential critics. The results are more dialectically complex thought-listing protocols, suggestive of active perspective taking and searching for viable syntheses of opposing perspectives ("On the one hand . . . on the other . . . on balance . . . "). A series of studies has also shown that predecisional accountability to unknown audiences is a reasonably effective de-biasing tool, at least for certain types of effects: "correspondence bias" in a Jones attitude attribution paradigm (Tetlock, 1985); primacy effects in judgments of guilt and innocence in simulated trials (Tetlock, 1983b); recency effects in auditing tasks (Kennedy, 1993); overconfidence in personality prediction tasks (Tetlock & Kim, 1987); and, most recently, the power of prior emotions to "contaminate" attributions of responsibility for completely unrelated events (Lerner, Goldberg, & Tetlock, 19987).

Encouraging self-critical, integratively complex thought does, however, have potential disadvantages. People who have been encouraged to think this way are more susceptible to the dilution effect (Tetlock & Boettger, 1989; Tetlock, Lerner, & Boettger, 1996)—a form of underconfidence in which people lose confidence in the predictive power of diagnostic cues when those cues are accompanied by irrelevant evidence (Nisbett, Zukier, & Lemley, 1981). Self-critical thinkers arguably try too hard to make good use of all the information at their disposal, even irrelevant evidence (the qualification "arguably" is important, because Tetlock, Lerner, & Boettger [1996], have shown that the dilution effect is in part a rational response to the conversational norm to assume that the information presented is indeed relevant to the task). Self-critical thinkers are also more prone to deviate from the strict prescriptions of rational models of choice in key respects, sticking with the status quo even when change is clearly in the overall interest of the collective (Tetlock & Boettger, 1994) and being swayed by the introduction of irrelevant (dominated) alternatives (Simonson, 1989). Here again, though, we need to be careful about labeling these accountability amplification effects "errors"; both may represent shrewd political adaptations designed to minimize criticism.

Whereas predecisional accountability to unknown audiences stimulates self-critical thought, postdecisional accountability to both known and unknown audiences stimulates defensive bolstering and self-justifying thought (Kiesler, 1971; Tetlock et al., 1989). The major cognitive goal for decision makers becomes generating as many thoughts as they can to demonstrate that they are correct and that would-be critics are wrong. Perhaps not surprisingly, this type of accountability amplifies efforts to recoup sunk costs and escalates commitment to failing policies (Simonson & Staw, 1992; Staw, 1980; Staw & Ross, 1989).

But it would be wrong to suppose that bolstering is inherently maladaptive. It may facilitate individual performance on tasks that require optimism and can-do confidence (Seligman, Nolen-Hoeksema, Thornton, & Thornton, 1990; Taylor & Brown, 1988), and it may inspire subordinates in work settings that require tenacious persistence.

Finally, when people are accountable to conflicting standards or audiences, and there appears to be little or no hope of reconciling the opposing perspectives, there is a marked increase of interest in the decision evasion tactics of buckpassing, procrastination, and obfuscation (cf. Janis & Mann, 1977; Tetlock, 1998b). Consider, for example, the predicament that Tetlock and Boettger (1994) created in a laboratory simulation of Food and Drug Administration decision making on the admissibility of a controversial drug into the U.S. pharmaceuticals market—a drug that would benefit some and harm others. Confronted by pressures to take a stand one way or the other that was guaranteed to earn them the enmity of an influential constituency, subjects often sought out response options that allowed them to avoid taking any stand. This was true, moreover, even when the buckpassing and procrastination options were relatively unattractive. For instance, subjects buckpassed even when they were told that the agency to which they could refer the decision had no more information than they themselves possessed, and even when there was little or no prospect that additional useful evidence would materialize in the permissible delayed-action period (Tetlock & Boettger, 1994).

DEMONSTRATING THE IMPACT OF ACCOUNTABILITY ON COGNITIVE PROCESSING

In addition to documenting the precise preconditions for activating coping strategies, laboratory studies are well designed for answering perennial level-of-analysis questions on whether accountability (or, more generally, institutional context) merely affects public posturing or also shapes underlying cognitive processes. Converging evidence now strongly suggests that both classes of effects occur (see Chen & Chaiken, Chapter 4, this volume). Skeptics who want to depict all accountability

effects as mere public posturing are hard pressed to explain five classes of evidence, discussed below.

Manipulations of Preexposure versus Postexposure Accountability

When people learn of being accountable—before or after exposure to the evidence on which they must base their judgments—is a critical moderator of whether accountability attenuates judgmental biases. Preexposure accountability is a more potent de-biasing manipulation than postexposure accountability; this result strongly suggests that accountability affects the initial encoding and interpretation of evidence, and not merely post hoc adjustments of response thresholds.

For instance, Tetlock (1983b) replicated the primacy effect (the tendency to overweight evidence received early in a sequence in a simulated criminal case) among subjects who did not feel accountable for their judgments of guilt and among subjects who learned of being accountable only after exposure to the evidence. The primacy effect disappeared, however, among subjects who learned that they would have to justify their judgments prior to exposure to the information on which they would be basing their judgments. The opposite bias—the recency effect—is also open to correction by preexposure accountability. Using as subjects MBA students working on an auditing task, Kennedy (1993) found that the recency effect disappeared among subjects with preexposure accountability, but was quite robust among both subjects with postexposure accountability and subjects who were not held accountable.

Tetlock and Kim (1987) found that the accuracy of personality prediction improved among subjects who learned that they were accountable prior to exposure to the information, but not among those who learned this after exposure to that information. Moreover, participants in the preexposure accountability condition became more accurate judges of their own states of knowledge, as reflected in stronger associations between the accuracy of personality predictions and confidence in those predictions. Unaccountable and postexposure accountability subjects who were not held accountable fell prey to the usual overconfidence effect (Fischhoff, 1982), whereas preexposure accountable subjects did not. Mediational analysis offered partial support for the hypothesis that preexposure accountability improved both predictive performance and confidence calibration by motivating subjects to attend to incongruities and contradictions in the personality profiles of the target individuals whose behavior was being predicted. These subjects showed greater awareness of inconsistencies in targets' answers to questions designed to measure the same trait ("This person is outgoing in this situation but introverted in that situation"), as well as greater sensitivity to the problems of integrating information across trait dimensions ("This person is ambitious but still wants a social life, so it is hard to say how he'd respond to item 27").

Tetlock (1985) found that preexposure accountability, but not postexposure accountability, made subjects more cautious about drawing strong dispositional conclusions about the "true attitudes" of essay writers in an essay attribution paradigm originally developed by Jones (1979). Subjects in the preexposure accountability condition did not, moreover, become indiscriminately cautious. Like postexposue accountability subjects, they drew extreme conclusions about essay writers in the high-choice conditions, in which the writers were free to take whatever stand they wanted; observers' reticence about making dispositional attributions was confined to the low-choice conditions, in which writers were required by an authority figure to advocate a certain position. Here a rational observer arguably should be maximally uncertain about the true causes of the essay writers' conduct.

Taken together, the evidence is hard to reconcile with simple models of response threshold adjustment, in which, for example, people are transformed into timid fence sitters unwilling to commit to any position. The effects of accountability are too dependent on when people learn of being accountable—on whether people have been given an opportunity to form a thoughtful, nuanced, and balanced assessment of the initial evidence.

Manipulations of Audience Cancellation

Certain accountability effects persist even after the anticipated interview with the evaluative audience has been canceled. Cialdini et al. (1976) found that elastic "snap-back" effects occur when subjects expect to discuss low-involvement relevant issues and then learn that the interview has either been canceled or been delayed for a week. A different pattern emerges, however, when subjects expect to engage in an immediate discussion of a personally relevant issue. Under these circumstances, anticipatory shifts are resistant to the "snap-back" effect even when the interview is canceled. The tendency to generate proattitudinal thoughts in justification of the new stance may explain why these circumstances lead to relatively more durable attitudes.

Pennington and Schlenker (1996) found a similar pattern of results on personally relevant issues. When students expected to justify their decisions to punish a fellow student accused of cheating to an honor court official, they recommended more severe punishments than did subjects expecting to justify their views either to the accused student or to control subjects who did not expect to justify their views. Even when subjects thought that the anticipated meeting had been canceled, these opinion shifts endured. Similarly, subjects accountable to the accused student viewed the cheating violation as less severe, and expressed greater sympathy for the student. Once again, these perspectival shifts held regardless of whether subjects thought that the anticipated accountability session had been canceled. Pennington and Schlenker also point, however, to evidence that "expediency concerns" influenced thought. Content analyses of the justifications subjects provided for their judgments revealed that subjects accountable to the honor court official were less sympathetic toward the accused student only when the meeting had not been canceled. Similarly, subjects accountable to the honor court expressed more one-sided views for punishment than subjects in other conditions only when the meeting was not canceled.

Differential Impact on Confidential Thought-Listing Protocols and Public Attitude Scales

Certain accountability effects appear on dependent measures that subjects have been assured will be completely confidential; other effects only appear on public measures. For instance, accountability to an audience known to be liberal or conservative often produces attitude shifting toward the audience's stance on "public" semantic-differential scales, but the same type of accountability has little impact on the number of liberal or conservative thoughts that subjects generate on private thought-listing protocols. It is tempting to dismiss this finding as an artifact of the unreliability or insensitivity of open-ended content-analytic measures. But the thought-listing protocols prove highly sensitive to the impact of accountability to audiences with unknown views on the integrative complexity of the thoughts reported; they pick up on the hypothesized tendency of these subjects to engage in preemptively self-critical patterns of thinking, designed to prepare themselves for interaction with either a liberal or a conservative audience. These thought protocols are much more likely to have a dialectical "point–counterpoint–synthesis" character, with more "buts," "howevers," and "althoughs," and more references to the need to strike reasonable balances, compromises, and tradeoffs.

The thought-listing protocols also prove sensitive to shifting patterns of within-cell correlations between public attitudes and private cognitive structure. For instance, subjects who resist shifting their attitudes toward known audiences generate more integratively complex and self-critical protocols than do subjects who avail themselves of the low-effort attitude-shifting option (Tetlock, 1983a; Tetlock et al., 1989). People presumably feel a need to "arm themselves" for conversational combat in defense of unpopular positions they are unwilling to abandon. The implicit message seems to be this: "I may believe X, but I am no fool. I know counterarguments Y and Z."

Interactions of Accountability with Cognitive Load

Insofar as the underlying cognitive processes activated by accountability manipulations require minimal cognitive effort and conscious monitoring, these processes should be relatively unaffected by manipulations of cognitive load (such as distraction or time pressure) that siphon off or otherwise constrain the mental resources that can be devoted to the task (cf. Kahneman & Tversky, 1973); but insofar as these underlying processes do require substantial cognitive effort, these processes should be severely impaired (see also Chen & Chaiken, Chapter 4, this volume; Fiske et al., Chapter 11, this volume; Gilbert, Chapter 1, this volume; Smith & DeCoster, Chapter 16, this volume). Available evidence—and it is scarce—favors the latter interpretation. Accountability manipulations interact with cognitive-load manipulations in ways that suggest that the underlying cognitive processes do indeed require attention and effort. Kruglanski and Freund (1983) found that whereas unaccountable subjects demonstrated a primacy effect when predicting a candidate's future success on the job, accountable subjects were far less susceptible to the bias—but only if they were not under time pressure. Under time pressure, any protective benefit conferred by accountability was entirely wiped out. Kruglanski and Freund (1983) replicated this same pattern of effects on the tendency to rely on numerical anchors, as well as on the tendency to use stereotypical category labels.

Differentiated Effects on Logically Complex Dependent Variables

Accountability often has rather subtle and differentiated effects on dependent variables that are difficult to reproduce through simple models of response threshold adjustment. Results from two studies suggest that preexposure accountability to an audience with unknown views improves the calibration of the confidence ratings that subjects assign to their predictions (Siegel-Jacobs & Yates, 1996; Tetlock & Kim, 1987). "Calibration" is statistically defined as the weighted average of the mean square differences between the proportion of correct predictions in each subjective probability category and the probability value of that category. One self-assessments of one's knowledge are well calibrated to the degree that all answers to which one assigns 100% confidence are correct, 80% of answers assigned 80% confidence are correct, and so forth. As such, it is hard to imagine improving calibration by indiscriminately lowering or raising one's threshold for expressing confidence. Rather, it requires either careful monitoring of the correspondence between one's probability estimates and "hit" rates or careful attention to the evidential support for particular predictions. It is also noteworthy that improvement in calibration occurs without cost to resolution (the variance of correct predictions across the confidence categories). These results directly challenge the notion that subjects are simply bunching up all of their confidence ratings at the low end of the subjective probability scale to avoid the embarrassment of being wrong when they claim to be 90% or 100% confident that they are correct. Subjects actually seem to become better judges of the limits of their knowledge—a valuable metacognitive skill.

Differential effects also appear when researchers partition the accuracy scores in person perception tasks (cf. Cronbach, 1955). Especially important here is the concept of "differential accuracy"—the ability of judges to predict shifting patterns of individual differences across situational contexts. Mero and Motowidlo (1995) found that holding raters accountable for their ratings and rewarding raters on the basis of ratees' performance improved this kind of judgmental accuracy. Similarly, in a personality prediction study, Tetlock and Kim (1987) decomposed predictive accuracy into the Cronbach components. This analysis revealed not only that subjects with preexposure accountability made more accurate predictions than did either subjects with no accountability or subjects with postexposure accountability, but also that it improved both differential accuracy (accuracy in predicting particular combinations of test takers and items) and stereotype accuracy (accuracy in predicting responses to particular items). As noted earlier, mediational analysis revealed that the increase in accuracy was partly produced by the tendency of subjects with preexposure accountability to form more integratively complex impressions of test takers that allowed for situational exceptions to trait generalizations, and that even occasionally confronted the classic (Allportian) problem of gauging how different traits interact to produce behavioral outcomes.

Reprise

When the totality of the evidence is weighed, the scales of plausibility now rather decisively favor the view that accountability effects cannot be dismissed as mere adjustments of response thresholds. An integral function of thought is preparation for conversations in which one expects to be called upon to explain, justify, and excuse one's opinions and decisions.

It is also worth commenting on a minor irony of intellectual history. Standards of evidence and proof in social psychology can shift quite dramatically, depending on whether a claim is consistent with the conventional wisdom. In the 1970s and early 1980s, advocates of impression management explanations had a "challenger" status and bore the burden of proof as they advanced reinterpretations of standard dissonance, reactance, equity, attribution, and group polarization effects. Tetlock and Manstead (1985) reviewed the methodological strategies deployed to demonstrate that impression management effects could not be easily reduced to intrapsychic processes, and demonstrated in each case that plausible intrapsychic mediational accounts could not be completely ruled out (although such accounts could be made to appear rather contrived). In the late 1980s and 1990s, the argument "Accountability shapes cognitive processing, not just public posturing" runs against the grain of the conventional wisdom that the more "basic" the cognitive process (the more "hard-wired" the process in neurologically grounded laws of perception or memory networks), the less likely the process is to be affected by institutional context (cf. Arkes, 1991). And we suspect that this is why the burden of proof is now borne by those who argue that some accountability effects cannot be attributed to strategic impression management and simple adjustments of response thresholds.

THE REDUCTIONIST CHALLENGE: CAN ACCOUNTABILITY EFFECTS BE ASSIMILATED TO SOME OTHER (MORE BASIC) EXPLANATORY CONSTRUCT?

Accountability is a logically complex bundle of causal constructs, perhaps too complex for the epistemological tastes of those experimental social psychologists who put a premium on isolating exact causal pathways. To paraphrase William James, there are, in principle, as many distinct forms of accountability as there are distinctive relationships among people. Pursuers of parsimony may find it tempting to try to reduce accountability to some combination of putatively more fundamental processes, and there is no shortage of plausible candidates. Accountability bears a family resemblance to a host of other independent variables in the literature, including (1) the mere presence of fellow members of one's species, (2) cognitive tuning, (3) reason giving/introspection, (4) incentives/involvement/importance, and (5) conformity pressure. Nevertheless, efforts to "reduce" all accountability effects to these "more fundamental" causal constructs run aground on some stubborn empirical anomalies.

1. *Mere presence.* The physical or symbolic presence of at least one other human being is a necessary condition for any kind of accountability. Although some accountability studies do find support for the prediction of social facilitation and drive theory (cf. Zajonc, 1965) that the mere presence of a conspecific amplifies dominant responses (Weigold & Schlenker, 1991), other studies report quite the opposite pattern. Far from enhancing theoretically dominant responses such as low-effort heuristics in social cognition experiments, loafing in group tasks, or aggression in electric shock paradigms, accountability often stimulates self-critical forms of thought, motivates individual work effort, and attenuates aggression in response to provocation (Prentice-Dunn & Rogers, 1982; Tetlock, 1992; Weldon & Gargano, 1988).

2. *Cognitive tuning.* Zajonc (1960) argued that expecting to communicate one's impressions of an event—a "transmission set"—places a premium on one's ability to generate succinct and readily comprehensible descriptions of that event, thus polarizing and simplifying thought. By contrast, accountability research finds that expecting to justify one's views often places a premium not only on communicating one's opinions, but also on defending those opinions against reasonable counterarguments (see Tetlock, 1992). The former manipulation encourages people to suppress ambiguity and to present issues in sharp, polarized terms. The latter manipulation encourages people to express complex, many-sided opinions that are difficult to refute and easy to justify. Research on over-attribution illustrates the diverging predictions. Subjects in transmission sets form more extreme dispositional attributions in an essay attribution paradigm than do subjects in a no-set control condition (Harvey, Harkins, & Kagehiro, 1976). By contrast, subjects given accountability instructions make less extreme and more discriminating patterns of causal attributions (Tetlock, 1985).

3. *Reason giving/introspection.* Introspective searches for reasons often disrupt the relation between attitudes and behavior, and decrease awareness of the true sources of subjects' preferences and choices (Wilson, Hodges, & LaFleur, 1995; Wilson, Kraft, & Dunn, 1989). When people try to explain their feelings, they focus on cognitively accessible reasons that only loosely correspond to the actual causes for their feelings. By contrast, accountability has repeatedly been found to strengthen the covariation between the cues that subjects say they are using to make choices and the cues that regression models suggest subjects are using (Cvetkovich, 1978; Hagafors & Brehmer, 1983; Weldon & Gargano, 1988). In one case, less self-awareness of judgment processes is observed; in the other, more is observed. One possibility worth investigating is that this divergence reflects the types of tasks used in the different research programs. Search for reasons may be both futile and disruptive in domains where an implicit de gustibus norm prevails stipulating that matters of taste do not require reasons. By contrast, search for reasons may promote awareness of cognitive processing in analytical or problem-solving tasks, such as multiple-cue probability learning. Another possibility is that the divergence reflects important but yet not identified functional differences between processes of private introspection and public justification.

4. *Incentives/decision importance.* The de-biasing effects of accountability on overconfidence (Kassin et al., 1991; Tetlock & Kim, 1987) are very different from the null effects generally found for monetary incentives (Fischhoff, 1982) and the bias-amplifying effects sometimes found for task importance manipulations (Sieber, 1974). One possibility worth exploring is that accountability and money activate qualitatively distinct modes of processing. Monetary incentives may convey a host of unintended messages: "The task is boring, so I must be bribed to do it" (eroding intrinsic motivation), or "The task is competitive, so I should look for an angle that others

won't see to maximize my chances of winning" (encouraging a search for a usually nonexistent trick solution). By contrast, accountability, especially preexposure/predecisional accountability to unknown audiences, may motivate people to become more self-reflective and self-critical—not because people think that it is the "best way to think" (the cognitive equivalent of putting on one's "Sunday best"), but rather because self-critical thought is a relatively well-rehearsed response to unfamiliar or normatively ambiguous situations in which people are unsure of how they should act.

Task importance and accountability manipulations also differ in a multiplicity of ways, so it should not be surprising that their effects are sometimes strikingly similar (McAllister et al., 1979) and sometimes strikingly divergent (Sieber, 1974). Consider, for example, the de-biasing effects of accountability reported by Tetlock and Kim (1987) and the bias-amplifying effects of task importance in Sieber (1974). She explains her results by invoking Hull–Spence drive theory and the tendency for drive/arousal to increase the likelihood of dominant responses. Given the many differences between the Sieber (1974) and Tetlock and Kim (1987) studies, it is logically possible that the two manipulations simply placed subjects on different points of the infamous arousal–performance curve. Perhaps Siebert's task importance manipulation (course grades were thought to be at stake) was more powerful than the Tetlock and Kim (1987) accountability manipulation and produced levels of arousal that interfered with, rather than facilitated, self-critical thought. Arousal has repeatedly been found to be related in a curvilinear fashion to integrative complexity, with moderate levels most conducive to complex functioning (Schroder, Driver, & Streufert, 1967). Tetlock and Kim's manipulation may have created optimum arousal, and Sieber's may have created a superoptimal level. It is also possible, however, that the two manipulations may have differed in qualitative ways. More important than the general arousing properties of accountability may be the specific coping responses activated by the need to justify one's views. Accountability may serve as a signal to subjects to take the role of the other toward

their own mental processes and to give serious weight to the possibility that their preferred answers might be wrong. In this view, accountability does not simply motivate thought; it functions as a social brake on easy-to-execute heuristics and automatic forms of social inference that people rely upon in their less reflective moments.

5. *Conformity pressure.* As we have seen, conformity or attitude shifting is a relatively popular strategy of dealing with predecisional accountability to audiences with well-defined views. But as the earlier review of the response threshold argument has revealed, it is implausible to insist that all accountability effects can be modeled as mindless conformity adjustments to the anticipated audience. The importance of accountability timing; the persistence of certain effects after audience cancellation; the emergence of effects even on confidential thought-listing protocols; the interactions of accountability with cognitive load; and the complexity of accountability effects on subtle, difficult-to-influence-mindlessly dependent measures (calibration, differential accuracy, correspondence between statistical models of cue utilization and self-reported judgmental policy)—all these lines of evidence point to the power of accountability to induce more self-reflective, self-critical, and effort-demanding patterns of thinking than those that typically occur when people do not feel their judgments are under evaluative scrutiny.

CONCLUDING THOUGHTS

Accountability is a multidimensional construct with a correspondingly multidimensional array of effects. It shapes what people are willing to say as well as how people think. Disentangling these effects is not always easy and may sometimes be impossible; nevertheless, there has been empirical progress. We know more than we did before about the types of accountability that trigger attitude shifting and the types of accountability that activate more effort-demanding processing, which may in turn take either self-critical or self-justifying forms.

Although many of the findings reviewed here fit nicely within the emerging emphasis on dual-process models, there are some cautionary caveats. The most important is that there is nothing inherently superior about the effort-demanding "second tier" of thought. We have repeatedly seen that neither self-justifying nor self-critical thought automatically improves or degrades judgment. Much hinges on both the social context and the goals that we posit people are trying to achieve. Self-justifying thought arguably improves judgment when efforts to recoup sunk costs elicit political applause for a principled stand (staying the course). Economic irrationality may sometimes be politically rational. But self-justifying thought arguably degrades judgment in settings that place a premium on flexible adjustment, awareness of tradeoffs, and rapidly writing off sunk costs. Normative assessments of self-critical thought need to be equally qualified. Self-criticism may improve judgment when anticipating potential critics leads people to incorporate valid objections into their assessment of a problem, thereby correcting overconfidence and belief perseverance. But it may degrade judgment when self-criticism shades into chronic vacillation (buckpassing and procrastination), or into inferential wild-goose chases (as in the dilution effect) in which people bend over backwards to make sense of nonsense. But the key term here is "may." What one political observer denounces as cowardly decision evasion tactics, another may praise as an appropriately circumspect approach to the exercise of authority. And whereas scholars who view people as intuitive statisticians may not hesitate to label the dilution effect a bias (why lose confidence in a genuinely predictive cue simply because it is surrounded by nonpredictive cues?), scholars who stress the importance of conversational norms in guiding social thought may spring to the defense of dilution, arguing that attentive conversational partners presume relevance and try hard to glean useful information from even the most opaque cues.

Accountability effects are thus both descriptively and normatively complex. They are descriptively complex because different types of accountability can elicit very different social and cognitive coping responses. They are normatively complex because accountability links previously isolated laboratory subjects to the world of institutions, politics, and power—a world in which labeling something a mistake almost never goes uncontested.

ACKNOWLEDGMENTS

Support for this project came in part from a National Science Foundation grant (SRB No. 9696162) to Philip E. Tetlock and a National Science Foundation graduate fellowship to Jennifer S. Lerner.

NOTE

1. Of course, social systems also cannot rely exclusively on external modes of social control for maintaining order. The transaction costs of monitoring everybody all the time would quickly become prohibitive. The SCM recognizes that a large measure of trust and self-accountability is necessary for the smooth functioning of institutions, but affirms that self-accountability by itself is insufficient.

REFERENCES

Allport, G. W. (1985). The historical background of social psychology. In G. Lindzey & E. Aronson (Eds.), *Handbook of social psychology* (3rd ed., Vol. 1, pp. 5–42). New York: Random.

Aronson, E. (1976). *The social animal* (2nd ed.). San Francisco: W.H. Freeman.

Arkes, H. (1991). Costs and benefits of judgment errors: Implications for debiasing. *Psychological Bulletin, 110,* 486–498.

Baumeister, R. F., & Leary, M. F. (1995). The need to belong: Desire for interpersonal attachments as a fundamental human motive. *Psychological Bulletin, 117,* 497–529.

Blau, P. M. (1964). *Exchange and power in social life.* New York: Wiley.

Brockner, J., & Rubin, J. Z. (1985). *Entrapment in escalating conflicts: A social psychological analysis.* New York: Springer-Verlag.

Camerer, C. (1995). Individual decision making. In J. H. Hagel & A. E. Roth (Eds.), *The handbook of experimental economics* (pp. 587–704). Princeton, NJ: Princeton University Press.

Chaiken, S. (1980). Heuristic versus systematic information processing and the use of source versus message cues in persuasion. *Journal of Personality and Social Psychology, 40,* 111–120.

Chen, S., Schecter, D., & Chaiken, S. (1996). Getting at the truth or getting along: Accuracy versus impression-motivated heuristic and systematic processing. *Journal of Personality and Social Psychology, 71,* 262–275.

Cialdini, R. B., Levy, A., Herman, C. P., Kozlowski, I. T., & Petty, R. E. (1976). Elastic shifts of opinion: Determinants of direction and durability. *Journal of Personality and Social Psychology, 34,* 663–672.

Cronbach, L. J. (1955). Processes affecting scores on "understanding others" and "assumed similarity." *Psychological Bulletin, 52,* 177–193.

Cvetkovich, G. (1978). Cognitive accommodation, language, and social responsibility. *Social Psychology, 2.*

Fischhoff, B. (1982). "Debiasing." In D. Kahneman, P. Slovic, & A. Tversky (Eds.), *Judgment under uncertainty* (pp. 237–262). Cambridge, MA: Cambridge University Press.

Fiske, S. T., & Neuberg, S. L. (1990). A continuum of impression formation, from category-based to individuating processes: Influences of information and motivation on attention and interpretations. In M. P. Zanna (Ed.), *Advances in experimental social psychology* (Vol. 23, pp. 1–74). San Diego, CA: Academic Press.

Fiske, S. T., & Taylor, S. (1991). *Social cognition* (2nd ed.). New York: McGraw-Hill.

Hagafors, R., & Brehmer, B. (1983). Does having to justify one's judgments change the nature of the judgment process? *Organizational Behavior and Human Performance, 31,* 223–232.

Hare, A. P. (1976). *Handbook of small group research* (2nd ed.). New York: Free Press.

Harvey, J. H., Harkins, S. G., & Kagehiro, D. K. (1976). Cognitive tuning and the attribution of causality. *Journal of Personality and Social Psychology, 34,* 708–715.

Heider, F. (1958). *The psychology of interpersonal relations.* New York: Wiley.

Janis, I. L., & Mann, L. (1977). *Decision making: A psychological analysis of conflict, choice, and commitment.* New York: Free Press.

Jones, E. E. (1979). The rocky road from acts to dispositions. *American Psychologist, 34,* 107–117.

Jones, E. E., & Wortman, C. (1973). *Ingratiation: An attributional approach.* Morristown, NJ: General Learning Press.

Kahneman, D., & Tversky, A. (1973). On the psychology of prediction. *Psychological Review, 80,* 237–251.

Kassin, S. M., Castillo, S. R., & Rigby, S. (1991). The accuracy–confidence correlation in eyewitness testimony: Limits and extensions of the retrospective self-awareness effect. *Journal of Personality and Social Psychology, 5,* 698–707.

Kelley, H. H. (1967). Attribution theory in social psychology. In D. Levine (Ed.), *Nebraska Symposium on Motivation* (Vol. 15, pp. 192–240). Lincoln: University of Nebraska Press.

Kelley, H. H., & Thibaut, J. W. (1978). *Interpersonal relations: A theory of interdependence.* New York: Wiley.

Kennedy, J. (1993). Debiasing audit judgment with accountability: A framework and experimental results. *Journal of Accounting Research, 31,* 231–245.

Kiesler, C. A. (1971). *The psychology of commitment: Experiments linking behavior to belief.* New York: Academic Press.

Kruglanski, A. W. (1990). Lay epistemic theory in social-cognitive psychology. *Psychological Inquiry, 1,* 181–197.

Kruglanski, A. W., & Freund, T. (1983). The freezing and unfreezing of lay-inferences: Effects on impressional primacy, ethnic stereotyping and numerical anchoring.

Journal of Experimental Social Psychology, 19, 448–468.

Lerner, J. S., Goldberg, J. H., & Tetlock, P. E., (1996, July). *Accountability and punitive bias.* Poster session presented at the annual meeting of the American Psychological Society, San Francisco.

Lerner, J. S., Goldberg, J. H., & Tetlock, P. E. (1998). Sober second thought: The effects of accountability, anger and authoritarianism on attributions of responsibility. *Personality and Social Psychology Bulletin, 24,* 563–574.

Lerner, J. S., & Tetlock, P. E. (in press). Accounting for the effects of accountability. *Psychological Bulletin.*

Levi, A., & Tetlock, P. E. (1980). A cognitive analysis of Japan's 1941 decision for war. *Journal of Conflict Resolution, 24,* 195–211.

Loevinger, J. (1976). *Ego development: Conceptions and theories.* San Francisco: Jossey-Bass.

March, J. G., & Olsen, J. P. (1995). *Democratic governance.* New York: Free Press.

McAllister, D. W., Mitchell, T. R., & Beach, L. R. (1979). The contingency model for the selection of decision strategies: An empirical test of the effects of significance, accountability, and reversibility. *Organizational Behavior and Human Performance, 24,* 228–244.

Mead, G. H. (1934). *Mind, self, and society from the standpoint of a social behaviorist* (Vol. 1). Chicago: University of Chicago Press.

Mero, N., & Motowidlo, S. (1995). Effects of rater accountability on the accuracy and favorability of performance ratings. *Journal of Applied Psychology, 80*(4), 517–524.

Nisbett, R. E., Zukier, H., & Lemley, R. (1981). The dilution effect: Nondiagnostic information weakens the implications of diagnostic information. *Cognitive Psychology, 13,* 248–277.

Pennington, J., & Schlenker, B. R. (1996). *Accountability for consequential decisions: justifying ethical judgments to audiences.* Manuscript submitted for publication.

Petty, R. E., & Cacioppo, J. T. (1986). The elaboration likelihood model of persuasion. In L. Berkowitz (Ed.), *Advances in experimental social psychology* (Vol. 19, pp. 123–205). New York: Academic Press.

Prentice-Dunn, S., & Rogers, R. W. (1982). Effects of public and private self-awareness on deindividuation and aggression. *Journal of Personality and Social Psychology, 43*(3), 503–513.

Rozelle, R. M., & Baxter, J.C. (1981). *Impression formation under conditions of accountability and self salience.* Unpublished manuscript, University of Houston.

Rusbult, C. E., Insko, C. A., Lin, Y. W., & Smith, W. J. (1990). Social motives underlying rational selective exploitation: The impact of instrumental versus social-emotional allocator orientation on the distribution of rewards in groups. *Journal of Applied Social Psychology, 20,* 1984–1025.

Schlenker, B. R. (1980). *Impression management: The self-concept, social identity, and interpersonal relations.* Monterey, CA: Brooks/Cole.

Schlenker, B. R. (1982). Translating actions into attitudes: An identity-analytic approach to the explanation of social conduct. In L. Berkowitz (Ed.), *Advances in experimental social psychology* (Vol 15, pp. 194–248). New York: Academic Press.

Schlenker, B. R. (Ed.). (1985). *The self and social life.* New York: McGraw-Hill.

Schroder, H. M., Driver, M., & Streufert, S. (1967). *Human information processing.* New York: Holt, Rinehart & Winston.

Seligman, M. E., Nolen-Hoeksema, S., Thornton, N., & Thornton, K. M. (1990). Explanatory style as a mechanism of disappointing athletic performance. *Psychological Science, 1,* 143–146.

Sieber, J. E. (1974). Effects of decision importance on ability to generate warranted subjective uncertainty. *Journal of Personality and Social Psychology, 30,* 688–694.

Siegel-Jacobs, K., & Yates, J. F. (1996). Effects of procedural and outcome accountability on judgment quality. *Organizational Behavior and Human Decision Processes, 1,* 1–17.

Simonson, I. (1989). Choices based on reasons: The case of attribution and compromise effects. *Journal of Consumer Research, 16,* 158–174.

Simonson, I., & Staw, B. M. (1992). Deescalation strategies: A comparison of techniques for reducing commitment to losing courses of action. *Journal of Applied Psychology, 77,* 419–426.

Staw, B. M. (Ed.). (1980). *Rationality and justification in organizational life* (Vol. 2). Greenwich, CT: JAI Press.

Staw, B. M., & Ross, J. (1989). Understanding behavior in escalation situations. *Science, 246,* 216–220.

Steele, C., Spencer, S., & Lynch, M. (1993). Self-image resilience and dissonance: The role of affirmational resources. *Journal of Personality and Social Psychology, 64,* 885–896.

Stone, D. N., & Ziebart, D. A. (1995). A model of financial incentive effects in decision making. *Organizational Behavior and Human Decision Processes, 61,* 250–261.

Taylor, S. E., & Brown, J. D. (1988). Illusion and well-being: A social psychological perspective on mental health. *Psychological Bulletin, 103,* 193–210.

Tetlock, P. E. (1983a). Accountability and complexity of thought. *Journal of Personality and Social Psychology, 45*(1), 74–83.

Tetlock, P. E. (1983b). Accountability and the perseverance of first impressions. *Social Psychology Quarterly, 46,* 285–292.

Tetlock, P. E. (1985). Accountability: A social check on the fundamental attribution error. *Social Psychology Quarterly, 48,* 227–236.

Tetlock, P. E. (1992). The impact of accountability on judgment and choice: Toward a social contingency model. *Advances in Experimental Social Psychology, 25,* 331–376.

Tetlock, P. E. (1998a). Losing our religion: On the collapse of precise normative standards in complex accountability systems. In R. Kramer & M. Neale (Eds.), *Influence processes in organizations.* Thousand Oaks, CA: Sage.

Tetlock, P. E. (1998b). Accountability theory: Mixing properties of human agents with properties of social systems. In L. Thompson, D. Messick, & J. Levine (Eds.), *Shared cognition in organizations: The management of knowledge.* Mahwah, NJ: Erlbaum.

Tetlock, P. E. (1998c). *Cognitive biases and organizational correctives: Do both disease and cure depend on the political beholder?* Unpublished manuscript, Ohio State University.

Tetlock, P. E., & Boettger, R. (1989). Accountability: A social magnifier of the dilution effect. *Journal of Personality and Social Psychology, 57,* 388–398.

Tetlock, P. E., & Boettger, R. (1994). Accountability amplifies the status quo effect when change creates victims. *Journal of Behavioral Decision Making, 7,* 1–23.

Tetlock, P. E., & Kim, J. I. (1987). Accountability and judgment processes in a personality prediction task. *Journal of Personality and Social Psychology, 52,* 700–709.

Tetlock, P. E., Lerner, J. S., & Boettger, R. (1996). The dilution effect: Judgmental bias, conversational convention, or a bit of both? *European Journal of Social Psychology, 26,* 915–934.

Tetlock, P. E., & Manstead, A. S. R. (1985). Impression management versus intrapsychic explanations in social psychology: A useful dichotomy? *Psychological Review, 92,* 59–77.

Tetlock, P. E., Skitka, L., & Boettger, R. (1989). Social and cognitive strategies for coping with accountability: Conformity, complexity, and bolstering. *Journal of Personality and Social Psychology, 57,* 632–640.

Weigold, M. F., & Schlenker, B. R. (1991). Accountability and risk taking. *Personality and Social Psychology Bulletin, 17,* 25–29.

Weldon, E., & Gargano, G. M. (1988). Cognitive loafing: The effects of accountability and shared responsibility on cognitive effort. *Personality and Social Psychology Bulletin, 14,* 159–171.

Wilson, T. D., Hodges, S. D., & LaFleur, S. J. (1995). Effects of introspecting about reasons: Inferring attitudes from accessible thoughts. *Journal of Personality and Social Psychology, 69,* 16–28.

Wilson, T. D., Kraft, D., & Dunn, D. S. (1989). The disruptive effects of explaining attitudes: The moderating effect of knowledge about the attitude object. *Journal of Experimental Social Psychology, 25,* 379–400.

Zajonc, R. B. (1960). The process of cognitive tuning in communication. *Journal of Abnormal and Social Psychology, 61,* 159–167.

Zajonc, R. B. (1965). Social facilitation. *Science, 149,* 269–274.

29

On the Relationship between Social and Cognitive Modes of Organization

REUBEN M. BARON
STEPHEN J. MISOVICH

The general objective of this chapter is an exploration of the effect of social factors such as group size and group organization on the operation of social knowing, and the reciprocal effects of social knowing on the social properties of groups. From the present perspective, social knowing is assumed to range from stimulus-constrained social perception based on the detection of social affordances (e.g., Baron & Misovich, 1993a) to increasingly schema-driven, cognitive processes rooted in categorical-inferential thinking (e.g., stereotyping and other "top-down" processes). A basic theme involves the relationship between social and epistemic organization, with our argument being that social complexity has functioned evolutionarily as an environmental challenge requiring cognitive adaptations, in regard to whether perceptual or conceptual modes of processing are more functional. We propose that at a process level social complexity is in effect the "mind's environment" (Caporael & Baron, 1996), in the sense that as social complexity increases, there are critical values where a small change in complexity creates a phase transition in epistemic mode from stimulus-driven social perception to schema-driven conceptual processes. To the extent that such processes occur, we may assume that organizational changes may be modeled as involving principles of complex, dynamic systems (Nicolis & Prigogene, 1988).

A brief example will set the stage for our systematic exposition. Given that people join groups for adaptive advantage in terms of protection from environmental threats ranging from large animals to hostile groups (i.e., to increase inclusive fitness), the necessities of group living become a constraint on the relative prepotency of different epistemic modes. For example, for an individual operating alone, the act of picking a pear may involve predominantly perceptual activities related to perceiving the affordances of the accessibility of the piece of fruit, in terms of its distance and the length of the person's arm. In contrast, for a group of individuals, the act of attacking a large animal requires complex social coordination of roles. Such an activity may be an antecedent of category-based distributed cognition as a mediator of complex social coordination. Similarly, individual problem solving (e.g., detecting whether a piece of fruit is edible) may entail more perception-based strategies than would be effective with a social group that is attempting to solve a group problem (e.g., determining together whether an individual is well suited to join the group).

We begin this chapter with an effort to establish the primacy of social organization over epistemic modes. This is not because we believe there is a general unidirectional relationship between social organization and epistemic activity (such as affect's having primacy over cognition; e.g., Zajonc, 1984), but rather because this side of what we believe is a circular causal relationship (such that social constraints shape cognitive organization, which in turn limits subsequent types of social organization) has been so neglected. In this context, although we begin with the path from social to cognitive organization, we eventually explore the reciprocal impact of cognition on social organization.

THE CASE FOR THE PRIMACY OF SOCIAL CONSTRAINTS

General Antecedents

It is perhaps fitting, given the broad net cast by our introductory remarks, that the most general support for sociality as a constraint on epistemic modes comes from one of the leading historical figures in cognitive development, Lev Vygotsky (see Baron & Misovich, 1993b). Vygotsky (1978) has explicitly focused on the relationship between social and cognitive modes of organization. For example, he describes a "zone of proximal development" (ZPD), wherein through social guidance or scaffolding by a person with more developed ability, an ability may appear in a child earlier than it would have if the child had been tested without such social guidance. The ZPD is the difference between "the actual developmental level as determined by individual problem solving, and the level of problem solving under adult guidance or in collaboration with more capable peers" (Vygotsky, 1978, p. 86). This suggests that social interaction may exert a strong effect on cognitive functioning. Furthermore, Vygotsky states in his two-plane view of the course of social-cognitive development that individual knowing arises from, and is refracted through, social interaction. Specifically, "the very mechanism underlying the higher mental functions

is a copy of the social" (Vygotsky, 1978/1991, p. 40).

An evolutionary illustration of the link between social and cognitive structure comes from Cosmides (1989). In her examination of how the constraints of social exchange may shape aspects of human reasoning in the Johnson-Laird and Wason (1970) selection problem, Cosmides (1989) provides data that are strongly consistent with the present position. Specifically, Cosmides proposes that the ability to detect the correct disconfirmation rule—that is, the card containing the information necessary to falsify the rule—may have evolved out of the importance of detecting cheaters (i.e., people who do not reciprocate social benefits received) in social exchange processes. To appreciate this interpretation of Cosmides's work, consider the following hypothetical evolutionary scenario. It may be hypothesized that the ability to grasp transitivity—that is, if A is greater than B, and B is greater than C, then A is greater than C—can be linked to the essential social skill of being able to detect one's place in a dominance hierarchy. Finally, a general rationale for the link between shared social and cognitive structure has been advanced by a prominent cognitive psychologist, Jennifer Freyd (1983), who describes what she refers to as the "shareability constraint." Freyd states that the weak form of this constraint is that "many cognitive or linguistic structures have the form they do because they must be shared . . . the stronger argument is that only in sharing do these forms exist" (1983, p. 192).

Social-Psychological Antecedents

Interestingly, a social psychologist, Robert Zajonc (1960), was perhaps the first to demonstrate experimentally the effect of social demands on cognitive processing. In his investigation of cognitive tuning, he found that individuals set to transmit trait information to others created more polarized cognitive organizations than people set to receive such information (see also Hoffman, Mischel, & Mazze, 1981). Earlier work in social psychology also explored the relationships between social and cognitive modes of organization. Specifically, Heider (1958, 1990), as summarized in Baron (1991), proposed that the preference for cognitive balance derives from principles of interpersonal preferences and stable social organization, embodied in Newcomb's (1953) *A-B-X* model of social communication. In this regard, a person is uncomfortable when two other people the person likes disagree with each other about an issue or dislike each other, because such a pattern of interpersonal conflict may force the person to take sides and perhaps lose a friend (see also Abelson, 1983). In addition, if we scale the primacy issue up to the small-group level, it can be argued that Sherif's (1936/1966) classic study of norm formation demonstrates that norm formation begins as a problem of the social coordination of differing judgments, and ends with individuals' internalizing the group norm. This finding is very much in line with Vygotsky's two-plane principle of how the social is refracted at the individual cognitive level.

It is also proposed that people's anthropomorphic interpretations of the movements of geometric forms in the classic Heider and Simmel (1944) bully–victim–rescuer triad derive from their prior attunements to patterns of actual social movements, which may be learned or evolutionarily driven. For example, properly attuned observers with a prior history of violent crimes are able to differentiate accurately people who have and have not been mugged, simply by viewing videos of these people walking (Grayson & Stein, 1981). In this case, being able to detect vulnerability may transfer to being able to categorize abstract geometric movements. Further support for this line of reasoning may be found in the work of Aronoff, Woike, and Hyman (1992), who found that so-called "evil" characters in ballet move in a jagged, linear fashion, whereas the "good" characters are given rounded patterns of movements. Thus, contrary to the prevailing nominalism in social cognition (cf. Fiske & Taylor, 1991), it is proposed that social organization may not typically be driven in a top-down manner by social categories. Rather, as proposed by Heider (1990), the cognitive units (e.g., labels or cognitive categories) may be constrained by natural social units, with those cognitive units persisting that correspond to actual patterns of social action and interaction. For example, the "Big Five" personality trait categories may reflect adaptive strategies that have evolved in response to persistent social problems, such as finding a mate, fitting into a group, and being able to detect when to boss others as opposed to being led by them (Buss, 1996; Baron & Misovich, 1993b).

Similarly, the possibility that social categories arise from direct encounters with social actions that afford the success of certain social goals (the reverse of nominalism) may account at least in part for the accuracy of the detection of social dispositions based on brief observations of other people (Ambady & Rosenthal, 1992). For example, under suitable circumstances, shy people meeting strangers may adopt highly informative bodily postures (e.g., compensatory body lean) designed to minimize the closeness of social encounters. In this view, the act of labeling persons as "shy" reflects the fact that shy behaviors appear visibly in their social interactions, and also increases the likelihood that individuals so labeled will continue to act shyly. That is, although initially the label is socially constrained, once in place it becomes a kind of self-fulfilling prophecy (e.g., Snyder, 1984).

Having established the possibility that social and cognitive organization are linked at both the evolutionary level and the level of individual development and social interaction, we now explore in more depth the distinctive nature of social organization and cognitive organization, before describing further how they reciprocally influence each other.

COGNITIVE AND SOCIAL ORGANIZATION

At this point we draw upon Caporael and Baron (1996) and Baron (1995) to clarify what is meant by cognitive and social organization, given a common framework of dynamic, complex systems. We also explore sociality and cognition at a process level, in regard to representative group and epistemic processes at different levels of group size (i.e., the "mind's environment" metaphor).

Cognitive Organization

Before we detail the nature of social organization, it is necessary to clarify the present use of the term "cognitive organization" in regard to its dynamic properties, involving temporally organized shifts in the mode of information processing.

Perceptual versus Conceptual Modes of Organization

Baron (1988) has argued that a meaningful distinction between modes of cognitive organization lies in the difference between conceptual and perceptual epistemic modes—distinct epistemic modes that have evolved to solve different problems of social knowing. In this vein, Baron (1988) has proposed that perception enables people to know more and more about less and less, whereas conceptual processes tell people less and less about more and more (via categorical inference and default values).

This approach draws upon the work of Gibson (1979), who distinguishes between direct and indirect knowing. Specifically, he

> treats direct perception as in need of *neither* stages of processing *nor* centrally mediated constructive processes. For Gibson it is not necessary to go "beyond the information given" (Bruner, 1957) to acquire useful knowledge about the environment. Specifically, under natural conditions the stimulation available to the sensory modalities has been systematically deformed or constrained by the . . . properties of environmental entities. That is, there is information potentially available to be detected by our sensory systems, in the form of higher-order stimulus properties (e.g. Gibson's formless invariants), which specifies the functional utilities or affordances of environmental entities or constellations of entities. (Baron, 1988, p. 50; emphasis in original)

This approach rests upon the assumption that "perception is for doing" (Gibson, 1979). In the present context, it is primarily through *doing* that structure is unlocked. The yoking of perception to active exploration and manipulation of the world make it possible for perceptual-level meaning to be data-driven—a matter of *detecting and preserving* knowledge, rather than constructing it from the top down. In Bertrand Russell's (1912) apt terms, perception is limited to firsthand knowledge or "knowledge by acquaintance," as opposed to "knowledge by description"— indirect or conceptually mediated knowing,

as in the secondhand pickup of knowledge through processes ranging from reading to group discussions. It is in the latter context that the perceiver is forced to use interpretive structures to go beyond the information given by verbal descriptions (Russell's "knowledge by description").

The value of such a dual-mode view is that it allows us to appreciate better how the perceptual and conceptual epistemic systems become integrated in the context of specific phenomena, be they the decision that a piece of fruit is edible, the forming of a dyadic relationship, or socialization into a group. Thus, as in Zajonc's (1984) distinction between cognition and emotion, there can be simple direct perception unconfounded by categorical processes. Indeed, in certain instances labeling may impoverish the information picked up at a direct perceptual level, as in the proposition *Seeing is Forgetting the Name of the Thing Seen* (Weschler, 1982). Recent experimental data from Ambady (1997) directly support the proposition that categorical thinking may lower perception-based accuracy. However, in most cases of adult social encounters, we are dealing with what Baron (1980) has referred to as "mixed-mode processing." Such mixed-mode processing can take various forms. It can consist of direct perception followed by cognitive elaboration (e.g., trying to communicate to someone *about* an emotional encounter with another person). Or it can begin with the priming of a category as described by Neisser (1976), where schemas guide perception by directing selectivity of attention, thereby creating a change in the *object of judgment*—as opposed to changing the meaning of a constant environmental target, which is a schema-based change in the *judgment of the object* (Asch, 1952).

Moreover, these different epistemic modes may cycle back and forth, as during an extended interaction. That is, people may detect certain dispositional properties directly through nonverbal inputs, which lead them to act in ways that elicit strong actions from others, which in turn make certain stereotypes salient. It is also possible that there are parallel processes taking place. For example, during impression formation, aspects of the impression may be a matter of the direct perception of certain social affordances, while at the same time a person is categorically processing a complex self-presentation of another person. These parallel processes may be contrasted with Gilbert's model of serial process correction (Gilbert, Pelham, & Krull, 1988), in which categorical processing is viewed as invariably taking place first, with corrections made only when cognitive load is low. A more differentiated view of dual processes that allows derivations similar to the ecological perspective is described in Trope's integration model (e.g., Trope & Gaunt, Chapter 8, this volume). The integration model argues, in essence, that highly salient (as opposed to nonsalient) perceptual information relevant to situational discounting will be processed even under overload conditions. This state of affairs is in effect analogous to the type of mixed-mode, parallel-processing situation described above. For Trope, but not for Gilbert, contextual information is important both during identification and during the causal-attribution, interpretive stage. Thus Trope's use of trait dispositions is nearer to the ecological concept of a social affordance, given that the actions, the person, and the situation are syncretically merged in the ecological view of an affordance. Furthermore, unlike Gilbert model's, Trope's model does not assume that people always proceed beyond identification to higher-order trait inference. This framing of the dual-mode process (assuming that identification is a perception-type process) is more compatible with the current ecological claim that conceptual-level processing is optional, depending on the occurrence of certain social constraints such as increases in group size. The present view seeks to avoid reductionism at either end; we do not reduce perception to a lower level of constructive processing (e.g., Gilbert et al., 1988) or treat cognition as parasitic on perception (Gibson, 1979). Rather, as we examine the effect of social organization on epistemic organization, we seek to clarify the complexity of the entanglements of perceptual and conceptual epistemic modes.

The relation between perceptual and conceptual modes may also be treated in terms of a continuum, given the distinctions being made in the literature on implicit memory regarding shallow levels of processing (perceptual processing) versus deep levels (conceptual processing). As summarized by Roediger and McDermott (1993), we may observe shifts from shallow to deep processing. Complexity

in this framework emphasizes differential drains on cognitive capacity. Furthermore, it should be noted that there is strong evidence for the validity of a distinction between perceptual and conceptual processes in the implicit-memory literature (cf. Roediger & McDermott, 1993) based on Daniel Schacter's (1989) double-dissociation paradigm. In this paradigm, presumed manipulations of perceptual- or conceptual-level processes are only considered successful if effects selectively cross over at the dependent-variable level. Thus perceptual activity is established if effects occur in regard to perceptually sensitive indices but not to conceptual ones, whereas the reverse would have to obtain to demonstrate the operation of conceptual processes. In social psychology, Zajonc's (1984) finding that frequency-of-exposure effects are found on indices of implicit liking, but not on indices of explicit recognition, is illustrative.

Other Distinctions in Cognitive Organization

It should also be noted that the basic distinction between perceptual and conceptual modes of organization does not exhaust the ways that cognitive organization can be parsed at a functional level. Specifically, the peripheral–central distinction (e.g., Petty & Cacioppo, 1984; Petty & Wegener, Chapter 3, this volume) and the related heuristic-systematic differentiation (e.g., Chaiken, 1980; Chen & Chaiken, Chapter 4, this volume; Chen, Schechter, & Chaiken, 1996) may also be utilized in illustrating how changes in social organization constrain cognitive organization. In this regard, the peripheral–central distinction is perhaps closer to the perceptual–conceptual split, because peripheral processing encompasses affective conditioning effects; these are likely to be heavily linked to direct perception, in that the perception of affordances probably precedes affective reactions. There is also a link to the heuristic–systematic distinction in the sense that both direct perception and heuristic processing occur at an automatic, noncontrolled level. Moreover, heuristics may be a substitute for direct perception when direct encounters are not possible in a domain. For example, both direct perception and heuristics allow on-line, quick responding. However, whereas increases in group size are likely to *decrease* the likelihood of impression formation's being based on direct perception, such increases may *increase* the likelihood of heuristics' being used as a substitute.

We have now summarized various modes of parsing the process of social knowing, ranging from direct, unelaborated detection of information about other people (as in the nonverbal discerning of different emotions and intentions) to highly categorical knowing (as in stereotyping, the extreme form of knowing by description). Given that in our view the ordering of such epistemic modes is significantly constrained by social organization, we introduce principles of complex, dynamic systems at this point.

Social Organization

Overview

We use the term "social organization" to refer to two different but related foci. First, we pro-

pose that there is a hierarchy of social units that constrains different epistemic processes (see Table 29.1). Second, at a process level, we use "social organization" to refer to relations between parts and wholes, involving both issues of coordination and the emergence of collective properties that may not be equal to the sum of the parts. Specifically, we deal with the repeated assembly of lower-order social units into higher-order organizations and with the circular causality between these levels of organization.

The group parameter that we take as driving such organizations is group size, viewed in terms of its functional and structural constraints in regard to what we might designate as "social complexity." Thus, at one level the conceptual challenge is one of relating social complexity of organization to complexity of cognitive organization. Presumed molar mediators of social complexity involve internal modes of organization, such as specifying the roles that constitute group power and communication structures in regard to carrying out modal group tasks (Caporael &

TABLE 29.1. Configurations of Social Systems

Core configurations	Group size	Modal task	Representative processes of social and cognitive coordination
Dyad	2	Mating; infant interaction with adults and older children; expert–novice relations (e.g., ZPD)	Microcoordination, including affective synchrony, mutual perceiving–acting cycles, predominance of perceptual over conceptual processes
Team	5	Foraging, hunting/gathering; contemporary work teams in organizations (e.g., study groups)	Distributed cognition, including both pooled cognition (e.g., dividing a memory task among group members) and emergent knowledge structures; shareability as constraint on cognition
Deme (band)	10-30	Maintenance of group stability, movement from place to place; building coalitions between primary units, dyads, families, etc.; building group cohesion	Emergence of categorical information processing, including sex typing, in-group typing, and outgroup stereotyping; shared construction of reality; minority views as divergent thinking versus groupthink
Macrodeme (macroband)	150+	Maintenance of secondary group cohesion through seasonal gatherings; exchange of individuals, resources, information	Stabilizing and standardizing language, creation of policing body beyond kinship and affinity bonds; relevance of Brewer's optimal-distinctiveness model and Barker's staffing theory to subgroup formation; building intergroup relations through loosening within-group ties

Note. The estimated sizes beyond the dyad are modal approximations based on anthropological sources described in Caporael and Baron (1997). Adapted and expanded from Caporael and Baron (1997). Copyright 1997 by Lawrence Erlbaum Associates. Adapted by permission.

Baron, 1996). These structural constraints in turn create qualitative shifts in epistemic mode, as detailed below.

Dynamic Modes of Social Organization

There are two basic properties of dynamic social organization. First, such systems evolve in a bottom-up fashion over time, such that the interactions at the local level among discrete entities (e.g., individuals) give rise to novel or emergent properties at the collective level. Such emergent properties cannot be predicted from the individual properties of the entities that aggregate; for example, the individuals forming a study group generate a group knowledge structure that exceeds the summation of each participant's individual knowledge. Such groups are self-organized in the sense that the nature of this emergent structure—group-level expertise or group norms— are not specified by external executive programs or scripts. Rather, the nature of the property is the product of a contingent sequence of local interactions. Dynamically, the actions of the system are influenced by feedback from previous states of the system. That is, outputs from one level of organization (e.g., the forming or storming phases of the

evolution of a group) provide outputs that are inputs to the norming phase, which involves individuals' accepting role assignments that cannot be predicted from knowledge of their individual personalities or goals (Tuckman, 1965). Furthermore, this feedback is circular. Once this global or collective structure has emerged, it feeds back and influences subsequent individual members' behavior; for example, members of the study group can deal with a level of exam complexity well beyond their initial capabilities. This process is somewhat similar to that observed with Vygotsky's ZPD (see Figure 29.1).

Further properties of such systems can be specified. The changes in contingent local organization over time are nonlinear: Small changes in input, such as one additional person's favoring consensus, create qualitative phase transitions, as when the group goes from storming (or conflict) to norming (or a state of rule-regulated behavior). Such changes in self-organized systems are driven by continuously changing variables called "control parameters." These may involve external inputs (as when closeness to the date of an exam initiates a shift from individual studying to forming a study group) and/or internal parameters (as when states of increasing group cohesiveness affect the transition from storming to norming to performing) (cf. Tuckman, 1965). Such changes do not involve intermediate states, but occur abruptly when the control parameter exceeds a critical threshold.

Another powerful use of the control parameter concept is "hysteresis": There is an asymmetry between the level of a control parameter that elicits a phase transition and attempts to restore the initial phase state by reversing the level of the control parameter. For example, if a certain level of pay decrease triggers the formation of a union, restoring the original wage level will not break the union; instead, a considerably higher wage increase may be needed. Similarly, if a certain increase in group size instigates a shift from perceptually to categorically based knowing, dropping the group size to that initial level will not wipe out the dominance of categorical/conceptual processing. A very radical reduction in group size will have to take place, and even if it does, mixed-mode processing is likely to occur.

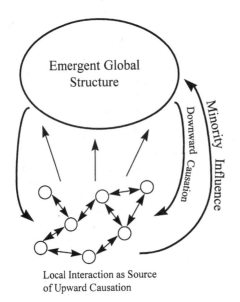

FIGURE 29.1. The self-organization of local and global dynamics within a social system.

The nested, hierarchical system we now describe (see Table 29.1) allows for circular causality, in the sense that the highest levels of social and cognitive organization feed back and modify lower levels in ways that would not be true of isolated dyads or teams. At issue here is a relation designated by Donald Campbell (1990) as "downward causation." This principle is best illustrated in social psychology by Sherif's (1936/1966) study of norm formation. This study showed that the local social dynamics of coordinating individual judgments of movement give rise to the global dynamics of norm formation, which in turn constrain subsequent individual judgments (see Figure 29.1). This analysis also allows us to claim that the relationship between social and epistemic modes of organization can be modeled by aspects of how bottom-up, self-organized, dynamic systems function.

Finally, it should be noted that complex systems are multistable. "Stability" here involves the idea that a system changes its preferred state of organization (the attractor) as it needs to deal with different types of environmental challenges. For example, when an exam is far off, the study group may be attracted to a loose level of organization with little in the way of strict role assignment. However, as the exam gets closer, a more formal role differentiation and rules of operating become enforced by the group. A classic group example of multistability is the regular cycling of groups from a task to a social-emotional orientation (Bales, 1965). This cycling involves what is referred to as a "periodic-attractor regime" (see Beek & Hopkins, 1992). Within the domain of group dynamics, multistability can be used to distinguish single-attractor regimes such as groupthink (Janis, 1982) from groups where minority influence is a potent force. Epistemically, in turn, there is a shift from convergent to divergent processes, which allow a much greater role for the individual to contribute perception-based knowledge (e.g., Nemeth, 1986).

Processes of Self-Organization

Within the model of dynamic systems, self-organization can be instigated either extrinsically or intrinsically. In either case there is self-organization, in the sense that the collective structures or states that emerge are not scripted from the top down—as, for example, the Communist collective farm was, in contradistinction to the kibbutz movement in Israel. That is, whether or not the events triggering self-organization are exogenous or endogenous, they merely set into motion the aggregation process without determining its form; for example, the rules or norms under which the Soviet collective operated were prescribed by the Communist party, while in Israel each kibbutz generated its own norms and rules.

Given this difference, we can still distinguish between extrinsic and intrinsic processes of self-organization. Consider, for example, building intergroup cooperation (see Figure 29.2). The classic Sherif (1966) "robber's cave" model involves triggering the intergroup organization process from the top down by creating a joint external threat. Since the groups are allowed to work out their own reactions to this threat, this situation may qualify as self-organization, much as workers' forming a union when they receive pay cuts below a certain level illustrates such a process.

The external-threat route to self-organization may be contrasted with a codetermination model. The classic physical case example occurs in a chemical-clock type of physical-chemical reaction known as the Belousov–Zhabotinski (BZ) effect.

> In the BZ reaction, the system has the potential to exist in two different states. Assuming that an iron catalyst is used, one state appears red and the other blue. If the reaction is allowed to run in a continuously stirred breaker and the concentration of the reactants crosses a critical threshold, it will oscillate every few minutes (or even seconds) between the red state and the blue at regular intervals. Unlike other chemical reactions it does not move toward a static equilibrium; change is sudden and discontinuous. This occurs because the chemical processes that result in the red state coming into existence become linked to the processes resulting in the blue. When this happens, the two states codetermine one another in a cyclical, nonlinear fashion. (Barton, 1994, p. 7)

The alternation of attractor states described above reflects what might be called temporal self-organization, in that the discontinuous, sudden changes in color emerge not

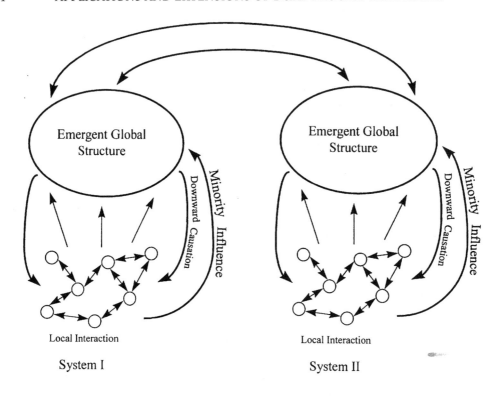

FIGURE 29.2. Building intergroup relations.

because of any specifications from outside the system, but because of local dynamics within the system that self-catalyze the reactions. Specifically, a collective property of the system—which phase state predominates (e.g., which color predominates)—can be viewed as a temporally contingent process of outputs' becoming inputs in a regular cycle of circular causality.

Within social phenomena this principle is of particular importance, because it allows us to treat processes that are typically treated as mutually exclusive as part of a higher-order system. For example, treating minority and majority influence as involving processes of codetermination allows us to see that such processes are interdependent, as are their concomitant cognitive modes of organization. Specifically, minority influence is necessary for divergent thinking, lest a groupthink mentality develop (cf. Janis, 1982). The distinction between minority-based divergent thinking and majority-based convergent thinking can be mapped onto our earlier differential

between perceptual and conceptual modes of knowing. In support of this reinterpretation, we draw upon Wood and her colleagues' persuasive demonstration (based on a meta-analysis) that minority influence is a species of informational social influence, whereas majority influence is rooted in convergent, normative social influence (Wood, Lundgren, Ouellette, Busceme, & Blackstone, 1994).

To see how such processes may codetermine one another, consider how, following Campbell (1990), information-based group processes may evolve in a bottom-up manner. They are data-driven by each person's attempts to know the world accurately. This description fits the present view of perception as the direct detection of information about the world acquired "hands-on." On the other hand, majority influence is probably a top down attempt to make group members accept the wisdom of the majority, in lieu of their own investigation of a problem. That is, normative frameworks replace individual exploration. Group size enters as a control parameter in the sense that as the size of the deviant faction increases, there is a phase transition from disagreement as a deviant viewpoint to deviation as minority influence that needs to be taken seriously (e.g., the shift from one deviant to two or more dissenters).

Furthermore, this description also provides a framework for more perception-based knowing to occur at an intergroup level. Thus, such minority-based feedback processes produce a certain lessening of within-group ties, which is necessary for communication bridges to be built to outside groups (Granovetter, 1973) so as to accomplish cooperative, intergroup problem solving (Sherif, 1966; Aronson, Stephan, Sikes, Barney, & Snapp, 1978). That is, epistemically, members of the ingroup may begin to perceive the actual individual characteristics of outgroup members, as opposed to treating them categorically as evil and/or incompetent. These processes are depicted in Figure 29.2. However, if the within-group ties become too loose, processes are likely to be instigated that strengthen majority influence as a way of maintaining group boundaries. For example, metacontrast may increase; that is, high cohesiveness may motivate members to exaggerate ingroup similarities and outgroup differences (Turner, Hogg, Oakes, Reicher, & Wetherell, 1987). Furthermore, the inhibition of stereotypes may be decreased, because stereotyping facilitates metacontrast (Devine, 1989). This process analysis illustrates the possible circular paths between changes in social organization and the nature of the cognitive mode that is instigated to help resolve the social crisis (see Figure 29.2).

In sum, whether the social system involves the cycling between task and social-emotional processes in group problem solving, or the relative primacy of minority and majority influences, the basic codetermination processes are postulated to be the same. Specifically, the output of dissipative processes from one phase state becomes the input for future levels of organization of the system; literally, there are group dynamics. For example, task-level problem-solving frustration engenders a phase transition to social-emotional processes, which in turn give rise to task focus after a certain level of social bonding is achieved, or *Zeigarnik* processes (task completion tension) build up. Similarly, too strong

a majority influence may arouse reactance and/or a motive for distinctiveness (e.g., Brewer, 1991); too strong a minority influence may instigate a threat to group identity, which serves to restore a better balance between minority and majority influence. As noted earlier, such examples of cycles of intrinsic self-organization, where the triggering or control parameter takes its values from earlier phase states, can be contrasted with self-organization instigated by extrinsic control parameters—such as when the threat of starvation instigates the aggregation of amoebas into a multicellular organism, the slime mold (Garfinkel, 1987); or when the threat of an exam leads to the formation of a study group; or when common external threat leads to intergroup cooperation (Sherif, 1966).

It is also possible that perceptual and conceptual processes directly codetermine each other in a cyclical manner. For example, at a dyadic level, perception-based knowing may generate too much particularistic information; people can't see the forest for the trees. Specifically, when such data-based knowledge gets "too thick," categorical thinking may be instigated. Similarly, the divergent thinking stimulated by minority influence may after a while involve too great a drain on capacity and leave people willing to let others think for them. There is an analogy to such cyclic epistemic shifts in modern art history that will perhaps highlight this point. The excessive perceptual preoccupations of impressionism (as exemplified by Monet) led to the more conceptually oriented paintings of Cezanne, which in turn helped give rise to the conceptual rigors of cubism (cf. Golding, 1994).

What should hold in all cases is certain standard properties of nonlinear, dynamic systems. Thus, whether or not change is a matter of self-organized criticality (Bak & Chen, 1991) or an extrinsic control parameter, it should be nonlinear, such that a small change in the triggering control variable is able to produce a qualitative change or phase transition all at once (i.e., without moving through intermediate stages), and that many such changes will evidence hysteresis. In order to illustrate such claims in greater depth, we are proposing that group size is such a control parameter and that shifts from perceptual to conceptual modes are phase transitions, as would be shifts from heuristic to systematic modes of processing.

Group Size and the Coordination of Social and Cognitive Processes

Table 29.1 summarizes how (based on anthropological data) it is possible to define levels of group size that moderate shifts in social problem solving in ways that require different types of epistemic mediation. Despite the ordering implied in this table, there is more than a simple hierarchical organization. That is, once a higher-level organization appears, the constraints from this level of feedback (downward causation) serve to modify epistemic modes at the level of smaller units, so as to stabilize the higher-level type of organization. For example, relatively isolated dyads may function at a level of microcoordination involving affective synchrony (i.e., coordination of moods or emotions) and may demonstrate the general predominance of perceptual over conceptual processes. However, if a dyad is nested in a team or a band, even dyadic coordination becomes more conceptual. For example, partners may begin to treat each other as types, in terms of more categorical linguistic forms of communication. Such relations may also show evidence of hysteresis, in that once such a shift to conceptually oriented processes has occurred, it is difficult ever to achieve a dominance of perception-based knowing even when the partners are alone (Baron, 1988). Similarly, the nature of epistemic organization at the level of a team may be different, depending on whether the team or study group acts in isolation or is embedded in a larger group context (the band). For example, there are different ways that shareability of information can be structured. At the simplest level, pooled cognition may involve a division of cognitive labor, such as dividing up a phone number so that different people remember different segments. At a more complex level, pooled cognition can involve emergent properties and circular causality, as in Sherif's study of norm formation. This latter mode of organization is naturalistically more likely if the team is nested in a band or larger group (10–30). Specifically, a nested work team is at the cusp of the boundary between intra- and intergroup effects, in that norm formation can be viewed as a significant step toward increased group cohesiveness. Moreover, the Sherif study illustrates how social construction can be treated within a self-organization paradigm involving the interplay of group-level and individual-level processes that form a system of circular causality including downward causation, as illustrated in Figure 29.1. More generally, at the level of group problem solving, the early stages of group development prior to norm formation are assumed to allow a greater role for perception-based knowing.

One of the particularly useful aspects of group size as a control parameter is that it gives us a principled way of describing the transition from within-group to intergroup processes, as well as their interrelationship (see Figure 29.2). Specifically, we assume that certain ingroup problems of power and control, as well as social identity, constrain the evolution of cognitive processes that are needed to cope with these problems of increasing social complexity. For example, as we move from team/study group units (with approximate sizes of 5 members; see Table 29.1) to bands (10–30 members), power-role-type structures are likely to arise, along with minority groups that deviate from the majority. The group modal task (Caporael & Baron, 1996) is likely to involve building group cohesion. Epistemically, we should see the emergence of categorical information processing so that others are treated as types, beginning perhaps with the emergence of gender as a functional status distinction. For example, there is anthropological evidence that forager peoples in Zaire who live in small groups minimize sex typing, whereas groups in Zaire whose farming lifestyle allows for greater population density have a more highly sex-differentiated society (cited in Harris, 1995, p. 471).

Characteristics of Larger Social Groups

Specifically, as group size increases, there is likely to be increased difficulty of direct perception-based social bookkeeping and an increased treatment of others as types, such as "the quiet one" or "the aggressive one" (see Dunbar, 1993, for supporting evidence). The emergence of minority groups is likely to accelerate this process of increased *within-*

group social stereotyping. With the emergence of ingroup inequalities in power, one way to get people to accept such power differentials is to create a strong social identity in terms of the group as a major source of self-esteem. Thus we see the emergence of social-categorical thinking as a mechanism leading to the emergence of ingroup favoritism and eventually to outgroup hostility (see Figure 29.2). For example, the group will use outgroup threat to maintain an ingroup power hierarchy (see Table 29.1). In terms of our own basic epistemic distinctions, individuals are increasingly treated as category types, as opposed to complex particulars whose properties are directly encountered.

Furthermore, group size itself is a deterrent to group loyalty and identity, forcing high-status groups to seek further differentiation into subgroups (Brewer, 1991). As noted in Table 29.1, unless larger social organizations evince subgroup formation, with the concomitant building of cohesiveness, formal rule-enforcing mechanisms develop as a substitute for the self-organized regulation by shared affinity bonds. It is in this context that Brewer's optimal-distinctiveness theory—the balancing of distinctiveness and assimilation motives—predicts that numerically smaller groupings such as minority groups will evince stronger group identity and loyalty. If to Brewer's theory we add Barker's (1968) and Barker and Gump's (1964) over- and understaffing model of the relationship between the number of roles to be filled and the number of participants available, some clear predictions can be made regarding the relationship between larger social units and epistemic mode. For example, supportive of Brewer's predictions about group identity and group loyalty are the findings reported in the book *Big School, Small School* (Barker & Gump, 1964); that is, in understaffed settings, where roles exceed participants, people will engage in more activities, expend more effort, feel more committed, be more attracted to the group, and in general feel more involved and important. Large, overstaffed groups handle deviant individuals qualitatively differently than small, understaffed groups do. In overstaffed groups deviates are expelled, whereas in understaffed groups they are rehabilitated. Rehabilitation requires a good deal more perception-based, particularistic epistemic treatment than expelling; that is, stereotyping or demonizing the deviant will be more likely with larger group size and overstaffing.

In sum, in such contexts, size–involvement relations are likely to be reflected in more "hands-on," perception-based knowledge of other people. Moreover, because in small-group behavior settings the same person plays more than one role, it becomes possible to treat impression formation as the detection of invariants in a "bottom-up" epistemic mode. In such contexts, categorization enters at the level of stabilizing and communicating impressions, as opposed to the generation of the impression (e.g., Hoffman et al., 1981).

Epistemic Mode in Small versus Large Groups

With regard to task-level group activities, level of involvement has been specified by Eagly and Chaiken (1993) as a key moderator of whether heuristic or systematic processing will be the preferred epistemic mode for problem solving. It can thus generally be predicted that smaller groups are more likely to utilize systematic than heuristic processing. In this context, the fact that investigators such as Nemeth (1986) find that minority factions generate more divergent thinking in groups than majority factions do can be attributed at least in part to group size variations between minority and majority groupings. That is, minorities, which are smaller and often more involved than majorities, are more likely to engage in systematic thinking. Finally, as can be seen from Table 29.1, the prediction regarding the behavior of macrobands can be reframed in these terms. For example, the fact that macro-band level groupings (150–300 or larger) regularly schedule seasonal meetings (e.g., those of the American Psychological Association and the American Psychological Society) fits Brewer's (1991) derivations from optimal-distinctiveness theory, as does the occurrence of regional meetings. At issue in all of these instances is the attempt to increase secondary group cohesion by generating subgroup organizations.

This general line of reasoning can also be applied to the U.S. political system of two large parties, versus the multiparty system favored by other countries such as Italy, France, and Israel. The basic hypothesis follows from the general arguments adduced thus far regarding the relationships between size and conceptual epistemic mode. Specifically, the two-party system, although it has national, regional, and local subgroupings, in general is likely to involve larger groups than a multiparty system. For example, understaffing is more likely to be a problem with multiple political parties. However, in a multiparty system given smaller sized parties, there is likely to be greater within-group cohesiveness and, if we are correct, greater possibilities for divergent thinking, since in effect each party is a minority group. In support of this line of reasoning, a far larger proportion of the electorate votes in national elections in these countries. Furthermore, we would predict that a content analysis of political speeches in these countries, as opposed to the United States, would find far more examples of systematic as opposed to heuristic thinking.

A rather unsettling implication of this analysis is the hypothesis that increased heuristic processing is what is presently supporting the U.S. two-party system (including Baron's own heuristic for presidential elections, which is to vote for the party more likely to keep the Supreme Court from becoming too conservative). Furthermore, this hypothesis can be seen to derive from the circular relations that are postulated to be at the heart of our approach: Group size parameters constrain epistemic mode, which in turn constrains the stability of the mode of political organization that exists in this country. Finally, when the country was smaller it is possible that systematic processing was more possible within the two-party framework, given such traditions as town meetings.

Given the speculative nature of this section, it is perhaps appropriate that in the next section of this chapter we deal with a more classic problem in personality and social psychology—the achievement of accuracy in social knowing. Consistent with the present approach to modeling the relationship between social and cognitive organization, we treat accuracy as an epistemic achievement that is validated pragmatically at a collective, social level.

IMPLICATIONS FOR THE STUDY OF SOCIAL ACCURACY

We choose to use social accuracy to illustrate (1) how the size of the social unit influences the meaning of accuracy in regard to the nature of the epistemic mode; and (2) how once we view different-sized units as nested, accuracy becomes constrained by broader principles of dynamic self-organization, such that one cannot evaluate accuracy at the lower level independently of the higher level—a special case of Campbell's (1990) downward causation. For example, this interpretation provides a systematic context for Steiner's (1955) seminal insight that accuracy at the dyadic level can be counterproductive at the level of the larger group or organization.

Following Steiner's (1955) early analysis of accuracy in organizational settings, it appears that the success of individual perceiving may be nested in the success of the larger social unit, be it the dyad, group, or organization. That is, dyadic accuracy is relational and perception-based. For example, if a person is operating in a dyad (see Table 29.1), we propose that the accuracy of a particular perceived attribute is an extension of the basic Gibsonian proposition that perceiving is for doing, or in this case for social doing. Thus, we can test the accuracy of a perceiver's prediction that a target is high in agreeableness by seeing whether the other person is willing to be agreeable in suitable circumstances. Specifically, it is hypothesized that accuracy is a matter of social pragmatics: If people are asked for help that is increasingly demanding in nature, highly agreeable people will probably continue to agree longer before refusing than less agreeable people will.

At the small-group level, the test of an accurate perception of another's agreeableness is whether people selected, for example, to be part of a study group actually work well with the other people, in the sense of being able to coordinate their efforts to divide up a complex task situation. In effect, accuracy is as accuracy does. At the level of larger groups and organizations, including behavioral settings, accuracy becomes a matter of reciprocal self-selection. Specifically, what is at issue is getting the right people into the right roles, into the right subgroups, in the right behavior settings. For example, do people with different dispositions who select themselves into particular behavior settings succeed in these settings? Conversely, how well do gatekeepers in a setting do in selecting people along the correct dimensions to keep the setting functioning properly, whether it is an athletic team or church (see Kenrick, McCreath, Govern, King, & Bordin, 1990)?

Determinants of Social Accuracy

The Face-to-Face Encounter

The prototype of the face-to-face encounter (see Table 29.1) is the mother–child interaction. This is perhaps the purest example of reciprocal direct perception that is validated online. For example, the infant's smile directly elicits a reciprocal response by the mother; she smiles back. Or a cry of distress elicits a nurturing response by the mother, which, if appropriate, leads to the cessation of crying. Here we can indeed observe that perception is for social doing, within this microcoordination view of accuracy.

Observability

The relationship between observability and accuracy is well documented (Kenrick & Funder, 1988). The particular "spin" we wish to put on this finding is that such results are supportive of the ecological claim that perceptual-level processes mediate the detection of individual differences in adults that have high adaptive significance. Specifically, observability means that there is rich information available regarding the presence of certain dispositions (or social affordances, in terms of the ecological framework of McArthur & Baron, 1983). Indeed, the range of information available to the perceptual detection of dispositional affordances is so great that consensual perceptions of affective and motivational dispositions have been demonstrated with protosocial stimuli limited to the movement patterns (individual and reciprocal) of differently shaped geometric entities (Heider & Simmel, 1944; Michotte, 1963; Misovich, 1995). The boundary conditions for consensual judgments, as well as evidence regarding the operative epistemic mode (perceptual vs. conceptual), has recently been demonstrated in a line of research using the original Heider

and Simmel (1944) film (e.g., Berry & Misovich, 1994; Berry, Misovich, Kean, & Baron, 1992; Misovich, 1995). Specifically, perceivers' dispositional judgments regarding the film's triangles and circle are highly sensitive to procedures that interfere with movement information (Berry et al., 1992). However, they are relatively unaffected by conceptual-interference operations (e.g., counting backwards), unless a level of perceptual interference is also present (Misovich, 1995).

Consistent with the importance of perceptually relevant information for accuracy of dispositional judgment is the importance of the observability of dispositionally relevant information. In this context, aggression is more accurately detected than conscientiousness (Wright & Mischel, 1987), because it is more observable and hence becomes grist for the perceptual apparatus. On the other hand, conscientiousness is largely a culturally constrained category that is probably inferred from the top down, rather than detected from the bottom up. Dimensions such as conscientiousness are hypothesized to lack consistent, observable referents that people are preattuned to detect because of the attribute's relative lack of evolutionary significance. That is, it is more important to diagnose aggressive intent correctly than steady work habits, given the consequences of mistakes in each case.

Event–Activity Tests

Sometimes, however, observability does not suffice, because socially skilled others learn to hide socially undesirable dispositions. We (Baron & Misovich, 1993a) have proposed, in the spirit of King Solomon's test for diagnosing which woman claiming to be the mother of an infant is authentic, that in such contexts competent perceivers create diagnostic conditions for detecting dispositional variations. Such tests are directly relevant to our distinction between perceptual and conceptual processes. It is proposed that event–activity tests (EATs) mediate observability, thereby turning the detection of dispositions into a more direct perceptual mode. For example, when confronted by a stranger in an evaluative situation, shy people manifest a number of detectable nonverbal signs of social anxiety (Cheek & Buss, 1981). Similarly, when scarce, valued resources are open for control, high-dominance people are likely to engage in easily perceivable verbal and nonverbal acts of an assertive nature, such as looming over the other, controlling pause patterns, and looking while speaking as opposed to looking while listening (e.g., Ellyson & Dovidio, 1985). Specifically, just as the solubility of salt is revealed under suitable circumstances, such as placing the suspected entity in a solvent such as water (as opposed to exposing it to flame to test its solubility), so many personality dispositions have suitable circumstances that will function to reveal an individual's standing on that disposition. For example, shy people are uniquely likely to be more withdrawn when encountering strangers than when they are meeting friends. Similarly, dominance-seeking people are more likely to assert control when a scarce, valued resource is being competed for than when they are enjoying plentiful resources.

Viewed from this perspective, the use of EATs can be treated as a good means of observing the interaction of perceptual and conceptual modes, because it is analogous to diagnosticity under high salience in Trope and Gaunt's (Chapter 8, this volume) integration model. For example, the use of EATs may proceed from a conceptual to a perceptual level, becoming, in effect, an interpersonal extension of Neisser's (1976) insight that schemas may function to guide perception. Moreover, such EATs either may function as heuristics and hence run automatically, or, in other contexts and perhaps for other people, may involve systematic processing. For example, socially skilled persons may use such tests automatically, whereas in other contexts such as personnel selection, these are carefully thought-out processes. In either case, the data yielded by such tests may be detected perceptually, particularly in regard to leakage occurring in nonverbal channels.

Recently we carried out research designed to investigate the first part of this conceptualization of EATs—the availability of diagnostic schemas—on the assumption that these schemas have important implications for the problem of accuracy. Certain schemas improve accuracy because they attune people more selectively to the relevant social variables; in such cases, cognition directs the process of perception. For instance, Misovich

(1992) found that college women who had more extensive experience with infants made greater use of diagnostic information about dynamic synchrony when judging whether an infant was interacting with its mother or a stranger. Women with relatively little experience used this information less and appeared to make use of less diagnostic affective cues. Consequently, they were less accurate in their judgments of who was the actual mother.

Following from the ideas presented within event-test theory, we conducted a study to investigate the relationships between participants' social competence scores and the diagnosticity of their self-generated EATs. Specifically, we attempted to demonstrate that socially skilled people are better at creating circumstances that yield diagnostic information, in the sense that on-line such information is likely to capitalize on the nonverbal leakage of "true" intentions. Participants were given hypothetical situations that required the selection of an individual who possessed a certain trait (i.e., one of the "Big Five"). The task for the participants was to describe a situation they could set up that would allow them to determine whether the person did indeed possess the trait that the situation required. Essentially, by describing these situations, subjects created their own EATs for all of the Big Five traits (extraversion, agreeableness, conscientiousness, emotional stability, and openness). In this context, it was assumed that generating the tests might be a conceptual process, whereas the data they reveal might be detected perceptually. Trained raters then categorized participants' EATs as consisting of one or more of the following behaviors: (1) observing the target person alone; (2) observing the target interacting with others; (3) interacting with the target oneself; or (4) directly asking the target whether he or she possessed the trait of interest. An overall diagnosticity score was also assigned to each of the EATs, which was based on three criteria: practicality (could the EAT actually be carried out?), correspondence (did the EAT contain behaviors that were relevant to the trait?), and extent (did the EAT elicit behaviors or situations that related to the trait?).

The category type and overall diagnosticity were then correlated with participants' self-reported social competence scores. The

Social Skills Inventory (e.g., Riggio, 1986) yields an overall social competence score and six individual subscale scores measuring the more specific emotional and social skills that characterize social competence. The results indicated the following relationships: For women, high scores on Social Control (one of the subscales of the Social Skills Inventory) were associated with greater diagnosticity in their EATs across all of the traits ($r = .36$, $p < .05$). Also, women scoring higher on Social Control generated more diagnostic tests of emotional stability ($r = .34$, $p < .05$) and were higher in the diagnosticity of their tests for extraversion ($r = .33$, $p < .05$). Consistent with these findings, Ambady, Hallahan, and Rosenthal (1995) found that participants high in self-monitoring were more accurate than those low in self-monitoring in judging the dimension of emotional stability.

Our finding that women high in social control achieved greater diagnosticity across traits and on specific traits is supported by previous findings that women are more accurate than men on tasks involving sensitivity to the emotions, nonverbal cues, and verbal implications of others (Costanzo & Archer, 1989; Sullins, 1992; Thompson, 1967). Specifically, a woman high in social control is someone who interacts with many people, accepts a leadership role readily, and feels comfortable with a diverse range of people (Riggio, 1986). This ability to adapt and respond to the current cues of the social environment probably provided our high-social-control participants with experience and information that were very useful to them in creating EATs. Since the underlying goal of EAT theory is to constrain the behaviors of others in ways that will reveal relevant dispositional information, we propose that women higher in social control are better able both to generate the situations cognitively and to perceive the diagnostic information thus obtained (the latter hypothesis remains to be tested).

Accuracy in Larger-Group Settings

First we must distinguish between accuracy in larger-group settings where tests akin to EATs are possible, and accuracy in situations where it cannot be constrained by information generated through face-to-face interaction. Spe-cifically, at the larger-group level it is likely that gatekeepers perform such tests. Indeed, the whole field of personnel selection can be viewed as an attempt to devise such tests. EATs are, in effect, the mechanisms through which various behavior settings recruit appropriate role occupants (Kenrick et al., 1990). Furthermore, it is likely that the motivation for selecting the appropriate recruit in a given setting, group, or organization increases as the cohesiveness of the group increases. EATs become devices for shaping ingroup–outgroup differences—often with tragic consequences, as these tests become ever more superficial and destructive, such as the genocidal gatekeeping of Hitler's Germany. Indeed, in Denmark, the country most protective of its Jewish population, the Danes tried to eliminate all cues that might discriminate between Jews and non-Jews, with the King going so far as to wear a yellow armband (Baron vividly recalls a Danish family telling him that they first and foremost looked at their Jews as Danes).

Moreover, often schemas do not function as attunements designed to increase accurate accommodation to the environment. Rather, they function as expectations, replete with a confirmation bias that is indifferent to disconfirming information. Specifically, such schemas function to construct a selective reality. For example, groupthink organizations, in their attempts to solidify ingroup biases, are likely to ignore disconfirming information altogether, as when John F. Kennedy's CIA advisors ignored evidence that the Cuban population was not about to rise up against Castro if there was an invasion (Janis, 1982).

On the other hand, as Baron (1995) has proposed elsewhere, certain stereotypes may facilitate accuracy in social perception. For example, suppose an academic family is changing jobs and moving to a rural school. The teenage children of this family may enter the local high school with an urban–rural stereotype that rural teens are naive, "big into football," and so on. Furthermore, suppose there are two high schools in town—one that has largely the offspring of faculty as students, the other the children of local towns-people. Depending on which school this family sends the children to, the country bumpkin stereotype may or may not be accurate or useful, in the sense that when the stereotype matches the modal school social structure, the children's initial socializing is likely to be more successful than not, in choices of conversational topics and other social behaviors. At issue here is the problem of matching the right stereotype to the right referent, rather than whether or not a stereotype is correct or incorrect per se. That is, in the right setting, schemas may facilitate appropriate attunements and *environmentally appropriate actions*—our major criteria for accuracy.

The Problem of Nested Levels of Social Units

Given that in certain settings, social organization is largely a problem of nested levels of social units (see Table 29.1), two other refinements are needed in relating social constraints to the accuracy of cognitive units. First, it is possible that different types of persons are needed at different phases of the evolution of a group or organization. For example, certain stages of problem solving require a task leader, while others require a social-emotional leader. In this case, accuracy is the degree to which the role is well filled in regard to solving the problem—for example, building the atomic bomb versus reducing task-based frustration. A good example was the firing of a coach of the New York Knicks basketball team for being too "laid back" (a more successful previous coach was extremely task-oriented). In this context, this lack-of-fit outcome could probably have been correctly predicted.

Accuracy, then is relational; it is a matter of the reciprocal fit between cognitive and social units or modes of organization. Such synergisms evolve because they stabilize the highest level of organization of the systems, thereby allowing the social unit to function effectively in the external environment. This reasoning fits Steiner's (1955) proposal that dyadic accuracy may be dysfunctional at the organizational level. That is, being a good boss from the individual subordinate's point of view may involve different criteria than being a good supervisor from top management's perspective may. For example, what appears distant and cold at the dyadic level may involve the supervisor's following his or her role prescriptions, and thereby providing a good fit at the broader social level.

Because we usually decontextualize accuracy, we miss the broader constraints on what are appropriate actions. In this regard, Fiedler's (1978) contingency model of leadership—which proposes that the type of leader who will be most effective (e.g., task-oriented and distant vs. relationship-sensitive) depends on the situation—also becomes a guide to accuracy. That is, accuracy is circumscribed at more than the interpersonal level proposed in Swann's (1984) analysis. Similarly, Wright and Mischel's (1987) if–then contingencies appear to be local and one-way; in our view, accuracy reflects a broader, nested set of constraints. Moreover, the lesson at the lower level is to disambiguate whether the coldness of the supervisor is a role-prescribed leadership style (the supervisor treats subordinates the way all subordinates are supposed to be treated), is a general personality trait (the supervisor even treats his or her equals in power coldly), or is circumscribed dyadically (as in Swann's [1984] or Kenny's [1988] relationship effect).

These situations, in turn, involve different types of relationships between conceptual and perceptual bases of knowing. For example, perceptual-level knowing requires face-to-face encounters (ideally, extended over time) and the ability to see the other person in multiple contexts. As group size increases, such possibilities first increase and then sharply decrease. For example, dyads may be more informative than individual actions, and small groups allow people to establish relationship effects by observing when certain actions hold across different partners or are partner-specific (Kenny, 1988). Beyond a certain size, however, accuracy becomes largely a matter of categorical fits and the accuracy of stereotypes.

Finally, we suggest that accuracy itself should be viewed at the level of a complex system. From this perspective, the lack of accuracy is not a matter of deficits in human information-processing capabilities; rather, it reflects states of dissynchrony among the units of the system. That is, individuals who are inaccurate, groups that foster inaccuracy (e.g., groupthink), and organizations that read their task environment inaccurately (e.g., IBM's initial response to the emergence of small personal-computer companies) lack bridges to the broader social environment

(Granovetter, 1973) that could provide accurate, if unsettling, information from outgroups. At the process level, the reason why groups become able to cooperate with outgroups may have to do with a loosening of local cohesiveness, which enables a shift from schema-based functioning aimed at avoiding disconfirmation to schema-based functioning aimed at better attuning the ingroup to the outgroup. Here accuracy probably emerges from a loosening of social ties, based on the ascendance to power of previous minorities who favored alliances based on a more accurate reading of the outgroup properties. That is, cohesiveness, because it both stifles within-group divergent thinking and encourages inappropriate outgroup stereotypes, is a strong deterrent to accuracy in collective social judgment.

CONCLUDING COMMENTS

The proposal that cohesiveness may interfere with the particularistic epistemic processes necessary for group-level accuracy epitomizes the central thrust of this analysis. The type of epistemic mode that emerges is, to paraphrase Vygotsky (1978), refracted through the type of social organization that occurs, thereby offering us a new perspective on group mind. For us, "group mind" means that the group is the mind's environment, and that, reciprocally, the nature of the epistemic mode actively constrains what type of social organizations are likely to emerge and become stabilized. Treating the group in this manner makes it very difficult to maintain the standard individualistic interpretation of social cognition. Indeed, what is called for is no less than a paradigm shift, in order to encompass both the sociality constraint and the concomitant claim that the relations between social and epistemic modes of organization be conceptualized in terms of principles derived from the operation of nonlinear, dynamic systems of a complex nature. In sum, we are attempting to go beyond critiquing the traditional interpretation of social cognition by proposing that sociality and cognition mutually constrain each other in ways that are derivable from the principles of how complex, dynamic systems build higher-order levels of organization.

REFERENCES

Abelson, R. P. (1983). Whatever became of consistency theory? *Personality and Social Psychology Bulletin, 9,* 37–54.

Ambady, N. (1997). *Accuracy of thin slice judgments: Judging sexual orientation.* Paper presented at the annual meeting of the Society of Experimental Social Psychology, Toronto.

Ambady, N., Hallahan, M., & Rosenthal, R. (1995). On judging and being judged accurately in zero-acquaintance situations. *Journal of Personality and Social Psychology, 69,* 518–529.

Ambady, N., & Rosenthal, R. (1992). Thin slices of expressive behavior as predictors of interpersonal consequences: A meta-analysis. *Psychological Bulletin, 111,* 256–274.

Aronoff, J., Woike, B. A., & Hyman, L. M. (1992). Which are the stimuli in facial displays of anger and happiness? *Journal of Personality and Social Psychology, 62,* 1050–1066.

Aronson, E., Stephan, C., Sikes, J., Barney, N., & Snapp, M. (1978). *The jigsaw classroom.* Beverly Hills, CA: Sage.

Asch, S. (1952). *Social psychology.* Englewood Cliffs, NJ: Prentice-Hall.

Bak, P., & Chen, K. (1991). Self-organized criticality. *Scientific American, 264,* 46–53.

Bales, R. (1965). The equilibrium problem in small groups. In A. P. Hare, E. F. Borgotta, & R. F. Bales (Eds.), *Small groups: Studies in social interaction* (pp. 111–161). New York: Knopf.

Barker, R. G. (1968). *Ecological psychology.* Stanford, CA: Stanford University Press.

Barker, R. G., & Gump, P. (1964). *Big school, small school.* Stanford, CA: Stanford University Press.

Baron, R. M. (1980). Contrasting approaches to social knowing: An ecological perspective. *Personality and Social Psychology Bulletin, 6,* 591–600.

Baron, R. M. (1988). An ecological framework for establishing a dual mode theory of social knowing. In D. Bar-Tal & A. W. Kruglanski (Eds.), *The social psychology of knowledge* (pp. 48–82). New York: Cambridge University Press.

Baron, R. M. (1991). A meditation on levels of structure. *Contemporary Psychology, 36,* 566–568.

Baron, R. M. (1995). An ecological view of stereotype accuracy. In Y. T. Lee, L. Jussim, & C. R. McCauley (Eds.), *Stereotype accuracy: Toward appreciating group differences* (pp. 115–140). Washington, DC: American Psychological Association.

Baron, R. M., & Misovich, S. J. (1993a). Dispositional knowing from an ecological perspective. *Personality and Social Psychology Bulletin, 19,* 541–552.

Baron, R. M., & Misovich, S. J. (1993b). An integration of Gibsonian and Vygotskian perspectives on changing attitudes in group contexts. *British Journal of Social Psychology, 32,* 53–70.

Barton, S. (1994). Chaos, self-organization and psychology. *American Psychologist, 49,* 5–14.

Beek, P. J., & Hopkins, B. (1992). Four requirements for a dynamical systems approach to the development of social coordination. *Human Movement Science, 11,* 425–442.

Berry, D. S., & Misovich, S. J. (1994). Methodological

approaches to the study of social event perception. *Personality and Social Psychology Bulletin, 20,* 139–152.

Berry, D. S., Misovich, S. J., Kean, K. J., & Baron, R. M. (1992). The effects of disruption of structure and motion on perceptions of social causality. *Personality and Social Psychology Bulletin, 18,* 237–244.

Brewer, M. (1991). The social self: On being the same and different at same time. *Personality and Social Psychology Bulletin, 17,* 475–482.

Bruner, J. S. (1957). Going beyond the information given. In J. Bruner (Ed.), *Contemporary approaches to cognition: The Colorado Symposium* (p. 473). Cambridge, MA: Harvard University Press.

Buss, D. M. (1996). Social adaptation and five major factors of personality. In J. S. Wiggins (Ed.), *The five-factor model of personality: Theoretical perspectives* (pp. 180–207). New York: Guilford Press.

Campbell, D. T. (1990). Levels of organizations downward causation and the selection theory approach to evolutionary epistemology. In G. Greenberg & E. Tobach (Eds.), *Theories of the evolution of knowing* (pp. 1–17). Hillsdale, NJ: Erlbaum.

Caporael, L. R., & Baron, R. M. (1997). Groups as mind's natural environment. In J. Simpson & D. Kenrick (Eds.), *Evolutionary approaches in personality and social psychology* (pp. 313–339). Hillsdale, NJ: Erlbaum.

Chaiken, S. (1980). Heuristic versus systematic processing and the use of source versus message cues in persuasion. *Journal of Personality and Social Psychology, 39,* 752–766.

Cheek, J. M., & Buss, A. H. (1981). Shyness and sociability. *Journal of Personality and Social Psychology, 41,* 330–339.

Chen, S., Schechter, D., & Chaiken, S. (1996). Getting at the truth or getting along: Accuracy- versus impression-motivated heuristic and systematic processing. *Journal of Personality and Social Psychology, 71,* 262–275.

Cosmides, L. (1989). The logic of social exchange: Has natural selection shaped how humans reason? *Cognition, 31,* 187–276.

Costanzo, M., & Archer, D. (1989). Interpreting the expressive behaviors of others: The Interpersonal Perception Task. *Journal of Nonverbal Behavior, 13,* 225–245.

Devine, P. G. (1989). Stereotypes and prejudice: Their automatic and controlled components. *Journal of Personality and Social Psychology, 56,* 5–15.

Dunbar, R. I. M. (1993). Coevolution of neocortical size, group size, and language in humans. *Behavioral and Brain Sciences, 16,* 681–735.

Eagly, A. E., & Chaiken, S. (1993). *The psychology of attitudes.* Fort Worth, TX: Harcourt Brace Jovanovich.

Ellyson, S. L., & Dovidio, J. F. (1985). Power, dominance and nonverbal behavior: Basic conceptual issues. In S. L. Ellyson & J. F. Dovidio (Eds.), *Power, dominance and nonverbal behavior* (pp. 1–28). New York: Springer-Verlag.

Fiedler, F. E. (1978).The contingency model and the dynamics of the leadership process. In L. Berkowitz (Ed.), *Advances in experimental social psychology* (Vol. 12, pp. 59–112). New York: Academic Press.

Fiske, S. T., & Taylor, S. E. (1991). *Social cognition* (2nd ed.). New York: McGraw-Hill.

Freyd, J. J. (1983). Shareability: The social psychology of epistemology. *Cognitive Science, 7,* 191–210.

Garfinkel, A. (1987). The slime mold *Dictyostelium* as a model of self-organization in social systems. In F. E. Yates (Ed.), *Self-organizing systems: The emergence of order* (pp. 181–212). New York: Plenum Press.

Gibson, J. (1979). *The ecological approach to visual perception.* Boston: Houghton Mifflin.

Gilbert, D. T., Pelham, B. W., & Krull, D. S. (1988). On cognition busyness: When person perceivers meet persons perceived. *Journal of Personality and Social Psychology, 54,* 733–739.

Golding, J. (1994). Cubism. In N. Stangos (Ed.), *Concepts of modern art: From Fauvism to postmodernism* (pp. 50–78). New York: Thames & Hudson.

Granovetter, M. S. (1973). The strength of weak ties. *American Journal of Sociology, 78,* 1360–1380.

Grayson, B., & Stein, M. J. (1981). Attracting assault: Victims' nonverbal cues. *Journal of Communication, 31,* 68–75.

Harris, J. R. (1995). Where is the child's environment?: A group socialization theory of development. *Psychological Bulletin, 102,* 458–489.

Heider, F. (1958). *The psychology of interpersonal relations.* New York: Wiley.

Heider, F. (1990). *The notebooks: Vol. 6. Units and coinciding units.* Munich: Psychologie Verlags Union.

Heider, F., & Simmel, M. (1944). An experimental study of apparent behavior. *American Journal of Psychology, 57,* 243–259.

Hoffman, C., Mischel, W., & Mazze, K. (1981). The role of purpose in the organization of information about behavior: Trait-based versus goal-based categories in person cognition. *Journal of Personality and Social Psychology, 40,* 211–221.

Janis, I. (1982). *Victims of groupthink* (2nd ed.). Boston: Houghton Mifflin.

Johnson-Laird, P. N., & Wason, P. C. (1970). Insight into a logical relation. *Quarterly Journal of Experimental Psychology, 22,* 49–61.

Kenny, D. A. (1988). Interpersonal perception: A social relations analysis. *Journal of Social and Personal Relationships, 5,* 247–261.

Kenrick, D. T., & Funder, D. C. (1988). Profiting from controversy: Lessons from the person–situation debate. *American Psychologist, 43,* 23–34.

Kenrick, D. T., McCreath, H. E., Govern, J., King, R., & Bordin, J. (1990). Person–environment interactions: Everyday setting and common trait dynamics. *Journal of Personality and Social Psychology, 58,* 685–698.

McArthur, L. Z., & Baron, R. M. (1983). Toward an ecological theory of social perception. *Psychological Review, 90,* 215–238.

Michotte, A. (1963). *The perception of causality.* New York: Basic Books.

Misovich, S. J. (1992). *The effect of dyadic synchrony and behavioral experience on detection of maternal relationship and judgments of a daycare worker.* Unpublished manuscript, University of Connecticut.

Misovich, S. J. (1995). *The effects of stimulus disruption and cognitive busyness on the tendency to describe the Heider and Simmel film in anthropomorphic terms.* Unpublished doctoral dissertation, University of Connecticut.

Neisser, U. (1976). *Cognition and reality.* San Francisco: Freeman.

Nemeth, C. J. (1986). Differential contributions of majority and minority influence. *Psychological Review, 93*, 23–32.

Newcomb, T. M. (1953). An approach to the study of communicative acts. *Psychological Review, 60*, 393–404.

Nicolis, G., & Prigogene, I. (1988). *Exploring complexity: An introduction.* New York: Freeman.

Petty, R. E., & Cacioppo, J. (1984). The effects of involvement on responses to argument quantity and quality: Central and peripheral routes to persuasion. *Journal of Personality and Social Psychology, 46*, 69–81.

Riggio, R. E. (1986). Assessment of basic social skills. *Journal of Personality and Social Psychology, 51*, 649–660.

Roediger, H. L., & McDermott, K. B. (1993). Implicit memory in normal human subjects. In F. Boller & J. Grafman (Eds.), *Handbook of neuropsychology* (Vol. 8, pp. 63–128). Amsterdam: Elsevier.

Russell, B. (1912). *Problems of philosophy.* New York: Oxford University Press.

Schacter, D. L. (1989). On the relation between memory and consciousness: Dissociable interactions and conscious experience. In H. L. Roediger & F. Craik (Eds.), *Varieties of memory and consciousness: Essays in honor of Endid Tulving* (pp. 355–389). Hillsdale, NJ: Erlbaum.

Sherif, M. (1966). *The psychology of social norms.* New York: Harper & Row. (Original work published 1936)

Sherif, M. (1966). *In common predicament: Social psychology of intergroup conflict and cooperation.* Boston: Houghton Mifflin.

Snyder, M. (1984). When belief creates reality. In L. Berkowitz (Ed.), *Advances in experimental social psychology* (Vol. 18, pp. 185–208). New York: Academic Press.

Steiner, I. D. (1955). Interpersonal behavior as influenced by accuracy of social perception. *Psychological Review, 62*, 268–274.

Sullins, E. (1992). Interpersonal perception between same-sex friends. *Journal of Social Behavior and Personality, 7*, 395–414.

Swann, W. B. (1984). Quest for accuracy in person perception: A matter of pragmatics. *Psychological Review, 91*, 457–477.

Thompson, W. N. (1967). *Quantitative research in public address and communication.* New York: Random House.

Tuckman, B. W. (1965). Developmental sequences in small groups. *Psychological Bulletin, 63*, 384–399.

Turner, J. C., Hogg, M., Oakes, P., Reicher, S., & Wetherell, M. (1987). *Rediscovering the group: A self-categorization theory.* Oxford: Blackwell.

Vygotsky, L. S. (1978). *Mind in society.* Cambridge, MA: Harvard University Press.

Vygotsky, L. S. (1991). Genesis of higher mental functions. In P. Light, S. Sheldon, & M. Woodhead (Eds.), *Learning to think* (pp. 32–41). London: Open University Press. (Original work published 1978)

Weschler, L. (1982). *Seeing is forgetting the name of the thing one sees.* Berkeley: University of California Press.

Wood, W., Lundgren, S., Ouellette, J. A., Busceme, S., & Blackstone, T. (1994). Minority influence: A meta-analytic review of social influence processes. *Psychological Bulletin, 115*, 323–345.

Wright, J. C., & Mischel, W. (1987). A conditional approach to dispositional constructs: The local predictability of social behavior. *Journal of Personality and Social Psychology, 53*, 1158–1177.

Zajonc, R. B. (1960). The process of cognitive tuning in communication. *Journal of Abnormal and Social Psychology, 61*, 159–167.

Zajonc, R. B. (1984). On the primacy of affect. *American Psychologist, 39*, 117–123.

30

Dualities and Continua

IMPLICATIONS FOR UNDERSTANDING
PERCEPTIONS OF PERSONS AND GROUPS

DAVID L. HAMILTON
STEVEN J. SHERMAN
KEITH B. MADDOX

When we were asked to write a chapter concerning our work on impression formation processes for individual and group targets (Hamilton & Sherman, 1996; Hamilton, Sherman, & Lickel, 1998) for a book on dual-process models in social psychology, we were naturally flattered and enthusiastic. But we were also somewhat surprised. What could we say about dual processes in the formation of impressions of social targets? Did our analysis of the mechanisms involved in social perception and stereotype development qualify as a dual-process analysis? Although we had considered at great length the processes and mechanisms thought to underlie the development of impressions of individuals and groups, we had not framed the discussion specifically in terms of a dual-process approach. We had employed the important distinction between impressions that are formed on-line, as the relevant information about the target is received, and impressions that are memory-based, developed long after the initial target information was presented. But we were not convinced that this distinction truly qualified as a dual-process model of impression formation.

At this point, we stepped back a little to ask ourselves what the purpose of the present book really was. We looked at the titles of other chapters that had been proposed for the book, and we tried to see how our work would fit with or complement these other chapters. We wanted to gain some insight into what these chapters had in common and what the "glue" was that held these chapters together as descriptions of dual-process models in social psychology. The glue proved to be quite elusive to capture. More questions were raised than were answered. It was here that we came to a rather embarrassing realization: We were not sure exactly what constituted a dual-process model or why! How could we write a chapter about our work under the rubric of a dual-process model without having a clear understanding of the conditions necessary for an approach to qualify as such a model?

So we did what any good scientist would do: We asked our friends who should know the answers. These were primarily cognitive psychologists who had done work that, in our minds, clearly fell into the category of dual-process models. Surely they would have the answers for us. At least they would be able to steer us in the right direction. As surprising as our revelation about our own ignorance was, the answers from our friends and colleagues were even more surprising. In a nutshell, we were told that the questions had not been answered and perhaps should not even be asked. The response from one prominent cognitive psychologist is both typical and revealing:

> I wish I could help, but the field provides no answer. Every possible cut point to define "two processes" has been used by someone or other. Furthermore, the imprecision involved has caused no end of needless debate and irrelevant experimentation. Finally, I don't think it is possible to come up with any satisfactory global and generally agreed-upon definition. All you can do is try to be as precise as you can be—define what you mean by two processes, and give examples where possible.

Not to be deterred, we at least tried to frame some of the important issues. We attempted to identify the questions that should be asked and the criteria that should be used in determining whether or not an approach qualifies as a dual-process model. At the worst, this exercise might give us a way to see where our work on impression formation fits in the overall scheme of things. In this chapter, we first present some of these issues and questions; we then discuss our own conceptual and empirical work, using these issues and questions as a framework for our discussion.

WHAT IS A DUAL-PROCESS MODEL, ANYWAY?

Distinctions among Dual-Process Approaches

As the many chapters in this book indicate, there is no dearth of dual-process approaches that have been employed to help understand and explain a wide variety of social-psychological phenomena. The content areas range from mood to relationship formation, from attitudes to social identity. Abelson (1994) has noted this rapid growth of what he refers to as "coacting central subsystems." Interestingly, he distinguishes between two types of dual-system dichotomies within models that have been applied to social-psychological phenomena. First, he identifies those models that are based on *process* distinctions—that propose an automatic/affective/arational process on the one hand, and a controlled/cognitive/rational process on the other hand. Examples of these models exist in the areas of affect (Zajonc, 1980), stereotypes (Banaji & Greenwald, 1993; Devine, 1989), and attitudes (Dovidio & Fazio, 1992; Herek, 1987), as well as in other content areas. The reasoning model of Sloman (1996), which we soon consider in some detail, is also an example of this kind of dual-process distinction.

The other type of dual-system dichotomy considered by Abelson is based on a distinction in the type of *content* that is processed. This typically involves processes that operate on general or abstract content on the one hand, and processes operating on specific, concrete content on the other hand. These content dichotomies include the category-based versus individualistic judgment systems proposed by Brewer (1988), Fiske and Neuberg (1990), and Jones and McGillis (1976), as well as other models that distinguish between the levels of generality of stimulus objects.

As we considered these different approaches and models, one of the first questions that occurred to us was whether the two processes proposed in each of these dual-process accounts are truly separate and distinct processes, or whether there exists a continuum of process with an arbitrary cutoff point, such that any level above that point is considered one process and any level below the point is considered the other process. Using examples outside the domain of social psychology, we realized that this distinction is far from simple and straightforward. In fact, we quickly thought of examples in which (1) an underlying continuum becomes associated with a dual-process mechanism, and (2) an underlying dual-process distinction generates the appearance of a continuous phenomenon.

For example, temperature is obviously a continuous function. Yet one can arbitrarily choose a temperature level on a thermostat and designate this point as a cutoff, such that any temperature below that point will cause a heater to be turned on, and any temperature above that point will cause an air conditioner to go into action. In this case, what drives the underlying mechanisms falls along a continuum, but the processes generate *outputs* (heating and cooling) that are quite distinct and separate, are represented by different structures, and are governed by different functions. Can we consider them dual processes of temperature control?

In contrast, walking and running are clearly identifiable as two separate processes of locomotion, each with its own distinguishable set of mechanics. Technically speaking, walking involves having one foot in contact with the ground at all times, whereas in running there are times when both feet are off the ground at the same time. In addition, compared to walking, running involves more forward body lean; shorter takeoff, flight, and landing distances; and a foot strike that is closer to the middle of the foot. However, the *output* of these two processes of locomotion—speed of movement—falls along a continuum. And although the distribution of speeds that results from walking versus running is not totally overlapping (the maximum speed for walking is far less than the maximum speed for running), the distributions do overlap to some extent (one can walk at a pace that is faster than many people may choose to run). Thus, the output alone (speed) cannot indicate which process is engaged. Moreover, the same output level can be achieved by any combination of underlying processes. For example, an output of traversing 4 miles in an hour can be achieved solely by walking at a brisk pace, solely by running at a slow pace, or by a combination of leisurely walking and fast running. Thus, although the two processes of walking and running can always be distinguished by the mechanics involved, the output measure of speed is only a crude indicator of which locomotion process is more likely.

Similar concerns are important in conceptualizing about psychological processes. For example, through categorization we refer to "warm days" and "cold days," in each case grouping a range of temperatures into categories defined by a single term. Thus a continuous phenomenon is referred to in terms of distinct categories. The same process is observed in many psychological judgments. On the other hand, Kelly (1955) postulated that people construe events in terms of dichotomous

(not continuous) constructs, but that through simultaneous use of multiple constructs (including some pertaining to quantity), the resulting judgments can generate the appearance of reflecting an underlying continuum. Thus, in social-psychological dual-process models, too, it is important to determine whether any of the output measures (e.g., memory, judgment, latency, persuasion) can truly distinguish between the two proposed underlying processes.

The example of walking and running as dual processes of locomotion raises a second important question with regard to dual-process models. This question concerns the extent to which the two proposed processes can occur simultaneously. Running and walking cannot both be engaged at the same time. They operate by using the same equipment (primarily the legs) in different ways, such that this equipment can be used in either one way or the other way at any given time. Thus, running and walking must proceed sequentially rather than simultaneously if both are to be done within a certain time frame. In contrast, heating and cooling employ different equipment, and thus theoretically both can be engaged at the same time. Certain forms of dual processes in psychology have been proposed as having, at least in principle, the capability of occurring simultaneously (e.g., visual and verbal processing, Paivio, 1971; implicit and explicit memory, Jacoby, 1991). The simultaneous versus sequential operation of the two proposed processes is important to specify for any process model, and as we shall see (Sloman, 1996), this distinction has recently been used as a criterion for identifying the existence of a true dual-process account.

In social-psychological models, the issue of simultaneous versus sequential dual-processing systems has also been raised. For example, the model of systematic–heuristic processing proposed by Chaiken (1980) and the model of central–peripheral processing proposed by Petty and Cacioppo (1986) to explain persuasive-message effectiveness have typically been depicted as quite similar in nature. However, these models have at least one important difference. Chaiken proposes that the two routes to persuasion can operate simultaneously and that the two processes should be viewed as complementary rather than competing. Petty and Cacioppo, on the other hand, argue that the central and peripheral processes of persuasion are mutually exclusive and do not operate at the same time. The outcome in terms of attitude change may well look the same whether the two processes operate in parallel or whether there is rapid switching from one mode of processing to the other, but the underlying mechanism will look quite different in the two cases, with important implications.

Properties of Dual-Processing Systems: Sloman's Thinking

Although many attempts have been made to outline the features or criteria necessary for the identification of a dual-process model (Curran & Hintzman, 1995; Farah, 1994; Townsend, 1990), a recent approach by Sloman (1996) is worth considering in some detail. Sloman offers a unique perspective on dual-process models, and his ideas can serve as a fruitful basis for discussing our own work in particular and social-psychological dual-process models more generally.

Sloman (1996) has argued for the existence of a dual-process system of reasoning. One system of reasoning is referred to as the "associative" system, and the other is referred to as the "rule-based" system. The associative system employs computations that reflect similarity structure and relations of temporal contiguity. This system is rapid and automatic, deals with things at a more concrete level, and entails parallel processing. Importantly, the associative system produces responses in such a way that a person is aware only of the results of processing, but not of the underlying process itself. The rule-based system, on the other hand, operates on structures that have logical content and variables. The computation involves rules, and the system is analytic, symbolic, and sequential. Rule-based reasoning is further characterized as being very slow, complex, and controlled. In rule-based judgments, unlike associative reasoning, the thinker is aware of both the underlying processes and the output of those processes.

In short, Sloman argues that human reasoning is performed by two systems—two algorithms that are designed to achieve very different computational goals. One is associative, and it operates reflexively, using knowledge of similarity relations as well as the kinds of general knowledge contained in images and stereotypes. The other system is rule-based, and it describes the world by employing a structure that is logical, hierarchical, and causal-mechanical.

What is most important for the current chapter is that Sloman maintains that his two systems of reasoning are not either–or systems. Rather, they are thought to operate simultaneously and to operate independently of each other. Because they can operate simultaneously, the two systems have the potential for leading to quite different and opposite solutions to the very same reasoning problem— different solutions that are then held in one's head at the same time. That is, the rule-based and associative systems can address the same judgment at the same time, and can arrive at separate, independent, and possibly contradictory conclusions that have their origins in two different reasoning systems. Therefore, under Sloman's proposal, one can both believe in and not believe in a proposition at the same moment in time.

In fact, it is precisely this simultaneous existence of two contradictory answers that is taken by Sloman as proof of the existence of a dual-processing system. He refers to this simultaneous representation as "Criterion S." Sloman thus argues that the Müller–Lyer illusion, the conjunction fallacy (Tversky & Kahneman, 1983), and the Wason four-card selection task (Wason, 1966) all qualify as involving dual processes because in each case the reasoner is (or at least can be) simultaneously aware of two contradictory solutions to the problem. One of the solutions is provided by the associative system, the other by the rule-based system.

Also important for the current chapter is Sloman's claim that both systems, the associative and the rule-based, are psychologically real. That is, people may choose to make judgments by employing simple associative processes such as similarity and availability assessments, as well as by employing logical and statistical rules. The psychological reality of associative versus rule-based systems has also been recognized by several social psychologists in their analyses of trait inferences, hypothesis testing, and category membership judgments (Ginossar & Trope, 1987; Nisbett, Krantz, Jepson, & Kunda, 1983; Trope & Liberman, 1996).

Following a summary of our own work concerning impression formation processes for individual and group social targets, we return to some of the issues raised by Sloman's (1996) analysis for a discussion of our conceptual and empirical work, as well as a discussion of dual-processing models in social psychology more generally. We consider what, if any, aspects of our own model might qualify as involving dual processes. In doing so, we consider both the benefits and the constraints of Sloman's approach to identifying and evaluating dual-process distinctions. Finally, we use Sloman's approach as a framework for discussing some important process issues that should be addressed in analyzing the nature and role of dual-processing models in social psychology. In doing so, we consider the possibility that dual-process models in social psychology (including our own model) do not meet Sloman's Criterion S (or other aspects of his conditions) but are still usefully conceived of in dual-process terms, and we point out the important similarities and differences among these models.

COMPARING INDIVIDUAL AND GROUP IMPRESSION FORMATION

The specific context in which we confronted this question of dual-process mechanisms was in a comparison of the processes underlying individual and group perception (Hamilton & Sherman, 1996). Traditionally, the study of individual impression formation has remained quite distinct from the study of group impression formation in the social-psychological literature. At first glance, this individual–group distinction seems to be a likely candidate for a situation where two separate processes are involved in making social judgments.

In contrast, Hamilton and Sherman (1996) argued that this distinction is at least in part illusory. Their general thesis was that forming impressions of individuals and forming impressions of groups are driven by the same fundamental information-processing system. However, the processes involved can appear to be different for individual and group targets—not because people process information about individuals and groups differently, but because the expectations that people generally hold about these two targets

differ in a way that is fundamental to the impression formation process.

Hamilton and Sherman proposed that, other things being equal, perceivers expect different levels of unity and organization in individuals and groups; specifically, they expect more unity in individual than in group targets. It is the degree of perceived unity, not the individual or group nature of the social target, that drives the impression formation process. Because individuals and groups are seen as possessing different degrees of unity or entitativity (Campbell, 1958), specific perceptual and processing outcomes may differ for individual and group targets. These differences, however, derive from an *a priori* difference in expected or perceived unity and hence do not reflect qualitatively different processing systems for the two targets.

How did Hamilton and Sherman (1996) arrive at this conclusion? From a review of the literature on forming impressions of individuals, they developed a fundamental postulate and a series of principles about the impression formation process. They then applied this framework to research that has compared the processes of impression formation for individuals and groups. Their goal was to examine each principle and its manifestations where the social target was described as an individual, and to compare it to the nearly identical situation where the same information described a group of persons. Because the same information is used to describe an individual or group target, this comparison allows an analysis of the role of the nature of the social target—individual or group—in the various processes underlying impression formation.

Hamilton and Sherman's (1996) fundamental postulate was that perceivers assume unity in the personalities of other individuals. Because persons are seen as coherent entities, impressions of them should reflect this unity and coherence. Furthermore, this expectation of unity drives a number of processes that are central to the impression formation process for *all* social targets. Therefore, regardless of whether the target is an individual or a group, any variation in the perceived unity or "entitativity" of the target will lead to variation in impression processes. Importantly, Hamilton and Sherman (1996) proposed that perceivers do not expect the same degree of unity in group targets as they do in individual targets. Therefore, because the expected level of unity drives impression formation processes, differences in impression outcomes for individual and group targets can occur.

Hamilton and Sherman (1996) used this framework to account for many differences in the impressions of individuals and groups that had been reported in the literature. For example, the tendency for perceivers to make spontaneous trait inferences while forming impressions of individuals is greatly attenuated when the target is a group. This was demonstrated in studies that reported distinctiveness-based illusory correlations when the impression targets were groups, but not when the targets of impression were individuals (McConnell, Sherman, & Hamilton, 1994; Sanbonmatsu, Sherman, & Hamilton, 1987).

The explanation for this difference rests in the type of processing that the different targets elicit. Previous evidence supports the hypothesis that the distinctiveness-based illusory correlation is largely a memory-based effect (Hamilton, Dugan, & Trolier, 1985; Johnson & Mullen, 1994; Stroessner, Hamilton, & Mackie, 1992); it is attributable due to the enhanced accessibility of distinctive information in memory, which in turn has a disproportionate influence on subsequent judgments (e.g., frequency estimates, liking). In contrast, illusory correlations do not develop for individual targets because the impression of the individual is formed on-line, as the information is presented (Sanbonmatsu et al., 1987). Infrequent or inconsistent information is made to fit with the predominant impression of the individual, through assimilating it into the overall impression or discounting it as nondiagnostic. This on-line judgment, rather than the information upon which it is based, is then used for subsequent judgments, and no illusory correlation emerges. Within this interpretative framework, the relative lack of illusory correlations for individual versus group targets is consistent with the idea that perceivers extract dispositional information as they are learning about an individual target person to a greater extent than they do when learning about individual members of a group.

In addition, perceivers expect more consistency when learning about individual rather than group targets. For example, Weisz

and Jones (1993) found that impressions derived from information about an individual (target-based expectancies) were more stable than impressions derived from information about individual members of a social category (category-based expectancies). Hence, perceivers' expectations of consistency in the individual target buffered their impressions against the effects of an expectancy-violating episode (see also Park, DeKay, & Kraus, 1994). Moreover, participants in another study rated individual targets as more coherent and organized than they rated group targets (Susskind, Maurer, Thakkar, Hamilton, & Sherman, in press), and also rated a set of behaviors describing an individual as fitting a meaningful pattern to a greater extent than when those behaviors described members of a group.

In another study, Stroessner, Hamilton, Acorn, Czyzewska, and Sherman (1989) presented participants with information that either described four individuals or described persons belonging to four different groups. Results showed that in free recall these participants clustered information by target more in the individual-target than in the group-target condition. Participants also recalled more information in the individual-target than in the group-target condition (a result subsequently replicated by McConnell et al., 1994). In general, then, these results are consistent with the view that perceivers are more inclined to organize information for individual than for to group targets.

Finally, several studies have found differences in the influence of inconsistent information in impression formation as a function of the individual or group nature of the target. For example, participants who learn about individual targets spend more time looking at inconsistent versus consistent information, but this difference does not exist when they learn about group targets (Stern, Marrs, Millar, & Cole, 1984). Furthermore, when asked to write continuations for descriptions of an individual target's behavior, participants write explanatory continuations to a greater extent for inconsistent behaviors than for consistent behaviors (Hastie, 1984). However, this difference is less evident when participants learn about group targets (Susskind et al., in press). Finally, the recall advantage for inconsistent behaviors typically found in studies using the person memory paradigm (see Srull & Wyer, 1989, for a review) holds for individual-target conditions, but not for group-target conditions (Srull, 1981; Srull, Lichtenstein, & Rothbart, 1985; Stern et al., 1984; Wyer, Bodenhausen, & Srull, 1984; see Stangor & McMillan, 1992, for a meta-analysis). Hamilton and Sherman (1996) interpreted these findings as evidence that the relative lack of perceived unity in groups as compared to individuals renders inconsistencies much less troubling to perceivers, and hence less in need of explanation.

In summary, Hamilton and Sherman's (1996) review outlined several important differences in impression outcomes for individual and group targets. However, they argued that the individual or group nature of the social target is *not* the key factor in determining the variations in the impression formation process. Rather, it is the level of (perceived or expected) entitativity in the social target that is crucial. The concept of entitativity is largely correlated with the individual–group distinction because, other things being equal, individuals tend to be seen as more entitative than groups.

As stated elsewhere (Hamilton & Sherman, 1996; Hamilton et al., 1998), we see entitativity as a continuum on which any social target can be found relative to another. With respect to this entitativity continuum, groups *in general* are perceived as having less entitativity than individuals. However, because both individual and group targets vary along the entitativity continuum, it is also true that some individual targets are perceived as having less entitativity than some group targets. For example, if a perceiver learns that a person is erratic and inconsistent, the expectation of unity is lessened. If a particular individual is seen as less entitative than a particular group, the typical differences in processing engaged in the impression formation process may actually be reversed.

Support for this interpretation has been obtained in two different ways. First, McConnell et al. (1994) manipulated the processing strategies that participants used when presented with information about an individual or a group target. In one condition, participants were given instructions that encouraged forming on-line impressions of both individual and group targets during informa-

tion presentation. Results here showed evidence of on-line processing and were similar for individual and group targets. In another condition, on-line processing for both types of targets was discouraged by instructing participants to attend to the comprehensibility of the stimulus sentences. Again, results were similar for both targets, but showed evidence of memory-based processing.

Second, McConnell, Sherman, and Hamilton (1997) manipulated instructions in a manner designed to enhance or to undermine baseline expectations of entitativity for both individual and group targets. When participants expected a high-entitativity target (a target that was consistent and predictable), results showed evidence of on-line processing for both individual and group targets. When participants expected a low-entitativity target (a target that was inconsistent and unpredictable), results suggested memory-based processing for both targets.

Although the Hamilton and Sherman (1996) review of the literature strongly suggested the existence of the entitativity continuum, the McConnell et al. (1994, 1997) studies provide empirical support for its theoretical importance. With an expectation of high entitativity, or encouragement of on-line processing, results mimic those found typically for individual targets. An expectation of low entitativity, or discouragement of on-line processing, leads to results consistent with those found typically for group targets.

The preceding analysis has illuminated two important points. The first is that the same general processes are involved in forming first impressions of individuals and groups. The second is that the observed differences in impression outcomes for individual and group targets are not a function of these targets per se, but rather derive from the level of unity or entitativity perceived in those targets. In general, individuals are perceived to be more entitative than groups, leading to differences in information processing. The implication of this analysis, then, is that the individual–group distinction is not a candidate for a dual-process distinction, because the theoretically important dimension is the expectation of entitativity in a social target. If this analysis is correct, then the next question becomes whether differences in perceived entitativity can lead to any differences in information processing that might qualify as a dual-process distinction.

THE ENTITATIVITY CONTINUUM AND INTEGRATIVE PROCESSING

What are the processing differences associated with variations along the entitativity continuum? We refer to this continuum as representing increasing degrees of "integrative processing" as information is acquired, used, and stored in memory. As indicated earlier, integrative processing in our view includes several components, each of which involves "going beyond the information given" (Bruner, 1957) as it is encoded. Integrative processing occurs to the extent that these component processes take place on-line, as information is acquired. We can briefly characterize these component processes as follows:

1. *Spontaneous dispositional inferences.* Integrative processing involves spontaneous dispositional inferences about a target based on the specific information acquired. These inferences, which involve elaborations of available evidence, may pertain to the traits, goals, motives, and so on of the target person or group.

2. *Organization of information.* Information acquired about social targets is often organized as it is processed and stored in memory according to prominent themes (traits, goals, etc.) that inform a perceiver about a target.[1]

3. *Evaluations.* Social perception is notoriously evaluative in nature; it is difficult for perceivers to remain totally neutral about the people they encounter. Nevertheless, perceivers engage in evaluation of social targets to varying degrees, according to the situational context and demands. Integrative processing involves actively engaging in evaluative judgment as information is acquired.

4. *Causal analysis.* Social perceivers often (but not always) engage in causal analysis, attempting to determine the causal basis for some observed behavior. When they do, they make attributional inferences; such inferences, if made on-line, contribute to integrative processing.

Terminological Distinctions

Prior to continuing our analysis of integrative processing, a comment on terminology is in order. The term "on-line" is used in more than one sense in the social-psychological literature. For some authors, anything that happens in cognitive processing as information is processed can be characterized as an on-line process. When we refer to "integrative processing," we are referring to processes that occur on-line in this sense. A second and more focused use of the term derives from a classic paper by Hastie and Park (1986), in which they differentiated between on-line and memory-based *judgments*. Their analysis was specifically concerned with the question of the time when social judgments are made, and on-line and memory-based judgments differ explicitly in when such a judgment is formed. If the judgment is formed when the information on which it is based is being acquired and processed, it is an on-line judgment. In contrast, if the judgment is not made at the time of information acquisition, but rather is formed at a later time, it is based on information that can be retrieved from memory at that time; hence it is a memory-based judgment.

The Hastie and Park (1986) use of the term "on-line" is a more restrictive one, in that it is limited to the process of forming judgments. Processes other than forming social judgments can occur as the information is processed (e.g., organization and representation of information in memory—Hamilton, Driscoll, & Worth, 1989; Hamilton, Katz, & Leirer, 1980; retrieval of previously acquired information into working memory—Sherman & Hamilton, 1994). These processes might qualify as being on-line in the general sense, but not in the more restrictive sense of Hastie and Park. We believe that conceptual clarity will be enhanced by limiting the use of the term "on-line" to the specific question of when judgments are formed, following Hastie and Park (1986). Therefore, we use the term "integrative processing" to refer to the more inclusive set of processes that may (or may not) occur as information about social targets is acquired and processed. For the same reasons, later in this chapter we use the term "retrospective processing" as a more general term to refer to the use of information at a later time, which includes but is broader than the term "memory-based judgments."

Components of Integrative Processing

To this point, we have argued that the distinction between perceptions of individual and group targets is not a case of dual-process mechanisms, but rather reflects an underlying entitativity continuum along which both individual and group targets are perceived. The variation in perceived entitativity in turn generates corresponding variation in the extent to which integrative processing becomes engaged.

In addition, we have identified the various components of integrative processing. These components include spontaneous dispositional inferences, organization of information, evaluative judgments, and causal attributions. Having identified the various components of integrative processing, we could now ask whether, and to what extent, each of those component processes reflects a dual-mechanism distinction versus continuous gradations in the degree of engaging a particular mechanism. However, such a discussion would distract us from the primary goal of this chapter, and thus a detailed account of the component processes is not presented. No doubt each of these processes might be construed either as one part of a dual-process system or as a unitary process that varies along a continuum.

For example, implicit in correspondent inference theory (Jones & Davis, 1965) and attribution theory (Kelley, 1967), and more explicit in research that started with Winter and Uleman's (1984) classic paper (see Uleman, Newman, & Moskowitz, 1996, for a review), is the suggestion that trait inferences are made almost automatically during the reception of the behavioral information. On the other hand, Bassili and Smith (1986) suggest that dispositional inferences do not always meet the criteria for an automatic process. Perhaps dual processes, one automatic and one thoughtful, are involved. Or perhaps, as Uleman (1987, 1989) suggested, there is a continuum of trait inference processing that varies in the extent to which judgments reflect the properties of automatic versus controlled processes.

In the realm of attitudinal evaluations,

there are approaches that view such evaluations as automatic. Fazio (1995) discusses the automatic formation and activation of links between objects and evaluations, which require little or no critical thinking. On the other hand, Ajzen and Fishbein (1973, 1980) present a theory of reasoned action for the development and application of attitudes, which is a rule-based perspective and involves controlled, reasoned processing. Fazio (1990) suggests that the operation of attitudes represents dual processes, one automatic and one controlled, that seem similar to Sloman's (1996) associative and rule-based systems. Unlike Sloman, however, Fazio does not assume that the two processes operate simultaneously or interactively. Rather, whether automatic attitude activation or a process of reasoned action is evoked will depend upon the motivation for accurate responding and the opportunity to engage in time-consuming processing.

Suffice it to say that integrative processing reflects the combined effects of underlying mechanisms that themselves may be continua or may be dual processes. What is important is that "integrative processing" refers to impression formation of social targets that occurs as target information is received, that uses this information to arrive at a variety of conclusions about the target, that integrates this information as it is encoded, and that goes beyond the information provided. In addition, the expectation and perception of the social target along the entitativity continuum are what influence whether or not and to what extent integrative processing is engaged. Thus it is the degree of perceived entitativity of the social target that serves as the main driving force behind the engagement of integrative processing.

However, other factors aside from entitativity can also have an effect on whether or not and to what extent integrative processing operates as information about a social target is received. Obviously the perceiver's momentary goals in processing information about the target will have a direct bearing on the way information is processed and used. For example, learning about a potential date or coworker will invoke greater integrative processing than will a brief encounter with a stranger; information about members of a group will be processed more integratively if one is considering joining that group than if one is not. In addition, external constraints, such as cognitive load and time pressure, can influence the extent to which information will be processed integratively. Presumably the perception of target entitativity is an independent determinant of integrative processing, though it may interact with these other determinants as well.

Relations among Components of Integrative Processing

Another interesting question concerns the relationships among the various components of integrative processing. Of particular interest are any different patterns of integrative processing as a function of target entitativity. That is, in identifying the various components of integrative processing, we have suggested that increasing target entitativity should generate increased integrative processing. The possibility being considered here is that there may be circumstances where this effect is more true for one component than for another. In other words, we do not assume that target entitativity will in all cases have equivalent effects on all components of integrative processing. This point can be elucidated with some possible examples of differential patterns of response.

A plausible case is one where circumstances induce a high degree of integrative processing of a particular kind, but not of the other components. For example, certain perceiver goals or motivations may generate extensive processing of information solely for its evaluative implications, with little concern for developing an organized impression or for understanding the causal bases of the target's behaviors.

A second possible case is one where some circumstance may have differing impacts on different components of integrative processing. For example, we know that for high-entitativity targets, perceivers are quite sensitive to the consistency or inconsistency of behavioral information with *a priori* expectancies about a target. Behavioral information that is consistent with expectancies is likely to generate correspondent dispositional inferences, but unlikely to produce attributional analysis of causes for such behavior. In contrast, expectancy-inconsistent behavior is a primary catalyst for attributional thinking, but seems less likely to generate correspondent dispositional inferences (cf. Hamilton, 1998). Thus the same property of behavioral information can have differing impact on two different components of integrative processing. It is important to note that in our analysis both effects— dispositional inferences from expectancy-consistent behavior, and attributional analysis triggered by expectancy-inconsistent behavior—are more likely to occur for high-entitativity than for low-entitativity targets, reflecting the overall effect of perceived entitativity on integrative processing. The specific *form* of that processing, however, can differ as a function of other properties, such as behavioral consistency.

Finally, a third possible case takes us back to Sloman's analysis of a dual-response system. Under some conditions, can two components of integrative processing operate to produce simultaneously different outcomes? Consider, for example, the well-known Kohlberg (1981) moral dilemma of the man who steals drugs that will aid his ailing wife. This scenario represents a dilemma specifically because of the simultaneous operation of two components of integrative processing: dispositional inference (stealing is a felony; the man is a criminal) and causal analysis (his behavior is motivated by caring for his wife; the man is an altruist). If we assume further that spontaneous dispositional inferences correspond to Sloman's associative responding and that causal analysis corresponds to Sloman's rule-based responding, then this illustration may provide our best example of the operation of dual responding. Interestingly, in our analysis these dual-response modes are two components of one larger system, which we call integrative processing.

RETROSPECTIVE PROCESSING

To this point we have discussed the nature of integrative processing and its relationship to the entitativity continuum, and we have identified the important components of integrative processing. In focusing on integrative processing, we have been dealing explicitly with processes that are engaged as information is being encoded, interpreted, and represented in memory. These processes include on-line judgments, organization of information as it is encoded, and immediate resolution of inconsistencies. We have argued that these processes are more likely to be engaged, and are engaged to a greater extent, when the target is perceived as being high in entitativity.

What is the nature of processing when targets are perceived as low in entitativity? Clearly, one answer is that there is less integrative processing; perceivers do less of the stuff that makes for integration during information acquisition. Certainly our inclination to view the extent of integrative processing as varying along a continuum—one that is closely associated with the entitativity continuum—fosters such an answer. At the same time, however, the processing that characterizes the lower portion of the entitativity continuum takes on sufficiently different properties that it warrants discussion in its own right. In this section we consider these differences, and in doing so we distinguish between integrative and retrospective processing.

To the extent that information is *not* processed integratively, perceivers will not, at the time that this information is acquired, make evaluative and descriptive inferences about the target; they will not organize the information according to meaningful themes; and they will not seek causal understanding. Rather, the information will be stored in memory in a diffuse and relatively unorganized way. Some of this information will be lost through forgetting, and the rest can be retrieved from memory at a later time when judgments are required. It is important to note that these judgments, made after the relevant information is received, are the same in nature as the kinds of judgments that are made through integrative processing, which occurs during information reception. That is, target judgments made through retrospective processing will involve impression formation, and there will be some organization of the information into a coherent picture, some evaluation, and some causal attribution. As in integrative processing, these impressions may go beyond the information provided. It is the degree of perceived entitativity that will determine whether these judgments are made at the time the behavioral information is received or at a later time. Importantly, this retrospective processing of information will differ in significant ways from integrative processing.

Part of this difference is related to the *content* on which the impressions are based. Recall that Abelson (1994) has distinguished between dual-processing systems that represent process dichotomies and dual-processing systems that represent content dichotomies. Because there is some overlap in the processes that are involved in integrative and retrospective processing, we focus first on the important content differences. Integrative processing involves the encoding and integration of behavioral information about the target as that information is received. Most, if not all, of the information is used for the impression, and this information is integrated in an on-line fashion. Inconsistent behaviors are attended to especially carefully and are explained in a way that allows the predominant impression to be maintained. Thus primacy is important for the impression, as the initial information lays the groundwork for the impression and provides the framework within which later information is interpreted. As the information is received, encoded, and integrated, an abstract or schematic representation of the target is developed and stored—to be used for subsequent judgments.

However, integrative processing may not occur for a variety of reasons: a lack of perceived entitativity of the target; a lack of cognitive resources at the time of information reception; or processing goals (e.g., the judgment of grammatical correctness) that would prevent a focus on the meaning of the information. Under these conditions, when an impression of the target is called for at a later time, this judgment must necessarily be based on retrospective processing. Here, it is *not* the totality of the information received that is involved in the judgment, and it is not a previously stored abstract representation of the target that is used for the judgment. Rather, a sample or subset of the original information is used—whatever information can be recalled, or whatever information is most salient or accessible at the time of judgment. In addition, whereas integrative processing uses only information that is actually presented (although various interpretations of this information are likely), retrospective processing can involve information that is not actually presented. Intrusions, distortions of information, false memories, and elaborations of the retrieved information can all be available during retrospective processing. Moreover, during integrative processing inconsistent information is rendered sensible in the light of other facts, and is either integrated into the predominant impression or is discounted; thus the overall impression of the target is heavily weighted toward the predominant behavioral information. For retrospective processing, it is likely that inconsistent (or infrequent) information is strongly represented in memory because of its initial salience, is accessed quickly and easily, and thus gets much weight in the impression of the target. This is why illusory-correlation formation occurs only when judgments of the target are made retrospectively (Hamilton & Sherman, 1996), in which case the distinctive information plays an especially strong role in the impressions.

In addition, whereas primacy is evident for impressions based on integrative processing, it is more likely that recency effects emerge when judgments involve retrospective processing (McConnell et al., 1997). In the absence of integrative processing, recent events are most strongly represented in memory, and these easily accessible recent behaviors will thus play a stronger role in impression judgments. In addition, integrative processing is sensitive to attentional effects at input, to clear dispositional implications of behavioral information, and to inconsistencies in the information being processed. In contrast, retrospective processing is sensitive to all of the variables that make information easily accessible from memory (strength of encoding, distinctiveness of information, recency of input, recently activated relevant categories, etc.). Finally, as Hastie and Park (1986) noted, the fact that retrospective processing requires a judgment explicitly based on the content of memory means that memory–judgment correlations will be stronger when retrospective processing is engaged (McConnell et al., 1994).

In short, the content upon which impressions are based is quite different for integrative and retrospective processing—the veridical behavioral information as it is received in the case of integrative processing, and the content of memory at the time of judgment in the case of retrospective processing. Important outcome differences can be expected, depending upon which process is engaged. Integrative processing leads to primacy effects in judgments, with heavy weight being given to information that is frequent and consistent with the overall theme, and low memory–judgment correlations. Retrospective processing leads to recency effects in judgments, a heavy weight for infrequent information or information that is inconsistent with the predominant theme, and high memory–judgment correlations. Thus, the amount and type of information used for the two judgment processes differ substantially, and impressions and judgments of the target are likely to differ, depending upon whether these judgments are based on integrative processing or on retrospective processing. And it is important to note that the behavioral information provided is of course identical. This tendency for two processes to lead to different conclusions, depending on the processing system that is engaged, is the hallmark of dual-processing systems and is embodied in Sloman's Criterion S. We return to this point later.

In addition to content differences in the information that is used for integrative versus retrospective processing, differences in processes are apparent. From the discussion just presented, it should be clear that integrative processing involves primarily attentional and encoding processes, whereas retrospective processing involves primarily retrieval and memory processes. These differences have been explored in the research, summarized earlier in this chapter, comparing conditions in which targets are perceived as being high or low in entitativity (McConnell et al., 1994, 1997; Susskind et al., in press). As reviewed earlier, this research has found differences in processing the same information when it describes individual and group targets—except when the perceived entitativity of the group is enhanced or that of the individual is diminished. The research has also shown differences in illusory-correlation effects for individual and group targets. Differences as a function of perceived entitativity have been found on a variety of process measures, including strength and latency of judgments, primacy–recency effects in recall, sensitivity to distinctive stimuli, spontaneous generation of explanations for expectancy-inconsistent behaviors, and recall of stimulus information (for a full discussion, see Hamilton & Sherman, 1996).

In addition, even though there is some overlap in the component processes of integrative processing and retrospective processing (e.g., impression formation, evaluation, causal attribution, organization), these component processes are likely to differ in certain respects. There is less overall information used during retrospective processing, and the impression is less likely to represent a careful integration of this information. Thus, with retrospective processing as opposed to integrative processing, one is less likely to see organizational processes, causal analyses, or attempts to come to grips with inconsistent information. Moreover, retrospective processing typically occurs in response to a specific question about what the target is like. Retrospective processing thus represents a rather controlled and reasoned process in answer to a question. There is less likely to be evidence of spontaneous processes, which are so prevalent in integrative processing, that involve quick evaluations and spontaneous trait inferences.

Another important difference between integrative and retrospective processing is that integrative processing should produce an impression with far greater stability and far greater resistance to change. This should occur for several reasons:

1. There are differences in content, such that integrative processing uses more of the original information than retrospective processing does. This should lead to a more stable and confident impression.

2. Integrative processing involves more organization of the information and greater assimilation of inconsistent information, as well as causal attribution and evaluation. These should all suggest a more unified and coherent impression.

3. As we have indicated, the major determinant of whether or not integrative processing is engaged is the expectation of a high level of entitativity for the social target. This expectation of high coherence should encourage the formation of impressions that are indeed highly entitative, and thus are more stable and more resistant to subsequent change.

In short, in terms of several important features, integrative and retrospective processing appear to be distinct modes of responding: They clearly occur at different times (either as the information is being processed or not until some later time); they are likely to rely on different aspects of the original information; they involve different mechanisms and processes; and they can produce different outcomes. These questions then arise: Do integrative and retrospective processing constitute a dual-process system, as we have discussed in previous sections? If so, how does this system fit into the overall theoretical framework regarding the role of entitativity in the perception of social targets?

A Dual-Process System?

Given the distinguishing features enumerated above, we view integrative and retrospective processing to be distinct, independent means of processing information and generating judgments about social targets. However, in terms of the analysis of dual-process systems that we have presented at the beginning of this chapter, does the distinction between integrative processing and retrospective processing qualify as a dual-processing distinction? In our earlier presentation, we focused heavily on Sloman's (1996) analysis of dual-process systems and on his distinction between associative and rule-based processing modes. In light of Sloman's account, two questions arise concerning whether the distinction between integrative and retrospective processing qualifies as a dual-process system. First, integrative and retrospective processing do not seem to map easily onto Sloman's distinction between associative processing, which is characterized as intuitive, figural, and automatic, and rule-based processing, which is characterized as analytic, deliberative, reasoned, and controlled.

For example, we have noted that integrative processing involves spontaneous trait inferences and automatic evaluations (as in Sloman's associative mode), but that it may also entail careful, thoughtful judgments when inconsistent information is analyzed and assimilated or when causal attributions are made (as in Sloman's rule-based approach). Similarly, retrospective responding may involve oversensitivity to distinctive and easily accessible information (associative), as well as judgments and decisions that are based on a thorough, thoughtful analysis following extensive retrieval of relevant information (rule-based). Nevertheless, it is not clear to us that, in a dual-process system, the two systems must be divided in a nonoverlapping way between automatic and controlled processes. Most processes in fact represent a mixture of associative and rule-based mechanisms, and it is difficult to conceive of a purely automatic or purely controlled process. For example, in Fazio's (1990) analysis of the activation and application of attitudes, the two mechanisms of attitude processing are seen as complex mixtures of automatic and controlled processes, although one is clearly far more associative in nature and the other is far more rule-based. Similarly, we have noted that retrospective processing involves less that is automatic and spontaneous than does integrative processing. Thus, we suggest that a dual-process system can exist without either mode's representing a purely associative or a purely rule-based process.

The second question that Sloman's analysis raises with regard to the dual-process nature of integrative versus retrospective processing concerns his Criterion S—the capacity for the systems to produce conflicting responses *simultaneously*. Clearly, integrative processing and retrospective processing do not occur contemporaneously. Integrative processing by definition occurs as the information is being processed; retrospective processing by definition consists of the analysis of previously processed information. Processing systems that necessarily occur at different points in time cannot *simultaneously* generate conflicting responses.

However, it is not at all clear that Sloman's Criterion S requires the parallel or contemporaneous operation of the two processes. All that would appear to be necessary is the ultimate *simultaneous belief* in the two contradictory responses—regardless of whether the processes leading to these two responses actually occur at the same time or not. In fact, Sloman (1996, p. 11) claims that evidence would exist for two forms of reasoning "if, and only if, the tendency to provide the first response continues to be compelling irrespective of belief in the second answer, irrespective even of certainty in the second answer." This would not seem to us to require the simultaneous operation of the two underlying processes leading to the two responses. In fact, even for Sloman's model of reasoning, completely parallel and contemporaneous processing seems unlikely. One process is automatic and fast, whereas the other is controlled and time-consuming; thus the rule-based process is likely to extend longer in time than is the associative process.

Can integrative and retrospective processing lead to the simultaneous belief in two contradictory responses? The answer is clearly "no" if only one or the other system is engaged during the judgment of a social target. However, we believe that it is likely that both systems can be operative during the judgment. Consider the instance where an impression of a social target is formed integratively, as behavioral information is received. In the strongest case, this processing involves an organization of the information, trait inferences, an evaluative response, some causal analysis, and an assimilation of inconsistent information. The outcome is an abstract, schematic representation of the social target. At a subsequent time, a judgment of this social target may be requested. In response to this request, our social perceiver can use either or both processes to render a judgment. The use of both processes is more likely when it is important for the judgment to be accurate, when there is high accountability for decisions based on the judgment, or when the judgment based on previous integrative processing now seems unexpected or surprising. That is, the perceiver can consult the abstract representation that was arrived at through integrative processing. In addition, he or she can consult the content of memory and use this episodic information in order to arrive at the judgment. Because the current content of memory may imply different qualities and attributes of the target from those that have been stored as an abstract representation, retrospective processing will lead to a different judgment. If both processes are used in making the judgments, there may indeed be two simultaneous conflicting judgments in the person's head at the same time. And this would meet Sloman's Criterion S.

It is also important to recognize that the two kinds of processing can intersect in generating the products of processing. Specifically, the abstractions, summary judgments, and representations that are the products of integrative processing are stored in memory and become a part of the information base that is potentially available for retrieval if and when retrospective processing is engaged (Lingle & Ostrom, 1981). These abstractions can then combine with the specific instances and exemplars that are stored in memory to produce new judgments, decisions, evaluations, and causal attributions. The inferences, evaluations, and so forth that were formed on-line may of course be compatible with or contradictory to the implications of the specific items of information retrieved at a later time. In this way, the two independent processing systems may work in concert toward the same end, or they may generate conflicting outcomes. In the latter case, these discrepancies may or may not be resolved as a part of the retrospective analysis (a point to be discussed further in a later section of the chapter).

In addition to Sloman's analysis of dual-process systems and his criteria for the identification of such systems, it seems to us that there are other important criteria to consider as well. Perhaps a fundamental criterion for the operation of dual-process systems would be evidence for the differential effects of theoretically relevant independent variables on measures of the two processes. Much work by Kahneman and Tversky (Kahneman, Slovic, & Tversky, 1982; Kahneman & Tversky, 1973; Tversky & Kahneman, 1983) has suggested this criterion in demonstrating that formal considerations are irrelevant to informal thinking and vice versa.

In terms of this criterion for the operation of dual processes, there are many cases where manipulations do indeed seem to have different effects on integrative and retrospective processing. For example, McConnell et al. (1997) have manipulated expectancies of entitativity for individual and group targets. Inducing an expectancy of high entitativity has a significant effect on the processing of information about group targets, but has no effect on the processing of information about individual targets. This is because an expectancy of high entitativity induces integrative processing for forming impressions of groups (which would otherwise operate through retrospective processing). However, because impressions of individuals already entail integrative processing, expectations of high entitativity will have no effect. Similarly, ex-

pectancies of low target entitativity affect only the processing of individuals but not groups. Moreover, we would suggest that a manipulation of cognitive load should interfere with integrative processing, but should not interfere with retrospective processing. Manipulating the amount of inconsistent information about the target should also affect the two modes of processing differently, because integrative processing involves an assimilation of inconsistent information, whereas retrospective processing does not. Finally, when the behavioral information consists of both desirable and undesirable acts, presenting one kind of behavior early and the other kind of behavior late in the stimulus presentation should have different effects, depending on whether integrative processing or retrospective processing is operative. Primacy effects in impressions are likely with integrative processing, but recency effects are likely with retrospective processing (McConnell et al., 1994, 1997).

We have tried to make the case that integrative and retrospective processing meet the criteria for a dual-process system and that they are distinct and independent processes. On the other hand, we are equally comfortable with the notion that integrative processing represents a continuum. That is, more or less integrative processing occurs during the formation of an impression of a social target, depending upon expectations of entitativity, processing goals, and cognitive resources. To the extent that not much integrative processing is accomplished and no abstract representation of the social target is formed, one necessarily has to depend more on the retrieval of behavioral episodes in order to arrive at a judgment required subsequently.

This view is consistent with recent work by Sherman (1996) on the development of stereotypes. Sherman suggests that social perceivers are always trying to form abstract representations of social targets. However, more information and experience are necessary in certain cases—when cognitive resources are low or when the target is not a coherent entity. In the absence of an abstract representation, target impressions will be based on exemplar information. However, with higher levels of experience and a chance for more integrative processing, an abstract representation will ultimately be formed and will be stored and retrieved independently of the exemplars on which it is based. Thus integrative processing is always occurring, but the development of an abstract representation requires a certain level of experience. This approach and its implications for the use of previously formed abstract representations versus episodic, exemplar information based on recall have been explored across a variety of social targets, including individuals, groups, and the self (Klein & Loftus, 1993; Klein, Loftus, Trafton, & Fuhrman, 1992; Sherman & Klein, 1994).

A similar approach can be taken with other dual-process models in social psychology. Central or systematic processing of persuasive information occurs along a continuum. Without a sufficient amount of such processing, heuristic or peripheral cues will have to be relied on in order to judge the validity of the message (Chaiken, 1980; Petty & Cacioppo, 1986). Similarly, attitude activation by the presence of an object occurs along a continuum (Fazio, 1995). To the extent that only low levels of activation occur, a more controlled and reason-based process will be necessary to render an evaluation of the object (Ajzen & Fishbein, 1973, 1980).

The Entitativity Continuum and Dual Processing

Now that we have distinguished between integrative and retrospective processing, we can ask how these two modes of processing relate to our earlier, continuum-based notions regarding the perception of entitativity in social targets. As we have indicated earlier, we do not view different social targets (persons, groups) as inherently initiating qualitatively different forms of information processing. In our view, the empirical differences often observed in comparisons of individual and group targets derive primarily from perceivers' *a priori* expectations that these targets differ in their unity or entitativity. However, our research has shown that when these targets are equated in their perceived entitativity, the results indicate very similar manifestations of underlying processing mechanisms. Moreover, despite these "default" differences, both individual and group targets are distributed across an entitativity continuum that has important implications for the nature of the

information processing that will be engaged. The more entitativity a target is perceived as possessing, the more the processing will be characterized by the components of integrative processing discussed earlier. The lower the level of perceived entitativity, the less integrative processing will occur. In addition, the greater the perceived entitativity and the greater the degree of integrative processing, in general the less need there will be for retrospective processing at the time of judgment. With low levels of perceived entitativity and little integrative processing at encoding, the level of retrospective processing at the time of judgment, based on the retrieval of original information, will be greater. Thus both integrative and retrospective processing operate along a continuum, and in general these two types of processing are inversely related.

Finally, it is crucial to recognize an important consequence of this relationship between perceived entitativity and integrative processing. When the target is perceived as highly entitative, integrative processing will occur. Thus spontaneous trait inferences and evaluations will be made; organized representations of the information will be established; and inconsistencies will be resolved. To the extent that these processes do *not* transpire as information about the target is acquired, these analyses will need to be performed if those issues become important at a later time. In other words, integrative and retrospective processing are in this sense in a synergistic relationship: The more these forms of processing occur as the information is received, the less retrospective processing is needed later; the less integrative processing occurs, the more likely it is that similar forms of retrospective processing will be required later.

IMPLICATIONS FOR DUAL-PROCESS MODELS IN SOCIAL PSYCHOLOGY

Having analyzed our own model of integrative versus retrospective processing in terms of Sloman's (1996) framework as well as other criteria for identifying dual-process models, we now turn to a consideration of other dual-process models in social psychology. Among social-psychological dual-process models, perhaps the one closest to Sloman's approach is Epstein's cognitive–experiential self-theory (Epstein, 1983, 1985). In fact, this is the only social-psychological model that Sloman refers to in his article.

Epstein proposes that people have two systems for processing information—a rational system and an experiential system. The attributes of these systems are very similar in nature to the attributes of Sloman's rule-based and associative systems, respectively. The rational system is slow, employing rules governed by logical principles. It is deliberative, verbally mediated, conscious, and analytical. On the other hand, the experiential system is quick and simple, and relies heavily on the "feel" of the information. This system operates in an automatic way, is associated with affective experience, and often operates below the level of consciousness. Like Sloman, Epstein assumes that the two systems operate in parallel, that they can interact, and (most importantly) that this can lead to the simultaneous existence of incompatible judgments. For example, in one experiment (Denes-Raj & Epstein, 1994), subjects were given two bowls; their task was to pick one of the bowls from which to draw one bean blindfolded, and they were to try to pick a red bean. One bowl had 1 red bean out of a total of 10 beans, whereas the other bowl had 7 red beans out of a total of 100. Although subjects knew at the rational level that the former bowl provided a better opportunity, at the same time they felt that the latter bowl was a better choice.

As we have seen, consideration of our own process model for the formation of impressions of social targets has led us to conclude that this model may not precisely fit Sloman's criteria for a dual-process model. It is not clear that the timing of our processes, the distinction of the processes in terms of associative versus rule-based reasoning, or the outcome in terms of the simultaneous existence of incompatible judgments will allow us to conclude that two distinct processes are in operation.

In general, though, our kind of dual-process approach seems fairly typical of the dual-process models that have been developed in social psychology. For example, in Fiske and Neuberg's (1990) continuum model of impression formation, the two processes (categorical vs. piecemeal judgments) are not assumed to occur simultaneously. Rather, a sequential operation of the two processes is assumed, and although the outcome may represent an integration of the two processes, there is no assumption of simultaneous incompatible judgments.

Similarly, Petty and Cacioppo (1986), in their model of the persuasive impact of messages, try to identify conditions where the processing is central and other conditions under which the processing is peripheral. Their goal is to identify the circumstances under which one or the other process will predominate. In fact, when such factors as self-relevance are manipulated, the same message will be processed centrally by high-self-relevance subjects and peripherally by low-self-relevance subjects. Thus, if the peripheral cue is positive (e.g., high source credibility) and yet the arguments are weak, different conclusions from the message will be arrived at by the two groups (Petty, Cacioppo, & Goldman, 1981). However, there is no assumption of simultaneous incompatible conclusions within any subject's head. On the other hand, Chaiken (1980) has argued for the simultaneous operation of her two message-analytic processes, heuristic and systematic. However, she does not consider the possibility that this could entail the simultaneous belief in contradictory conclusions. In fact, such evidence that systematic and heuristic processing could produce simultaneously conflicting responses would constitute strong evidence of a dual-process system for Chaiken, from Sloman's (1996) point of view. Rather, she considers how the two processes work together, simultaneously and in a complementary way, to arrive at a single integrated judgment that represents the combined operation of the two processes.

Interestingly, Abelson (1994) has recently addressed this issue of cooperative parallel processing versus antagonistic parallel processing. He concludes that social-psychological models, such as cognitive-consistency theories, have been too quick to assume that inconsistencies, once engaged and detected, must be resolved. Abelson suggests that antagonistic systems can lead to chronically held inconsistencies. Furthermore, he proposes that this is not necessarily bad. Humans may be well served by maintaining simultaneous incompatible judgments, so that the appropriate decision will be available to emerge under the right circumstances. This kind of notion seems implicit in Sloman's (1996) model, as he does not discuss any need or mechanism for resolving the incompatible responses that are the consequence of the operation of dual processes. The idea that the existence of simultaneous incompatible answers to a reasoning or judgment problem is a normal and functional state is one from which many dual-process models in social psychology might benefit.

Despite the fact that most current social-psychological dual-process models do not precisely fit Sloman's Criterion S, the existence of simultaneous incompatible beliefs seems natural in the social world. Consider, for example, people's beliefs about the ability of astrology to make predictions about the quality of the upcoming day or to capture the personality characteristics of individuals born under a certain zodiac sign. People seem both to disbelieve horoscopes (perhaps through rule-based reasoning), and yet at the same time to be drawn to them, to see some truth value in them, and even to look to them for guidance (perhaps through associative reasoning). People's attraction to astrology has, for us, the feel of the simultaneous existence of two incompatible beliefs.

In a more serious and relevant domain, stereotypes and beliefs in them seem to have a similar quality. People both believe in and disbelieve stereotypes at the same time. Many individuals hold egalitarian beliefs and claim not to believe in stereotypes regarding gender, race, or nationality. Such beliefs are expressed under a wide variety of circumstances (e.g., filling out an attitude questionnaire) and are strongly held. And yet, for many of these individuals, there exists a simultaneous belief in the (at least partial) truth value of these stereotypes. These beliefs may emerge in such behaviors as choosing a seat in a classroom, crossing the street to walk on the other side when being followed by persons of a certain race or nationality, or nonverbal behaviors such as eye contact (see Devine & Monteith, 1993, for a discussion of these kinds of beliefs and their consequences). It is possible that in many circumstances, people both believe in and do not believe in the truth value of social stereotypes.

As indicated earlier, social-psychological models (e.g., dissonance theory) typically assume that individuals will become aware of the simultaneous existence of such incompatible beliefs, and that such awareness will lead to the strengthening or adoption of one of these beliefs at the expense of the other. However, the long duration of both belief and disbelief in social phenomena such as horoscopes and stereotypes may support Abelson's (1994) and Sloman's (1996) suggestion that holding incompatible beliefs and judgments in one's head at the same time may in fact be both a natural and a functional state of affairs.

CONCLUSION

We have tried to achieve several goals in writing this chapter. We have begun by addressing the broad question of what a dual-process model is. In so doing, we have outlined the difficulties in answering this question and presented one recent attempt to provide a set of criteria for the identification of the operation of dual processes (Sloman, 1996). Next, we have outlined our own work in the area of impression formation of groups and individuals. We have considered the dual process implications of this work in several different respects. First, our early work indicated large differences in the impressions of social targets from identical information, depending only on whether the target is a group or an individual. This led to the question of whether these differences indicated that different types of processing are involved merely as a function of the type of target. More recent work (McConnell et al., 1994, 1997) indicates strongly that this is not the case. Rather, we conclude that the perceived entitativity of the target is critical: The greater the degree of perceived entitativity, the greater the extent of integrative processing. In general, individuals are perceived as higher in entitativity than groups, and thus integrative processing is more characteristic of the impression formation of individual targets. However, when the level of perceived entitativity of individual and group targets is equalized by information about specific targets, the same type of processing and the same impressions are observed for the two types of targets.

Second, we have considered the aspects

of integrative processing that are engaged by high levels of perceived entitativity. We have identified the mechanisms involved in integrative processing, as well as some of the important outcomes. Finally, we have considered the alternative mode of impression formation to integrative processing—retrospective processing that is carried out at a later time, such as when a judgment about the target is subsequently required. We have outlined the similarities and differences between integrative and retrospective processing. In addition, we have concluded that even if these processes do not strictly meet Sloman's (1996) criteria for dual processes, it is useful to consider them as alternative processes for forming impressions of social targets.

Our analysis leads us to the conclusion that questions about dual-processing mechanisms in social psychology are complex, and that some of the most critical questions about the nature of the dual processes that have been proposed have seldom been seriously addressed. Among these questions are those of what the criteria for a true dual-process model are, whether the two proposed processes operate in parallel or are sequential, whether the processes fall along a single continuum or represent different mechanisms and structures, and under what conditions one or the other process is more likely to predominate. One particularly interesting question arises when the model assumes a parallel operation of the two processes and when the outcome of the two processes is a pair of inconsistent and incompatible judgments. In that case, is it likely that the output of the two processes will be integrated and the conflict will be resolved, or is it more likely that the incompatible judgments will both remain strongly represented in memory, each one to be used according to the requirements of each situation? This is certainly a question that is worth pursuing, and one that strikes at the heart of many of the standard assumptions made in social-psychological theories.

We feel that it would be extremely useful to consider all the dual-processing models presented in the current volume with regard to these questions and issues. It would, in addition, be beneficial to analyze where these various models fit according to the distinctions made by Abelson (1994), Sloman (1996), and some of the other important distinctions that we have discussed. Such an exercise would have the dual benefits of arriving at a better understanding of dual-processing models in general, as well as an enhanced understanding of the specific content area addressed by each of the models.

ACKNOWLEDGMENT

Preparation of this chapter was supported in part by National Institute of Mental Health Grant No. 40058.

NOTE

1. It is assumed that this organization occurs as the information is being processed. Others (e.g., Klein & Loftus, 1990) have argued that such organization, as reflected in free-recall data, does not characterize the representation in memory but rather emerges only later, as the retrieval of information is guided by trait cues. Of course, it may be that both mechanisms can contribute to organization in recall.

REFERENCES

Abelson, R. P. (1994). A personal perspective on social cognition. In P. G. Devine, D. L. Hamilton, & T. M. Ostrom (Eds.), *Social cognition: Impact on social psychology* (pp. 15–37). San Diego, CA: Academic Press.

Ajzen, I., & Fishbein, M. (1973). Attitudinal and normative variables as predictors of specific behaviors. *Journal of Personality and social Psychology, 27*, 41–57.

Ajzen, I., & Fishbein, M. (1980). *Understanding attitudes and predicting social behavior relation.* Englewood Cliffs, NJ: Prentice-Hall.

Banaji, M. R., & Greenwald, A. G. (1993). Implicit stereotyping and prejudice. In M. P. Zanna & J. M. Olson (Eds.), *The psychology of prejudice: The Ontario Symposium* (Vol. 7). Hillsdale, NJ: Erlbaum.

Bassili, J. N., & Smith, M. C. (1986). On the spontaneity of trait attribution: Converging evidence for the role of cognitive strategy. *Journal of Personality and Social Psychology, 50*, 239–245.

Brewer, M. B. (1988). A dual process model of impression formation. In T. K. Srull & R. S. Wyer, Jr. (Eds.), *Advances in social cognition* (Vol. 1, pp. 1–36). Hillsdale, NJ: Erlbaum.

Bruner, J. S. (1957). On perceptual readiness. *Psychological Review, 64*, 123–152.

Campbell, D. T. (1958). Common fate, similarity, and other indices of the status of aggregates of persons as social entities. *Behavioral Science, 3*, 14–25.

Chaiken, S. (1980). Heuristic versus systematic information processing and the use of source versus message cues in persuasion. *Journal of Personality and Social Psychology, 39*, 752–756.

Curran, T., & Hintzman, D. L. (1995). Violations of the independence assumption in process dissociation.

Journal of Experimental Psychology: Learning, Memory, and Cognition, 21, 531–547.

Denes-Raj, V., & Epstein, S. (1994). Conflict between intuitive and rational processing: When people behave against their better judgment. *Journal of Personality and Social Psychology, 66*, 819–829.

Devine, P. G. (1989). Stereotypes and prejudice: Their automatic and controlled components. *Journal of Personality and Social Psychology, 56*, 5–18.

Devine, P. G., & Monteith, M. J. (1993). The role of discrepancy-associated affect in prejudice reduction. In D. M. Mackie & D. L. Hamilton (Eds.), *Affect, cognition, and stereotyping: Interactive processes in intergroup perception* (pp. 317–344). San Diego, CA: Academic Press.

Dovidio, J., & Fazio, R. (1992). New technologies for the direct and indirect assessment of attitudes. In J. Tanur (Ed.), *Questions about survey questions* (pp. 204–237). New York: Russell Sage.

Epstein, S. (1983). The unconscious, the preconscious, and the self-concept. In J. Suls & A. Greenwald (Eds.), *Psychological perspectives on the self* (Vol. 2, pp. 219–247). Hillsdale, NJ: Erlbaum.

Epstein, S. (1985). The implications of cognitive–experiential self-theory for research in social psychology and personality. *Journal of the Theory of Social Behavior, 15*, 283–310.

Farah, M. J. (1994). Neuropsychological inference with an interactive brain: A critique of the "locality" assumption. *Behavioral and Brain Sciences, 17*, 43–104.

Fazio, R. H. (1990). Multiple processes by which attitudes guide behavior: The MODE model as an integrative framework. In M. P. Zanna (Ed.), *Advances in experimental social psychology* (Vol. 23, pp. 75–109). New York: Academic Press.

Fazio, R. H. (1995). Attitudes as object–evaluation associations: Determinants, consequences, and correlates of attitude accessibility. In R. E. Petty & J. A. Krosnick (Eds.), *Attitude strength: Antecedents and consequences* (pp. 197–216). Hillsdale, NJ: Erlbaum.

Fiske, S. T., & Neuberg, S. L. (1990). A continuum of impression formation, from category-based to individuating processes: Influences of information and motivation on attention and interpretation. In M. P. Zanna (Ed.), *Advances in experimental social psychology* (Vol. 23, pp. 1–74). New York: Academic Press.

Ginossar, A., & Trope, Y. (1987). Problem solving in judgment under uncertainty. *Journal of Personality and Social Psychology, 52*, 464–476.

Hamilton, D. L. (1998). Dispositional and attributional inferences in person perception. In J. M. Darley & J. Cooper (Eds.), *Attribution processes and social interaction: The legacy of Edward E. Jones* (pp. 99–114). Washington, DC: American Psychological Association.

Hamilton, D. L., Dugan, P. M., & Trolier, T. K. (1985). The formation of stereotypic beliefs: Further evidence for distinctiveness-based illusory correlations. *Journal of Personality and Social Psychology, 48*, 5–17.

Hamilton, D. L., Katz, L. B., & Leirer, V. O. (1980). Cognitive representation of personality impressions: Organizational processes in first impression formation. *Journal of Personality and Social Psychology, 39*, 1050–1063.

Hamilton, D. L., & Sherman, S. J. (1996). Perceiving persons and groups. *Psychological Review, 103*, 336–355.

Hamilton, D. L., Sherman, S. J., & Lickel, B. (1998). Perceptions of groups: The importance of the entitativity continuum. In C. Sedikides, J. Schopler, & C. A. Insko (Eds.), *Intergroup cognition and intergroup behavior* (pp. 47–74). Mahwah, NJ: Erlbaum.

Hastie, R. (1984). Causes and effects of causal attribution. *Journal of Personality and Social Psychology, 46*, 44–56.

Hastie, R., & Park, B. (1986). The relationship between memory and judgment depends on whether the judgment task is memory-based or on-line. *Psychological Review, 93*, 258–268.

Herek, G. M. (1987). Can functions be measured?: A new perspective on the functional approach to attitudes. *Social Psychology Quarterly, 50*, 285–303.

Jacoby, L. L. (1991). A process dissociation framework: Separating automatic from intentional uses of memory. *Journal of Memory and Language, 30*, 513–541.

Johnson, C., & Mullen, B. (1994). Evidence for the accessibility of paired distinctiveness in distinctiveness-based illusory correlation in stereotyping. *Personality and Social Psychology Bulletin, 20*, 65–70.

Jones, E. E., & Davis, K. E. (1965). From acts to dispositions: The attribution process in person perception. In L. Berkowitz (Ed.), *Advances in experimental social psychology* (Vol. 2, pp. 220–266). New York: Academic Press.

Jones, E. E., & McGillis, D. (1976). Correspondent inferences and the attribution cube: A comparative reappraisal. In J. H. Harvey, W. J. Ickes, & R. F. Kidd (Eds.), *New directions in attribution research* (Vol. 1, pp. 389–420). Hillsdale, NJ: Erlbaum.

Kahneman, D., Slovic, P., & Tversky, A. (1982). *Judgment under uncertainty: Heuristics and biases.* Cambridge, England: Cambridge University Press.

Kahneman, D., & Tversky, A. (1973). On the psychology of prediction. *Psychological Review, 80*, 237–251.

Kelley, H. H. (1967). Attribution theory in social psychology. In D. Levine (Ed.), *Nebraska Symposium on Motivation* (Vol. 15, pp. 192–240). Lincoln: University of Nebraska Press.

Kelly, G. A. (1955). *The psychology of personal constructs.* New York: Norton.

Klein, S. B., & Loftus, J. (1990). Rethinking the role of organization in person memory: An independent trace storage model. *Journal of Personality and Social Psychology, 59*, 400–410.

Klein, S. B., & Loftus, J. (1993). The mental representation of trait and autobiographical knowledge about the self. In T. K. Srull & R. S. Wyer, Jr. (Eds.), *Advances in social cognition* (Vol. 5, pp. 1–49). Hillsdale, NJ: Erlbaum.

Klein, S. B., Loftus, J., Trafton, J. G., & Fuhrman, R. W. (1992). Use of exemplars and abstractions in trait judgments: A model of trait knowledge about the self and others. *Journal of Personality and Social Psychology, 63*, 739–753.

Kohlberg, L. (1981). *The philosophy of moral development.* San Francisco: Harper & Row.

Lingle, J. H., & Ostrom, T. M. (1981). Principles of memory and cognition in attitude formation. In R. E. Petty, T. M. Ostrom, & T. C. Brock (Eds.), *Cognitive responses in persuasive communications: A text in attitude change* (pp. 399–420). Hillsdale, NJ: Erlbaum.

McConnell, A. R., Sherman, S. J., & Hamilton, D. L. (1994). On-line and memory-based aspects of individual and group target judgments. *Journal of Personality and Social Psychology, 67,* 173–185.

McConnell, A. R., Sherman, S. J., & Hamilton, D. L. (1997). Target cohesiveness: Implications for information processing about individual and group targets. *Journal of Personality and Social Psychology, 72,* 750–762.

Nisbett, R. E., Krantz, D. H., Jepson, C., & Kunda, Z. (1983). The use of statistical heuristics in everyday inductive reasoning. *Psychological Review, 90,* 339–363.

Paivio, A. (1971). *Imagery and verbal processes.* New York: Holt, Rinehart & Winston.

Park, B., DeKay, M. L., & Kraus, S. (1994). Aggregating social behavior into person models: Perceiver-induced consistency. *Journal of Personality and Social Psychology, 66,* 437–459.

Petty, R. E., & Cacioppo, J. T. (1986). The elaboration likelihood model of persuasion. In L. Berkowitz (Ed.), *Advances in experimental social psychology* (Vol. 19, pp. 123–205). New York: Academic Press.

Petty, R. E., Cacioppo, J. T., & Goldman, R. (1981). Personal involvement as a determinant of argument-based persuasion. *Journal of Personality and Social Psychology, 41,* 847–855.

Sanbonmatsu, D. M., Sherman, S. J., & Hamilton, D. L. (1987). Illusory correlation in the perception of individuals and groups. *Social Cognition, 5,* 1–25.

Sherman, J. W. (1996). Development and mental representation of stereotypes. *Journal of Personality and Social Psychology, 70,* 1126–1141.

Sherman, J. W., & Hamilton, D. L. (1994). On the formation of interitem associative links in person memory. *Journal of Experimental Social Psychology, 30,* 203–217.

Sherman, J. W., & Klein, S. B. (1994). Information-gathering processes: Diagnosticity, hypothesis-confirmatory strategies, and perceived hypothesis confirmation. *Journal of Experimental Social Psychology, 67,* 972–983.

Sloman, S. A. (1996). The empirical case for two systems of reasoning. *Psychological Bulletin, 119,* 3–22.

Srull, T. K. (1981). Person memory: Some tests of associative storage and retrieval models. *Journal of Experimental Psychology: Human Learning and Memory, 7,* 440–462.

Srull, T. K., Lichtenstein, M., & Rothbart, M. (1985). Associative storage and retrieval processes in person memory. *Journal of Experimental Psychology: Learning, Memory, and Cognition, 11,* 316–345.

Srull, T. K., & Wyer, R. S., Jr. (1989). Person memory and judgment. *Psychological Review, 96,* 58–83.

Stangor, C., & McMillan, D. (1992). Memory for expectancy-congruent and expectancy-incongruent social information: A meta-analytic review of the social psychological and social developmental literatures. *Psychological Bulletin, 111,* 42–61.

Stern, L. D., Marrs, S., Millar, M. G., & Cole, E. (1984). Processing time and the recall of inconsistent and consistent behaviors of individuals and groups. *Journal of Personality and Social Psychology, 47,* 253–262.

Stroessner, S. J., Hamilton, D. L., Acorn, D. A., Czyzewska, M., & Sherman, S. J. (1989). *Representational differences in impressions of groups and individuals.* Paper presented at the annual convention of the American Psychological Association, New Orleans, LA.

Stroessner, S. J., Hamilton, D. L., & Mackie, D. M. (1992). Affect and stereotyping: Effect of induced mood on distinctiveness-based illusory correlations. *Journal of Personality and Social Psychology, 62,* 564–576.

Susskind, J., Maurer, K., Thakkar, V., Hamilton, D. L., & Sherman, J. W. (in press). Perceiving individuals and groups: Expectancies, dispositional inferences, and causal attributions. *Journal of Personality and Social Psychology.*

Townsend, J. T. (1990). Serial vs. parallel processing: Sometimes they look like Tweedledum and Tweedledee but they can (and should) be distinguished. *Psychological Science, 1,* 46–54.

Trope, Y., & Liberman, A. (1996). Social hypothesis testing: Cognitive and motivational mechanisms. In E. T. Higgins & A. W. Kruglanski (Eds.), *Social psychology: Handbook of basic principles* (pp. 239–270). New York: Guilford Press.

Tversky, A., & Kahneman, D. (1983). Extensional versus intuitive reasoning: The conjunction fallacy in probability judgment. *Psychological Review, 90,* 293–315.

Uleman, J. S. (1987). Consciousness and control: The case of spontaneous trait inferences. *Personality and Social Psychology Bulletin, 13,* 337–354.

Uleman, J. S., Newman, L. S., & Moskowitz, G. B. (1996). Unintended social inference: The case of spontaneous trait inference. In M. P. Zanna (Ed.), *Advances in experimental social psychology* (Vol. 28, pp. 211–280). San Diego, CA: Academic Press.

Wason, P. C. (1966). Reasoning. In B. Foss (Ed.), *New horizons in psychology* (Vol. 1, pp. 135–151). Harmondsworth, England: Penguin.

Weisz, C., & Jones, E. E. (1993). Expectancy disconfirmation and dispositional inference: Latent strength of target-based and category-based expectancies. *Personality and Social Psychology Bulletin, 19,* 563–573.

Winter, L., & Uleman, J. S. (1984). When are social judgments made?: Evidence for the spontaneousness of trait inferences. *Journal of Personality and Social Psychology, 47,* 237–252.

Wyer, R. S., Jr., Bodenhausen, G. V., & Srull, T. K. (1984). The cognitive representation of persons and groups and its effect on recall and recognition memory. *Journal of Experimental Social Psychology, 20,* 445–469.

Zajonc, R. B. (1980). Feeling and thinking: Preferences need no inferences. *American Psychologist, 35,* 151–175.

31

When Do Decent People Blame Victims?

THE DIFFERING EFFECTS OF THE EXPLICIT/RATIONAL AND IMPLICIT/EXPERIENTIAL COGNITIVE SYSTEMS

MELVIN J. LERNER
JULIE H. GOLDBERG

The current political dialogues in the United States and those that took place in the 1960s have in common a focus on issues of welfare and victimization. Both then and now, the leading political figures turned the public's attention to the poverty-stricken minorities living in crime-ridden neighborhoods. But there the resemblance ends. The then widely accepted "war on poverty" policies of the Johnson administration portrayed these people as innocent victims needing vast governmental aid to break through the culture of poverty and overcome the effects of generations of economic and social discrimination. However, the emerging political consensus today proposes to radically reduce publicly funded aid, blaming these welfare programs for eroding the beneficiaries' moral fiber and sustaining their dependence on the support of hardworking taxpayers. It appears that people living in poverty, who would have been described as victimized minorities in the 1960s, have now become indolent exploiters of the publicly financed welfare system. A key issue at the core of these radically different policies is the social-psychological question of what determines where observers, citizens, and taxpayers place the blame for the victims' suffering and deprivation: Do they primarily blame a hostile economic and social environment or the victims' flawed characters?

The most familiar answers to this question of blame emphasize either the observing citizens' self-interest or their political ideology. Supporting the political-ideology hypothesis, research shows that politically right-wing citizens are more likely to attribute economic victims' fates to their presumed personal failings of will or character, whereas more liberal, politically left-wing constituents place more blame on environmental forces (Skitka & Tetlock, 1992, 1993). Alternatively, the self-interest explanation attributes both political orientations and the blaming of victims or the environment to people's efforts to enhance their own economic resources, status, or political power. According to this theory, victims and their advocates place the blame on the environment rather than themselves in order to excuse their own failings, to justify their demands for aid, and to gain political advantages. On the other hand, the privileged sectors of society blame the victims in order to reduce their own taxes, keep wages low, and maintain their superior status.

THE COMMITMENT TO DESERVING AND THE BELIEF IN A JUST WORLD

The research Lerner and his colleagues began in the 1960s set out to test an alternative explanation to self-interest and political ideology—one that began with the observation that people's reactions to victims, regardless of their political posture, follow from their judgments of deserving. Observers, whatever their political orientation, primarily want to know whether or not the victims did or did not deserve to suffer. Lerner's theory proposed that people want to believe they live in a world in which everyone gets his or her just deserts in the long run, or at least a world in which terrible things do not happen to good people. Maintaining this belief is so important, and the awareness of undeserved suffering is so threatening to people, that they may resort to condemning and blaming objectively innocent victims—victims whom, under other circumstances, they would try to rescue and compensate because of their obvious innocence. Lerner's hypothesis then led to many critical questions, not the least of which was this: If people are committed to seeing that justice prevails, why do they tolerate the continuing suffering of the many obviously innocent victims in their world?

The Initial Research: Simple Defenses

The initial program of research designed to answer this question revealed the ironic, often tragic effects of people's efforts to maintain their faith in a just world. Experiments demonstrated that if people had the needed resources and were given the opportunity to use them, they would try to restore justice by coming to the aid of the innocent victims. But if they were unable to intervene on behalf of the victims and unable to emotionally remove themselves from the event, they might resort to blaming or derogating those same innocent victims. As revealed in a series of experiments, both helping and derogating the same victims appeared to be driven by the observers' need to restore their faith in the justness of their world; the greater the injustice, the more severe the victim-blaming reactions (Lerner, 1980). Observers did not want to believe that "bad" things could happen to "good" people in their world. Later research

confirmed that even the innocent victims of something as obviously random as the draft lottery of the last Vietnam War years might blame themselves rather than give up the sense of security that the belief in a just world provided (Rubin & Peplau, 1973).

Further research showed that in situations where observers were unable to eliminate a victim's suffering, and the victim's innocence and virtue were virtually impossible to question, they did not derogate the victim. Instead, they felt compelled to leave the scene. The assumption that injustices to others threatened the observers' security led to the further prediction that the more similar a victim was to the observers, the greater the experienced threat. Subsequent experiments confirmed the counterintuitive hypothesis that if observers had no other way of restoring justice in the situation, they would try to avoid the awareness of the undeserved suffering of someone who was very much like them. However, the suffering of someone who was rather different posed relatively little threat, and was therefore more easily tolerated (Lerner & Agar, 1972; Novak & Lerner, 1968). It was not nearly so frightening when something "bad" happened to one of "them."

More Sophisticated Expressions of the Justice Motive

Later research considered the ways people maintained their belief in a just world, in spite of evidence of widespread undeserved suffering and deprivation that could not be denied or avoided. These just-world-maintaining defenses included adopting belief systems that promised the ultimate triumph of justice, regardless of what injustices appeared to be occurring. Participants believed that in the next life, if not the present one, the victims would be compensated and the villains punished (Lerner, 1980). Evidence was also found of even more elaborate defenses. The identification of one such defense arose out of the observation that many people insist both to themselves and publicly that they have no responsibility beyond that of charitable taxpayers for others' victimization. Moreover, they even deny having faith in a just world. Contrary to what one might expect from their professed detachment from issues of justice and innocent victims, they remain emotionally vulnerable to witnessing injustices and highly responsive to any opportunities to help victims. However, they will act upon the desire to help only if in so doing they do not jeopardize their own deserving.

The "Exchange Fiction"

Holmes (see Lerner, Miller, & Holmes, 1976) termed one such sophisticated defense the "exchange fiction" and demonstrated its presence in an experiment that sent university students into the neighboring community to sell decorator candles and solicit donations for various causes. The findings of this field study revealed that when people in the community were asked for direct donations, they gave very little to the worthy cause of either helping emotionally disabled children to receive therapy or providing athletic equipment for neighborhood organized sports. However, when given the opportunity to buy rather expensive decorator candles, the profits of which would be used to help the disabled children, similar community members were remarkably responsive. By contrast, the opportunity to buy these expensive candles for neighborhood children's athletic equipment created virtually no appeal.

The reasoning behind the Holmes experiment assumed that in the normal course of development, most people, at some point in their lives, recognize that they are emotionally vulnerable to the suffering of innocent victims. But their experiences also teach them that because there are so many truly innocent victims in their world capable of eliciting those emotions, they would quickly exhaust their resources and become emotionally overwhelmed if they were to act upon their feelings. As a consequence of this need to control their own emotions, they train themselves to respond to victims only under conditions that allow them to be good citizens while maintaining their separateness from the hopeless world of victims. Holmes reasoned that the opportunity to buy the decorator candles in the field study would enable the purchasers to portray their caring for the children as the desire for an impersonal economic exchange, rather than an admission to themselves and others that they cared about the children's suffering. In other words, they could both

help the children and continue to maintain their separateness from the world of victims— all those innocently deprived and suffering people who could elicit strong feelings of compassion and caring and the impulse to help.

The "exchange fiction," as Holmes termed this fascinatingly complex defense, assumes that what is ultimately threatened by people's emotional responsiveness to victims is the observers' own ability to get and keep what they deserve. In the field study, allowing the donors to pretend to themselves as well as others that they were simply engaging in an economic exchange (i.e., buying decorator candles) enabled the donors to maintain their emotional separateness from these victims and, more importantly, from innocent victims in general, while still relieving the victims' suffering.

A Contemporary Dilemma: "My Deserving" versus "Justice for Them"

Miller (1975, 1977) constructed a rather compelling experimental demonstration of this internal conflict between one's own deserving and justice for others. He gave male undergraduates the opportunity to earn money for part-time work under varying incentive conditions, including, in some cases, the opportunity to share part of their pay with a family in desperate need of money. By comparing the effects of a variety of incentives, he was able to show that these young men were rather reluctant to accept the job if sharing some of their pay with the family meant that their own resultant earnings would be less than a fair return for their effortsHowever, if their pay was slightly larger, so that after 33% was deducted for the family their own share would still be a fair wage, they were highly motivated to work. In fact, they were considerably more motivated by the opportunity to work for a fair wage and help the needy family than if they could keep all the money, including the additional 33%, for themselves.

Those findings took on added significance when compared with the predictions of role-playing participants. When presented with these various incentive conditions, similar young men came up with a radically different set of reactions, and the pattern of their predictions was particularly revealing. The role-playing participants predicted that their own and other students' motivation to work would be entirely dependent upon how much money they could keep for themselves (i.e., their own profits). They believed that allocating any of their wages for the needy family would create a strong deterrent to accepting the job.

Obviously, these predictions reflected the role-playing participants' conscious understanding of the reasons people work: to earn money for themselves, and the more money the better. As expected, they were entirely unaware of the preconscious conflict between their own strong impulses to help victims and to protect what they felt they deserved for themselves. These role-playing participants could not predict the behavior of their peers in the actual situation and would probably have had difficulty believing or explaining their actions. These systematic discrepancies between the responses of the role-playing participants and those who were actually involved as full participants in the situations Miller created for them have very important implications both for our theories of human motivation and for the methods we employ to test them.

Theoretical Assumptions: Preconscious and Conscious Reactions

Although it was not specifically articulated at the time, it is obvious in retrospect that elaborating upon the justice motive hypothesis to explain the various ways people respond to victims led to important theoretical assumptions concerning how people process and respond to emotionally arousing information. The emerging model portrayed an observer as having conscious thoughts about a victim that take the form of conventional understandings of what matters to people. This understanding reflects normative rules for making rational decisions and evaluating behavioral alternatives—for example, "No, I'm sorry, but I already gave to the United Fund and to my church charities," and "Why, yes, those are very attractive candles, and that seems like an excellent price; I'll take two" (and, as an afterthought, "It is nice that you are trying to help those chil-

dren get the treatment they need". However, Lerner and his colleagues also found reason to believe that at the same time, observers are also pre- or subconsciously processing information, and that this processing is guided by rather nonrational and unconventional rules. Moreover, this nonrational processing greatly influences the way observers reacted—what they think and say, as well as what they do. Although there was considerably less explicit understanding of those preconscious processes, it seemed fairly clear that they include affect-laden concerns about the victims and the impulse to help, as well as specific fears of the dangers of helping. The offer to purchase the candles, in the Holmes study, served to neutralize the fear in this preconscious internal dialogue, thus enabling the impulse to help the victims.

Perhaps the most compelling evidence for this dual-level model of information processing and dynamics can be found not only in the experimental data—such as the remarkable increase in the candle purchases when these were paired with the disabled children, or the equally remarkable increase in the young men's desire to work for fair wages and to help the desperate family—but more importantly in the fact that the participants in these studies were not aware of what was driving their reactions. For all intents and purposes, in the critical conditions they had simply discovered how much they wanted or needed those particular expensive decorator candles, or how much they wanted to work. Although they might express pleasure that the profits from the economic exchange would go to such a worthy cause, they would genuinely insist that this was not the reason for their decisions. Nor would they be able to articulate why they would buy expensive candles, or why the job seemed so attractive to them when associated with relief for the victims, while on other occasions they would not donate directly to help those very same victims.

To summarize, by that point it appeared to Lerner and his colleagues that people may be strongly committed to eliminating injustices to others, but they may also be even more committed to protecting what they have earned in the past and hope to deserve in the future. It also seemed that for the most part, this continuing management of their own deserving in a world of many injustices takes place out of people's awareness. Although their conscious thoughts are couched in conventional terms and reflect normatively acceptable ways of making sense out of, or "rationalizing," what they are supposed to be feeling and doing, internal dynamics operating out of their awareness may lead them to help, avoid, or derogate an innocent victim.

RECENT THEORETICAL ADVANCES: MODES OF INFORMATION PROCESSING

As this volume indicates, developments throughout numerous areas of psychology have spawned a family of dual-processing theories with similar general assumptions (see, e.g., Bargh, Chapter 18, this volume; Chen & Chaiken, Chapter 4, this volume; Devine & Monteith, Chapter 17, this volume; Fiske, Lin, & Neuberg, Chapter 11, this volume). Greenwald and Banaji (1995) present considerable evidence documenting the importance of "implicit" cognitions in shaping people's social judgments. The characteristic feature of implicit cognitive processes is that past experiences affect a person's reactions, even though they are not available to self-report or introspection. According to Greenwald and Banaji, it is important to interpret social judgments from the perspective of an interaction between not consciously retrievable "implicit" cognitions and introspectively available "explicit" social cognitions.

Similarly, the personality theorist Epstein (see, e.g., Epstein, Lipson, Holstein, & Huh, 1992, Epstein & Pacini, Chapter 23, this volume) describes the psychological properties of the "experiential system" and the "rational system." The rational system has the properties of conventional, logical thought and operates primarily at the conscious level. In contrast, Epstein characterizes the experiential system as a passive and preconscious, "relatively crude system that provides a quick and dirty way of assessing and responding to reality," especially when people are seized by their emotions (Epstein et al., 1992, p. 328). Although these systems exist and operate in parallel, they often interact to shape a person's reactions.

Shweder and Haidt (1993), in their essay "The Future of Moral Psychology," describe theories of "cognitive intuitionism" that have many important elements in common with Epstein's and Greenwald and Banaji's distinctions. According to Shweder and Haidt (1993), moral reasoning is characterized by relatively slow, *ex post facto*, conscious thoughts, whereas moral intuitions typically involve rapid, automatically elicited appraisals of events. They argue that though the appraisal process in moral intuitions is "introspectively opaque," the person consciously experiences the consequences of this appraisal as emotions of anger, shame and guilt, which Shweder and Haidt (1993) term "self-evident truths of morality" (p. 364). These truths refer to "injustice, the right, and the good".

The dynamics underlying the initial research on the justice motive and reactions to victims, described above, fit very nicely within these recent theoretical models. Epstein (Epstein et al., 1992; Epstein & Pacini, Chapter 23, this volume) proposes that people's fundamental assumptions about themselves and their world reside in their preconscious "experiential system." Similarly, Shweder and Haidt (1993) locate the rules for what is just, right, and good, and thus the sources of the emotions of anger, guilt, and shame, in a person's "introspectively opaque" moral intuitions. Finally, Greenwald and Banaji (1995) provide extensive documentation of the influence that "implicit" cognitions have on a person's reactions to others, especially social judgments and decisions.

In line with these conceptual frameworks, and consistent with most of the dual-process theories in this volume, it should be no surprise to find that people who care deeply about justice experience strong emotions when confronted with a victim. The important dynamics underlying those emotions should take place in the experiential system and involve implicit cognitions, such as the moral intuitions concerning what is just and good. At the same time, people's conscious thought processes, rather than directly reflecting these preconscious dynamics, should correspond to the conventional understanding of what most people care about and why—making rational decisions about how to maximize their own benefits and minimize their costs, in ways that will not get them into trouble with their conscience or their community. Although people are initially driven by their preconscious moral intuitions, they will, if given the time and opportunity, frame their reactions and shape their behavior in ways that are conventionally rational and normatively appropriate (Lerner, 1987).

BLAMING THE VICTIM: THE INFLUENCE OF AUTOMATIC AND MOTIVATED PROCESSES

Even with the support of these recent theoretical advances and experimental evidence, it is not easy to accept this portrayal of people as so committed to simple, intuitive rules of justice that they will reject or avoid objectively innocent victims, without being aware of what they are doing or why. Considerable evidence seems to directly contradict this explanation of victim blaming. For example, everyday observations and the results of several experimental demonstrations clearly reveal that people feel sympathy for innocent victims and would like to help them, and that they only condemn victims who have brought about their own suffering through some moral failing. No social agency could legitimately deny aid to truly innocent victims, nor would it knowingly support victims who were morally corrupt. It is easy to document the assertion that no sane, reasonable person would ever knowingly condemn a victim who was not blameworthy (Weiner, 1993).

These apparent contradictions may be resolved by first recognizing that human beings' normative systems and conscious thought processes, as well as their preconscious moral intuitions, all concur on the importance of justice and on these simple propositions: People should get what they deserve; bad things should not happen to good people; people who have caused harm to themselves or others should be condemned. Where the preconscious and conscious systems differ is in the process by which people arrive at judgments of harm doing and thus blameworthiness. The conscious, normatively based, moral reasoning system assumes that people decide blameworthiness after examining and weighing the evidence concerning the person's intentions and/or negligence. By contrast, the more complex implicit/experiential model offered here recognizes that people consciously think this way, and that at times this rational process

does shape their reactions. However, there are many other occasions when implicit cognitive processes and moral intuitions elicit a blaming response, not at all based upon a rational analysis of the evidence, for which people then find a normatively acceptable reason to justify that response.

But is that possible? What is the evidence concerning how this nonrational blaming of innocent victims can occur? Several lines of recent research, falling roughly into two general categories, converge to describe how preconscious processes can influence blaming reactions. Some of these occur automatically, with no accompanying forethought or direct awareness. They appear in the absence of any particular affect, and are most often understood as descriptions of "That's simply the way our minds work," without any deeper explanation for why this is the case. These types of processes include "correspondence bias" and "hindsight bias." A second subset of preconscious, implicit processes appears to be affect-driven: A person's perception of an event and subsequent reactions are shaped by the affect the person is experiencing at the time, often, but not exclusively, because of the motivational implications of what is taking place. Let us consider some of these processes that can contribute to the blaming of innocent victims.

Automatic Processes

Correspondence Biases

The normatively appropriate, rational approach to determining blameworthiness begins with the attribution of a causal relation between the person and an undesirable outcome. Both common-sense understanding and several psychological theories (Shaver, 1985; Weiner, 1993) assume that people recognize that most outcomes have multiple causes, including those that are more or less proximal or distal, and those that are most reasonably attributed to the person or to situational influences. Did a person perform badly on a test because of lack of ability or lack of preparation, and/or because of the difficulty of the test or the threatening environment in which it took place? Presumably, before blaming the person for the bad grade rather than praising him or her for a good effort, an observer will attempt to answer this question by examining the relevant evidence. In particular, the observer should consider the person's intentions and abilities, and the environmental barriers, such as how well other students did on the test.

Gilbert and Malone (1995) have presented a review of the extensive research documenting the prevalence of a much simpler attribution pattern, the "correspondence bias," which does not conform with this common-sense, rational model. Apparently, given the expectations with which people enter most encounters, they typically assign responsibility for an event by reasoning backward from the outcomes to the proximal personal causal agent. It then takes special effort and time for them to explain away and undo this initial reaction by considering the influence of other causal factors, such as situational influences. The recognition of this process, at some level of awareness, may account for why people are reluctant to be the bearers of bad news (Tesser & Rosen, 1972). It may also explain why people who have caused harm, clearly by accident, nevertheless may feel terribly guilty (Freedman, Wallington, & Bless, 1967; McGraw, 1987).

Hindsight Bias

A similar automatic reaction has been termed the "hindsight bias" (Fischhoff, 1975). This reaction is characterized by an increase in the subjective belief in the probability of an event, simply as a function of knowing that the outcome has occurred. Although this bias has been documented in a variety of contexts, Janoff-Bulman, Timko, and Carli (1985) conducted an experiment with particular relevance to the issue of reactions to victims. In their experiment, participants learned of various events that took place between a young man and a woman during a date that lasted through an afternoon and evening, and ended in either his raping her or his simply taking her home. Those participants who believed that she had been raped rated her prior behaviors as more foolhardy and irresponsible, thus contributing to her victimization, than did those who evaluated the very same acts but who did not believe she had been assaulted at the end of the evening. The evi-

dence clearly indicates that this form of "I knew it all along" or "She should have known it all along" thinking is a very common source of bias and is probably involved in some instances of victim blaming. However, it is important to remember that describing and categorizing the phenomenon of victim blaming as an instance of hindsight bias is not the same as explaining the dynamics underlying this systematic bias.

Affect-Generated Processes

The greatest preponderance of evidence illustrating the influence of the preconscious/implicit/experiential system appears in the recent research on the cognitive consequences of engaging a person's emotions and motivation (Forgas, 1995). Some of the major findings can be briefly summarized here as documenting the influence of "affect as information" and "motivated cognitive constructions."

Affect as Information

Misattribution Effects. One very productive line of research has shown that an emotion elicited by one source may be generalized or simply attributed to another. When that occurs, people's subsequent reactions will reflect how they interpret the emotions they are experiencing. For example, Wyer, Bodenhausen, and Gorman (1985) reported that as a consequence of showing participants slides dramatically depicting rather horrible acts of aggression, the participants subsequently attributed greater responsibility to a rape victim for her fate. Similarly, Thornton (1984) found that when he raised the anxiety level of his experimental participants by the subtle technique of making them more objectively self-aware, they attributed greater characterological and behavioral blame to a rape victim. Conversely, when he gave other participants an alternative explanation for the anxiety they were experiencing (i.e., he attributed it to the novelty of participating in an experiment), they judged the rape victim to be considerably less blameworthy.

Apparently people can misinterpret the anxiety they experience from witnessing a victim's undeserved suffering. They may, in their search for an explanation of what they are experiencing, use their feelings and emotions as information about the victim. Preconsciously, at the experiential level, the participants are distressed by the injustice of the victim's suffering, but they may attribute the distress they are experiencing to the victim's irresponsible behavior and bad character. The tacit internal dialogue can be described as follows: "I am upset, not only because of the terrible thing that was done to you, but also because of how irresponsibly and immorally you behaved."

This intrusion of implicit/experiential processes into a person's explicit conscious responses has been dramatically documented by Rozin and his colleagues. For example, in a typical experiment (Rozin, Markwith, & McCauley, 1994), their participants were reluctant to have contact with various items when they believed that a victim of AIDS, an accident, or murder had had prior contact with them. The items included wearing a sweater, sleeping in a bed, or driving an automobile. Although the nature of the victimization made a difference in their responses, in all cases the participants' aversive reactions were significantly stronger than if the prior "owner" had not been victimized. Even when participants were assured that the items were now sanitary, the items, by their mere association with a victim, had been "contaminated" and elicited emotionally based, irrational, aversive reactions. Although the participants were aware of wanting to avoid those contaminated items, they were unable to consciously retrieve the introspectively opaque, preconscious dynamics that created the feelings of aversion. They had no rational explanation for their emotional reactions to the victims' "contaminated" objects. Apparently people may interpret their intuitively based emotional reactions to undeserved suffering as feelings of revulsion to the victims and anything associated with them.

Emotion-Specific Attributions. Ellsworth and her colleagues (Keltner, Ellsworth, & Edwards, 1993; Smith & Ellsworth, 1985) generated considerable evidence directly linking the perception of an injustice to the emotion of anger and to the attribution of responsibility to persons rather than to their circumstances. They demonstrated, for example, that when participants in an experiment were

primed to reexperience anger stemming from an injustice, in the very next situation they manifested the residual effects of that emotion in the form of blaming a person rather than a situational factor for a variety of outcomes (missing a flight, losing a friend in a plane crash, losing most of one's money, suffering health problems, etc.) (Keltner et al., 1993). The design of this research enabled the investigators to rule out various alternative explanations and thus provided support for the basic hypothesis that whenever a person feels angry (for whatever reason), the perception of other people as causally responsible agents becomes highly salient. Ellsworth's group's findings suggest that anger is one important consequence of witnessing an injustice that preconsciously threatens the observer's sense of security. This emotion increases the probability that the observer will find someone to blame—either the harm doer, the victim, or both.

Goldberg, Lerner, and Tetlock (1996) discovered some important elaborations on this relationship between anger and blaming. In their experiment, they first elicited the emotion of anger in participants by having them view a video clip of excerpts from a film in which a teenage boy was beaten up and humiliated by a bully (Gross & Levenson, 1995). Goldberg et al. varied whether the participants believed that justice was served and the bully was appropriately punished, or that justice failed and the bully got away on a technicality. In a seemingly unrelated second study, the participants were then asked to assign blame and punishment to negligent workers described in brief vignettes. The results indicated that simply witnessing the bullying event made the participants angry. And, consistent with prior research, in the condition where the bully was not punished, the participants' level of anger predicted the degree to which they blamed and punished the negligent workers. However, in the condition where the bully was appropriately punished, the participants' anger was unrelated to their subsequent blaming and punishment responses. When they believed that the bully was punished (i.e., that justice was served), the participants' subsequent blaming reactions followed the normative, rational process of first considering whether the workers intended to do harm and then determining the appropriate level of punishment (Shaver, 1985). However, when the participants believed that the bully went unpunished, their reactions followed what one would expect from the experiential mode of information processing: They subsequently disregarded how intentional the workers' behavior had been, as described in the vignettes, and punished them according to how angry they felt.

Motive-Directed Cognitive Constructions: Ideology and Self-Interest

Attribution theorists have amply demonstrated the tendency for people to construe and recall events in ways that are self-esteem-maintaining (Miller & Ross, 1975). More contemporary evidence has revealed that people's commitments to certain beliefs about their world can also lead to what appears to be motivated biasing of attributions of responsibility and blame. Skitka and Tetlock (1992, 1993) have shown that people's political ideology is highly predictive of their view of victims in need of public assistance. Those with right-wing, conservative ideologies are more likely to blame victims for their state of dependence, whereas those with left-wing ideologies are more likely to find environmental factors responsible. Even more general effects have been found for the belief in a just world. A large body of evidence demonstrates that people who are strongly committed to believing that they live in a just world are likely to find virtually all victims relatively responsible for their fates, compared to people who are less committed to that belief (Furnham & Procter, 1989).

Bruno Bettelheim's Description of the German Citizens' Dilemma. Although it may not be possible to empirically establish, in the strictest sense, that people's motives produce these observed associations between systems of belief and blaming (see Tetlock & Levi, 1982), one can find persuasive personal descriptions of this dynamic. Bruno Bettelheim (1943) provides a compelling example of this process in his account of how many German citizens resolved their psychological conflicts during the early stages of the Nazi regime. According to Bettelheim, when they learned that some of their highly respected friends and neighbors had been arrested, publicly accused of horrible crimes against the German people, and sent off to prison camps, they had two choices. They could acknowledge that these people they knew so well were innocent victims of what must be a mad, tyrannical government. Or they could accept their government's portrayal of what was happening as actually rescuing the German people from these congenitally criminal elements in their midst, the Jews. Of course, this latter construction was much more comforting than recognizing that a group of sadistic monsters had taken charge of their government, and it was therefore much easier to accept. And, so, according to Bettelheim, many of them did accept it.

Becoming aware that something "bad" has happened to a "good" person is upsetting in many ways. Besides the anger or sadness stemming from the violation of one's moral intuitions, it implies that one is living in a dangerous world where being virtuous provides no assurance of freedom from terrible harm. But the resultant anger, sadness, fear, insecurity, helplessness, and even grief can be relieved if one adopts a belief system that redefines what occurred so that an injustice has not taken place: Either the victim is not really a "good" person, or something "bad" has not happened. Religious beliefs often provide this comforting redefinition by promising that everything will be set right in the next life, invariably and absolutely, the wicked will be punished and the good rewarded.

Mario Cuomo's: Reactions to a Nephew's Accidental Death. Given the potentially devastating consequences of witnessing an injustice, it is no surprise that the adoption of these comforting beliefs appears among all social strata and levels of education. Former Governor Mario Cuomo of New York provided a compelling illustration of this when asked whether the death of his brother's child, who had fallen through the ice in a canal behind their house, led him to question the existence of God:

What my brother, my sister-in-law, my whole family concluded then, is that either there is some explanation that eludes me at the moment, or there is none. If there is utterly no rationale then I'm not sure I can deal with the rest of my life. I'm not sure I can make myself sufficiently comfortable in this environment to go forward in it. Therefore I must accept the thesis that there is some justification. That in the long run it does work out, even if I don't understand at the moment. (Quoted in Rosenbaum, 1995, p. 58)

As important as this belief is to Mario Cuomo and his family, neither he nor anyone else can provide a rational explanation for the accidental death or the emotions they experienced following the serious violations of their moral intuitions. Those emotions were the automatic consequences of their implicit processing of the events. The preconscious processing in the experiential system led to horror, grief, outrage, and pity, from which they tried to find relief in the faith that "there is some justification."

Summary

By way of summary, at this point several important issues have been addressed. First, people do seem to process information about important events in their lives at two levels of awareness. Second, the information processing that occurs at these two levels follows different rules and scripts. In brief, consistent with Epstein's model (Epstein et al., 1992; Epstein & Pacini, Chapter 23, this volume), the consciously represented and retrievable level appears to be a direct representation of cultural forms. These forms include normatively based contents, such as ideas and concepts, and the means by which these contents are combined to produce conventionally rational thoughts. Considerably less, but some, is known about the scripts, schemas, prototypes, and information processing of the moral intuitions contained in the implicit, introspectively opaque, preconscious level (Lerner et al., 1976). Enough is known about the automatic and the motivated processing of information to describe some of the implicit processes that appear in people who are frightened, angered, and repulsed by witnessing an injustice. The evidence indicates that these emotions and the associated preconscious processes may lead observers to blame the suffering victim instead of, or along with, the perpetrator. At the same time, people consciously adhere to the conventional rules of

discourse and societal norms. As Shweder and Haidt (1993) have indicated, for the most part people are unable either to retrieve or to understand the dynamics that are elicited when they or others are actually confronted with events that violate their moral intuitions and their sense of justice.

COMPARING THE REACTIONS OF NORMATIVELY INSTRUCTED AND EMOTIONALLY ENGAGED OBSERVERS

Simons and Piliavin (1972) provided an early demonstration of some of the conditions under which these two modes of responding to victims are likely to appear. They compared the evaluative reactions of observers who thought they were watching an experimental participant receiving electric shocks while participating in a learning experiment. Their main finding, which replicated previous research (see Lerner, 1980), was that observers assigned more negative characteristics to the victim in those conditions where they believed her suffering was greater. More suffering from unavoidable shocks led to more derogation. However, in another condition, Simons and Piliavin (1972) informed observers in advance that they were participating in a study of how people react to victims of misfortune: "This experiment studies the way people react to other people who, through no fault of their own, fall victim to some uncontrollable outside force or action. Victims of a hurricane or earthquake are examples, another would be a person attacked by a stranger on a city street" (Simons, 1968). In other conditions, they told observers that they were watching "some students in the psychology department acting as though they were victims of misfortune" (Simons, 1968, p. 2 Appendix). The "actors" they were observing were playing the part of participants who were receiving electric shocks in a learning experiment. The findings revealed that both of these sets of instructions eliminated the victim derogation. This was also true in a role-playing condition where the participants were explicitly asked to react as if they were watching a victim who was actually suffering, not merely pretending to suffer.

In effect, Simons and Piliavin (1972) demonstrated that participants in an experiment who thought they were actually witnessing a vivid instance of undeserved suffering might resort to derogating that victim. However, if the participants were explicitly reminded of the norms associated with how people are supposed to respond to "innocent victims of misfortune," they would not openly derogate such a victim. To do so would have made them appear irrational and unkind. Similarly, observers would not derogate someone who was only pretending to suffer, whether or not the appropriate norms were made explicit. Since there was no actual innocent, suffering victim, they experienced no threat or fear and had no need to derogate or blame anyone. Finally, and of most importance here, the introspectively opaque aspect of the preconscious process of threat leading to derogation was documented by the failure of role-playing participants to anticipate that they or other observers would derogate an innocent, suffering victim. That failure followed from their having available only the normative expectations upon which to base their responses.

The reactions of the role-playing observers confirmed what everyone knows: Nice, rational people do not derogate innocent victims. And those responses are exactly what one can expect to elicit in any situation that does not include a threat to the participants' sense of justice, or any experimental situation that reminds observers of their normative obligations as good, concerned citizens to innocent victims of misfortune. But as also demonstrated in this experiment, nice, rational people who become upset by vivid signs of undeserved suffering, and who are not reminded of how good citizens are supposed to react, may very well resort to finding the victim contemptible in order to restore their own sense of security, even though they may sincerely deny ever doing anything like that. At least, they may not be conscious of doing it.

MANAGERS AND FILIAL CAREGIVERS AS VICTIMS OF THEIR MORAL INTUITIONS

The failure to recognize and anticipate the potential influence of the preconscious, experiential system can create a serious hazard for people faced with critical decisions. This is most readily observed in the differences be-

tween decisions made under thoughtful, detached circumstances and those that occur when a person is emotionally involved. It is well recognized that when people make decisions while angry or frightened, they may have subsequent doubts, if not regrets. Recent studies have also documented the less commonly recognized alternative: People who have carefully thought out the alternatives and made objectively sensible and appropriate decisions may then, after having acted upon them, experience unexpected, irrational emotional reactions, including elements of serious regret and guilt.

One very current example of this can be found among the managers in many corporations. It has now become common practice for corporations in both the public and private sectors to engage in what is euphemistically described as "restructuring." This typically requires discharging large numbers of otherwise adequate employees. The managers play a critically important—and, as it turns out, often rather tragic—role in this process (Smith, 1994). Societal norms, as well as their contractual obligations, clearly require the managers to make the most rational decisions concerning the ultimate welfare of the stakeholders, including the workforce. Since the need to discharge a certain number of employees is blamed on the demands of the competitive marketplace, and the procedures employed in deciding whom to discharge are thoughtfully arrived at and normatively appropriate, the managers should feel reasonably content with (if not actually proud of) their participation in the restructuring of the organization. However, as they implement and experience the consequences of those decisions, they often experience feelings of guilt and demoralization (Levenson, 1994; Smith, 1994).

Professional consultants have recognized the prevalence of these strong, unanticipated emotional reactions to corporate restructuring as a serious management problem. In his address upon receiving an award from the American Psychological Association, Harry Levenson (1994) noted: "The conscious guilt any manager of conscience has about terminating someone else without cause is compounded by the unconscious guilt that arises from the sense that he or she is destroying the other" (p. 429). Levenson's observation implies the important and obviously unanticipated influence of preconscious moral intuitions. At the time of their conscious, eminently rational decision making, the managers do not have conscious access to these introspectively opaque experiential processes. However, once the managers are confronted with the cues signaling that they are causing their discharged employees and their families serious suffering and deprivation, their preconscious moral intuitions automatically produce the irrational guilt feelings. Whatever justifications the societal norms and their conscious moral reasoning may have provided them with, they view themselves preconsciously as harm doers. As the anthropologist M. Thurner has observed (personal communication June 5, 1994), it appears that in the unconscious "the lesser of two evils is still evil."

Similar dynamics may account for the unanticipated emotional experiences that have been observed among filial caregivers, particularly daughters, subsequent to institutionalizing their parents. Brody (1985) has reported that often such daughters experience irrational degrees of guilt and remorse. This guilt appears even though the decisions to institutionalize the parents have been arrived at only after the alternatives have been carefully considered and the family members and health professionals have agreed that for the sake of all concerned, institutionalization is the only sensible thing to do. Apparently the parents' suffering following institutionalization provides cues that automatically elicit the daughters' nonrational perceptions of themselves as insufficiently grateful and caring children. Regardless of what the rational analysis of the situation has demanded, the signs of their parents' suffering make them feel terribly guilty. Their emotions tell them that they have let their parents down and caused them to suffer.

CONCLUSION

This chapter begins, as Lerner's research began in the 1960s, with the question of what determines how people react to victims. The political dialogues raging both then and now provide an added incentive for wanting to know whether reasonably sane and decent people will condemn and derogate "objectively" innocent victims, and if so, why. The pursuit of the answers to those questions leads very quickly to the importance we all attach to deserving and justice.

Most of us would like to believe that we live in a just world, but we are continually confronted with experiences that tell us this is not the case. Even though we may pretend to have given up this comforting fairy tale for a more realistic appraisal of our world, our continuing preconscious, irrational investment in this belief can lead to elaborate psychological defenses, including a deep, abiding, and entirely nonrational faith that everything will be set right and justice will prevail in the future, in heaven if not on earth. Ironically, the evidence reveals that when our faith in ultimate justice is not operative, and an injustice elicits strong emotions, we may blame innocent victims, or avoid them as a way of maintaining our confidence that, by and large, we live in a world where people get what they deserve. Nevertheless, if asked, we may honestly state that we will only reject or avoid victims who deserve their suffering, and that we will react with compassion if the evidence indicates that someone is a truly innocent victim. No decent, sane person would do otherwise.

In truth, the evidence needed to document the central role of deservingness in people's reactions to victims is as easily available as our own introspections. We respond to victims with compassion and caring when we believe they do not deserve their suffering, and with indifference or even condemnation if, by virtue of their character or behavior, we believe they deserve their suffering and deprivation. But then the important question becomes this: How do we arrive at this judgment? Do we dispassionately and rationally search for evidence concerning sufficient and necessary causation, as well as evaluate the victims' intentions and foresight, or do we automatically and intuitively sense when victims have violated fundamental rules of decency and wrongfully caused themselves or others to suffer? The evidence indicates that we do both of these at various times, and that they can often lead to greatly discrepant judgments. What we may reason to be normatively and rationally justifiable we may intuitively experience as fundamentally "wrong," "bad," or "evil." The evidence points to the conclusion that our normatively based moral reasoning and our moral intuitions may follow different rules and can contradict each other. The dual-process theories offered by Epstein (Epstein et al., 1992; Epstein & Pacini, Chapter 23, this volume) and Shweder and Haidt (1993), as well as several others presented in this volume, are rich sources of hypotheses concerning when and under what circumstances the implicit/intuitive/experiential or the explicit/conscious/rational processes are more likely to influence people's reactions. Let us hope that the next generation of research not only will add to our understanding of the relatively uninvestigated experiential processes, but will also explore the more complex issue of how the two systems interact to influence the ongoing stream of experiences and behavior.

In the meantime, it is important to realize that although it is often highly functional for people to engage in thoughtful, conventionally rational causal analyses, and employ moral reasoning to shape their reactions, there are serious risks contingent upon failing to recognize the extent to which automatically elicited, preconscious moral intuitions influence people's emotions and subsequent reactions to critical events (see Bargh, Chapter 18, this volume). These risks include conducting research that misconstrues people's conventional understanding of their motives and beliefs as directly revealing their reactions, when in actuality their preconscious intuitions and scripts are engaged. People cannot recall and consciously represent these introspectively opaque processes. The main scientific risk is that social psychologists will infer that they have an adequate representation of human motivation—what people care about and why—from their participants' thoughtful efforts to imagine how they would respond to an important event.

The second set of risks arises from the problematic, often tragic consequences of people's making decisions on the basis of their conventional understanding of normatively acceptable rules for determining responsibility and morality. One common form of this at the individual level can be found in situations where societal norms require decision makers to select a course of action that promises the least harm and most benefit for all, even if it

means knowingly causing some to suffer. The evidence cited here reveals that the postdecisional consequences of these normatively justified decisions may cause the decision makers to experience guilt based upon the intuitive, "irrational" reaction of perceiving themselves as harm doers. It is as if, preconsciously, whatever normative justifications are present, people believe that "the lesser of two evils is still evil." And they choose to do that "evil."

In all probability, there is not much that can be done to alter our "moral intuitions." Nor would it be necessarily desirable to let those intuitions and preconscious agendas, including the justice motive, dominate our lives. However, it is just as clear that the more we know about the ways implicit/experiential processes influence our thoughts and emotions, the better prepared we will be to understand ourselves and the behavior of others. And possibly, eventually, we may not have to blame and avoid victims, but rather can help them without having to pretend that we want to buy decorator candles.

ACKNOWLEDGMENTS

Major portions of this chapter were first presented in the plenary address at the International Conference on Social Justice Research V, Reno, Nevada, June 1995. We want to thank Dan Batson, Peter Degoey, Ron Dillehay, John G. Holmes, and Dale T. Miller, as well as our colleagues at the Institute for Personality and Social Research, the University of California at Berkeley, and Clark University, for their helpful comments on earlier versions of the ideas presented in this chapter.

REFERENCES

Bettelheim, B. (1943). Individual and mass behavior in extreme situations. *Journal of Abnormal and Social Psychology*, 38, 417–452.

Brody, E. (1985). Parent care as normative family stress. *The Gerontologist*, 25, 19–29.

Epstein, S., Lipson, A., Holstein, C., & Huh, E. (1992). Irrational reactions to negative outcomes: Evidence for two conceptual systems. *Journal of Personality and Social Psychology*, 62, 328–339.

Fischhoff, B. (1975). Hindsight (does not equal) foresight: The effects of outcome knowledge on judgments under uncertainty. *Journal of Experimental Psychology: Human Perception and Performance*, 1, 288–299.

Forgas, J. P. (1995). Mood and judgment: The affect infusion model (AIM). *Psychological Bulletin*, 117, 39–66.

Freedman, J. L., Wallington, S. A., & Bless, E. (1967).

Compliance without pressure: The effects of guilt. *Journal of Personality and Social Psychology, 7,* 117–124.

Furnham, A., & Procter, E. (1989). Belief in a just world: Review and critique of the individual difference literature. *British Journal of Social Psychology, 28,* 365–384.

Gilbert, D. T., & Malone, S. P. (1995). The correspondence bias. *Psychological Bulletin, 117,* 21–38.

Goldberg, J., Lerner, J., & Tetlock, P. (1996, April). *The psychology of punitive bias in judgments of responsibility.* Paper presented at the meeting of the Western Psychological Association, San Jose, CA.

Greenwald, A. G., & Banaji, M. R. (1995). Implicit social cognition: Attitudes, self-esteem, and stereotypes. *Psychological Review, 102,* 4–27.

Gross, J., & Levenson, R. (1995). Emotion elicitation using films. *Cognition and Emotion, 9*(1), 87–108.

Janoff-Bulman, R., Timko, C., & Carli, L. L. (1985). Cognitive biases in blaming the victim. *Journal of Experimental Social Psychology, 21,* 161–177.

Keltner, D., Ellsworth, P. C., & Edwards, K. (1993). Beyond simple pessimism: Effects of sadness and anger on social perception. *Journal of Personality and Social Psychology, 64,* 740–752.

Lerner, M. J. (1980). *The belief in a just world: A fundamental delusion.* New York: Plenum Press.

Lerner, M. J. (1987). Integrating societal and psychological rules of entitlement: The basic task of each social actor and fundamental problem for the social sciences. *Social Justice Research, 1,* 107–125.

Lerner, M. J., & Agar, E. (1972). The consequences of perceived similarity: Attraction and rejection, approach and avoidance. *Journal of Experimental Research in Personality, 6,* 69–75.

Lerner, M. J., Miller, D. T., & Holmes, J. G. (1976). Deserving and the emergence of forms of justice. In L. Berkowitz & E. Walster (Eds.), *Advances in experimental social psychology* (Vol. 9, pp. 133–162), New York: Academic Press.

Levenson, H. (1994). Why the behemoths fell: Psychological roots of corporate failure. *American Psychologist, 49,* 428–436.

McGraw, K. M. (1987). Guilt following transgression: An attribution of responsibility approach. *Journal of Personality and Social Psychology, 53,* 247–256.

Miller, D. T. (1975). *Personal deserving versus justice for others: An exploration of the justice motive.* Unpublished doctoral dissertation, University of Waterloo, Waterloo, Ontario, Canada.

Miller, D. T. (1977). Personal deserving and justice for others: An exploration of the justice motive. *Journal of Experimental Social Psychology, 13,* 1–13.

Miller, D. T., & Ross, M. (1975). Self-serving biases in the attribution of causality : Fact or fiction? *Psychological Bulletin, 82,* 213–225.

Novak, D. W., & Lerner, M. J. (1968). Rejection as a consequence of perceived similarity. *Journal of Personality and Social Psychology, 9,* 147–152.

Rosenbaum, R. (1995, June 4). Staring into the heart of darkness. *New York Times Magazine,* pp. 36–46.

Rozin, P., Markwith, M., & McCauley, C. (1994). Sensitivity to indirect contacts with other persons: AIDS aversion as a composite of aversion to strangers, infection, moral taint, and misfortune. *Journal of Abnormal Psychology, 103,* 495–504.

Rubin, Z., & Peplau, L. A. (1973). Belief in a just world and reaction to another's lot: A study of participants in the national draft lottery. *Journal of Social Issues, 29,* 73–93.

Shaver, K. G. (1985). *The attribution of blame: Causality, responsibility, and blameworthiness.* New York: Springer-Verlag.

Shweder, R. A., & Haidt, J. (1993). The future of moral psychology: Truth, intuition, and the pluralist way. *Psychological Science, 4,* 360–365.

Simons, C. (1968). *The effects of deception manipulations within an experiment on reactions to victims of misfortune.* Unpublished master's thesis, University of Pennsylvania.

Simons, C., & Piliavin, J. A. (1972). The effect of deception on reactions to a victim. *Journal of Personality and Social Psychology, 21,* 56–60.

Skitka, L. J., & Tetlock, P. E. (1992). Allocating aid: The roles of scarcity, ideology, causal attributions, and distributive norms. *Journal of Experimental Social Psychology, 29,* 397–409.

Skitka, L. J., & Tetlock, P. E. (1993). Providing public assistance: Cognitive and motivational processes underlying liberal and conservative policy preferences. *Journal of Personality and Social Psychology, 65,* 1205–1223.

Smith, C. A., & Ellsworth, P. C. (1985). Patterns of cognitive appraisal in emotion. *Journal of Personality and Social Psychology, 48,* 813–838.

Smith, L. (1994, July 25). Burned-out bosses. *Fortune,* pp. 44–52.

Tesser, A., & Rosen, S. (1972). Similarity of objective fate as a determinant of the reluctance to transmit unpleasant information: The MUM effect. *Journal of Personality and Social Psychology, 23,* 46–53.

Tetlock, P., & Levi, A. (1982). On the inconclusiveness of the cognition–motivation debate. *Journal of Experimental Social Psychology, 18,* 68–88.

Thornton, B. (1984). Defensive attribution of responsibility: Evidence for an arousal-based motivational bias. *Journal of Personality and Social Psychology, 46,* 721–734.

Weiner, B. (1993). On sin versus sickness: A theory of perceived responsibility and social motivation. *American Psychologist, 48,* 957–965.

Wyer, R. S., Bodenhausen, G. V., & Gorman, T. F. (1985). Cognitive mediators of reactions to rape. *Journal of Personality and Social Psychology, 48,* 324–338.

Author Index

Subject Index